Clinical Pain Management

Acute Pain

LEAD EDITOR

Andrew SC Rice MB BS MD FRCA
Reader in Pain Research, Department of Anaesthetics, Pain Medicine and Intensive Care
Imperial College London; and Honorary Consultant in Pain Medicine, Chelsea and
Westminster Hospital Foundation NHS Trust, London, UK

SERIES EDITORS

Douglas Justins MB BS FRCA
Fellow of the Faculty of Pain Medicine of the Royal College of Anaesthetists
Consultant in Pain Medicine and Anaesthesia
Pain Management Centre
St Thomas' Hospital
London, UK

Toby Newton-John BA(Hons) MPsych(Clin) PhD
Consultant Clinical Psychologist and Program Director
Innervate Pain Program and
Faculty of Medicine, University of Sydney
Australia

Richard F Howard BSc MB ChB FRCA
Fellow of the Faculty of Pain Medicine of the Royal College of Anaesthetists
Consultant in Paediatric Anaesthesia and Pain Management
Great Ormond Street Hospital for Children
London, UK

Christine A Miaskowski RN PhD FAAN
Professor and Associate Dean for Academic Affairs
Department of Physiological Nursing
UCSF School of Nursing
San Francisco, CA, USA

Acute Pain
Edited by Pamela E Macintyre, Suellen M Walker, and
David J Rowbotham

Chronic Pain
Edited by Peter R Wilson, Paul J Watson, Jennifer A Haythornthwaite, and
Troels S Jensen

Cancer Pain
Edited by Nigel Sykes, Michael I Bennett, and
Chun-Su Yuan

Practice and Procedures
Edited by Harald Breivik, William I Campbell, and
Michael K Nicholas

Clinical Pain Management

Acute Pain

2nd edition

Edited by

Pamela E Macintyre BMEDSC MBBS FANZCA MHA FFPMANZCA
Consultant Anaesthetist; and Director, Acute Pain Service
Department of Anaesthesia, Pain Medicine and Hyperbaric Medicine
Royal Adelaide Hospital and University of Adelaide
Adelaide, Australia

Suellen M Walker MBBS MM(PM) MSC PHD FANZCA FFPMANZCA
Clinical Senior Lecturer in Paediatric Anaesthesia and Pain Medicine
UCL Institute of Child Health and Great Ormond Street Hospital NHS Trust
London, UK

David J Rowbotham MB CHB MD MRCP FRCA
Professor of Anaesthesia and Pain Management; and
Head, Clinical Division of Anaesthesia, Critical Care and Pain Management, University of Leicester
Leicester, UK

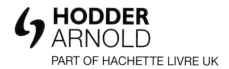

HODDER
ARNOLD
PART OF HACHETTE LIVRE UK

First published in Great Britain in 2003
This second edition published in 2008 by
Hodder Arnold, an imprint of Hodder Education,
part of Hachette Livre UK, 338 Euston Road, London NW1 3BH

http://www.hoddereducation.com

British Library Cataloguing in Publication Data
A catalogue record for this book is available from the British Library

Library of Congress Cataloging-in-Publication Data
A catalog record for this book is available from the Library of Congress

ISBN 978-0-340-94009-9 (Acute Pain)
ISBN 978-0-340-94008-2 (Chronic Pain)
ISBN 978-0-340-94007-5 (Cancer Pain)
ISBN 978-0-340-94006-8 (Practice and Procedures)
ISBN 978-0-340-93992-5 (4 vol set: Acute Pain/Chronic Pain/Cancer Pain/Practice and Procedures/Web edition)

1 2 3 4 5 6 7 8 9 10

Commissioning Editor: Joanna Koster
Project Editor: Zelah Pengilley
Production Controller: Joanna Walker
Cover Design: Helen Townson

Typeset in 10 pt Minion by Macmillan India
Printed and bound in the UK by MPG Books, Bodmin, Cornwall
Text printed on FSC accredited material

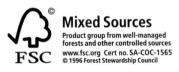

What do you think about this book? Or any other Hodder Arnold title?
Please visit our website: **www.hoddereducation.com**

Contents

Please note: The table of contents and a combined index for all four volumes in the series can be found on the Clinical Pain Management website at: www.clinicalpainmanagement.co.uk.

Contributors

Pedram Aleshi MD
Clinical Fellow
Harvard Medical School, Department of Anaesthesia
Beth Israel Deaconess Medical Center
Boston, MA, USA

Pierre Beaulieu MD PhD FRCA
Associate Professor
Department of Anesthesiology and Pharmacology, CHUM
Montreal, Canada

Julie Bruce RGN BSc MSc PhD
MRC Senior Research Fellow
Department of Public Health, School of Medicine
University of Aberdeen, Aberdeen, UK

Chester C Buckenmaier III MD
Assistant Professor, Uniformed Services University Chief
Army Regional Anesthesia and Pain Management Initiative
Walter Reed Army Medical Center, Washington, DC, USA

Jeremy Cashman BA BSc MB BS MD FRCA
Fellow of the Faculty of Pain Medicine of the
Royal College of Anaesthetists
Consultant Anaesthetist
St George's Hospital
London, UK

Hance Clarke Msc MD
Department of Anesthesia
University of Toronto
Toronto, Canada

Milton L Cohen MB BS MD FRACP FFPMANZCA
Associate Professor
Rheumatology and Pain Medicine, St Vincent's Campus, Sydney
Darlinghurst, NSW, Australia

Julia Coldrey MBBS(Hons) FANZCA
Consultant Anaesthetist
Department of Anaesthesia, Hyperbaric Medicine and Pain
Medicine, Royal Adelaide Hospital
Adelaide, Australia

H Clare Daniel BSc (Hons) D Clin Psych
Consultant Clinical Psychologist
Pain Management Centre
The National Hospital for Neurology and Neurosurgery
London, UK

Linda S Franck PhD RN RGN RSCN FRCPCH FAAN
Professor and Chair
Children's Nursing Research, Patient Care Research and
Innovation Centre, UCL Institute of Child Health, Great Ormond
Street Hospital for Children NHS Trust, London, UK

C Roger Goucke MB ChB FANZCA FFPMANZCA
Head
Department of Pain Management, Sir Charles Gairdner Hospital
Nedlands, Western Australia

Sina Grape MD
Senior Registrar
Department of Anaesthesia and Pain Medicine
Royal Perth Hospital
Perth, Australia

Barry D Gunn MBBS FACEM
Emergency Physician
Western Health, Footscray, Victoria, Australia

William Harrop-Griffiths MA MB BS FRCA
Consultant Anaesthetist
Department of Anaesthesia, St Mary's Hospital
London, UK

Anne Heffernan MB MSc MD FFARCSI
Consultant
Department of Anaesthesia and Pain Medicine, Tallaght Hospital
Dublin 24, Ireland

Philip Hess MD
Assistant Professor of Anesthesia
Anesthesia and Critical Care
Beth Israel Deaconess Medical Center
Boston, MA, USA

Richard F Howard BSc MB ChB FRCA
Fellow of the Faculty of Pain Medicine of the
Royal College of Anaesthetists
Consultant in Anaesthesia and Pain Management
Great Ormond Street Hospital for Children
London, UK

Mark I Johnson BSc (Hons) PhD
Professor of Pain and Analgesia, Faculty of Health
Leeds Metropolitan University; and
Leeds Pallium Research Group, Leeds, UK

Stephen F Jones MB BS FRCA
Consultant Anaesthetist
Department of Anaesthesia, Waikato Hospital
Hamilton, New Zealand

Girish P Joshi MB BS MD FFARCSI
Professor of Anesthesiology and Pain Management, Director of
Perioperative Medicine and Ambulatory Anesthesia
University of Texas Southwestern Medical Center
Dallas, Texas, USA

Joel Katz PhD
Acute Pain Research Unit, Department of Anesthesia and
Pain Management, Toronto General Hospital and
Mount Sinai Hospital; and
Professor
Department of Anesthesia, University of Toronto; and
Professor and Canada Research Chair
Department of Psychology, York University
Toronto, ON, Canada

Anne-Maree Kelly MD MClinED FACEM
Academic Head, Emergency Medicine and Director
Joseph Einstein Centre for Emergency Medicine Resarch
Western Health, Footscray
Victoria, Australia; and
Professorial Fellow
The University of Melbourne, Australia

John Kinsella MB BS MD FRCA
Professor and Head of Section of Anaesthesia
Pain and Critical Care Medicine
University of Glasgow
Glasgow Royal Infirmary
Glasgow, UK

Christina Liossi BA (Hons) MPhil MSc DPsych CPsychol
Senior Lecturer in Health Psychology
School of Psychology, University of Southampton
Southampton, UK; and
Honorary Consultant Clinical Psychologist
Great Ormond Street Hospital for Children NHS Trust
London, UK

Pamela E Macintyre BMedSc MBBS FANZCA MHA FFPMANZCA
Director, Acute Pain Service, Consultant Anesthetist
Department of Anaesthesia, Hyperbaric Medicine and Pain
Medicine
Royal Adelaide Hospital and University of Adelaide
Adelaide, Australia

William A Macrae MB ChB FRCA
Consultant in Pain Medicine, Honorary Senior Lecturer
Ninewells Hospital and Medical School
Dundee, UK

Wendy M McDonald RN BN Grad Dip (Crit Care)
Acute Pain Nurse
Department of Anaesthesia, St Vincent's Hospital
Melbourne, Australia

Jonathan McGhie MB ChB FRCA FFPMANZCA
Consultant in Anaesthesia and Pain Medicine
Department of Anaesthesia, Western Infirmary
Glasgow, UK

Aidan M O'Donnell BSc MB ChB FRCA
Consultant Anaesthetist
St John's Hospital, Livingston, UK

Stephen G Oxberry MBChB BSc MRCP
Specialist Registrar in Palliative Medicine
Yorkshire Deanery, Leeds, UK

Leo Pinczewski
Orthopaedic Surgeon
North Sydney Orthopaedic and Sports Medicine Centre
Sydney, Australia

Alison E Powell MA PhD
Health Services Researcher
Centre for Public Policy and Management
University of St Andrews, St Andrews, UK

Ian Power BSc (Hons) MD FRCA FFPMANZCA FANZCA FRCSEd FRCP Edin
Professor of Anaesthesia
Critical Care and Pain Medicine, The University of Edinburgh
Edinburgh, UK

Colin P Rae MBChB FRCA (Lond)
Fellow of the Faculty of Pain Medicine of the
Royal College of Anaesthetists
Consultant in Anesthesia and Pain Management
Department of Anesthesia, Glasgow Royal Infirmary
Glasgow, UK

Lindy J Roberts MB BS (Hons) BMedSci (Hons) FANZCA FFPMANZCA
Staff Specialist and Director Acute Pain Service
Departments of Anaesthesia and Pain Management,
Sir Charles Gairdner Hospital, Nedlands, Australia

David J Rowbotham MB ChB MD MRCP FRCA
Professor of Anaesthesia and Pain Management
University of Leicester, Leicester, UK

Kim E Russon MBchB FRCA
Consultant Anaesthetist
Rotherham General Hospital, Rotherham, UK

Stephan A Schug MD FANZCA FFPMANZCA
Chair of Anaesthesiology
School of Medicine and Pharmacology
Faculty of Medicine Dentistry and Health Sciences
University of Western Australia; and
Director of Pain Medicine
Department of Anaesthesia and Pain Medicine
Royal Perth Hospital
Perth, Australia

David A Scott MB BS PhD FANZCA FFPMANZCA
Associate Professor and Deputy Director
Department of Anaesthesia, St Vincent's Hospital
Melbourne, Australia

Michael G Serpell MBChB FRCA
Fellow of the Faculty of Pain Medicine of the
Royal College of Anaesthetists
Consultant and Senior Lecturer
University Department of Anaesthesia, Western Infirmary
Glasgow, UK

Alcira Serrano-Gomez FRCA
Honorary Lecturer in Anaesthesia
University of Leicester, Leicester, UK

R Scott Simpson MB BS DA(UK) FANZCA FFPMANZCA FJFICM
Staff Specialist
Intensive Care Unit, The Townsville Hospital
North Queensland, Australia

Karen H Simpson MBCHB FRCA
Consultant in Anaesthesia and Pain Medicine
Pain Management Service
Leeds Teaching Hospitals Trust; and
Leeds Pallium Research Group
Leeds, UK

Matthew HJ Size MBChB BMedSci FRCA
SpR in Anaesthesia
University College Hospital NHS Trust
London, UK

Louise Tulloh MB BS FACSP
Sports Physician
North Sydney Orthopaedic and Sports Medicine Centre
Sydney, Australia

Evangelos Tziavrangos BMBS FANZCA FFPMANZCA
Staff Specialist
Department of Anaesthesia and Pain Medicine
Royal Perth Hospital
Perth, Australia

Richard Upton BSc PhD
Principal Medical Scientist, Senior Lecturer
Royal Adelaide Hospital and University of Adelaide
Adelaide, Australia

Eric J Visser MBBS FANZCA FFPMANZCA
Pain Medicine Specialist and Anaesthetist
Department of Anaesthesia and Pain Medicine
Royal Perth Hospital
Western, Australia

Suellen M Walker MBBS MM(PM) MSc PhD FANZCA FFPMANZCA
Clinical Senior Lecturer and Consultant in Paediatric Anaesthesia
and Pain Medicine
UCL Institute of Child Health and Great Ormond St Hospital
NHS Trust
London, UK

Phil Wiffen MSc MRPhamS
Co-ordinating Editor
Cochrane Pain and Palliative Care Group
Pain Relief Unit, Churchill Hospital, Oxford, UK

Iain H Wilson MB ChB FRCA
Consultant in Anaesthesia
Royal Devon and Exeter NHS Foundation Trust
Exeter, UK

Series preface

Since the successful first edition of *Clinical Pain Management* was published in 2002, the evidence base in many areas of pain medicine has changed substantially, thus creating the need for this second edition. We have retained the central ethos of the first volume in that we have continued to provide comprehensive coverage of pain medicine, with the text geared predominantly to the requirements of those training and practicing in pain medicine and related specialties. The emphasis continues to be on delivering this coverage in a format that is easily accessed and digested by the busy clinician in practice.

As before, *Clinical Pain Management* comprises four volumes. The first three cover the main disciplines of acute, chronic, and cancer pain management, and the fourth volume covers the practical aspects of clinical practice and research. The four volumes can be used independently, while together they give readers all they need to know to deliver a successful pain management service.

Of the 161 chapters in the four volumes, almost a third are brand new to this edition while the chapters that have been retained have been completely revised, in many cases under new authorship. This degree of change reflects ongoing progress in this broad field, where research and development provide a rapidly evolving evidence base. The international flavor of *Clinical Pain Management* remains an important feature, and perusal of the contributor pages will reveal that authors and editors are drawn from a total of 16 countries.

A particularly popular aspect of the first edition was the practice of including a system of simple evidence scoring in most of the chapters. This enables the reader to understand quickly the strength of evidence which supports a particular therapeutic statement or recommendation. This has been retained for the first three volumes, where appropriate. We have, however, improved the system used for scoring evidence from a three point scale used in the first edition and adopted the five point Bandolier system which is in widespread use and will be instantly familiar to many readers (www.jr2.ox.ac.uk/bandolier/band6/b6-5.html).

We have also retained the practice of asking authors to highlight the key references in each chapter. Following feedback from our readers we have added two new features for this edition: first, there are key learning points at the head of each chapter summarizing the most salient points within the chapter; and second, the series is accompanied by a companion website with downloadable figures.

This project would not have been possible without the hard work and commitment of the chapter authors and we are deeply indebted to all of them for their contributions. The volume editors have done a sterling job in diligently editing a large number of chapters, and to them we are also most grateful. Any project of this magnitude would be impossible without substantial support from the publishers – in particular we would like to acknowledge our debt to Jo Koster and Zelah Pengilley at Hodder. They have delivered the project on a tight deadline and ensured that a large number of authors and editors were kept gently, but firmly, "on track."

Andrew SC Rice, Douglas Justins, Toby Newton-John,
Richard F Howard, Christine A Miaskowski
London, Newcastle, and San Francisco

I would also like to add my personal thanks to the Series Editors who have given their time generously and made invaluable contributions through the whole editorial process from the very outset of discussions regarding a second edition in deciding upon the content of each volume and in selecting Volume Editors. More recently, they have provided an important second view in the consideration of all submitted chapters, not to mention stepping in and assisting with first edits where needed. The timely completion of the second edition would not have been possible without this invaluable input.

Andrew SC Rice
Lead Editor

Introduction to Clinical Pain Management: Acute Pain

Since publication of the first edition of *Clinical Pain Management: Acute Pain*, there has been a significant increase in the amount and quality of evidence relating to the treatment of acute pain. There has also been increasing recognition of the need to improve the management of acute pain, with key international bodies such as the World Health Organization (WHO) and the International Association for the Study of Pain (IASP) stating that appropriate pain relief, including relief of acute pain, ". . . should be a human right."

A better understanding that acute pain is just one end of the pain spectrum and that many patients do not fit neatly into either an acute pain or chronic pain category, has led to an expansion of the traditional patient treatment groups (mainly postoperative, obstetric, and trauma patients) to include those with acute-on-chronic pain, acute cancer pain, or acute pain from a large number of medical conditions. There has also been a progressive increase in the number of patients who are opioid-tolerant and in whom effective management of acute pain can be more problematic. Increased knowledge about acute neuropathic pain, and the recognition that it can occur within hours of a nerve injury and that patients undergoing particular types of surgery are at greater risk of developing persistent postoperative pain, continues to suggest that better treatment of acute pain could reduce this risk.

As a result of all these developments, pain therapies more traditionally used for the management of chronic pain are now also used in the acute pain setting. The second edition of *Clinical Pain Management: Acute Pain* aims to reflect these changes and the progress made in the management of acute pain.

The first part has therefore been expanded. As well as reviews of some of the basic aspects of acute pain management (now including developmental biology of nociception) and many of the drugs traditionally used in the management of acute pain, it now includes a chapter on the pharmacology of other adjuvant drugs, including those used for the management of acute neuropathic pain. Up-to-date information on preventive analgesia is also given.

The second part of the volume again considers some of the techniques used for the treatment of acute pain. Methods of drug delivery and routes by which drugs can be given are described and the importance of non-drug treatment is again recognized, both in adults and children. The chapter on nerve blocks now concentrates on continuous peripheral neural blockade – an increasingly common method of pain relief after surgery and one that may be continued once the patient has left hospital.

The third and final part reflects the increasing complexity of acute pain management in some patients. As before, it looks at a number of the many clinical situations in which acute pain can arise and the methods of treatment that may be suitable in these circumstances, whether the patient is young or old, or has pain due to surgery, trauma, medical illnesses, or childbirth. New chapters have been added to provide information on acute pain management in emergency departments, field and disaster situations, and the developing world, as well as the increasingly common problem of acute pain management in the opioid-tolerant patient, and the risk and possible prevention of persistent postsurgical pain.

Many authors kindly contributed to this volume (as with the other volumes in this series) and they were invited to present their information in a practical and evidence-based manner. It is hoped that this second edition of *Clinical Pain Management: Acute Pain* will be of value to all who are involved in the management of acute pain.

Pamela E Macintyre, Suellen Walker, and David J Rowbotham
Adelaide, London, and Leicester

How to use this book

SPECIAL FEATURES

The four volumes of *Clinical Pain Management* incorporate the following special features to aid the readers' understanding and navigation of the text.

Key learning points

Each chapter opens with a set of key learning points which provide readers with an overview of the most salient points within the chapter.

Cross-references

Throughout the chapters in this volume you will find cross-references to chapters in other volumes in the *Clinical Pain Management* series. Each cross-reference will indicate the volume in which the chapter referred to is to be found.

Evidence scoring

In chapters where recommendations for surgical, medical, psychological, and complementary treatment and diagnostic tests are presented, the quality of evidence supporting authors' statements relating to clinical interventions, or the papers themselves, are graded following the Oxford Bandolier system by insertion of the following symbols into the text:

[I]   Strong evidence from at least one published systematic review of multiple well-designed randomized controlled trials
[II]   Strong evidence from at least one published properly designed randomized controlled trial of appropriate size and in an appropriate clinical setting
[III]   Evidence from published well-designed trials without randomization, single group pre-post, cohort, time series, or matched case-controlled studies
[IV]   Evidence from well-designed non-experimental studies from more than one center or research group
[V]   Opinions of respected authorities, based on clinical evidence, descriptive studies or reports of expert consensus committees.

Oxford Bandolier system used by kind permission of Bandolier: www.jr2.ox.ac.uk/Bandolier

Where no grade is inserted, the quality of supporting evidence, if any exists, is of low grade only (e.g. case reports, clinical experience, etc).

Other textbooks devoted to the subject of pain include a tremendous amount of anecdotal and personal recommendations, and it is often difficult to distinguish these from those with an established evidence base. This text is thus unique in allowing the reader the opportunity to do this with confidence.

Reference annotation

The reference lists are annotated with asterisks, where appropriate, to guide readers to key primary papers, major review articles (which contain extensive reference lists), and clinical guidelines. We hope that this feature will render extensive lists of references more useful to the reader and will help to encourage self-directed learning among both trainees and practicing physicians.

A NOTE ON DRUG NAMES

The authors have used the international nonproprietary name (INN) for drugs where possible. If the INN name differs from the US or UK name, authors have used the INN name followed by the US and/or UK name in brackets on first use within a chapter.

Abbreviations

5-HT	5-hydroxytryptamine	CBT	cognitive-behavioral therapy
6-MAM	6-monoacetyl morphine	CCI	chronic constriction injury
6-MNA	6-methoxy-2-naphthylacetic acid	CCK	cholecystokinin
		CEA	continuous epidural analgesia
a-PC	activated protein C	CGRP	calcitonin gene-related peptide
AA	arachidonic acid	CHEOPS	Children's Hospital of Eastern Ontario
AAG	alpha-acid glycoprotein		Pain Score
AAMPGG	Australian Acute Musculoskeletal Pain	CHIP	Checklist for Interpersonal Pain
	Guidelines Group		Behavior
AC1/AC8	adenylyl cyclase 1 and 8	CI	confidence interval
ACC	Accident Rehabilitation and Compensation	CNS	central nervous system
	Insurance Corporation; or arterior cingulate	COMT	catecholamine-O-methyltransferase
	cortex	CONSORT	Consolidated Standards for Reporting
AIDS	acquired immune deficiency syndrome		Trials
AL-TENS	acupuncture-like TENS	COX	cyclooxygenase
ALA	aminolaevulinic acid	CPNB	continuous peripheral nerve block
ALOS	average length of stay	CPSP	chronic postsurgical pain
ALT	aminotransferase	CREB	cyclic AMP response element binding
AM	abdominal migraine		protein
AMPA	α-amino-3-hydroxy-5-methyl-4-isaxazole	CRIES	CRying, Increased vital signs, Expression,
	propionic acid; or α-amino-3-hydroxy-5-		and Sleeplessness
	methylisoxazole-4-propionic acid	CRP	C-reactive protein
AP	action potential	CRPS	complex regional pain syndrome
APRV	airway pressure release settings	CRRT	continuous renal replacement therapy
APS	acute pain service	CSA	continuous spinal analgesia
ARDS	acute respiratory distress syndrome	CSAG	Clinical Standards Advisory Group
ASIC	acid sensing ion channel	CSE	combined spinal-epidural
ASR	abdominal skin reflex	CSF	cerebrospinal fluid
ATP	adenosine triphosphate	CSH	combat support hospital
AUC	area under the concentration-time curve; or	CT	computed tomography
	area under the curve	CTS	carpal tunnel syndrome
		CVS	cardiovascular system
B1/B2	bradykinin receptors		
BAB	butyl amino-benzoate	DAG	1,2-diacylglycerol
BAN	British Approved Name	DAGb	diacyglycerol
BDNF	brain-derived neurotrophic factor	DCD	donation after cardiac death
BIS	bispectral analysis	DH	dorsal horn
BK	bradykinin	DLF	dorsolateral funiculus
BPI	brief pain inventory	DNIC	diffuse noxious inhibitory controls
BPI-SF	short form of the BPI	DRASH	deployable rapid assembly shelter and
			surgical hospital
CaMK	calcium-calmodulin-dependent kinase	DRG	dorsal root ganglion
CaMKII	calcium calmodulin kinase II	DS-DAT	Discomfort Scale for Dementia of the
cAMP	cyclic AMP		Alzheimer Type

DSP	distal symmetrical polyneuropathy	INR	international normalized ratio
EA	electroacupuncture	IP3	inositol triphosphate
ECG	electrocardiogram	IPSC	inhibitory post-synaptic currents
ECM	extracellular matrix	ISAP	International Society for the Prevention of Pain
ECMO	extracorporeal membrane oxygenation	IUPHAR	International Union of Pharmacology
ED	emergency departments	i.v.	intravenous
EDA	electronic dental anesthesia	IVRA	intravenous regional anesthesia
EDTA	ethylenediaminetetracetate		
EEG	electroencephalogram	JCAHO	Joint Commission for Accreditation of Healthcare Organizations
EMG	electromyography	JRA	juvenile rheumatoid arthritis
EMLA	eutectic mixture of local anesthetics		
ENT	ear, nose, and throat	KCC2	potassium-chloride cotransporter
EPSP	excitatory postsynaptic potentials		
ER	emergency room	LA	local anesthetic
EREM	extended-release epidural morphine	LBP	low back pain
ERK	extracellular signal-regulated kinase	LIF	leukemia inhibitory factor
ESR	erythrocyte sedimentation rate	LMWH	low molecular weight heparin
ESWT	extracorporeal shock wave treatment	LOS	length of stay
		LT	low-threshold
FAS	functional activity scale	LTD	long-term depression
FBD	functional bowel disorders	LTP	long-term potentiation
FDA	Food and Drug Administration		
FEB	fentanyl effervescent buccal	M3G	morphine-3-glucuronide
FLACC	Face, Legs, Arms, Cry, Consolability	M6G	morphine-6-glucuronide
fMRI	functional magnetic resonance imaging	MAPK	mitogen-activated protein kinases
FPS	faces pain scale	MARAA	Military Advanced Regional Anesthesia and Analgesia
GABA	gamma-aminobutyric acid	MEAC	minimum effective analgesic concentration
GBS	Guillain–Barré syndrome		
GDNF	glial cell line-derived neurotrophic factor	mEPSC	mini-excitatory postsynaptic current
GI	gastrointestinal	mGluR	metabotropic glutamate receptor
GlyR	glycine receptor	MIS	minimal intervention strategy
GPCR	G-proteins coupled receptor	MLAC	minimum local analgesic concentration; or minimum local anesthetic concentration
GRECC	Geriatric Research Education Clinical Centre		
GRS	graphic rating scale	MMT	methadone maintenance treatment
		MOR	μ-opioid receptor
H2RA	histamine H2 receptor antagonist	MPQ	McGill Pain Questionnaire
HBOT	hyperbaric oxygen therapy	MRI	magnetic resonance imaging
HCP	healthcare providers	MRP	multidrug resistance protein
HDU	high-dependency unit	MS	multiple sclerosis
HIV	human immunodeficiency virus	MSD	maximum safe dose
HPA	hypothalamic–pituitary axis	MSF	Médicins Sans Frontières
HS	harvest site		
		N/OFQ	Nociceptin/orphanin FQ
i.a.	intra-articular	N_2O	nitrous oxide
IASP	International Association for the Study of Pain	NBC	nuclear, biological, or chemical
IBS	irritable bowel syndrome	NCA	nurse-controlled analgesia
IC Ca	intracellular calcium	NCCPC	Noncommunicating Children's Pain Checklist
ICU	intensive care unit		
IHD	intermittent hemodialysis and filtration	NFCS	Neonatal Facial Coding System
IL	interleukin	NGC	nucleus reticularis gigantocellularis
i.m.	intramuscular	NGF	nerve growth factor
i.n.	intranasal	NIRS	near-infrared spectroscopy
INCB	International Narcotics Control Board	NK1	neurokinin 1
INN	International Nonproprietary Name		

NMDA	*N*-methyl-D-aspartic acid		QST	quantitative sensory testing
NNH	numbers-needed-to-harm			
NNT	number needed to treat		RA	rheumatoid arthritis
NO	nitric oxide		RCT	randomized controlled trial
NOS	nitric oxide synthase		RICE	rest, ice, compression, elevation
NRM	nucleus raphe magnus		RTA	road traffic accidents
NRS	numerical rating scale		RVM	rostroventromedial medulla
NS	nociceptive-specific		Ry1	ryanodine
NSAID	nonsteroidal anti-inflammatory drug		s.c.	subcutaneous
NT-3	neurotrophin-3		SAD	substance abuse disorder
NT-4/5	neurotrophin-4/5		SCS	spinal cord stimulation
NTS	nucleus tractus solitarius		SEP	somatosensory evoked potential
NUD	non-ulcer dyspepsia		SF-MPQ	short form MPQ
NYHA	New York Heart Association		SIRS	systemic inflammatory response syndrome
			SLED	slow low efficiency dialysis
OA	osteoarthritis		SNI	spared nerve injury
OIH	opioid-induced hyperalgesia		SNP	single nucleotide polymorphism
OP	occiput–posterior		SNRI	serotonin and norepinephrine reuptake inhibitor
OR	odds ratio			
OSA	obstructive sleep apnea		SOM	somatostatin
OTC	over-the-counter		SP	substance P
OTFC	oral transmucosal fentanyl citrate		SPID	summed pain intensity difference
			STAI	State-Trait Anxiety Inventory
PACU	postanesthesia care unit		STRICTA	Standards for Reporting Interventions in Controlled Trials of Acupuncture
PAG	periaqueductal gray			
PAINAD	Pain Assessment in Advanced Dementia		STT	spinothalamic tract
PAR	proteinase-activated receptors		T4	fourth thoracic
PAR2	proteinase-activated receptor-2		TCA	tricyclic antidepressants
PBN	parabrachial nucleus		TCM	traditional Chinese medicine
PCA	patient-controlled analgesia; or postconceptional age		TEA	thoracic epidural analgesia
			TENS	transcutaneous electrical nerve stimulation
PCEA	patient-controlled epidural analgesia		TNFα	tumor necrosis factor-alpha
PCINA	patient-controlled intranasal analgesia		TNF	tumor necrosis factor
pCREB	phosphoCREB		TNS	transient neurologic symptom
PCTS	patient-controlled transdermal system		TOTPAR	total pain relief
PD	primary dysmenorrhea		TPBV	thoracic paravertebral block
PDPH	postdural puncture headache		TRI	transient radicular irritation
PET	positron emission tomography		trk	tyrosine kinase
PG	prostaglandin		trkA	tyrosine kinase A
PGE2	prostaglandin E_2		TRP	transient receptor potential
PID	pain intensity difference		TTX	tetrodotoxin
PIPP	Premature Infant Pain Profile		TTX-R	tetrodotoxin-resistant
PKA	protein kinase A		TTX-S	tetrodotoxin-sensitive
PKC	protein kinase C			
PLA$_2$	phospholipase A_2		USAA	Uniformed Services Society of Anesthesiologists
PLC	phoshpolipase C			
PNB	peripheral nerve block		USAN	US Approved Name
PONV	postoperative nausea and vomiting		USP	United States Pharmacopeia
PPI	proton pump inhibitor		VA	Veterans Administration
PPP	Pediatric Pain Profile		VAP	ventilator-associated pneumonia
PRI	pain rating index		VAS	visual analog scale
PRID	pain relief and intensity difference		VDS	verbal descriptor scale
PROSPECT	Procedure-specific Postoperative Pain Management		VGCC	voltage-gated calcium channels
			VNRS	Verbal Numerical Rating Scale

VR1	vanilloid receptor 1	WDR	wide dynamic range
VRS	verbal rating scale	WFSA	World Federation of Societies of Anaesthesiologists
WADA	World Anti-doping Agency	WHO	World Health Organization
WBPQ	Wisconsin Brief Pain Questionnaire	WMD	weighted mean difference

PART I

GENERAL CONSIDERATIONS

1a

Applied physiology of nociception

PIERRE BEAULIEU

KEY LEARNING POINTS

- The somatosensory system processes four broadly distinct sensory modalities: tactile, proprioceptive, thermal sensations, and pain.
- Four distinct processes can be identified between the delivery of a noxious stimulus and the subjective experience of pain: transduction, transmission, modulation, and perception.
- There are two types of primary afferent fiber involved in nociception: $A\delta$- and C-fibers. The two principal functions of primary afferent neurons are stimulus transduction and transmission of encoded stimulus information to the central nervous system (CNS).
- In nociceptive signaling in the dorsal horn, three major categories of neuronal cells can be identified: projection neurons, and inhibitory and excitatory interneurons utilizing a variety of neurotransmitters.

- Nociceptive input to the dorsal horn is relayed to higher centers in the brain via several ascending pathways: the spinothalamic tract being classically considered as the major pain pathway.
- Multiple cortical areas are activated by painful stimuli including: the primary and secondary somatosensory cortices, the insula, the anterior cingulate cortex, and the prefrontal cortex.
- The modulation of nociceptive messages in spinal cord neurons is dependent on the balance of inputs from primary afferent nociceptors, intrinsic spinal cord neurons, and descending systems projecting from supraspinal sites.

INTRODUCTION

The somatosensory system processes four broadly distinct sensory modalities: tactile, proprioceptive, thermal sensations, and pain.[1] According to the specificity theory, each sensory modality is mediated by a separate class of receptor and a distinct neuroanatomical pathway. However, while this classification is by no means as rigid as first thought, it does hold under most physiological conditions. Sherrington[2] proposed that cutaneous receptors responding selectively to tissue-damaging (noxious) stimuli should be designated nociceptors. When noxious thermal or mechanical stimuli are applied to the skin, a chain of events is set in motion that usually results in perception of the sensation of pain.

Interspersed between the delivery of a noxious stimulus and the subjective experience of pain is a series of complex electrical and chemical events during which four distinct processes can be identified: transduction, transmission, modulation, and perception. Transduction, or receptor activation, is the process by which external noxious energy is converted into electrophysiological activity in nociceptive primary afferent neurons. Transmission refers to the process by which this coded information is relayed to those structures of the central nervous system (CNS) concerned with pain. The first stage of transmission is the conduction of impulses in primary afferent neurons to the dorsal horn of the spinal cord, from where a network of neurons ascends in the spinal cord to the brain stem and thalamus. Finally, reciprocal connections are made between the thalamus and the multiple higher areas of the brain concerned with the perceptive and affective responses associated with pain. However, nociceptive activity does not always result in pain perception (equally, pain may be perceived in the absence of nociception). Therefore, a process of signal modulation must be introduced into this system that is capable of interfering in this "pathway;" the modulatory site about which most is known is the dorsal horn of the spinal cord. The final process is perception, in which the pain message is relayed to the brain, producing an unpleasant sensory experience, which has affective, defensive, and perceptive components.

PERIPHERAL ASPECTS OF NOCICEPTION

Neurons in peripheral nerves can be classified according to morphological, electrophysiological, and biochemical characteristics (**Table 1a.1** and **Figure 1a.1**).[3, 4, 5, 6] There are two types of primary afferent fiber involved in nociception: Aδ- and C-fibers (**Table 1a.2**). The two principal functions of primary afferent neurons are stimulus transduction and transmission of encoded stimulus information to the CNS. The cell body of such a neuron is located in the dorsal root ganglion of a spinal nerve (or trigeminal ganglion for the trigeminal nerve), and the smaller diameter cell bodies are associated with nociception. Each axon possesses two branches, one projecting to the periphery (peripheral process), where its terminal is sensitive to noxious stimuli, and

one projecting to the CNS (central process), where it synapses with CNS neurons. Eighty percent of nociceptor primary afferents are nonmyelinated C-fibers.

Classification of somatic nociceptors

Primary afferent nociceptors have more recently been classified according to their neurochemical characteristics and spinal connections, although the precise implications of these findings for physiological function are at present unclear (**Figure 1a.1a**).[7] Using a genetic transneuronal tracing analysis, it has recently been suggested that parallel and largely independent circuits are engaged by the two major primary afferent nociceptor populations (peptidergic and nonpeptidergic). Furthermore, motor as well as limbic targets predominate in the circuits that originate from the nonpeptide population (**Figure 1a.1b**).

The elaborate cutaneous receptors associated with large myelinated neurons have no identifiable counterpart in the nociceptive domain. Nociceptors in the skin and other somatic tissues are morphologically free nerve endings or very simple receptor structures and are widespread in the superficial layers of the skin and also in certain deeper somatic tissues (e.g. periosteum and joint surfaces).

C polymodal nociceptors are the most numerous of somatic nociceptors and respond to the full range of mechanical, thermal, and chemical noxious stimuli, including, characteristically, the pungent ingredient of chilli peppers, capsaicin,[8] as well as various molecules associated with tissue injury and inflammation (**Table 1a.3**).[9] The more rapidly conducting (5–30 m/s) Aδ nociceptors form a more heterogeneous group and generally respond to thermal and/or mechanical stimuli.

PRIMARY AFFERENT RECEPTORS

A noxious stimulus activates the nociceptor by distorting and depolarizing the membrane of the sensory nerve ending. The exact cellular mechanisms by which various stimuli depolarize free sensory endings and trigger an action potential are not known, but it is suggested that the transduction

Table 1a.1 Classification of neurons.

Type	Conduction velocity (m/s)	Neuron diameter (μm)	Characteristics
Aα	60–120	12–22	Skeletal motor (M)
Aβ	50–70	4–12	Touch, vibration, light pressure (M)
Aγ	35–70	4–12	Intrafusal proprioception (M)
Aδ	5–30	1–5	Primary nociceptive afferent (M)
B	3–30	1.5–4	Autonomic preganglionic (M)
C	<3	<1.5	Primary nociceptive afferent (unM)
			Autonomic postganglionic (unM)

M, myelinated fibers; unM, unmyelinated fibers.

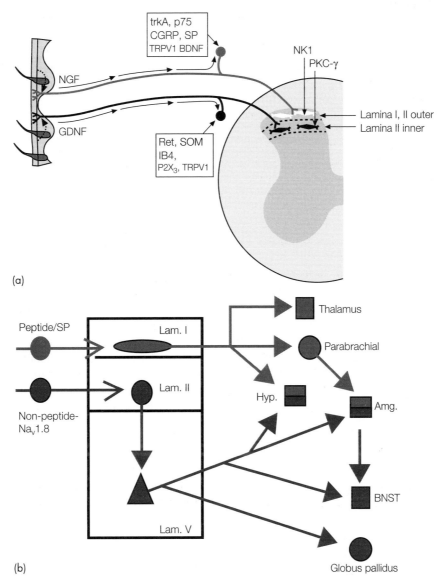

(a)

(b)

Figure 1a.1 (a) Many primary afferent nociceptors are sensitive to the effects of capsaicin, which exerts its effects via an interaction with the transient receptor potential vanilloid 1 (TRPV1) receptor, but can be subdivided according to their dependence on various growth factors and neurochemical composition. This can be ascertained by immunohistochemical study of the cell bodies of primary afferent nociceptors in the dorsal root ganglion (DRG) and dorsal horn of the spinal cord. In fetal life, 75 percent of DRG cells are dependent on the neurotrophin nerve growth factor (NGF) for survival and express the high-affinity receptor for NGF, trkA (tyrosine kinase A). However, during early postnatal life, this growth factor dependency alters, so that in adult life only 45 percent of DRG cells express trkA. Therefore, to date, two major classes of unmyelinated primary afferent nociceptors have been identified. The peptidergic population which in addition to its NGF dependency also expresses the neuropeptides substance P (SP) and calcitonin gene-related peptide (CGRP) and low levels of another neurotrophin brain-derived neurotrophic factor (BDNF). They project to dorsal horn lamina I and the outer part of lamina II, in which the neurokinin 1 (NK1) (agonist, substance P) receptor is found. The nonpeptidergic population comprises the 30 percent of DRG cells which lose trkA and can be identified by their expression of the lectin IB4 and the enzyme FRAP. They become sensitive to glial cell line-derived neurotrophic factor (GDNF) and express the high-affinity receptor for GDNF, Ret. They also express the purine receptor P2X₃. A subset of these cells contains the neuromodulator somatostatin (SOM). These neurons terminate in the inner aspect of dorsal horn lamina II, an area characterized by its specific expression of protein kinase C-γ (PKC-γ). The fundamental differences in the pattern of primary afferent termination has recently been suggested to account for two parallel ascending pain pathways in the central nervous system. This figure was published in Snider WD, McMahon SB. Tackling pain at the source: new ideas about nociceptors. *Neuron.* 1998; **20**: 629–32, Copyright Elsevier.[3] (b) Using genetic tracing of ascending nociceptive circuits, the nonpeptidergic population of neurons (that expresses the sodium channel Na$_v$1.8) project to several limbic and striatal regions including the globus pallidus. As the latter is involved in regulating motor functions, this newly discovered pain target may explain why noxious stimuli almost always induce changes in motor behaviors. In contrast, the peptidergic population projects heavily to the brain stem and thalamus. The two populations of neurons may converge at supraspinal levels in the hypothalamus and amygdala (Amg, amygdala; BNST, bed nucleus of the stria terminalis; Hyp, hypothalamus). This figure was published in Braz JM, Nassar MA, Wood JN, Basbaum AI. Parallel "pain" pathways arise from subpopulations of primary afferent nociceptor. *Neuron.* 2005; **47**: 787–93, Copyright Elsevier.[4]

Table 1a.2 Nociceptors.

Receptor type	Fiber group	Quality
Polymodal (mechanical, heat, chemical)	C	Slow, burning pain
Thermal and mechanothermal	Aδ	Sharp, pricking pain

C polymodal nociceptors respond to a broad range of tissue-damaging energy (chemical, thermal, and mechanical). In the peripheral nerve, they are coupled to slowly conducting unmyelinated C-fibers. Human microneurography experiments have demonstrated that primary afferent neuronal traffic associated with C polymodal nociceptor activity relates to the perception of a prolonged "burning" pain. Aδ mechanoheat receptors form a more heterogeneous group, generally responding only to noxious mechanical and thermal stimuli. They are coupled to the more rapidly conducting Aδ thinly myelinated axons. Microneurography has shown that activity in these axons is associated with the perception of a brief "sharp" pain.

Table 1a.3 Some of the endogenous molecules that activate nociceptors.

Substance	Source	Enzyme involved in synthesis	Effect on primary afferent fibers
Potassium	Damaged cells		Activation
Protons	Hypoxic cells		Activation
Serotonin	Platelets	Tryptophan hydroxylase	Activation
Bradykinin	Plasma kininogen	Kallikrein	Activation
Histamine	Mast cells		Activation
Prostaglandins	AA-damaged cells	Cyclooxygenase	Sensitization
Leukotrienes	AA-damaged cells	5-Lipoxygenase	Sensitization
Substance P	Primary afferents		Sensitization

After Basbaum and Jessel.[9] AA, arachidonic acid.

mechanism for each type of noxious stimulus is distinct. A number of specialized ion channels have been identified that underlie transduction. These include thermoreceptors, mechanoreceptors, and chemoreceptors. Electrophysiologically, the mechanoreceptors can be divided into two major groups: (1) the low-threshold mechanoreceptors that all robustly respond to the ramp phase of a stimulus and (2) nociceptive mechanoreceptors (or mechanonociceptors) that respond primarily to the static phase of a stimulus.[10] Mechanonociceptors can form free nerve endings in the dermis or epidermis and typically form synapses in the superficial dorsal horn. The molecular mechanisms by which sensory neurons detect mechanical stimuli are not fully understood, but may involve subtypes of Na^+, K^+, transient receptor potential (TRP), or acid-sensing ion channels.[10, 11] Acid-sensing ion channels (ASIC) are almost ubiquitous in the mammalian nervous system, especially in the periphery where they are involved in mechanoreception and nociception.[12]

At any given moment, we can experience a wide range of temperatures, when a thermal stimulus excites primary afferent sensory neurons. Once activated, these cells relay signals, through action potentials, from peripheral tissues to the spinal cord and brain, where they are integrated and interpreted to trigger appropriate reflexive and cognitive responses.[13] Psychophysically, we perceive heat to be uncomfortable or pain-producing (noxious) when temperatures exceed around 43°C, whereas the threshold for noxious cold is in the vicinity of 15°C. The proteins that enable sensory neurons to convey temperature information are mainly ion channels activated by specific changes in temperature and belonging to the TRP family (**Figure 1a.2**).[14] Several TRP channels are temperature sensitive and, when activated, depolarize nociceptor terminals. The TRPV1 channel, originally named the vanilloid receptor 1 (VR1), is a calcium permeable ion channel, which is gated directly by heat at temperatures around 43°C, but is also activated by capsaicin and protons.[14]

Many nociceptors express ionotropic (P2X) and G-protein-coupled (P2Y) receptors that are responsive to adenosine triphosphate (ATP). All cells in the body contain millimolar concentrations of ATP, which is released if cells are lysed during injury and can then activate nociceptors. $P2X_3$ receptors are selectively expressed predominantly on small-diameter nociceptive sensory neurons.[15, 16] Serotonin (5-hydroxytryptamine (5-HT)) is released from platelets and mast cells after tissue injury. Receptors of the $5-HT_3$[17] and $5-HT_{2A}$ subtype are present on C-fibers, acting with other inflammatory mediators to excite and sensitize afferent nerve fibers (see Chapter 1b, Mechanisms of inflammatory hyperalgesia).[18]

Nociception: somatic versus visceral

For obvious reasons, the physiology of nociception has traditionally been elucidated by the examination of responses to ephemeral stimuli delivered to the skin.

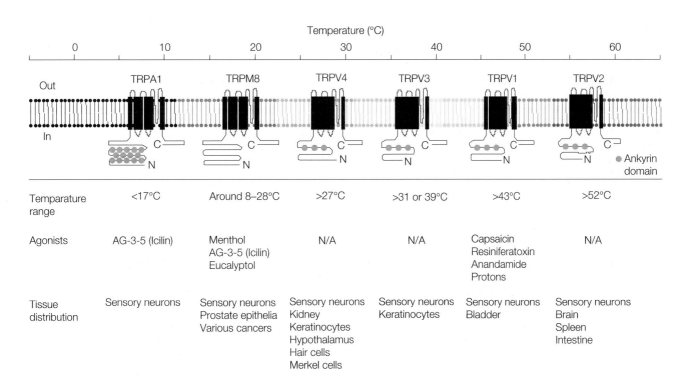

	TRPA1	TRPM8	TRPV4	TRPV3	TRPV1	TRPV2
Temparature range	<17°C	Around 8–28°C	>27°C	>31 or 39°C	>43°C	>52°C
Agonists	AG-3-5 (Icilin)	Menthol AG-3-5 (Icilin) Eucalyptol	N/A	N/A	Capsaicin Resiniferatoxin Anandamide Protons	N/A
Tissue distribution	Sensory neurons	Sensory neurons Prostate epithelia Various cancers	Sensory neurons Kidney Keratinocytes Hypothalamus Hair cells Merkel cells	Sensory neurons Keratinocytes	Sensory neurons Bladder	Sensory neurons Brain Spleen Intestine

Figure 1a.2 Capsaicin, the pungent ingredient of chili peppers, hydrogen ions, and noxious heat can activate the TRPV1 receptor. The involvement of TRPV1 in thermal nociception has been demonstrated by multiple methods, including the analysis of TRPV1-deficient mice. TRPV2, TRPM8, and TRPA1 are also very likely to be involved in thermal nociception, because their activation thresholds are within the noxious range of temperature. In addition to the TRP family K^+ channels, other membrane proteins such as Na^+/K^+ ATPase, members of degenerin/epithelial sodium channels (DEG/ENaC), and $P2X_3$ receptors have been reported to be thermosensitive.[14] However, the involvement of those proteins in thermonociception remains to be established. This figure was published in Jordt S-E, McKemy DD, Julius D. Lessons from peppers and peppermint: the molecular logic of thermosensation. *Current Opinion in Neurobiology*. 2003; **13**: 487–92, Copyright Elsevier.

Nevertheless, pain of visceral origin is an important clinical problem, and visceral and somatic nociception differ in several fundamental respects (**Table 1a.4**).[19] This is unsurprising when the biological functions of the sensory innervation of skin and viscera are considered: the somatic system warns of external threats, whereas the visceral system alerts the organism to the danger of internal disease. This functional difference is most obvious when the "effective stimuli" for exciting somatic and visceral nociceptors are considered. The thermal and mechanical stimuli referred to above as exciting somatic nociceptors are generally ineffective in evoking pain when delivered to internal organs. Indeed, sensory stimuli applied to certain parenchymatous internal organs, such as healthy lung, liver, and kidney, appear not to result in perception of any sensation. Pathological distension or contraction of the smooth muscle walls of hollow viscera and the capsules of parenchymatous organs does evoke pain, for example ureteric colic or labor pain, as does ischemia or inflammation. The precise localization of the source of injury is biologically important for cutaneous injury, but not for the viscera, and the activities of patients in this regard reflect this.[20]

Visceral afferents projecting into the spinal cord represent less than 10 percent of all spinal afferent input. Each viscus is innervated by two different nerves, typically the vagus nerve and a spinal ("splanchnic") nerve. Second-order spinal neurons upon which visceral afferents terminate also receive convergent nonvisceral input, as well as input from other viscera. Visceral nociceptors have been identified in most internal organs and are usually classified according to their mechanical properties. However, it is likely that their chemical sensitivity by locally acting agents play a more important role in the signaling of clinically relevant pain states than their mechanosensitivity. There is also increasing evidence for a major role of some nonneural elements in the signaling and transduction of visceral nociceptive events: for example, it has been demonstrated that ATP and nitric oxide (NO) released from urothelial cells modifies the activity of bladder sensory afferents. Molecular substrates underlying sensitivity of different viscera include acid-sensing ion channel (ASIC), TRPV1 and purinergic (P2X) receptors, voltage-gated Na^+ channels ($Na_v1.8$) and neuropeptides of the tachykinin family.[21] Finally, emerging evidence suggests that one visceral sensory cell soma in the dorsal root ganglion may generate axons that innervate different organs,

Table 1a.4 A comparison of the features of somatic and visceral pain.

	Visceral	Cutaneous
Effective stimuli	Direct trauma ineffective	Direct trauma effective
	Distension and ischemia effective	
Localization of site of injury	Poor	Precise
Primary hyperalgesia	Yes	Yes
Secondary hyperalgesia	Yes, at site of referral	Yes, around site of damage
Associated autonomic symptoms	Usual	Unusual

The transduction mechanisms for pain of visceral origin differ from those of the cutaneous system, reflecting the dissimilar biological roles of the cutaneous and visceral innervations. The function of the visceral system is to warn of internal disease rather than external threats. Thus, high-intensity thermal and mechanical stimuli are generally ineffectual, whereas visceral distension, inflammation, or ischemia and smooth muscle contraction evoke perception of pain.
Redrawn from McMahon SB. Are there fundamental differences in the peripheral mechanisms of visceral and somatic pain. *Behavioral and Brain Sciences.* 1997; **20**: 381–91, with permission from Cambridge University Press.[19]

and that silent visceral nociceptors appear to represent a greater proportion of the visceral innervation than has been reported in the skin.

THE SPINAL CORD

The central processes of the vast majority of primary afferent neurons enter the spinal cord via the dorsal roots, those associated with nociception lying in the ventrolateral portion of the root.[22] While most nociceptive neurons immediately enter the dorsal horn at the same segmental level, a significant proportion course caudally or rostrally for a few segments in the Lissauer's tract. The primary afferent neurons synapse with CNS (second order) neurons in the dorsal horn (**Figure 1a.3a**). In addition, descending axons from the brain stem synapse in the dorsal horn and modulate nociceptive transmission.

Anatomy: Rexed's laminae

The dorsal horn of the spinal cord is the first relay point for sensory information conveyed to the brain from the periphery. The spinal gray matter contains the nerve cell bodies of spinal neurons and the white matter contains axons that ascend to or descend from the brain. In 1952, based on neuronal cytoarchitecture, Rexed subdivided the gray matter into 10 laminae (**Figure 1a.3b**).[23] Laminae I–VI correspond to the dorsal horn and contain interneurons and projection neurons that relay incoming sensory information to the brain.[24]

Nociceptive fibers terminate primarily in the superficial dorsal horn, which comprises the marginal zone (lamina I) and the substantia gelatinosa (lamina II). Some Aδ-fibers also project more deeply and terminate in lamina V. In the dorsal horn, nociceptive afferents form connections with projection neurons or local excitatory

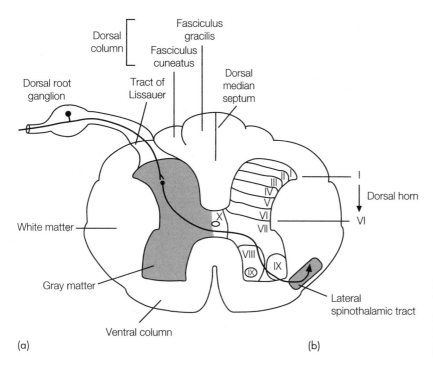

(a)   (b)

Figure 1a.3 Anatomy of the spinal cord. (a) The columnar organization of the white matter of the spinal cord is shown. (b) Rexed's scheme for lamination of the spinal gray matter (after Rexed[23]).

(glutamatergic) or inhibitory (GABAergic and/or glyci-nergic) interneurons to regulate the flow of nociceptive information to higher centers. These neurons are also located in laminae V and VI (**Figure 1a.4**). Under normal physiological conditions, tactile afferents (light touch) synapse in layers III and IV. Both nociceptive and tactile afferent neurons also have a convergent input into lamina V neurons, either directly or via interneurons.

Three major categories of neuronal cells can be identified in the dorsal horn: projection neurons and inhibitory and excitatory interneurons. Projection neurons are responsible for the forwarding of afferent traffic to higher centers, and three physiologically distinct neuronal types can be identified:

1. Nociceptive-specific (NS) cells respond exclusively to noxious stimuli, have small receptive fields, and predominate in lamina I, but are also found in laminae II and V.
2. Low-threshold (LT) neurons respond solely to innocuous stimuli and predominate in laminae III and IV.
3. Wide dynamic range (WDR) neurons respond to a range of sensory stimuli. WDR neurons receive converging inputs from a large number and diverse range of primary afferent neurons of disparate sensory modalities and consequentially possess large receptive fields. WDR neurons are predominantly in lamina V.

Compared with somatic fibers, visceral nociceptors are fewer, more widely distributed, proportionately activate a larger number of spinal neurons, and are not as well organized somatotopically. Visceral afferents terminate primarily in lamina V and to a lesser extent in lamina I. These two laminae represent points of central convergence between somatic and visceral inputs, an important feature

for the physiology of "referred" pain associated with visceral injury (see Mechanisms of referred pain).

Neurotransmitters in the dorsal horn

A variety of neurotransmitters have been implicated in nociceptive signaling in the dorsal horn (**Table 1a.5**).[25, 26, 27, 28, 29, 30, 31] While certain amino acids and neuropeptides play a predominant role, there is no convincing evidence for the existence of a single "pain neurotransmitter." In fact, the identification of a specific peptide with a specific physiological class of sensory receptor is unlikely in view of the coexistence, in various combinations, of up to four peptides in single dorsal root ganglia neurons. Furthermore, the distribution of neuropeptides in various types of tissue can be quite different. For example, in general, dorsal root ganglia neurons that innervate visceral targets are rich in substance P (SP) and calcitonin gene-related peptide (CGRP) compared with those innervating the skin. The concentrations of peptides in dorsal root ganglia neurons change after tissue injury and these changes outlast the pain behavior evoked by the pain stimulus. This indicates that tissue injury can alter the biochemical phenotype of the primary afferent neuron.

In addition to the interactions between peptides, there are also interactions between peptides and excitatory amino acid transmitters on dorsal horn neurons. Noxious stimulation evokes the release of glutamate and other amino acids that co-occur with the peptides in primary afferent terminals.[32] The amino acids glutamate and aspartate are the major participants in excitatory transmission at a spinal level. These substances are stored in the terminals of primary afferent nociceptors and are released in response to nociceptive activity. Exogenous application of these amino acids replicates spinal nociception and antagonists have analgesic qualities. The fast excitatory

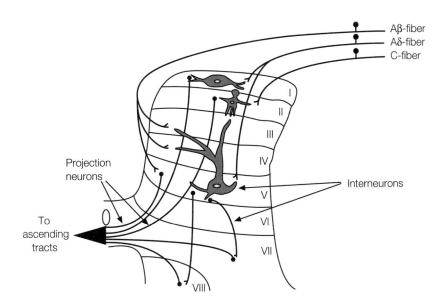

Figure 1a.4 Termination of primary afferent neurons in the dorsal horn of the spinal cord. Projection neurons in lamina I receive direct input from myelinated Aδ nociceptors and indirect input from unmyelinated C nociceptors via stalk cell interneurons terminating in lamina II. Lamina V neurons are predominantly of the wide dynamic range type. They receive low-threshold input from large-diameter myelinated Aα-fibers of mechanoreceptors, as well as both direct and indirect input from Aδ and C nociceptive afferents. (Redrawn with permission from Fields HL. *Pain*. The McGraw-Hill Companies, Inc., 1987, Copyright).[1]

Table 1a.5 Neurotransmitters in the dorsal horn mediating/modulating pain.

Neurotransmitter	Receptor	Effect on nociception
Nonpeptides		
Monoamines		
Norepinephrine	α_2	Inhibitory
5-HT	5-HT$_1$, (5-HT$_2$), (5-HT$_3$)	Inhibitory
Amino acids		
Inhibitory		
GABA	GABA$_A$, GABA$_B$	Inhibitory
Glycine		Inhibitory
Excitatory		
Glutamate	NMDA, AMPA, kainate, mGluR	Excitatory
Aspartate	NMDA, AMPA, kainate, mGluR	Excitatory
NO	cGMP	Excitatory
Acetylcholine	Muscarinic	Inhibitory
Peptides		
Opioids		
Enkephalins	δ (DOR), κ (KOR), μ (MOR)	Inhibitory
β-Endorphins	δ (DOR), κ (KOR), μ (MOR)	Inhibitory
Nociceptin	Nociceptin/orphanin F/Q, NOP (OP$_4$)	Excitatory/inhibitory
Nonopioids		
Substance P	NK1	Excitatory
CGRP	CGRP	Excitatory
CCK	CCK$_B$	Antagonist[a]
Galanin	GAL	Inhibitory
Somatostatin	sst	Inhibitory
Neuropeptide Y	Y$_1$, (Y$_2$)	Inhibitory
Neurotensin	NTS$_1$	Inhibitory
Bradykinin	B$_2$ (B$_1$)	Excitatory
Other		
Adenosine	A$_1$	Inhibitory
Purines	P2X$_3$	Excitatory
Cytokines		Excitatory
Capsaicin	TRPV1	Excitatory
Cannabinoids	CB$_1$, CB$_2$	Inhibitory

[a]Functional antagonist of opioid-induced analgesia.
Norepinephrine (noradrenaline). 5-HT, 5-hydroxytryptamine; AMPA, α-amino-3-hydroxy-5-methyl-4-isaxazole propionic acid; CCK, cholecystokinin; cGMP, cyclic guanosine monophosphate; CGRP, calcitonin gene-related peptide; DOR, delta opioid receptor; GABA, gamma-aminobutyric acid; KOR, kappa opioid receptor; mGluR, metabotropic glutamate receptor; MOR, mu opioid receptor; NK, neurokinin; NMDA, *N*-methyl-D-aspartate; NO, nitric oxide.

postsynaptic potentials generated by glutamate at the α-amino-3-hydroxy-5-methyl-4-isaxazole propionic acid (AMPA) subtype of glutamate receptor are principally involved in the onward transmission of nociceptive information under physiological conditions. The conditions required for glutamate-induced *N*-methyl-D-aspartate (NMDA) receptor activation are complex and only seem to be achieved after sustained activity in C-fiber primary afferent neurons. Neuropeptides such as SP and CGRP are costored in glutamatergic neurons and are also released from the spinal terminals of nociceptors in response to

afferent activity. These neuropeptides probably play a facilitatory role (neuromodulators) to the excitatory amino acids.

In addition to effects of GABA- and/or glycinergic interneurons, there are a number of other inhibitory neurotransmitters which modulate nociception at the dorsal horn segmental level. Somatostatin plays an important role in pain modulation at both central and peripheral sites. Studies have shown that peripheral somatostatin receptor activation on primary afferents prevents peripheral sensitization, modulates TRPV1 receptor, provides phasic and tonic inhibitory control of nociceptors, and contributes to counterirritation-induced analgesia.[33] One role of the endogenous opioids at a spinal level is to hyperpolarize primary afferent neurons and thus to attenuate neurotransmitter release in response to a nociceptive stimulus. A number of other molecules play a role in spinal modulation of nociception, e.g. adenosine, α_2-adrenergics, taurine, and endogenous cannabinoids (see **Table 1a.5** and below under Modulation of nociceptive messages). Neurotrophic factors, which support neuronal survival and growth during development of the nervous system, have been shown to play significant roles in the transmission of physiologic and pathologic pain. Brain-derived neurotrophic factor (BDNF), synthesized in the primary sensory neurons, is anterogradely transported to the central terminals of the primary afferents in the spinal dorsal horn, where it is involved in the modulation of painful stimuli.[34]

Microglia, oligodendrocytes, and astrocytes form a large group of CNS glial cells. These are not activated under basal conditions and appear not to influence pain sensitivity. However, microglia are activated by events such as CNS injury, microbial invasion, and some pain states, which leads to an increase in the production of various inflammatory cytokines, chemokines, and other potentially pain-producing substances (see Chapter 1b, Mechanisms of inflammatory hyperalgesia).[35]

Mechanisms of referred pain

A clinical characteristic of the pain which accompanies visceral injury is that it is often perceived by the sufferer as arising from a distinct somatic structure. A classic example is the pain that develops shortly after myocardial ischemia which is most often perceived as diffuse along the left arm. Such "referred pain" tends to be perceived as arising from somatic structures sharing an embryologically common spinal segmental origin with the injured viscus. Although the physiological mechanism of referred pain remains obscure, the weight of evidence suggests that it is a spinally mediated phenomenon. There are three major theories of referred pain: (1) the axon convergence (or axon reflex) theory, (2) the projection theories, (3) and a thalamic theory. None of these is mutually exclusive (**Figure 1a.5**).[19, 36]

Referred pain from viscera is partly due to central sensitization of viscerosomatic convergent neurons (triggered by the massive afferent visceral barrage), but also probably results from a reflex arc activation (the visceral input triggers reflex muscle contraction in turn responsible for sensitization of muscle nociceptors). However, referred pain from deep somatic structures is not explained by the mechanism of central sensitization of convergent neurons in its original form, since there is little convergence from deep tissues in the dorsal horn neurons. It has been proposed that these connections, not

present from the beginning, are opened by nociceptive input from skeletal muscle, and that referral to myotomes outside the lesion results from the spread of central sensitization to adjacent spinal segments.[37]

FROM THE SPINAL CORD TO THE BRAIN

Nociceptive input to the dorsal horn is relayed to higher centers in the brain via several ascending pathways: the spinothalamic tract, classically considered as the major pain pathway; spinomedullary and spinobulbar projections to regions of the medulla and brain stem that are important for homeostatic control; and the spinohypothalamic tract to the hypothalamus and ventral forebrain. Spinal projections to other sites, such as the cerebellum or lateral reticular nucleus, are more involved in sensorimotor integration than direct nociceptive transmission.[9] Evidence suggests that there may be other pathways, i.e. a spinopontoamygdaloid pathway and an additional pathway for visceral pain ascending in the posterior funiculus.[38]

Spinothalamic pathways

The spinothalamic tract (STT) originates from neurons in laminae I and V–VII, and is composed of the axons of nociceptive-specific and wide dynamic range neurons. The majority (85 percent) of spinothalamic tract axons cross and ascend contralaterally. Lamina I cells form the lateral STT and project to the thalamus (particularly the posterior part of the ventral medial nucleus (Vmpo)), and then to the insular cortex, and mediate the autonomic and unpleasant emotional perceptions of pain. Deeper laminae neurons form the anterior STT and project to the ventral posterolateral nucleus of the thalamus and carry the discriminative aspect of pain (e.g. location, intensity, duration).[39] Some spinothalamic fibers also project to the periaqueductal gray matter (creating a link with descending pathways), reticular activating system, and hypothalamus (probably contributing to the arousal response to pain).

Spinobulbar pathways

Ascending spinobulbar pathways project to several sites within the brain stem, that include the parabrachial nucleus, periaqueductal gray (PAG), catecholamine cell groups (A1–A7), and the brain stem reticular formation.[9, 40] The spinoparabrachial pathway originates largely from lamina I neurons that express the NK1 receptor, and the parabrachial area is a major site for nociceptive and homeostatic integration in the brain stem.[40, 41] This pathway signals the intensity of noxious stimuli, has large receptive fields, and provides input to parts of the brain involved in the emotional or affective components of pain.[42] From

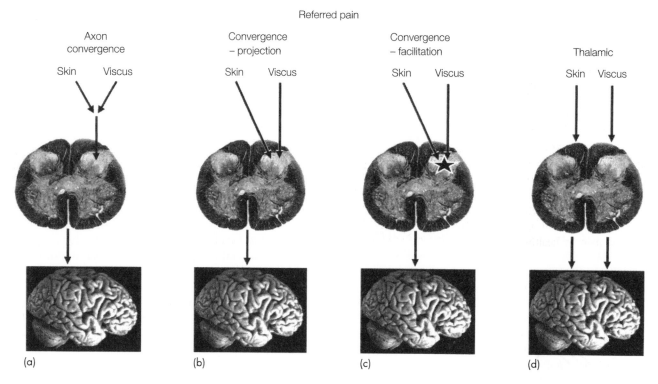

Figure 1a.5 Various theoretical mechanisms of referred pain. (a) Axon convergence/reflex theory. Primary sensory neurons possess bifurcating axons which innervate both somatic and visceral targets. The central nervous system (CNS) is unable to differentiate between such inputs and misinterprets visceral nociceptive input as somatic in origin. While there is some experimental evidence to support this hypothesis, it is not generally accepted as explaining referred pain. (b,c) Convergence theories. There are two variants of this theory, projection (b) and facilitation (c). They both require the convergence of somatic and visceral afferent signals on single dorsal horn neurons. In general, the greater proportion of afferent neurons is of somatic origin and, therefore, visceral afferent information is perceived as somatic in origin. Indeed, there may be an inherent lack of capability of visceral pain perception in the absence of a somatic input. (b) Convergence-projection theory. Visceral afferent neurons converge on the same spinal pain-projection neurons as the nociceptive afferent neurons from the somatic structures in which the pain is perceived. The brain is unable to discriminate between visceral and somatic inputs and mistakenly "projects" the sensation to the somatic structure. (c) Convergence–facilitation theory. Sustained activity in visceral afferent fibers alters the excitability states of dorsal horn neurons with convergent visceral and somatic afferent input. This creates an "irritable focus" which facilitates the onward progress of normally subliminal traffic of somatic origin, so that other, segmentally appropriate, somatic inputs can now produce abnormal and, of course, referred pain sensations. While both these theories (b) and (c) explain the segmental rule, the convergence–facilitation theory has the advantage of explaining the phenomenon of referred hyperalgesia and the concept of central sensitization, which adds weight to its credence. (d) Thalamic theory. Interactions at supraspinal levels (thalamus) lead to the phenomenon of referred pain. Although the thalamic theory was regarded as improbable, the existence of distinct spinal ascending pathways for visceral nociceptors have lent support for this hypothesis. However, referred hyperalgesia and the segmental nature of referred pain are hard to account for by the thalamic theory alone. (Redrawn from McMahon SB. Are there fundamental differences in the peripheral mechanisms of visceral and somatic pain. *Behavioral and Brain Sciences.* 1997; **20**: 381–91, with permission from Cambridge University Press).[19]

the parabrachial area, neurons project to the hypothalamus and to amygdala components of the limbic system (**Figure 1a.1b**).

Projections to catecholamine cell groups, such as the locus coeruleus or A7, are involved in integration of cardiorespiratory and autonomic function, and link with descending modulatory mechanisms.[9] The PAG also receives spinal input (predominantly lamina I cells, but also lamina VII), is involved in homeostatic control, and is integrated with descending modulatory pathways, particularly via projections to the rostroventromedial medulla (RVM).[9]

IN THE BRAIN

By following the projection pathways originating in the nociceptive areas of the spinal cord dorsal horn (laminae I and V), it is possible to associate brain regions with nociceptive function. By doing so, several nuclei in the lateral thalamus (ventral posterior lateral nucleus, ventral posterior medial nucleus, ventral posterior inferior nucleus, posterior part of ventromedial nucleus) and in the medial thalamus (centrolateral thalamus, ventrocaudal part of medial dorsal nucleus, parafascicular nucleus) have been identified, which in turn project to the cortical areas. The list of cortical areas that may subserve nociceptive functions includes: primary somatosensory cortex (S1), secondary somatosensory cortex (S2), and its vicinity in the parietal operculum, insula, anterior cingulate cortex, and prefrontal cortex.[38, 43, 44] Thus, multiple cortical areas are activated by painful stimuli (**Figure 1a.6**).[45]

Pain is a multidimensional experience including sensory–discriminative and affective–motivational components. A recent major advance in the understanding of the central mechanisms of pain processing has evolved from application of brain imaging with positron emission tomography (PET) and functional magnetic resonance imaging (fMRI). The results from several groups working on experimentally induced pain in healthy volunteers have shown decreased

global blood flow, as well as increased regional cerebral blood flow in those areas of the brain subserving nociceptive functions (see also **Figure 1a.6**).[46, 47] One important new aspect of correlating PET imaging with psychological assessment is the possibility of attributing the processing of specific pain dimensions to an anatomical substrate in the brain's pain circuitry: (1) the gating function reflected by the pain threshold appeared to be related to the anterior cingulate cortex, the frontal inferior cortex, and the thalamus; (2) the coding of pain intensity to the periventricular gray and the posterior cingulate cortex; (3) the encoding of pain unpleasantness to the posterior sector of the anterior cingulate cortex.[48] Furthermore, investigators are now considering the impact of individual traits and of the context of the pain experience (e.g. attention or distraction) on

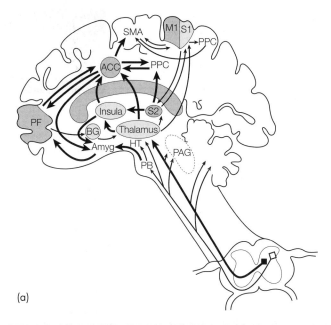

(a)

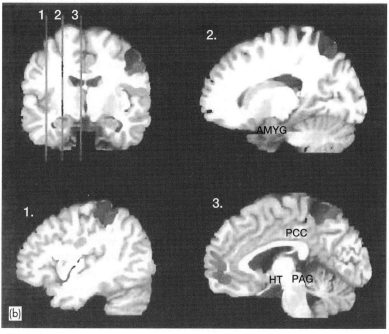

(b)

Figure 1a.6   (a) Afferent pathways and their interconnectivity of cortical and subcortical regions of the brain involved in pain perception. (b) Coronal and sagittal slices of a magnetic resonance image showing the areas corresponding to those shown in (a). ACC, anterior cingulate cortex; Amyg, amygdala; BG, basal ganglia; HT, hypothalamus; M1, primary motor cortex; PAG, periaqueductal gray; PB, parabrachial nuclei; PCC, posterior cingulate cortex; PPC, posterior parietal cortex; PF, prefrontal cortex; S1 and S2, primary and secondary somatosensory cortices; SMA, supplementary motor cortex. This figure was published in Apkarian AV, Bushnell MC, Treede RD, Zubieta JK. Human brain mechanisms of pain perception and regulation in health and disease. *European Journal of Pain.* 2005; **9**: 463–84, Copyright Elsevier.[45]

forebrain activity evoked by noxious stimuli.[49, 50] Finally, it has recently been suggested that cortical activity must be highly dependent on reciprocal interactions with thalamic relays as there are nearly ten times as many fibers projecting back from S1 to the ventrobasal thalamus as there are in the forward direction from thalamus to cortex. Thus, heightened activity in corticofugal S1 neurons may create a zone of enhanced activity within the thalamocortical loop that mediates discrimination between tactile and painful sensations.[48]

MODULATION OF NOCICEPTIVE MESSAGES

It is a common observation that, under certain circumstances, pain perception is not necessarily a consequence of tissue injury and nociception. To explain this finding, it is necessary to hypothesize that the "pain pathway" has a

more complex role than the mere relaying of sensory information from nociceptor to brain, but can also regulate the passage of nociceptive activity information. There are a number of sites where such modulation might take place, but most is known about the major interface between the peripheral and central nervous systems at the dorsal horn of the spinal cord. The excitability of spinal cord neurons is dependent on the balance of inputs from primary afferent nociceptors, intrinsic spinal cord neurons, and descending systems projecting from supraspinal sites.[27, 51]

Segmental (spinal) control

Spinal modulation of nociceptive activity involves the endogenous opioid system, segmental inhibition, the balance of activity between nociceptive and other afferent inputs, and a descending control operative mechanism (**Figure 1a.7**).[9, 51]

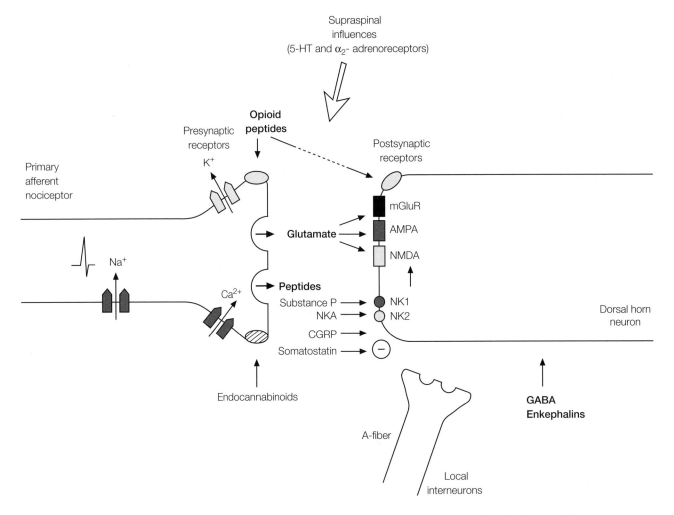

Figure 1a.7 A schematic diagram illustrating the release of neurotransmitters and neuropeptides from C-fibers and the subsequent effects and interactions between different excitatory and inhibitory systems on a dorsal horn neuron. The primary afferent neuron releases a variety of co-occurring neuropeptides and excitatory amino acids in response to noxious stimuli. These act at several postsynaptic receptors. In addition, opioid peptides act upon both pre- and postsynaptic opioid receptors (presynaptic action being predominant) to modulate transmitter release and the firing of second-order nociceptors. (Reprinted with permission from Elsevier (*The Lancet*. 1999; **353**, 1610–15)).[51]

Opioid receptors in the spinal cord are a key site for the production of analgesia. There are four classes of opioid receptors: delta, δ (DOR); kappa, κ (KOR); mu, μ (MOR); and nociceptin/orphanin F/Q, NOP (also previously known as ORL1 or OP4). Numerous endogenous opioid peptides are derived from one of the genes that encode the large glycoprotein precursors of the physiologically active peptides.[52] Members of each family are located at sites associated with the processing or modulation of nociception, and, in particular, in laminae I and II of the dorsal horn of the spinal cord. At this level, the principal analgesic mechanism of opioids is by presynaptic inhibition of injury-evoked neurotransmitter release from the primary afferent nociceptive neurons (over 70 percent of the total spinal μ receptor sites are located on the primary afferent terminals).[53] Endogenous opioids also appear to cause some direct postsynaptic inhibition of dorsal horn nociresponsive neurons, including identified projection cells. In summary, each of the four major classes of opioid receptor may contribute to the opioid-induced modulation of transmission of nociceptive information in the dorsal horn.

Transmission of nociceptive input in the spinal cord can be inhibited by segmental activity in the cord itself, as well as descending neural activity from supraspinal centers (see below under Supraspinal/descending control).[54] Inhibitory interneurons release GABA and glycine and play an important role in segmental inhibition of pain in the spinal cord. GABA is well situated to modulate the afferent transmission of nociceptive information by presynaptic and postsynaptic mechanisms. The concentration of GABA is the highest in the dorsal horn of the spinal cord, where it is a major inhibitory transmitter. Studies of acute nociception suggest that the afferent transmission of nociceptive information in the spinal cord is subject to modulation by endogenously released GABA acting at either $GABA_A$ or $GABA_B$ receptors. GABA and glycine colocalize in many neurons in the dorsal horn, and in fact nearly every glycine-immunoreactive neuron in laminae I–III also contains GABA. The mechanism by which glycine modulates afferent transmission in the dorsal horn is one of postsynaptic inhibition; glycine receptors are predominantly postsynaptic in the dorsal horn.

Our understanding of the activity of cannabis started with the isolation and synthesis of Δ^9-tetrahydrocannabinol, its main psychoactive constituent. Two subtypes of the cannabinoid receptor, CB_1 and CB_2, have been identified and cloned.[30] Synthetic cannabinoids have been described and an endocannabinoid system identified (anandamide and 2-arachidonyl glycerol).[55, 56, 57] The potential antinociceptive action of cannabinoids is now well demonstrated in animal studies and in some clinical trials. More studies are necessary to fully appreciate the analgesic potential of cannabinoids in humans.[58] The mechanisms of action for cannabinoid antinociception include both spinal and supraspinal actions,[59] as well as a more recently

recognized peripheral mechanism. Cannabinoid CB_1 receptors have been identified in the spinal cord and on primary afferent neurons, where they are ideally located to modulate dorsal horn neuron activity. Evidence suggests that cannabinoids and endocannabinoids may act on spinal interneurons to modulate the release of neurotransmitters and thus pain transmission. Finally, cannabinoid CB_2 receptors have been found in the immune system and participate in the anti-inflammatory and antinociceptive effects of cannabinoids.[60]

Other modulators in nociception – one gas (nitric oxide) and two peptides (cholecystokinin and galanin) – have also been studied extensively. Nitric oxide has been recognized to have a prominent role in the nervous system, both as an intracellular second messenger and as a presynaptically formed neurotransmitter.[61] NO takes part in many aspects of pain perception process (inflammation, neuronal transmission). Hence, NO has been shown to have a pronociceptive or antinociceptive role in pain perception.[62, 63] NO plays a facilitating role in the neuronal process of pain transmission especially in the spinal cord. This had been confirmed by the fact that NOS inhibitors could reduce pain behavior in different pain models.[64] However, the NO/cGMP pathway is involved in the mechanisms of action of some analgesic drugs and donors of NO (nitroglycerine, L-arginine) have been shown to have antinociceptive properties, especially in the periphery.

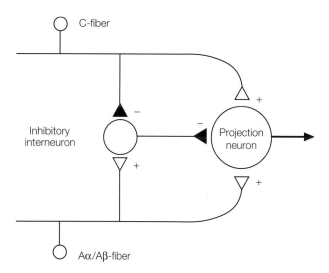

Figure 1a.8 The dorsal horn is not merely a pathway for transmission of nociceptive information, but also the site of considerable signal modulation. In 1965, in attempting to explain the clinical observation that tissue damage and the activation of peripheral nociceptors does not necessarily result in the perception of pain, Melzack and Wall[70] formulated the gate control theory of pain. They proposed that, within the spinal cord, a physiological "gate" existed and, depending on the degree of opening of this gate, nociceptive information was permitted or prevented from ascending to the brain.

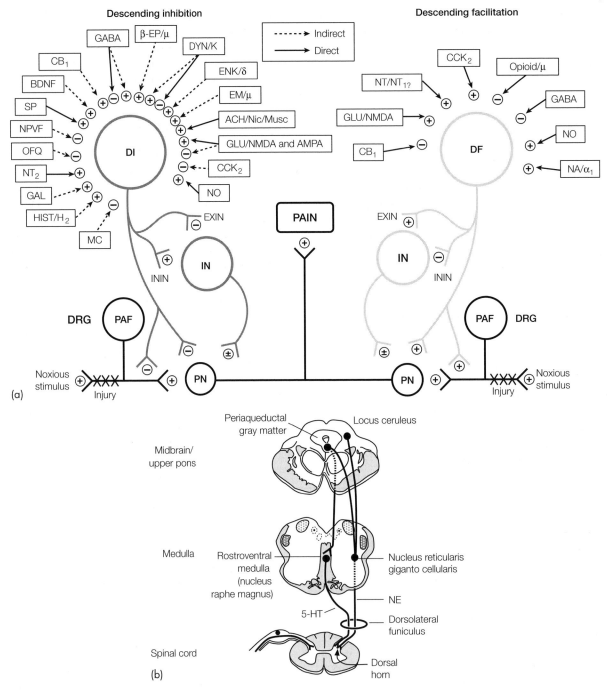

Figure 1a.9 (a) Overview of the multiplicity of mechanisms involved in the modulation of the activity of pathways mediating descending inhibition (DI) as compared to descending facilitation (DF). Certain act directly and others indirectly via intervening neurones. For mechanisms modulating DI, in many cases, actions at "OFF" cells in the rostroventromedial medulla and at serotonergic and noradrenergic neurones are involved, but additional mechanisms are certainly implicated. For mechanisms modulating DF, actions at "ON" cells in the rostroventromedial medulla and at descending pathways releasing transmitters are likely implicated but they remain poorly defined. At the level of the dorsal horn, note that pathways mediating DI and DF exert opposite patterns of influence upon primary afferent fiber (PAF) terminals, projection neurones (PNs), excitatory interneurones (EXINs) and inhibitory interneurones (ININs). ACh, acetylcholine; β-EP, β-endorphin; CB, cannabinoid; CCK, cholecystokinin; DRG, dorsal root ganglion; DYN, dynorphin; EM, endomorphin; ENK, enkephalin; GABA, gamma-hydroxy-butyric acid; GLU, glutamate; Hist, histamine; musc, muscarinic; NA, noradrenaline; NE, norepinephrine; nic, nicotinic; NMDA, N-methyl-D-aspartate; NO, nitric oxide; NPVF, neuropeptide VF; NT, neurotensin; OFQ, orphanin FQ (nociceptin); SP, substance P. (This figure was published in Millan MJ. Descending control of pain. *Progress in Neurobiology*. 2002; **66**: 355–474, Copyright Elsevier).[72] (b) Descending control system showing postulated sites of action of opioids on pain transmission. Each of these locations contains neurons that are potentially capable of modulating the firing of nociceptive projection neurons. 5-HT, 5-hydroxytryptamine.

Cholecystokinin (CCK) belongs to the gastrin family of peptides and is widely distributed in the nervous system, where it has been shown to be a neurotransmitter mediating many important functions. CCK appears to have an important but complex involvement in nociceptive transmission and modulation. The most well-defined and apparently physiological role for CCK is that it is a functional antagonist of opioid-induced analgesia.[65] The sites of interaction between CCK and opioids are clearly multiple, but the spinal cord is an important site. It has been suggested that CCK does not alter baseline pain threshold but reduces the binding affinity of MOR (μ opioid receptor) ligands and also counteracts intracellular events subsequent to opioid receptor activation. Thus, CCK antagonists are a potential interesting target to enhance opioid analgesia.[66]

Galanin is a neuropeptide widely distributed in the nervous system and occurs in a small population of primary sensory neurons and also in spinal interneurons.[67] Overwhelming evidence supporting an antinociceptive role for galanin has been obtained from electrophysiological studies in which galanin hyperpolarizes the majority of dorsal horn neurons. Under normal conditions, galanin is released upon C-fiber stimulation and plays an inhibitory role in mediating spinal cord excitability. Studies on the interaction between galanin and morphine support an antinociceptive role for galanin: it is suggested that the spinal effect of morphine is mediated in part by the inhibitory action of galanin.[68]

Proteinases, such as thrombin, trypsin, and tryptase, released during trauma and inflammation, exert many of their effects by activating proteinase-activated receptors (PAR). Proteinase-activated receptor-2 (PAR2) is expressed by primary spinal afferent neurons, and PAR2 agonists (such as trypsin or tryptase) stimulate release of substance P and CGRP in peripheral tissues. Recent evidence has shown that agonists of PAR2 signal to primary afferent neurons to cause marked and sustained hyperalgesia.[69] These agonists induce sensitization of dorsal horn neurons and the release of prostaglandins. Therefore, it is suggested that proteinases, acting in part through PAR2, have a role to play in pain transmission.

Purines, such as adenosine and ATP, are endogenous ligands involved in modulating pain transmission by acting on P1 and P2 purinoceptors, respectively, at sites both in peripheral tissues and in the CNS. The most well-known of the P2 receptors is the $P2X_3$ subtype, which is found in primary sensory neurons (only in nonpeptidergic neurons). Multiple subtypes of purinoceptors are potential molecular targets for the treatment of pain.[15]

In summary, segmental modulation of nociception has been studied extensively and many neurotransmitters and receptors (**Table 1a.5**) located in the dorsal horn of the spinal cord have been identified, but the role of some of these substances remains obscure, whereas the involvement of others in pain processes has been relatively established. This is further complicated by the fact that some of the peptides implicated are localized not only in primary afferent neuron terminals, but also in intrinsic neurons and descending fibers. Finally, additional complexity is provided by the coexistence of several peptides and classic neurotransmitters in the same neuron.

Supraspinal/descending control

The activity of neurons in the spinal cord that receive input from nociceptive fibers may be modified by inputs from other nonnociceptive afferent neurons.[11] This concept led to the introduction by Melzack and Wall in 1965 of the gate control theory (**Figure 1a.8**).[70] According to this model, activity in Aβ afferents inhibits dorsal horn neurons from responding to Aδ- and C-fiber inputs. Thus, pain may be relieved by stimulation of the myelinated afferent fibers. The use of transcutaneous electrical nerve stimulation to relieve pain in clinical practice is based in part on this theory (see Chapter 14, Transcutaneous electrical nerve stimulation (TENS) and acupuncture for acute pain, for further details).

A network of descending pathways projecting from cerebral structures to the dorsal horn plays a complex and crucial role. Early studies established that descending influences were tonically active and principally inhibitory in function.[71] However, we now know that specific centrifugal pathways either suppress (descending inhibition) or potentiate (descending facilitation) passage of nociceptive messages to the brain (**Figure 1a.9**).[72] Accumulating evidence suggests that descending facilitatory influences may contribute to the development and maintenance of chronic pain states.[71, 73]

REFERENCES

1. Fields HL. *Pain*. New York: McGraw-Hill, 1987.
2. Sherrington CS. *The integrative action of the nervous system*. New York: Scribner, 1906.
3. Snider WD, McMahon SB. Tackling pain at the source: new ideas about nociceptors. *Neuron*. 1998; **20**: 629–32.
4. Braz JM, Nassar MA, Wood JN, Basbaum AI. Parallel "pain" pathways arise from subpopulations of primary afferent nociceptor. *Neuron*. 2005; **47**: 787–93.
5. Gardner EP, Martin JH, Jessell TM. The bodily senses. In: Kandel ER, Schwartz JH, Jessell TM (eds). *Principles of neural science*. New York: McGraw-Hill, 2000: 430–50.
6. Julius D, Basbaum AI. Molecular mechanisms of nociception. *Nature*. 2001; **413**: 203–10.
7. Meyer RA, Ringkamp M, Campbell JN, Raja SN. Peripheral mechanisms of cutaneous nociception. In: McMahon BS, Koltzenburg M (eds). *Textbook of pain*. Philadelphia, PA: Elsevier, Churchill Livingstone, 2006: 3–34.
8. Caterina MJ, Schumacher MA, Tominaga M *et al*. The capsaicin receptor: a heat-activated ion channel in the pain pathway. *Nature*. 1997; **389**: 816–24.

9. Dostrovsky J, Craig A. Ascending projection systems. In: McMahon SB, Koltzenburg M (eds). *Wall and Melzack's textbook of pain*, 5th edn. New York: Elsevier, Churchill Livingstone, 2006: 187–203.

10. Lewin GR, Moshourab R. Mechanosensation and pain. *Journal of Neurobiology.* 2004; **61**: 30–44.

11. Gold MS. Ion channels: Recent advances and clinical applications. In: Flor H, Kalso E, Dostrovsky JO (eds). *Proceedings of the 11th World Congress on Pain.* Seattle, WA: IASP Press, 2006: 73–92.

12. Krishtal O. The ASICs: signaling molecules? Modulators? *Trends in Neuroscience.* 2003; **26**: 477–83.

* 13. Jordt S-E, McKemy DD, Julius D. Lessons from peppers and peppermint: the molecular logic of thermosensation. *Current Opinion in Neurobiology.* 2003; **13**: 487–92.

14. Tominaga M, Caterina MJ. Thermosensation and pain. *Journal of Neurobiology.* 2004; **61**: 3–12.

* 15. Liu XJ, Salter MW. Purines and pain mechanisms: recent developments. *Current Opinion in Investigational Drugs.* 2005; **6**: 65–75.

* 16. Burnstock G. Purinergic P2 receptors as targets for novel analgesics. *Pharmacology and Therapeutics.* 2006; **110**: 433–54.

17. Zeitz KP, Guy N, Malmberg AB *et al.* The 5-HT₃ subtype of serotonin receptor contributes to nociceptive processing via a novel subset of myelinated and unmyelinated nociceptors. *Journal of Neuroscience.* 2002; **22**: 1010–9.

18. Sommer C. Serotonin in pain and analgesia: actions in the periphery. *Molecular Neurobiology.* 2004; **30**: 117–25.

19. McMahon SB. Are there fundamental differences in the peripheral mechanisms of visceral and somatic pain. *Behavioral and Brain Sciences.* 1997; **20**: 381–91.

20. Cervero F, Laird JMA. Understanding the signaling and transmission of visceral nociceptive events. *Journal of Neurobiology.* 2004; **61**: 45–54.

21. Gebhart GF, Bielefeldt K, Dang K *et al.* Visceral pain and visceral hypersensitivity. In: Flor H, Kalso E, Dostrovsky JO (eds). *Proceedings of the 11th World Congress on Pain.* Seattle, WA: IASP Press, 2006: 285–300.

22. Amaral DG. The functional organization of perception and movement. In: Kandel ER, Schwartz JH, Jessell TM (eds). *Principles of neural science.* New York: McGraw-Hill, 2000: 337–48.

23. Rexed B. The cytoarchitectonic organization of the spinal cord in the cat. *Journal of Comparative Neurology.* 1952; **96**: 415–95.

24. Parent A. *Carpenter's human neuroanatomy.* Baltimore, MD: Williams & Wilkins, 1996.

25. Levine JD, Fields HL, Basbaum AI. Peptides and the primary afferent nociceptor. *Journal of Neuroscience.* 1993; **13**: 2273–86.

26. Dickenson AH. Spinal cord pharmacology of pain. *British Journal of Anaesthesia.* 1995; **75**: 193–200.

27. Fürst S. Transmitters involved in antinociception in the spinal cord. *Brain Research Bulletin.* 1999; **48**: 129–41.

28. Chizh BA, Illes P. P2X receptors and nociception. *Pharmacological Reviews.* 2001; **53**: 553–68.

29. Couture R, Harrisson M, Vianna RM, Cloutier F. Kinin receptors in pain and inflammation. *European Journal of Pharmacology.* 2001; **429**: 161–76.

30. Pertwee RG. Cannabinoid receptors and pain. *Progress in Neurobiology.* 2001; **63**: 569–611.

31. Dobner PR. Neurotensin and pain modulation. *Peptides.* 2006; **27**: 2405–14.

32. Horvath G, Kekesi G. Interaction of endogenous ligands mediating antinociception. *Brain Research Reviews.* 2006; **52**: 69–92.

33. Ji GC, Zhou ST, Shapiro G *et al.* Analgesic activity of a non-peptide imidazolidinedione somatostatin agonist: *In vitro* and *in vivo* studies in rat. *Pain.* 2006; **124**: 34–49.

34. Obata K, Noguchi K. BDNF in sensory neurons and chronic pain. *Neuroscience Research.* 2006; **55**: 1–10.

35. Marchand F, Perretti M, McMahon SB. Role of the immune system in chronic pain. *Nature Reviews Neuroscience.* 2005; **6**: 521–32.

36. Bielefeldt K, Gebhart GF. Visceral pain: basic mechanisms. In: McMahon SB, Koltzenburg M (eds). *Wall and Melzack's textbook of pain.* New York: Elsevier, Churchill Livingstone, 2006: 721–36.

37. Giamberardino MA. Referred muscle pain/hyperalgesia and central sensitisation. *Journal of Rehabilitation Medicine.* 2003; **41** (Suppl.): 85–8.

38. Bushnell MC, Apkarian AV. Representation of pain in the brain. In: McMahon SB, Koltzenburg M (eds). *Wall and Melzack's textbook of pain.* New York: Elsevier Churchill Livingstone, 2006: 107–24.

39. Craig AD. Pain mechanisms: labeled lines versus convergence in central processing. *Annual Review of Neuroscience.* 2003; **26**: 1–30.

* 40. Mantyh PW, Hunt SP. Setting the tone: superficial dorsal horn projection neurons regulate pain sensitivity. *Trends in Neuroscience.* 2004; **27**: 582–4.

41. Bester H, Chapman V, Besson JM, Bernard JF. Physiological properties of the lamina I spinoparabrachial neurons in the rat. *Journal of Neurophysiology.* 2000; **83**: 2239–59.

42. Hunt SP, Mantyh PW. The molecular dynamics of pain control. *Nature Reviews. Neuroscience.* 2001; **2**: 83–91.

43. Treede R-D, Kenshalo DR, Gracely RH, Jones AKP. The cortical representation of pain. *Pain.* 1999; **79**: 105–11.

44. Craig AD, Chen K, Bandy D, Reiman EM. Thermosensory activation of insular cortex. *Nature Neuroscience.* 2000; **3**: 184–90.

45. Apkarian AV, Bushnell MC, Treede RD, Zubieta JK. Human brain mechanisms of pain perception and regulation in health and disease. *European Journal of Pain.* 2005; **9**: 463–84.

* 46. Tracey I. Nociceptive processing in the human brain. *Current Opinion in Neurobiology.* 2005; **15**: 478–87.

47. Schweinhardt P, Lee M, Tracey I. Imaging pain in patients: is it meaningful? *Current Opinion in Neurology.* 2006; **19**: 392–400.

48. Montconduit L, Lopez-Avila A, Molat J-L *et al.* Corticothalamic feedback from the primary somatosensory cortex: A link for bottom-up and top-down processing of

innocuous and noxious inputs. In: Flor H, Kalso E, Dostrovsky JO (eds). *Proceedings of the 11th World Congress on Pain.* Seattle, WA: IASP Press, 2006: 321–9.

49. Rainville P. Brain mechanisms of pain affect and pain modulation. *Current Opinion in Neurobiology.* 2002; **12**: 195–204.

50. Raij TT, Numminen J, Narvanen S et al. Brain correlates of subjective reality of physically and psychologically induced pain. *Proceedings of the National Academy of Sciences of the United States of America.* 2005; **102**: 2147–51.

51. Besson JM. Neurobiology of pain. *Lancet.* 1999; **353**: 1610–15.

52. Eguchi M. Recent advances in selective opioid receptor agonists and antagonists. *Medical Research Reviews.* 2004; **24**: 182–212.

53. Fields H. State-dependent opioid control of pain. *Nature Reviews Neuroscience.* 2004; **5**: 565–75.

54. Hammond DL. Inhibitory neurotransmitters and nociception: role of GABA and glycine. In: Dickinson AH, Besson JM (eds). *The pharmacology of pain.* Berlin: Springer-Verlag, 1997: 361–83.

55. Hohmann AG. Spinal and peripheral mechanisms of cannabinoid antinociception: behavioral. Neurophysiological and neuroanatomical perspectives. *Chemistry and Physics of Lipids.* 2002; **121**: 173–90.

56. Rice AS, Farquhar-Smith WP, Nagy I. Endocannabinoids and pain: spinal and peripheral analgesia in inflammation and neuropathy. *Prostaglandins, Leukotrienes, and Essential Fatty Acids.* 2002; **66**: 243–56.

57. Pacher P, Batkai S, Kunos G. The endocannabinoid system as an emerging target of pharmacotherapy. *Pharmacological Reviews.* 2006; **58**: 389–462.

58. Beaulieu P, Ware M. Reassessment of the role of cannabinoids in the management of pain. *Current Opinion in Anaesthesiology.* 2007; **20**: 473–7.

59. Hohmann AG, Suplita RL, Bolton NM et al. An endocannabinoid mechanism for stress-induced analgesia. *Nature.* 2005; **435**: 1108–12.

60. Ibrahim MM, Rude ML, Stagg NJ et al. CB2 cannabinoid receptor mediation of antinociception. *Pain.* 2006; **122**: 36–42.

61. Meller ST, Gebhart GF. Nitric oxide (NO) and nociceptive processing in the spinal cord. *Pain.* 1993; **52**: 127–36.

62. Sousa AM, Prado WA. The dual effect of a nitric oxide donor in nociception. *Brain Research.* 2001; **897**: 9–19.

63. Vivancos GG, Parada CA, Ferreira SH. Opposite nociceptive effects of the arginine/NO/cGMP pathway stimulation in dermal and subcutaneous tissues. *British Journal of Pharmacology.* 2003; **138**: 1351–7.

64. Aronov S, Ben-Abraham R, Givati-Divshi D, Katz Y. Involvement of nitric oxide in clonidine-induced spinal analgesia. *Drug Metabolism and Drug Interactions.* 2005; **21**: 41–53.

65. Stanfa LC, Dickenson AH, Xu XJ, Wiesenfeld Hallin Z. Cholecystokinin and morphine analgesia: variations on a theme. *Trends in Pharmacological Sciences.* 1994; **15**: 65–6.

66. Le Guen S, Mas Nieto M, Canestrelli C et al. Pain management by a new series of dual inhibitors of enkephalin degrading enzymes: long lasting antinociceptive properties and potentiation by CCK2 antagonist or methadone. *Pain.* 2003; **104**: 139–48.

67. Wiesenfeld-Hallin Z, Xu XJ, Crawley JN, Hökfelt T. Galanin and spinal nociceptive mechanisms: recent results from transgenic and knock-out models. *Neuropeptides.* 2005; **39**: 207–10.

68. Liu HX, Hokfelt T. The participation of galanin in pain processing at the spinal level. *Trends in Pharmacological Sciences.* 2002; **23**: 468–74.

69. Vergnolle N, Bunnett NW, Sharkley KA et al. Proteinase-activated receptor-2 and hyperalgesia: a novel pain pathway. *Nature Medicine.* 2001; **7**: 821–6.

70. Melzack R, Wall PD. Pain mechanisms: a new theory. *Science.* 1965; **150**: 971–9.

71. Gebhart GF. Descending modulation of pain. *Neuroscience and Biobehavioral Reviews.* 2004; **27**: 729–37.

∗ 72. Millan MJ. Descending control of pain. *Progress in Neurobiology.* 2002; **66**: 355–474.

73. Hunt SP, Suzuki R, Rahman W, Dickenson AH. Chronic pain and descending facilitation. In: Flor H, Kalso E, Dostrovsky JO (eds). *Proceedings of the 11th World Congress on Pain.* Seattle, WA: IASP Press, 2006: 349–63.

Mechanisms of inflammatory hyperalgesia

SUELLEN M WALKER

KEY LEARNING POINTS

- Hyperalgesia is defined as an increased sensitivity to noxious stimuli. Allodynia refers to pain evoked by previously non-noxious or subthreshold stimuli.
- Primary hyperalgesia is increased sensitivity within the area of injury and is produced by changes in peripheral nociceptor function.
- Secondary hyperalgesia occurs in undamaged skin around an injury site and is due to centrally mediated changes in sensitivity.
- Enhanced sensitivity in dorsal horn nociceptive processing is described by the general term central sensitization.
- Changes in the electrophysiological properties of dorsal horn neurons may contribute to central sensitization. Wind up is evoked by low frequency stimuli and manifest as an enhanced postsynaptic response during a

train of stimuli. Long-term potentiation (LTP) is usually generated by higher frequency stimuli and outlasts the conditioning stimulus.
- Intracellular signaling cascades contribute to sensitization by (1) posttranslational modification of channels and receptors and (2) more long-term changes in gene expression and transcription of new protein.
- Descending pathways from the brain stem can have facilitatory or inhibitory effects on nociceptive transmission in the dorsal horn.
- Interactions between nociceptive pathways and the immune system occur in association with the inflammatory response and sensitization of peripheral nociceptors, and the central activation of glial cells (microglia and astrocytes) in the dorsal horn can also modify nociceptive sensitivity.

INTRODUCTION

Nociceptive pathways convert external stimuli into sensory signals and can provide a warning of potential tissue damage. If an acute stimulus is severe or associated with tissue injury and inflammation, sensitivity to sensory stimuli is increased, and this may act as a protective function that promotes rest and healing of the injured part.[1] In many chronic or persistent pain states, the relationship between the intensity of the peripheral stimulus and the evoked response is significantly altered due

to the plasticity of the nervous system and to intercurrent environmental and psychological factors.

DEFINITION OF HYPERALGESIA AND ALLODYNIA

Hyperalgesia is defined as a leftward shift of the stimulus response function that relates the magnitude of pain to stimulus intensity (see **Figure 1b.1**).[1] Electrophysiological features include a decrease in threshold (response evoked

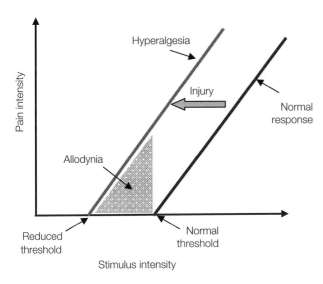

Figure 1b.1 Relationship between pain and stimulus intensity. Tissue injury produces a leftward shift in the stimulus–response function and is associated with an increase in response to both suprathreshold (i.e. hyperalgesia) and previously subthreshold stimuli (i.e. allodynia).

by less intense stimulus), an increased response to suprathreshold stimuli, and the onset of spontaneous activity. The behavioral correlates include increased pain sensitivity and pain evoked by previously nonnoxious stimuli (i.e. allodynia). Although allodynia specifically describes a painful response to a previously nonnoxious stimulus (i.e. a reduction in threshold), it has been suggested that hyperalgesia be used as an umbrella term for all phenomena of increased pain sensitivity.[2] Therefore, in the following sections, hyperalgesia will be used to denote an increased response to nociceptive stimuli and/or a reduction in threshold.

Hyperalgesia that occurs within the area of injury is referred to as primary hyperalgesia and is associated with increased sensitivity to thermal and mechanical stimuli.[1] Primary hyperalgesia is produced by changes in peripheral nociceptor function, which may also be described as peripheral sensitization.

Secondary hyperalgesia occurs in undamaged skin around an injury site and is characterized by a leftward shift of the stimulus–response function for mechanical stimuli.[1, 3] Secondary mechanical hyperalgesia is mediated by central changes in sensitivity and/or in the functional connectivity of myelinated fibers.[4]

MECHANISMS OF PERIPHERAL SENSITIZATION

A-delta and C-fiber primary nociceptive afferents are activated by a range of noxious mechanical, thermal, and chemical stimuli. Nociceptive sensory neurons transduce external stimuli into electrical action potentials that can be transmitted to the spinal cord and signal the onset,

duration, intensity, and location of a stimulus.[5] While transducing ion channels primarily determine response specificity, voltage-gated ion channels in nociceptors are involved in determining the timing and extent of action potential firing. Therefore, peripheral responses can be sensitized by either (1) increasing the efficacy of transducing ion channels or (2) by modifying voltage-gated channels to reduce firing thresholds and increase the response to suprathreshold stimuli.[6]

Tissue injury initiates an inflammatory response that is characterized by:

- redness and warmth due to vasodilation;
- edema due to increased vascular permeability and recruitment of inflammatory cells;
- pain due to activation of sensory afferents.

Release of substance P (SP) and calcitonin gene-related peptide (CGRP) from peripheral primary afferent terminals contributes to these changes, and is termed neurogenic edema. Inflammation induces a complex interaction between damaged endothelial cells, white blood cells, platelets, sympathetic efferents, and primary sensory afferent neurons that contributes to peripheral sensitization (more details can be found in recent reviews[7, 8, 9]).

Inflammatory mediators (including endothelin, prostaglandin E_2 (PGE$_2$), leukotrienes, cytokines, bradykinin, serotonin, adrenaline) and neurotrophic factors (e.g. nerve growth factor (NGF)) released during tissue damage activate and/or sensitize the nociceptor terminal leading to increased excitability.[5, 6] Inflammatory mediators initiate signaling cascades (see **Box 1b.1**), leading to acute modulation of the protein structure (i.e. posttranslational change) of transducing and voltage-gated ion channels, which alter function and enhance responsiveness via the action of protein kinases. The sensitizing actions of several inflammatory mediators, including prostaglandins, require protein kinase A (PKA) activation. Protein kinase C (PKC) is activated by mediators such as BK, and the PKC-ε subtype is important for heat, NGF, adrenaline, and carrageenan-mediated hypersensitivity.[6] Extracellular signal-regulated kinase (ERK) is involved in signaling capsaicin, adrenaline, and P2X$_3$ receptor-mediated hypersensitivity.[15, 16] Increased expression of the active phosphorylated (pERK) form is found in peripheral fibers and terminals in skin, as well as DRG neurons following capsaicin injection, and thermal hyperalgesia is attenuated by ERK inhibitors (**Figure 1b.2**).[16]

Changes in gene expression and protein synthesis (i.e. translational changes) contribute to more persistent alterations in sensitivity[7, 14] and may include:

- increased peptide expression (e.g. CGRP, SP);
- increased receptor expression (e.g. increased TRPV1 and BK receptors);
- phenotypic changes in sensory neurons (e.g. subpopulation of A fibers now release SP).[17]

Box 1b.1 Intracellular signaling

Neuronal responses to neurotransmitters are determined by the type and density of receptor expression. The resultant activation of ion channels, enzymes, and intracellular signaling pathways not only mediate the effects of the transmitter but can also alter the stimulus–response characteristics of the cell. Postsynaptic receptor systems include:[10]

- ligand-gated ion channels (e.g. AMPA). Binding of transmitter to the receptor results in rapid activation and deactivation of ion channels (within 10 msec) and provides a rapid response system;
- receptor tyrosine kinases (e.g. trkB). These receptors typically respond to growth and trophic factors (e.g. nerve growth factor (NGF); brain-derived neurotrophic factor (BDNF)) and produce changes in growth, differentiation, and survival of neurons. In addition, these receptors and factors have important modulatory effects and may produce sensitizing effects of peripheral and/or central components of nociceptive pathways;
- G-protein-linked receptors (e.g. mGluR). Activation of these receptors generates a second messenger in the cell which then activates a number of enzymes, including protein kinases, that modify cellular processes. As several steps are required, the response is relatively slow (100–300 msec to many minutes), but the diversity of signaling pathways allows for significant plasticity in the response.

G-proteins coupled receptor (GPCR) activation changes the activity of effector enzymes, which can directly modulate ion channels, but also regulate the activity of protein kinases that phosphorylate intracellular proteins, ion channels, enzymes, and transcription factors.[11, 12] Neural activity and pathophysiological states can influence the function of GPCR by altering the degree of trafficking and insertion of the receptor at the membrane surface.[13] Signaling pathways include:

- G_s stimulates and G_i or G_o inhibit adenylate cyclases which synthesize cyclic AMP (cAMP). Cyclic AMP activates protein kinase A (PKA);
- phospholipase C (PLC) generates diacyglycerol (DAG) and also inositol triphosphate (IP_3) which releases intracellular stores of calcium. Calcium not only acts as a carrier of electrical current, but also as a second messenger by activating kinases such as protein kinase C (PKC) and calcium-calmodulin-dependent kinase (CaMK).

The degree of protein phosphorylation and dephosphorylation is controlled by the action of kinases and phosphatases, respectively. Protein kinases catalyze phosphorylation of proteins, leading to changes in a protein's charge and conformation that can rapidly modify the function of enzymes (i.e. posttranslational modification), receptors and ion channels without requiring any change in the level of protein expression.[12] In addition, intracellular pathways involving phosphorylation can regulate gene expression by interaction with transcription factors. For example, the activated form of extracellular signal-regulated kinase (phosphorylated ERK) translocates to the nucleus, interacts with a transcription factor (cyclic AMP response element binding protein (CREB)), and activates immediate–early genes (e.g. c-fos, c-jun). As a result, the expression of mRNA and proteins are increased (i.e. transcriptional modification) and long-term alterations in cellular function may be produced.[5, 11, 14] As genes, such as c-fos, are strongly and rapidly induced by noxious stimuli, it can be used as a marker of activated nociceptive pathways.

Chemical mediators

ARACHIDONIC ACID METABOLITES

Tissue damage releases arachidonic acid, which is metabolized to a number of active compounds including prostaglandins via cyclooxygenase (COX) enzymes and leukotrienes via lipoxygenases. In general, COX-1 is constitutively expressed and COX-2 expression is induced in cells following inflammation; however COX-2 is also constitutively expressed in the central nervous system (CNS).[9]

Prostaglandin E_2 (PGE_2) is the principal proinflammatory prostanoid and effects are mediated by four G-protein coupled EP receptors (EP1–4). Levels of EP4 receptor, but not other forms, increase in the DRG following peripheral inflammation and therefore may represent a specific target for inflammatory pain.[18] PGE_2 sensitizes nociceptors to noxious thermal and chemical stimuli.[8, 9] This is mediated in part by phosphorylation of

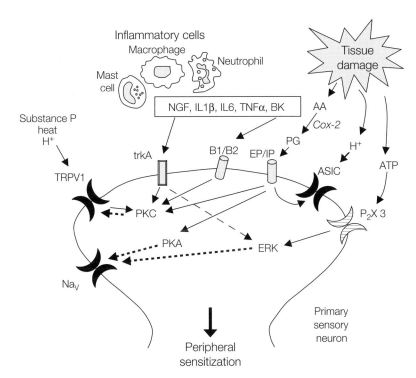

Figure 1b.2 Inflammatory mediators, receptors and intracellular messengers associated with sensitization of peripheral nociceptors. Modified from Samad et al.,[9] Bhave and Gereau,[6] and Marchand et al.[7] AA, arachidonic acid; ASIC, acid sensing ion channel; ATP, adenosine triphosphate; B1/B2, bradykinin receptors; BK, bradykinin; ERK, extracellular-signal regulated kinase; IL, interleukin; NGF, nerve growth factor; PG, prostaglandin; PKA, protein kinase A; PKC, protein kinase C; TNF, tumor necrosis factor; trkA, tyrosine kinase A; TRP, transient receptor potential.

TRP channels and voltage-gated sodium channels, leading to a reduction in threshold and increased excitability, respectively.[18] PGE_2 also has central excitatory actions on nociceptive transmission, which include increased transmitter release, direct depolarization via a cation channel, and reduction in glycine-mediated inhibition.[9]

BRADYKININ

Bradykinin and kallidin are kinins that act via the constitutively expressed G-protein coupled B2 receptor; whereas cleavage of these peptides produces smaller compounds that act through the inducible B1 receptor. Bradykinin acts via multiple intracellular signaling pathways and alters nociceptor excitability by:[19]

- decreasing the threshold of transducing ion channels;
- altering the threshold and kinetics of voltage-gated sodium channels;
- reducing activity in voltage-gated potassium channels.

In addition, when nociceptors are sensitized by BK, TRPV1 receptors are activated by much lower temperatures, and sensitivity to noxious cold is also enhanced due to activation of TRPA1.[19]

CYTOKINES

Cytokines are small, secreted proteins (e.g. interleukins IL-1 and IL-6; tumor necrosis factor-alpha (TNFα); leukemia inhibitory factor (LIF)) which bind to specific receptors expressed by nociceptor terminals and alter sensitivity. Immune cells involved in the peripheral inflammatory response release a range of cytokines, chemokines, and mediators that include the following:[7]

- mast cells release NGF, TNFα, histamine, chemokines;
- activated macrophages release TNFα, IL-1β, NGF, nitric oxide, prostanoids;
- neutrophils release lipoxygenase products, nitric oxide, cytokines, chemokines.

Sodium channels

Voltage-gated sodium channels transmit action potentials, but different forms can also modulate the sensitivity of primary afferent terminals. These channels can be broadly divided into tetrodotoxin-sensitive (TTX-S) channels with fast kinetics and tetrodotoxin-resistant (TTX-R) channels with slow kinetics. TTX-R sodium channels regulate nociceptor excitability by altering action potential generation, repetitive firing, and resting membrane potential.[6] As the kinetics of these channels allow prolonged membrane depolarizations, they can mediate the repetitive discharge associated with hyperalgesia.[20]

Nine subtypes of voltage-gated sodium channel have been identified ($Na_v1.1$–$Na_v1.9$), which vary in their distribution, electrophysiologic properties (threshold and kinetics of channel opening and inactivation), and the response to injury.[21, 22] The subtypes $Na_v1.8$ and $Na_v1.9$ are selectively expressed in nociceptors, and in about half of unmyelinated C-fibers. $Na_v1.8$ is also expressed in a small subset of myelinated A fibers.[6, 22, 23] Recently, a mutation in the gene encoding a subunit of the $Na_v1.7$ channel was identified in a family with congenital insensitivity to pain,[24] suggesting this subtype is important for pain sensation.

Posttranslational modifications enhance the excitability of TTX-R channels and contribute to peripheral nociceptor sensitization. Inflammatory mediators (e.g. PGE_2, adenosine, serotonin, NGF, and adenosine) activate intracellular second messengers (e.g. PKA, PKC, and ERK), leading to phosphorylation of the channel and an increase in $Na_v1.8$-mediated currents.[21] NGF not only acutely enhances TTX-R currents, but also produces a longer-term effect via upregulation of $Na_v1.8$ in small DRG cells.[23] Similarly, inflammatory mediators such as PGE_2 increase phosphorylation and activity of $Na_v1.9$, and expression of the channel is increased by GDNF.[21, 23]

Neurotrophic factors

Neurotrophins are a family of related proteins that interact with the low-affinity p75 receptor and with specific high-affinity tyrosine kinase (trk) receptors. Nerve growth factor (NGF) is the preferred ligand for trkA, brain-derived neurotrophic factor (BDNF) and neurotrophin-4/5 (NT-4/5) for trkB, and neurotrophin-3 (NT-3) has the highest affinity for trkC.[8] As their name suggests, neurotrophins have an important role in the growth and survival of different subsets of sensory neurons, but also have an ongoing role in nociception.[25] Levels of NGF are increased in inflammatory states and injection of NGF induces hyperalgesia in both clinical and laboratory studies.[25, 26, 27] NGF alters the expression of a number of mediators involved in peripheral sensitization, including:[25]

- increased production of the proteins sP and CGRP;
- increased receptor expression (TRPV1, P2X3, ASIC3, B2);
- altered voltage-gated ion channel expression (Ca, K, Na) which impacts on the excitability of the neuron.

NGF also has indirect effects on inflammatory hyperalgesia by increasing cytokine expression in mast cells and producing mast cell degranulation.[8]

BDNF mRNA and protein is upregulated in an NGF-dependent manner following inflammation.[25] BDNF is released from the central terminals of nociceptors and enhances nociceptive transmission by multiple mechanisms, including modulation of NMDA receptor activity and activation of ERK.[28, 29]

Peripheral opioid receptors

In addition to the excitatory hyperalgesia produced by inflammation, peripheral inhibitory mechanisms may produce a partial compensatory effect. In the presence of inflammation, opioid receptors are expressed in the periphery[30] and peripherally administered morphine reduces inflammatory hyperalgesia in behavioral models.[31] Although morphine has no effect on the electrophysiological properties of nerves from normal skin, morphine produced dose-dependent reductions in thermal and mechanical hyperalgesia in inflamed skin.[32]

MECHANISMS OF CENTRAL SENSITIZATION

Intense peripheral noxious stimuli, tissue damage, or nerve injury, produce centrally mediated increases in sensitivity (i.e. central sensitization). Behaviorally, central sensitization manifests as a heightened sensitivity to sensory input, spread of sensitivity to uninjured sites (i.e. secondary hyperalgesia), and generation of pain by low threshold stimuli (i.e. allodynia).[33]

Electrophysiological correlates of dorsal horn plasticity

WIND UP

Wind up is a form of activity-dependent plasticity identified in wide dynamic range (WDR) neurons in the deep dorsal horn.[34, 35, 36] Wind up is an electrophysiological phenomenon and has the following features:

- it is produced by a slow train of repeated low-frequency C-fiber stimuli of the same intensity (e.g. up to 16 stimuli at 1–2 Hz);[33]
- there is a progressive increase in the electrophysiological response in the postsynaptic dorsal horn neuron;[5, 37]
- it may be viewed as a normal feature of the coding properties of WDR neurons;[38]
- activation of the NMDA receptor is a prerequisite;[39]
- it is not produced by A-fiber stimulation;
- it is manifest only during a train of repetitive inputs and rarely outlasts the stimulus period;[35]
- in human studies, repeated noxious heat stimuli produce successive increases in reported pain.[40]

LONG-TERM POTENTIATION

Long-term potentiation (LTP) is an experimental phenomenon that demonstrates the capability for more long-lasting activity-dependent modification of individual synapses.[41] LTP was first demonstrated in the hippocampus[42] and is thought to be important in modifications of brain function by previous experience, such as learning and memory.[41] Parallels have been drawn between the mechanisms underlying LTP in the hippocampus and the synaptic plasticity in the dorsal horn that results in hyperalgesia.[37, 43] Features of LTP include the following:

- it is produced by a brief high frequency input;
- electrical stimulation of fine primary afferents (100–400 pulses at 2–100 Hz) induces LTP at A-delta and C-fiber synapses in the superficial dorsal horn;[43, 44]
- it occurs particularly at synapses of lamina I neurons that express the NK1 receptor;[45]
- LTP manifests as a potentiated response to subsequent inputs for a prolonged period (i.e. long outlasts the conditioning stimulus);[36, 43]
- descending pathways may inhibit the development of LTP in the dorsal horn as noxious stimuli such as heat, pinch and formalin do not produce LTP in intact animals, but the same stimulus is effective following spinalization.[38]

Although such high-frequency stimuli may not have a clear physiological correlate, LTP has also been induced by relatively low-frequency afferent input associated with peripheral inflammation in animal models.[46] In addition, electrical stimulus conditioning protocols that reliably elicit LTP in intact animals produce long-term increases in pain perception in human studies. Responses to stimuli at the site of the conditioning stimulus (i.e. homosynaptic perceptual LTP) and also to punctate mechanical and light tactile stimuli in the surrounding area (i.e. secondary mechanical hyperalgesia or heterosynaptic perceptual LTP) were increased for several hours following brief conditioning stimuli.[47, 48]

Central sensitization

Fast excitatory synaptic transmission is mediated by glutamate acting on AMPA and kainate ligand-gated ion channels to generate excitatory postsynaptic potentials (EPSPs) that signal the onset, duration, intensity, and location of a noxious stimulus.[5] In the presence of ongoing or persistent activity, cumulative depolarization leads to removal of the magnesium block from the NMDA receptor and calcium influx through the open channel.[5] Alterations in the stimulus-response profile of dorsal horn neurons ensue, with a generalized increased responsiveness termed **central sensitization**. Wind up, LTP and secondary hyperalgesia may all contribute to central sensitization and may share some of the same cellular mechanisms, but are different and independent phenomena.[33, 36]

Centrally mediated alterations in nociceptive processing were initially demonstrated in laboratory experiments, and the following changes were noted:

- reduction in threshold and increased sensitivity of spinal cord neurons;[49, 50, 51]

- increased excitability of the withdrawal reflex without prolonged changes in primary afferent or motoneuron activity;[52]
- expansion of the receptive field of dorsal horn neurons;[53]
- increased response to both C- and A-fiber inputs following injury;
- duration of increased excitability greatly outlasts the initiating stimulus by minutes to hours, days, or weeks.[54, 55, 56]

Dorsal horn plasticity is initiated by an increase in intracellular calcium, which triggers a range of intracellular messengers that mediate or modulate the intracellular response (see **Figure 1b.3**).[37, 41] Ongoing nociceptive input activates ligand-gated ion channels (AMPA, NMDA, and/or kainate) and G-protein coupled metabotropic receptors (NK1, mGluR, trkB, and Eph) in dorsal horn neurons.[37] Intracellular calcium is increased via direct influx through the NMDA channel, activation of voltage-gated calcium channels (VGCCs), and release of calcium from intracellular stores via G-protein coupled receptors (e.g. mGluR).[33, 43, 59] Subsequent kinase activation and posttranslational changes in receptors contribute to persistent increases in response. Phosphorylation of ionotropic glutamate receptors alters channel kinetics and further increases calcium influx.[37]

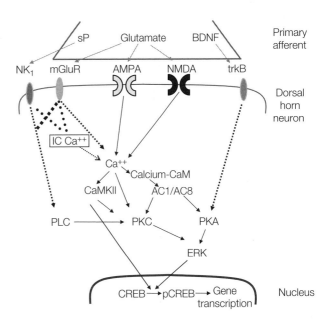

Figure 1b.3 Intracellular events associated with sensitization of dorsal horn neurons. Modified from Ji *et al.*,[11] Ji *et al.*,[37] Kawasaki *et al.*,[57] Wei *et al.*[58] AC1/AC8, adenylyl cyclase 1 and 8; BDNF, brain derived neurotrophic factor; CaMKII, calcium calmodulin kinase II; CREB, cAMP responsive element binding protein; ERK, extracellular-signal regulated kinase; IC Ca, intracellular calcium; mGluR, metabotropic glutamate receptor; NK1, neurokinin1; PKA, protein kinase A; PKC, protein kinase C; PLC, phospholipase C; sP, substance P.

Phosphorylation of NMDA NR1 subunits occurs within 30 minutes of capsaicin injection[60] and rapid and prolonged increases in phosphorylation of the NR2B subunit occur in association with CFA inflammation,[61] leading to increases in the postsynaptic response. The tyrosine kinase Src is activated by trkB and EphB receptors, and also enhances NMDA currents.[62]

Protein kinases and sensitization

Protein kinases are involved in changes associated with peripheral and central sensitization (see **Box 1b.1**). As inhibitors of kinase activation reduce hyperalgesia,[57, 63] these enzymes may represent potential therapeutic targets.

PKA AND PKC

Protein kinase A (PKA; also referred to as cAMP-dependent protein kinases) is involved in both peripheral and central sensitization. PKA is required for the second phase of the formalin response and capsaicin-induced mechanical allodynia.[11] The protein kinase C (PKC) family has been divided into three groups of isozymes based on their sequence homology and activation by calcium and/or 1,2-diacylglycerol (DAG). The subtypes most involved in nociceptive processing are PKCε (Ca^{2+}-independent, DAG-dependent) and PKCγ (Ca^{2+}-dependent, DAG-dependent). PKCε is present in primary afferents that terminate in the superficial dorsal horn, and PKCγ is located in lamina IIi of the dorsal horn.[11] Noxious stimuli activate PKC in the dorsal horn, and PKC acts via Src to phosphorylate the NMDA receptor.[11] Activity-dependent trafficking of AMPA receptors to the synapse is important for hippocampal LTP[41] and may also contribute to conversion of "silent" to active synapses in the dorsal horn.[64] PKC may be the trigger for increased expression and insertion of AMPA receptors into the postsynaptic membrane of DH neurons.[64]

Capsaicin induces PKA and PKC activation in the spinal cord.[57] Inflammatory mediators such as PGE_2, serotonin, adrenaline, and NGF also activate PKA or PKC.[65] Both PKA and PKC mediate CGRP-induced sensitization of dorsal horn neurons.[66]

CaMKII

Calcium/calmodulin-dependent protein kinase (CaMKII) is involved in activity-induced synaptic changes throughout the CNS.[41] CaMKII is expressed in small diameter DRG neurons, and in lamina I and II neurons in the dorsal horn.[67] Activation of CaMKII enhances AMPA and NMDA inward currents,[43] but the role of CaMKII in pain processing and central sensitization may vary depending on the intensity of the stimulus and the type of injury. Capsaicin injection has been shown to increase expression and

phosphorylation of CaMKII in DH neurons, and enhance phosphorylation of AMPA GluR1 subunits.[68] Experiments in mice with a mutation that prevents autophosphorylation of the enzyme suggest that activated CaMKII is not required for stimulus-evoked threshold changes after injury (i.e. no difference is seen between mutant and wild-type mice in mechanical and thermal thresholds after CFA), but it is necessary for the persistence of spontaneous pain behavior in the setting of tissue injury (e.g. reduction in second-phase formalin injection).[67]

MAPK AND ERK

Mitogen-activated protein kinases (MAPK) are a family of protein kinases that transduce extracellular stimuli into intracellular posttranslational and transcriptional responses, and are widely expressed in the CNS.[65] Extracellular signal-regulated kinases (ERK) and p38 MAPK are members of the MAPK family.

Noxious stimuli induce intensity-dependent phosphorylation and activation of ERK in DRG neurons, and this may contribute to peripheral sensitization.[16] Inflammation also induces p38 MAPK in DRG neurons, which operates through a separate intracellular cascade and functions as a mediator of cellular stresses.[65] Whereas ERK is primarily activated by neural activity, p38 MAPK is mainly activated by cytokines and is required for NGF-induced increases in TRPV1 expression in the periphery.[69]

Activation of ERK is activity-dependent and nociceptive specific in dorsal horn neurons. Increases in activated phospho-ERK (pERK) positive neurons in lamina I and IIo of the dorsal horn are seen within minutes of C-fiber electrical stimuli,[70] capsaicin injection,[57] and formalin injection.[65] ERK is also activated by peripheral inflammation induced by CFA and carrageenan.[71] Multiple primary afferent transmitters (NMDA, sP, and BDNF) and receptors (ionotropic NMDA and AMPA/kainate receptors, mGluR1, NK-1 receptor, trk receptors) contribute to activation of ERK by capsaicin or electrical stimulation.[57]

PKA and PKC activators have an additive effect on the induction of pERK and are likely to act via independent parallel pathways. CaMK has been implicated in ERK activation in the cortex, but an inhibitor of CaMK had no effect on pERK activation by capsaicin or electrical stimulation.[57] The adenylyl cyclase subtypes 1 and 8 (AC1 and AC8) are also upstream activators of ERK (see **Figure 1b.3**).[58]

ERK is also involved in longer-term transcriptional changes. Activated ERK can translocate from the cytoplasm to the nucleus and activates Rsk2, which then phosphorylates cAMP-response-element binding protein (CREB). PhosphoCREB (pCREB) binds to CRE sites in the promoter regions of DNA and initiates the transcription of genes.[11, 65] This results in increased expression of immediate–early genes (e.g. c-fos, Cox-2) and later response genes encoding neuropeptides and receptors (e.g. prodynorphin, NK1, trkB).[11, 37] C-fiber stimulation increases pCREB in superficial dorsal horn neurons, where it is colocalized with pERK.[57] It is suggested that ERK and CaMK act via parallel pathways leading to CREB phosphorylation, but that the ERK pathway is more important for C-fiber-mediated phosphorylation of CREB in dorsal horn neurons.[57]

DESCENDING MODULATION OF HYPERALGESIA

Activity in spinobulbospinal pathways and brain stem sites are important for modulation of pain processing in the spinal cord. Bidirectional control via both descending inhibitory and facilitatory pathways modulate nociceptive transmission in the dorsal horn. The relative balance between these two systems varies with stimulus modality, stimulus intensity, and time, and is subject to considerable plasticity following injury.[72, 73, 74, 75]

The rostroventromedial medulla (RVM) is an important site for integration of descending input to the spinal cord. It is composed of a number of nuclei including the nucleus raphe magnus (NRM), nucleus reticularis gigantocellularis (NGC), nucleus reticularis paragigantocellularis lateralis, and nucleus gigantocellularis pars alpha.[76, 77] Afferent input includes pathways from the periaqueductal gray (PAG), parabrachial nucleus (PBN), and nucleus tractus solitarius (NTS).[77] The RVM and adjacent areas also receive direct afferent input from the superficial dorsal horn and in turn send descending projections to the cord, thus forming spinobulbospinal loops.

The RVM contains three classes of cells with differing and distinct functions which provide the cellular mechanisms for both inhibitory and facilitatory effects.[72, 75, 78] RVM ON- and OFF-cells project to laminae I–II and V in the spinal cord of the rat and are thus well placed to modulate nociception.[78] ON-cells are characterized by a burst of activity immediately before nociceptive reflexes, are inhibited by opioids, and contribute to descending facilitation. OFF-cells exhibit an abrupt pause in ongoing activity immediately before nociceptive reflexes, their activity is indirectly increased by opioids, and they contribute to descending inhibition. Neutral cells do not change their activity with nociception, but may undergo an NMDA-dependent phenotypic switch to ON- or OFF-cell characteristics in the presence of inflammation.[79] ON, OFF, and neutral cells are intermixed and not anatomically separate and therefore manipulations at the same site can produce opposing effects.[72, 73] Low-intensity electrical stimulation and low concentrations of glutamate in the RVM have been shown to facilitate spinal behavioral and dorsal horn neuron responses to noxious stimulation;[76, 80] whereas high-intensity electrical stimulation and high concentrations of glutamate produce inhibitory effects.[74]

The net effect of RVM activation also relates to activation of subsets of neurons with different connections and different combinations of neurotransmitter receptors.[81] Projections of RVM ON and OFF-cells are diffusely rather than topographically organized as collateral branches enter several segments of the spinal cord, and terminate in laminae I, II, and V. Inhibitory pathways tend to descend in the dorsolateral funiculus, while facilitatory pathways are predominantly in the ventral and ventrolateral funiculi.[74, 78] Descending facilitatory pathways from the RVM have an important role in the development of C-fiber-induced secondary hyperalgesia,[72, 82, 83] but descending facilitatory effects have also been recognized following formalin injection and nerve injury.[73, 84] Descending facilitation has been noted in early stages of inflammation, but inhibitory effects gradually build up and become the dominant effect.[73] This inhibition limits the expansion of receptive fields and inflammatory hyperalgesia.[75] Serotonergic and noradrenergic pathways in the dorsolateral funiculus (DLF) contribute to descending inhibitory effects[77] and serotonergic pathways have more recently been implicated in facilitatory effects.[85]

INTERACTIONS WITH THE IMMUNE SYSTEM

Interactions between nociceptive mechanisms and the immune system are possible at multiple sites in the peripheral and CNS, and can have a major influence on inflammatory hyperalgesia.[7, 86, 87] As previously discussed, recruitment of immune cells (e.g. macrophages, T lymphocytes, mast cells) into areas of injury are an important component of the inflammatory response, and peripheral nerve terminals express receptors for immune products which contribute to peripheral sensitization. Within the CNS, the main role of glia (astrocytes and microglia) was thought to be maintenance of the extracellular environment (e.g. pH, levels of ions and transmitters, removal of debris), but it is now clear that there are more dynamic interactions with neurons.[7, 88] In the DRG, satellite glial cells ensheath and modulate the function of adjacent neuronal cell bodies, and electrophysiological connections between glia and neurons are enhanced following inflammation.[89]

In the spinal cord, glia form dynamic networks and can modify the function of nociceptive neurons in dorsal horn. Although normally quiescent, glia can be activated by:[88]

- sP, EAAs, fractalkine, and ATP released by A-delta or C-fiber presynaptic terminals (fractalkine is a presumed neuron-to-glia signal as it can be released and diffuse away from neurons and microglia have receptors for fractalkine);
- nitric oxide, prostaglandins, and fractalkine released by second-order nociceptive neurons.

Glial activation results in:[88, 90, 91]

- central release of proinflammatory cytokines (e.g. IL-1, IL-6, TNF, NGF);
- indirect effects via release of PGE_2 or nitric oxide;
- acute increases in neuronal excitability via multiple intracellular pathways, but particularly p38 MAP kinase;
- long-term changes in gene expression.

Dorsal horn activation of microglia has an important role in the induction and maintenance of nerve injury-induced allodynia.[92, 93, 94] Activation of glia can also occur in response to inflammation or infection, although the mechanisms of glial involvement in inflammatory pain are not as well established.[90] Opioid receptors are expressed on glia, and morphine can activate glia causing release of nitric oxide and proinflammatory cytokines, and it has been postulated that glial activation contributes to morphine tolerance.[91]

CONCLUSIONS

Inflammation induces increased sensitivity within nociceptive pathways, both in the peripheral and central nervous system. Understanding the mechanisms of inflammatory hyperalgesia is essential for further identification of effective and potentially novel analgesic targets.

ACKNOWLEDGMENTS

This chapter is updated and expanded from Nagy I and Rice ASC. Applied physiology of inflammatory pain. In: Rowbotham DJ and Macintyre PE (eds). *Clinical Pain Management: Acute Pain*, 1st edn. London: Hodder Arnold, 2003: 17–41.

REFERENCES

* 1. Treede RD, Meyer RA, Raja SN, Campbell JN. Peripheral and central mechanisms of cutaneous hyperalgesia. *Progress in Neurobiology.* 1992; **38**: 397–421.

2. Treede R, Handwerker HO, Baumgartner U *et al.* The nomenclature of hyperexcitability. In: Brune K, Handwerker HO (eds). *Hyperalgesia: molecular mechanisms and clinical implications.* Seattle: IASP Press, 2004: 3–15.

3. Treede RD, Magerl W. Multiple mechanisms of secondary hyperalgesia. *Progress in Brain Research.* 2000; **129**: 331–41.

* 4. Lewin GR, Moshourab R. Mechanosensation and pain. *Journal of Neurobiology.* 2004; **61**: 30–44.

5. Woolf CJ, Salter MW. Neuronal plasticity: increasing the gain in pain. *Science.* 2000; **288**: 1765–9.

* 6. Bhave G, Gereau 4th RW. Posttranslational mechanisms of peripheral sensitization. *Journal of Neurobiology.* 2004; **61**: 88–106.

* 7. Marchand F, Perretti M, McMahon SB. Role of the immune system in chronic pain. Nature Reviews. *Neuroscience.* 2005; **6**: 521–32.

8. McMahon SB, Bennett DL, Bevan S. Inflammatory mediators and modulators of pain. In: McMahon SB, Koltzenburg M (eds). *Wall and Melzack's textbook of pain*, 5th edn. London: Elsevier Churchill Livingstone, 2006: 49–72.

* 9. Samad TA, Sapirstein A, Woolf CJ. Prostanoids and pain: unraveling mechanisms and revealing therapeutic targets. *Trends in Molecular Medicine.* 2002; **8**: 390–6.

10. Zigmond M, Bloom F, Landis S *et al. Fundamental neuroscience.* San Diego: Academic Press, 1999: 1–1600.

* 11. Ji RR, Woolf CJ. Neuronal plasticity and signal transduction in nociceptive neurons: implications for the initiation and maintenance of pathological pain. *Neurobiology of Disease.* 2001; **8**: 1–10.

12. Lodish H, Berk A, Zipursky S *et al. Molecular cell biology*, 4th edn. New York: WH Freeman, 2000.

13. Cahill CM, Holdridge SV, Morinville A. Trafficking of delta-opioid receptors and other G-protein-coupled receptors: implications for pain and analgesia. *Trends in Pharmacological Sciences.* 2007; **28**: 23–31.

14. Woolf CJ, Costigan M. Transcriptional and posttranslational plasticity and the generation of inflammatory pain. *Proceedings of the National Academy of Sciences of the United States of America.* 1999; **96**: 7723–30.

15. Dai Y, Fukuoka T, Wang H *et al.* Contribution of sensitized P2X receptors in inflamed tissue to the mechanical hypersensitivity revealed by phosphorylated ERK in DRG neurons. *Pain.* 2004; **108**: 258–66.

16. Dai Y, Iwata K, Fukuoka T *et al.* Phosphorylation of extracellular signal-regulated kinase in primary afferent neurons by noxious stimuli and its involvement in peripheral sensitization. *Journal of Neuroscience.* 2002; **22**: 7737–45.

17. Neumann S, Doubell TP, Leslie T, Woolf CJ. Inflammatory pain hypersensitivity mediated by phenotypic switch in myelinated primary sensory neurons. *Nature.* 1996; **384**: 360–4.

18. Lin CR, Amaya F, Barrett LB *et al.* Prostaglandin E2 receptor EP4 contributes to inflammatory pain hypersensitivity. *Journal of Pharmacology and Experimental Therapeutics.* 2006; **319**: 1096–103.

* 19. Wang H, Ehnert C, Brenner GJ, Woolf CJ. Bradykinin and peripheral sensitization. *Biological Chemistry.* 2006; **387**: 11–4.

20. Gold MS. Tetrodotoxin-resistant Na+ currents and inflammatory hyperalgesia. *Proceedings of the National Academy of Sciences of the United States of America.* 1999; **96**: 7645–9.

21. Amir R, Argoff CE, Bennett GJ et al. The role of sodium channels in chronic inflammatory and neuropathic pain. *Journal of Pain*. 2006; **7**: S1–29.

 * 22. Wood JN, Boorman JP, Okuse K, Baker MD. Voltage-gated sodium channels and pain pathways. *Journal of Neurobiology*. 2004; **61**: 55–71.

 * 23. Lai J, Porreca F, Hunter JC, Gold MS. Voltage-gated sodium channels and hyperalgesia. *Annual Review of Pharmacology and Toxicology*. 2004; **44**: 371–97.

24. Cox JJ, Reimann F, Nicholas AK et al. An SCN9A channelopathy causes congenital inability to experience pain. *Nature*. 2006; **444**: 894–8.

 * 25. Pezet S, McMahon SB. Neurotrophins: mediators and modulators of pain. *Annual Review of Neuroscience*. 2006; **29**: 507–38.

26. Svensson P, Cairns BE, Wang K, Arendt-Nielsen L. Injection of nerve growth factor into human masseter muscle evokes long-lasting mechanical allodynia and hyperalgesia. *Pain*. 2003; **104**: 241–7.

27. Hathway GJ, Fitzgerald M. Time course and dose-dependence of nerve growth factor-induced secondary hyperalgesia in the mouse. *Journal of Pain*. 2006; **7**: 57–61.

28. Pezet S, Malcangio M, Lever IJ et al. Noxious stimulation induces Trk receptor and downstream ERK phosphorylation in spinal dorsal horn. *Molecular and Cellular Neurosciences*. 2002; **21**: 684–95.

29. Zhao J, Seereeram A, Nassar MA et al. Nociceptor-derived brain-derived neurotrophic factor regulates acute and inflammatory but not neuropathic pain. *Molecular and Cellular Neurosciences*. 2006; **31**: 539–48.

30. Stein C, Hassan AH, Przewlocki R et al. Opioids from immunocytes interact with receptors on sensory nerves to inhibit nociception in inflammation. *Proceedings of the National Academy of Sciences of the United States of America*. 1990; **87**: 5935–9.

31. Stein C. The control of pain in peripheral tissue by opioids. *New England Journal of Medicine*. 1995; **332**: 1685–90.

32. Wenk HN, Brederson JD, Honda CN. Morphine directly inhibits nociceptors in inflamed skin. *Journal of Neurophysiology*. 2006; **95**: 2083–97.

33. Woolf CJ. Windup and central sensitization are not equivalent. *Pain*. 1996; **66**: 105–08.

34. Dickenson AH, Sullivan AF. Electrophysiological studies on the effects of intrathecal morphine on nociceptive neurones in the rat dorsal horn. *Pain*. 1986; **24**: 211–22.

35. Woolf CJ, Thompson SW, King AE. Prolonged primary afferent induced alterations in dorsal horn neurones, an intracellular analysis *in vivo* and *in vitro*. *Journal de Physiologie*. 1988; **83**: 255–66.

36. Herrero JF, Laird JM, Lopez-Garcia JA. Wind-up of spinal cord neurones and pain sensation: much ado about something? *Progress in Neurobiology*. 2000; **61**: 169–203.

 * 37. Ji RR, Kohno T, Moore KA, Woolf CJ. Central sensitization and LTP: do pain and memory share similar mechanisms? *Trends in Neurosciences*. 2003; **26**: 696–705.

38. Sandkuhler J, Liu X. Induction of long-term potentiation at spinal synapses by noxious stimulation or nerve injury. *European Journal of Neuroscience*. 1998; **10**: 2476–80.

39. Dickenson AH, Sullivan AF. Evidence for a role of the NMDA receptor in the frequency dependent potentiation of deep rat dorsal horn nociceptive neurones following C fibre stimulation. *Neuropharmacology*. 1987; **26**: 1235–8.

40. Price DD, Hu JW, Dubner R, Gracely RH. Peripheral suppression of first pain and central summation of second pain evoked by noxious heat pulses. *Pain*. 1977; **3**: 57–68.

41. Malenka RC, Bear MF. LTP and LTD: an embarrassment of riches. *Neuron*. 2004; **44**: 5–21.

42. Bliss TV, Lomo T. Long-lasting potentiation of synaptic transmission in the dentate area of the anaesthetized rabbit following stimulation of the perforant path. *Journal de Physiologie*. 1973; **232**: 331–56.

43. Sandkuhler J. Learning and memory in pain pathways. *Pain*. 2000; **88**: 113–8.

44. Randic M, Jiang MC, Cerne R. Long-term potentiation and long-term depression of primary afferent neurotransmission in the rat spinal cord. *Journal of Neuroscience*. 1993; **13**: 5228–41.

45. Ikeda H, Heinke B, Ruscheweyh R, Sandkuhler J. Synaptic plasticity in spinal lamina I projection neurons that mediate hyperalgesia. *Science*. 2003; **299**: 1237–40.

46. Ikeda H, Stark J, Fischer H et al. Synaptic amplifier of inflammatory pain in the spinal dorsal horn. *Science*. 2006; **312**: 1659–62.

47. Klein T, Magerl W, Mantzke U et al. Perceptual correlates of long-term potentiation in the spinal cord. In: Dostrovsky J, Carr D, Koltzenburg M (eds). *Proceedings of the 10th World Congress on Pain*. Seattle: IASP Press, 2003: 407–15.

48. Klein T, Magerl W, Hopf HC et al. Perceptual correlates of nociceptive long-term potentiation and long-term depression in humans. *Journal of Neuroscience*. 2004; **24**: 964–71.

49. Cook AJ, Woolf CJ, Wall PD, McMahon SB. Dynamic receptive field plasticity in rat spinal cord dorsal horn following C-primary afferent input. *Nature*. 1987; **325**: 151–3.

50. Woolf CJ, King AE. Dynamic alterations in the cutaneous mechanoreceptive fields of dorsal horn neurons in the rat spinal cord. *Journal of Neuroscience*. 1990; **10**: 2717–26.

51. Woolf CJ, Shortland P, Sivilotti LG. Sensitization of high mechanothreshold superficial dorsal horn and flexor motor neurones following chemosensitive primary afferent activation. *Pain*. 1994; **58**: 141–55.

52. Cook AJ, Woolf CJ, Wall PD. Prolonged C-fibre mediated facilitation of the flexion reflex in the rat is not due to changes in afferent terminal or motoneurone excitability. *Neuroscience Letters*. 1986; **70**: 91–6.

53. Woolf CJ. Evidence for a central component of post-injury pain hypersensitivity. *Nature*. 1983; **306**: 686–8.

54. Wall PD, Woolf CJ. Muscle but not cutaneous C-afferent input produces prolonged increases in the excitability of

the flexion reflex in the rat. *Journal de Physiologie*. 1984; **356**: 443–58.

55. Woolf CJ, Wall PD. Relative effectiveness of C primary afferent fibers of different origins in evoking a prolonged facilitation of the flexor reflex in the rat. *Journal of Neuroscience*. 1986; **6**: 1433–42.

56. Woolf CJ. Long term alterations in the excitability of the flexion reflex produced by peripheral tissue injury in the chronic decerebrate rat. *Pain*. 1984; **18**: 325–43.

57. Kawasaki Y, Kohno T, Zhuang ZY *et al.* Ionotropic and metabotropic receptors, protein kinase A, protein kinase C, and Src contribute to C-fiber-induced ERK activation and cAMP response element-binding protein phosphorylation in dorsal horn neurons, leading to central sensitization. *Journal of Neuroscience*. 2004; **24**: 8310–21.

58. Wei F, Vadakkan KI, Toyoda H *et al.* Calcium calmodulin-stimulated adenylyl cyclases contribute to activation of extracellular signal-regulated kinase in spinal dorsal horn neurons in adult rats and mice. *Journal of Neuroscience*. 2006; **26**: 851–61.

59. Heinke B, Balzer E, Sandkuhler J. Pre- and postsynaptic contributions of voltage-dependent Ca2+ channels to nociceptive transmission in rat spinal lamina I neurons. *European Journal of Neuroscience*. 2004; **19**: 103–11.

60. Zou X, Lin Q, Willis WD. Enhanced phosphorylation of NMDA receptor 1 subunits in spinal cord dorsal horn and spinothalamic tract neurons after intradermal injection of capsaicin in rats. *Journal of Neuroscience*. 2000; **20**: 6989–97.

61. Guo W, Zou S, Guan Y *et al.* Tyrosine phosphorylation of the NR2B subunit of the NMDA receptor in the spinal cord during the development and maintenance of inflammatory hyperalgesia. *Journal of Neuroscience*. 2002; **22**: 6208–17.

62. Yu XM, Askalan R, Keil 2nd GJ, Salter MW. NMDA channel regulation by channel-associated protein tyrosine kinase Src. *Science*. 1997; **275**: 674–8.

63. Walker SM, Meredith-Middleton J, Lickiss T *et al.* Primary and secondary hyperalgesia can be differentiated by postnatal age and ERK activation in the spinal dorsal horn of the rat pup. *Pain*. 2007; **128**: 157–68.

64. Li P, Kerchner GA, Sala C *et al.* AMPA receptor-PDZ interactions in facilitation of spinal sensory synapses. *Nature Neuroscience*. 1999; **2**: 972–7.

* 65. Obata K, Noguchi K. MAPK activation in nociceptive neurons and pain hypersensitivity. *Life Sciences*. 2004; **74**: 2643–53.

66. Sun RQ, Tu YJ, Lawand NB *et al.* Calcitonin gene-related peptide receptor activation produces PKA- and PKC-dependent mechanical hyperalgesia and central sensitization. *Journal of Neurophysiology*. 2004; **92**: 2859–66.

67. Zeitz KP, Giese KP, Silva AJ, Basbaum AI. The contribution of autophosphorylated alpha-calcium-calmodulin kinase II to injury-induced persistent pain. *Neuroscience*. 2004; **128**: 889–98.

68. Fang L, Wu J, Lin Q, Willis WD. Calcium-calmodulin-dependent protein kinase II contributes to spinal cord central sensitization. *Journal of Neuroscience*. 2002; **22**: 4196–204.

69. Ji RR, Samad TA, Jin SX *et al.* p38 MAPK activation by NGF in primary sensory neurons after inflammation increases TRPV1 levels and maintains heat hyperalgesia. *Neuron*. 2002; **36**: 57–68.

70. Ji RR, Baba H, Brenner GJ, Woolf CJ. Nociceptive-specific activation of ERK in spinal neurons contributes to pain hypersensitivity. *Nature Neuroscience*. 1999; **2**: 1114–9.

71. Ji RR, Befort K, Brenner GJ, Woolf CJ. ERK MAP kinase activation in superficial spinal cord neurons induces prodynorphin and NK-1 upregulation and contributes to persistent inflammatory pain hypersensitivity. *Journal of Neuroscience*. 2002; **22**: 478–85.

72. Urban MO, Gebhart GF. Supraspinal contributions to hyperalgesia. *Proceedings of the National Academy of Sciences of the United States of America*. 1999; **96**: 7687–92.

* 73. Ren K, Dubner R. Descending modulation in persistent pain: an update. *Pain*. 2002; **100**: 1–6.

* 74. Gebhart GF. Descending modulation of pain. *Neuroscience and Biobehavioral Reviews*. 2004; **27**: 729–37.

* 75. Vanegas H, Schaible HG. Descending control of persistent pain: inhibitory or facilitatory? *Brain Research. Brain Research Reviews*. 2004; **46**: 295–309.

76. Urban MO, Jiang MC, Gebhart GF. Participation of central descending nociceptive facilitatory systems in secondary hyperalgesia produced by mustard oil. *Brain Research*. 1996; **737**: 83–91.

* 77. Millan MJ. Descending control of pain. *Progress in Neurobiology*. 2002; **66**: 355–474.

78. Fields HL, Malick A, Burstein R. Dorsal horn projection targets of on and off cells in the rostral ventromedial medulla. *Journal of Neurophysiology*. 1995; **74**: 1742–59.

79. Miki K, Zhou QQ, Guo W *et al.* Changes in gene expression and neuronal phenotype in brain stem pain modulatory circuitry after inflammation. *Journal of Neurophysiology*. 2002; **87**: 750–60.

80. Zhuo M, Gebhart GF. Characterization of descending inhibition and facilitation from the nuclei reticularis gigantocellularis and gigantocellularis pars alpha in the rat. *Pain*. 1990; **42**: 337–50.

81. Ren K, Zhuo M, Willis W. Multiplicity and plasticity of descending modulation of nociception: implications for persistent pain. In: Devor M, Rowbotham M, Wiesenfeld-Hallin Z (eds). *Proceedings of the 9th World Congress on Pain*. Seattle: IASP Press, 2000: 387–400.

82. Mansikka H, Pertovaara A. Supraspinal influence on hindlimb withdrawal thresholds and mustard oil-induced secondary allodynia in rats. *Brain Research Bulletin*. 1997; **42**: 359–65.

83. Pertovaara A. A neuronal correlate of secondary hyperalgesia in the rat spinal dorsal horn is submodality selective and facilitated by supraspinal influence. *Experimental Neurology*. 1998; **149**: 193–202.

84. Urban MO, Zahn PK, Gebhart GF. Descending facilitatory influences from the rostral medial medulla mediate secondary, but not primary hyperalgesia in the rat. *Neuroscience.* 1999; **90**: 349–52.

∗ 85. Suzuki R, Rygh LJ, Dickenson AH. Bad news from the brain: descending 5-HT pathways that control spinal pain processing. *Trends in Pharmacological Sciences.* 2004; **25**: 613–7.

86. Watkins LR. Immune and glial regulation of pain. *Brain, Behavior, and Immunity.* 2007; **21**: 519–21.

87. Watkins LR, Maier SF. Beyond neurons: evidence that immune and glial cells contribute to pathological pain states. *Physiological Reviews.* 2002; **82**: 981–1011.

∗ 88. Watkins LR, Maier SF. Glia: a novel drug discovery target for clinical pain. *Nature Reviews. Drug Discovery.* 2003; **2**: 973–85.

89. Dublin P, Hanani M. Satellite glial cells in sensory ganglia: Their possible contribution to inflammatory pain. *Brain, Behavior, and Immunity.* 2007; **21**: 592–8.

∗ 90. McMahon SB, Cafferty WB, Marchand F. Immune and glial cell factors as pain mediators and modulators. *Experimental Neurology.* 2005; **192**: 444–62.

∗ 91. Watkins LR, Hutchinson MR, Johnston IN, Maier SF. Glia: novel counter-regulators of opioid analgesia. *Trends in Neurosciences.* 2005; **28**: 661–9.

92. Beggs S, Salter MW. Stereological and somatotopic analysis of the spinal microglial response to peripheral nerve injury. *Brain, Behavior, and Immunity.* 2007; **21**: 624–33.

93. Coull JA, Beggs S, Boudreau D *et al.* BDNF from microglia causes the shift in neuronal anion gradient underlying neuropathic pain. *Nature.* 2005; **438**: 1017–21.

94. Tsuda M, Inoue K, Salter MW. Neuropathic pain and spinal microglia: a big problem from molecules in "small" glia. *Trends in Neurosciences.* 2005; **28**: 101–7.

Developmental neurobiology of nociception

SUELLEN M WALKER

KEY LEARNING POINTS

- Behavioral, neurophysiological, and molecular nociceptive processes undergo important changes throughout early development that impact on the response to noxious stimuli, injury, and analgesia.
- Due to the enhanced plasticity of the developing nervous system, early pain and injury can produce effects not seen in the adult, which may also be associated with long-term changes in sensory function and/or the response to future injury.

- Peripheral nociceptive responses mature early, but there is a tendency to increased excitatory and reduced inhibitory modulation in the spinal cord during early development.
- Changes in receptor distribution, neurotransmitter levels, and nociceptive pathways can have a significant impact on the pharmacodynamic profile of analgesic agents at different postnatal ages.

INTRODUCTION

Responses to noxious stimuli, and to different forms of injury and analgesics, can differ significantly in early life. Many aspects of nociceptive processing cannot be directly correlated with those seen in the adult as behavioral, neurophysiological, and molecular nociceptive processes undergo important postnatal changes.[1, 2, 3] Activity within sensory pathways is required for normal development, but abnormal or excessive activity related to pain and injury during the neonatal period may produce structural and functional changes not seen following the same injury in adults. In addition, there may be associated long-term changes in sensory processing and/or the response to future injury.[4, 5, 6] Effective, developmentally appropriate, pain management strategies have not been developed for all clinical situations,[7] and advances in knowledge and treatment depend on research which encompasses both clinical trials and preclinical studies in infant animal surrogate models.[8] Providing a neurobiological basis for treatment in early life,[1] rather than empirically basing treatment on data from older children and adults, is necessary to further improve both acute and long-term outcomes for children experiencing pain in early life.

NOCICEPTIVE PROCESSING

During the first weeks and months of life, there are significant functional and structural changes in the developing nervous system that influence nociceptive transmission. The expression of a number of molecules and channels involved in nociception are developmentally regulated, there are changes in the distribution and density of many important receptors, and the levels and effects of several neurotransmitters alter significantly during the postnatal period.[1, 2, 9]

The rat pup is born at a relatively immature stage and is an established model for investigation of developmental changes. Data collected from human tissue and rat pups show a comparable pattern of progression throughout development, and approximate age correlations can be made across the two species.[10] The development of peripheral and spinal cord somatosensory function during the first postnatal week in the rat pup corresponds to preterm development from 24 weeks until full-term birth at 40 postconceptional weeks. Rat pups are weaned around the 21st postnatal day (P21) and by this age may be considered developmentally comparable to human adolescents.[10, 11] Rather than representing absolute correlations, these timelines provide a framework for assessing progressive changes in function throughout development.

Peripheral responses to noxious stimuli

The cell bodies of peripheral sensory neurons are located in the dorsal root ganglia (DRG) and send axons both peripherally to innervate target organs such as skin and centrally to synapse within the spinal cord. In the periphery, large A-fibers innervate the skin before C-fibers, but by birth in the rat and the second trimester in man, sensory fibers are distributed to all body regions.[1, 12] Peripheral cutaneous receptors respond to a range of mechanical, thermal, and chemical stimuli from early development.[13, 14] Many different receptors mediate responses to peripheral stimuli, but the developmental profile of relatively few have been investigated. Both the TRPV1 receptor, which is activated by capsaicin, protons, and thermal stimuli ($>43°C$), and the TRPA1 receptor, which responds to pungent compounds such as mustard oil, are functional from early development.[14, 15] TRPV1-positive nerve terminals are present in cutaneous structures at P10, but at reduced density compared with adults.[16] In the DRG, the percentage of cells that contain TRPV1 remains relatively constant (around 60 percent) from P2 to P45, but the distribution on C-fiber subpopulations changes: the percentage that are colocalized with non-peptidergic IB4-positive fibers increases, while those with peptidergic trkA-positive fibers decreases.[16] This is influenced by the normal postnatal increase in IB4-positive DRG cells.[17] Both TTX-sensitive and TTX-resistant Na channels can be identified from birth in rat DRG, and their kinetic properties do not change significantly throughout development.[18] The sensory neuron-specific tetrodotoxin-resistant sodium channels $Na_v1.8$ and $Na_v1.9$ are expressed on C-fibers at birth and reach adult levels by P7.[19]

Pain transmission in the spinal cord

AFFERENT INPUT

In the adult, C-fiber polymodal nociceptors project to the superficial dorsal horn (lamina I and II), while larger myelinated A-beta fibers which subserve light touch and pressure, project to deeper layers of the dorsal horn (lamina III and IV). However, during development the functional and anatomical relationships between C and A fibers change, leading to age-related changes in the processing of sensory inputs. A-beta fibers enter the cord earlier than C-fibers, initially project throughout lamina I–V of the dorsal horn, and then gradually withdraw to the adult pattern of distribution in lamina III–IV over the first three postnatal weeks.[12, 20, 21, 22] As C-fiber function matures, there is a progressive reduction in A-fiber input and increase in C-fiber input in the superficial dorsal horn.[23, 24]

A-fibers form synaptic contacts in the superficial laminae in the neonate,[25] and A-fiber stimulation produces sensitization in dorsal horn cells in the first postnatal week.[26, 27] Although the intrinsic excitability of superficial dorsal horn neurons is stable throughout development,[28] these changes in synaptic input during the period of overlap between A and C fiber projections increase the degree of central activation produced by peripheral stimuli.[26, 29, 30]

Functional contacts between C-fiber terminals and dorsal horn neurons can be demonstrated in spinal cord slice preparations as capsaicin: (1) evokes glutamate release,[31] (2) dose-dependently increases mini-excitatory postsynaptic current (mEPSC) frequency from P0, and (3) evokes action potentials from P1.[32] However, these immature synapses lack the ability to synchronously release large amounts of transmitter, and *in vivo*, C-fiber stimulation does not evoke postsynaptic responses in the dorsal horn during the first postnatal week.[26, 33] By P10, C-fiber stimulation produces centrally mediated secondary hyperalgesia,[34] and repetitive C fiber stimulation produces wind up, which is seen in an increased proportion of cells with further increases in age.[26, 27, 30]

EXCITATORY MODULATION

The balance between excitatory and inhibitory neurotransmission in the dorsal horn alters during postnatal development (see **Table 2.1**).[2] Enhanced excitatory mechanisms are important for activity-dependent changes[4] and there is a tendency for more delayed development of inhibitory mechanisms.[49]

Developmental changes in the distribution and subunit composition of glutamate receptors in the spinal cord contribute to the increased excitability of the neonatal dorsal horn.[2] AMPA, kainate, and NMDA receptors are activated by glutamate to produce inward cation currents and depolarization of the postsynaptic cell. Several factors contribute to an enhanced excitability in early development including (see **Table 2.1**):

- increased density and distribution of receptors throughout the dorsal horn;
- increased affinity for agonist;
- changes in subunit expression that alter channel kinetics and increase the calcium permeability of the receptor.

Table 2.1 Excitatory and inhibitory modulation in the spinal cord during early development.

	Structure	Function
Excitation		
C fiber	Last primary afferents to project into cord[12]	Frequency of mEPSCs initially low: asynchronous glutamate release[32]
	C-fiber markers trkA, IB4 and CGRP are expressed in the spinal cord from early development[12, 35, 36]	No postsynaptic response to C-fiber electrical stimuli[26, 33]
	TRPV1-immunoreactivity detectable in lamina I of the dorsal horn at P2; diffusely distributed in lamina II also by P10; density increased by P20; two distinct zones in lamina I and inner lamina II by P30[16]	Reduced spontaneous reflex activity to chemical C-fiber stimuli[34, 37] Reduced secondary hyperalgesia[34, 38, 39]
A fiber	Initially project throughout and form functional synapses in superficial DH[25]	Activity in A-beta fibers evokes monosynaptic responses in laminae I and II[23, 24]
	Overlap with C fibers Withdraw as C fiber function matures[12, 20, 21, 22]	Prolonged after discharge and mediate central sensitization[26, 27]
DH input	Initial overlap between A and C-fiber inputs in superficial DH[12]	Reduced mechanical threshold of DH neurons[29]
	Large receptive field[40]	Increased central activation for given peripheral input[26, 29, 30] Reflex response has low threshold and poorly directed
AMPA receptor	Highly expressed in newborn cord GluR1, 2, and 4 more highly expressed[41, 42]	Increased excitability Ca permeability (no Ca flux in adult)
NMDA receptor	Highly expressed and more widespread distribution[42, 43] Increased expression of NR2D subunit[2] Increased affinity for agonist[44] May not be colocalized with AMPA[47, 48]	Increased excitability Slower offset time, increased Ca influx Repeat stimuli can activate in absence of AMPA[45, 46]
mGluR	mGluR3 and mGluR5 highly expressed at birth[2]	Functional effects not elucidated
Inhibition		
GABA$_A$ receptor	Altered subunit composition[2]	Reduced spontaneous IPSCs[49] Some neurons depolarize rather than hyperpolarize following GABA activation but insufficient for action potential[49] Intrinsic spinal GABAergic inhibition functional[50]
KCC2	Reduced expression K$^+$-Cl$^-$ cotransporter[51]	High intracellular chloride Progressively more neurons hyperpolarize to GABA[49] Inhibition progressively enhanced throughout first week
GlyR	Altered subunit composition[2] Expression of postsynaptic scaffolding protein required for anchoring of GABA and glycine receptors	Reduced channel opening time No glycine mediated spontaneous IPSCs in superficial DH initially: altered balance and temporal relationship of excitatory and inhibitory inputs[49]
Interneurons	Axodendritic growth occurs postnatally[52]	Reduced local inhibition
Descending inhibition	Fibers in DLF do not project into cord[53]	Stimulation of DLF:no DH inhibition[53] Activation of PAG:no DH inhibition[54] DNIC immature[55]

DH, dorsal horn; DLF, dorsolateral funiculus; DNIC, diffuse noxious inhibitory controls; GABA, gamma-aminobutyric acid; GlyR, glycine receptor; IPSC, inhibitory post-synaptic currents; KCC2, potassium-chloride cotransporter; mGluR, metabotropic glutamate receptor; NMDA, N-methyl-D-aspartate; PAG, periaqueductal gray. Further details in recent reviews and chapters.[1, 2, 3]

INTRACELLULAR CASCADES

The influx of calcium ions following NMDA receptor opening activates a number of protein kinases and intracellular enzyme cascades, leading to rapid onset posttranslational and longer-term transcriptional changes (see Chapter 1a, Applied physiology of nociception). In adult animals, induction of nitric oxide synthase (NOS) and increased production of nitric oxide (NO) in the spinal cord has been associated with hyperalgesia following a number of stimuli.[56] NOS expression is not seen in lamina II before P5 and does not reach adult levels until P20.[56, 57] Developmental changes in a number of intracellular cascades contribute to the differential maturation of peripheral and central sensitization mechanisms. Whereas C-fiber stimuli produce primary hyperalgesia or peripheral sensitization at all postnatal ages, the maturation of central responses to C-fiber stimuli is delayed (see **Table 2.2**). The protein kinase C isoform PKC-ε is present in DRG and modulates responses to formalin throughout development. However, there are relatively few PKC-γ-positive cells in the dorsal horn in early life and inhibition of this enzyme has little effect on the response to formalin until P21.[31] Extracellular signal-regulated kinase (ERK) protein can be identified in the dorsal horn in early development but at lower levels than in older animals, and the degree and distribution of capsaicin-induced activation of ERK in the spinal cord also increases with postnatal age.[34] Identification of age-related changes in the cellular responses to different stimuli is necessary to identify developmentally appropriate analgesic targets.

INHIBITORY MODULATION

Inhibitory mechanisms may not be fully mature in early life (see **Table 2.1**). Fast inhibitory transmission is mediated by gamma-aminobutyric acid (GABA) and glycine receptors, both of which undergo developmental changes in subunit expression that influence channel kinetics.[2] In the hippocampus, GABA initially produces depolarizing rather than hyperpolarizing currents, as the intracellular chloride concentration remains high until the potassium-chloride cotransporter KCC2 is upregulated later in development.[51, 59] However, GABAergic inhibition may mature earlier in the spinal cord. In dorsal horn slices, although GABA produced depolarization in a proportion of cells at P0–2 this was insufficient to produce action potentials, and by P6-7 only the adult pattern of

Table 2.2 Postnatal changes in intracellular kinases.

Enzyme	Site	Developmental profile	Function	Effect of inhibition
PKCε[31]	DRG	Expressed by increasing proportion of DRG cells 41% at P7, 60% at P20; 90% in adult	Mediates peripheral response to formalin Effect independent of age	Reduces both phases of formalin response at all postnatal ages Reduces CGRP and glutamate release from spinal cord
PKCγ[31]	Dorsal horn	Relatively few cells at P7 Number of cells increases with age Becomes localized to lamina II	Effect increases with postnatal age Activation by formalin at P21, no effect at P7 or P15	Attenuates second phase of formalin response at P21 and P15 No effect at P7
CaMK II[58]	Dorsal horn	Low levels at P0, upregulation of expression to P14	Required for normal activity-dependent development of sensory circuits	Mutation at autophosphorylation site: deficit in A-fiber input and increased receptive field size
ERK[34]	Dorsal horn	Significant increase in ERK protein from P3 to P21	Mediates central C-fiber induced secondary hyperalgesia Minimal activation in cord by capsaicin at P3 Increased degree and distribution of activated phosphoERK in cord at P21	Blocks secondary hyperalgesia at P21 No effect on primary hyperalgesia at P3 or P21 (IT PD98059)

CaMK, calcium calmodulin kinase; ERK, extracellular signal-regulated kinase; P, postnatal day; PKC, protein kinase C.

hyperpolarizing responses was recorded.[49] Application of the GABA$_A$-antagonist gabazine to the spinal cord *in vivo* produced a similar degree of increased firing at P3 and P21, suggesting that intrinsic spinal GABAergic inhibition is functional during early life.[50] Although GABA does not appear to have significant direct excitatory effects in the spinal cord, the overall response to GABA activation is also influenced by descending inputs.[60] Although local inhibition within the spinal cord can be demonstrated in early life, modulation by descending inputs may initially result in an overall facilitatory effect.

Withdrawal reflexes

Withdrawal reflexes are important models for the investigation of nociceptive processing at all ages in both laboratory and clinical studies.[61, 62] Measuring reflex thresholds allow quantification of responses to different forms of injury[63, 64] and assessment of analgesic efficacy in preclinical studies.[65, 66, 67, 68] Similarly, changes in reflex thresholds in infants can provide additional objective evaluation of responses to injury and analgesia in clinical studies.[69, 70]

LABORATORY STUDIES

Flexor-withdrawal responses to mechanical and thermal stimuli can be measured from birth, but thresholds are lower, and the reflex response has greater amplitude, longer latency, and a higher degree of variability.[2, 37, 71, 72] The increase in withdrawal reflex thresholds with age reflects a gradual decrease in the excitability of spinal cord neurons, increased inhibitory input, and reorganization of sensory connections that reduce the size of the receptive field.[26] Reflex responses are initially less organized, can be evoked by both noxious and innocuous stimuli, and may result in inappropriate generalized movements. Maturation of sensory and motor inputs, and an activity-dependent process that involves strengthening of appropriate connections and suppression of erroneous movements, leads to tuning of the receptive fields of each withdrawal reflex module. As a result, more specific motor responses develop that selectively move the stimulated area away from the stimulus.[73, 74, 75]

CLINICAL STUDIES

In clinical studies, changes in reflex thresholds, receptive field size, and the specificity of withdrawal responses have been demonstrated that correlate with the developmental pattern seen in laboratory investigations (**Figure 2.1**). The mechanical threshold of the hindlimb flexion withdrawal reflex is initially low and increases with postconceptional age (PCA) in preterm neonates, but is still well below adult levels at term (40 weeks PCA).[76, 77] Electromyography (EMG) responses of the biceps femoris to mechanical, electrical, and noxious (heel stick for routine blood sampling) stimuli confirmed lower reflex thresholds in infants aged 28–42 weeks PCA, and there was good correlation between stimulus intensity and the amplitude of the reflex at all ages.[78] Reflex movements are also less synchronized in premature neonates. The receptive field of the hindlimb reflex is large in early development, as withdrawal can be elicited by low intensity stimuli over the whole limb at 27 weeks PCA. As age increases, withdrawal is more specifically produced by stimuli on the foot, and there is now a gradient of increasing threshold from distal to proximal sites on the limb.[77] A mechanical stimulus (von Frey hair) applied perpendicular to the abdomen produces a brisk contraction of the ipsilateral abdominal musculature in infants (abdominal skin reflex). In preterm neonates, a more generalized response that includes hip flexion is evoked, but the incidence and degree of hip flexion decreases sharply from 30 to 42 weeks PCA.[70] Erroneous reflex

Figure 2.1 Characteristics of withdrawal reflexes in infant rats (a–d) and human neonates (e–f). The mechanical threshold of both the hind limb withdrawal reflex in the rat pup (a) and the abdominal skin reflex assessed in the neonate (f) can be determined by application of graded nylon monofilaments (von Frey hairs) which apply a logarithmically increasing force. The threshold increases with age in rat pups aged 3, 10, and 21 postnatal days (b) and in preterm and term neonates and infants aged from 32 weeks postconceptional age to 2 years (f). Reflexes are generalized and not well-tuned in early life. In the rat pup, the withdrawal in the extensor digitorum longus muscle is elicited by multiple sites on the paw (strongest response from dark area drawn on hind paw), but in the adult is localized to the skin on the toes (i.e. maximal response evoked from the skin area that is most effectively withdrawn as the muscle contracts) (c). In the youngest infants, the response to mechanical stimuli on the abdomen produces a generalized response which includes bilateral hip flexion, but becomes more focused to abdominal muscles alone with increasing age (g). Electromyography recordings in biceps femoris from a rat pup (d) and human neonate (h) show that the magnitude of the response increases with increasing stimulus intensity. (c) Reprinted from Holmberg H, Schouenborg J. Postnatal development of the nociceptive withdrawal reflexes in the rat: a behavioural and electromyographic study. *Journal of Physiology*. 1996; **493**: 239–52; (e–g) modified from Andrews K, Fitzgerald M. Wound sensitivity as a measure of analgesic effects following surgery in human neonates and infants. *Pain*. 2002; **99**: 185–95; (h) reprinted from Andrews K, Fitzgerald M. Cutaneous flexion reflex in human neonates: a quantitative study of threshold and stimulus-response characteristics after single and repeated stimuli. *Developmental Medicine and Child Neurology*. 1999; **41**: 696–703.

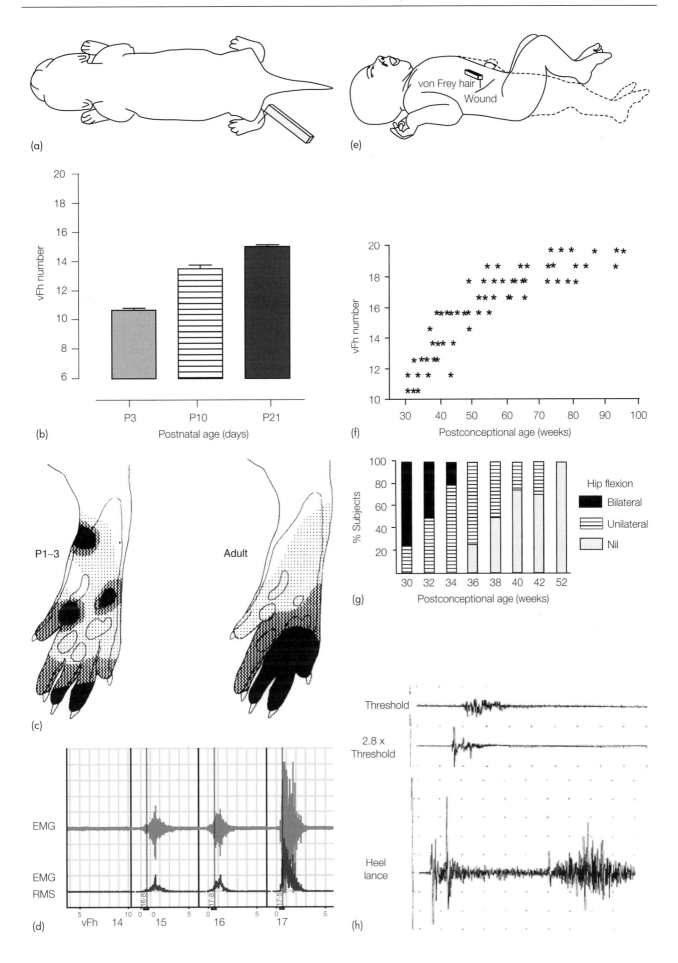

movements have also been demonstrated in clinical studies. In an adult, stimulation of the plantar surface of the heel produces plantar flexion of the toes and no response in tibialis anterior (which produces dorsiflexion of toes). However, in neonates aged 30–39.5 weeks PCA, low intensity mechanical (von Frey hairs) or electrical stimuli on the plantar surface of the foot produced an EMG response in tibialis anterior.[62] This leads to inappropriate movement towards the stimulus, which resolves with further maturation and tuning of the reflex response.

Higher centers

ASCENDING PATHWAYS

Nociceptive sensory discriminative information ascends from the dorsal horn to the thalamus in the spinothalamic pathways. By birth in the rat, afferents from the spinal cord have reached the thalamus and functional thalamocortical synaptic connections have been formed.[3]

Ascending fibers from lamina I of the dorsal horn (spinoparabrachial pathways) ascend to the amygdala (affective components of pain) and the hypothalamus (autonomic function),[79, 80] but as yet there is little information on the structure and function of these pathways during development.

DESCENDING MODULATION

Descending pathways from the brain stem modulate pain transmission in the spinal cord.[81, 82] The periaqueductal gray (PAG) receives inputs from the dorsal horn and a wide range of higher centers including the amygdala and cortex, and projects to the rostroventromedial medulla (RVM) which exerts bidirectional inhibitory and facilitatory control on the spinal cord (see Chapter 1b, Mechanisms of inflammatory hyperalgesia). Many pathways projecting from the brain stem are anatomically present in early life, including descending pathways in the dorsolateral funiculus, but may not be fully functional. Inhibition of dorsal horn cell responses by stimulation of the dorsolateral funiculus is not present until P10–12, and until P22–24 is only activated by high-intensity stimulation.[53] Diffuse noxious inhibitory controls are also not functional in the first two postnatal weeks[55] and stimulus-produced analgesia from the PAG is not apparent until P21.[54] The effect of developmental age on descending facilitatory pathways, and on the balance between inhibitory and facilitatory activity, is currently being investigated.

In adults, fibers from noradrenergic cell groups in the brain stem descend to the dorsal horn.[83] Noradrenergic-immunoreactive fibers are visible in the dorsal horn at all spinal levels at P3, but the density of immunoreactive fibers progressively increases until adult levels are reached at P30.[84] However, binding sites for alpha2-adrenergic agonists and messenger RNA for the alpha2A receptor are present in the dorsal horn in early life.[85, 86, 87] Laboratory studies show increased sensitivity to the analgesic effects of spinally administered dexmedetomidine (an alpha2-adrenergic agonist), and to the cardiovascular and sedative effects of epidural or systemic dexmedetomidine in early life.[68, 88, 89]

Descending serotonergic fibers are present in the dorsal horn at birth, but the adult distribution and density are not achieved until P21.[90] Effects of serotonin are difficult to delineate due to the number of receptor subtypes involved and the presence of both descending inhibitory and facilitatory pathways.[91] Intrathecal alpha-methyl-5-hydroxytryptamine (5HT 2A/2C receptor agonist) produces dose-dependent suppression of the formalin response in adult rats.[92] In rat pups, intrathecal 2-methylserotonin did not suppress the formalin response before P10 and dose requirements were initially higher than in older animals.[93]

CORTICAL FUNCTION IN HUMAN NEONATES

The reflex responses and alterations in stress hormones associated with noxious procedures in neonates are indicators of functional nociceptive and hypothalamo–pituitary–adrenal axis pathways, but do not directly equate with cortical activation or pain perception.[94] Emphasis has previously been placed on the presence of thalamocortical fibers as a minimum requirement for pain perception and, although these pathways are anatomically present from 23 to 30 weeks gestational age in the human,[95] functional maturity has only recently been confirmed. Electroencephalographic (EEG) activity can be detected from 24 weeks, and synchronous activity suggesting wakefulness from 30 weeks PCA in premature neonates.[95]

Cortical activation in association with painful procedural interventions has recently been investigated using near-infrared spectroscopy (NIRS) in premature neonates. Heel prick for blood sampling produces changes in cerebral oxygenation over the contralateral somatosensory cortex indicative of cortical activation. These changes could be observed as early as 25 weeks postmenstrual age, the magnitude of response increased and latency decreased with age, and greater responses were recorded in awake neonates.[96] A later study reported bilateral increases in blood flow over the somatosensory cortex following venepuncture, and a negative correlation was found between cortical activity and gestational age (28 to 36 weeks).[97] Although some results vary due to differing methodology (brief heel lance versus more prolonged venepuncture and squeeze, duration of recordings, time after birth), both studies show that noxious stimuli produce functional activation of the somatosensory cortex in premature neonates.[98]

DEVELOPMENTAL AGE AND THE RESPONSE TO INJURY

Developmental changes in nociceptive pathways can alter the degree and/or pattern of hyperalgesia following injury in early life. In addition, the enhanced plasticity of the developing nervous system[1] can result in effects not seen following the same injury in adults, which may be associated with long-term changes in sensory function and/or the response to future injury. In the following section, responses to different forms of laboratory injury are described, and where possible compared with results from clinical studies. Long-term effects following different laboratory models of early injury are further outlined in **Table 2.3**.

Primary and secondary hyperalgesia

LABORATORY INVESTIGATIONS

Primary hyperalgesia is characterized by a decrease in pain threshold and increased response to suprathreshold stimuli due to sensitization of nociceptors within an area of injury[114] and can be demonstrated in a number of early developmental models.[34, 115] Peripheral application of mustard oil, which activates C-fibers via the TRPA1 receptor, enhances the response to subsequent brushing or pinching within the receptive field of dorsal horn neurons.[10] Although hind paw mustard oil application evokes less immediate reflex activity at P3 than in older pups, the reflex response to mechanical hind paw stimuli is increased ten minutes later (i.e. primary hyperalgesia is induced) at all postnatal ages.[34, 37]

In addition to primary hyperalgesia at the site of injury, noxious C-fiber stimulation produces a surrounding zone of secondary mechanical hyperalgesia in adult animals.[116, 117] However, minimal C-fiber-induced secondary hyperalgesia is observed in early development,[34, 38, 39] suggesting that the necessary spinal cord and/or supraspinal mechanisms are not mature in the first postnatal week.

CLINICAL STUDIES

C-fiber-induced primary and secondary hyperalgesia can be clearly demonstrated and quantified in adult human volunteers.[118, 119] Tissue injury due to repeated heel prick blood sampling in neonates results in primary hyperalgesia, as reflected by a reduction in the mechanical threshold for hind limb withdrawal.[120, 121] Changes in withdrawal threshold in the contralateral limb, suggestive of secondary hyperalgesia, have been reported with more extensive injury.[78] Therefore, secondary hyperalgesia may be mediated by pathways other than C-fibers in early life, and analgesic agents that specifically target C-fiber

mechanisms may be advantageous in adults, but less so in early development. The abdominal skin reflex (ASR) has also been used to assess the response to injury in neonates and infants. The mechanical threshold (von Frey hairs) for evoking this reflex is significantly lower for at least 24 hours following abdominal surgery, and can be returned towards baseline values by analgesia.[69]

Inflammation

Hind paw inflammation produces hyperalgesia at all postnatal ages in the rat pup, but the degree of acute change varies with age, and long-term changes are critically dependent on the severity of injury.[6, 68] Severe neonatal inflammation produces permanent structural alterations in primary afferent projections in the dorsal horn that are associated with increased behavioral and electrophysiological responses to subsequent painful stimuli.[99, 100] As these changes are only seen in association with chronic inflammation they may be of limited clinical significance, but even relatively mild inflammation in neonatal animals produces acute reversible structural changes that are not seen following a similar injury in the adult.[6]

Recent studies have reported a dual pattern of long-term response following mild neonatal inflammation.[105] A generalized increase in basal sensory thresholds or hypoalgesia is seen in all paws when these animals reach adulthood, possibly due to stress-induced alterations in the hypothalamic–pituitary axis (HPA). By contrast, repeated injury in the previously inflamed hind paw seems to unmask segmental changes of long term sensitization and produces a greater degree of local hyperalgesia.[105, 122] These changes only occur if inflammation is induced in the first postnatal week in the rodent, and therefore this represents a critical period of susceptibility for long-term effects following inflammation.

Surgical incision

LABORATORY INVESTIGATIONS

As responses to inflammation, skin wounding and nerve injury have different developmental profiles, but may all contribute to surgical injury,[123] developmentally regulated responses to surgery need to be specifically investigated. Plantar hind paw incision through skin, fascia, and muscle layers is increasingly used as a model of postoperative pain in adult animals.[124] This incision produces acute hyperalgesia in two-week-old rats, which resolves more rapidly than when the same procedure is performed in 4- and 16-week-old animals.[125] Effects at earlier stages of development require evaluation. Laparotomy in neonatal mice (P0) produces both acute behavioral responses indicative of pain and distress, as well as long-term changes in sensory function.[110]

Table 2.3 Long-term effects of neonatal injury in laboratory models.

	Structural changes	Behavioral/functional changes	Response to repeat injury in adult	Developmental profile
Severe inflammation 25 μL CFA at P0–1	*Periphery:* Chronic inflammation[6] No cell death or change in cell number in DRG[6] *Dorsal horn:* Brief (3–6 days) alterations in mRNA expression in DRG[103] Expanded sciatic terminal field[99] (not seen with less severe inflammation)[6] Increase density CGRP[99]	*Dorsal horn:* Increased spontaneous and evoked firing (adult)[99, 100]	*Formalin:*[99] *CFA:*[101] *Capsaicin:*[102] Late phase earlier Increased Fos in DH Increased thermal and mechanical hyperalgesia Increased Fos expression in DH	Long-term effects if inflammation at P0, no effect at P14[99] Response to capsaicin enhanced if inflammation at P0 not P14[102]
Mild inflammation 1 μL/g (8–10 g) 0.25–1% carrageenan	*Dorsal horn:* Altered gene expression at baseline and differing pattern with reinflammation[104] Acute, but reversible change in sciatic afferent terminal field[6]	*Generalized:* Increased threshold all paws emerges at P34[105] Reduced response to stress (swim test; plus-maze)[106]	*CFA:*[105] Increased mechanical and thermal hyperalgesia Present at all time points after injection	Inflammation in first postnatal week (P0, P1, P3, P5) produces dual pattern of baseline hypoalgesia and enhanced response to repeat injury[105] No effect if inflammation at P8 or beyond)[105] *(Continued over)*

	Brain: Increased 5HT receptor expression in PAG[106]		Reduced baseline and stress induced neuroendocrine response[106]		Only if injection in same paw: no contralateral effect	Gene changes following inflammation at P3 differ from P12[104]
		Dorsal horn:	No persistent change in receptive field size or spontaneous or evoked activity[40]	*Colonic distension:*[107]	Decreased response	Visceral effects (colon) after inflammation at P3 not P14[107]
Full thickness skin wound	*Periphery:* Hyperinnervation (up to 12 weeks)[108] Down-regulation ephrin-A4[109]	*Generalized:*	Persistent mechanical hyperalgesia at 3 weeks[108]		Relatively greater response following colonic inflammation	Effect if wound at P0 or P7 Not seen at P14 or P21[108]
		Dorsal horn:	Increased receptive field size at 3 and 6 weeks;[40] no persistent change in DH threshold, spontaneous or evoked activity[40]			
Laparotomy (mice) P0[110]	Hypoalgesia to thermal and mechanical stimuli Thermal tail latency and AC effects prevented by post-procedure morphine Thermal paw effects also after sham surgery stress			*Acetic acid abdominal constriction (AC):*	Decreased response	Laparotomy only performed at P0 No comparison with surgery at older ages

(Continued over)

Table 2.3 Long-term effects of neonatal injury in laboratory models (continued).

	Structural changes	Behavioral/ functional changes		Response to repeat injury in adult		Developmental profile
Intramuscular injection pH4 (gastrocnemius daily P12–20)[111]	*Periphery:* No detectable changes in muscle histology	*Periphery:* Decreased threshold for withdrawal following muscle pinch		*Colonic distension:* Enhanced response		Effect if injections P12–20 No long-term effect following injections in adult
		Dorsal horn: Neurons responding to colonic distension (short latency sustained): increased spontaneous activity and increased response to distension				
Colonic irritation[112] (mechanical or mustard oil)	*Periphery:* No detectable changes in bowel histology	*Dorsal horn:* Increased neuronal firing		*Colonic distension:* Enhanced response		Effect if repeat injury from P8 to P20 No effect if repeat injury from P21 to P42
Bladder inflammation (intravesical zymosan)[113]		Increased spontaneous micturition frequency		Reinflammation of bladder[113] Increased response to distension Increased extravasation		Effect if injury P14–16 No effect if injury P28–30

Multiple noninjury-related factors may influence the response to interventions in early life, including:

- **Maternal separation**. Maternal separation (for prolonged periods in some studies) can have multiple effects on subsequent behaviors, including responses to visceral stimuli[126] and analgesic agents.[127]
- **Maternal behavior**. An initial increase in maternal contact but later neglect was reported after hind paw inflammation,[106] but no change in maternal behavior was seen in mice whose pups had undergone laparotomy.[110, 128]
- **Intercurrent infection**. Early exposure to an immune challenge (intraperitoneal lipopolysaccharide at P14) produces long-term changes in nociceptive thresholds in later life.[129, 130]
- **Stress response**. Neonatal handling and interventions may evoke stress responses, but there is conflicting data on the effects of early injury on the stress response when animals reach adulthood. Repeated paw needle prick has been reported to either increase[131] or have no effect[132] on subsequent measures of anxiety and humoral stress responses. Mild inflammation during the first postnatal week[106] and daily handling of pups during the neonatal period[128] have been associated with decreased stress responsiveness on reaching adulthood.

To evaluate specific injury-related effects in developmental studies it is therefore crucial that comparisons are made with appropriate control groups. For example, an increased threshold for hind limb withdrawal was observed in both the neonatal laparotomy and sham group who had the same degree of stress (anesthesia, maternal separation, placebo injection).[110] Changes in subsequent visceral sensitivity have been found following both sham and inflammatory neonatal injections.[107] Controls may need to include include both animals with the same degree of neonatal stress and a naive group.

CLINICAL STUDIES

Clinical evidence for long-term effects following early injury is compelling but incomplete, as both increases and decreases in pain sensitivity have been reported following surgery and/or intensive care in the neonatal period. Examples include:

- **Alterations in pain-related behavior in ex-neonatal intensive care unit (NICU) patients.**[5, 133] The cognitive and behavioral impairments reported in large cohorts of ex-premature infants[134, 135] may confound the interpretation of alterations in pain behavior[133, 136] and it is difficult to attribute effects specifically to pain.

- **Increased mechanical sensitivity 12–18 years following NICU.** The number of tender points was increased and the tenderness threshold was reduced when assessed by dolorimeter.[137]
- **Significant changes in heat pain sensitivity in ex-NICU children.**[138] Quantitative sensory testing (QST) demonstrated hypoalgesia to brief heat pain stimuli (i.e. increased threshold), but enhanced perceptual sensitization to prolonged tonic heat.[138]
- **Changes in mechanical thresholds following neonatal surgery.** Ten years following neonatal thoracotomy, QST demonstrated higher mechanical thresholds both at the site of surgery and at a distant reference point (thenar eminence) when compared to an age-matched nonoperated control group.[139]
- **Enhanced response to subsequent surgery.** Surgery during the first three months of life has been associated with higher pain scores and increased perioperative analgesic requirements when subsequent surgery is performed in the same dermatome.[140]

These studies are suggestive of the dual profile of response also seen following neonatal inflammation in the rat pup, i.e. generalized baseline hypoalgesia, but an enhanced response to repeated injury in the same area.[105] Further clinical studies following surgery performed at different ages are required to determine if there is a specific age range during which surgery in children produces long-term changes in sensory function.[64]

Analgesia at the time of the initial painful stimulus may modulate long-term effects. Male neonates circumcised without analgesia show an increased behavioral pain response to immunization several months later, but this is reduced if local anesthetic is used before the initial surgery.[141] Infants who had undergone surgery in the neonatal period with perioperative morphine did not show any increase in later response to immunization when compared with infants without significant previous pain experience.[142] Further research is required to evaluate the ability of different analgesic regimes to modulate or prevent long-term changes in sensory function and responses to pain.

Visceral injury

LABORATORY INVESTIGATIONS

Rat pups subjected to repeated mechanical or chemical (mustard oil) colonic irritation from P8 to P20 had behavioral and electrophysiological changes in the dorsal horn when adult, suggestive of persistent hyperalgesia, despite recovery of peripheral tissues and no detectable changes in bowel histology. Prolonged effects were not seen when the same degree of irritation was performed from P21 to P42, suggesting that this is a specific developmental effect (although older animals were sedated during treatment).[112] Similarly, early bladder inflammation (at P14–16) increased the response to subsequent inflammation, whereas injury at P28–30 was not associated with persistent effects.[113]

As spinal neurons receive convergent input from both somatic and visceral afferents, it has also been postulated that early somatic injury may influence subsequent visceral responses. Neonatal hind paw inflammation decreases the response to colonic distension in adults, but there is a relatively greater response to colonic inflammation by mustard oil.[107] Repeated intramuscular injection of low pH 4.0 saline from P8 to P20 produces long-term deep somatic hyperalgesia and visceral (colonic) hyperalgesia, which is not seen when the same stimulus is applied in adults.[111]

CLINICAL STUDIES

In infants with unilateral hydronephrosis, the threshold of the abdominal skin reflex was reduced ipsilaterally reflecting referred visceral hyperalgesia. In addition, the reflex threshold did not follow the normal developmental pattern of increasing threshold with increasing postnatal age and remained lower than in control infants even after corrective surgery.[70] This suggests that long-term alterations in sensory processing may occur following early visceral injury.

Given the link between early somatic insults and subsequent visceral sensitivity, it has been postulated that early insults may predispose children to future functional bowel disorders (FBD). An association between neonatal gastric suctioning and subsequent FBD has been reported.[143] However, as noted in an accompanying editorial, it is difficult to clearly define an association, let alone causation, between early injury and subsequent clinical conditions.[144]

Full thickness skin wounding

The response to full thickness skin wounds on the hind paw differs markedly in neonatal and adult animals. When performed in the first postnatal week, skin wounding results in a reduction in withdrawal threshold that persists well beyond the period of wound healing,[108, 145] and which is not prevented by a brief sciatic nerve block at the time of injury.[146] Central changes in sensory connections contribute to this persistent sensitivity, as the receptive field size of dorsal horn neurons is significantly greater in wounded compared with control animals three and six weeks later.[40] In addition, marked peripheral hyperinnervation occurs within the wounded area, mediated by local release of neurotrophic factors[147] and changes in short-range inhibitory cues.[109] Ephrins act as contact-mediated guidance molecules during development and repair, and ephrin-A4 inhibits neurite outgrowth. However, following neonatal skin wounding this inhibition is reduced as ephrin-A4 expression is down-regulated, allowing an increase in innervation density.[109]

Nerve injury

LABORATORY INVESTIGATIONS

In early development, peripheral sensory neurons are dependent on neurotrophins from the target area of innervation.[3] Axotomy produces marked cell death within the dorsal root ganglion[148] that is not seen with other forms of injury, such as severe inflammation.[6] Sciatic nerve axotomy during the first postnatal week leads to a reduction in the central terminal field of these primary afferents, but adjacent saphenous neurons project into the denervated area[149, 150] and form functional connections.[151] Therefore, despite cell death, central inputs are maintained.

Several different forms of peripheral nerve injury have been used to investigate the pathophysiology of neuropathic pain. Responses during early development differ significantly from those seen when the same injury occurs in adults. Ligation of the spinal nerve roots (L5 and L6) produces significant and prolonged allodynia in adult animals, but changes are of shorter duration if performed at one or two weeks of age.[152, 153] Partial sciatic ligation produced minimal difference in threshold from control animals in two-week-old rat pups, but when performed in four- or 16-week-old animals a greater degree and duration of allodynia was observed.[153] The spared nerve injury (SNI) model (i.e. division of tibial and common peroneal branches of sciatic nerve, while leaving sural nerve intact) produces marked allodynia in adult animals.[154] When performed at 3, 7, 10, and 21 days of age, SNI did not produce significant mechanical allodynia at any time in the next four weeks, whereas when performed at P33 allodynia occurred, but to a lesser degree than in adult animals. Similarly, chronic constriction injury (CCI) lesion at P10 did not produce the prolonged allodynia seen in adults.[155]

Activation of spinal microglia play a key role in neuropathic pain in adults,[156] but significant differences in the degree and pattern of glial activation is seen in early life. In the adult, microglial activation is evoked at five days and glial activation seven days after spared nerve injury, but in young animals a weak microglial but robust astrocytic response is seen initially (day one) followed by a second activation at seven days.[157] Although spinal microglia are capable of being activated by exogenous stimuli in young pups, minimal microglial response is triggered by nerve injury at P10 when compared with adult animals.[158] These age-related differences in the glial response to nerve injury may contribute to the lack of neuropathic allodynia in early life.

CLINICAL STUDIES

Age-related changes in pain following nerve injury are supported by clinical studies, but further prospective trials with long-term follow up are required. Traumatic injury to the brachial plexus in adults is frequently followed by severe neuropathic pain.[159] By contrast, brachial plexus injury at the time of birth is not associated with chronic neuropathic pain, and restoration of normal sensation and ability to localize stimuli was seen following early surgical repair.[160] It has also been postulated that the reduced sensitivity following nerve injury in early life correlates with clinical experience in children with complex regional pain syndrome (CRPS), which is rare before eight years of age.[161] In older children and adolescents, neuropathic pain is recognized. Phantom pain is much more common following surgery or trauma than in children with congenital absence of a limb[162, 163] and can be of moderate to severe intensity (6.43 on 0–10 rating scale).[164] Phantom pain also occurs following amputations for burn injury[165] or cancer treatment.[166] As 75 percent of children with phantom pain also had preoperative limb pain,[166] it has been suggested that preoperative regional anesthesia may be beneficial, but no prospective trials have been conducted in children.

DEVELOPMENTAL CHANGES IN ANALGESIC PHARMACODYNAMICS

Changes in nociceptive mechanisms not only alter responses to noxious stimuli, but can also have a significant impact on the response to analgesic agents. The pharmacokinetic profile of drugs changes rapidly during the first weeks of life, but can be readily investigated in clinical studies. Understanding age-related changes in pharmacokinetics (e.g. morphine and paracetamol) has allowed refinement of dose recommendations based on age, as well as weight.[167, 168, 169, 170, 171] However, plasma concentrations often target doses that either: (1) avoid side effects (such as respiratory depression), or (2) are associated with analgesia in older children. Whereas pharmacokinetic data can be readily obtained by measuring plasma concentrations in clinical studies, there is much less data relating to the effect of age on the efficacy and developmental pharmacodynamics of analgesics in common use. Analgesic efficacy trials are difficult to conduct in neonates and infants. As pain outcome measures have reduced specificity and sensitivity at this age and it is difficult to recruit large homogeneous samples, studies may not be adequately powered to demonstrate a difference between types or doses of analgesic agent.

Information from laboratory studies can improve our knowledge of developmentally regulated changes in analgesic efficacy. Ensuring that different analgesic mechanisms are functional in early life, and if there is an increase or decrease in sensitivity to the drug in question, can improve the design of subsequent clinical trials.[11] In addition to functional studies, the mechanisms underlying age-related differences can also be investigated in the laboratory. Clinical aspects of analgesia and pain management in children are covered in Chapter 27, Acute pain management in children. Some examples of laboratory experiments evaluating developmental analgesic pharmacodynamics are included here.

Age-related changes in analgesic efficacy

Dose-dependent effects of drugs on the sensory thresholds of the hind limb withdrawal reflex can be used to evaluate analgesic efficacy. Both antinociceptive effects (i.e. increased threshold above baseline) and the ability to reverse injury-induced sensitivity (i.e. antihyperalgesia) can be assessed (**Figure 2.2**). The sensitivity to epidural bupivacaine is increased in early life, as the concentration required to reverse inflammatory hyperalgesia is lower in younger rat pups. In addition, at all postnatal ages, selective reversal of hyperalgesia could be achieved at concentrations that had no effect on the threshold of the contralateral limb.[67]

Changes in receptor expression

Significant changes in mu opioid receptor distribution in DRG neurons and the spinal cord occur during postnatal development, contributing to the increased sensitivity to morphine in early life.[172, 173] Lower doses of epidural morphine increase withdrawal reflex thresholds (i.e. antinociceptive effect)[65] and reverse the hyperalgesic effect of hindpaw inflammation[174] in younger pups, and systemic morphine effectively suppresses the response to formalin soon after birth.[175, 176] In the first postnatal week, opioid receptors are expressed by both small (C-fiber) and large (A-fiber) cell bodies in the DRG, but by P21 the adult pattern of expression in predominantly small diameter neurons is seen.[177] Receptors on large A-fibers are functional and contribute to the increased sensitivity of mechanical thresholds to morphine in early life.[178] In the spinal cord, mu receptor binding sites are initially spread diffusely through the dorsal horn, overall binding peaks at P7, and by P21 binding sites are reduced and localized to the superficial dorsal horn.[179] In addition to the established differences in the pharmacokinetic profile of morphine,[167, 170, 180] these pharmacodynamic differences are likely to contribute to the age-related changes in morphine requirements seen in neonates and infants in clinical studies.[181]

Changes in transmitter function

Neurotransmitters may have differing roles throughout development. Noradrenaline has a trophic role in the

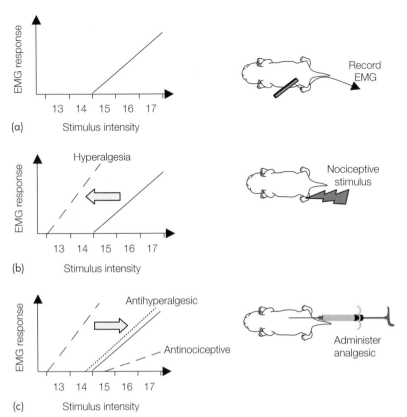

Figure 2.2 Quantification of the hind limb withdrawal reflex allows evaluation of the response to injury and analgesia. (a) In anesthetized rat pups, the biceps femoris response to graded mechanical stimuli (von Frey hairs) on the hind paw are recorded and values used to construct a stimulus–response curve. (b) Following noxious stimulation (e.g. inflammation or application of mustard oil), there is a leftward shift of the stimulus–response curve with reduction in threshold and increased response to suprathreshold stimuli. (c) The effect of analgesics on the reflex response can be evaluated to determine the dose that brings the reflex back to baseline (i.e. antihyperalgesia). Higher doses may suppress the reflex response and increase the withdrawal threshold (i.e. have an antinociceptive effect).

developing nervous system, and alpha$_2$-adrenergic receptors are highly expressed in the brain stem during the early postnatal period in the rat.[87, 182] These changes may underlie the increased susceptibility to centrally mediated sedative and cardiovascular effects of the alpha2 agonist dexmedetomidine seen in younger rat pups.[68, 88, 89] Similarly, binding of [3H]para-aminoclonidine is higher in the brain stem of human neonates than infants,[183] and sedative effects have been reported in neonates following doses of caudal clonidine that are well tolerated in older infants.[184, 185, 186]

Age-related changes in metabolic function and analgesic efficacy

Analgesic effects of codeine are dependent on metabolism to morphine by the cytochrome P450 enzyme CYP2D6. As activity of this enzyme is developmentally regulated and increases with age, the efficacy of codeine is reduced in early life.[66] In addition, there is significant genetic variation in the activity of this enzyme, and a significant proportion of children (47 percent in a UK study)[187] have reduced metabolic capacity, which reduces the incidence of side effects but also analgesic efficacy. Tramadol is also metabolized by CYP2D6. Activity of the enzyme has been demonstrated in neonates and clearance of tramadol increases with age,[188] but age- and genotype-related changes in pharmacodynamics require further evaluation.

CONCLUSIONS

Significant advances have been made in our understanding of responses to pain and injury in early life. Nociceptive pathways are functional following birth even in the most premature neonate, but changes in the developing nervous system have a significant impact on the type and degree of response to painful stimuli, and on the efficacy of analgesic interventions. Alterations in levels of neural activity due to pain and injury have the potential to produce responses not seen in the adult, and may result in long-term changes in sensory function. Further elucidation of the mechanisms underlying developmental changes in nociceptive processing and the response to injury will inform future translational clinical trials directed at developmentally appropriate treatments.

REFERENCES

* 1. Fitzgerald M. The development of nociceptive circuits. *Nature Reviews. Neuroscience.* 2005; **6**: 507–20.

 2. Pattinson D, Fitzgerald M. The neurobiology of infant pain: development of excitatory and inhibitory neurotransmission in the spinal dorsal horn. *Regional Anesthesia and Pain Medicine.* 2004; **29**: 36–44.

 3. Baccei M, Fitzgerald M. Development of pain pathways and mechanisms. In: McMahon SB, Koltzenburg M (eds).

Wall and Melzack's textbook of pain, 5th edn. London: Elsevier Churchill Livingstone, 2006: 143–58.

4. Fitzgerald M, Walker S. The role of activity in developing pain pathways. In: Dostrovsky J, Carr D, Koltzenburg M (eds). *Proceedings of the 10th World Congress on Pain. Progress in Pain Research and Management*, Vol. 24. Seattle: IASP Press, 2003: 185–96.

5. Grunau RE, Tu M. Long-term consequences of pain in human neonates. In: Anand KJS, Stevens BJ, McGrath PJ (eds). *Pain in neonates and infants*, 3rd edn. *Pain research and clinical management*. Edinburgh: Elsevier, 2007: 45–55.

6. Walker SM, Meredith-Middleton J, Cooke-Yarborough C, Fitzgerald M. Neonatal inflammation and primary afferent terminal plasticity in the rat dorsal horn. *Pain*. 2003; **105**: 185–95.

7. Anand KJ, Aranda JV, Berde CB *et al*. Analgesia and anesthesia for neonates: study design and ethical issues. *Clinical Therapeutics*. 2005; **27**: 814–43.

8. Berde CB, Jaksic T, Lynn AM *et al*. Anesthesia and analgesia during and after surgery in neonates. *Clinical Therapeutics*. 2005; **27**: 900–21.

9. Alvares D, Fitzgerald M. Building blocks of pain: the regulation of key molecules in spinal sensory neurones during development and following peripheral axotomy. *Pain*. 1999; (Suppl. 6): S71–85.

10. Fitzgerald M. The developmental neurobiology of pain. In: Bond M, Charlton JE, Woolf CJ (eds). *Proceedings of the VIth World Congress on Pain. Pain Research and Clinical Management*, Vol. 4. Amsterdam: Elsevier, 1991: 253–61.

11. Berde C, Cairns B. Developmental pharmacology across species: promise and problems. *Anesthesia and Analgesia*. 2000; **91**: 1–5.

12. Jackman A, Fitzgerald M. Development of peripheral hindlimb and central spinal cord innervation by subpopulations of dorsal root ganglion cells in the embryonic rat. *Journal of Comparative Neurology*. 2000; **418**: 281–98.

13. Fitzgerald M. Spontaneous and evoked activity of fetal primary afferents *in vivo*. *Nature*. 1987; **326**: 603–5.

14. Fitzgerald M. Cutaneous primary afferent properties in the hind limb of the neonatal rat. *Journal of Physiology*. 1987; **383**: 79–92.

15. Zhu W, Galoyan SM, Petruska JC *et al*. A developmental switch in acute sensitization of small dorsal root ganglion (DRG) neurons to capsaicin or noxious heating by NGF. *Journal of Neurophysiology*. 2004; **92**: 3148–52.

16. Guo A, Simone DA, Stone LS *et al*. Developmental shift of vanilloid receptor 1 (VR1) terminals into deeper regions of the superficial dorsal horn: correlation with a shift from TrkA to Ret expression by dorsal root ganglion neurons. *European Journal of Neuroscience*. 2001; **14**: 293–304.

17. Beland B, Fitzgerald M. Influence of peripheral inflammation on the postnatal maturation of primary sensory neuron phenotype in rats. *Journal of Pain*. 2001; **2**: 36–45.

18. Ogata N, Tatebayashi H. Ontogenic development of the TTX-sensitive and TTX-insensitive Na+ channels in neurons of the rat dorsal root ganglia. *Brain Research. Developmental Brain Research*. 1992; **65**: 93–100.

19. Benn SC, Costigan M, Tate S *et al*. Developmental expression of the TTX-resistant voltage-gated sodium channels Nav1.8 (SNS) and Nav1.9 (SNS2) in primary sensory neurons. *Journal of Neuroscience*. 2001; **21**: 6077–85.

20. Fitzgerald M, Butcher T, Shortland P. Developmental changes in the laminar termination of A fibre cutaneous sensory afferents in the rat spinal cord dorsal horn. *Journal of Comparative Neurology*. 1994; **348**: 225–33.

21. Mirnics K, Koerber HR. Prenatal development of rat primary afferent fibers: II. Central projections. *Journal of Comparative Neurology*. 1995; **355**: 601–14.

22. Torsney C, Meredith-Middleton J, Fitzgerald M. Neonatal capsaicin treatment prevents the normal postnatal withdrawal of A fibres from lamina II without affecting fos responses to innocuous peripheral stimulation. *Brain Research. Developmental Brain Research*. 2000; **121**: 55–65.

23. Park JS, Nakatsuka T, Nagata K *et al*. Reorganization of the primary afferent termination in the rat spinal dorsal horn during post-natal development. *Brain Research. Developmental Brain Research*. 1999; **113**: 29–36.

24. Nakatsuka T, Ataka T, Kumamoto E *et al*. Alteration in synaptic inputs through C-afferent fibers to substantia gelatinosa neurons of the rat spinal dorsal horn during postnatal development. *Neuroscience*. 2000; **99**: 549–56.

25. Coggeshall RE, Jennings EA, Fitzgerald M. Evidence that large myelinated primary afferent fibers make synaptic contacts in lamina II of neonatal rats. *Brain Research. Developmental Brain Research*. 1996; **92**: 81–90.

26. Fitzgerald M, Jennings E. The postnatal development of spinal sensory processing. *Proceedings of the National Academy of Sciences of the United States of America*. 1999; **96**: 7719–22.

27. Jennings E, Fitzgerald M. Postnatal changes in responses of rat dorsal horn cells to afferent stimulation: a fibre-induced sensitization. *Journal of Physiology*. 1998; **509**: 859–68.

28. Baccei ML, Fitzgerald M. Intrinsic firing properties of developing rat superficial dorsal horn neurons. *Neuroreport*. 2005; **16**: 1325–8.

29. Torsney C, Fitzgerald M. Age-dependent effects of peripheral inflammation on the electrophysiological properties of neonatal rat dorsal horn neurons. *Journal of Neurophysiology*. 2002; **87**: 1311–7.

30. Fitzgerald M. The post-natal development of cutaneous afferent fibre input and receptive field organization in the rat dorsal horn. *Journal of Physiology*. 1985; **364**: 1–18.

31. Sweitzer SM, Wong SM, Peters MC *et al*. Protein kinase C epsilon and gamma: involvement in formalin-induced nociception in neonatal rats. *Journal of Pharmacology and Experimental Therapeutics*. 2004; **309**: 616–25.

32. Baccei ML, Bardoni R, Fitzgerald M. Development of nociceptive synaptic inputs to the neonatal rat dorsal horn: glutamate release by capsaicin and menthol. *Journal of Physiology*. 2003; **549**: 231–42.

33. Fitzgerald M. The development of activity evoked by fine diameter cutaneous fibres in the spinal cord of the newborn rat. *Neuroscience Letters*. 1988; **86**: 161–6.

34. Walker SM, Meredith-Middleton J, Lickiss T *et al.* Primary and secondary hyperalgesia can be differentiated by postnatal age and ERK activation in the spinal dorsal horn of the rat pup. *Pain*. 2007; **128**: 157–68.

35. Bennett DL, Averill S, Clary DO *et al.* Postnatal changes in the expression of the trkA high-affinity NGF receptor in primary sensory neurons. *European Journal of Neuroscience*. 1996; **8**: 2204–8.

36. Reynolds ML, Fitzgerald M. Neonatal sciatic nerve section results in thiamine monophosphate but not substance P or calcitonin gene-related peptide depletion from the terminal field in the dorsal horn of the rat: the role of collateral sprouting. *Neuroscience*. 1992; **51**: 191–202.

37. Fitzgerald M, Gibson S. The postnatal physiological and neurochemical development of peripheral sensory C fibres. *Neuroscience*. 1984; **13**: 933–44.

38. Chen JH, Weng HR, Dougherty PM. Sensitization of dorsal root reflexes *in vitro* and hyperalgesia in neonatal rats produced by capsaicin. *Neuroscience*. 2004; **126**: 743–51.

39. Jiang MC, Gebhart GF. Development of mustard oil-induced hyperalgesia in rats. *Pain*. 1998; **77**: 305–13.

40. Torsney C, Fitzgerald M. Spinal dorsal horn cell receptive field size is increased in adult rats following neonatal hindpaw skin injury. *Journal of Physiology*. 2003; **550**: 255–61.

41. Jakowec MW, Fox AJ, Martin LJ, Kalb RG. Quantitative and qualitative changes in AMPA receptor expression during spinal cord development. *Neuroscience*. 1995; **67**: 893–907.

42. Brown KM, Wrathall JR, Yasuda RP, Wolfe BB. Quantitative measurement of glutamate receptor subunit protein expression in the postnatal rat spinal cord. *Brain Research. Developmental Brain Research*. 2002; **137**: 127–33.

43. Gonzalez DL, Fuchs JL, Droge MH. Distribution of NMDA receptor binding in developing mouse spinal cord. *Neuroscience Letters*. 1993; **151**: 134–7.

44. Hori Y, Kanda K. Developmental alterations in NMDA receptor-mediated [Ca2+]$_i$ elevation in substantia gelatinosa neurons of neonatal rat spinal cord. *Brain Research. Developmental Brain Research*. 1994; **80**: 141–8.

45. Bardoni R. Excitatory synaptic transmission in neonatal dorsal horn: NMDA and ATP receptors. *News in Physiological Sciences*. 2001; **16**: 95–100.

46. Bardoni R, Magherini PC, MacDermott AB. Activation of NMDA receptors drives action potentials in superficial dorsal horn from neonatal rats. *Neuroreport*. 2000; **11**: 1721–7.

47. Bardoni R, Magherini PC, MacDermott AB. NMDA EPSCs at glutamatergic synapses in the spinal cord dorsal horn of the postnatal rat. *Journal of Neuroscience*. 1998; **18**: 6558–67.

48. Li P, Zhuo M. Silent glutamatergic synapses and nociception in mammalian spinal cord. *Nature*. 1998; **393**: 695–8.

49. Baccei ML, Fitzgerald M. Development of GABAergic and glycinergic transmission in the neonatal rat dorsal horn. *Journal of Neuroscience*. 2004; **24**: 4749–57.

50. Bremner L, Fitzgerald M, Baccei M. Functional GABA(A)-receptor-mediated inhibition in the neonatal dorsal horn. *Journal of Neurophysiology*. 2006; **95**: 3893–7.

51. Ben-Ari Y. Excitatory actions of gaba during development: the nature of the nurture. *Nature Reviews. Neuroscience*. 2002; **3**: 728–39.

52. Bicknell Jr HR, Beal JA. Axonal and dendritic development of substantia gelatinosa neurons in the lumbosacral spinal cord of the rat. *Journal of Comparative Neurology*. 1984; **226**: 508–22.

53. Fitzgerald M, Koltzenburg M. The functional development of descending inhibitory pathways in the dorsolateral funiculus of the newborn rat spinal cord. *Brain Research*. 1986; **389**: 261–70.

54. van Praag H, Frenk H. The development of stimulation-produced analgesia (SPA) in the rat. *Brain Research. Developmental Brain Research*. 1991; **64**: 71–6.

55. Boucher T, Jennings E, Fitzgerald M. The onset of diffuse noxious inhibitory controls in postnatal rat pups: a C-Fos study. *Neuroscience Letters*. 1998; **257**: 9–12.

56. Soyguder Z, Schmidt HH, Morris R. Postnatal development of nitric oxide synthase type 1 expression in the lumbar spinal cord of the rat: a comparison with the induction of c-fos in response to peripheral application of mustard oil. *Neuroscience Letters*. 1994; **180**: 188–92.

57. Vizzard MA, Erdman SL, Forstermann U, de Groat WC. Ontogeny of nitric oxide synthase in the lumbosacral spinal cord of the neonatal rat. *Brain Research. Developmental Brain Research*. 1994; **81**: 201–17.

58. Pattinson D, Baccei M, Karadottir R *et al.* Aberrant dendritic branching and sensory inputs in the superficial dorsal horn of mice lacking CaMKIIalpha autophosphorylation. *Molecular and Cellular Neurosciences*. 2006; **33**: 88–95.

59. Rivera C, Voipio J, Payne JA *et al.* The K+/Cl- co-transporter KCC2 renders GABA hyperpolarizing during neuronal maturation. *Nature*. 1999; **397**: 251–5.

60. Hathway G, Harrop E, Baccei M *et al.* A postnatal switch in GABAergic control of spinal cutaneous reflexes. *European Journal of Neuroscience*. 2006; **23**: 112–8.

61. Woolf CJ. Long term alterations in the excitability of the flexion reflex produced by peripheral tissue injury in the chronic decerebrate rat. *Pain*. 1984; **18**: 325–43.

62. Andrews K, Fitzgerald M. Flexion reflex responses in biceps femoris and tibialis anterior in human neonates. *Early Human Development*. 2000; **57**: 105–10.

63. Fitzgerald M, de Lima J. Hyperalgesia and allodynia in infants. In: Finley G, McGrath P (eds). *Acute and procedure*

pain in infants and children. Progress in pain research and management. Seattle: IASP Press, 2001: 1–12.

64. Fitzgerald M, Walker S. Infant pain traces. *Pain.* 2006; **125**: 204–5.

65. Marsh D, Dickenson A, Hatch D, Fitzgerald M. Epidural opioid analgesia in infant rats. I: Mechanical and heat responses. *Pain.* 1999; **82**: 23–32.

66. Williams DG, Dickenson A, Fitzgerald M, Howard RF. Developmental regulation of codeine analgesia in the rat. *Anesthesiology.* 2004; **100**: 92–7.

67. Howard RF, Hatch DJ, Cole TJ, Fitzgerald M. Inflammatory pain and hypersensitivity are selectively reversed by epidural bupivacaine and are developmentally regulated. *Anesthesiology.* 2001; **95**: 421–7.

68. Walker SM, Howard RF, Keay KA, Fitzgerald M. Developmental age influences the effect of epidural dexmedetomidine on inflammatory hyperalgesia in rat pups. *Anesthesiology.* 2005; **102**: 1226–34.

69. Andrews K, Fitzgerald M. Wound sensitivity as a measure of analgesic effects following surgery in human neonates and infants. *Pain.* 2002; **99**: 185–95.

70. Andrews KA, Desai D, Dhillon HK *et al.* Abdominal sensitivity in the first year of life: comparison of infants with and without prenatally diagnosed unilateral hydronephrosis. *Pain.* 2002; **100**: 35–46.

71. Holmberg H, Schouenborg J. Postnatal development of the nociceptive withdrawal reflexes in the rat: a behavioural and electromyographic study. *Journal of Physiology.* 1996; **493**: 239–52.

72. Falcon M, Guendellman D, Stolberg A *et al.* Development of thermal nociception in rats. *Pain.* 1996; **67**: 203–8.

73. Schouenborg J. Modular organisation and spinal somatosensory imprinting. *Brain Research. Brain Research Reviews.* 2002; **40**: 80–91.

74. Waldenstrom A, Thelin J, Thimansson E *et al.* Developmental learning in a pain-related system: evidence for a cross-modality mechanism. *Journal of Neuroscience.* 2003; **23**: 7719–25.

75. Petersson P, Waldenstrom A, Fahraeus C, Schouenborg J. Spontaneous muscle twitches during sleep guide spinal self-organization. *Nature.* 2003; **424**: 72–5.

76. Fitzgerald M, Shaw A, MacIntosh N. Postnatal development of the cutaneous flexor reflex: comparative study of preterm infants and newborn rat pups. *Developmental Medicine and Child Neurology.* 1988; **30**: 520–6.

77. Andrews K, Fitzgerald M. The cutaneous withdrawal reflex in human neonates: sensitization, receptive fields, and the effects of contralateral stimulation. *Pain.* 1994; **56**: 95–101.

78. Andrews K, Fitzgerald M. Cutaneous flexion reflex in human neonates: a quantitative study of threshold and stimulus-response characteristics after single and repeated stimuli. *Developmental Medicine and Child Neurology.* 1999; **41**: 696–703.

79. Mantyh PW, Hunt SP. Setting the tone: superficial dorsal horn projection neurons regulate pain sensitivity. *Trends in Neurosciences.* 2004; **27**: 582–4.

80. Hunt SP, Mantyh PW. The molecular dynamics of pain control. *Nature Reviews. Neuroscience.* 2001; **2**: 83–91.

81. Millan MJ. Descending control of pain. *Progress in Neurobiology.* 2002; **66**: 355–474.

82. Ren K, Dubner R. Descending modulation in persistent pain: an update. *Pain.* 2002; **100**: 1–6.

83. Kwiat GC, Basbaum AI. The origin of brainstem noradrenergic and serotonergic projections to the spinal cord dorsal horn in the rat. *Somatosensory and Motor Research.* 1992; **9**: 157–73.

84. Rajaofetra N, Poulat P, Marlier L *et al.* Pre- and postnatal development of noradrenergic projections to the rat spinal cord: an immunocytochemical study. *Brain Research. Developmental Brain Research.* 1992; **67**: 237–46.

85. Savola MK, Savola JM. Alpha 2A/D-Adrenoceptor subtype predominates also in the neonatal rat spinal cord. *Brain Research. Developmental Brain Research.* 1996; **94**: 106–8.

86. Huang Y, Stamer WD, Anthony TL *et al.* Expression of alpha(2)-adrenergic receptor subtypes in prenatal rat spinal cord. *Brain Research. Developmental Brain Research.* 2002; **133**: 93–104.

87. Winzer-Serhan UH, Raymon HK, Broide RS *et al.* Expression of alpha 2 adrenoceptors during rat brain development – I. Alpha 2A messenger RNA expression. *Neuroscience.* 1997; **76**: 241–60.

88. Walker SM, Fitzgerald M. Characterisation of spinal alpha-adrenergic modulation of nociceptive transmission and hyperalgesia throughout postnatal development. *British Journal of Pharmacology.* 2007; **151**: 1334–42.

89. Sanders RD, Giombini M, Ma D *et al.* Dexmedetomidine exerts dose-dependent age-independent antinociception but age-dependent hypnosis in Fischer rats. *Anesthesia and Analgesia.* 2005; **100**: 1295–302.

90. Rajaofetra N, Sandillon F, Geffard M, Privat A. Pre- and post-natal ontogeny of serotonergic projections to the rat spinal cord. *Journal of Neuroscience Research.* 1989; **22**: 305–21.

91. Suzuki R, Rygh LJ, Dickenson AH. Bad news from the brain: descending 5-HT pathways that control spinal pain processing. *Trends in Pharmacological Sciences.* 2004; **25**: 613–7.

92. Sasaki M, Obata H, Saito S, Goto F. Antinociception with intrathecal alpha-methyl-5-hydroxytryptamine, a 5-hydroxytryptamine 2A/2C receptor agonist, in two rat models of sustained pain. *Anesthesia and Analgesia.* 2003; **96**: 1072–8.

93. Giordano J. Antinociceptive effects of intrathecally administered 2-methylserotonin in developing rats. *Brain Research. Developmental Brain Research.* 1997; **98**: 142–4.

94. Derbyshire SW. Can fetuses feel pain? *British Medical Journal.* 2006; **332**: 909–12.

95. Lee SJ, Ralston HJ, Drey EA *et al.* Fetal pain: a systematic multidisciplinary review of the evidence. *Journal of the American Medical Association.* 2005; **294**: 947–54.

96. Slater R, Cantarella A, Gallella S *et al.* Cortical pain responses in human infants. *Journal of Neuroscience.* 2006; **26**: 3662–6.

97. Bartocci M, Bergqvist LL, Lagercrantz H, Anand KJ. Pain activates cortical areas in the preterm newborn brain. *Pain*. 2006; **122**: 109–17.

98. Slater R, Boyd S, Meek J, Fitzgerald M. Cortical pain responses in the infant brain. *Pain*. 2006; **123**: 332; author reply 332–4.

99. Ruda MA, Ling QD, Hohmann AG et al. Altered nociceptive neuronal circuits after neonatal peripheral inflammation. *Science*. 2000; **289**: 628–31.

100. Peng YB, Ling QD, Ruda MA, Kenshalo DR. Electrophysiological changes in adult rat dorsal horn neurons after neonatal peripheral inflammation. *Journal of Neurophysiology*. 2003; **90**: 73–80.

101. Tachibana T, Ling QD, Ruda MA. Increased Fos induction in adult rats that experienced neonatal peripheral inflammation. *Neuroreport*. 2001; **12**: 925–7.

102. Hohmann AG, Neely MH, Pina J, Nackley AG. Neonatal chronic hind paw inflammation alters sensitization to intradermal capsaicin in adult rats: a behavioral and immunocytochemical study. *Journal of Pain*. 2005; **6**: 798–808.

103. Chien CC, Fu WM, Huang HI et al. Expression of neurotrophic factors in neonatal rats after peripheral inflammation. *Journal of Pain*. 2007; **8**: 161–7.

104. Ren K, Novikova SI, He F et al. Neonatal local noxious insult affects gene expression in the spinal dorsal horn of adult rats. *Molecular Pain*. 2005; **1**: 27.

105. Ren K, Anseloni V, Zou SP et al. Characterization of basal and re-inflammation-associated long-term alteration in pain responsivity following short-lasting neonatal local inflammatory insult. *Pain*. 2004; **110**: 588–96.

106. Anseloni VC, He F, Novikova SI et al. Alterations in stress-associated behaviors and neurochemical markers in adult rats after neonatal short-lasting local inflammatory insult. *Neuroscience*. 2005; **131**: 635–45.

107. Wang G, Ji Y, Lidow MS, Traub RJ. Neonatal hind paw injury alters processing of visceral and somatic nociceptive stimuli in the adult rat. *Journal of Pain*. 2004; **5**: 440–9.

108. Reynolds ML, Fitzgerald M. Long-term sensory hyperinnervation following neonatal skin wounds. *Journal of Comparative Neurology*. 1995; **358**: 487–98.

109. Moss A, Alvares D, Meredith-Middleton J et al. Ephrin-A4 inhibits sensory neurite outgrowth and is regulated by neonatal skin wounding. *European Journal of Neuroscience*. 2005; **22**: 2413–21.

110. Sternberg WF, Scorr L, Smith LD et al. Long-term effects of neonatal surgery on adulthood pain behavior. *Pain*. 2005; **113**: 347–53.

111. Miranda A, Peles S, Shaker R et al. Neonatal nociceptive somatic stimulation differentially modifies the activity of spinal neurons in rats and results in altered somatic and visceral sensation. *Journal of Physiology*. 2006; **572**: 775–87.

112. Al-Chaer ED, Kawasaki M, Pasricha PJ. A new model of chronic visceral hypersensitivity in adult rats induced by colon irritation during postnatal development. *Gastroenterology*. 2000; **119**: 1276–85.

113. Randich A, Uzzell T, DeBerry JJ, Ness TJ. Neonatal urinary bladder inflammation produces adult bladder hypersensitivity. *Journal of Pain*. 2006; **7**: 469–79.

114. Treede RD, Meyer RA, Raja SN, Campbell JN. Peripheral and central mechanisms of cutaneous hyperalgesia. *Progress in Neurobiology*. 1992; **38**: 397–421.

115. Koltzenburg M, Lewin GR. Receptive properties of embryonic chick sensory neurons innervating skin. *Journal of Neurophysiology*. 1997; **78**: 2560–8.

116. Simone DA, Sorkin LS, Oh U et al. Neurogenic hyperalgesia: central neural correlates in responses of spinothalamic tract neurons. *Journal of Neurophysiology*. 1991; **66**: 228–46.

117. Reeh PW, Kocher L, Jung S. Does neurogenic inflammation alter the sensitivity of unmyelinated nociceptors in the rat? *Brain Research*. 1986; **384**: 42–50.

118. LaMotte RH, Lundberg LE, Torebjork HE. Pain, hyperalgesia and activity in nociceptive C units in humans after intradermal injection of capsaicin. *Journal of Physiology*. 1992; **448**: 749–64.

119. Koltzenburg M, Lundberg LE, Torebjork HE. Dynamic and static components of mechanical hyperalgesia in human hairy skin. *Pain*. 1992; **51**: 207–19.

120. Fitzgerald M, Millard C, MacIntosh N. Hyperalgesia in premature infants. *Lancet*. 1988; **1**: 292.

121. Fitzgerald M, Millard C, McIntosh N. Cutaneous hypersensitivity following peripheral tissue damage in newborn infants and its reversal with topical anaesthesia. *Pain*. 1989; **39**: 31–6.

122. Fitzgerald M. Painful beginnings. *Pain*. 2004; **110**: 508–9.

123. Kehlet H, Jensen TS, Woolf CJ. Persistent postsurgical pain: risk factors and prevention. *Lancet*. 2006; **367**: 1618–25.

124. Brennan TJ, Vandermeulen EP, Gebhart GF. Characterization of a rat model of incisional pain. *Pain*. 1996; **64**: 493–501.

125. Ririe DG, Vernon TL, Tobin JR, Eisenach JC. Age-dependent responses to thermal hyperalgesia and mechanical allodynia in a rat model of acute postoperative pain. *Anesthesiology*. 2003; **99**: 443–8.

126. Schwetz I, McRoberts JA, Coutinho SV et al. Corticotropin-releasing factor receptor 1 mediates acute and delayed stress-induced visceral hyperalgesia in maternally separated Long-Evans rats. *American Journal of Physiology. Gastrointestinal and Liver Physiology*. 2005; **289**: G704–12.

127. Kalinichev M, Easterling KW, Holtzman SG. Early neonatal experience of Long–Evans rats results in long-lasting changes in reactivity to a novel environment and morphine-induced sensitization and tolerance. *Neuropsychopharmacology*. 2002; **27**: 518–33.

128. Sternberg WF, Ridgway CG. Effects of gestational stress and neonatal handling on pain, analgesia, and stress behavior of adult mice. *Physiology and Behavior*. 2003; **78**: 375–83.

129. Boisse L, Spencer SJ, Mouihate A et al. Neonatal immune challenge alters nociception in the adult rat. *Pain*. 2005; **119**: 133–41.

130. Spencer SJ, Boisse L, Mouihate A, Pittman QJ. Long term alterations in neuroimmune responses of female rats after neonatal exposure to lipopolysaccharide. *Brain, Behavior, and Immunity.* 2006; **20**: 325–30.

131. Anand KJ, Coskun V, Thrivikraman KV *et al.* Long-term behavioral effects of repetitive pain in neonatal rat pups. *Physiology and Behavior.* 1999; **66**: 627–37.

132. Walker CD, Kudreikis K, Sherrard A, Johnston CC. Repeated neonatal pain influences maternal behavior, but not stress responsiveness in rat offspring. *Brain Research. Developmental Brain Research.* 2003; **140**: 253–61.

133. Grunau RE, Holsti L, Peters JW. Long-term consequences of pain in human neonates. *Seminars in Fetal and Neonatal Medicine.* 2006; **11**: 268–75.

134. Marlow N, Wolke D, Bracewell MA, Samara M. Neurologic and developmental disability at six years of age after extremely preterm birth. *New England Journal of Medicine.* 2005; **352**: 9–19.

135. Bhutta AT, Cleves MA, Casey PH *et al.* Cognitive and behavioral outcomes of school-aged children who were born preterm: a meta-analysis. *Journal of the American Medical Association.* 2002; **288**: 728–37.

136. Porter FL, Grunau RE, Anand KJ. Long-term effects of pain in infants. *Journal of Developmental and Behavioral Pediatrics.* 1999; **20**: 253–61.

137. Buskila D, Neumann L, Zmora E *et al.* Pain sensitivity in prematurely born adolescents. *Archives of Pediatrics and Adolescent Medicine.* 2003; **157**: 1079–82.

138. Hermann C, Hohmeister J, Demirakca S *et al.* Long-term alteration of pain sensitivity in school-aged children with early pain experiences. *Pain.* 2006; **125**: 278–85.

139. Schmelzle-Lubiecki BM, Campbell KA, Howard RH *et al.* Long-term consequences of early infant injury and trauma upon somatosensory processing. *European Journal of Pain.* 2007; **11**: 799–809.

140. Peters JW, Schouw R, Anand KJ *et al.* Does neonatal surgery lead to increased pain sensitivity in later childhood? *Pain.* 2005; **114**: 444–54.

141. Taddio A, Katz J, Ilersich AL, Koren G. Effect of neonatal circumcision on pain response during subsequent routine vaccination. *Lancet.* 1997; **349**: 599–603.

142. Peters JW, Koot HM, de Boer JB *et al.* Major surgery within the first 3 months of life and subsequent biobehavioral pain responses to immunization at later age: a case comparison study. *Pediatrics.* 2003; **111**: 129–35.

143. Anand KJ, Runeson B, Jacobson B. Gastric suction at birth associated with long-term risk for functional intestinal disorders in later life. *Journal of Pediatrics.* 2004; **144**: 449–54.

144. Di Lorenzo C, Saps M. Gastric suction in newborns: guilty as charged or innocent bystander? *Journal of Pediatrics.* 2004; **144**: 417–20.

145. Alvares D, Torsney C, Beland B *et al.* Modelling the prolonged effects of neonatal pain. *Progress in Brain Research.* 2000; **129**: 365–73.

146. De Lima J, Alvares D, Hatch DJ, Fitzgerald M. Sensory hyperinnervation after neonatal skin wounding: effect of

147. Reynolds M, Alvares D, Middleton J, Fitzgerald M. Neonatally wounded skin induces NGF-independent sensory neurite outgrowth *in vitro*. *Brain Research. Developmental Brain Research.* 1997; **102**: 275–83.

148. Himes BT, Tessler A. Death of some dorsal root ganglion neurons and plasticity of others following sciatic nerve section in adult and neonatal rats. *Journal of Comparative Neurology.* 1989; **284**: 215–30.

149. Fitzgerald M, Woolf CJ, Shortland P. Collateral sprouting of the central terminals of cutaneous primary afferent neurons in the rat spinal cord: pattern, morphology, and influence of targets. *Journal of Comparative Neurology.* 1990; **300**: 370–85.

150. Shortland P, Fitzgerald M. Neonatal sciatic nerve section results in a rearrangement of the central terminals of saphenous and axotomized sciatic nerve afferents in the dorsal horn of the spinal cord of the adult rat. *European Journal of Neuroscience.* 1994; **6**: 75–86.

151. Shortland P, Fitzgerald M. Functional connections formed by saphenous nerve terminal sprouts in the dorsal horn following neonatal sciatic nerve section. *European Journal of Neuroscience.* 1991; **3**: 383–96.

152. Lee DH, Chung JM. Neuropathic pain in neonatal rats. *Neuroscience Letters.* 1996; **209**: 140–2.

153. Ririe DG, Eisenach JC. Age-dependent responses to nerve injury-induced mechanical allodynia. *Anesthesiology.* 2006; **104**: 344–50.

154. Decosterd I, Woolf CJ. Spared nerve injury: an animal model of persistent peripheral neuropathic pain. *Pain.* 2000; **87**: 149–58.

155. Howard RF, Walker SM, Michael Mota P, Fitzgerald M. The ontogeny of neuropathic pain: Postnatal onset of mechanical allodynia in rat spared nerve injury (SNI) and chronic constriction injury (CCI) models. *Pain.* 2005; **115**: 382–9.

156. Tsuda M, Inoue K, Salter MW. Neuropathic pain and spinal microglia: a big problem from molecules in "small" glia. *Trends in Neurosciences.* 2005; **28**: 101–7.

157. Vega-Avelaira D, Moss A, Fitzgerald M. Age-related changes in the spinal cord microglial and astrocytic response profile to nerve injury. *Brain, Behavior, and Immunity.* 2007; **21**: 617–23.

158. Moss A, Beggs S, Vega-Avelaira D *et al.* Spinal microglia and neuropathic pain in young rats. *Pain.* 2007; **128**: 215–24.

159. Kato N, Htut M, Taggart M *et al.* The effects of operative delay on the relief of neuropathic pain after injury to the brachial plexus: a review of 148 cases. *Journal of Bone and Joint Surgery.* 2006; **88**: 756–9.

160. Anand P, Birch R. Restoration of sensory function and lack of long-term chronic pain syndromes after brachial plexus injury in human neonates. *Brain.* 2002; **125**: 113–22.

161. Berde CB, Lebel A. Complex regional pain syndromes in children and adolescents. *Anesthesiology.* 2005; **102**: 252–5.

bupivacaine sciatic nerve block. *British Journal of Anaesthesia.* 1999; **83**: 662–4.

162. Wilkins KL, McGrath PJ, Finley GA, Katz J. Phantom limb sensations and phantom limb pain in child and adolescent amputees. *Pain.* 1998; **78**: 7–12.

163. Melzack R, Israel R, Lacroix R, Schultz G. Phantom limbs in people with congenital limb deficiency or amputation in early childhood. *Brain.* 1997; **120**: 1603–20.

164. Wilkins KL, McGrath PJ, Finley GA, Katz J. Prospective diary study of nonpainful and painful phantom sensations in a preselected sample of child and adolescent amputees reporting phantom limbs. *Clinical Journal of Pain.* 2004; **20**: 293–301.

165. Thomas CR, Brazeal BA, Rosenberg L et al. Phantom limb pain in pediatric burn survivors. *Burns.* 2003; **29**: 139–42.

166. Krane EJ, Heller LB. The prevalence of phantom sensation and pain in pediatric amputees. *Journal of Pain and Symptom Management.* 1995; **10**: 21–9.

167. Kart T, Christrup LL, Rasmussen M. Recommended use of morphine in neonates, infants and children based on a literature review. Part 1: Pharmacokinetics. *Paediatric Anaesthesia.* 1997; **7**: 5–11.

168. Kart T, Christrup LL, Rasmussen M. Recommended use of morphine in neonates, infants and children based on a literature review. Part 2: Clinical use. *Paediatric Anaesthesia.* 1997; **7**: 93–101.

169. Anderson BJ, van Lingen RA, Hansen TG et al. Acetaminophen developmental pharmacokinetics in premature neonates and infants: a pooled population analysis. *Anesthesiology.* 2002; **96**: 1336–45.

170. Bouwmeester NJ, Anderson BJ, Tibboel D, Holford NH. Developmental pharmacokinetics of morphine and its metabolites in neonates, infants and young children. *British Journal of Anaesthesia.* 2004; **92**: 208–17.

171. Lynn AM, Nespeca MK, Bratton SL, Shen DD. Intravenous morphine in postoperative infants: intermittent bolus dosing versus targeted continuous infusions. *Pain.* 2000; **88**: 89–95.

172. Nandi R, Fitzgerald M. Opioid analgesia in the newborn. *European Journal of Pain.* 2005; **9**: 105–8.

173. Rahman W, Dickenson AH. Development of spinal opioid systems. *Regional Anesthesia and Pain Medicine.* 1999; **24**: 383–5.

174. Marsh D, Dickenson A, Hatch D, Fitzgerald M. Epidural opioid analgesia in infant rats. II: Responses to carrageenan and capsaicin. *Pain.* 1999; **82**: 33–8.

175. Abbott FV, Guy ER. Effects of morphine, pentobarbital and amphetamine on formalin-induced behaviours in infant rats: sedation versus specific suppression of pain. *Pain.* 1995; **62**: 303–12.

176. Gupta A, Cheng J, Wang S, Barr GA. Analgesic efficacy of ketorolac and morphine in neonatal rats. *Pharmacology, Biochemistry, and Behavior.* 2001; **68**: 635–40.

177. Beland B, Fitzgerald M. Mu- and delta-opioid receptors are downregulated in the largest diameter primary sensory neurons during postnatal development in rats. *Pain.* 2001; **90**: 143–50.

178. Nandi R, Beacham D, Middleton J et al. The functional expression of mu opioid receptors on sensory neurons is developmentally regulated; morphine analgesia is less selective in the neonate. *Pain.* 2004; **111**: 38–50.

179. Rahman W, Dashwood MR, Fitzgerald M et al. Postnatal development of multiple opioid receptors in the spinal cord and development of spinal morphine analgesia. *Brain Research. Developmental Brain Research.* 1998; **108**: 239–54.

180. Lynn AM, Slattery JT. Morphine pharmacokinetics in early infancy. *Anesthesiology.* 1987; **66**: 136–9.

181. Bouwmeester NJ, Hop WC, van Dijk M et al. Postoperative pain in the neonate: age-related differences in morphine requirements and metabolism. *Intensive Care Medicine.* 2003; **29**: 2009–15.

182. Happe HK, Coulter CL, Gerety ME et al. Alpha-2 adrenergic receptor development in rat CNS: an autoradiographic study. *Neuroscience.* 2004; **123**: 167–78.

183. Mansouri J, Panigrahy A, Assmann SF, Kinney HC. Distribution of alpha 2-adrenergic receptor binding in the developing human brain stem. *Pediatric and Developmental Pathology.* 2001; **4**: 222–36.

184. Bouchut JC, Dubois R, Godard J. Clonidine in preterm-infant caudal anesthesia may be responsible for postoperative apnea. *Regional Anesthesia and Pain Medicine.* 2001; **26**: 83–5.

185. Breschan C, Krumpholz R, Likar R et al. Can a dose of 2 microg.kg^{-1} caudal clonidine cause respiratory depression in neonates? *Paediatric Anaesthesia.* 1999; **9**: 81–3.

186. Fellmann C, Gerber AC, Weiss M. Apnoea in a former preterm infant after caudal bupivacaine with clonidine for inguinal herniorrhaphy. *Paediatric Anaesthesia.* 2002; **12**: 637–40.

187. Williams DG, Patel A, Howard RF. Pharmacogenetics of codeine metabolism in an urban population of children and its implications for analgesic reliability. *British Journal of Anaesthesia.* 2002; **89**: 839–45.

188. Allegaert K, Anderson BJ, Verbesselt R et al. Tramadol disposition in the very young: an attempt to assess *in vivo* cytochrome P-450 2D6 activity. *British Journal of Anaesthesia.* 2005; **95**: 231–9.

Clinical pharmacology: opioids

DAVID J ROWBOTHAM, ALCIRA SERRANO-GOMEZ, AND ANNE HEFFERNAN

KEY LEARNING POINTS

- Worldwide, opioids remain the mainstay for the treatment of moderate to severe acute pain.
- Fears of addiction should not limit the appropriate use of opioids for acute pain.
- An opioid is any substance with a pharmacological action at the opioid receptor; an opiate is a naturally occurring opioid.
- Efficacy describes the magnitude of the maximal pharmacological response to an opioid. Potency is related to the dose of the opioid needed to produce an effect, not its magnitude.
- The classical opioid receptors are μ, κ, and δ. No subreceptors of these have been identified but many receptor gene polymorphisms have been discovered; these may be responsible for clinically important differences in receptor expression and function.
- The nociceptin/orphanin FQ receptor is an opioid-like receptor; agents acting at this site have the potential to produce analgesia without respiratory depression.

- Opioid pharmacodynamic and pharmacokinetic variables vary widely between patients and the therapeutic index is narrow. This necessitates the need for close observation and titration of dose to effect in every patient receiving opioids for acute pain.
- Nausea and vomiting are predictable and significant side effect of opioids when used to treat opioid-naive patients in acute pain; prophylactic antiemetics are often administered routinely.
- Oral bioavailability of opioids used for acute pain is low and varied.
- Morphine is metabolized to two major metabolites that are excreted by the kidney. Morphine-6-glucuronide is a full agonist at the μ receptor; morphine-3-glucuronide may have an anti-opioid effect in some situations.

INTRODUCTION

Despite years of extensive research to identify effective alternatives, opioids remain the mainstay of treatment for moderate to severe acute pain. Many opioids are available worldwide for medical use, but the pharmacological action of all of them is very similar. They differ only in respect of their relative efficacy at each type of opioid receptor (and therefore relative clinical efficacy and specific side-effect profile), their pharmacokinetics, and their actions other than those at the opioid receptor. The choice of opioid is also influenced by the traditional prescribing practices prevailing in each country. For example, diamorphine is never used medically in the USA and many European countries, but it is administered frequently in the UK. There is no logical pharmacological reason for this – it is simply tradition.

An opioid is defined as a compound (endogenous or administered, naturally occurring or synthetic) which has pharmacological activity at an opioid receptor. An important property of this interaction is that it is reversed by an opioid antagonist (e.g. naloxone).[1] Opium contains a variety of naturally occurring opioids and is obtained from the seeds of the poppy plant Papaver somniferum; it has been available for thousands of years, perhaps even to the Pharaohs of Egypt. The term "opium" is derived from Greek (opioin, poppy juice) and is used to describe more than 20 pharmacologically active or inactive alkaloids, including morphine, codeine, and papaverine.[2] An "opiate" is a naturally occurring opioid. The Greek word for "to benumb" is narkoo, from which the term "narcotic" is derived. Originally used to describe any sleep-inducing substance, narcotic has no strict medical definition. The term may be employed to describe any illegal, abused substance and it is used in some countries synonymously with the term opioid.

OPIOID EFFICACY AND POTENCY

The pharmacology of commonly used opioids is described in this chapter. However, it is important to clarify the precise pharmacological definitions of two terms that often cause confusion when comparing the properties of opioids: efficacy and potency.

Efficacy (or intrinsic activity) is a concept which describes the magnitude of the maximal response of a tissue arising from a drug–receptor interaction.[3] Potency is an expression of the activity of the drug, in terms of the amount needed to produce a defined effect.[3] The relationship between these terms is best illustrated by considering morphine, fentanyl, and buprenorphine. Morphine has the same efficacy as fentanyl (both can cause respiratory arrest). Unfortunately, the term potency is often used in general conversation synonymously with the term efficacy, i.e. "morphine is just as potent as fentanyl." In pharmacological terms, this is incorrect because fentanyl is more potent than morphine as the ED_{50} (the dose that is effective in 50 percent of patients for any defined effect) is less than that of morphine. Under normal circumstances, buprenorphine does not cause respiratory depression. Therefore, it is less efficacious (in terms of effect on the respiratory system) than morphine. It is also less efficacious as an analgesic (see below under Buprenorphine). However, because the dose of buprenorphine is far smaller than morphine (e.g. 0.3–0.6 mg intramuscularly (i.m.)), it has a smaller ED_{50}. Therefore, buprenorphine is more potent than morphine.

OPIOID RECEPTORS

Martin and colleagues[4] were the first to classify opioid receptors. In 1976, they described the mu (μ), kappa (κ), and sigma receptors (σ). This was based on the specificity of three agents acting at these receptors, i.e. morphine, ketazocine (ketocyclazocine), and SKF10047, respectively. The delta (δ) and epsilon (ε) receptors were identified shortly after this, based on their responses to enkephalins and β-endorphins (but not morphine), respectively.[5, 6] However, data from later studies demonstrated conclusively that sigma and epsilon receptors were not opioid receptors.[7, 8] It has taken a long time for these findings to be appreciated by some, particularly with respect to the sigma receptor. From the 1980s, only three opioid receptors (μ, κ, and δ) were recognized.

For some years, data have suggested the possibility of receptor subtypes for the opioid receptors. For example, it was postulated that $μ_1$ receptors were responsible for analgesia and $μ_2$ for respiratory depression.[9] However, no receptor subtype has been identified following the cloning of the classical opioid receptors (μ, κ, and δ) in the early 1990s.[10, 11, 12, 13]

Recent studies in knockout mice (deletion of the gene coding for μ receptors) showed that they did not demonstrate opioid-induced analgesia or respiratory depression,[14] supporting the notion that a single μ-opioid receptor mediate these effects.

Despite the failure to identify opioid receptor subtypes, recent work has discovered that there are a number of polymorphisms in the μ opioid receptor gene (OPRM1) that may be responsible for some of the variation in response to opioid therapy. Gene polymorphism refers to differences in the DNA sequence that may affect the expression or structure of the receptor. About 100 variants in the μ-opioid receptor gene have been identified,[15] more than 20 involving amino-acid changes.[16] The most commonly studied single nucleotide polymorphism (SNP) so far is A118G, where the nucleotide adenine is replaced by guanine in the position 118 of the OPRM1 gene. This results in an amino-acid exchange (asparagine for aspartate) in the extracellular region of the receptor at position 40 (Asn40Asp or N40D).[15] The frequency of the A118G variant differs according to the population, e.g. approximately 45 percent in the Asian population and 5–25 percent in African-Americans.[17]

The clinical significance of the defined SNPs with respect to response to opioid therapy is yet to be clarified. Several studies suggest that polymorphism in the OPRM1 gene may contribute to the wide variation in opioid sensitivity, tolerance, and addiction.[18, 19, 20] It has been reported from in vitro studies that differences in the expression, transduction systems, and receptor trafficking of the A118G polymorphism can affect potency and efficacy.[21, 22, 23] Studies have demonstrated a reduced response to opioids in acute, chronic, and cancer pain, and a reduced incidence of side effects (e.g. miosis, nausea and vomiting, respiratory depression) in subjects with the A118G variant.[24, 25, 26, 27]

Work on opioid receptor polymorphism continues; it has the potential to have a major influence on future advances in opioid therapy.

Location and mechanism of action of opioid receptors

It has been known for some time that opioid receptors are abundant throughout the central nervous system (CNS).[28] Mu and kappa receptors are present in the cerebral cortex, amygdala, hippocampal formation, thalamus, mesencephalon, pons, medulla, and spinal cord.[13, 29] Kappa receptors are found also in the hypothalamus. Delta receptors are present throughout the telencephalon and the spinal cord.

High densities of μ-opioid receptors are found in the descending inhibitory control pathway, the periaqueductal gray (PAG) in the midbrain.[30] Efferent outflow from the PAG descends via the rostroventromedial medulla (RVM) to the dorsal horn of the spinal cord synapsing with the inhibitory interneurons in laminae II. In the spinal cord, opioid receptors are found at the presynaptic terminals of primary afferent sensory neurons (Aδ and C-fibers), primarily in lamina I and the substantia gelatinosa (laminae II). These presynaptic receptors inhibit the release of excitatory neurotransmitters (e.g. substance P, glutamate), and hence transmission of nociceptive stimuli. Although δ receptors are classically considered to be spinal, μ receptors still predominate (e.g. 70 percent μ, 24 percent δ, and 6 percent κ in the rat).[28, 31]

Opioid receptors and ligands have been identified in peripheral tissue. For example, enkephalins have been described in periosteum, synovium, bone marrow, and juxta-articular bone.[32] Furthermore, analgesic effects of peripherally administered opioids have been demonstrated in the laboratory and the clinic.[33, 34, 35] However, a recent review identified the poor quality and inconsistency of the available clinical data on efficacy and a significant number of studies failing to show an effect.[36]

Opioid receptors inhibit the conduction of signals in the nociceptive pathways by inhibiting the release of, and response to, neurotransmitters. This is achieved by:

- preventing calcium influx at presynaptic voltage-gated calcium channels;[37]
- inhibiting the response of the postsynaptic membrane to neurotransmitters by activating potassium channels and consequently hyperpolarizing the membrane;
- negative receptor coupling by inhibitory G-protein to adenylyl cyclase, thus reducing cAMP formation.[38, 39, 40]

Endogenous ligands acting at opioid receptors include enkephalins (δ receptor), dynorphins (κ receptor), endorphins (high affinity, but poor selectivity for μ receptors),[41]

and nociceptin/orphanin FQ (NOP receptor, see below under Nociceptin/orphanin FQ receptor). The endogenous selective ligands for the μ receptor (endomorphins) were first identified in 1997.[29] Both endomorphin 1 and endomorphin 2 are peptides of four amino acids and intimately involved in nociceptive pathways.[42] Unlike the other recognized peptides, precursors for endomorphin 1 and 2 have not been identified.

Nomenclature of opioid receptors

Since the discovery of opioid receptors, there has been considerable debate around their nomenclature. In 1996, the guidelines of the International Union of Pharmacology (IUPHAR) Committee on Receptor Nomenclature and Drug Classification recommended that the Greek terms μ, δ, and κ should be replaced with OP_3, OP_1, and OP_2, respectively[43] (numbered with respect to the order in which they were cloned). The use of MOP, DOP, and KOP has also been recommended. However, the Greek letter nomenclature (μ, δ, κ) is well established and, in 2005, IUPHAR considered that their use should be accepted (see **Table 3.1**).[44]

Nociceptin/orphanin FQ receptor

Attempts to clone the known opioid receptors led to the accidental cloning of a new, previously unidentified opioid-like receptor. This was christened the orphan receptor because no ligand was known at that time.[43] However, a year later, the endogenous ligand was discovered simultaneously by two groups, who named the agonist orphanin F/Q (owing to its terminal amino acids) or nociceptin.[45, 46] Nociceptin/orphanin FQ (N/OFQ) is a heptadecapeptide cleaved from prepronociceptin and shows similarity to dynorphin A.[47] The "orphan" receptor has been given numerous names: ORL-1 (opioid receptor like), NCR (nociceptin receptor), or OP_4. However, latest guidelines from IUPHAR recommend that, because of the structural relationship between this receptor and μ, κ, and

Table 3.1 Nomenclature of opioid receptors.

Conventional nomenclature	Official IUPHAR nomenclature	Other names	Ligand
Mu	μ	MOP, MOR, OP_3	Endomorphins
Delta	δ	DOP, DOR, OP_1	β-Endorphin
Kappa	κ	KOP, KOR, OP_2	Dynorphin A
Orphan	NOP	ORL1, OP_4	Nociceptin/ orphanin FQ

IUPHAR, International Union of Pharmacology; ORL, opioid receptor like.

δ receptors, it should be considered as a nonopioid branch of the opioid family of receptors. They propose the abbreviation NOP for this receptor.[48]

The system is involved in several physiological processes, including pain modulation.[49] The receptor is distributed widely throughout the CNS, e.g. cortex, hippocampus, hypothalamus, PAG, locus ceruleus, and spinal cord (laminae I, II, and X). Spinally, nociceptin produces analgesia; this prevails over the supraspinal actions that produce hyperalgesia or anti-opioid actions.[47, 50]

The NOP receptor functions in similar ways to the other opioid receptors, e.g. enhances outward potassium flow from the cell and inhibits voltage-gated calcium channels.[47] It is not implicated in respiratory depression.[47] It may be that drugs acting at this receptor will provide good analgesia with no respiratory depression and investigations into selective antagonists at this receptor are in progress.[51] Novel ligands (e.g. UFP-112) have shown similar spinal antinociceptive and supraspinal pronociceptive actions, with higher potency and longer-lasting effects than the natural peptide N/OFQ.[52]

The effects of orphanin FQ on other systems is complex, depend on mode of administration, and are not yet fully understood. The cardiovascular and renal effects render the receptor a possible candidate for the treatment of heart failure,[53] anxiety and depression,[54] and eating disorders;[55] it is also involved in learning and memory processes.[56]

CLASSIFICATION OF OPIOID DRUGS

Traditionally, opioids have been classified as strong, intermediate, and weak, according to their perceived analgesic properties and propensity to addiction (**Table 3.2**). For example, codeine is described as "weak"; partial μ-agonists (less efficacy than morphine) or mixed agonist–antagonist opioids (κ agonist, μ antagonist) are often referred to as "intermediate" opioids; and pure opioid agonists (e.g. morphine, pethidine (meperidine), oxycodone, hydromorphone, diamorphine, fentanyl) are described as "strong." Although this approach has been useful (e.g. the adoption of the World Health Organization analgesic ladder), it can

be misleading. It implies that the "weak" opioids, such as codeine, are less dangerous despite the fact that codeine is simply less potent than morphine and can cause respiratory depression if given in a sufficient dose.[57]

Opioids can also be classified according to their structure, but this is not helpful to the clinician. Perhaps the best way of classifying opioids is by adopting a functional approach (**Table 3.2**). As described below, pure agonists (e.g. morphine, fentanyl) have predictable pharmacological properties, as do partial agonists (e.g. buprenorphine), and agonists–antagonists (e.g. pentazocine). Some opioids have mixed actions because they are also active at other receptors or systems. For example, pethidine is an antagonist at the cholinergic receptor (cardiovascular effects) and also has a membrane-stabilizing effect (local anesthetic action);[58] tramadol inhibits reuptake of norepinephrine and 5-HT (another mechanism for analgesia).[59]

OPIOID PHARMACODYNAMICS

The general pharmacodynamic effects of opioids are summarized in **Table 3.3**. Effects on the central nervous system include analgesia, sedation, respiratory depression, miosis, nausea, and vomiting. No other class of drug has equivalent efficacy for moderate to severe nociceptive pain.

As well as being antinociceptive, opioids often reduce the affective components of pain. Nausea and vomiting is a predictable and significant side effect in many patients, especially in acute pain when prophylactic antiemetics are often administered routinely. The mechanism of action is thought to be stimulation of opioid receptors within the chemoreceptor trigger zone in the area postrema of the medulla. However, effects on the gastrointestinal tract (e.g. delayed gastric emptying, altered intestinal tone and motility) and vestibular function probably play a significant role as well.

Euphoria is often reported but dysphoria may occur, particularly with κ agonists. Morphine and most μ and κ agonists cause constriction of the pupil by an excitatory action on the parasympathetic nerve innervating the pupil.[60]

Table 3.2 Classification of opioid drugs.

Traditional	Structural	Functional
Strong	Morphinans	Pure agonists
Morphine, diamorphine, fentanyl	Morphine, codeine	Morphine, fentanyl
Intermediate	Phenylperidines	Partial agonists
Partial agonists, mixed agonist–antagonist	Pethidine, fentanyl	Buprenorphine
Weak	Diphenylpropylamines	Agonist–antagonist
Codeine	Methadone, dextropropoxyphene	Pentazocine, nalbuphine, butorphanol
	Esters	Mixed action
	Remifentanil	Pethidine, tramadol

Pethidine (meperidine).

Table 3.3 Opioid pharmacodynamics.

System	
Central nervous system	Analgesia
	Influence-affective dimensions of pain
	Nausea and vomiting
	Sedation
	Euphoria
	Miosis
	Dysphoria (particularly κ)
	Loss of REM sleep
	Tolerance
	Physical dependence
Respiratory (not κ)	Decreased tidal volume
	Decreased respiratory rate
	Right shift CO_2 response curve
	Upper respiratory tract obstruction
	Decreased response to hypoxemia
	Synergy with general anesthetic agents
Cardiovascular system	Bradycardia
	Hypotension
Gastrointestinal	Reduced gastric emptying
	Increased intestinal transit time
	Reduced intestinal propulsive contractions
	Increased intestinal tone
	Increased tone of sphincter of Oddi
Urogenital tract	Inhibition of voiding reflex
	Increased detrusor muscle tone
	Polyuria (κ only)

Inhibition of the brain stem respiratory centers causes respiratory depression; both respiratory rate and tidal volume are reduced.[60] However, respiratory rate is often a poor indicator of the degree of opioid-induced respiratory depression. The effect of opioids on respiratory function is profound; some effects are discernible even with doses too small to disturb consciousness. There may be periods of prolonged apnea and upper respiratory tract obstruction, particularly during sleep. The respiratory center becomes less responsive to carbon dioxide,[60] and the carbon dioxide response curve is shifted to the right and the slope is decreased. Opioids also inhibit the respiratory response to hypoxemia – a particularly important issue in the post-operative patient. Opioid toxicity is an important cause of hypoxemia and impaired consciousness levels in the acute pain situation.

Standard doses of opioids have little effect on blood pressure, heart rate, and rhythm in reasonably fit supine patients. However, they are associated with peripheral vasodilatation, decreased peripheral resistance, and baroreceptor inhibition. Therefore, hypotension may occur on rising from the supine position.[60] Intravenous administration is most often associated with significant hypotension, particularly if blood pressure is dependent on a high sympathetic tone or if cardiac reserve is poor.[60] Bradycardia is common, especially after large doses.

Opioids reduce the rate of gastric emptying significantly, interfering with fluid and solid intake and the absorption of orally administered drugs. Intestinal tone is increased and propulsive contractions are reduced,[61] resulting in constipation; this is often the limiting factor when opioids are used for chronic pain. Biliary, pancreatic, and intestinal secretions are reduced and food digestion in the small intestine is inhibited.[61] Pressure within the biliary tract is increased owing to an increase in the tone of the sphincter of Oddi, an effect which may be prolonged.[61]

Therapeutic doses of morphine increase the tone and amplitude of ureteric contractions but the clinical significance of this is uncertain.[60] Inhibition of the voiding reflex and increased tone in the detrusor and external sphincter of the bladder may cause urinary retention.[62] Kappa stimulation is associated with polyuria, which can be clinically significant.

Opioid administration is often associated with dilatation of cutaneous blood vessels and flushing of the neck, face, and thorax.[60] In part, this is due to the release of histamine; it is a particular property of morphine and pethidine, especially when given intravenously. Histamine release is also thought to account for urticaria commonly seen at the site of injection. This is not mediated by opioid receptors and is not prevented by naloxone. Pruritus is a recognized complication of acute opioid therapy, particularly after neuraxial administration. This is not likely to be due to histamine release as it is reversed by naloxone.[63] Other systems may be involved in its etiology including dopamine D_2 and seretonin receptors, prostaglandins, and spinal inhibitory pathways.[64]

Rapid intravenous administration of large doses of opioids can cause muscular rigidity, which may interfere with attempts at manual ventilation during anesthesia or resuscitation.[65] The precise cause of this is uncertain, but it can be alleviated by muscle relaxants administered by those trained in advanced airway management, e.g. anesthesiologists.

Hyperalgesia is a recognized symptom during opioid withdrawal. However, recent work has suggested that, paradoxically, opioids may themselves cause hypersensitivity to pain, i.e. opioid-induced hyperalgesia. This concept has arisen from a considerable amount of animal work and some human studies in patients receiving chronic opioid therapy, patients undergoing surgery, and volunteers in laboratory pain models. It is particularly associated with the use of high and very low doses of opioids. The literature on this complex subject has been well reviewed recently by Angst and Clark.[66] With respect to acute clinical pain, a few studies have shown that the use of high-dose intraoperative opioids may lead to increased postoperative pain and opioid consumption. It is not clear if this represents opioid-induced hyperalgesia or acute opioid tolerance. Considerably more work is required before the clinical relevance of this phenomenon is clarified and whether it should influence the use of opioids in the acute pain situation.

PHARMACOKINETICS OF OPIOIDS

Oral bioavailability

The oral bioavailability of commonly used opioids varies but tends to be poor (**Table 3.4**). Methadone is an exception (approximately 80 percent); this opioid is not suitable for the treatment of acute pain because of its prolonged half-life (see below under Half-life and volume of distribution). However, patients may present with acute pain who are taking regular methadone because of chronic pain or opioid addiction. Oral opioids can be used effectively in some acute pain situations if they are titrated to effect and gastric emptying is not inhibited.

Half-life and volume of distribution

Half-life ($T_{1/2}$) is a consequence of clearance (Cl) and volume of distribution (V_d), as given by the equation:

$$T_{1/2} = \log_e 2 \times V_d/Cl$$

Most opioids have a large volume of distribution and many have similar half-lives (**Table 3.5**).

Remifentanil and alfentanil have relatively small volumes of distribution but are not used frequently for relief of acute pain. The rapid clearance and the small volume of distribution of remifentanil is responsible for its very short half-life.[67] Methadone has a low clearance

Table 3.4 Approximate oral bioavailabilities of commonly used opioids.

	Oral bioavailability (%)
Morphine	25
Pethidine	52
Codeine	50
Oxycodone	60
Hydromorphone	25
Tramadol	75
Methadone	80
Nalbuphine	16
Pentazocine	47
Buprenorphine	30[a]

[a]After sublingual administration.

and a large volume of distribution, resulting in a very prolonged half-life.[68] Duration of action is often related to half-life, but not if the opioid has a pharmacologically active metabolite (e.g. morphine, tramadol, codeine), has a relatively high receptor affinity (e.g. buprenorphine), or tends to accumulate in peripheral compartments.

Context-sensitive half-time

When terminating an infusion of a drug, the time taken for the plasma concentration to fall by 50 percent is known as the context-sensitive half-time or half-life. Context refers to the duration of the infusion. Many opioids accumulate in peripheral tissues during infusion so that, when the infusion is stopped, drug continues to be released into the blood, thus reducing the expected rate of fall of blood concentration and pharmacological effect. For example, the time necessary for the plasma concentration of fentanyl to drop by 50 percent is very much dependent on the duration of the infusion; this is due to its high lipid solubility and large volume of distribution. The context-sensitive half-time of sufentanil is less affected by duration of infusion compared with fentanyl. Alfentanil shows this effect, but less so than sufentanil and fentanyl. In contrast, the context-sensitive half-time of remifentanil is largely independent of the duration of the infusion. The context-sensitive half-times after a three-hour infusion of alfentanil and remifentanil is approximately 55 minutes and 3 minutes, respectively.[69, 70] Remifentanil does not accumulate because of rapid metabolism by tissue esterases.

VARIABILITY IN PHARMACOKINETICS AND PHARMACODYNAMICS

In general, there is a large variation between individuals with respect to opioid pharmacokinetics and pharmacodynamics; it should be emphasized that the pharmacokinetic values given in **Table 3.5** represent mean values. For example, the elimination half-life of morphine in a group of normal volunteers varied from 101 to 442 minutes.[71] Considerable variation is also observed in pharmacodynamic parameters. For example, the minimum effective analgesic plasma concentrations of pethidine in patients after surgery ranged from 0.24 to 0.76 μg/mL.[72] Some, but not all, of the variability of opioid pharmacological values has been shown to be related to coexisting pathology,[73] age,[74] and sex.[75] The possible role of receptor gene polymorphisms is discussed under Opioid receptors above. This variability, and the narrow therapeutic index of all opioids, is responsible for the need for close observation and titration of dose to effect in each patient and the development of techniques such as patient-controlled analgesia.

Table 3.5 Approximate pharmacokinetic values of commonly used opioids.

	Volume of distribution (L/kg)	Clearance (mL/min/kg)	Elimination half-life (hours)
Morphine	3.5	15.0	3.0
Pethidine	4.0	12.0	4.0
Codeine	2.6	11.0	2.9
Oxycodone	2.6	9.7	3.7
Hydromorphone	4.1	22.0	3.1
Fentanyl	4.0	13.0	3.5
Alfentanil	0.8	6.0	1.6
Sufentanil	1.7	12.7	2.7
Remifentanil	0.4	40.0	0.1
Tramadol	2.9	6.0	7.0
Methadone	3.8	1.4	35.0
Nalbuphine	3.8	22.0	2.3
Pentazocine	7.1	17.0	4.6
Buprenorphine	7.0	70.0	2.5

Pethidine (meperidine).

PHARMACOLOGY OF COMMONLY USED OPIOIDS

Full agonists

MORPHINE

Morphine (Morpheus, the Greek god of dreams) is still the most commonly used opioid for acute pain; it remains the gold standard with which other opioids are compared. Opium contains morphine 9–17 percent, and it was first isolated from this source in 1806. It was first synthesized in 1952.

Morphine is commonly administered intramuscularly, intravenously, or orally (bioavailability approximately 25 percent); it can also be administered per rectum and into the epidural space or spinal cerebrospinal fluid (CSF). Unlike most other opioids, it is relatively water soluble. Metabolism is by hepatic conjugation and its major metabolites are morphine-3-glucuronide (M3G) and morphine-6-glucuronide (M6G), which are excreted in the urine.[61] Small amounts of normorphine are produced by demethylation. Although morphine is relatively selective for μ-receptors, it does have activity at the κ- and δ-receptors, particularly in large doses. The half-life of morphine is about two to three hours.

M6G is a full agonist at the μ opioid receptor and accumulates if renal function is impaired. Initial work indicated that it was a potent analgesic and possibly associated with less respiratory depression and emesis compared with morphine.[76, 77] These and other data gave rise to several studies and investigations in order to identify the potential use of M6G for acute and chronic pain. This work is reviewed by van Dorp et al.[78] Early clinical studies have shown a prolonged, well-tolerated,

relatively delayed analgesic effect with a similar inhibitory effect on the carbon dioxide response curve. However, M6G may have a reduced effect on the ventilatory response to hypoxemia. In addition, there is some evidence confirming a reduced association with nausea and vomiting. It is still early days in the development of this compound and further work is ongoing. The literature is inconsistent at present with respect to relative potency of M6G and morphine.

The main metabolite of morphine (M3G) is a mild opioid antagonist.[79] Therefore, it is postulated that accumulation of M3G may reduce the efficacy of morphine administration and gives some theoretical basis for changing to another opioid if this occurs. There is some evidence that M3G has excitatory effects, but this is not substantial.

DIAMORPHINE

Diamorphine (3,6-diacetyl morphine, heroin) is a semisynthetic opioid with no activity at the μ-receptor.[80] It is converted rapidly to the active metabolite 6-monoacetyl morphine (6-MAM), which is metabolized further to morphine. These metabolites are responsible for the pharmacological actions of heroin.[81] It is likely that there are no significant differences in the pharmacodynamics of diamorphine compared with morphine when used for acute pain,[82] despite the common belief that diamorphine is associated with more euphoria and less nausea and vomiting. Diamorphine is used therapeutically in only a few countries.

Diamorphine can also be given intrathecally and epidurally. For example, diamorphine 0.25 mg intrathecally has been shown to produce the same duration and quality of postoperative analgesia as 5 mg of epidural diamorphine for elective cesarean section.[83]

CODEINE

Codeine (3-methoxy morphine) has an oral bioavailability of approximately 50 percent. Like diamorphine, it is a prodrug. It is metabolized in the liver primarily by glucuronidation and also by N-demethylation to norcodeine.[60] However, approximately 10 percent is metabolized to morphine by O-demethylation, and it is this activity which accounts for the analgesic effects of codeine because codeine itself has a low affinity for opioid receptors. The polymorphic CYP2D6 enzyme is responsible for this transformation and it is absent in some individuals (e.g. 7 percent of the white population), suggesting that these patients will derive no benefit[84] from codeine. Heterozygotes may have a reduced response. The incidence of poor and intermediate metabolizers in a British pediatric population was 47 percent.[85]

OXYCODONE

Oxycodone (14-hydroxy-7,8-dihydrocodeinone) is a full opioid agonist with a half-life of 2.6 hours. It is a semisynthetic derivative of thebaine. It may be given intramuscularly, intravenously, subcutaneously, orally, or rectally. Oxycodone is more bioavailable (60 percent) than morphine (25 percent) when given orally.[86] A high proportion of oxycodone is N-dealkylated to noroxycodone during the first pass, and approximately 8–14 percent of the dose is excreted as free oxycodone over 24 hours after administration.[86]

The affinity of oxycodone for the μ-receptor is 1:10 to 1:40 of that of morphine and four times that of pethidine.[87] In analgesic efficacy[88] and addictive potential,[89] it is similar to that of morphine.

HYDROMORPHONE

Hydromorphone is a semisynthetic opioid used primarily for the treatment of pain in cancer,[90] but it may have a place for acute pain. It is a hydrogenated ketone analog of morphine and is an effective alternative to morphine in the treatment of moderate to severe pain.[91]

It can be administered intravenously, orally, and rectally.[90] Hydromorphone is five times as potent as morphine when given by the oral route and 8.5 times as potent when given intravenously,[90] with a similar duration of action. The liver is the principal site of metabolism. In contrast to morphine, the 6-glucuronide metabolite is not produced in any significant amount; the major metabolite being hydromorphone-3-glucuronide. Some metabolites are active but they are present in such small amounts that they are unlikely to have significant effects, except perhaps in renal failure.[92]

FENTANYL

Fentanyl is approximately 100 times more potent than morphine[60] and is primarily a μ agonist. Metabolism is by N-dealkylation to the inactive norfentanyl and then to other inactive compounds, which are excreted in urine.[93] It was one of the first opioids developed specifically for use in anesthesia because of its relatively rapid, but short, duration of action.[94] High doses of fentanyl produce marked muscular rigidity, possibly as a result of the effects of opioids on dopaminergic transmission in the striatum.[95]

Fentanyl is very lipid soluble, has a low molecular weight, and is highly potent. These properties make it very suitable for transdermal administration, a technique which is used extensively for the management of chronic pain.[96] Time from application to minimum effective and maximum plasma concentrations is 1.2–40 and 12–48 hours, respectively.[97] Steady state is reached on the third day and the terminal half-life after removal of the patch is 13–25 hours.[98] These properties of the standard transdermal device make it unsuitable for acute pain and its use is not recommended.

However, transdermal administration of fentanyl utilizing iontophoresis is now available for acute pain management. Ionized molecules of fentanyl are transported along a potential difference into the skin and circulation when a button is pressed on the device which delivers a pulse of electrical current. This results in a relatively rapid bolus administration of fentanyl to the bloodstream and the technique is not associated with the accumulation of a fentanyl depot within the skin.[99] Clinical data are now becoming available; for example, the fentanyl iontophoretic transdermal system has been shown to be comparable with morphine patient-controlled analgesia for postoperative pain relief.[100]

Fentanyl has been used for intravenous patient-controlled analgesia (PCA).[101] It has also been administered as a lollipop preparation in children.[102]

ALFENTANIL

Alfentanil is less potent than fentanyl, but its half-life is shorter.[93] It is metabolized by N-dealkylation and O-demethylation to inactive metabolites.[93] Alfentanil is more rapid in onset than fentanyl, despite being less lipid soluble.[103] This is because 89 percent of the unbound drug in plasma is unionized, thus generating a large concentration gradient for diffusion across the blood–brain barrier. Although the half-life of alfentanil after bolus administration is short, the drug accumulates during infusion and the plasma half-life increases with duration of infusion.[104]

SUFENTANIL

Sufentanil is an analog of fentanyl and has been used for anesthesia and postoperative analgesia.[104] It is specific for the μ-receptor site[105] and its half-life is 2.7 hours. It is highly lipophilic and is rapidly distributed throughout the tissues.[104] It is metabolized by dealkylation and demethylation to inactive metabolites and is eliminated in the urine.[105]

REMIFENTANIL

Remifentanil is a μ-opioid receptor agonist with an analgesic potency similar to that of fentanyl.[106] It is a fentanyl derivative which is broken down by blood and tissue esterases.[106] Its speed of onset is similar to that of alfentanil.[107] It has a short and predictable half-life which is not affected by hepatic or renal function[108] or plasma cholinesterase (butyrylcholinesterase or pseudocholinesterase) deficiency. The main metabolic product of ester hydrolysis is a carboxylic acid derivative (GI-90291) which is excreted by the kidneys (elimination half-life approximately 100 minutes).[109] Although its elimination is delayed in renal failure, significant pharmacological effects are unlikely as its potency relative to remifentanil is only 0.1–0.3 percent.[110]

Unlike all other opioids, the plasma half-life of remifentanil (approximately five minutes) is independent of the duration of infusion – no matter how long. Its short half-life offers some advantages, but makes it difficult to use for acute pain relief and bolus administration is not recommended. However, remifentanil infusions which are controlled by patient feedback systems similar to PCA (i.e. patient-controlled infusions) are now being utilized in some centers There is a paucity of data in the literature on the efficacy and safety of this technique, but some have demonstrated good pain relief after surgery[111, 112] and during labor.[113] Patients receiving postoperative remifentanil infusions should be monitored very closely and care should be taken to avoid inadvertent bolus administration.

METHADONE

Methadone is a synthetic opioid used commonly as a maintenance drug for opioid addicts, but it is being used increasingly for cancer pain. It is rapidly absorbed after oral administration with measurable concentrations in plasma within 30 minutes after oral administration,[114] and its oral bioavailability is approximately 80 percent.[115] It is extensively metabolized in the liver to inactive metabolites via N-demethylation.[115] It has a relatively high lipid solubility and is highly protein bound (α_1-acid glycoprotein).

The duration of action of a single dose is similar to that of morphine. However, this is entirely the result of redistribution.[116] The elimination half-life of methadone is 20–45 hours and, with regular administration, steady-state plasma concentration may not be reached for ten days.[117] There is some suggestion that the analgesic efficacy of methadone is greater than that of morphine, particularly in some patients with cancer pain. It is postulated that this may be due to activity at the N-methyl-D-aspartate (NMDA) receptor.[118, 119]

Methadone is not suitable for the treatment of acute pain. However, many patients presenting with an acute exacerbation of chronic pain will be taking this drug, and an appreciation of its unique pharmacology is essential for good and safe management.

Partial agonists

BUPRENORPHINE

Buprenorphine is a semisynthetic derivative of thebaine and closely related chemically to the pure agonist etorphine.[120] However, buprenorphine is a partial μ-agonist with less analgesic efficacy and respiratory depression than the full agonists.

Buprenorphine is 30 times more potent than morphine and, despite being a partial agonist only, its receptor affinity is high.[121] This means that it dissociates from the receptor very slowly.[122] Thus, peak effect after administration may be as long as three hours, with a duration of action of approximately ten hours. In theory, a partial agonist may stimulate the receptor sufficiently to produce analgesia but not enough for respiratory depression, with less potential for abuse.[123] However, respiratory depression can occur with buprenorphine; if it does occur, it may be difficult to reverse with naloxone alone because of receptor kinetics.[124] For this reason, it is not recommended in labor as its effects on the fetus cannot be readily reversed.[125]

Buprenorphine can be given intramuscularly, intravenously, sublingually, and transdermally.[126] It is generally accepted that buprenorphine is not as effective as morphine for acute pain and it is not devoid of other opioid side effects, such as constipation and nausea and vomiting.[124] In theory, because of its high receptor affinity and partial agonist activity, it may reduce the efficacy of coadministered pure opioid agonists. It may precipitate physical withdrawal symptoms when given to opioid-dependent patients.[125] The transdermal preparation has recently become available for chronic pain; it is not indicated for the treatment of acute pain.

Mixed agonist–antagonist opioids

Drugs in this class include pentazocine, butorphanol, and nalbuphine. They act as partial agonists at the κ-receptor and weak antagonists at the μ-receptor.[120] Consequently, they may cause withdrawal symptoms in patients tolerant to other opioids.

Pentazocine is one-sixth as potent as morphine, nalbuphine is slightly less potent than morphine, and butorphanol is between five and nine times as potent.[120] The duration of analgesia is similar to that of morphine (three to four hours).[127] In terms of analgesia, mixed agonist–antagonist opioids are not as efficacious as pure μ agonists, but have less effect on respiratory function and there is less risk of abuse.[127] Unlike morphine, there appears to be a ceiling to both the respiratory depression and analgesic action.[120] However, dysphoria (κ-receptor) and nausea are relatively common side effects.

Although useful in some patients, the pharmacological properties of this class of opioids are responsible for the fact that they have found little use in the routine treatment of severe acute pain. Several new κ-agonists have been developed and tested recently, but they have been associated with limited analgesia and unpleasant side effects.

Opioids with actions on other systems

PETHIDINE

Pethidine (meperidine; bioavailability 52 percent, half-life four hours) was discovered in 1939 during a search for atropine-like compounds.[128] Its use as a treatment for asthma was abandoned when its opioid agonist properties were appreciated. It is primarily a μ agonist and exerts it chief pharmacological actions on the CNS and the neural elements in the bowel. In general, 75–100 mg given parenterally is approximately equivalent to 10 mg of morphine.

Pethidine is metabolized in the liver by hydrolysis to several inactive compounds and by N-demethylation to norpethidine (normeperidine).[60] Norpethidine causes central excitation and, eventually, convulsions, particularly after prolonged, high-dose administration. These effects have been reported in patients receiving pethidine by PCA. Patients with liver impairment are particularly sensitive to pethidine: its oral bioavailability is increased to as much as 80 percent, and the half-lives of both pethidine and norpethidine are prolonged. Pethidine is contraindicated in patients taking monoamine oxidase inhibitors.[65]

Pethidine has two further specific pharmacological actions. It is an anticholinergic agent, presumably because of its structural similarity to atropine. Furthermore, pethidine has a local anesthetic effect; its use as a spinal anesthetic has been reported for a number of surgical procedures.[129]

TRAMADOL

Tramadol is presented as a mixture of two stereoisomers (+)tramadol and (−)tramadol.[130] It is a centrally acting analgesic with relatively weak μ opioid receptor activity. However, it also inhibits norepinephrine and 5-HT uptake within the nervous sytem,[131] which is thought to account for some of its analgesic activity.

It is extensively metabolized by O- and N-demethylation, glucuronidation, and sulfation.[132] O-desmethyltramadol production is dependent on the cytochrome CYP2D6 (see above under Codeine); it is an active μ-agonist with a greater receptor affinity than the parent molecule. Advantages over traditional opioids are reduced likelihood of tolerance and addiction and less respiratory depression. It is less efficacious than morphine for postoperative pain

and has a significant incidence of nausea. Other side effects include vomiting, dizziness, sedation (less than morphine), dry mouth, sweating, and headache.[133]

TOLERANCE, DEPENDENCE, AND ADDICTION

The fear of healthcare staff and patients about opioid addiction following treatment of acute pain has been, and continues to be, responsible for their reluctance to administer or request appropriate amounts of opioids. Those involved in the management of acute pain should understand the precise definitions and clinical relevance of tolerance, dependence, and addiction.

Tolerance

Tolerance is a common response to the repetitive use of a drug acting at a receptor. It can be defined as a reduction in response to the same dose of drug after repeated administration. Tolerance occurs in a number of clinical situations and is not specific to opioids. It is a normal pharmacological phenomenon and does not indicate addiction.

Dependence

Dependence is a state in which an abstinence syndrome may occur following abrupt withdrawal, reduction in dose, or administration of an antagonist. Again, this can be associated with a number of drugs, but is common during prolonged opioid use. This complication simply means that, if a patient has been receiving an opioid for some time for severe pain, the opioid should be withdrawn slowly and in a controlled manner. It does not mean that the patient has become a drug addict.

Addiction

Addiction is defined as a behavioral pattern of drug use, characterized by compulsive self-administration on a continuous or periodic basis in order to experience its psychic effects and sometimes to avoid discomfort of its absence, often securing supply by deceptive or illegal means. The development of addiction is extremely rare in patients receiving opioids for severe acute pain; it should not limit their use for this indication.

REFERENCES

1. Rang HP, Dale MM, Ritter JM, Flower R. *Rang and Dale's pharmacology*, 6th edn. Edinburgh: Churchill Livingstone, 2007.
2. Ayyangar NR, Bhide SR. Separation of eight alkaloids and meconic acid and quantitation of five principal alkaloids in

gum opium by gradient reversed-phase high-performance liquid chromatography. *Journal of Chromatography.* 1988; **463**: 455–65.

3. Girdlestone D (ed.). Terms and symbols in quantitative pharmacology. In: *The IUPHAR compendium of receptor characterization and classification.* London: IUPHAR Media, 1998: 9–11.

4. Martin WR, Eades CG, Thompson JA *et al.* The effects of morphine- and nalorphine-like drugs in the nondependent and morphine-dependent chronic spinal dog. *Journal of Pharmacology and Experimental Therapeutics.* 1976; **197**: 517–32.

5. Lord JAH, Waterfield AA, Hughes J, Kosterlitz HW. Endogenous opioid peptides: multiple agonists and receptors. *Nature.* 1977; **276**: 495–699.

6. Wuster M, Schulz R, Herz A. Specificity of opioids towards the μ, δ and opiate receptors. *Neuroscience Letters.* 1979; **36**: 291–8.

7. Largent BL, Wikstrom H, Gundlach AL, Snyder SH. Structural determinants of sigma receptor affinity. *Molecular Pharmacology.* 1987; **32**: 772–84.

8. Shook JE, Kazmierski W, Wire WS *et al.* Opioid receptor selectivity of β-endorphin in vitro and in vivo: mu, delta, and epsilon receptors. *Journal of Pharmacology and Experimental Therapeutics.* 1988; **246**: 1018–25.

9. Pasternak GW, Wood PJ. Multiple mu opiate receptors. *Life Sciences.* 1986; **38**: 1889–98.

10. Simonin F, Befort K, Gaveriaux-Ruff C *et al.* The human delta-opioid receptor: genomic organization, cDNA cloning, functional expression, and distribution in human brain. *Molecular Pharmacology.* 1994; **4**: 1015–21.

∗ 11. Evans CJ, Keith DE, Morrison H *et al.* Cloning of a delta-opioid receptor by functional expression. *Science.* 1992; **258**: 1952–5.

12. Yasuda K, Raynor K, Kong H *et al.* Cloning and functional comparison of kappa-opioid and delta-opioid receptors from mouse-brain. *Proceedings of the National Academy of Sciences of the United States of America.* 1993; **90**: 6736–40.

13. Thompson RC, Mansour A, Akil H, Watson SJ. Cloning and pharmacological characterization of a rat μ-opioid receptor. *Neuron.* 1993; **11**: 903–13.

∗ 14. Inturrisi CE. Clinical pharmacology of opioids for pain. *Clinical Journal of Pain.* 2002; **18**: S3–13.

15. Ikeda K, Ide S, Han W *et al.* How individual sensitivity to opiates can be predicted by gene analyses. *Trends in Pharmacological Sciences.* 2005; **26**: 311–7.

∗ 16. Lotsch J, Geisslinger G. Are mu-opioid receptor polymorphisms important for clinical opioid therapy? *Trends in Molecular Medicine.* 2005; **11**: 82–9.

∗ 17. Bond C, LaForge KS, Tian M *et al.* Single-nucleotide polymorphism in the human mu opioid receptor gene alters beta-endorphin binding and activity: possible implications for opiate addiction. *Proceedings of the National Academy of Sciences of the United States of America.* 1998; **95**: 9608–13.

18. Han W, Ide S, Sora I *et al.* A possible genetic mechanism underlying individual and interstrain differences in opioid actions: focus on the mu opioid receptor gene. *Annals of the New York Academy of Sciences.* 2004; **1025**: 370–5.

19. Mogil JS. The genetic mediation of individual differences in sensitivity to pain and its inhibition. *Proceedings of the National Academy of Sciences of the United States of America.* 1999; **96**: 7744–51.

∗ 20. Uhl GR, Sora I, Wang Z. The mu opiate receptor as a candidate gene for pain: polymorphisms, variations in expression, nociception, and opiate responses. *Proceedings of the National Academy of Sciences of the United States of America.* 1999; **96**: 7752–5.

∗ 21. Landau R. One size does not fit all: genetic variability of mu-opioid receptor and postoperative morphine consumption. *Anesthesiology.* 2006; **105**: 235–7.

22. Beyer A, Koch T, Schroder H *et al.* Effect of the A118G polymorphism on binding affinity, potency and agonist-mediated endocytosis, desensitization, and resensitization of the human mu-opioid receptor. *Journal of Neurochemistry.* 2004; **89**: 553–60.

23. Befort K, Filliol D, Decaillot FM *et al.* A single nucleotide polymorphic mutation in the human mu-opioid receptor severely impairs receptor signaling. *Journal of Biological Chemistry.* 2001; **276**: 3130–7.

∗ 24. Reyes-Gibby CC, Shete S, Rakvag T *et al.* Exploring joint effects of genes and the clinical efficacy of morphine for cancer pain: OPRM1 and COMT gene. *Pain.* 2007; **130**: 25–30.

25. Lotsch J, Skarke C, Grosch S *et al.* The polymorphism A118G of the human mu-opioid receptor gene decreases the pupil constrictory effect of morphine-6-glucuronide but not that of morphine. *Pharmacogenetics.* 2002; **12**: 3–9.

26. Skarke C, Darimont J, Schmidt H *et al.* Analgesic effects of morphine and morphine-6-glucuronide in a transcutaneous electrical pain model in healthy volunteers. *Clinical Pharmacology and Therapeutics.* 2003; **73**: 107–21.

27. Romberg R, Olofsen E, Sarton E *et al.* Pharmacokinetic-pharmacodynamic modeling of morphine-6-glucuronide-induced analgesia in healthy volunteers: absence of sex differences. *Anesthesiology.* 2004; **100**: 120–33.

28. Mansour A, Khachaturian H, Lewis ME *et al.* Anatomy of CNS opioid receptors. *Trends in Neurosciences.* 1988; **11**: 308–14.

29. Zadina JE, Hackler L, Ge LJ, Kastin AJ. A potent and selective endogenous agonist for the μ-opioid receptor. *Nature.* 1997; **386**: 499–502.

∗ 30. McDonald J, Lambert DG. Opioid receptors. Continuing education in anaesthesia. *Critical Care and Pain.* 2005; **5**: 22–5.

∗ 31. Stein C, Yassouridis A. Peripheral morphine analgesia. *Pain.* 1997; **71**: 119–21.

32. Bergstrom J, Ahmed M, Li J *et al.* Opioid peptides and receptors in joint tissues: study in the rat. *Journal of Orthopaedic Research.* 2006; **24**: 1193–9.

33. Stein C, Comisel K, Haimerl E et al. Analgesic effect of intraarticular morphine after arthroscopic knee surgery. New England Journal of Medicine. 1991; 325: 1123–6.

∗ 34. Picard PR, Tramer MR, McQuay HJ, Moore RA. Analgesic efficacy of peripheral opioids (all except intra-articular): a qualitative systematic review of randomised controlled trials. Pain. 1997; 72: 309–18.

35. Coggeshall RE, Zhou S, Carlton SM. Opioid receptors on peripheral sensory axons. Brain Research. 1997; 764: 126–32.

∗ 36. Rosseland LA. No evidence for analgesic effect of intra-articular morphine after knee arthroscopy: a qualitative systematic review. Regional Anesthesia and Pain Medicine. 2005; 30: 83–98.

∗ 37. Law PY, Wong Y-H, Loh HH. Molecular mechanisms and regulation of opioid receptor signalling. Annual Review of Pharmacology and Toxicology. 2000; 40: 389–430.

38. Smart D, Hirst RA, Hirota K et al. The effects of recombinant rat μ-opioid receptor activation in CHO cells on phospholipase C and adenylyl cyclase. British Journal of Pharmacology. 1997; 120: 1165–71.

39. Hirst RA, Hirota K, Grandy DK, Lambert DG. Coupling of the cloned rat κ receptor to adenylyl cyclase is dependent on receptor expression. Neuroscience Letters. 1997; 232: 119–22.

40. Hirst RA, Smart D, Devi LA, Lambert DG. Effects of C-terminal truncation of the recombinant δ-opioid receptor on phospholipase C and adenylyl cyclase coupling. Journal of Neurochemistry. 1998; 70: 2273–8.

41. Pleuvry BJ. Opioid receptors and their ligands – natural and unnatural. British Journal of Anaesthesia. 1991; 66: 370–80.

∗ 42. Horvath G. Endomorphin-1 and endomorphin-2: pharmacology of the selective endogenous mu-opioid receptor agonists. Pharmacology and Therapeutics. 2000; 88: 437–63.

43. Dhawan BN, Celsselin F, Raghubir R et al. International Union of Pharmacology. 12. Classification of opioid receptors. Pharmacological Reviews. 1996; 48: 567–92.

∗ 44. Foord SM, Bonner TI, Neubig RR. International Union of Pharmacology. XLVI. G protein-coupled receptor list. Pharmacology Review. 2005; 57: 279–88.

45. Meunier JC, Mollereau C, Toll L et al. Isolation and structure of the endogenous agonist of opioid receptor-like ORL(1) receptor. Nature. 1995; 377: 523–35.

46. Reinscheid RK, Northacker HP, Bourson A et al. Orphanin-FQ – a neuropeptide that activates an opioid-like G-protein-coupled receptor. Science. 1995; 270: 792–4.

47. Calo G, Guerrini R, Rizzi A et al. Pharmacology of nociceptin and its receptor: a novel therapeutic target. British Journal of Pharmacology. 2000; 129: 1261–83.

48. Cox B, Chavkin C, McDonald C et al. Revised IUPHAR Opioid Receptor Nomenclature Subcommittee Proposals. Tulsa, USA: International Narcotics Research Conference, last updated July 2001, cited February 2008. Available from: www.inrcworld.org/statements.htm.

∗ 49. Darland T, Heinricher MM, Grandy DK. Orphanin FQ/nociceptin: a role in pain and analgesia, but so much more. Trends in Neurosciences. 1998; 21: 215–21.

∗ 50. Rizzi A, Nazzaro C, Marzola GG et al. Endogenous nociceptin/orphanin FQ signalling produces opposite spinal antinociceptive and supraspinal pronociceptive effects in the mouse formalin test: pharmacological and genetic evidences. Pain. 2006; 124: 100–08.

51. Calo G, Guerrini R, Bigoni R et al. Characterisation of [Nphe (1)]nociceptin (1–13)NH2, a new selective nociceptin receptor antagonist. British Journal of Pharmacology. 2000; 129: 1183–93.

∗ 52. Rizzi A, Spagnolo B, Wainford RD et al. In vitro and in vivo studies on UFP-112, a novel potent and long lasting agonist selective for the nociceptin/orphanin FQ receptor. Peptides. 2007; 28: 1240–51.

53. Doggrell SA. Cardiovascular and renal effects of nociceptin/orphanin FQ: a new mediator to target? Current Opinion in Investigational Drugs. 2007; 8: 742–9.

∗ 54. Gavioli EC, Calo' G. Antidepressant- and anxiolytic-like effects of nociceptin/orphanin FQ receptor ligands. Naunyn-Schmiedebergs Archives of Pharmacology. 2006; 372: 319–30.

∗ 55. Ciccocioppo R, Cippitelli A, Economidou D et al. Nociceptin/orphanin FQ acts as a functional antagonist of corticotropin-releasing factor to inhibit its anorectic effect. Physiology and Behavior. 2004; 82: 63–8.

56. Sandin J, Ogren SO, Terenius L. Nociceptin/orphanin FQ modulates spatial learning via ORL-1 receptors in the dorsal hippocampus of the rat. Brain Research. 2004; 997: 222–33.

57. Redpath JB, Pleuvry BJ. Double-blind comparison of the respiratory and sedative effects of codeine phosphate and (±)-glausine phosphate in human volunteers. British Journal of Clinical Pharmacology. 1982; 14: 555–8.

58. Mehta VL. Cholinergic mechanisms in narcotic analgesics. Neuropharmacology. 1975; 14: 893–1.

59. Raffa RB, Friderichs E, Reimann W et al. Opioid and non-opioid components independently contribute to the mechanism of action of tramadol, an "atypical" opioid analgesic. Journal of Pharmacology and Experimental Therapeutics. 1992; 260: 275–85.

60. Reisine T, Pasternak G. Opioid analgesics and antagonists. In: Goodman, Gillman (eds). Goodman and Gillman's the pharmacological basis of therapeutics, 9th edn. New York: McGraw Hill, 1996: 521–55.

∗ 61. Martin WR. Pharmacology of opioids. Pharmacological Reviews. 1983; 35: 283–323.

62. Dray A, Nunan L. Supraspinal and spinal mechanisms in induced inhibition of reflex urinary bladder contractions in the rat. Neuroscience. 1987; 22: 281–7.

63. Ballantyne JC, Loach AB, Carr DB. Itching after epidural spinal opiates. Pain. 1988; 33: 149–60.

64. Ganesh A, Maxwell LG. Pathophysiology and management of opioid-induced pruritus. Drugs. 2007; 67: 2323–33.

65. Duthie DJR, Nimmo WS. Adverse effects of opioid analgesic drugs. *British Journal of Anaesthesia.* 1987; **59**: 61–77.

∗ 66. Angst MS, Clark JD. Opioid-induced hyperalgesia: a qualitative systematic review. *Anesthesiology.* 2006; **104**: 570–87.

67. Glass PS, Gan TJ, Howell S. A review of the pharmacokinetics and pharmacodynamics of remifentanil. *Anesthesia and Analgesia,* **89** Suppl. 4: 1999: S7–14.

∗ 68. Nicholson AB. Methadone for cancer pain. *Cochrane Database of Systematic Reviews.* 2004; **CD00397**.

∗ 69. Kapila A, Glass PS, Jacobs JR *et al.* Measured context-sensitive half-times of remifentanil and alfentanil. *Anesthesiology.* 1995; **83**: 968–75.

70. Shafer SL, Varvel JR. Pharmacokinetics, pharmacodynamics, and rational opioid selection. *Anesthesiology.* 1991; **74**: 53–63.

71. Aitkenhead AR, Vater M, Achola K. Pharmacokinetics of single-dose i.v. morphine in normal volunteers and patients with end-stage renal failure. *British Journal of Anaesthesia.* 1984; **56**: 813–19.

72. Austin KL, Stapleton JV, Mather LE. Relationship between blood meperidine concentrations and analgesic response: a preliminary report. *Anesthesiology.* 1980; **53**: 460–6.

73. Glare PA, Walsh TD. Clinical pharmacokinetics of morphine. *Therapeutic Drug Monitoring.* 1991; **13**: 1–23.

74. Baillie SP, Bateman DN, Coates PE, Woodhouse KW. Age and the pharmacokinetics of morphine. *Age and Ageing.* 1989; **18**: 258–62.

75. Gear RW, Miaskowski C, Gordon NC *et al.* Kappa-opioids produce significantly greater analgesia in women than in men. *Nature Medicine.* 1996; **2**: 1248–50.

76. Hill RG. Analgesic drugs in development. In: McMahon SB, Koltzenburg MK (eds). *Wall and Melzack's textbook of pain*, 5th edn. Amsterdam: Elsevier, 2005: 541–52.

∗ 77. Christrup LL. Morphine metabolites. *Acta Anaesthesiologica Scandinavica.* 1997; **41**: 116–22.

∗ 78. van Dorp ELA, Romberg R, Sarton E *et al.* Morphine-6-glucuronide: morphine's successor for postoperative pain relief? *Anesthesia and Analgesia.* 2006; **102**: 1789–97.

79. Mazoit JX, Butscher K, Samii K. Morphine in postoperative patients: pharmacokinetics and pharmacodynamics of metabolites. *Anesthesia and Analgesia.* 2007; **105**: 70–8.

80. Smith CF. Morphine, but not diacetyl morphine (heroin), possess opiate analgesic activity in the mouse vas deferens. *Neuropeptides.* 1984; **5**: 173–6.

∗ 81. Sawynok J. The therapeutic uses of heroin: a review of the pharmacological literature. *Canadian Journal of Physiology and Pharmacology.* 1986; **64**: 1–6.

82. Robinson SL, Rowbotham DJ, Smith G. Morphine compared with diamorphine: a comparison of dose requirements and side-effects after hip surgery. *Anaesthesia.* 1991; **46**: 538–40.

83. Hallworth SP, Fernando R, Bell R *et al.* Comparison of intrathecal and epidural diamorphine for elective caesarean section using a combined spinal-epidural technique. *British Journal of Anaesthesia.* 1999; **82**: 228–32.

84. Henthorn TK, Spina E, Dumort E, conBahr C. In vitro inhibition of a polymorphic human liver P-450 isoenzyme by narcotic analgesics. *Anesthesiology.* 1989; **70**: 339–42.

85. Williams DG, Patel A, Howard RF. Pharmacogenetics of codeine metabolism in an urban population of children and its implications for analgesic reliability. *British Journal of Anaesthesia.* 2002; **89**: 839–45.

86. Poyhia R, Seppala T, Olkkola KT, Kalso E. The pharmacokinetics and metabolism of oxycodone after intramuscular and oral administration to healthy subjects. *British Journal of Clinical Pharmacology.* 1992; **33**: 617–21.

87. Chen ZR, Irvine RJ, Somogyi AA, Bochner F. Mu receptor binding of some commonly used opioids and their metabolites. *Life Science.* 1991; **48**: 2165–71.

∗ 88. Poyahia R, Vainio A, Kalso E. A review of oxycodone's clinical pharmacokinetics and pharmacodynamics. *Journal of Pain and Symptom Management.* 1993; **8**: 63–7.

89. Maruta T, Swanson DW. Problems with the use of oxycodone compound in patients with chronic pain. *Pain.* 1981; **11**: 389–96.

90. Sarhill N, Walsh D, Nelson K. Hydromorphone: pharmacology and clinical applications in cancer patients. *Supportive Care Cancer.* 2001; **9**: 84–96.

91. Cherny NJ, Chang V, Frager G *et al.* Opioid pharmacotherapy in the management of cancer pain: a survey of strategies used by pain physicians for the selection of analgesic drugs and routes of administration. *Cancer.* 1995; **76**: 1283–93.

92. Babul N, Darke AC, Hagen N. Hydromorphone metabolite accumulation in renal failure. *Journal of Pain and Symptom Management.* 1995; **10**: 184–6.

∗ 93. Davis PJ, Cook DR. Clinical pharmacokinetics of the newer intravenous anaesthetic agents. *Clinical Pharmacokinetics.* 1986; **11**: 18–35.

94. Clotz MA, Nahota MC. Clinical uses of fentanyl, sufentanil and alfentanil. *Clinical Pharmacology.* 1991; **10**: 581–93.

95. Viscomi CM, Bailey PL. Opioid-induced rigidity after intravenous fentanyl. *Obstetrics and Gynecology.* 1997; **89**: 822–4.

96. Muijsers RB, Wagstaff AJ. Transdermal fentanyl: an updated review of its pharmacological properties and therapeutic efficacy in chronic cancer pain control. *Drugs.* 2001; **61**: 2289–307.

97. Grond S, Radbruch L, Lehmann KA. Clinical pharmacokinetics of transdermal opioids: focus on transdermal fentanyl. *Clinical Pharmacokinetics.* 2000; **38**: 59–89.

98. Milligan KA, Campbell C. Transdermal fentanyl in patients with chronic, nonmalignant pain: a case study series. *Advances in Therapy.* 1999; **16**: 73–7.

99. Power I. Fentanyl HCl iontophoretic transdermal system (ITS): clinical application of iontophoretic technology in

the management of acute postoperative pain. *British Journal of Anaesthesia*. 2007; **98**: 4–11.

*100. Grond S, Hall J, Spacek A *et al*. Iontophoretic transdermal system using fentanyl compared with patient-controlled intravenous analgesia using morphine for postoperative pain management. *British Journal of Anaesthesia*. 2007; **98**: 806–15.

101. Nikkola EM, Ekblad UU, Kero PO *et al*. Intravenous fentanyl PCA during labour. *Canadian Journal of Anesthesia*. 1997; **44**: 1248–55.

102. Feld LH, Champeau MW, van Steennis CA, Scott JC. Preanaesthetic medication in children: a comparison of oral transmucosal fentanyl citrate versus placebo. *Anesthesiology*. 1989; **71**: 374–7.

103. Bower S, Hull CJ. Comparative pharmacokinetics of fentanyl and alfentanil. *British Journal of Anaesthesia*. 1982; **54**: 871–7.

*104. Monk JP, Beresford R, Ward A. Sufentanil: a review of its pharmacological properties and therapeutic uses. *Drugs*. 1988; **36**: 286–313.

105. Meuldermans W, Hendrickx J, Lauwers W *et al*. Excretion and biotransformation of sufentanil in rats and dogs. *Drug Metabolism and Disposition*. 1987; **15**: 905–13.

106. Burkle H, Dunbar S, Van Aken H. Remifentanil: a novel, short-acting, μ-opioid. *Anesthesia and Analgesia*. 1996; **83**: 646–51.

107. Glass PS, Hardman D, Kamiyama Y *et al*. Preliminary pharmacokinetics and pharmacodynamics of an ultrashort acting opioid remifentanil. (GI87084B). *Anesthesia and Analgesia*. 1993; **77**: 1031–40.

108. Dershwitz M, Hoke JF, Rosow CE *et al*. Pharmacokinetics and pharmacodynamics of remifentanil in volunteer subjects with severe liver disease. *Anesthesiology*. 1996; **84**: 812–20.

109. Westmoreland CL, Hoke JF, Sebel PS *et al*. Pharmacokinetics of remifentanil (GI87084B) and its major metabolite (GI90291) in patients undergoing elective in-patient surgery. *Anesthesiology*. 1993; **79**: 893–903.

110. Hoke JF, Shlugman D, Dershwitz M *et al*. Pharmacokinetics and pharmacodynamics of remifentanil in persons with renal failure compared with healthy volunteers. *Anesthesiology*. 1997; **87**: 533–41.

111. Krishnan K, Elliot SC, Berridge JC, Mallick A. Remifentanil patient-controlled analgesia following cardiac surgery. *Acta Anaesthesiologica Scandinavica*. 2005; **49**: 876–9.

112. Yarmush J, D'Angelo R, Kirkhart B *et al*. A comparison of remifentanil and morphine sulfate for acute postoperative analgesia after total intravenous anesthesia with remifentanil and propofol. *Anesthesiology*. 1997; **87**: 235–43.

*113. Balki M, Kasodekar S, Dhumne S *et al*. Remifentanil patient-controlled analgesia for labour: optimizing drug delivery regimens. *Canadian Journal of Anaesthesia*. 2007; **54**: 626–33.

114. Garrido MJ, Troconiz IF. Methadone: a review of its pharmacokinetic/pharmacodynamic properties. *Journal of Pharmacological and Toxicological Methods*. 1999; **42**: 61–6.

115. Nilsson MI, Mersaar U, Anngard E *et al*. Clinical pharmacokinetics of methadone. *Acta Anaesthesiologica Scandinavica*. 1982; **S74**: 66–9.

116. Sawe J. High-dose morphine and methadone in cancer patients: clinical pharmacokinetic considerations of oral treatment. *Clinical Pharmacokinetics*. 1986; **11**: 87–106.

117. Inturrisi CE, Colburn WA, Kaiko RF *et al*. Pharmacokinetics and pharmacodynamics of methadone in patients with chronic pain. *Clinical Pharmacology and Therapeutics*. 1987; **41**: 392–401.

118. Inturrisi CE, Portenoy RK, Max MB *et al*. Pharmacokinetic–pharmacodynamic relationships of methadone infusions in patients with cancer pain. *Clinical Pharmacology and Therapeutics*. 1990; **47**: 565–77.

119. Levy M. Pain management in advanced cancer. *Seminars in Oncology*. 1985; **12**: 394–410.

120. Hoskin PJ, Hanks GW. Opioid agonist–antagonist drugs in acute and chronic pain states. *Drugs*. 1991; **41**: 326–44.

121. Boas RA, Villiger JW. Clinical actions of fentanyl and buprenorphine: the significance of receptor binding. *British Journal of Anaesthesia*. 1985; **57**: 192–6.

122. Yassen A, Olofsen E, Dahan A, Danhof M. Pharmacokinetic–pharmacodynamic modeling of the antinociceptive effect of buprenorphine and fentanyl in rats: role of receptor equilibration kinetics. *Journal of Pharmacology and Experimental Therapeutics*. 2005; **313**: 1136–49.

123. Heel RC, Brogden RN, Speight TM, Avery GS. Buprenorphine: a review of its pharmacological properties and therapeutic efficacy. *Drugs*. 1979; **17**: 81–110.

124. Maunuksela EL, Korpela R, Olkkola KT. Comparison of buprenorphine with morphine in the treatment of postoperative pain in children. *Anesthesia and Analgesia*. 1988; **67**: 233–9.

125. Wallenstein SL, Kaiko RF, Rogers AG, Houde RW. Crossover trials in clinical analgesic assays: studies of buprenorphine. *Pharmacotherapy*. 1986; **6**: 228–35.

126. Sittl R. Transdermal buprenorphine in cancer pain and palliative care: review. *Palliative Medicine*. 2006; **20**: s25–30.

127. Tammisto T, Tigerstedt I. Comparison of the analgesic effects of intravenous nalbuphine and pentazocine in patients with postoperative pain. *Acta Anaesthesiologica Scandinavica*. 1977; **21**: 390–4.

128. Kirvela OA, Kanto JH. Clinical and metabolic responses to different types of premedication. *Anesthesia and Analgesia*. 1991; **73**: 49–53.

129. Ngan Kee WD. Intrathecal pethidine: pharmacology and clinical applications. *Anaesthesia and Intensive Care*. 1998; **26**: 137–46.

130. Eggers KA, Power I. Editorial: tramadol. *British Journal of Anaesthesia*. 1995; **74**: 247–9.

131. Raffa RB, Friderichs E, Reimann W *et al.* Opioid and non-opioid components independently contribute to the mechanism of action of tramadol, and "atypical" opioid analgesic. *Journal of Pharmacology and Experimental Therapeutics.* 1992; **260**: 275–85.

132. Sevcik J, Nieber K, Driessen B, Illes P. Effects of the central analgesic tramadol and its main metabolite, O-desmethyl-tramadol, on rat locus coeruleus neurones. *British Journal of Pharmacology.* 1993; **110**: 169–76.

∗133. Scott LJ, Perry CM. Tramadol: a review of its use in perioperative pain. *Drugs.* 2000; **60**: 139–76.

4

Clinical pharmacology: traditional NSAIDs and selective COX-2 inhibitors

STEPHEN F JONES AND AIDAN M O'DONNELL

KEY LEARNING POINTS

- Nonsteroidal anti-inflammatory drugs (NSAIDs) are highly effective analgesics for moderate to severe pain.
- Co-administration of NSAIDs and opioids is more appropriate for severe pain, with opioid sparing and potential for reduction in opioid-related adverse effects.
- Non-selective NSAIDs and cyclooxygenase (COX)-2 inhibitors have similar analgesic efficacy.
- There are many cautionary considerations to be made before prescribing NSAIDs, especially in the elderly and in the postoperative period.
- Safety considerations with short-term use after major trauma or surgery are different from those that apply to chronic administration.

- The neurohumoral stress response to major surgery or trauma makes renal function more prostaglandin dependent and thus more influenced by NSAIDs.
- Nonselective NSAIDs can increase the risk of bleeding.
- Co-administration of aspirin increases the gastrointestinal (GI) toxicity of nonselective NSAIDs, negates any gastrointestinal advantage of COX-2 inhibitors, and does not prevent increased cardiovascular morbidity.
- Traditional NSAIDs may cause similar increase in cardiovascular morbidity to COX-2 inhibitors.
- Ibuprofen may impede the cardioprotection of low-dose aspirin.

INTRODUCTION

The most commonly used nonopioid drugs for acute pain therapy are the NSAIDs and paracetamol (see Chapter 5, Clinical pharmacology: paracetamol and compound analgesics). The long history of use, relative paucity of serious adverse events with short-term use, and lack of tolerance or abuse potential make them comfortable choices for most physicians. Considering the widely differing chemical structures, it is perhaps the similarity of their effects that is the most remarkable.

TERMINOLOGY

No formal nomenclature exists for the various divisions within this class of drug. In this review, the term "NSAID" is used to describe any nonsteroidal anti-inflammatory drug acting through COX inhibition. It thus includes selective COX-2 inhibitors and full-dose aspirin, but excludes low-dose aspirin and paracetamol. The term "COX-2 inhibitor" implies moderate to high selectivity with little or no activity on the COX-1 enzyme.

INDICATIONS

NSAIDs have analgesic, anti-inflammatory, and anti-pyretic properties. They are indicated in the relief of mild to moderate pain associated with injury, inflammation or malignancy in skin, ligaments, muscles or bone, post-operative pain, dysmenorrhea, headache, and renal or biliary colic. They can be used in conjunction with opioids for more severe pain. With the exception of aspirin and other salicylates, they are also used to treat acute gouty arthritis.

MECHANISMS OF ACTION

The cell is the basic building block of mammalian tissues. Through the action of the enzyme phospholipase-A2, the phospholipids within the cell membranes release arachidonic acid, which serves as the substrate for the ubiquitous COX enzymes, generating a variety of biologically active metabolites throughout the body. These thromboxanes (from platelets) and prostaglandins exert diverse and often mutually opposing influences on local cellular function (**Table 4.1**). The principal actions of NSAIDs are through inhibition of COX and the consequences are seen in many organ systems. Arachidonic acid may alternatively be metabolized via the lipoxygenase pathway to produce proinflammatory leukotrienes (from leukocytes). There is an obligatory facilitation of this pathway associated with nonselective NSAIDs due to substrate diversion, though this is less significant with selective COX-2 inhibition as the COX-1 pathway remains intact. Two isoenzymes have been identified with certainty; the existence of a third (COX-3) remains controversial.[1]

In general, COX-1 is the "constitutive" or "housekeeping" enzyme producing prostaglandins responsible for many homeostatic functions, whereas the "inducible" COX-2 mediates the vascular response to inflammation and sensitizes nociceptors to the action of bradykinin, thus increasing the sensation of pain through the phenomenon of peripheral hyperalgesia (Chapter 1b, Mechanisms of inflammatory hyperalgesia). However, COX-2 is now also recognized to have low level constitutive expression in many tissues including the central nervous system (CNS), lung, female reproductive tract, and kidneys. COX-2, induced in the vascular endothelium by hemodynamic shear forces and atheromatous inflammatory processes, is responsible for much of the local prostacyclin synthesis.

The COX-2 enzyme differs structurally from COX-1 in having a smaller amino acid (valine) at position 523, permitting access to a side pocket and thereby accommodating the larger COX-2 inhibitors. Corticosteroids stimulate lipocortin which inhibits phospholipase A2, thus limiting arachidonic acid release. In addition, they also inhibit transcription of COX-2 RNA. The arachidonic acid cascade is described in detail in standard pharmacology texts.[2]

General pharmacology of NSAIDs

ABSORPTION

Absorption of NSAIDs is rapid and almost complete. It occurs primarily in the upper small intestine and, to a lesser extent, from the stomach. Food intake or gastrostasis associated with acute pain can delay the delivery of drug to the small intestine leading to slower onset of analgesia. However, absorption can occur across any mucous membrane, therefore several NSAIDs (and paracetamol) can be given in suppository form. Salt forms of the NSAIDs generally have faster absorption profiles than the poorly soluble acid forms.[3] Consequently, many oral NSAIDs are prepared as the sodium or potassium salts. Diclofenac potassium was developed for faster onset in migraine pain and naproxen sodium was developed as an improvement over the acidic form.[4]

DISTRIBUTION

NSAIDs (or their active metabolites) are generally weak acids (pK_a 3–5), or salts thereof, and are fully ionized at physiological pH (7.4). Ion trapping of NSAID molecules occurs in inflamed synovium, injured tissue, the gastrointestinal tract, the kidney, or the bone marrow, and may

Table 4.1 Main actions of principal eicosanoids.

Eicosanoid	Action
PGE_2	Hyperalgesia, vasodilatation, production of cytoprotective gastric mucus, decreased gastric acid synthesis, pyrexia
PGI_2	Hyperalgesia, vasodilatation, inhibition of platelet aggregation, production of cytoprotective gastric mucus, renin release, natriuresis
$PGF_{2\alpha}$	Bronchoconstriction, uterine contraction
TXA_2	Vasoconstriction, platelet aggregation

prolong their duration of action in these areas.[5] They have a low apparent volume of distribution, predominantly reflecting a high degree of binding to plasma proteins (see below under Protein binding).

PROTEIN BINDING

Most NSAIDs are > 98 percent bound to plasma proteins, except for piroxicam, salicylates, and paracetamol, which are < 20 percent bound.[6] Extensive protein binding, with consequent reduction in free active drug, is problematic in patients with hypoalbuminemia (< 30 g/dL) combined with liver insufficiency, or where renal insufficiency (serum creatinine > 20 mg/L) is present. A lower than usual initial dose should be given to these patients and careful follow up scheduled. Even at normal plasma protein concentrations, extensive protein binding accounts for many drug–drug interactions as NSAIDs can displace other agents from plasma proteins, e.g. warfarin.

Metabolism and elimination

NSAIDs are extensively metabolized in the liver, resulting in inactivation.[6] One exception is nabumetone, which is activated by hepatic metabolism.[7] NSAID clearance is dependent upon protein binding and not hepatic blood flow. Aspirin and diclofenac have a high first-pass clearance resulting in bioavailability of 60 and 54 percent, respectively.[6]

NSAIDs that are metabolized to inactive acyl glucuronides (e.g. ketoprofen, diflunisal, indometacin (indomethacin), naproxen) are normally eliminated by the kidney.[6, 8, 9, 10] However, a reduction in renal function can result in accumulation of these conjugates leading to a "futile cycle" in which the glucuronide metabolites are hydrolyzed in the vascular compartment back to active drug.[11] This reactivation is especially important in the elderly, in whom reduced renal function can lead to increased levels of glucuronides.[9] The renal excretion of unmetabolized NSAID is generally not a major pathway of elimination (even when the urine is alkaline), except for azapropazone (apazone), and salicylates. Small increases in urinary pH that can occur with antacid therapy can significantly lower the plasma concentrations of salicylates.

ANALGESIC EFFICACY AND THERAPEUTIC BENEFITS

NSAIDs are effective analgesics in a variety of acute pain conditions, including low back pain, renal colic,[12][I] dysmenorrhea,[13][I] tension headache,[14][II] and surgery[14][I], [15][V] They are superior to opioids for treating biliary colic and may prevent the progression to cholecystitis.[14] [II] Comparative studies in postoperative pain found that

maximal recommended doses of NSAIDs are comparable with standard, though not necessarily full, therapeutic doses of opioids. However, NSAIDs have a ceiling of analgesic efficacy and increasing the dose adds to adverse effects, rather than pain relief. COX-2 inhibitors achieve this maximal efficacy with less inhibition of COX-1, but they are not significantly more efficacious.[16][I]

Multimodal pain therapy using NSAIDs and opioids has been described as near optimal for the management of mild to moderate pain states.[17][V] Numerous studies have shown NSAIDs improve analgesia, reduce opioid requirement, typically by 30–50 percent,[18][I], [19] or both. Morphine sparing *per se* is of limited value and relatively few studies have shown significant reductions in opioid-related adverse events.[19] It has been suggested that NSAIDs, by reducing renal excretion of active opioid metabolites, may simply be prolonging the opioid effect in some situations.[20] However, a recent meta-analysis found co-administration of NSAIDs significantly decreased nausea, vomiting, and sedation with nonsignificant reductions in pruritus, urinary retention, and respiratory depression.[18][I]

NSAIDs are an important component of day surgical analgesia and facilitate fast-tracking. The updated US practice guidelines recommend that "unless contraindicated, all patients should receive an around-the-clock regimen of NSAID, coxib, or paracetamol."[21][V]

In view of the risks of major adverse events associated with NSAIDs, it is useful to recognize a number of other established or putative outcome benefits in the postoperative setting. Traditional NSAIDs reduce heterotopic bone formation after certain orthopedic procedures,[22][I] although they are not indicated for routine use following hip arthroplasty.[23][II] A large retrospective cohort study has shown a 50 percent reduction in the incidence of postoperative myocardial infarction with ketorolac,[24] possibly mediated through the antiplatelet mechanism or via improved hemodynamics consequent upon better analgesia.[25] Preservation of immune competence via enhanced natural killer cell activity has been shown[26] and animal studies have shown a reduction in adhesion formation.[27] Finally, NSAIDs are an important component of effective acute pain relief, widely held to be important in preventing the transition to chronic pain states (Chapter 31, Preventing chronic pain after surgery). Although earlier reviews concluded no significant preemptive or preventive analgesia,[28] two recent studies have shown a reduction in chronic pain following 5 or 14 days treatment with celecoxib.[29, 30][II]

ADVERSE EFFECTS AND THEIR MANAGEMENT

Gastrointestinal

NSAIDs cause a variety of adverse upper and lower gastrointestinal effects including dyspeptic pain, ulceration, hemorrhage, and perforation. This is primarily due to an increase in gastric acid production and inhibition of cytoprotective mucus production, but impairment of platelet function also contributes to gastrointestinal hemorrhage. Gastrointestinal ulcer complications are more likely in patients with previous gastrointestinal ulceration; the elderly; patients on corticosteroids, high-dose or multiple NSAIDs (including low-dose aspirin); substantial users of alcohol or tobacco; and patients with inherited, pathological, or iatrogenic impairment of hemostasis. While dyspeptic symptoms and endoscopic evidence of mucosal ulceration are common and early, there is little, if any, increase in severe adverse effects with short-term NSAID therapy in clinical studies or retrospective cohort studies, though increases were seen in the elderly, with higher doses and with therapy exceeding five days.[31][III]

Selective COX-2 inhibitors have shown a reduction in major gastrointestinal adverse events in only a few studies,[32][II], [33][II] possibly as a result of inhibition of COX-2-mediated ulcer healing. Any reduced gastrointestinal toxicity of COX-2 inhibitors appears to be lost with concomitant administration of low-dose aspirin.[33, 34][V]

Misoprostol, proton pump inhibitors (PPIs), and histamine H2 receptor antagonists (H2RAs) all prevent duodenal ulcers, but high doses of H2RAs are required to reduce the risk of gastric ulceration. Only misoprostol has been directly shown to reduce ulcer complications,[35][I] but it is less well tolerated. The incidence of dyspeptic symptoms is lower with a PPI plus traditional NSAID than with a COX-2 inhibitor.[36][I] Avoidance of the oral route does not eliminate these adverse effects, which are systemically mediated.[14][I] Experimental and clinical data both suggest that enteric-coated or sustained-release preparations may reduce gastroduodenal toxicity, but at the expense of increasing exposure to the distal gut mucosa, where endoscopic monitoring and diagnosis is more difficult and complications may be more severe.

Hepatic

Slight elevations in serum transaminases are not uncommon with NSAIDs, especially diclofenac and lumiracoxib;[33] however, a review of epidemiological studies of acute hepatitis requiring hospital admission suggests the additional risk from NSAIDs is low and only significantly associated with nimesulide or sulindac.[37][III] Significant elevation in transaminases (e.g. to three times upper limit of normal) should prompt drug withdrawal or substitution. However, there are case reports of recurrent hepatitis with a second NSAID.[38]

Renal

Prostaglandins have little effect on renal function under normal circumstances, but preserve renal blood flow in the presence of high levels of vasoconstrictors, e.g. hypovolemia, congestive heart failure, major surgery. They also affect intrarenal distribution of perfusion in favor of the more poorly perfused medulla and facilitate salt and water excretion. Inhibition by NSAIDs causes edema, exacerbates or precipitates hypertension and heart failure (see below under Cardiovascular), and may cause hyponatremia, hyperkalemia, or acute renal failure.[39][II]

Despite a large number of case reports of NSAID-associated postoperative renal failure, there are few instances of this in prospective studies. A large retrospective cohort study found no increased risk with ketorolac given for less than five days, but a two-fold increase if duration of therapy was longer.[40][III] A Cochrane analysis of 19 trials, including 1204 adults with normal preoperative renal function, found a mean reduction in creatinine clearance of 18 percent on the first postoperative day, but no cases requiring dialysis. The authors concluded, "NSAIDs caused a clinically unimportant transient reduction in renal function in the early postoperative period in patients with normal preoperative renal function."[41][I] Judicious patient selection with adequate fluid replacement and appropriate monitoring are important if these results are to be replicated in clinical practice.

The risk of renal failure is higher in the elderly, in hypovolemic or dehydrated patients (including aggressive diuretic therapy), those with preexisting renal impairment or medical conditions predisposing to this, for example, diabetes, peripheral vascular disease, heart failure, cirrhosis with ascites, co-administration of nephrotoxic drugs (especially aminoglycosides), ACE inhibitors, radiocontrast media. Major surgery increases the risk through myocardial depression, fluid shifts, and activation of a vasoconstrictive neurohumoral stress response. Laparoscopy may increase the risk through increased intra-abdominal pressure.[42] COX-2 inhibitors and traditional NSAIDs have similar adverse effects on renal function.[43][I]

Asthma

Between 8 and 20 percent of adult asthmatics have a specific syndrome of aspirin-induced allergy, characterized by rhinitis, nasal polyps, asthma, and aspirin intolerance.[44] There is marked cross-sensitivity to most traditional NSAIDs,[44] but less so to COX-2 inhibitors.[14] Patients with documented aspirin-induced asthma tolerate supramaximal doses of celecoxib without bronchospasm.[45][III] COX-2 inhibitors allow metabolism of arachidonic acid by COX-1, whereas nonselective inhibitors increase metabolism through the lipoxygenase pathway. The safety of COX-2 inhibitors during acute exacerbations is unproven.[45]

Cardiovascular

Thromboxane, generated by COX-1 within platelets, is a powerful vasoconstrictor and promoter of platelet aggregation facilitating hemostasis, but also pathological vascular occlusion. On the other hand, prostacyclin, synthesized largely through COX-2, is a vasodilator and inhibits platelet aggregation, protecting the integrity of the vascular lumen. Low-dose aspirin (see below under Hemostasis) exerts a uniquely selective, though incomplete inhibition of platelet aggregation, totally blocking thromboxane synthesis despite near complete preservation of prostacyclin. Conversely, COX-2 inhibitors preserve platelet function but inhibit prostacyclin synthesis. NSAIDs inhibit both. This is the basis for the Fitzgerald hypothesis explaining the increased incidence of cardiovascular morbidity associated initially with rofecoxib, but increasingly with other COX-2 inhibitors and also traditional NSAIDs.[46][I], [47, 48] However, other mechanisms, including cardiorenal effects and inhibition of ischemic preconditioning, may also be involved.[49] A meta-analysis of 145,373 patients in 138 prospective trials has now shown that regular treatment for four weeks or more increases the risk of a serious vascular event by 42 percent for all COX-2 inhibitors (predominantly myocardial infarction), similar to the increased risk from traditional nonselective NSAIDs.[46][I] Naproxen was not cardioprotective but did not increase the risk.[46][I] A US Food and Drug Administration (FDA) review also concluded a similar risk with traditional NSAIDs and COX-2 inhibitors.[47][V] With respect to postoperative pain management, an increased cardiovascular risk from high-dose parecoxib/valdecoxib was found after coronary artery bypass grafting,[50][II], [51][II] but not after general or orthopedic surgery.[52] Low-dose aspirin by itself is undoubtedly effective for cardioprotection,[47, 53] but does not prevent the increased risk when used together with COX-2 inhibitors.[33, 50][II], [51][II] There is some evidence that ketorolac may be cardioprotective postoperatively,[24, 25][II] Regulatory authorities have required that COX-2 inhibitors be avoided in patients with established ischemic heart disease, stroke, or peripheral arterial disease, after cardiac or major vascular surgery or after other major surgery in patients with increased cardiovascular risk,[34][V] but concluded that there is otherwise no evidence for increased cardiovascular morbidity with short-term use for acute pain.[47][V] They should possibly also be avoided whenever an arterial anastomosis is created, e.g. free tissue transfer or solid organ transplantation surgery.[49][V] The American Heart Association has suggested naproxen as the preferred first choice in patients with overt or known risk factors for ischemic heart disease who require an NSAID.[54][V]

Nonselective NSAIDs increase supine mean blood pressure by an average of 5 mmHg.[55][I] COX-2 inhibitors, especially rofecoxib and etoricoxib, increase blood pressure more than nonselective agents.[56][I], [57][V] NSAIDs may precipitate or exacerbate congestive heart failure[58] and regulatory restrictions have now been extended to include moderate (New York Heart Association (NYHA) class II–IV), as well as more severe heart failure.[57][V]

Hemostasis

Because of the inhibition of vasoconstriction and platelet aggregation, low-dose aspirin and NSAIDs that inhibit COX-1 increase bleeding times and may increase the risk of postoperative bleeding,[14, 19, 23][II], [59][I], [60][I], [61][II] though the clinical significance remains controversial. In two meta-analyses of traditional NSAID administration for tonsillectomy, an increased risk of reoperation was found, with a number needed to harm (NNH) of 29[59][I] or 60.[60][I] However, a Cochrane review of pediatric tonsillectomies found smaller and statistically insignificant differences.[62][I] They should be avoided in patients with a coagulopathy or where the risk or consequences of hemorrhage are high, e.g. thyroidectomy, neurosurgery, possibly in association with epidural analgesia. Platelets do not express COX-2 and highly selective inhibitors do not increase the risk of bleeding[14][II] and so may be preferable in these situations. It is controversial whether or when low-dose aspirin should be discontinued. One must weigh the strength of the indication against the risk and consequence of hemorrhage. Although platelets remain inhibited for their lifespan of 10–12 days, fresh platelets are produced at the rate of approximately 35,000 per microliter per day and volunteer studies suggest substantially complete recovery of platelet function two to six days after stopping aspirin.[63, 64, 65] However, there are "hyperresponders" in whom hemostasis may remain impaired. The situation is further complicated by concerns about an increased propensity for thrombotic events in the days following cessation.[66] When starting aspirin acutely, complete platelet inhibition occurred in seven of ten subjects within 15 minutes, and in all subjects within 30 minutes of chewing a 325-mg enteric coated tablet.[64][III]

Central nervous system

Central adverse events of NSAIDs are not usually recognized, but can include dizziness and drowsiness as well as changes in mood, cognition, and perception.[67, 68, 69] They tend to be mild, but may be significant in the elderly. Psychosis has been reported with indometacin, sulindac, and the COX-2 inhibitors.[69] Aseptic meningitis has been reported, most commonly in young women with systemic lupus erythematosus who have had ibuprofen therapy reinstituted after a hiatus.[67]

Tissue healing

Prostaglandins facilitate bone remodelling through enhanced osteoblastic and osteoclastic activity,[70, 71] though the clinical significance of this is controversial. A retrospective study suggested that high-dose ketorolac therapy increases nonunion after spinal fusion, especially in cigarette smokers.[72]

Prostaglandins synthesized in injured tissue stimulate angiogenesis and other components of wound healing.[71] There are theoretical concerns supported by animal studies of impaired wound healing, though most clinical studies and extensive databases have not identified a major problem with either wound healing or anastomotic dehiscence. An increase in sternal wound complications was found (parecoxib/valdecoxib) in two CABG studies.[50, 51] [II] Piroxicam reduced the quality of pleurodesis in an animal study.[73]

Immunological

The anti-inflammatory action of NSAIDs is due in part to an inhibition of the infiltration of leukocytes into inflamed tissue. However, this mechanism may impair the response to soft tissue infections and NSAID therapy has been inconclusively linked to soft tissue infections, such as necrotizing fasciitis.[74] NSAIDs may enhance cell-mediated immunity.[26]

Miscellaneous

Occasional severe allergic reactions may occur, including Stevens–Johnson syndrome, Lyell syndrome, and shock. Aplastic anemia has been reported, most frequently with phenylbutazone and metamizole (dipyrone).

Special patient groups

CHILDREN

Not all preparations are licenced for use in children. NSAIDs are generally well tolerated, even in asthmatics.[75] [III] Aspirin should be avoided below the age of 12 years because of the risk of Reye's syndrome. There are concerns that NSAIDs may predispose to necrotizing fasciitis in children with varicella.[74]

PREGNANCY AND LACTATION

NSAIDs have not been associated with fetal malformations, but regular use in early pregnancy is associated with an increased risk of miscarriage.[14][III] They have been used as tocolytics and for the treatment of polyhydramnios, but can cause neonatal renal impairment and oligohydramnios. NSAID therapy in the third trimester may cause premature closure of the fetal ductus arteriosus. It will also delay and impair the progress of labor and increases the risk of hemorrhage from decreased uterine tone and platelet inhibition.

NSAIDs are not readily transferred to maternal milk and they are considered safe for short-term use. Aspirin should be avoided because of the risk of neonatal Reye's syndrome. Insufficient evidence is available for the COX-2 inhibitors.

ELDERLY

Because of reduced elimination capacity and a higher prevalence of comorbid disease, the risk from NSAIDs is increased in the elderly[19][IV]; they should be used with caution and appropriate dose adjustment. Routine monitoring of renal, hepatic, and hematologic function should be considered.

PORPHYRIA

Some NSAIDs have the potential to precipitate acute porphyria in predisposed individuals. The University of Capetown maintains an online database indicating relative safety.[76]

DRUG INTERACTIONS

Many interactions arise from the reduction in glomerular filtration induced by NSAIDs or competitive displacement of the second drug from protein-binding sites. These are summarized in **Table 4.2**.

CONTRAINDICATIONS AND MAJOR CAUTIONS

There are few absolute contraindications to the use of NSAIDs, rather an accumulation of relative contraindications against which must be weighed the need and likely benefit of using these drugs and the potential harm from alternative treatments including surgery. This is summarized in **Table 4.3**.

CHOICE OF DRUG AND MANAGEMENT

The choice of NSAID will be determined by factors including available formulations (e.g. parenteral, enteric-coated, topical, suppository), half-life, tolerability, cost, and product licence. Drugs with a short half-life will more quickly establish steady-state plasma concentrations and are more suitable for acute pain management. Immediate-release or soluble preparations work faster than enteric-coated or sustained-release preparations. COX-2 selectivity is another important determinant of choice (see **Table 4.4**) with the lack of platelet impairment particularly relevant in the postoperative setting. It is possible that some patients will obtain better relief from certain agents, but this is of little relevance to short-term therapy unless prior experience has identified a preferred agent.

The choice of pharmacological management for acute pain is influenced by the severity of the pain, the time

Table 4.2 Major drug:NSAID interactions.

Drug	Interactions
Corticosteroids	Increased risk of peptic ulceration
Aminoglycosides	Reduced renal excretion, enhanced nephrotoxicity.[77] Preliminary evidence suggests COX-2 inhibitors may be safer[78]
Lithium	Reduced renal excretion, potential lithium toxicity
Methotrexate	Reduced renal excretion, potential methotrexate toxicity
Ciclosporin	Increased nephrotoxicity
Digoxin	Competitive protein binding and reduced renal excretion, potential digoxin toxicity
ACE inhibitors	Decreased antihypertensive efficacy, hyperkalemia, renal impairment (especially in association with diuretics)
Beta-blockers	Decreased antihypertensive efficacy
Diuretics	Impaired diuresis, extracellular dehydration increases nephrotoxicity, risk of hyperkalemia with potassium sparing diuretics, especially triamterene
Radiographic contrast media	Increased renal risk
Warfarin	Competitive protein binding. Increased severity of gastrointestinal bleeding. COX-2 inhibitors may be no safer[79]
Aspirin	Ibuprofen may block the cardioprotection of aspirin[80, 81, 82]
Sulfonylureas	Enhanced hypoglycemic effect with pyrazoles, but not ibuprofen, diclofenac, naproxen, or sulindac[19]
Phenytoin	Competitive protein binding and, with pyrazole group, reduced metabolism

COX, cyclooxygenase; NSAID, nonsteroidal anti-inflammatory drugs.

Table 4.3 Contraindications and major cautions with NSAIDs.

Contraindications	Major cautions
Active peptic ulceration	Prior peptic ulceration
Advanced renal impairment	Risk factors for renal impairment (see above under Renal)
Hypovolemia	Severe hypertension
Aspirin-induced asthma (COX-2 inhibitors may be acceptable)	Hyperkalemia
Congestive heart failure	Bleeding disorders (COX-2 inhibitors may be acceptable)
Cardiac and major vascular surgery	Severe hepatic disease
Major surgery with prior myocardial infarction or stroke (COX-2 inhibitors)	Major surgery
	Pregnancy, especially third trimester
	Elderly
	Drug interactions, especially anticoagulants, aminoglycosides, methotrexate, ACE inhibitors, potassium-sparing diuretics, corticosteroids

COX, cyclooxygenase; NSAID, nonsteroidal anti-inflammatory drugs.

from injury or surgery, and the ability to take medications by mouth. Acute pain management should be multimodal and viewed as a continuum with early use of preventative analgesic agents, through the acute period where parenteral analgesics are frequently required and into the later recovery phase where oral analgesia can be established. NSAIDs are generally safe and effective for younger and healthy patients having painful procedures. In high-risk situations, it may be prudent to rely more on opioids initially, generally in conjunction with paracetamol.[83][V] NSAIDs can be introduced later when hemostasis has been consolidated, the stress response is attenuating, and fluid balance and cardiovascular stability have been confidently established. NSAIDs may be introduced earlier with due caution if satisfactory analgesia is not otherwise achieved. Comparative studies have documented a lack of association between anti-inflammatory and analgesic activity. NSAIDs can exhibit differential effects on pain and inflammation; therefore, some agents are better anti-inflammatory agents (indometacin, tolmetin), others are better analgesics (ibuprofen and etodolac), and others have balanced analgesic and anti-inflammatory actions (ketoprofen, diclofenac, naproxen).[84] Choices are then made based upon the condition to be treated. For example, osteoarthritis may be better treated with a pure analgesic, whereas acute injuries call for a different

Table 4.4 Characteristics of COX-2 selective versus traditional NSAIDs.

COX-2 selective versus traditional NSAIDs
Similar analgesic efficacy
No impairment of hemostasis
Probable modest reduction in serious gastrointestinal adverse events
Probably less bronchospasm in asthmatics
Similar renal toxicity
Possibly less nephrotoxicity with aminoglycosides
Generally much more expensive

COX, cyclooxygenase; NSAID, nonsteroidal anti-inflammatory drugs.

approach depending upon the amount of inflammation involved. When managing acute pain:

- consider paracetamol, possibly with an opioid as first-line therapy, especially in the elderly or higher risk patient;[83][V]
- there should be compelling reasons to choose a COX-2 inhibitor as a first-line NSAID;
- there is little justification for a COX-2 inhibitor if the patient is taking aspirin;[34][V]
- the combination of a non-aspirin NSAID and low-dose aspirin may be associated with an increased gastrointestinal risk and should only be used if absolutely necessary;[85][V]
- do not use more than one NSAID concurrently;[85][V]
- use the lowest dose of an NSAID for the shortest time required;[34][V], [47][V]
- consider ibuprofen as first line because of lower gastrotoxicity;[85][V], [86]

- consider naproxen as a first choice in patients at cardiovascular risk;[46][I], [54][V]
- use drugs with a short half-life for acute pain management;
- enteric-coated and sustained-release preparations have a slower onset;
- NSAIDs do not have a significant preemptive effect, therefore preoperative administration should only be to lower risk patients where early postoperative efficacy is required. Late intraoperative or early postoperative parenteral administration will also achieve this result;
- topical application of NSAID gels are effective against somatic pain from superficial tissues.[87][I]

Pharmaceutical considerations of selected NSAIDs

The properties of selected NSAIDs are listed in **Table 4.5**.

SALICYLATES

The salicylate family includes aspirin (acetylsalicylic acid), diflunisal, salsalate (salicyl salicylate), choline magnesium trisalicylate, and benorilate. Benorilate is an ester of aspirin and paracetamol which is hydrolyzed *in vivo* to the two parent drugs.

ASPIRIN (ACETYLSALICYLIC ACID)

In full doses, aspirin exhibits classical NSAID properties with a slight COX-1 selectivity. It is widely used as a sole agent or as a component of numerous proprietary analgesics or cold or influenza remedies. More recently, in very

Table 4.5 Properties of selected NSAIDs.

Drug	Half-life (hours)	Selectivity	Toxicity			
			GI	Renal	Hepatic	CNS
Ketorolac	2.4–8.6	High COX-1	Mod	High	Mod	Mod
Indometacin	4.5–6	Weak COX-1	High	Low	Mod	High
Aspirin	0.25	Weak COX-1	Mod	Low	Mod	Low
Naproxen	12–15	Weak COX-1	Mod	Mod	Mod	Mod
Ibuprofen	2–2.5	Weak COX-1	Low	Mod	Mod	Low
Nabumetone (6-MNA)	22.5–30	Nonselective	Low	Low	Low	Low
Mefenamic acid	3–4	Nonselective	Mod	Low	Low	High
Piroxicam	30–86	Weak COX-2	High	Mod	Mod	Low
Diclofenac	1–2	Weak COX-2	Mod	Mod	High	Low
Nimesulide	1.8–4.7	Mod COX-2	Low	Low	High	Low
Celecoxib	11–16	Mod COX-2	Mod	Low	Low	Mod
Meloxicam	13–20	Mod COX-2	High	Low	Low	Mod
Etodolac	7	Mod COX-2	Low	Low	Low	Low
Etoricoxib	22	High COX-2	Low	Low	Low	Low

CNS, central nervous system; COX, cyclooxygenase; GI, gastrointestinal; NSAID, nonsteroidal anti-inflammatory drugs.

low doses (typically 75–150 mg/day), aspirin has evolved a greater role in the prevention of cardiovascular disease.[53] Despite emerging evidence of increased cardiovascular risk with some traditional as well as newer NSAIDs, this benefit of aspirin is not in doubt.[47] The low dose means that the risk of side effects, other than those mediated through platelet inhibition, is very low for the majority of patients.

Unlike other NSAIDs, aspirin binds covalently to cyclooxygenase, acetylating the enzyme and causing permanent inhibition of thromboxane synthesis. As platelets have no nuclear material, they cannot synthesize further enzyme and remain inhibited for the remainder of their 10–12-day life span. Aspirin is thus an irreversible, though incomplete, inhibitor of platelet aggregation, as platelet activation may occur independently of thromboxane.[2] Platelet aggregation and vasoconstriction are opposed by prostacyclin (PGI2), synthesized in the vascular endothelium. After oral administration, aspirin is rapidly and completely absorbed from the stomach. Platelets are exposed in the portal circulation, after which aspirin undergoes substantial first-pass metabolism to low levels of the relatively weak COX inhibitor, salicylic acid. Endothelial prostacyclin is thus preserved.

Reye's syndrome is a potentially fatal mitochondrial disease affecting predominantly hepatic and cerebral function.[88] It is associated with viral infections (influenza A and B, varicella-zoster virus) and with aspirin administration; it is most common in children and adolescents.[89] Administration of aspirin during a viral illness may be followed several days later by acute encephalopathy associated with selective hepatic abnormality. Approximately one-third of cases are fatal; a further third are associated with long-term neurological and behavioral deficits.

An intravenous preparation of aspirin is available in some countries.

DIFLUNISAL

Diflunisal is a nonacetylated difluorophenyl derivative of salicylic acid (with a half-life of 8–12 hours). Only small quantities cross the blood–brain barrier, so it is not effective as an antipyretic. It has only slight antiplatelet effects at normal doses and has fewer gastrointestinal side effects than aspirin, although more than ibuprofen.[90] As with aspirin, diflunisal is subject to concentration-dependent pharmacokinetics. It is not metabolized into salicylate and the fluoride ions are not displaced from the difluorophenyl ring. A hypersensitivity syndrome has been described, with flu-like symptoms progressing to multi-organ involvement.

Pyrazoles

The pyrazole class includes metamizole, azapropazone, phenylbutazone, and oxyphenbutazone. They have largely been withdrawn for human use in the USA and Europe,

although continue to be important drugs worldwide. Oxyphenbutazone is the major metabolite of phenylbutazone, differing only in the substitution of a single hydroxyl group in place of a hydrogen atom. It has a longer half-life than the parent drug. All pyrazoles may cause skin reactions, bone marrow suppression and agranulocytosis, and anaphylactoid episodes.

METAMIZOLE (DIPYRONE)

Worldwide, metamizole is one of the most widely marketed over-the-counter NSAID preparations, along with aspirin, paracetamol, and ibuprofen.[91] The most common side effects are somnolence, nausea, and gastric discomfort, but it has beneficial antispasmodic effects. It was withdrawn in the 1970s in the UK and USA because of concerns over agranulocytosis. However, early studies probably overestimated the risk.[92]

AZAPROPAZONE (APAZONE)

Azapropazone is eliminated via the kidneys and may accumulate in renal failure.[90] It has weak anti-COX activity *in vitro*. It is associated with a very high rate of gastrointestinal side effects[86][I] and is therefore recommended as a second- or third-line drug in the treatment of inflammatory disorders, such as rheumatoid arthritis.

Arylpropionic acids

Propionic acid derivatives include ibuprofen, naproxen, ketoprofen, flurbiprofen, fenoprofen, and tiaprofenic acid. Most members of this class are weakly COX-1 selective.[93]

IBUPROFEN

Ibuprofen was developed in 1964 as a safer alternative to aspirin in the treatment of rheumatoid arthritis. It was the first NSAID after aspirin licenced for over-the-counter use in the UK (1983) and the USA (1984). In common with other drugs in this class, ibuprofen contains a chiral carbon in the alpha position of the propionate moiety, which gives rise to two enantiomers of the molecule. It has been found that (S)-(+)-ibuprofen (dexibuprofen) is the active enantiomer both *in vitro* and *in vivo*. However, further testing has revealed an isomerase which converts inactive (R)-ibuprofen to the active (S)-enantiomer *in vivo*. Despite this, dexibuprofen preparations are available in many countries. Enantiomeric conversion varies widely between individuals, which may partly explain why plasma concentrations do not equate to analgesic efficacy.[90]

Ibuprofen is associated with the lowest rates of gastrointestinal side effects of all NSAIDs at clinically useful doses.[86] Meta-analysis of studies evaluating over-the-counter preparations of ibuprofen showed incidences of adverse effects comparable with placebo.[94] At higher doses (>1200 mg/day), the risk of side effects increases in a dose-dependent fashion. In overdose, ibuprofen is comparatively benign, making it an attractive alternative to paracetamol.[95]

Some preparations (e.g. potassium, lysine, or arginine salts) offer increased speed of onset.[96] Ibuprofen antagonizes the irreversible platelet inhibition induced by aspirin by obstructing access to the enzyme, and long-term administration in those taking low-dose aspirin is not recommended.[81] However, the FDA has concluded that, in those taking long-term low-dose aspirin, there is minimal risk from occasional use of ibuprofen. It recommends that aspirin be taken at least eight hours after, or 30 minutes before, a dose of ibuprofen. It makes no recommendations about enteric-coated aspirin and cautions that other nonselective NSAIDs may have similar potential.[82]

KETOPROFEN

Ketoprofen is weakly COX-1 selective, and has been shown to have a high rate of gastrointestinal side-effects.[86] It may accumulate in renal failure due to its "futile cycling."[90, 97] Topical ketoprofen gel preparations and patches may be useful for local musculoskeletal symptoms, with a lower incidence of GI side effects. Injectable preparations of ketoprofen are highly irritant and may cause localized thrombosis, as well as skin necrosis;[98] there is a small but significant risk of photoallergic contact dermatitis.[99]

NAPROXEN

Naproxen is marketed as the pure active S-enantiomer. It is associated with intermediate risk of GI side effects,[86, 100] and may accumulate in renal failure.[90] Naproxen is also available as the sodium salt, which offers increased speed of onset. It has an effective duration of about eight hours.[101] Naproxen has weak COX-1 selectivity.[102] Long-term use is not associated with the increased risk of cardiovascular adverse events (such as myocardial infarction) seen with both COX-2 inhibitors and traditional NSAIDs. One explanation is that its long duration of action results in sustained inhibition of COX-1 (similar to aspirin) compared with the transient inhibition associated with agents with shorter half-lives.[46]

TIAPROFENIC ACID

Between 50 and 80 percent of a dose of tiaprofenic acid is excreted unchanged in urine. Its excretion may be impaired in patients with renal disease (information from manufacturer's data sheet). Tiaprofenic acid has been associated with severe cystitis, although typically this resolves upon its withdrawal. It is contraindicated in patients with urinary tract disorders.[103] Its main indication is in the treatment of arthritis.

Arylacetic acids

Arylacetic acid derivatives include diclofenac, ketorolac, etodolac, sulindac, bromfenac, felbinac, indometacin, tolmetin, and nabumetone. With the exception of etodolac, these drugs have little or no COX-2 selectivity.

DICLOFENAC

Diclofenac is an achiral molecule.[104] Some studies suggest a slight COX-2 selectivity.[93, 102] It also inhibits the lipoxygenase pathway, inhibiting the synthesis of leukotrienes. Diclofenac is available in several formulations, including tablets, suppositories, eye drops, topical gels, and injectable preparations. Its use carries a relatively low risk of gastrointestinal side effects,[86] although it is implicated in hepatocellular damage[38, 105] and long-term use of high doses is associated with increased cardiovascular risk.[48] Preparations of the potassium salt offer increased speed of onset without altering efficacy, duration of action, or side effects.

Injectable preparations of diclofenac are irritant; intramuscular injection may cause prolonged pain at the injection site and intravenous injection may cause local thrombosis. Inadvertent subcutaneous injection may cause skin necrosis. It is recommended that the intramuscular route is avoided.[98]

Aceclofenac is an ester of diclofenac with fewer gastrointestinal side effects. It has no intrinsic inhibitory effect on COX-1 or COX-2, and its mechanism of analgesic effect probably relies on its biotransformation into diclofenac.[106]

KETOROLAC TROMETAMOL

Ketorolac is available in an injectable preparation and has been widely used for postoperative analgesia. It has high COX-1 selectivity[93] and a half-life of 2.4–8.6 hours.[90] It does not cross the blood–brain barrier.[107] Regulatory authority reviews following reports of a number of deaths have led several countries to suspend the drug's licence, or impose dose restrictions, concluding that ketorolac has a narrow therapeutic margin. In the UK, the use of ketorolac (by any route) is limited to two days. In the USA, the limit is five days.[107]

ETODOLAC

Etodolac displays moderate selectivity for COX-2.[108] It has a low incidence of gastrointestinal side effects, and has minimal hepatic and renal effects.[109] It is used in the treatment of arthritis.

SULINDAC

Sulindac is a racemic NSAID with a chiral sulfur atom. Sulindac is inactive and is converted to its active sulfide metabolite in the liver, bypassing the gastrointestinal mucosa. It carries an intermediate risk of gastrointestinal side effects (lower than aspirin),[86] but has minimal effects on renal function[110] and the CNS. However, it is much more likely to cause pancreatitis[111] and hepatocellular damage[37, 105] than other NSAIDs.

INDOMETACIN

Indometacin is a methylated indole derivative with a half-life of 4.5–6 hours. It is recommended for the treatment of arthritis and gout, although has too many side effects to be used as the NSAID of first choice for analgesia (with the exception of some topical preparations). CNS symptoms are frequent and include headaches, dizziness, and depression. Its use in acute gout and dysmenorrhea is well tolerated because the duration of treatment is limited to a few days. Acemetacin is the glycolic acid ester of indometacin.[100]

NABUMETONE

Nabumetone is a nonacidic prodrug, which is rapidly metabolized to its active form, 6-methoxy-2-naphthyl-acetic acid (6-MNA), which has a long half-life (22.5–30 hours).[90] It has a better gastrointestinal safety profile than other NSAIDs (e.g. naproxen, diclofenac, piroxicam, aspirin, indometacin, ibuprofen) with a lower risk of causing ulcers, bleeding, and perforations.[112] It has minimal effects on renal function.[110]

Fenamates

The fenamates are derivatives of anthranilic acid. This class includes mefenamic acid, tolfenamic acid and flufenamic acid.

MEFENAMIC ACID

Mefenamic acid has a half-life of three to four hours.[90] It is traditionally prescribed for dysmenorrhea, although there is no evidence that it is superior to ibuprofen.[113] Thrombocytopenia, hemolytic anemia, and aplastic anemia have all been reported. It also causes CNS toxicity, particularly convulsions in overdose.[100]

Oxicams

The oxicam class includes piroxicam, meloxicam, and tenoxicam. All three have long-half-lives, which allows once-daily dosing. However, several days are required to reach steady state. Loading doses may be required.

PIROXICAM

Piroxicam has a very long half-life (30–86 hours).[90] It carries a high risk of gastrointestinal side effects[86] and is associated with a significant rate of skin reactions. Topical and injectable preparations are available, although the injectable preparation is irritant. Piroxicam betadex is a formulation of piroxicam in beta cyclodextrin, which offers enhanced speed of onset, but does not improve its gastrointestinal tolerability.[107]

MELOXICAM

Meloxicam is moderately preferential for COX-2[93, 114] and is therefore often considered alongside COX-2 inhibitors in advice issued by regulatory bodies. Meloxicam undergoes extensive biliary excretion and has a half-life of 13–20 hours.[90]

TENOXICAM

Tenoxicam has a half-life of 60 hours.[90] An injectable preparation is available. A randomized controlled trial showed that tenoxicam is well tolerated when used as a post-operative analgesic, but may slightly increase the risk of bleeding following otorhinolaryngological surgery.[61]

COX–2 selective agents

There is some evidence to suggest that administration of selective COX-2 inhibitors may be safe in patients who have displayed anaphylactoid reactions to traditional NSAIDs.[45, 115] Celecoxib, valdecoxib, and parecoxib all contain a sulfonamide moiety in their chemical structure, which may provoke allergic responses, especially in those who are allergic to other sulfonamides ("sulfa drugs").

ROFECOXIB

Rofecoxib was withdrawn worldwide by the manufacturer in September 2004 following the discovery of increased risk of cardiovascular events during long-term use.

VALDECOXIB

Valdecoxib was withdrawn in Europe and the USA by the manufacturer in 2005, following concerns about the comparatively high rates of adverse drug reactions, notably serious skin reactions including Stevens–Johnson syndrome and toxic epidermal necrolysis.[116]

PARECOXIB

Parecoxib is an injectable prodrug of valdecoxib. It is rapidly converted into valdecoxib by enzymatic hydrolysis in the liver. Cutaneous reactions are rare with short-term therapy. Parecoxib will precipitate if mixed with lactated Ringer's solution. The combined use of parecoxib and valdecoxib after coronary artery bypass grafting was associated with an increased risk of cardiovascular events, including myocardial infarction, cardiac arrest, stroke, and pulmonary embolism.[50] Parecoxib and valdecoxib are associated with a slightly increased risk of renal dysfunction, hypertension, and peripheral edema.[117]

ETORICOXIB

Etoricoxib has a long half-life (22 hours) and is suitable for once-daily dosing in the treatment of arthritic and musculoskeletal problems. It carries a low risk of gastro-intestinal side effects,[118] but may be associated with more frequent and severe effects on blood pressure than other COX-2 inhibitors, particularly at high dose.[57, 119]

CELECOXIB

Celecoxib displays only moderate COX-2 selectivity, similar to etodolac, meloxicam, and nimesulide.[102] Its gastrointestinal safety profile has not been consistently demonstrated to be better than that of diclofenac,[119, 120] but meta-analysis of trials suggests it is associated with a significantly lower risk of both renal dysfunction and hypertension compared with controls taking traditional NSAIDs.[117] Confusion, somnolence, and insomnia have all been reported with its use.[107]

LUMIRACOXIB

Lumiracoxib is an arylacetic acid derivative with a structure very similar to that of diclofenac and lacks the sulfur-containing group of the other coxibs. It binds to the COX-2 enzyme at a different site and displays very high COX-2 selectivity.[102] Lumiracoxib has fewer gastro-intestinal side effects than diclofenac, although its kinetics are similar. It has a rapid onset of activity and good analgesic properties. A large randomized controlled study of lumiracoxib versus ibuprofen and naproxen showed a three- to four-fold reduction in ulcer complications in the lumiracoxib group when compared with either of the other NSAIDs, without an increase in cardiovascular events. 2.6 percent of patients developed an increase in liver enzymes, although this proportion is lower than with diclofenac.[33] However, lumiracoxib has recently been withdrawn because of suspected adverse liver reactions.

NIMESULIDE

Nimesulide has moderate COX-2 selectivity;[102] however, it is a sulfonanilide derivative unrelated chemically to coxibs and NSAIDs. Although it is widely prescribed worldwide, many countries including the UK and USA have not approved or have withdrawn the drug amid concerns about its hepatotoxicity.[37]

ACKNOWLEDGMENTS

This chapter is adapted and expanded from Manning DC and Richer B. Clinical pharmacology: nonsteroidal anti-inflammatory drugs. In: Rowbotham DJ and Macintyre PE (eds). *Clinical Pain Management: Acute Pain*. London: Hodder Arnold, p. 55–72.

REFERENCES

1. Warner TD, Vojnovic I, Giuliano F *et al.* Cyclooxygenases 1, 2, and 3 and the production of prostaglandin I2: investigating the activities of acetaminophen and cyclooxygenase-2-selective inhibitors in rat tissues. *Journal of Pharmacology and Experimental Therapeutics.* 2004; **310**: 642–7.
2. Rang HP, Dale MM, Ritter JM, Moore PK. *Pharmacology*, 5th edn. London: Churchill Livingstone, 2003.
3. Todd PA, Sorkin EM. Diclofenac sodium: a reappraisal of its pharmacodynamic and pharmacokinetics properties and therapeutic efficacy. *Drugs.* 1988; **35**: 244–85.
4. Marzo A, Dal Bo L, Verga F *et al.* Pharmacokinetics of diclofenac after oral administration of its potassium salt in sachet and tablet formulations. *Ärztliche Forschung.* 2000; **50**: 43–7.
5. Brooks PM, Day RO. Nonsteroidal anti-inflammatory drugs: differences and similarities. *New England Journal of Medicine.* 1991; **324**: 1716–25.
6. Day RO, Graham GG, Williams KM *et al.* Clinical pharmacology of NSAIDs. *Pharmacology and Therapeutics.* 1987; **33**: 383–433.
7. Jeremy JY, Williams JD. Prodrugs: the answer to NSAID-induced gastropathy? *Journal of Drug Delivery.* 1990; **3**: 93–107.
8. Furst DE. Are there differences among nonsteroidal anti-inflammatory drugs? *Arthritis and Rheumatism.* 1994; **37**: 1–9.
9. Verbeck RK, Wallace SM, Loewen GR. Reduced elimination of ketoprofen in the elderly is not necessarily due to impaired glucuronidation. *British Journal of Clinical Pharmacology.* 1984; **17**: 783–8.
10. Meffin PJ. The effect of renal dysfunction on the disposition of nonsteroidal anti-inflammatory drugs forming acyl-glucuronides. *Agents and Actions.* 1985; **17** (Suppl.): 85–9.
11. Grubb NG, Rudy DW, Brater DC, Hall SD. Stereoselective pharmacokinetics of ketoprofen and ketoprofen glucuronide in end-stage renal disease: evidence for a "futile cycle" of elimination. *British Journal of Clinical Pharmacology.* 1999; **48**: 494–500.
12. Holdgate A, Pollock T. Nonsteroidal anti-inflammatory drugs (NSAIDs) versus opioids for acute renal colic. *Cochrane Database of Systematic Reviews.* 2005; **CD004137**.
13. Marjoribanks J, Procter ML, Farquar C. Non-steroidal anti-inflammatory drugs for primary dysmenorrhoea. *Cochrane Database of Systematic Reviews.* 2003; **CD001751**.

＊ 14. Australian and New Zealand College of Anaesthetists and Faculty of Pain Medicine. *Acute pain management: scientific evidence*, 2nd edn. Melbourne: Australian and New Zealand College of Anaesthetists and Faculty of Pain Medicine, 2005.

＊ 15. Royal College of Surgeons and College of Anaesthetists. *Report of the working party on pain after surgery.* London: Royal College of Surgeons and College of Anaesthetists, 1990.

＊ 16. Rømsing J, Møiniche S. A systematic review of COX-2 inhibitors compared with traditional NSAIDs or different COX-2 inhibitors for postoperative pain. *Acta Anaesthesiologica Scandinavica.* 2004; **48**: 525–46.

＊ 17. Kehlet H. Postoperative pain relief – what is the issue? *British Journal of Anaesthesia.* 1994; **72**: 375–8.

＊ 18. Marret E, Kurdi O, Zufferey P, Bonnet F. Effects of nonsteroidal anti-inflammatory drugs on patient-controlled analgesia morphine side effects: meta-analysis of randomized controlled trials. *Anesthesiology.* 2005; **102**: 1249–60.

＊ 19. Royal College of Anaesthetists. *Guidelines for the use of non-steroidal anti-inflammatory drugs in the perioperative period.* London: Royal College of Anaesthetists, 1998.

20. Tighe KE, Webb AM, Hobbs GJ. Persistently high plasma morphine-6-glucuronide levels despite decreased hourly patient-controlled analgesia morphine use after single dose diclofenac: Potential for opioid-related toxicity. *Anesthesia and Analgesia.* 1999; **88**: 1137–42.

＊ 21. American Society of Anesthesiologists Task Force on Acute Pain Management. Practice guidelines for acute pain management in the perioperative setting. An updated report by the American Society of Anesthesiologists Task Force on acute pain management. *Anesthesiology.* 2004; **100**: 1573–81.

＊ 22. Fransen M, Neal B. Non-steroidal anti-inflammatory drugs for preventing heterotopic bone formation after hip arthroplasty. *Cochrane Database of Systematic Reviews.* 2004; **CD001160**.

＊ 23. Fransen M, Anderson C, Douglas J *et al.* Safety and efficacy of routine postoperative ibuprofen for pain and disability related to heterotopic bone formation after hip replacement surgery (HIPAID): randomised controlled trial. *British Medical Journal (Clinical research ed.).* 2006; **333**: 519–23.

24. Kimmel SE, Berlin JA, Kinman JL *et al.* Parenteral ketorolac and risk of myocardial infarction. *Pharmacoepidemiology and Drug Safety.* 2002; **11**: 113–19.

25. Beattie WS, Warriner CB, Etches R *et al.* The addition of ketorolac to a patient-controlled analgetic morphine regime reduced postoperative myocardial ischaemia in patients undergoing elective total hip or knee arthroplasty. *Anesthesia and Analgesia.* 1997; **84**: 715–22.

26. Colacchio TA, Yeager MP, Hildebrandt LW. Perioperative immunomodulation in cancer surgery. *American Journal of Surgery.* 1994; **167**: 174–9.

27. LeGrand EK, Rodgers KE, Girgis W *et al.* Comparative efficacy of nonsteroidal anti-inflammatory drugs and anti-thromboxane agents in a rabbit adhesion-prevention model. *Journal of Investigative Surgery.* 1995; **8**: 187–94.

28. Katz J. Current status of preemptive analgesia. *Current Opinion in Anaesthesiology.* 2002; **15**: 435–41.

29. Reuben SS, Ekman EF, Raghunathan K *et al.* The effect of cyclooxygenase-2 inhibition on acute and chronic donor-site pain after spinal-fusion surgery. *Regional Anesthesia and Pain Medicine.* 2006; **31**: 6–13.

30. Reuben SS, Ekman EF, Charron D. Evaluating the analgesic efficacy of administering celecoxib as a component of multimodal analgesia for outpatient anterior cruciate ligament reconstruction surgery. *Anesthesia and Analgesia.* 2007; **105**: 222–7.

31. Strom BL, Berlin JA, Kinman JL *et al.* Parenteral ketorolac and the risk of gastrointestinal and operative site bleeding. A postmarketing surveillance study. *Journal of the American Medical Association.* 1996; **275**: 376–82.

＊ 32. Bombardier C, Laine L, Reicin A *et al.* Comparison of upper gastrointestinal toxicity of rofecoxib and naproxen in patients with rheumatoid arthritis. *New England Journal of Medicine.* 2000; **343**: 1520–8.

33. Schnitzer TJ, Burmester GR, Mysler E *et al.* Comparison of lumiracoxib with naproxen and ibuprofen in the Therapeutic Arthritis and Gastrointestinal Event Trial (TARGET), reduction in ulcer complications: randomised controlled trial. *Lancet.* 2004; **364**: 665–74.

34. European Medicines Agency. Press release. European Medicines Agency concludes action on COX-2 inhibitors. Last updated June 21, 2005, cited February 2008. Available from: www.cbg-meb.nl/NR/rdonlyres/4E7814FF-5EF3-4F6A-8938-B223C8215948/0/20050627pbcox2review.pdf.

＊ 35. Rostom A, Dube C, Wells G *et al.* Prevention of NSAID-induced gastroduodenal ulcers. *Cochrane Database of Systematic Reviews.* 2002; **CD002296**.

＊ 36. Spiegel BMR, Farid M, Dulai GS *et al.* Comparing rates of dyspepsia with coxibs vs NSAID+PPI: A meta-analysis. *American Journal of Medicine.* 2006; **119**: e27–36.

＊ 37. Rubenstein JH, Laine L. Systematic review: the hepatotoxicity of non-steroidal anti-inflammatory drugs. *Alimentary Pharmacology and Therapeutics.* 2004; **20**: 373–80.

38. Sallie RW, Quinlan MF, McKenzie T *et al.* Diclofenac hepatitis. *Australian and New Zealand Journal of Medicine.* 1991; **21**: 251–5.

＊ 39. Whelton A. Clinical implications of nonopioid analgesia for relief of mild-to-moderate pain in patients with or at risk for cardiovascular disease. *American Journal of Cardiology.* 2006; **97**: 3–9.

40. Feldman HI, Kinman JL, Berlin JA *et al.* Parenteral ketorolac: the risk for acute renal failure. *Annals of Internal Medicine.* 1997; **126**: 193–9.

＊ 41. Lee A, Cooper MC, Craig JC, Keneally JP. Effects of nonsteroidal anti-inflammatory drugs on postoperative renal function in adults with normal renal function.

Cochrane Database of Systematic Reviews. 2004;
CD002765.

42. Jones SF, Ulyatt D. Ketorolac and renal impairment.
Anaesthesia and Intensive Care. 1994; **22**: 113–14.

43. Curtis SP, Ng J, Yu QF *et al*. Renal effects of etoricoxib and
comparator nonsteroidal anti-inflammatory drugs in
controlled clinical trials. *Clinical Therapeutics*. 2004; **24**:
70–83.

∗ 44. Power I. Aspirin-induced asthma. *British Journal of
Anaesthesia*. 1993; **71**: 619–21.

45. Gyllfors P, Bochenek G, Overholt J *et al*. Biochemical and
clinical evidence that aspirin intolerant asthmatic subjects
tolerate the cyclooxygenase 2-selective analgetic drug
celecoxib. *Journal of Allergy and Clinical Immunology*.
2003; **111**: 1116–21.

∗ 46. Kearney PM, Baigent C, Godwin J *et al*. Do selective cyclo-
oxygenase-2 inhibitors and traditional non-steroidal anti-
inflammatory drugs increase the risk of atherothrombosis?
Meta-analysis of randomised trials. *British Medical
Journal (Clinical research ed.)*. 2006; **332**: 1302–05.

∗ 47. Food and Drug Administration. Analysis and
recommendations for Agency action regarding NSAIDs and
cardiovascular risk. Last updated April 6, 2005, cited
February 2008. Available from: www.fda.gov/cder/drug/
infopage/COX2/NSAIDdecisionMemo.pdf.

48. McGettigan P, Henry D. Cardiovascular risk and inhibition
of cyclooxygenase: a systematic review of the
observational studies of selective and non-selective
inibitors of cyclooxygenase 2. *Journal of the American
Medical Association*. 2006; **296**: 1633–44.

∗ 49. Jones SF, Power I. Postoperative NSAIDs and COX-2
inhibitors: cardiovascular risks and benefits. *British
Journal of Anaesthesia*. 2005; **95**: 281–4.

∗ 50. Nussmeier NA, Whelton AA, Brown MT *et al*.
Complications of the COX-2 inhibitors parecoxib and
valdecoxib after cardiac surgery. *New England Journal of
Medicine*. 2005; **352**: 1081–91.

51. Ott E, Nussmeier NA, Duke PC *et al*. Efficacy and safety of
the cyclooxygenase 2 inhibitors parecoxib and valdecoxib
in patients undergoing coronary artery bypass surgery.
Journal of Thoracic and Cardiovascular Surgery. 2003;
125: 1481–92.

∗ 52. Nussmeier NA, Whelton A, Brar MT *et al*. Safety and
efficacy of the cyclooxygenase-2 inhibitors parecoxib and
valdecoxib after noncardiac surgery. *Anesthesiology*. 2006;
104: 518–26.

∗ 53. Antithrombotic Trialists' Collaboration. Collaborative
meta-analysis of randomised trials of antiplatelet therapy
for prevention of death, myocardial infarction, and stroke
in high risk patients. *British Medical Journal (Clinical
research ed.)*. 2002; **324**: 71–86.

54. Antman EM, Bennett JS, Daugherty A *et al*. Use of
nonsteroidal antiinflammatory drugs. An update for
clinicians. A scientific statement from the American Heart
Association. *Circulation*. 2007; **115**: 1634–42.

∗ 55. Johnson AG, Nguyen TV, Day RO. Do non-steroidal anti-
inflammatory drugs affect blood pressure? A

meta-analysis. *Annals of Internal Medicine*. 1994; **121**:
289–300.

∗ 56. Aw TJ, Haas SJ, Liew D, Krum H. Meta-analysis of
cyclooxygenase-2 inhibitors and their effects on blood
pressure. *Archives of Internal Medicine*. 2005; **165**:
490–6.

∗ 57. Committee on Safety of Medicines. Updated advice on the
safety of selective COX-2 inhibitors. Last updated 17
February, 2005, cited February 2008. Available from:
www.mhra.gov.uk/Safetyinformation/
Safetywarningsalertsandrecalls/
Safetywarningsandmessagesformedicines/CON1004250.

58. Garcia Rodriguez LA, Hernandez-Diaz S. Non-steroidal
anti-inflammatory drugs as a trigger of clinical heart
failure. *Epidemiology*. 2003; **14**: 240–6.

∗ 59. Marret E, Flahault A, Samama CM, Bonnet F. Effects of
postoperative, nonsteroidal anti-inflammatory drugs on
bleeding risk after tonsillectomy: meta-analysis of
randomized controlled trials. *Anesthesiology*. 2003; **98**:
1497–502.

∗ 60. Møiniche S, Rømsing J, Dahl J *et al*. Non steroidal
antiinflammatory drugs and the risk of operative site
bleeding after tonsillectomy: a quantitative systematic
review. *Anesthesia and Analgesia*. 2003; **96**: 68–77.

61. Merry AF, Webster CS, Holland RL *et al*. Clinical tolerability
of perioperative tenoxicam in 1001 patients – a
prospective, controlled, double-blind, multi-centre study.
Pain. 2004; **111**: 313–22.

∗ 62. Cardwell M, Siviter G, Smith A. Non-steroidal anti-
inflammatory drugs and perioperative bleeding in
paediatric tonsillectomy. *Cochrane Database of
Systematic Reviews*. 2005; **CD003591**.

63. Sonksen JR, Kong KL, Holder R. Magnitude and time course
of impaired primary haemostasis after stopping chronic
low and medium dose aspirin in healthy volunteers. *British
Journal of Anaesthesia*. 1999; **82**: 360–5.

64. Jimenez AH, Stubbs ME, Tofler GH *et al*. Rapidity and
duration of platelet suppression by enteric coated aspirin
in healthy young men. *American Journal of Cardiology*.
1992; **69**: 258–62.

65. Cahill RA, McGreal GT, Crowe BH *et al*. Duration of
increased bleeding tendency after cessation of aspirin
therapy. *Journal of the American College of Surgeons*.
2005; **200**: 564–73.

66. Albaladejo P, Geeraerts T, Fady F *et al*. Aspirin withdrawal
and acute lower limb ischaemia. *Anesthesia and
Analgesia*. 2004; **99**: 440–3.

67. Hoppmann RA, Peden JG, Ober SK. Central nervous system
side effects of nonsteroidal anti-inflammatory
drugs: aseptic meningitis, psychosis and cognitive
dysfunction. *Archives of Internal Medicine*. 1991; **151**:
1309–13.

68. Marquette CH, Joseph M, Tonnel AB *et al*. The abnormal in
vitro response to aspirin of platelets from aspirin-sensitive
asthmatics is inhibited after inhalation of nedocromil
sodium but not of sodium cromoglycate. *British Journal of
Clinical Pharmacology*. 1990; **29**: 525–31.

* 69. Onder G, Pellicciotti F, Gambassi G, Bernabei R. NSAID-related psychiatric adverse events: who is at risk? Drugs. 2004; **64**: 2619–27.

* 70. Harder AT, An YH. The mechanisms of inhibitory effects of non-steroidal anti-inflammatory drugs on bone healing: a concise review. *Journal of Clinical Pharmacology*. 2003; **43**: 807–15.

* 71. Busti AJ, Hooper JS, Amaya CJ, Kazi S. Effects of perioperative antiinflammatory and immunomodulating therapy on surgical wound healing. *Pharmacotherapy*. 2005; **25**: 1566–91.

72. Reuben SS, Ablett D, Kaye R. High dose non-steroidal anti-inflammatory drugs compromise spinal fusion. *Canadian Journal of Anaesthesia*. 2005; **52**: 506–12.

73. Lardinois D, Vogt P, Yang L et al. Non-steroidal anti-inflammatory drugs decrease the quality of pleurodesis after mechanical pleural abrasion. *European Journal of Cardiothoracic Surgery*. 2004; **25**: 865–71.

74. Kahn LH, Styrt B. Necrotizing soft tissue infections reported with nonsteroidal anti-inflammatory drugs. *Annals of Pharmacotherapy*. 1997; **31**: 1034–9.

75. Short JA, Barr CA, Palmer CD et al. Use of diclofenac in children with asthma. *Anaesthesia*. 2000; **55**: 334–7.

76. University of Cape Town. Porphyria service. Available from: http://web.uct.ac.za/depts/porphyria/professional/prof-home.htm.

77. Jaquenod M, Ronnedh C, Cousins MJ et al. Factors influencing ketorolac-associated perioperative renal dysfunction. *Anesthesia and Analgesia*. 1998; **86**: 1090–7.

78. Hosaka EM, Braz J. Effect of cyclooxygenase inhibitors on gentamicin-induced nephrotoxicity in rats. *Brazilian Journal of Medical and Biological Research*. 2004; **37**: 979–85.

79. Battistella M, Mamdami MM, Juurlink DN et al. Risk of upper gastrointestinal hemorrhage in warfarin users treated with nonselective NSAIDs or COX-2 inhibitors. *Archives of Internal Medicine*. 2005; **165**: 189–92.

80. MacDonald TM, Wei L. Effect of ibuprofen on cardio-protective effect of aspirin. *Lancet*. 2003; **361**: 573–4.

* 81. Catella-Lawson F, Reilly MP, Kapoor SC et al. Cyclooxygenase inhibitors and the antiplatelet effects of aspirin. *New England Journal of Medicine*. 2001; **345**: 1809–17.

* 82. US Food and Drug Administration. New information for healthcare professionals. Concomitant use of ibuprofen and aspirin. Last updated 6 September 2006, cited February 2008. Available from: www.fda.gov/cder/drug/InfoSheets/HCP/ibuprofen_aspirinHCP.htm.

83. Hyllested M, Jones S, Pedersen JL, Kehlet H. Comparative effect of paracetamol, NSAIDs or their combination in postoperative pain management: a qualitative review. *British Journal of Anaesthesia*. 2002; **88**: 199–214.

* 84. McCormack K, Brune K. Dissociation between the antinociceptive and anti-inflammatory effects of the nonsteroidal anti-inflammatory drugs. *Drugs*. 1991; **41**: 533–47.

85. Medicines Control Agency/Committee on the Safety of Medicines. Nonsteroidal anti-inflammatory drugs and gastrointestinal safety. *Current Problems in Pharmacovigilance*. 2002; **28**: 5.

* 86. Henry D, Lim LLY, Garcia Rodriguez LA et al. Variability in risk of gastrointestinal complications with individual non-steroidal anti-inflammatory drugs: results of a collaborative meta-analysis. *British Medical Journal (Clinical research ed.)*. 1996; **312**: 1563–6.

* 87. McQuay H, Moore A. Topically applied non-steroidal anti-inflammatory drugs. In: McQuay H, Moore A (eds). *An evidence-based resource for pain relief*. Oxford: Oxford University Press, 1998: 102–17.

88. Goetz CG. *Textbook of clinical neurology*, 2nd edn. Philadelphia: Saunders, 2003.

89. McGovern MC, Glasgow JF, Stewart MC. Lesson of the week: Reye's syndrome and aspirin: lest we forget. *British Medical Journal (Clinical research ed.)*. 2001; **322**: 1591–2.

* 90. Davies NM, Skjodt NM. Choosing the right nonsteroidal anti-inflammatory drug for the right patient: A pharmacokinetic approach. *Clinical Pharmacokinetics*. 2000; **38**: 377–92.

91. Wong A. *A reappraisal of antipyretic and analgesic drugs. WHO Pharmaceuticals Newsletter No. 1*. Geneva: World Health Organization, 2002.

92. Doll R, Lunde PK, Moeschlin S. Analgesics, agranulocytosis and aplastic anaemia. *Lancet*. 1987; **1**: 101.

* 93. Warner TD, Giuliano F, Vojnovic I et al. Nonsteroid drug selectivities for cyclo-oxygenase-1 rather than cyclo-oxygenase-2 are associated with human gastrointestinal toxicity: A full in vitro analysis. *Proceedings of the National Academy of Sciences of the United States of America*. 1999; **96**: 7563–8.

94. Kellstein DE, Waksman JA, Furey SA et al. The safety profile of non-prescription ibuprofen in multiple-dose use: a meta-analysis. *Journal of Clinical Pharmacology*. 1999; **39**: 520–32.

95. Volans G, Monaghan J, Colbridge M. Ibuprofen overdose. *International Journal of Clinical Practice*. 2003; **135** (Suppl.): 54–60.

96. Beaver WT. Review of the analgesic efficacy of ibuprofen. *International Journal of Clinical Practice*. 2003; **135** (Suppl.): 13–17.

97. Grubb NG, Rudy DW, Brater DC et al. Stereoselective pharmacokinetics of ketoprofen and ketoprofen glucuronide in end-stage renal disease: evidence for a 'futile cycle' of elimination. *British Journal of Clinical Pharmacology*. 1999; **48**: 494–500.

98. McGee AM, Davison PM. Skin necrosis following injection of non-steroidal anti-inflammatory drug. *British Journal of Anaesthesia*. 2002; **88**: 139–40.

99. Hindsen M, Zimerson E, Bruze M. Photoallergic contact dermatitis from ketoprofen in southern Sweden. *Contact Dermatitis*. 2006; **54**: 150–7.

100. Mehta DK (ed.). *British National Formulary*, 52nd edn. London: RPS Publishing, 2006.

*101. Mason L, Edwards JE, Moore RA, McQuay HJ. Single dose oral naproxen and naproxen sodium for acute postoperative pain. *Cochrane Database of Systematic Reviews*. 2004; **CD004234**.

102. Esser R, Berry C, Du Z *et al.* Preclinical pharmacology of lumiracoxib: a novel selective inhibitor of cyclooxygenase-2. *British Journal of Pharmacology*. 2005; **144**: 538–50.

103. Crawford MLA, Waller PC, Wood SM. Severe cystitis associated with tiaprofenic acid. *British Journal of Urology*. 1997; **79**: 578–84.

104. Sasada M, Smith S. *Drugs in anaesthesia and intensive care*, 3rd edn. Oxford: Oxford University Press, 2003.

105. O'Connor N, Dargan PI, Jones AL. Hepatocellular damage from non-steroidal anti-inflammatory drugs. *Quarterly Journal of Medicine*. 2003; **96**: 787–91.

106. Hinz B, Rau T, Auge D *et al.* Aceclofenac spares cyclooxygenaseas a result of limited but sustained biotransformation to diclofenac. *Clinical Pharmacology and Therapeutics*. 2003; **74**: 222–35.

107. Sweetman SC (ed.). *Martindale: the complete drug reference*, 35th edn. London: Pharmaceutical Press, 2006.

108. Glaser KB. Cyclooxygenase selectivity and NSAIDs: Cyclooxygenase-2 selectivity of etodolac. *Inflammopharmacology*. 1995; **3**: 335–45.

109. Jones RA. Etodolac: An overview of a selective COX-2 inhibitor. *Inflammopharmacology*. 1999; **7**: 269–75.

110. Cangiano JL, Figueroa J, Palmer R. Renal hemodynamic effects of nabumetone, sulindac and placebo in patients with osteoarthritis. *Clinical Therapeutics*. 1999; **21**: 503–12.

111. Trivedi CD, Pitchumoni CS. Drug-induced pancreatitis: an update. *Journal of Clinical Gastroenterology*. 2005; **39**: 709–16.

112. Huang JQ, Sridhar S, Hunt RH. Gastrointestinal safety profile of nabumetone: a meta-analysis. *American Journal of Medicine*. 1999; **107**: 55S–64.

113. Moore A, Edwards J, Barden J, McQuay H. *Bandolier's little book of pain*. Oxford: Oxford University Press, 2003: 144–6.

114. Sharpe P, Thomson J. Non-steroidal anti-inflammatory drugs. *Royal College of Anaesthetists Bulletin*. 2001; **6**: 265–8.

115. Quiralte J, Delgado J, Saenz de San Pedro B *et al.* Safety of the new selective cyclo-oxygenase type 2 inhibitors rofecoxib and celecoxib in patients with anaphylactoid reactions to nonsteroidal anti-inflammatory drugs. *Annals of Allergy, Asthma and Immunology*. 2004; **93**: 360–4.

116. Medicines and Healthcare products Regulatory Agency. Voluntary suspension of valdecoxib by Pfizer Ltd. Last updated April 7 2005, cited February 2008. Available from: www.mhra.gov.uk/Safetyinformation/ Safetywarningsalertsandrecalls/ Safetywarningsandmessagesformedicines/CON1004244.

117. Zhang J, Ding EL, Song Y. Adverse effects of cyclooxygenase 2 inhibitors on renal and arrhythmia events- meta-analysis of randomized trials. *Journal of the American Medical Association*. 2006; **296**: 1619–32.

118. Cochrane DJ, Jarvis B, Keating GM. Etoricoxib. *Drugs*. 2002; **62**: 2637–51.

*119. Clinical Knowledge Summaries. PRODIGY guidance: nonsteroidal anti-inflammatory drugs (NSAIDs). Newcastle-upon-Tyne: CKS, last updated January 2008, cited February 2008. Available from: www.prodigy.nhs.uk/ nsaids/view_whole_guidance.

120. Ashcroft DM, Chapman SR, Clark WK *et al.* Upper gastroduodenal ulceration in arthritis patients treated with celecoxib. *Annals of Pharmacotherapy*. 2001; **35**: 829–34.

5

Clinical pharmacology: paracetamol and compound analgesics

PHIL WIFFEN

KEY LEARNING POINTS

- Paracetamol is widely used in the treatment of mild to moderate pain and fever.
- Paracetamol is remarkably safe when used at recommended doses; however, deliberate or accidental overdoses are not uncommon.
- Paracetamol is a major metabolite of phenacetin and acetanilide.
- Paracetamol is readily absorbed from the gastrointestinal tract, reaching peak plasma concentrations after approximately 30–60 minutes with a plasma half-life of about two hours.
- Many compound medicines contain paracetamol; patients can be unaware that a medicine contains paracetamol and inadvertently exceed the maximum dose.
- For oral paracetamol 1 g, the numbers needed to treat (NNT) for a 50 percent reduction in acute

pain is 3.8 (95 percent confidence intervals 3.4–4.4).
- Codeine 8 mg adds more to adverse effects than to the analgesic benefit. The addition of codeine at higher doses adds to the analgesia of both paracetamol and codeine synergistically. The NNT (95 percent CI) for at least 50 percent pain relief for paracetamol 1 g plus codeine 60 mg is 2.2 (1.7–2.9).
- There are two forms of paracetamol available for intravenous (i.v.) use. The oldest is propacetamol which provides a 1 g dose of paracetamol in a 2 g propacetamol dose. The second is a form of i.v. paracetamol. 1 g paracetamol i.v. is equivalent to 2 g propacetamol i.v.
- Rectal administration is unreliable.

INTRODUCTION

Paracetamol (acetaminophen) is a popular analgesic and antipyretic compound that is used for the relief of fever, headaches, and other minor aches and pains. It is remarkably safe when used at recommended doses; however, deliberate or accidental overdoses are not

uncommon, probably due to its wide availability. It is not restricted to either prescription or pharmacies in most countries. Paracetamol has no anti-inflammatory properties, unlike aspirin and ibuprofen, and so is not considered a member of the class of nonsteroidal anti-inflammatory drugs (NSAID). It does not cause euphoria or alter mood in any way and is free of the problems of addiction, dependence, tolerance, and withdrawal.

The US Approved Name (USAN) is acetaminophen; paracetamol is both the (International Nonproprietary Name (INN) and the British Approved Name (BAN)), the INN term paracetamol will be used in this chapter.

HISTORICAL INFORMATION

In the late nineteenth century, analgesics and antipyretics consisted of preparations of natural compounds such as cinchona bark (quinine) or medicines based on willow bark, the earliest source of salicylate. Cinchona bark was in short supply and so cheaper, synthetic agents were required. Alternatives that were developed included acetanilide in 1886 and phenacetin in 1887; both of these were considered superior to quinine as they demonstrated antipyretic and analgesic properties. Initially, paracetamol was found in the urine of patients who had taken phenacetin and, in 1889, it was demonstrated that paracetamol was a urinary metabolite of acetanilide. However, these discoveries failed to attract much attention and were largely ignored at the time.

In 1948, the work of Brodie and Axelrod[1] established that paracetamol was a major metabolite of both phenacetin and acetanilide. The words acetaminophen and paracetamol both come from the chemical names for the compound: N-*acety*l-para-*aminophen*ol and *para-acetyl-amin*o-phen*ol*. The product first went on sale in the USA in 1955 under the brand name Tylenol®. In 1956, 500 mg tablets of paracetamol went on sale in the UK under the trade name Panadol. It was originally available only by prescription for the relief of pain and fever. In June 1958, a children's formulation (Panadol Elixir) was released. Subsequent formulations included suppositories, melt tablets, rapid release preparations, and injectable forms. The profile of paracetamol is shown in **Table 5.1**.

AVAILABLE PREPARATIONS

Paracetamol is available worldwide. For example:

- North America:[2] Acetaminophen tablets (USA and Canada) 325 and 500 mg. Acetaminophen oral solution or suspension (USA and Canada) 160 mg/ 5 mL or drops 160 mg/1.6 mL. Acetaminophen suppositories: 120, 325, 650 mg.
- UK:[3] Paracetamol tablets 500 mg, paracetamol soluble tablets 500 mg, 120 mg (pediatric), paracetamol oral suspension 120 mg/5 mL and 250 mg/5 mL. Paracetamol suppositories 60, 125, 250, 500 mg. Paracetamol intravenous infusion 10 mg/mL, 100 mL.
- Australia:[4] Paracetamol tablets 120 mg, 500 mg, paracetamol, paracetamol oral suspension 120 mg/ 5 mL. Paracetamol suppositories 125 mg.

Table 5.1 Profile of paracetamol.

Paracetamol (INN, BAN)	
Acetaminophen (USAN)	
N-acetyl-para-aminophenol	
Chemical formula	$C_8H_9NO_2$
Molecular weight	151.17
Bioavailability	Almost 100%
Metabolism	Hepatic
Elimination half-life	1–4 hours
Excretion	Renal

INDICATIONS

Paracetamol is widely used in the treatment of mild to moderate pain and fever. This includes headache, migraine, feverish conditions, period pain, toothache and other dental pain, back pain, muscular and joint pains, neuralgia, pains associated with colds and flu, and as an antipyretic. Paracetamol is the analgesic of choice in children (over aspirin), as it is not associated with Reye's syndrome. It is also preferred in the elderly as it lacks the gastric erosion properties of many NSAIDs. Paracetamol is readily available in most countries in retail outlets and pharmacies, as well as a prescribed medication. There are over 900 individual branded products of paracetamol available worldwide.[5]

DOSE

- Adults or children over 12 years of age: normally 500 mg to 1 g every four to six hours with a maximum of 4 g in any 24-hour period. There is a recommendation that self-administration should not exceed a period of ten days for adults or five days for children without seeking medical advice.
- Children: dose recommendations vary from country to country so it is important to check relevant resources; in general the recommendations are as follows:
  - Infants aged two to three months: a 60-mg paracetamol dose, as a liquid formulation, is suitable for babies with fever or mild to moderate pain provided the infant weighs over 4 kg and was not born before 37 weeks gestation. Medical advice should be sought promptly if further doses are required or if the cause of the infant's fever or pain is not known.
  - Infants three months to under one year: 60–120 mg paracetamol, as a liquid formulation, repeated every four hours, if necessary, up to a maximum of four doses per 24 hours.
  - Children aged one to <six years: 120–240 mg paracetamol, repeated every four hours, if

necessary, up to a maximum of four doses per 24 hours.

– Children aged 6–12 years: 250–500 mg paracetamol, repeated every four hours, if necessary, up to a maximum of four doses per 24 hours.

PREGNANCY AND LACTATION

Paracetamol is considered to be the analgesic of choice in pregnancy and is widely considered to be safe at recommended doses, though most manufacturers provide various cautions about seeking medical advice. Two case control studies (over 7500 mothers) from Boston University have shown that up to 65 percent of pregnant women use paracetamol.[6] A UK-based study also demonstrated use of paracetamol during all stages of pregnancy.[7] Paracetamol is excreted in breast milk, but not in a clinically significant amount. Available published data do not contraindicate breast feeding.[3]

EXTENT OF USE

Prescribing data for the calendar year of 2005 in England reveal that prescriptions for approximately 1.3 billion tablets of paracetamol were dispensed.[8] This equates to approximately 40 tablets for every man, woman, and child. The same source shows that 0.5 billion co-codamol (paracetamol 500 mg and codeine 8 mg) and 0.3 billion co-proxamol were also dispensed. There will be an additional unknown volume for paracetamol and co-codamol as these are available as over-the-counter (OTC) products.

MECHANISM OF ACTION

Paracetamol is an analgesic and antipyretic agent with weak anti-inflammatory properties. The mechanism of action of paracetamol is poorly understood. There have been some reports that the action is linked to cyclooxygenase (COX) isoenzymes with recent postulation of paracetamol action on a COX-3 isoenzyme,[9] but this is uncertain.

PHARMACOKINETICS

Paracetamol is readily absorbed from the gastrointestinal tract, reaching peak plasma concentrations after approximately 30–60 minutes with a plasma half-life of about two hours. There are now several instant-release products available which produce faster plasma concentrations. Paracetamol is distributed widely, crossing the placenta and is found in breast milk. Plasma-protein

binding is negligible at usual normal concentrations. Over 90 percent is excreted in the urine in the first day after conjugation in the liver as the glucuronate and sulfate salts.[10]

CONTRAINDICATIONS

There are few contraindications to the use of paracetamol. It is contraindicated in patients with severe hepatic disease and patients with known hypersensitivity to paracetamol, or any of the components contained in the formulation. Soluble tablets of paracetamol 500 mg can contain over 400 mg of sodium, which is significant for those on a regular daily maximum dose.

DRUG INTERACTIONS

Warfarin

A case–control study was conducted at the Massachusetts General Hospital in Boston[11, 12] in 2000 patients attending the anticoagulant therapy unit over a single year who had been on warfarin for at least one month, had a target international normalized ratio (INR) of 2 to 3, and were able to participate in a telephone interview. The study included those with an INR of greater than 6 (an increased risk of major hemorrhage) reported within 24 hours, whose target INR was 2 to 3; results were verified with a duplicate test. Controls were randomly selected from patients with lower INRs. Paracetamol was associated with increased risk of elevated INR. Taken mainly for acute pain, the more used in the week before the test, the greater the chance of a raised INR (**Figure 5.1**). More than nine 500-g tablets a week gave an odds ratio of 7 and more than 18 tablets a week an odds ratio of 10.

The clinical significance of these findings is a subject of much debate. There is no doubt that analgesia for those on warfarin becomes more difficult if paracetamol is not to be used, nor aspirin, nor NSAIDs. Paracetamol is preferable to NSAIDs, but it is wise to monitor patients with concomitant warfarin therapy some seven to ten days after starting paracetamol.

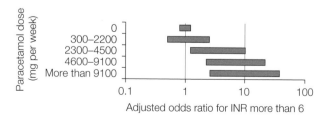

Figure 5.1 Paracetamol dose and risk of elevated INR above 6.

Alcohol

Some manufacturers and the FDA[13] recommend that patients who consume three units of alcohol per day or more are at greater risk of liver disease and should be advised accordingly. Over-the-counter preparations for analgesics in the USA have the following label: If you generally consume three or more alcohol-containing drinks per day you should consult your physician for advice on when and how you should take pain relievers.

Others

Caution may be needed with other medicines that are metabolized via the liver. These include antiepileptic agents and isoniazid.

ADVERSE EFFECTS

Adverse effects are rarely a problem. Drowsiness is regularly reported in randomized controlled trials (RCT) as an adverse effect, but often not mentioned in manufacturers' monographs.[14] A recent RCT[15] has demonstrated that a regular dose of paracetamol at 4 g daily is associated with raised aminotransferase (ALT).

EFFICACY OF ORAL ADMINISTRATION

Measuring efficacy

Efficacy is reported in a range of ways in RCTs. Probably the most unhelpful is the mean difference between two groups which only gives an indication of effect, but prevents useful measures such as NNTs being determined. In recent years, there has been an increasing trend to report a 50 percent reduction in total pain relief (TOTPAR). It was argued that this level was unlikely to be achieved by chance and that it was a significant outcome. A recent individual patient meta-analysis has added some validation to this outcome[16] and this measure of effectiveness is used where possible in this chapter.

Oral paracetamol as a single agent

Considering the amount of paracetamol consumed worldwide, the volume of high level evidence (type I or II) is modest, i.e. approximately 5000 participants in randomized controlled trials. Systematic review evidence is summarized in **Table 5.2**. The different numbers of participants in the reviews is due to different inclusion criteria set by the review authors.

Two systematic reviews[17, 19][I] look at single-dose studies of paracetamol compared to placebo. The later study[17] with stricter inclusion criteria provides NNTs (95 percent CI) as follows: 500 mg 3.5 (2.7–4.8), 650 mg 4.6 (3.9–5.5), 1 g 3.8 (3.4–4.4). The NNT for 1 g implies that for every four (actually 3.8) patients who receive a 1 g dose of paracetamol, one will get greater than 50 percent pain relief who would not have done so if they had received a placebo. It should be noted that the NNT for 500 mg is lower, but the confidence intervals are wider. This is simply a numbers issue – smaller studies give less certain results; the NNT for 500 mg will lie within the range of 2.7–4.8. Some additional reassurance about a dose response for paracetamol is provided by a systematic review by McQuay and Moore.[18][I]. This demonstrated that a greater number of patients gained benefit from a 1-g dose compared to a 600/650-mg dose (**Table 5.2**).

Three systematic reviews looked at osteoarthritis (OA) and rheumatoid arthritis (RA). These are included for completeness as both these chronic diseases have an acute pain component. One systematic review compares paracetamol with NSAIDs in rheumatoid arthritis.[21] It is not clear if the analgesic is for acute or chronic pain in this review. Apart from an expressed preference for NSAIDs, the studies are too small to draw firm conclusions. Two reviews[20, 22] demonstrate that, while paracetamol is better than placebo for pain relief of OA, the evidence is quite small and NSAIDs are in fact superior to paracetamol for pain relief.

There is also evidence from indirect comparisons. Systematic reviews have been used to build a league table of NNTs for a range of analgesics for mild or moderate pain; this puts paracetamol in the wider context and shows that NSAIDs and paracetamol with codeine perform better than paracetamol alone (**Table 5.3**). It should be remembered that there are associated disadvantages in terms of adverse effects with these agents compared with paracetamol.

Oral paracetamol and compound analgesics

Many compound medicines contain paracetamol and it regularly appears as an ingredient in cough and cold remedies. Patients can be unaware that a medicine contains paracetamol and inadvertently exceed the maximum dose by consuming more than one paracetamol-containing product. This needs to be remembered when taking medication histories. In developing countries, paracetamol is often combined with a wide range of other medicines limited only by the imagination of the manufacturer. Ten systematic reviews for combined paracetamol products have been identified (**Table 5.4**).

PARACETAMOL PLUS OPIOIDS

There are no known RCTs for the common formulation of paracetamol 500 mg and codeine 8 mg. There is general

Table 5.2 Systematic reviews of paracetamol as a single agent.

Author	Date of last search	Condition and doses used	Number of RCTs included and number of participants	Key findings
Barden et al.[17]	August 2001	Acute postoperative pain, single dose ranging from 325 mg to 1.5 g	47 RCTs, 2561 participants received paracetamol	NNTs (95% CI) for at least 50% pain relief were as follows: 325 mg: 3.8 (2.2–13.3); 500 mg: 3.5 (2.7–4.8); 600/650 mg: 4.6 (3.9–5.5) 1 g 3.8 (3.4–4.4) 1.5 g 3.7(2.3–9.5)
McQuay and Moor[18]	June 2005	Acute pain with direct comparisons of different doses of three analgesics: paracetamol, aspirin, and ibuprofen	50 RCTs (nine of paracetamol), paracetamol 4327 participants; aspirin 6056 participants; ibuprofen 6193 participants	Proportions achieving at least 50% pain relief were paracetamol 1 g: 62%; paracetamol 500 mg or 650 mg: 52%. The NNT (95% CI) for one additional patient to achieve more than 50% at the higher rather than the lower dose is 9 (6–29)
Moore et al.[19]	May 1996	Acute postoperative pain, moderate to severe. Single-dose paracetamol or paracetamol with codeine (see **Table 5.3**)	40 RCTs, 4171 participants	NNTs (95% CI) for at least 50% pain relief were as follows: paracetamol 1 g 4.6 (3.8–5.4) 600/650 mg: 5.3 (4.1–7.2)
Towheed et al.[20]	July 2005	Pain due to osteoarthritis. Effectiveness of paracetamol compared to placebo or NSAIDs	15 RCTs, 5986 participants. 7 compared paracetamol with placebo and 10 to NSAIDs. Median trial duration 6 weeks	NNT for paracetamol compared to placebo was 4–16 for improvement in pain. Paracetamol was less effective than NSAIDs
Wienecke and Gotzsche[21]	September 2003	Rheumatoid arthritis. Comparison of paracetamol and NSAIDs. Doses range	Four cross-over studies with 121 participants	Small numbers, so firm conclusions not possible. Generally NSAIDs were preferred by participants over paracetamol alone
Zhang et al.[22]	July 2003	Pain due to osteoarthritis. Effectiveness of paracetamol compared to placebo (two studies) or NSAIDs	10 RCTs 1712 participants, two studies compared paracetamol with placebo, eight compared paracetamol with NSAID	Paracetamol was superior to placebo, note wide CIs (effect size 0.21 (95% CI 0.02–0.41). NSAIDs were superior to paracetamol for pain relief (effect size 0.20 (95% CI 0.1–0.3)

consensus that the dose of codeine will add more to adverse effects than to the analgesic benefit. The addition of codeine at higher doses adds to the analgesia of both paracetamol and codeine synergistically. Codeine alone is a poor analgesic in acute pain;[32][I] however, when paracetamol 600/650 mg is combined with codeine 60 mg the NNT for 50 percent pain relief is 3.6 (2.9–4.5).[19][I] The NNT (95 percent CI) for at least 50 percent pain relief for paracetamol 1 g plus codeine 60 mg was 2.2 (1.7–2.9).[33] This compares well with NSAIDs, but participants reported significant constipation at these doses of codeine.

In 2005, the UK Medicine and Healthcare product Regulatory Agency[34] announced a gradual withdrawal of co-proxamol (dextropropoxyphene 32.5 mg and paracetamol 325 mg per tablet) from the UK market. This was done for safety and efficacy reasons. Fatal toxicity can occur with a small number of tablets (often as little as 15–20), particularly when taken with alcohol. Also, it was argued that the combination was no more effective than paracetamol alone. The combination is available in at least 15 other countries including the USA. There is no evidence of superiority over paracetamol 1 g in acute pain,[25] but it is preferred (anecdotally) by some patients for chronic use.

Table 5.3 Number needed to treat (NNT) for range of analgesics based on single-dose systematic reviews.

Analgesic (mg)	Number of patients in comparison	NNT	Lower confidence interval (95%)	Higher confidence interval (95%)
Aspirin 600/650	5061	4.4	4.0	4.9
Aspirin 650 and codeine 60	598	5.3	4.1	7.4
Codeine 60	1305	16.7	11.0	48.0
Diclofenac 100	411	1.9	1.6	2.2
Diclofenac 25	204	2.8	2.1	4.3
Diclofenac 50	738	2.3	2.0	2.7
Ibuprofen 200	1414	2.7	2.5	3.1
Ibuprofen 400	4703	2.4	2.3	2.6
Ibuprofen 600	203	2.4	2.0	4.2
Naproxen 440	257	2.3	2.0	2.9
Naproxen 550	500	2.6	2.2	3.2
Paracetamol 1000	2759	3.8	3.4	4.4
Paracetamol 1000 and codeine 60	197	2.2	1.7	2.9
Paracetamol 300 and codeine 30	379	5.7	4.0	9.8
Paracetamol 500	561	3.5	2.2	13.3
Paracetamol 600/650 and codeine 60	1123	4.2	3.4	5.3
Paracetamol 650 and dextropropoxyphene hydrochloride 65	963	4.4	3.5	5.6
Paracetamol 650 and tramadol 75	679	2.6	2.3	3.0
Piroxicam 20	280	2.7	2.1	3.8

Adapted from Ref. 23, with permission.

One systematic review[27] reports on the combination of paracetamol with oxycodone which seems to offer an improved NNT over paracetamol alone.

This combination is claimed to be the most popularly prescribed generic drug[35] in the USA. No systematic reviews of this combination could be identified. Four RCTs were identified.[36, 37, 38, 39] These include 230 participants receiving paracetamol 500 mg with hydrocodone 7.5 mg (two studies) and paracetamol 500 mg with hydrocodone 5 mg (two studies). The studies are small, but there is limited evidence to show that the combination is: (1) superior in terms of pain relief to tramadol 100 mg;[39][II] (2) superior to a paracetamol 300 mg plus codeine 30 mg combination;[38][II] (3) equivalent to a paracetamol 500 mg plus oxycodone 5 mg combination;[36] [II] and (4) inferior to an ibuprofen 400 mg plus oxycodone 5 mg combination.[37][II]

PARACETAMOL WITH NSAIDS

One systematic review included combinations of paracetamol with NSAIDs. The authors found eight studies comparing the combination with paracetamol alone and five studies comparing the combination with NSAID alone. Paracetamol was combined with either ketoprofen or diclofenac. The authors conclude that the combinations in general are superior to either single agent comparator, but data are sparse.[28][I]

Summary of evidence

Oral paracetamol can be an effective analgesic in dealing with mild to moderate acute pain. However, some patients will find this inadequate and will benefit from either the addition of an NSAID (if they can tolerate this) or a combination of paracetamol with codeine 30–60 mg. It seems reasonable therefore to start on paracetamol alone then add in another agent if pain relief is not achieved. This approach is developed further on the Bandolier website.[40]

OTHER ROUTES OF ADMINISTRATION

Intravenous

There are two forms of paracetamol available for intravenous use. The oldest is propacetamol which provides a 1 g dose of paracetamol in a 2 g propacetamol dose. The second is a form of i.v. paracetamol. No systematic reviews were identified, but 15 RCTs were found, two in children (223 participants) and 13 in a variety of postoperative pain settings in adults (1380 participants). In children, 1 g paracetamol i.v. was shown to be equivalent to 2 g propacetamol i.v.[41, 42] Children reported greater injection site pain with propacetamol.

Table 5.4 Systematic reviews of paracetamol in combination with other analgesics.

Author	Date of last search	Condition and doses used	No. RCTs included and no. participants	Key findings
Cepeda et al.[24]	August 2005	Osteoarthritis pain. Tramadol or tramadol 32.5 mg plus paracetamol 325 mg	11 RCTs and 1109 in total. 2 RCTs (350 participants) examined the combination	No clear results. All participants in these two studies were allowed to use COX-2 or NSAIDs. Authors conclude that paracetamol alone 1.5 g was superior to tramadol 150 mg
Collins et al.[25]	July 1998	Acute postoperative pain- moderate to severe. Single dose dextropropoxyphene with paracetamol 650 mg	6 RCTs (325 participants) and one individual patient meta-analysis (638 participants)	NNTs (95% CI) for at least 50% pain relief were as follows: 4.4 (3.5–5.6). Dextropropoxyphene (65 mg) alone: 7.7 (4.6–22)
De Craen et al.[26]	1995	Postoperative pain and pain in children. Paracetamol 400 to 1000 mg, codeine 10–60 mg	24 RCTs. No. participants not stated	Paracetamol plus codeine superior to paracetamol alone. Repeated use increases the occurrence of adverse effects. No studies were found on codeine 8 mg combined with paracetamol
Edwards et al.[27]	October 1999	Acute postoperative pain. Oxycodone or oxycodone with paracetamol. Paracetamol 325 mg with oxycodone 5 mg and paracetamol 650 mg (or 1000 mg) with oxycodone 10 mg included	7 RCTs. 483 participants on paracetamol and oxycodone	Paracetamol with oxycodone superior than placebo and associated with significantly more adverse effects. For single-dose oxycodone 5 mg plus paracetamol (325, 500, and 1000 mg) the NNT for at least 50% pain relief were 2.5 (2.0–3.4), 2.2 (1.7–3.2) and 3.9 (2.1–20), respectively, for moderate to severe postoperative pain over 4–6 hours. For single-dose oxycodone 10 mg plus paracetamol (650 or 1000 mg) the NNT for at least 50% pain relief were 2.5 (2.0–3.3) and 2.7 (1.7–5.6) for moderate to severe postoperative pain over 4–6 hours
Hyllested et al.[28]	January 2001	Postoperative pain. Paracetamol or NSAIDs or combination. Dose 1.3–4 g daily rectally, 500 mg–8 g daily orally and 2 g intravenously as propacetamol	36 double-blind RCTs. 3362 participants on active treatment	Combinations of paracetamol and NSAIDs were superior to paracetamol alone, but not to NSAIDs alone. No significant difference was shown between paracetamol alone and NSAID alone in major surgery or orthopedic surgery (8 RCTs, 668 participants). Note: doses of

(Continued over)

Source	Date	Focus	Trials/participants	Results
				different agents need to be considered; also some trials appear to be underpowered. Three studies looked at propacetamol (253 participants) but no results are presented.
Li Wan Po and Zhan[14]	March 1997	Post surgical pain, arthritis, and musculoskeletal pain. Paracetamol or paracetamol combined with dextropropoxyphene	27 trials, 2231 participants	In three trials (202 participants), the combination reduced pain intensity by 7% compared to paracetamol alone. The combination produced more dizziness (RR 3.1 95% CI 1.1–8.9) paracetamol alone produced more drowsiness (RR 1.8 95% CI 1.1–2.9)
McNicol et al.[29]	March 2003	NSAIDs or paracetamol alone combined with opioids for cancer pain	42 reports, 3084 participants	Little or no advantage of NSAIDs alone compared to NSAID plus opioid combinations. Six studies compared paracetamol alone or in combination with other treatments, but these are not analyzed separately
Moore et al.[19]	May 1996	Acute postoperative pain, moderate to severe. Single dose paracetamol with codeine	34 trials, 2200 participants	NNTs (95% CI) for at least 50% pain relief were as follows: paracetamol 600/650 mg plus codeine 60 mg 3.6 (2.9–4.5). Comparing paracetamol with the same dose of paracetamol plus codeine 60 mg the NNT was 7.7 (5.1–17). No studies were found on codeine 8 mg combined with paracetamol
Smith et al.[30]	March 2000	Acute postoperative pain. Single dose paracetamol 1 g with codeine 60 mg. High quality RCTs selected	Three trials, 197 participants	NNT (95% CI) for at least 50% pain relief for paracetamol 1 g plus codeine 60 mg 2.2 (1.7–2.9)
Zhang et al.[31]	May 1996	Postoperative pain. Paracetamol in combination with codeine and caffeine	Eighty trials containing 103 placebo comparisons and 26 head to head comparisons	Some evidence of the effects of combinations over paracetamol, but these may not be clinically significant. Caffeine was found to add little to the analgesic effect of paracetamol

NNT, number needed to treat; NSAID, nonsteroidal anti-inflammatory drugs; RCT, randomized controlled trials.

The key messages from the adult studies were: pro-pacetamol 2 g produces similar analgesia to intramuscular (i.m.) diclofenac 75 mg,[43] ketorolac 30 mg,[44] and morphine 10 mg i.m.[45] It produces a faster onset than oral paracetamol[46] and two doses of propacetamol 2 g were inferior to a single dose of parecoxib 40 mg i.v.[47]

Rectal

No systematic reviews were identified. Three RCTs (264 participants)[48, 49, 50] looked at postoperative pain in children. Evidence from larger studies suggests that paracetamol at a dose of 40 mg/kg rectally does not improve analgesia.[48, 50] Five RCTs[51, 52, 53, 54, 55] (420 participants) in adults suggests that paracetamol administered rectally (1 g dose) either during surgery or for postoperative pain is ineffective and inferior to other agents, such as diclofenac 75 mg rectally.[51]

OVERDOSE

Paracetamol toxicity is the leading cause of acute liver failure in a number of countries. A prospective cohort study in 2005 showed that of 275 case reports, 48 percent were unintentional, 44 percent were intentional and the rest unknown. The median dose ingested was 24 g, but constant use of as little as 7.5 g per day may be hazardous.[56][III]

Recommendations for treatment of acute paracetamol poisoning are more tried and tested, rather than evidence based. One Cochrane systematic review[57] (**Table 5.5**) assesses the evidence concluding that activated charcoal seems to have the best risk–benefit ratio, N-acetylcysteine is preferable to supportive treatment (dimercaprol and cysteamine). It is not clear whether N-acetylcysteine is superior to methionine. Several nomograms exist to asses the risk factors of a given ingested dose.[60, 61] Readers are advised to consult relevant poisons information centers for up to date information on treating acute paracetamol poisoning.

EVIDENCE RESOURCES

MEDLINE, EMBASE, and the Cochrane Library were used to search for relevant randomized controlled trials or systematic reviews.

Table 5.5 Systematic reviews of paracetamol: safety issues.

Author	Date of last search	Purpose of review	No. trials included and no. participants	Key findings
Brok et al.[57]	December 2005	Interventions for paracetamol overdose. Dose not applicable	10 small RCTs, 1 quasi-RCT and 48 observational trials. Includes some healthy volunteer studies. Approximately 850 participants in RCTs	Activated charcoal, gastric lavage and ipecacuanha are able to reduce absorption of paracetamol, but clinical benefit not demonstrated
Dart et al.[58]	November 1999	Assess the use of paracetamol in alcoholic patients to evaluate any hepatic injury. Dose 1–4 g daily	27 trials (2 RCTs, 1 prospective, rest were case studies). 315 participants excluding the case studies	RCTs: No deterioration in liver function or any clinical manifestations over 48-hour period. Prospective study: no adverse effects noted over 14-day period
Morgan and Majeed[59]	2003	Assessment of regulations issued in 1998 to restrict sales of paracetamol and their impact on poisoning	12 trials, all observational	There was an overall reduction in the volume of paracetamol sold. 3 studies in liver units reported a reduction in referrals; 3 studies reported a reduction in the severity of poisoning, while 5 studies reported no change; 5 studies reported a decrease in hospital admissions while 1 study reported no change. 2 studies reported no change in deaths due to paracetamol, 1 study reported a decrease

RCT, randomized controlled trials.

REFERENCES

1. Brodie B, Axelrod J. The fate of acetanilide in man. *Journal of Pharmacology and Experimental Therapeutics.* 1948; **94**: 29–38.

2. American Society of Health System Pharmacists. *AHFS drug information*, electronic version. 2006, Bethesda, MD: American Society of Health System Pharmacists. www.ashp.org/ahfs/index.cfm

3. Joint Formulary Committee. *British National Formulary 51st edn.* London: British Medical Association and Royal Pharmaceutical Society of Great Britain 2006.

4. Royal Australian College of General Practitioners (RACGP), Pharmaceutical Society of Australia (PSA), Australasian Society of Clinical and Experimental Pharmacologists and Toxicologists. *Australia medicines handbook, 2006 edition.* Adelaide: RACGP, 2006.

5. Sweetman S (ed.). *Martindale: the complete drug reference*, 34th edn. London: Pharmaceutical Press, 2004.

6. Werler M, Mitchell A, Hernandez-Diaz S, Honein M. Use of over-the-counter medications during pregnancy. *American Journal of Obstetrics and Gynecology.* 2005; **193**: 771–7.

7. Headley J, Northstone K, Simmons H *et al.* Medication use during pregnancy: data from the Avon Longitudinal Study of Parents and Children. *European Journal of Clinical Pharmacology.* 2004; **60**: 355–61.

8. Department of Health. Prescription statistics for England 2005. Cited September 2006. Available from: www.ic.nhs.uk/pubs/prescostanalysis2005.

9. Ayoub SC-N PR, Willoughby DA, Botting RM. The involvement of a cyclooxygenase 1 gene-derived protein in the antinociceptive action of paracetamol in mice. *European Journal of Pharmacology.* 2006; **538**: 57–65.

10. Brunton L, Parker K, Lazo J (eds). *Goodman and Gilman's pharmacological basis of therapeutics*, 11th edn. New York: McGraw-Hill, 2005.

11. Hylek EM, Heiman H, Skates SJ. Acetaminophen and other risk factors for excessive warfarin anticoagulation. *Journal of the American Medical Association.* 1998; **279**: 657–62.

12. Bell W. Acetaminophen and warfarin: undesirable synergy. *Journal of the American Medical Association.* 1998; **279**: 702–3.

13. Cruzan S. *FDA proposes alcohol warning for all OTC pain relievers.* Rockville MD: US Department of Health and Human Services, press release, 1997: P97–37.

14. Li Wan Po A, Zhang WY. Systematic overview of co-proxamol to assess analgesic effects of addition of dextropropoxyphene to paracetamol. *British Medical Journal.* 1997; **315**: 1565–71.

15. Watkins PB, Kaplowitz N, Slattery JT *et al.* Aminotransferase elevations in healthy adults receiving 4 grams of acetaminophen daily: a randomized controlled trial. *Journal of the American Medical Association.* 2006; **296**: 87–93.

16. Li Wan Po A, Petersen B. How high should total pain-relief score be to obviate the need for analgesic remedication in acute pain? Estimation using signal detection theory and individual patient meta-analysis. *Journal of Clinical Pharmacy and Therapeutics.* 2006; **31**: 161–5.

∗ 17. Barden J, Edwards J, Moore A, McQuay H. Single dose oral paracetamol (acetaminophen) for postoperative pain. *Cochrane Database of Systematic Reviews.* 2004; **CD004602.**

∗ 18. McQuay HJ, Moore RA. Dose-response in direct comparisons of different doses of aspirin, ibuprofen and paracetamol (acetaminophen) in analgesic studies. *British Journal of Clinical Pharmacy.* 2007; **63**: 271–8.

19. Moore A, Collins S, Carroll D, McQuay H. Paracetamol with and without codeine in acute pain: a quantitative systematic review. *Pain.* 1997; **70**: 193–201.

∗ 20. Towheed TE, Judd MJ, Hochberg MC, Wells G. Acetaminophen for osteoarthritis. *Cochrane Database of Systematic Reviews.* 2003; **CD004257.**

21. Wienecke T, Gotzsche PC. Paracetamol versus nonsteroidal anti-inflammatory drugs for rheumatoid arthritis. *Cochrane Database of Systematic Reviews.* 2004; **CD003789.**

22. Zhang W, Jones A, Doherty M. Does paracetamol (acetaminophen) reduce the pain of osteoarthritis? A meta-analysis of randomised controlled trials. *Annals of the Rheumatic Diseases.* 2004; **63**: 901–7.

∗ 23. Anon. Oxford league table of analgesics in acute pain. Oxford Pain Site, cited September 2006. Available from: www.jr2.ox.ac.uk/bandolier/booth/painpag/Acutrev/Analgesics/Leagtab.

24. Cepeda MS, Camargo F, Zea C, Valencia L. Tramadol for osteoarthritis. *Cochrane Database of Systematic Reviews.* 2006; **CD005522.**

25. Collins SL, Edwards JE, Moore RA, McQuay HJ. Single dose dextropropoxyphene, alone and with paracetamol (acetaminophen), for postoperative pain. *Cochrane Database of Systematic Reviews.* 2000; **CD001440.**

26. de Craen AJ, Di Giulio G, Lampe Schoenmaechers AJ *et al.* Analgesic efficacy and safety of paracetamol–codeine combinations versus paracetamol alone: a systematic review. *British Medical Journal.* 1996; **313**: 321–5.

27. Edwards JE, Moore RA, McQuay HJ. Single dose oxycodone and oxycodone plus paracetamol (acetominophen) for acute postoperative pain. *Cochrane Database of Systematic Reviews.* 2000; **CD002763.**

28. Hyllested M, Jones S, Pedersen JL, Kehlet H. Comparative effect of paracetamol, NSAIDs or their combination in postoperative pain management: a qualitative review. *British Journal of Anaesthesiology.* 2002; **88**: 199–214.

29. McNicol E, Strassels SA, Goudas L *et al.* NSAIDS or paracetamol, alone or combined with opioids, for cancer pain. *Cochrane Database of Systematic Reviews.* 2005; **CD005180.**

30. Smith LA, Moore RA, McQuay HJ, Gavaghan D. Using evidence from different sources: an example using paracetamol 1000 mg plus codeine 60 mg. *BMC Medical Research Methodology.* 2001; **1**: 1.

31. Zhang WY, Li Wan Po A. Analgesic efficacy of paracetamol and its combination with codeine and caffeine in surgical pain – a meta-analysis. *Journal of Clinical Pharmacy and Therapeutics.* 1996; **21**: 261–82.

32. Moore RA, McQuay HJ. Single-patient data meta-analysis of 3453 postoperative patients: oral tramadol versus placebo, codeine and combination analgesics. *Pain.* 1997; **69**: 287–94.

33. Smith LA, Moore RA, McQuay HJ, Gavaghan D. Using evidence from different sources: an example using paracetamol 1000 mg plus codeine 60 mg. *BMC Medical Research Methodology.* 2001; **1**: 1.

∗ 34. Medicines and Healthcare products Regulations Agency. Withdrawal of co-proxamol: reminder to prescribers. Cited September 2006. Available from: www.mhra.gov.uk.

35. Anonymous. Mallinckrodt pharamceuticals, generics. Cited September 2006. Available from: http://pharmaceuticals.mallinckrodt.com/GenericPharmaceuticals.

36. Marco CA, Plewa MC, Buderer N *et al.* Comparison of oxycodone and hydrocodone for the treatment of acute pain associated with fractures: a double-blind, randomized, controlled trial. *Academic Emergency Medicine.* 2005; **12**: 282–8.

37. Litkowski LJ, Christensen SE, Adamson DN *et al.* Analgesic efficacy and tolerability of oxycodone 5 mg/ibuprofen 400 mg compared with those of oxycodone 5 mg/acetaminophen 325 mg and hydrocodone 7.5 mg/acetaminophen 500 mg in patients with moderate to severe postoperative pain: a randomized, double-blind, placebo-controlled, single-dose, parallel-group study in a dental pain model. *Clinical Therapeutics.* 2005; **27**: 418–29.

38. Forbes JA, Bates JA, Edquist IA *et al.* Evaluation of two opioid–acetaminophen combinations and placebo in postoperative oral surgery pain. *Pharmacotherapy.* 1994; **14**: 139–46.

39. Turturro MA, Paris PM, Larkin GL. Tramadol versus hydrocodone-acetaminophen in acute musculoskeletal pain: a randomized, double-blind clinical trial. *Annals of Emergency Medicine.* 1998; **32**: 139–43.

40. McQuay H. Bandolier, three pot system. Cited September 2006. Available from: www.jr2.ox.ac.uk/bandolier/painres/combos/comboed.html#Heading6.

41. Murat I, Baujard C, Foussat C *et al.* Tolerance and analgesic efficacy of a new i.v. paracetamol solution in children after inguinal hernia repair. *Paediatric Anaesthesia.* 2005; **15**: 663–70.

42. Pendeville PE, Von Montigny S, Dort JP, Veyckemans F. Double-blind randomized study of tramadol vs. paracetamol in analgesia after day-case tonsillectomy in children. *European Journal of Anaesthesiology.* 2000; **17**: 576–82.

43. Hynes D, McCarroll M, Hiesse-Provost O. Analgesic efficacy of parenteral paracetamol (propacetamol) and diclofenac in post-operative orthopaedic pain. *Acta Anaesthesiologica Scandinavica.* 2006; **50**: 374–81.

44. Zhou TJ, Tang J, White PF. Propacetamol versus ketorolac for treatment of acute postoperative pain after total hip or knee replacement. *Anesthesia and Analgesia.* 2001; **92**: 1569–75.

45. Van Aken H, Thys L, Veekman L, Buerkle H. Assessing analgesia in single and repeated administrations of propacetamol for postoperative pain: comparison with morphine after dental surgery. *Anesthesia and Analgesia.* 2004; **98**: 159–65.

46. Moller PL, Juhl GI, Payen-Champenois C, Skoglund LA. Intravenous acetaminophen (paracetamol): comparable analgesic efficacy, but better local safety than its prodrug, propacetamol, for postoperative pain after third molar surgery. *Anesthesia and Analgesia.* 2005; **101**: 90–6.

47. Beaussier M, Weickmans H, Paugam C *et al.* A randomized, double-blind comparison between parecoxib sodium and propacetamol for parenteral postoperative analgesia after inguinal hernia repair in adult patients. *Anesthesia and Analgesia.* 2005; **100**: 1309–15.

48. Bremerich DH, Neidhart G, Heimann K *et al.* Prophylactically administered rectal acetaminophen does not reduce postoperative opioid requirements in infants and small children undergoing elective cleft palate repair. *Anesthesia and Analgesia.* 2001; **92**: 907–12.

49. Howell TK, Patel D. Plasma paracetamol concentrations after different doses of rectal paracetamol in older children A comparison of 1 g vs. 40 mg $\times$ kg^{-1}. *Anaesthesia.* 2003; **58**: 69–73.

50. Viitanen H, Tuominen N, Vaaraniemi H *et al.* Analgesic efficacy of rectal acetaminophen and ibuprofen alone or in combination for paediatric day-case adenoidectomy. *British Journal of Anaesthesiology.* 2003; **91**: 363–7.

51. Cobby TF, Crighton IM, Kyriakides K, Hobbs GJ. Rectal paracetamol has a significant morphine-sparing effect after hysterectomy. *British Journal of Anaesthesiology.* 1999; **83**: 253–6.

52. Hein A, Jakobsson J, Ryberg G. Paracetamol 1 g given rectally at the end of minor gynaecological surgery is not efficacious in reducing postoperative pain. *Acta Anaesthesiologica Scandinavica.* 1999; **43**: 248–51.

53. Kvalsvik O, Borchgrevink PC, Hagen L, Dale O. Randomized, double-blind, placebo-controlled study of the effect of rectal paracetamol on morphine consumption after abdominal hysterectomy. *Acta Anaesthesiologica Scandinavica.* 2003; **47**: 451–6.

54. Pluim MA, Wegener JT, Rupreht J, Vulto AG. Tramadol suppositories are less suitable for post-operative pain relief than rectal acetaminophen/codeine. *European Journal of Anaesthesiology.* 1999; **16**: 473–8.

55. Schmidt A, Bjorkman S, Akeson J. Preoperative rectal diclofenac versus paracetamol for tonsillectomy: effects on pain and blood loss. *Acta Anaesthesiologica Scandinavica.* 2001; **45**: 48–52.

56. Larson AM, Polson J, Fontana RJ *et al.* Acetaminophen-induced acute liver failure: results of a United States

multicenter, prospective study. *Hepatology.* 2005; **42**: 1364–72.

57. Brok J, Buckley N, Gluud C. Interventions for paracetamol (acetaminophen) overdoses. *Cochrane Database of Systematic Reviews.* 2006; **CD003328**.

58. Dart RC, Kuffner EK, Rumack BH. Treatment of pain or fever with paracetamol (acetaminophen) in the alcoholic patient: a systematic review (structured abstract). *American Journal of Therapeutics.* 2000; **7**: 123–34.

59. Morgan O, Majeed A. Restricting paracetamol in the United Kingdom to reduce poisoning: a systematic review. *Journal of Public Health.* 2004; **27**: 12–18.

60. Emergency-Med.info. Nomogram for paracetamol poisoning. Cited September 2006. Available from: www.emergency-med.info/index.

∗ 61. HyperTox. Nomogram for paracetamol poisoning. Cited September 2006. Available from: http:// members.ozemail.com.au/~ouad/doc/paracetamol.

Clinical pharmacology: other adjuvants

EVANGELOS TZIAVRANGOS AND STEPHAN A SCHUG

KEY LEARNING POINTS

- Nitrous oxide is a useful short-acting adjunct, which provides some analgesia in labor and is effective for procedural analgesia in adults and children in a wide variety of settings. Its adverse effects on vitamin B12, in particular with repeat exposure, require consideration and supplementation to avoid rare, but serious toxicity leading to bone marrow suppression and neuropathy.
- Continuous infusions of low doses of the *N*-methyl-D-aspartate (NMDA) receptor antagonist ketamine have opioid-sparing effects and reduce adverse effects of opioids in the acute pain setting. This approach also has a preventive analgesic effect, provides analgesia in pain poorly responsive to opioids, and may be particularly useful in settings of hyperalgesia, allodynia, and opioid tolerance.
- The alpha-2 adrenoreceptor agonists clonidine and dexmedetomidine have an opioid-sparing effect in the acute pain setting; however, they can lead to sedation and hypotension.
- Anticonvulsants, in particular the gabapentinoids gabapentin and pregabalin, are not only effective in acute neuropathic pain states, but also in reducing postoperative pain and opioid requirements. They may become an important component of multimodal analgesia.
- Antidepressants play no role as adjuvants in the treatment of acute pain, but have shown a preventive effect on the development of subsequent chronic pain states.
- Corticosteroids, in particular dexamethasone, are not only a very effective prophylaxis for postoperative nausea and vomiting, but also reduce pain and swelling in certain postoperative settings.
- Calcitonin is an effective treatment for the pain of vertebral crush fractures and for postamputation phantom limb pain.
- Systemic administration of lidocaine is an effective treatment of acute neuropathic pain of peripheral and central origin; due to its anti-inflammatory effect it might also be a useful adjuvant for perioperative pain treatment with benefits for analgesia and outcome.

INTRODUCTION

The pharmacological options for the treatment of acute pain are greater than ever, due in part to our better understanding of nociceptive pathways and their spinal and cerebral processing and driven by the ever-increasing demand to treat pain more effectively. Nonsteroidal anti-inflammatory drugs and opioids continue to be the mainstay analgesics for acute pain, but the role of other so-called adjuvant drugs is expanding rapidly, many with very clear indications for their use supported by scientific evidence from trials and meta-analyses. Mostly, these drugs are co-administered with standard analgesics as part of a multimodal regime, but in some instances, the literature suggests a more primary role for effective acute pain management. This chapter will discuss the current status of adjuvant drugs in the acute pain context, together with their clinical pharmacology.

NITROUS OXIDE

Introduction

The analgesic properties of nitrous oxide (N_2O) were recognized over 200 years ago,[1] and the use of this inorganic gas in anesthesia practice continues to date, although with the advent of newer, superior anesthetic and analgesic drugs with less potential for toxicity its popularity and routine use seems to be waning.[2] Nevertheless, its current role as a short-acting analgesic for a variety of indications persists, with sufficient evidence supporting its ongoing use. Its physical and chemical properties are briefly summarized in **Box 6.1** below.

Pharmacokinetics

In many countries, commercial preparations of N_2O for analgesic use are presented as gas mixtures containing 50 percent oxygen and 50 percent N_2O, contained in cylinders compressed to a pressure of 13,700 kPa. Delivery of this mixture to the patient is via a mask and pressure demand regulator that allows gas flow during inspiration.[5] The inhaled N_2O reaches the alveoli and here concentrations rapidly approach the inspired concentration because of its low solubility. The rate of uptake is increased by increased alveolar ventilation and decreased cardiac output. Subsequent distribution favors organs with relatively high blood flow particularly the brain and spinal cord, which are the predominant sites of action. N_2O is eliminated mostly via the lungs without undergoing any significant metabolism in humans, although minimal amounts are lost through the skin.[6]

Mechanism of action and clinical effects

Until recently, surprisingly little was known regarding the precise pharmacological mechanism of action of N_2O and its analgesic and anesthetic effects.[6] Animal studies and some human studies have begun to unravel these rather complex neurochemical mechanisms, and it seems likely that N_2O mediates antinociceptive effects in the central nervous system by first releasing opioid peptides in the peri-aqueductal gray area of the midbrain and in the noradrenergic nuclei of the pons. This then leads to activation of descending inhibitory neurons that release noradrenaline on alpha-2 adrenoreceptors in the dorsal horn of the spinal cord.[7] In essence, the net result is modulation of ascending pain transmission at the level of the spinal cord, i.e. "antinociception."

Side effects and toxicity of nitrous oxide

Euphoric and dysphoric experiences are relatively common with analgesic concentrations of N_2O,[8][II] although these are unlikely to depress consciousness unless other central nervous system depressants are used concomitantly. Cerebral blood flow, cerebral metabolic rate, and intracranial pressure are increased by nitrous oxide, and these effects can be significant.[9, 10][III] Mean arterial pressure is unchanged or slightly elevated, most likely due to its mild sympathomimetic effect increasing systemic vascular resistance. This effect offsets the mild, direct myocardial depressant actions, but also causes pulmonary vasoconstriction.[3] Respiration is well maintained with subanesthetic concentrations of N_2O, but ventilatory responses to hypoxia and hypercarbia are attenuated.[2] N_2O does not produce skeletal muscle or uterine relaxation, and is not a trigger for malignant hyperpyrexia, but is a significant cause of nausea and vomiting.[11][II]

N_2O is much more soluble than nitrogen in blood and will enter air-filled spaces in the body more rapidly than nitrogen can escape, leading to an increase in either volume or pressure in that space. This precludes its use in a number of clinical situations including pneumothorax, bowel obstruction, pneumoencephalon, pneumopericardium, and recent middle ear and eye surgery.[12, 13] One must also note that when N_2O is discontinued, this same physical phenomenon can also lead to its rapid movement into the alveoli lowering oxygen concentrations and can

---

> **Box 6.1 Physical–chemical properties of nitrous oxide**
>
> - Colorless inorganic gas
> - Sweet smelling
> - Nonflammable, but supports combustion
> - Specific gravity, 1.53
> - Boiling point, −88°C
> - Critical temperature, 36.5°C
> - Critical pressure, 71.7 atmospheres
> - Minimum alveolar concentration, 105
> - Oil:water solubility coefficient, 3.2
> - Blood:gas solubility coefficient, 0.47
> - Presented as a 50/50 mixture of oxygen and nitrous oxide for analgesic use
>
> Modified from multiple sources, including Refs 3, 4.

cause "diffusion hypoxia" unless supplemental oxygen is administered.[3]

Severe neurological and hematological complications can rarely occur with N_2O caused by its inhibition of vitamin B12, an essential coenzyme for methionine synthase. Methionine synthase itself is crucial in the formation of both methionine (involved in myelin formation) and tetrahydrofolate (involved in DNA synthesis).[14, 15] Risk factors for these complications include the length of exposure to N_2O (and this includes repeated short-term use), critically ill patients, the elderly, and underlying vitamin B12 and folate deficiency. Clinical manifestations include progressive but reversible bone marrow suppression, and progressive neuropathy and myelopathy that may be irreversible.[16]

Therefore, N_2O should not be used in patients with known vitamin B12 deficiency and only after screening for such in patients at risk. Prophylactic administration of vitamin B12, methionine, and folinic or folic acid, as well as monitoring for neuropathy, is recommended if repeated use of N_2O is contemplated.[14, 15][V] There are limited human data on this to guide best practice, nevertheless this practice is currently endorsed by clinical guidelines.[13][V]

N_2O has been shown to be teratogenic in animal studies, but similar effects in limited human studies have not been established.[17, 18]

Clinical use of N_2O in acute pain management

N_2O for short-term analgesia can potentially be utilized in a range of clinical situations and across different age groups. Its use for labor pain, for example, is well-described worldwide, with established safety (both maternal and newborn), provided that it is supervised by physicians, nurses, or midwives, and evidence for some analgesic efficacy.[19][I] It is typically used intermittently during the first stage of labor, but it can also be used at any time including late in the active second stage.[19]

In the pediatric population, effective procedural analgesia is essential to prevent undue distress (in children and parents) and longer-term emotional trauma. The current evidence supports the use of N_2O here, as it is efficacious and safe for a variety of emergencies, minor procedures, and other painful situations.[20][I] The most common emergency settings are suturing minor lacerations and the closed reduction of limb fractures,[21][IV] but N_2O can also be used to facilitate insertion of peripheral intravenous cannulas as an effective alternative to topical local anesthetics.[22, 23][II] Other pediatric procedures where N_2O has been evaluated for analgesia include lumbar punctures,[21][IV] dental treatments,[24][II] fiberoptic bronchoscopy,[25][II] and intra-articular injections.[26][IV]

Similarly, N_2O is also useful in adult acute pain management especially for short procedures, but also in the emergency setting, and even in the prehospital period by lay responders.[27] Among other settings, it provides effective analgesia for sigmoidoscopy,[28][II] bronchoscopy,[29][I] venous access port insertion,[30][II] as well as reducing the discomfort associated with elective cardiac defibrillation.[31][III]

Pain management in burn patients is notoriously difficult and the acute pain is usually due to the burn injury itself, but may also be associated with the multiple therapeutic procedures inevitably performed as part of its management.[32, 33] There may be a role for N_2O as an adjuvant for painful procedures, such as dressing changes and debridements.[34]

NMDA RECEPTOR ANTAGONISTS

Introduction

Drugs in this class include ketamine, dextromethorphan, memantine, and amantadine, although ketamine is by far the more widely studied and used drug of this group in both anesthesia and pain management. Indeed, substantial evidence from recent meta-analyses of randomized controlled trials (RCT) supports the emerging clinical use of ketamine as an adjuvant analgesic in acute pain management, in addition to its role in chronic pain and cancer pain settings.[35]

Physical and chemical properties

Ketamine hydrochloride is a phencyclidine derivative, usually prepared as a racemic mixture and formulated as an acid solution with an added preservative. This preservative component precludes neuraxial administration due to concerns regarding neurotoxicity, although preservative-free preparations are available. In some countries the more potent S(+)-ketamine enantiomer is used. Oral, sublingual (transmucosal), and transdermal preparations are used only experimentally.

Pharmacokinetics

These are briefly summarized in **Table 6.1**.

Mechanism of action and clinical effects

The nervous system is the primary pharmacological target for ketamine, via central and possibly even peripheral mechanisms involving various receptors (of which the NMDA receptor is considered pivotal) and where it interacts principally as a noncompetitive antagonist.[36, 37]

The NMDA receptor itself is a complex, ion channel-coupled receptor that is activated *in vivo* by glutamate, the predominant excitatory neurotransmitter of the central

Table 6.1 Ketamine pharmacokinetics.

	Ketamine
Absorption	Rapidly absorbed following sublingual, oral, and intramuscular administration
	Oral bioavailability approximately 20%
Distribution	Volume of distribution between 1–3 L/kg
	Distribution half-life 7–11 minutes
	20–50% plasma protein bound
Metabolism	Extensive hepatic metabolism occurs including dealkylation, hydroxylation, and conjugation reactions
	Norketamine, the major metabolite, is active as an NMDA antagonist
Excretion	Renal clearance 15 mL/min/kg
	90% excretion in the urine, mostly as metabolites, with about 2–4% unchanged
	5% excreted in feces

NMDA, *N*-methyl-D-aspartate.
Modified from multiple sources, including Ref. 3.

nervous system.[38] The importance of this receptor in the context of acute and chronic pain cannot be overstated. Following injury to peripheral tissues or nerves, nociception invariably results in NMDA receptor activation, especially in the dorsal horn of the spinal cord. It is particularly noteworthy that these dorsal horn NMDA receptors are also implicated in opioid tolerance,[39] opioid-induced hyperalgesia (a paradoxical phenomenon whereby opioid-treated patients develop greater sensitivity to pain),[40] and are fundamental to the processes of "wind up" and "long-term potentiation" which occur in the development of persistent and neuropathic pain states.[41]

Therefore, NMDA receptor antagonist drugs could play an important role as adjuvant analgesics in the acute pain setting, particularly so in patients who have developed or are at risk of developing opioid tolerance, hyperalgesia, or neuropathic pain. Of the currently registered drugs in this class, ketamine seems to possess the ideal potency and selectivity for NMDA receptors,[41] and appears, on balance, to be the most efficacious.[42, 43, 44, 45][I]

General anesthetic doses of ketamine characteristically induce a state of dissociative anesthesia, meaning that it causes a dissociation between the thalamoneocortical and limbic systems, preventing the higher centers from perceiving visual, auditory, or painful stimuli.[46] For the purposes of pain management (acute and chronic) however, much smaller subanesthetic amounts are used (see below under Perioperative pain management), and this applies to both bolus doses and continuous infusions. Additional clinical effects may be observed with ketamine, such as mild cardiovascular stimulation, bronchodilation, and excessive salivation although these are far less prominent with subanesthetic doses. Respiration and upper airway reflexes are relatively well maintained with ketamine, as is uterine and skeletal muscle tone.[46]

Side effects and toxicity

The widespread medical use of ketamine and other NMDA receptor antagonists has always been limited by

fears of undesirable side effects and concerns regarding abuse potential, as well as the uncertainty of possible long-term sequelae with chronic use.[47] By limiting the duration and using very low doses of ketamine for analgesic purposes, the overall incidence of many of these side effects is significantly attenuated.

Minor side effects include nausea and vomiting, as well as excessive salivation, and are rarely encountered and can be effectively managed with antiemetics and antisialogues as necessary. On this point, it is interesting to note that ketamine used concurrently with opioid-based postoperative analgesia actually reduces the incidence of nausea and vomiting, probably via its opioid sparing effects.[42][I]

Central nervous system side effects can include dizziness, dreams, diplopia, nystagmus, dysphoria, hallucinations, and sedation. With low-dose ketamine, the overall incidence is low in the range of less than 10 percent and can be further minimized with coadminstration of benzodiazepines or following general anesthesia.[43, 44]

Ketamine is a well-known substance of abuse, with reports of nonmedical use for its psychoactive effects dating back almost 40 years.[47, 48] For these reasons, it is a controlled drug in many countries including Australia and the United States. Long-term abuse may result in behavioral disturbances and altered memory function,[49] although this seems highly unlikely to be relevant in the current context of short-term, low-dose ketamine use in acute pain management.

Clinical use in acute pain management

Based on the current understanding of the mechanism of action of ketamine on the NMDA receptor in particular, and supported by extensive clinical data from randomized controlled trials and meta-analyses, the use of ketamine (in subanesthetic doses) is indicated in a number of clinical settings, as summarized in **Table 6.2**. The doses suggested are a guide only and reflect the significant heterogeneity amongst published data.

Table 6.2 The role of ketamine in acute pain management.

Acute procedural pain	Perioperative pain management	Acute neuropathic pain
In the emergency department, e.g. fracture reductions	As an opioid-sparing drug, e.g. in combination with opioid-based analgesia when treating severe postoperative pain in recovery rooms, on postoperative wards and in intensive care units	Medical conditions, e.g. acute zoster, poststroke, multiple sclerosis
In the burn unit, e.g. burn dressings	As a recovery room rescue co-analgesic postoperatively for severe pain	Surgical conditions or trauma, e.g. spinal cord injury, burns, postamputation
In oncology wards, e.g. lumbar puncture, bone marrow biopsy	For opioid-tolerant patients, e.g. chronic opioid use or abuse	
In radiology suites, e.g. contrast enemas	For opioid-resistant pain, e.g. opioid-induced hyperalgesia or allodynia in neuropathic pain as "preventive" analgesia	

Adapted from multiple sources, including Refs 35, 42, 43, 44, 45.

ACUTE PROCEDURAL PAIN

A wide range of painful procedures and interventions commonly encountered in emergency departments, burn units, and oncology wards can be managed effectively with ketamine, much in the same manner as described under Nitrous oxide above, and while there is greater clinical experience in pediatric patients its use can be extended to all age groups.[20][I], [50][V], [51][II]

Typically, intravenous doses less than 1 mg/kg are described in the literature, although higher doses can be used when sedation is also desirable, but this must be done with caution and only by practitioners who are appropriately trained in managing such patients in the correct environment.

PERIOPERATIVE PAIN MANAGEMENT

There is keen interest in the use of low-dose ketamine as an adjuvant to opioid-based analgesia in the perioperative period, and this potential role has been examined in three recent meta-analyses, demonstrating efficacy for at least 24 hours post operation, highlighted by improved pain scores, reduced opioid consumption, and decreased nausea and vomiting.[42, 43, 44][I] These meta-analyses also confirmed that in this context, adverse effects due to ketamine itself are either mild or absent, most likely a reflection of the small doses used.

Ketamine is similarly useful when coadministered with morphine as a bolus in the recovery room when treating severe pain that is initially recalcitrant to opioids alone.[52][II]

The most commonly utilized method of administration, however, is via a separate continuous intravenous infusion of ketamine (approximately 100–200 µg/kg per hour), administered concurrently with the opioid-based analgesic (via continuous infusion or patient-controlled analgesic (PCA) device); a fixed combination of ketamine and morphine via an intravenous PCA device has not been shown to be effective as a postoperative analgesic technique in five randomized controlled trials.[53, 54, 55, 56, 57][II]

The issues of opioid tolerance and opioid-induced hyperalgesia are extremely relevant to the current and future practice of acute pain management, the underlying key theme being lack of opioid potency leading to inadequately treated acute pain, especially in perioperative patients. Strategies which utilize multimodal analgesia, including adjuvants such as ketamine, are recommended in these patients.[58, 59, 60, 61][IV] Those considered at risk include all patients treated with long-term opioids (especially in high doses) regardless of indication, as well as those who chronically abuse illicit opioids.[40] It is of note that even opioid-naive patients can be at risk of these phenomena acutely and then benefit from ketamine, such as when high-dose remifentanil is used intraoperatively.[62][II]

A further useful property of ketamine in the perioperative period lies in its so-called preventive analgesic properties, whereby the reduction in postoperative pain intensity or analgesic consumption (or both), continues past the expected clinical duration of action of the drug.[63][I], [64] The implications of this phenomenon go beyond the superior analgesia and opioid-sparing effects observed in the acute phase and signify the ability of this drug to reduce peripheral and central sensitization that arises from noxious perioperative stimuli.[65] In a practical sense, wound hyperalgesia and residual pain is reduced, even after 12 months.[66][II] It remains to be seen if this application can be extended to the prevention of persistent postsurgical pain.[67]

ACUTE NEUROPATHIC PAIN

Neuropathic pain may be an early presenting feature in a wide range of conditions, in both surgical and nonsurgical settings. The true prevalence of acute neuropathic pain is unclear, although one Australian study suggested an incidence of 1–3 percent in an acute pain service.[68] Typically, this type of pain is not completely responsive to opioids at usual doses,[69, 70] and adjuvants are more likely to be needed. Ketamine might be such an adjuvant, although admittedly much of the data on this are either from experimental studies,[71] or are extrapolated from chronic pain studies.[72] There is currently only moderate evidence for the use of ketamine in neuropathic pain, but it might still be a reasonable option if other alternatives have been unsuccessful. This might be particularly true for acute neuropathic pain states, such as spinal cord injury pain,[73][II] central poststroke pain,[74][V] and ischemic pain.[75][II]

ALPHA-2 ADRENORECEPTOR AGONISTS

Introduction

Drugs such as clonidine and dexmedetomidine are included in this group of alpha-2 adrenoreceptor agonists that are useful adjuvants in acute pain management. Other newer drugs in this class that have even greater selectivity and fewer side effects have been developed, but as yet have not reached mainstream clinical use. Within the context of acute pain management and based on supportive evidence from clinical trials and reviews, it seems the main areas of clinical utility for these drugs lies in the perioperative period and in intensive care units. Furthermore, the role of these drugs in the management of selected chronic pain states, and in cancer pain management continues to evolve.

Physical and chemical properties

Clonidine and dexmedetomidine are both imidazole ring compounds. Clonidine is prepared for oral and parenteral administration (as well as for use in regional analgesia),

whereas dexmedetomidine is currently available for intravenous use only, typically prepared as an infusion in intensive care units. The relative selectivity of these two drugs for alpha-2 receptors compared to alpha-1 receptors differs, with clonidine being less selective (approximately 220:1) compared to dexmedetomidine (approximately 1620:1).[76]

Pharmacokinetics

These are briefly summarized in the **Table 6.3**.

Mechanism of action and clinical effects

Adrenoreceptors are ubiquitous in humans and mediate a vast range of complex homeostatic functions within the central nervous system, as well as peripheral organs. For example, in the central nervous system (i.e. brain and spinal cord) alpha-2 adrenoreceptors are involved in nociception, alertness, regulation of blood pressure, and sympathetic nerve function, whereas in the periphery these receptors control vascular and smooth muscle contraction, a range of gastrointestinal and metabolic functions, as well as endothelial and urogenital function.[78]

Pharmacological agonists at these receptors, such as clonidine and dexmedetomidine, exert their various effects by initially binding to this receptor and then activating inhibitory G-proteins.[78] Subsequent intracellular events and cascades include activation of second messengers, and actions directly on neuronal ion channel function, all of which ultimately lead to a targeted cellular response. Typically, the observed clinical effects of these drugs are analgesia, sedation, and sympatholysis, affecting the cardiovascular system in particular.[79]

With regards to analgesic mechanisms, the primary site of action is in the spinal cord, but it is recognized that supraspinal and even peripheral sites of action coexist,[80] although their relative importance is still to be

Table 6.3 Pharmacokinetics of selected alpha-2 adrenoceptor agonists.

	Clonidine	Dexmedetomidine
Absorption	Rapidly and well absorbed following oral and intramuscular administration; oral bioavailability 100%	N/A; prepared only for intravenous administration
Distribution	Volume of distribution between 1.7–2.5 L/kg; 20% plasma protein bound	Volume of distribution 1.33 L/kg; 94% plasma protein bound
Metabolism	Less than half the administered dose undergoes hepatic metabolism; five inactive metabolites identified	Quite extensive hepatic metabolism
Excretion	Approximately two-thirds of the administered dose excreted in urine (half of this unchanged) and the rest is excreted in the feces; clearance 1.9–4.3 mL/min/kg	95% excretion of metabolites in the urine with a small remainder excreted in the feces; clearance approximately 39 L/hour

Modified from multiple sources including Refs 4, 77.

determined.[77] The potential mechanisms of alpha-2 adrenoreceptor-mediated analgesia are multifactorial, but ultimately these effects are mediated by changes in neuronal ion channel function leading to modulation of nociception.[77] It is also of great interest that spinal alpha-2 receptors have been implicated in the development of neuropathic pain in experimental animal models, and that the administration of alpha-2 agonists results in antihyperalgesic effects.[80, 81, 82]

The sedative (and anxiolytic) actions are due to alpha-2 agonist actions in the locus ceruleus of the brain stem and are dose dependent in nature. When used intraoperatively they have significant anesthetic-sparing effects in the order of 30–40 percent.[83] In contrast to opioids, respiratory depression does not occur however, nor do these compounds potentiate opioid-induced respiratory depression.[84]

There are a number of dose-dependent cardiovascular effects that are due to central decreases in sympathetic tone, as well as peripheral actions on vasculature. Heart rate and blood pressure both decrease at clinically relevant doses of alpha-2 agonists, the effect more prominent in patients with higher resting sympathetic tone, and less prominent in healthy and physiologically unstressed individuals. Baroreceptor reflexes are not impaired and the responses to vasopressors are maintained.[84]

Other clinical effects include a dry mouth due to a decrease in salivation, an ability to decrease post-operative shivering, and a decrease in intraocular pressure by about 30 percent.[84]

Side effects and toxicity

The sedative effects are dose dependent and can result in an unrouseable patient if inappropriate doses are used; therefore titration of the drug is essential to achieve the desired clinical effects (see below under Clinical use in acute pain management). These drugs should be avoided in patients who are hypovolemic or hemodynamically unstable, in patients with underlying bradyarrhythmias, and where controlled hypotension is to be employed as part of the anaesthetic.[85] Other side effects include constipation and impairment of sexual function.

Clinical use in acute pain management

On the basis of evidence from clinical trials and recent reviews,[76, 83, 86, 87, 88] the use of clonidine (and to a lesser extent dexmedetomidine) is indicated in the following clinical settings.

PERIOPERATIVE SYSTEMIC USE

Clonidine administered either as a premedication or intraoperatively, in doses ranging from 2 to 5 µg/kg, has been extensively trialled in a wide range of pediatric and adult surgical populations with success achieving appropriate levels of anxiolysis and sedation, as well as reducing anesthetic requirements. In addition to this, intra- and postoperative opioid analgesic requirements were significantly reduced in the order of 30–50 percent, with an attendant decrease in opioid-related side effects such as nausea, vomiting, and pruritis.[89, 90, 91, 92, 93][II] Sedation and bradycardia are the most common side effects but rarely of clinical consequence, even in neonates when the drugs are administered to the mother prior to cesarean section.[89][II] In some situations, the sedative effects may actually be beneficial in preventing agitation in the recovery room, such as shown in pediatric patients following sevoflurane anesthesia.[94][II] In addition, by continuing the clonidine for four days postoperatively in high-risk patients undergoing noncardiac surgery, cardiac morbidity and mortality has been found to be reduced, even at two years.[95][II]

The addition of clonidine to an opioid-based PCA device does not achieve sustained analgesic benefits and does not reduce morphine consumption, a situation that bears similarity to ketamine as discussed above under NMDA receptor antagonists.[96][II]

As far as intraoperative dexmedetomidine is concerned, the limited data thus far do suggest similar benefits to clonidine with regards to postoperative analgesia and opioid-sparing effects,[97, 98][II] but further clinical studies are required.

USE IN THE INTENSIVE CARE UNIT

The importance of appropriate sedation and analgesia in intensive care patients cannot be overstated.[99] A number of different agents have been used over the years for this purpose including opioids, benzodiazepines, and propofol, but none of them are ideal and each has their own undesirable effects in critically ill patients. Dexmedetomidine is easily titratable as an intravenous infusion and possesses a number of desirable properties such as sedation and analgesia, but does not impair respiratory function, which is highly important to prevent prolonged mechanical ventilation.[100][II] In cardiac surgery patients, for example, postoperative analgesic requirements in the intensive care unit are reduced by about 50 percent.[101][II]

ACUTE NEUROPATHIC PAIN

Despite abundant animal data implicating adrenergic mechanisms in neuropathic pain models and the efficacy of alpha-2 agonists in these experiments, there is currently a notable lack of human data to support the use of these drugs for this indication. Even in chronic neuropathic pain states, the evidence for these drugs, either systemically or more commonly via neuraxial routes, is weak at best.[102] Further work is required in this field if the promising experimental results are to be extrapolated and realized in humans.

ANTICONVULSANTS

Introduction

The use of anticonvulsant drugs in chronic and neuropathic pain conditions is common and well supported by clinical evidence.[103, 104, 105] While the use of these drugs in acute pain management may seem quite novel, there is mounting experimental and clinical evidence supporting their inclusion in the multimodal analgesic mix.[106] In addition, some of these drugs may have a niche role as primary analgesics for specific indications. Of the numerous anticonvulsants currently available, only a few appear to have potential clinical utility in acute pain management and these include gabapentin, pregabalin, and valproate.

Physical and chemical properties

Anticonvulsants are chemically diverse and while gabapentin and pregabalin are structurally similar to the endogenous neurotransmitter gamma-aminobutyric acid (GABA), valproate (a carboxylic acid compound) does not share any such structural similarities. These drugs are all prepared for oral administration, although parenteral forms of valproate are available as well.

Pharmacokinetics

These are briefly summarized in **Table 6.4**.

Mechanism of action and clinical effects

Anticonvulsant drugs exert multiple pharmacological actions on the nervous system, with remarkable similarities between the antiseizure and analgesic mechanisms.[107] With regards to their specific analgesic mechanisms, it appears that gabapentin, pregabalin, and valproate all interact with voltage-gated calcium channels and suppress activity at NMDA and AMPA receptors as well.[106] Other anticonvulsants have significant voltage-gated sodium blocking effects, thought to be important in neuropathic pain mechanisms.

Experimental studies in animals have shown the ability of some (but not all) anticonvulsants to attenuate nociceptive processes in both inflammatory and neuropathic pain models.[107, 108] Furthermore, human studies with gabapentin and pregabalin, for example, show their ability to suppress experimentally induced skin hyperalgesia in otherwise healthy volunteers,[109] while also enhancing the analgesic effects of opioids.[110] These findings have forged the way towards a number of clinical trials in the perioperative setting.

Side effects and toxicity

Side effects are relatively common with all anticonvulsant drugs currently in use, some of which are dose dependent and others idiosyncratic.[107] Gabapentin and pregabalin both have similar side-effect profiles, with sedation, dizziness, ataxia, diplopia, nausea, and peripheral edema among some of the more common side effects.

Valproate causes similar central nervous system side effects, but in addition may result in blood dyscrasias, elevated liver function tests, and rare skin reactions. The teratogenic potential of these drugs in rats is established,

Table 6.4 Pharmacokinetics of selected anticonvulsants.

	Gabapentin	Pregabalin	Valproate
Absorption	Variable bioavailability dependent on dose; e.g. daily doses/bioavailability: 1200 mg/47%; 2400 mg/34%; 3600 mg/33%; 4800 mg/27%	Good oral absorption; oral bioavailability >90% independent of dose	Rapid and almost complete oral absorption
Distribution	Volume of distribution 58 L; less than 3% bound to plasma proteins	Volume of distribution 0.56 L/kg; not bound to plasma proteins	Nonlinear kinetics; concentration-dependent plasma protein binding (90%)
Metabolism	No significant metabolism in humans	No significant metabolism in humans	Complex metabolism, including glucuronidation and oxidation
Excretion	Eliminated via renal excretion, mostly as unchanged drug; elimination half life 5–7 hours	Eliminated via renal excretion, mostly as unchanged drug; elimination half-life 6.3 hours	Significant metabolism prior to excretion; half-life range 3.8–15.7 hours

Modified from multiple sources.

with some suggestions of potential adverse effects in pregnant women. In the context of acute pain management, particularly in the perioperative setting, it would be sensible to avoid these drugs in early pregnancy.

Clinical use in acute pain management

Specific anticonvulsants certainly have a potential role in acute pain management but thus far only for particular indications such as in the perioperative period, in acute neuropathic pain states, and in acute migraine.

PERIOPERATIVE USE: GABAPENTINOIDS

Anticonvulsants for perioperative pain management are currently only in the initial stages of clinical use. Preclinical data discussed above have suggested a role as an adjunct to opioids in particular, especially the perioperative setting, and this has now led to a significant number of very recent clinical trials evaluating the effect of gabapentin.

In these double-blinded randomized controlled trials, gabapentin was administered preoperatively in single doses ranging from 300 to 1200 mg, and in some cases continued into the early postoperative period. The types of surgery varied significantly, including gynecological surgery, orthopedic and spinal surgery, as well as oncological surgery, and even transplant surgery. There were even suggestions of improved postoperative pulmonary function following hysterectomy,[111][II] and enhanced functional recovery following knee surgery.[112][II]

Similar results were found in the few studies performed with pregabalin in the setting of dental pain[113][II] and after spinal fusion.[114][II]

A number of meta-analyses of these trials have been performed in 2006 and 2007.[115, 116, 117, 118, 119][I] Overall, they confirm the analgesic (at rest and with movement) and opioid-sparing effects of even single doses of gabapentin preoperatively, while leading to minor adverse effects, in particular increasing the incidence of sedation.[115, 116, 117, 118, 119][I] In parallel, the use of gabapentinoids perioperatively led to a decrease in nausea (number needed to treat (NNT) 25), vomiting (NNT 6), and urinary retention (NNT 7).[119][I] These effects were not dose-dependent in the dose range of 300–1200 mg investigated in the studies analyzed.[119][I]

It would seem from these data that gabapentinoids are establishing themselves in the paradigm of multimodal analgesia in the perioperative period; their role as "protective premedication" has been previously discussed in the literature.[120] However, the studies included in the above meta-analyses used a wide range of gabapentin and pregabalin doses and regimens of dosing. This means that any particular dosing regimen cannot be recommended currently; it is also unclear of which duration the perioperative intake of these compounds should be and if there are any long-term benefits such as reduced chronic pain from the perioperative use.

PERIOPERATIVE USE: OTHER ANTICONVULSANTS

In comparison to the gabapentinoids, other anticonvulsant drugs have received much less attention, with very few clinical studies examining their role in the perioperative period and no relevant findings. One study found no benefit in intravenous valproate administered postoperatively.[121][II]

Furthermore, a recent meta-analysis of carbamazepine in both acute and chronic pain concluded there was currently no role for this drug in acute pain management.[122][I]

ACUTE NEUROPATHIC PAIN

As outlined for ketamine and clonidine (see above under NMDA receptor antagonists and Alpha-2 adrenoreceptor agonists, respectively), neuropathic pain may be a significant presenting feature in various surgical and nonsurgical conditions, and the use of adjuvant drugs is more likely to result in effective analgesia. There are compelling data on the use of anticonvulsant drugs in a range of chronic neuropathic pain conditions.[103, 104, 105] By extrapolation, they could also be used in acute situations as well.[13] Specific acute neuropathic pain conditions where anticonvulsants have been used successfully include spinal cord injury (gabapentin),[123][II] Guillain–Barré syndrome (carbamazepine and gabapentin),[124, 125][II] and post-amputation phantom limb pain (gabapentin).[126][II]

ACUTE MIGRAINE HEADACHES – ABORTIVE THERAPY USING VALPROATE

Migraine refers to a common group of primary headache disorders, affecting nearly 20 percent of women and about 6 percent of men, but also affecting up to 3 percent of children.[127] Vast numbers of trials and reviews concerning pharmacological treatment and prevention of migraines have resulted in evidence-based guidelines.[13, 127, 128]

Valproate is not only considered beneficial in migraine prophylaxis,[129] but there are studies that also suggest intravenous valproate is beneficial in aborting acute episodes of migraine,[130][III], [131][II], [132][III], [133][II] although it is generally agreed that simple analgesics and triptans should be tried initially.[13, 134][I] Patients with acute migraine who have not responded to these initial measures commonly present to emergency departments,[135] and this is where additional treatments such as intravenous valproate may have a crucial role, particularly if nausea and vomiting (which is common in migraine) precludes administration of standard oral treatments. The effective doses used ranged from 300 mg to a maximum of 1200 mg in these studies, resulting in rapid improvements in pain and other migraine symptoms. To date, no trials have compared the relative efficacy of different valproate doses so it would seem reasonable to try to administer the minimum effective dose in clinical practice, until further studies clarifying this issue are published.

ANTIDEPRESSANTS

Introduction

While antidepressants, in particular the tricyclic compounds, are the most effective treatment of chronic neuropathic pain[136] and other chronic pain states, they play only a minor role as adjuncts for the treatment of acute pain.

Clinical use in acute pain management

Neither in experimental[137] nor in clinical acute pain after othopedic[138][II] and breast surgery[139][II] did tricyclic antidepressants show any analgesic effect.

However, antidepressants had a preventive effect on the development of neuropathic pain in a number of acute settings. Perioperative use of venlafaxine in breast surgery reduced the incidence of chronic pain assessed six months after the operation.[139][II] Similarly, amitriptyline given to patients with acute herpes zoster halved the incidence of postherpetic neuralgia at six months.[140]

In analogy to the effectiveness of tricyclic antidepressants in chronic neuropathic pain, there might also be a role for them in the treatment of acute neuropathic pain states.[13]

CORTICOSTEROIDS

Introduction

Synthetic corticosteroids have anti-inflammatory, analgesic, and antiemetic properties that are all potentially useful in acute pain management, notably in the perioperative setting.

Physical and chemical properties

The adrenal cortex produces steroid hormones that are involved in a vast number of physiological functions but, from a more simplistic pharmacological point of view, they can be considered either glucocorticoids or mineralocorticoids. The former are more relevant to the current discussion as they have important effects on inflammation. A range of synthetic drugs are available

clinically and they all share similarities in basic steroid composition; dexamethasone is most commonly studied in acute pain settings. Multiple formulations exist, but only the oral and parenteral forms are relevant to this discussion.

Pharmacokinetics

These are briefly summarized for dexamethasone in **Table 6.5**.

Mechanism of action and clinical effects

At a cellular level, all steroids bind to intracellular receptors and gain entry into the nucleus, subsequently altering gene expression and leading to tissue-specific effects. Glucocorticoids result in metabolic and immunosuppressive effects, as well as dramatic anti-inflammatory effects, the latter due to inhibition of phospholipase enzyme causing decreased production of prostaglandins and other eicosanoids. These fatty acid derivatives are normally induced following tissue injury (including surgery) and are pronociceptive. The more selective inhibition of these substances forms the basis for treatment with nonsteroidal anti-inflammatory drugs, and steroids therefore can be expected to result in similar responses.

Despite considerable advances in the understanding of mechanisms leading to nausea and vomiting, the mechanism of action of the antiemetic effects of corticosteroids remain unknown.[141]

Side effects and toxicity

Single dose and even short-term use of steroids in the acute pain management context is virtually devoid of significant adverse effects based on clinical experience in anesthesia and chemotherapy settings.

Table 6.5 Pharmacokinetics of dexamethasone.

	Dexamethasone
Absorption	Oral bioavailability 50–70%
	Rapidly absorbed following intramuscular injection
Distribution	Small amounts plasma protein bound
Metabolism	Predominantly hepatically metabolized
Excretion	Inactive metabolites excreted in the urine, mostly glucuronides and sulfates

Compiled from multiple sources.

Clinical use in acute pain management

The best described use of steroids in acute pain management is in the perioperative period, particularly in dental surgery,[142, 143] but also in laparoscopic cholecystectomy,[144] and to a lesser extent in orthopedic, ambulatory, and pediatric ear, nose, and throat (ENT) surgery.[76, 86, 145, 146] Steroids, such as betamethasone in doses 9–12 mg and dexamethasone in doses 8–10 mg, given either as a premedication or intraoperatively, resulted in reductions in pain and postoperative nausea and vomiting[142, 143, 145, 146][II], [147][I] and in the case of dental surgery, the incidence of severe postoperative swelling was less.[142, 143][II] Theoretical concerns regarding increased wound infections due to potential immune suppression have not eventuated. The use of steroids perioperatively as a prophylaxis against postoperative nausea and vomiting is widespread,[148] and their analgesic benefits are a welcome secondary effect.

CALCITONIN

Introduction

Calcitonin has analgesic effects that were realized over 30 years ago in both animal models and in humans, paving the way towards novel applications in pain management.[149] It has potential use in a number of acute and chronic pain conditions, but only some of these have been subjected to sufficiently rigorous trials and meta-analyses, thus limiting the present use of this useful drug.

Physical and chemical properties

Calcitonin is a 32 amino acid polypeptide hormone secreted by parafollicular cells in the thyroid gland. Salmon calcitonin (molecular weight, 3431) is synthesized for medical use, as it is considered significantly more potent than the human type. It is presented in various forms for administration via intranasal, rectal, subcutaneous, intramuscular, and intravenous routes.[149]

Pharmacokinetics

These are briefly summarized in **Table 6.6**.

Mechanism of action and clinical effects

Calcitonin binds to a transmembrane G-protein coupled receptor, resulting in actions by intracellular second messengers such as c-AMP and calcium. The primary physiological role of calcitonin appears to be calcium homeostasis, although this function is predominantly served by vitamin D and parathyroid hormone.[149]

The analgesic mechanisms are atypical, having been studied at length in animals and humans.[149] Calcitonin receptors are widespread in tissues and importantly they are found on central serotonergic neurons associated with pain pathways. The current hypothesis is that calcitonin produces antinociceptive effects via neuromodulation of central serotonergic pain pathways.

Side effects and toxicity

The more common side effects include nausea and vomiting, facial flushing, and dizziness. Antiemetics may significantly attenuate the nausea and vomiting, and are commonly co-administered. Less commonly, flu-like symptoms may occur (i.e. fevers, chills, arthralgias) and rashes may sometimes develop. Localized or generalized hypersensitivity reactions may occur in very rare cases.[149]

Long-term administration (up to five years) is considered safe and does not seem to cause any serious side effects.[150]

Clinical use in acute pain management

Calcitonin has found clinical utility in acute, chronic, and cancer pain management.[149] In the field of acute pain management, it is a useful adjuvant in vertebral fractures and in phantom limb pain.

Table 6.6 Pharmacokinetics of (salmon) calcitonin.

	Calcitonin
Absorption	Not administered orally as it is a protein, and would be inactivated in the gut; bioavailability after subcutaneous (s.c.) or intramuscular (i.m.) injection is about 70%; onset is immediate following intravenous administration, and 15 minutes following s.c. or i.m; peak plasma levels within one hour
Distribution	Volume of distribution 0.15–0.30 L/kg
Metabolism	Rapidly metabolized to unidentified and inactive metabolites, mainly in the kidneys, blood, and peripheral tissues
Excretion	95% excreted by the kidney; elimination half life 60–90 minutes

Modified from multiple sources, including Ref. 149.

ACUTE OSTEOPOROTIC VERTEBRAL CRUSH FRACTURES

Pain caused by acute osteoporotic vertebral fractures is intense and debilitating, typically lasting several weeks, and commonly persisting long term. A recent review examined 14 trials that have been undertaken to date, analyzing the effects of daily calcitonin (administered in various forms) in such patients.[150] The patients reported better analgesia at rest and with movement, used less additional analgesics, and perhaps most importantly, had significantly improved mobility and functional capacity.[150][I]

The doses used ranged from 50 to 200 IU depending on the route of administration and the duration of treatment was at least two weeks, and even up to one year in one study. Evidence-based clinical guidelines recommend the use of calcitonin as a first-line agent in the management of acute osteoporotic vertebral fractures.[151]

ACUTE PHANTOM LIMB PAIN

Phantom limb pain following amputations is very common with some suggestions as high as 60–70 percent in the first year.[152] Various treatments are reported in the literature for both acute and chronic phantom limb pain, yet consensus guidelines founded on a clear evidence base are notably lacking at this time. Nevertheless, treatment of acute phantom limb pain with calcitonin is a viable option, based on case series results[153, 154, 155][III] and one double-blinded randomized controlled trial;[156][II] patients experienced rapid and sustained pain relief, even after two years.

As noted with treatment of vertebral crush fractures, the optimal dose and route of administration for phantom pain is not known.

LIDOCAINE (SYSTEMIC ADMINISTRATION)

Introduction

Since the early 1950s, reports have appeared in the literature on the systemic, commonly intravenous, use of local anesthetics, specifically lidocaine (lignocaine) to provide pain relief.[157] In an elegant experiment, Boas *et al.*[158] could show very early that there was selectivity of the analgesic effect for neuropathic over nociceptive pain. The assumed mechanism of action is inhibition of ectopic discharge of damaged neurons,[159] mediated by blockade of sodium channels, which are overexpressed in these pathological states.[160] Clinically, this effect, which occurs at plasma concentration far below those to induce conduction blockade, has been utilized in a wide range of clinical settings.[161]

As physical and chemical properties, pharmacokinetics, mechanism of action, side effects, and toxicity of the local anesthetics for neural blockade are covered in Chapter 7, Clinical pharmacology: local anesthetics, only the clinical systemic use will be discussed here.

Clinical use in acute pain management

The effects of systemic lidocaine on neuropathic pain have been analyzed in detail in a recent meta-analysis of 13 RCTs.[161, 162] Overall, lidocaine, commonly administered in a single slow bolus dose of 5 mg/kg or as an infusion at a rate of 1–2 mg per minute, resulted in relief of neuropathic pain superior to placebo and equivalent to other compounds commonly used in this setting. Lidocaine was effective in neuropathic pain of central and peripheral origin.[162][I] Adverse effects were minor and included nausea, vomiting, drowsiness, and fatigue; the incidence of such adverse effects was again similar to other compounds used to treat neuropathic pain.[162][I] However, in an RCT, ketamine was superior to lidocaine in treating pain after spinal cord injury.[73][II] Systemic lidocaine has also been used in pain conditions other than neuropathic pain.

In the postoperative setting, parenteral lidocaine has been used as an adjunct to systemic analgesia under the hypothesis, that its anti-inflammatory effects might positively modulate the surgery-induced stress response. After major abdominal surgery, intravenous lidocaine as a bolus followed by infusion resulted in attenuated stress response leading to improved pain control and reduced opioid requirements, as well as faster bowel recovery and reduced hospital stay in a number of RCTs.[163, 164, 165][II]

For the treatment of burns pain, a Cochrane review found no published RCTs and use in this indication can only be based on case series or case reports.[166][V]

Subcutaneous administration of lidocaine can be an option in intractable terminal cancer pain.[167][IV]

In view of its parenteral route of administration and rapid onset of effect, parenteral lidocaine might be a useful compound in the treatment of acute neuropathic pain. It might also play a future role as an adjunct to other systemic analgesics in the perioperative setting.

CONCLUSIONS

Adjuvant analgesics comprise a large and pharmacologically diverse group of drugs that may be used to complement the standard multimodal analgesic regime in the treatment of acute pain. Their specific roles in acute pain management are rapidly expanding and there is sufficient evidence at present to guide their use in a variety of indications.

REFERENCES

1. Davy H. *Researches, chemical and philosophical chiefly concerning nitrous oxide or diphlogisticated air, and its respiration.* London: Johnson, 1800: 533.

✱ 2. Jahn UR, Berendes E. Nitrous oxide – an outdated anaesthetic. *Best Practice and Research. Clinical Anaesthesiology.* 2005; **19**: 391–7.

3. Stoelting RK. *Pharmacology and physiology in anesthetic practice*, 3rd edn. Philadelphia: Lippincott, Williams and Wilkins, 1998.

4. Sasada M, Smith S. *Drugs in anaesthesia and intensive care.* Oxford: Oxford Medical Publications, 2003.

5. Al-Shaikh B, Stacey S. *Essentials of anaesthetic equipment.* Philadelphia: Churchill Livingstone, 2002.

6. Evers AS, Koblin DD. Inhalational Anesthetics. In: Evers AS, Maze M (eds). *Anesthetic pharmacology – physiologic principles and clinical practice.* Philadelphia: Churchill Livingstone, 2003: 369–93.

7. Maze M, Fujinaga M. Pharmacology of nitrous oxide. *Baillière's Best Practice and Research. Clinical Anaesthesiology.* 2001; **15**: 339–48.

8. Galinkin JL, Janiszewski D, Young CJ et al. Subjective, psychomotor, cognitive, and analgesic effects of subanesthetic concentrations of sevoflurane and nitrous oxide. *Anesthesiology.* 1997; **87**: 1082–8.

9. Patel PM, Drummond JC. Cerebral physiology and the effects of anesthetics and techniques. In: Miller RD (ed.). *Miller's anesthesia*, 6th edn. Philadelphia: Churchill Livingstone, 2005: 813–57.

10. Reinstrup P, Ryding E, Algotsson L et al. Effects of nitrous oxide on human regional cerebral blood flow and isolated pial arteries. *Anesthesiology.* 1994; **81**: 396–402.

11. Gan TJ. Risk factors for postoperative nausea and vomiting. *Anesthesia and Analgesia.* 2006; **102**: 1884–98.

12. Berthoud MC, Reilly CS. Adverse effects of general anaesthetics. *Drug Safety.* 1992; **7**: 434–59.

✱ 13. Australian and New Zealand College of Anaesthetists. Faculty of Pain Medicine. *Acute pain management: scientific evidence*, 2nd edn. Melbourne: Australian and New Zealand College of Anaesthetists, 2005.

14. Takacs J. Toxicology of nitrous oxide. *Baillière's Best Practice and Research. Clinical Anaesthesiology.* 2001; **15**: 349–62.

✱ 15. Weimann J. Toxicity of nitrous oxide. *Best Practice and Research. Clinical Anaesthesiology.* 2003; **17**: 47–61.

16. Marie RM, Le Biez E, Busson P et al. Nitrous oxide anesthesia-associated myelopathy. *Archives of Neurology.* 2000; **57**: 380–2.

17. Fujinaga M. Teratogenicity of nitrous oxide. *Best Practice and Research. Clinical Anaesthesiology.* 2001; **15**: 363–75.

18. Burm AG. Occupational hazards of inhalational anaesthetics. *Best Practice and Research. Clinical Anaesthesiology.* 2003; **17**: 147–61.

19. Rosen MA. Nitrous oxide for relief of labor pain: a systematic review. *American Journal of Obstetrics and Gynecology.* 2002; **186**: S110–26.

✱ 20. Murat I, Gall O, Tourniaire B. Procedural pain in children: evidence-based best practice and guidelines. *Regional Anesthesia and Pain Medicine.* 2003; **28**: 561–72.

21. Annequin D, Carbajal R, Chauvin P et al. Fixed 50% nitrous oxide oxygen mixture for painful procedures: A French survey. *Pediatrics.* 2000; **105**: E47.

22. Hee HI, Goy RW, Ng AS. Effective reduction of anxiety and pain during venous cannulation in children: a comparison of analgesic efficacy conferred by nitrous oxide, EMLA and combination. *Paediatric Anaesthesia.* 2003; **13**: 210–6.

23. Paut O, Calmejane C, Delorme J et al. EMLA versus nitrous oxide for venous cannulation in children. *Anesthesia and Analgesia.* 2001; **93**: 590–3.

24. Lahoud GY, Averley PA. Comparison of sevoflurane and nitrous oxide mixture with nitrous oxide alone for inhalation conscious sedation in children having dental treatment: a randomised controlled trial. *Anaesthesia.* 2002; **57**: 446–50.

25. Fauroux B, Onody P, Gall O et al. The efficacy of premixed nitrous oxide and oxygen for fiberoptic bronchoscopy in pediatric patients: a randomized, double-blind, controlled study. *Chest.* 2004; **125**: 315–21.

26. Cleary AG, Ramanan AV, Baildam E et al. Nitrous oxide analgesia during intra-articular injection for juvenile idiopathic arthritis. *Archives of Disease in Childhood.* 2002; **86**: 416–8.

27. Faddy SC, Garlick SR. A systematic review of the safety of analgesia with 50% nitrous oxide: can lay responders use analgesic gases in the prehospital setting? *Emergency Medicine Journal.* 2005; **22**: 901–08.

28. Harding TA, Gibson JA. The use of inhaled nitrous oxide for flexible sigmoidoscopy: a placebo-controlled trial. *Endoscopy.* 2000; **32**: 457–60.

29. Atassi K, Mangiapan G, Fuhrman C et al. Prefixed equimolar nitrous oxide and oxygen mixture reduces discomfort during flexible bronchoscopy in adult patients: a randomized, controlled, double-blind trial. *Chest.* 2005; **128**: 863–8.

30. Douard MC, di Palma M, d'Agostino P et al. Prospective, double-blind, randomized trial of equimolar mixture of nitrous oxide/oxygen to prevent pain induced by insertion of venous access ports in cancer patients. *Supportive Care Cancer.* 2006; **14**: 161–6.

31. Ujhelyi M, Hoyt RH, Burns K et al. Nitrous oxide sedation reduces discomfort caused by atrial defibrillation shocks. *Pacing and Clinical Electrophysiology.* 2004; **27**: 485–91.

✱ 32. Abdi S, Zhou Y. Management of pain after burn injury. *Current Opinion in Anaesthesiology.* 2002; **15**: 563–7.

33. Montgomery RK. Pain management in burn injury. *Critical Care Nursing Clinics of North America.* 2004; **16**: 39–49.

34. Gallagher G, Rae CP, Kinsella J. Treatment of pain in severe burns. *American Journal of Clinical Dermatology.* 2000; **1**: 329–35.

✱ 35. Visser E, Schug SA. The role of ketamine in pain management. *Biomedicine and Pharmacotherapy.* 2006; **60**: 341–8.

36. Hirota K, Lambert DG. Ketamine: its mechanism(s) of action and unusual clinical uses. *British Journal of Anaesthesia.* 1996; **77**: 441–4.

37. Petrenko AB, Yamakura T, Baba H, Shimoji K. The role of N-methyl-D-aspartate (NMDA) receptors in pain: a review. *Anesthesia and Analgesia*. 2003; **97**: 1108–16.

38. Chen HS, Lipton SA. The chemical biology of clinically tolerated NMDA receptor antagonists. *Journal of Neurochemistry*. 2006; **97**: 1611–26.

39. Mao J. Opioid-induced abnormal pain sensitivity: implications in clinical opioid therapy. *Pain*. 2002; **100**: 213–7.

* 40. Angst MS, Clark JD. Opioid-induced hyperalgesia: a qualitative systematic review. *Anesthesiology*. 2006; **104**: 570–87.

41. Chizh BA, Headley PM. NMDA antagonists and neuropathic pain – multiple drug targets and multiple uses. *Current Pharmaceutical Design*. 2005; **11**: 2977–94.

42. Bell RF, Dahl JB, Moore RA, Kalso E. Peri-operative ketamine for acute post-operative pain: a quantitative and qualitative systematic review (Cochrane review). *Acta Anaesthesiologica Scandinavica*. 2005; **49**: 1405–28.

43. Elia N, Tramer MR. Ketamine and postoperative pain – a quantitative systematic review of randomised trials. *Pain*. 2005; **113**: 61–70.

44. Subramaniam K, Subramaniam B, Steinbrook RA. Ketamine as adjuvant analgesic to opioids: a quantitative and qualitative systematic review. *Anesthesia and Analgesia*. 2004; **99**: 482–95.

45. Duedahl TH, Romsing J, Moiniche S, Dahl JB. A qualitative systematic review of peri-operative dextromethorphan in post-operative pain. *Acta Anaesthesiologica Scandinavica*. 2006; **50**: 1–13.

46. White PF, Way WL, Trevor AJ. Ketamine – its pharmacology and therapeutic uses. *Anesthesiology*. 1982; **56**: 119–36.

47. Wolff K, Winstock AR. Ketamine: from medicine to misuse. *CNS Drugs*. 2006; **20**: 199–218.

48. Jansen KL, Darracot-Cankovic R. The nonmedical use of ketamine, part two: A review of problem use and dependence. *Journal of Psychoactive Drugs*. 2001; **33**: 151–8.

49. Narendran R, Frankle WG, Keefe R *et al*. Altered prefrontal dopaminergic function in chronic recreational ketamine users. *American Journal of Psychiatry*. 2005; **162**: 2352–9.

50. Bahn EL, Holt KR. Procedural sedation and analgesia: a review and new concepts. *Emergency Medicine Clinics of North America*. 2005; **23**: 503–17.

51. Evans D, Turnham L, Barbour K *et al*. Intravenous ketamine sedation for painful oncology procedures. *Paediatric Anaesthesia*. 2005; **15**: 131–8.

52. Weinbroum AA. A single small dose of postoperative ketamine provides rapid and sustained improvement in morphine analgesia in the presence of morphine-resistant pain. *Anesthesia and Analgesia*. 2003; **96**: 789–95.

53. Reeves M, Lindholm DE, Myles PS *et al*. Adding ketamine to morphine for patient-controlled analgesia after major abdominal surgery: a double-blinded, randomized controlled trial. *Anesthesia and Analgesia*. 2001; **93**: 116–20.

54. Hercock T, Gillham MJ, Sleigh J, Jones SF. The addition of ketamine to patient controlled morphine analgesia does not improve quality of analgesia after total abdominal hysterectomy. *Acute Pain*. 1999; **2**: 68–72.

55. Murdoch CJ, Crooks BA, Miller CD. Effect of the addition of ketamine to morphine in patient-controlled analgesia. *Anaesthesia*. 2002; **57**: 484–8.

56. Burstal R, Danjoux G, Hayes C, Lantry G. PCA ketamine and morphine after abdominal hysterectomy. *Anaesthesia and Intensive Care*. 2001; **29**: 246–51.

57. Unlugenc H, Ozalevli M, Guler T, Isik G. Postoperative pain management with intravenous patient-controlled morphine: comparison of the effect of adding magnesium or ketamine. *European Journal of Anaesthesiology*. 2003; **20**: 416–21.

58. Carroll IR, Angst MS, Clark JD. Management of perioperative pain in patients chronically consuming opioids. *Regional Anesthesia and Pain Medicine*. 2004; **29**: 576–91.

59. Swenson JD, Davis JJ, Johnson KB. Postoperative care of the chronic opioid-consuming patient. *Anesthesiology Clinics of North America*. 2005; **23**: 37–48.

60. Mitra S, Sinatra RS. Perioperative management of acute pain in the opioid-dependent patient. *Anesthesiology*. 2004; **101**: 212–27.

* 61. Brill S, Ginosar Y, Davidson EM. Perioperative management of chronic pain patients with opioid dependency. *Current Opinion in Anaesthesiology*. 2006; **19**: 325–31.

62. Joly V, Richebe P, Guignard B *et al*. Remifentanil-induced postoperative hyperalgesia and its prevention with small-dose ketamine. *Anesthesiology*. 2005; **103**: 147–55.

63. McCartney CJ, Sinha A, Katz J. A qualitative systematic review of the role of N-methyl-D-aspartate receptor antagonists in preventive analgesia. *Anesthesia and Analgesia*. 2004; **98**: 1385–400.

* 64. Pogatzki-Zahn EM, Zahn PK. From preemptive to preventive analgesia. *Current Opinion in Anaesthesiology*. 2006; **19**: 551–5.

65. Katz J, McCartney CJ. Current status of pre-emptive analgesia. *Current Opinion in Anaesthesiology*. 2002; **15**: 435–41.

66. De Kock M, Lavand'homme P, Waterloos H. 'Balanced analgesia' in the perioperative period: is there a place for ketamine? *Pain*. 2001; **92**: 373–80.

* 67. Kehlet H, Jensen TS, Woolf CJ. Persistent postsurgical pain: risk factors and prevention. *Lancet*. 2006; **367**: 1618–25.

68. Hayes C, Browne S, Lantry G, Burstal R. Neuropathic pain in the acute pain service: a prospective survey. *Acute Pain*. 2002; **4**: 45–8.

69. Eisenberg E, McNicol ED, Carr DB. Efficacy and safety of opioid agonists in the treatment of neuropathic pain of nonmalignant origin: systematic review and meta-analysis of randomized controlled trials. *Journal of the American Medical Association*. 2005; **293**: 3043–52.

70. Przewlocki R, Przewlocka B. Opioids in neuropathic pain. *Current Pharmaceutical Design*. 2005; **11**: 3013–25.

71. Sang CN. NMDA-receptor antagonists in neuropathic pain: experimental methods to clinical trials. *Journal of Pain and Symptom Management*. 2000; **19**: S21–5.

* 72. Hocking G, Cousins MJ. Ketamine in chronic pain management: an evidence-based review. *Anesthesia and Analgesia*. 2003; **97**: 1730–9.

73. Kvarnstrom A, Karlsten R, Quiding H, Gordh T. The analgesic effect of intravenous ketamine and lidocaine on pain after spinal cord injury. *Acta Anaesthesiologica Scandinavica*. 2004; **48**: 498–506.

74. Vick PG, Lamer TJ. Treatment of central post-stroke pain with oral ketamine. *Pain*. 2001; **92**: 311–3.

75. Mitchell AC, Fallon MT. A single infusion of intravenous ketamine improves pain relief in patients with critical limb ischaemia: results of a double blind randomised controlled trial. *Pain*. 2002; **97**: 275–81.

76. Habib AS, Gan TJ. Role of analgesic adjuncts in postoperative pain management. *Anesthesiology Clinics of North America*. 2005; **23**: 85–107.

77. Smith H, Elliott J. Alpha2 receptors and agonists in pain management. *Current Opinion in Anaesthesiology*. 2001; **14**: 513–8.

78. Scheinin M, Pihlavisto M. Molecular pharmacology of alpha2-adrenoceptor agonists. *Baillière's Best Practice and Research. Clinical Anaesthesiology*. 2000; **14**: 247–60.

79. Kamibayashi T, Maze M. Clinical uses of alpha2-adrenergic agonists. *Anesthesiology*. 2000; **93**: 1345–9.

80. Buerkle H. Peripheral anti-nociceptive action of alpha2-adrenoceptor agonists. *Baillière's Best Practice and Research. Clinical Anaesthesiology*. 2000; **14**: 411–8.

81. Lavand'homme PM, Ma W, De Kock M, Eisenach JC. Perineural alpha(2A)-adrenoceptor activation inhibits spinal cord neuroplasticity and tactile allodynia after nerve injury. *Anesthesiology*. 2002; **97**: 972–80.

82. Shi TS, Winzer-Serhan U, Leslie F, Hokfelt T. Distribution and regulation of alpha(2)-adrenoceptors in rat dorsal root ganglia. *Pain*. 2000; **84**: 319–30.

83. Jaakola M-L. Intra-operative use of alpha2-adrenoceptor agonists. *Baillière's Best Practice and Research. Clinical Anaesthesiology*. 2000; **14**: 335–45.

84. Talke PO. Pharmacodynamics of alpha2-adrenoceptor agonists. *Baillière's Best Practice and Research. Clinical Anaesthesiology*. 2000; **14**: 271–83.

85. Quintin L, Ghigone M. Risks associated with peri-operative use of alpha2-adrenoceptor agonists. *Baillière's Best Practice and Research. Clinical Anaesthesiology*. 2000; **14**: 347–68.

86. Dahl V, Raeder JC. Non-opioid postoperative analgesia. *Acta Anaesthesiologica Scandinavica*. 2000; **44**: 1191–203.

87. Tryba M, Gehling M. Clonidine – a potent analgesic adjuvant. *Current Opinion in Anaesthesiology*. 2002; **15**: 511–7.

88. Tonner PH, Scholz J. Pre-anaesthetic administration of alpha2-adrenoceptor agonists. *Baillière's Best Practice and Research. Clinical Anaesthesiology*. 2000; **14**: 305–20.

89. Yanagidate F, Hamaya Y, Dohi S. Clonidine premedication reduces maternal requirement for intravenous morphine after cesarean delivery without affecting newborn's outcome. *Regional Anesthesia and Pain Medicine*. 2001; **26**: 461–7.

90. Park J, Forrest J, Kolesar R *et al*. Oral clonidine reduces postoperative PCA morphine requirements. *Canadian Journal of Anaesthesia*. 1996; **43**: 900–6.

91. Marinangeli F, Ciccozzi A, Donatelli F *et al*. Clonidine for treatment of postoperative pain: a dose-finding study. *European Journal of Pain*. 2002; **6**: 35–42.

92. Bergendahl HT, Lonnqvist PA, Eksborg S *et al*. Clonidine vs. midazolam as premedication in children undergoing adeno-tonsillectomy: a prospective, randomized, controlled clinical trial. *Acta Anaesthesiologica Scandinavica*. 2004; **48**: 1292–300.

93. De Kock MF, Pichon G, Scholtes JL. Intraoperative clonidine enhances postoperative morphine patient-controlled analgesia. *Canadian Journal of Anaesthesia*. 1992; **39**: 537–44.

94. Bock M, Kunz P, Schreckenberger R *et al*. Comparison of caudal and intravenous clonidine in the prevention of agitation after sevoflurane in children. *British Journal of Anaesthesia*. 2002; **88**: 790–6.

95. Wallace AW, Galindez D, Salahieh A *et al*. Effect of clonidine on cardiovascular morbidity and mortality after noncardiac surgery. *Anesthesiology*. 2004; **101**: 284–93.

96. Jeffs SA, Hall JE, Morris S. Comparison of morphine alone with morphine plus clonidine for postoperative patient-controlled analgesia. *British Journal of Anaesthesia*. 2002; **89**: 424–7.

97. Aho MS, Erkola OA, Scheinin H *et al*. Effect of intravenously administered dexmedetomidine on pain after laparoscopic tubal ligation. *Anesthesia and Analgesia*. 1991; **73**: 112–8.

98. Arain SR, Ruehlow RM, Uhrich TD, Ebert TJ. The efficacy of dexmedetomidine versus morphine for postoperative analgesia after major inpatient surgery. *Anesthesia and Analgesia*. 2004; **98**: 153–8.

99. Ramsay MAE. Intensive care: problems of over- and undersedation. *Baillière's Best Practice and Research. Clinical Anaesthesiology*. 2000; **14**: 419–32.

100. Martin E, Ramsay G, Mantz J, Sum-Ping ST. The role of the alpha2-adrenoceptor agonist dexmedetomidine in postsurgical sedation in the intensive care unit. *Journal of Intensive Care Medicine*. 2003; **18**: 29–41.

101. Venn RM, Bradshaw CJ, Spencer R *et al*. Preliminary UK experience of dexmedetomidine, a novel agent for postoperative sedation in the intensive care unit. *Anaesthesia*. 1999; **54**: 1136–42.

102. Dunbar SA. Alpha2-adrenoceptor agonists in the management of chronic pain. *Baillière's Best Practice and Research. Clinical Anaesthesiology*. 2000; **14**: 471–81.

103. Jensen TS. Anticonvulsants in neuropathic pain: rationale and clinical evidence. *European Journal of Pain*. 2002; **6** (Suppl A): 61–8.

*104. Attal N, Cruccu G, Haanpaa M et al. EFNS guidelines on pharmacological treatment of neuropathic pain. European Journal of Neurology. 2006; 13: 1153–69.

*105. Finnerup NB, Otto M, McQuay HJ et al. Algorithm for neuropathic pain treatment: an evidence based proposal. Pain. 2005; 118: 289–305.

106. Gilron I. Review article: the role of anticonvulsant drugs in postoperative pain management: a bench-to-bedside perspective. Canadian Journal of Anaesthesia. 2006; 53: 562–71.

107. Perucca E. An introduction to antiepileptic drugs. Epilepsia. 2005; 46 (Suppl. 4): 31–7.

108. Hurley RW, Chatterjea D, Rose Feng M et al. Gabapentin and pregabalin can interact synergistically with naproxen to produce antihyperalgesia. Anesthesiology. 2002; 97: 1263–73.

109. Dirks J, Petersen KL, Rowbotham MC, Dahl JB. Gabapentin suppresses cutaneous hyperalgesia following heat-capsaicin sensitization. Anesthesiology. 2002; 97: 102–7.

110. Eckhardt K, Ammon S, Hofmann U et al. Gabapentin enhances the analgesic effect of morphine in healthy volunteers. Anesthesia and Analgesia. 2001; 91: 185–91.

111. Gilron I, Orr E, Tu D et al. A placebo-controlled randomized clinical trial of perioperative administration of gabapentin, rofecoxib and their combination for spontaneous and movement-evoked pain after abdominal hysterectomy. Pain. 2005; 113: 191–200.

112. Menigaux C, Adam F, Guignard B et al. Preoperative gabapentin decreases anxiety and improves early functional recovery from knee surgery. Anesthesia and Analgesia. 2005; 100: 1394–9.

113. Hill CM, Balkenohl M, Thomas DW et al. Pregabalin in patients with postoperative dental pain. European Journal of Pain. 2001; 5: 119–24.

114. Reuben SS, Buvanendran A, Kroin JS, Raghunathan K. The analgesic efficacy of celecoxib, pregabalin, and their combination for spinal fusion surgery. Anesthesia and Analgesia. 2006; 103: 1271–7.

115. Ho KY, Gan TJ, Habib AS. Gabapentin and postoperative pain – a systematic review of randomized controlled trials. Pain. 2006; 126: 91–101.

116. Seib RK, Paul JE. Preoperative gabapentin for postoperative analgesia: a meta-analysis. Canadian Journal of Anaesthesia. 2006; 53: 461–9.

117. Hurley RW, Cohen SP, Williams KA et al. The analgesic effects of perioperative gabapentin on postoperative pain: a meta-analysis. Regional Anesthesia and Pain Medicine. 2006; 31: 237–47.

118. Peng PW, Wijeysundera DN, Li CC. Use of gabapentin for perioperative pain control – a meta-analysis. Pain Research and Management. 2007; 12: 85–92.

*119. Tiippana EM, Hamunen K, Kontinen VK, Kalso E. Do surgical patients benefit from perioperative gabapentin/pregabalin? A systematic review of efficacy and safety. Anesthesia and Analgesia. 2007; 104: 1545–56.

120. Dahl JB, Mathiesen O, Moiniche S. 'Protective premedication': an option with gabapentin and related drugs? A review of gabapentin and pregabalin in in the treatment of post-operative pain. Acta Anaesthesiologica Scandinavica. 2004; 48: 1130–6.

121. Martin C, Martin A, Rud C, Valli M. [Comparative study of sodium valproate and ketoprofen in the treatment of postoperative pain]. Annales Françaises d'Anesthésie et de Rèanimation. 1988; 7: 387–92.

122. Wiffen PJ, McQuay HJ, Moore RA. Carbamazepine for acute and chronic pain. Cochrane Database of Systematic Reviews. 2005; CD005451.

123. Levendoglu F, Ogun CO, Ozerbil O et al. Gabapentin is a first line drug for the treatment of neuropathic pain in spinal cord injury. Spine. 2004; 29: 743–51.

124. Tripathi M, Kaushik S. Carbamezapine for pain management in Guillain-Barré syndrome patients in the intensive care unit. Critical Care Medicine. 2000; 28: 655–8.

125. Pandey CK, Bose N, Garg G et al. Gabapentin for the treatment of pain in Guillain-Barré syndrome: a double-blinded, placebo-controlled, crossover study. Anesthesia and Analgesia. 2002; 95: 1719–23.

126. Bone M, Critchley P, Buggy DJ. Gabapentin in postamputation phantom limb pain: A randomized, double-blind, placebo-controlled, cross-over study. Regional Anesthesia and Pain Medicine. 2002; 27: 481–6.

127. Oldman AD, Smith LA, McQuay HJ, Moore RA. Pharmacological treatments for acute migraine: quantitative systematic review. Pain. 2002; 97: 247–57.

128. Damen L, Bruijn JK, Verhagen AP et al. Symptomatic treatment of migraine in children: a systematic review of medication trials. Pediatrics. 2005; 116: e295–302.

129. Chronicle E, Mulleners W. Anticonvulsant drugs for migraine prophylaxis. Cochrane Database of Systematic Reviews. 2004; CD003226.

130. Stillman MJ, Zajac D, Rybicki LA. Treatment of primary headache disorders with intravenous valproate: initial outpatient experience. Headache. 2004; 44: 65–9.

131. Leniger T, Pageler L, Stude P et al. Comparison of intravenous valproate with intravenous lysine-acetylsalicylic acid in acute migraine attacks. Headache. 2005; 45: 42–6.

132. Mathew NT, Kailasam J, Meadors L et al. Intravenous valproate sodium (depacon) aborts migraine rapidly: a preliminary report. Headache. 2000; 40: 720–3.

133. Norton J. Use of intravenous valproate sodium in status migraine. Headache. 2000; 40: 755–7.

134. Tfelt-Hansen P. A review of evidence-based medicine and meta-analytic reviews in migraine. Cephalalgia. 2006; 26: 1265–74.

135. Cerbo R, Villani V, Bruti G et al. Primary headache in Emergency Department: prevalence, clinical features and therapeutical approach. Journal of Headache and Pain. 2005; 6: 287–9.

136. Sindrup SH, Otto M, Finnerup NB, Jensen TS. Antidepressants in the treatment of neuropathic pain. Basic and Clinical Pharmacology and Toxicology. 2005; 96: 399–409.

137. Wallace MS, Barger D, Schulteis G. The effect of chronic oral desipramine on capsaicin-induced allodynia and hyperalgesia: a double-blinded, placebo-controlled, crossover study. *Anesthesia and Analgesia*. 2002; **95**: 973–8.

138. Kerrick JM, Fine PG, Lipman AG, Love G. Low-dose amitriptyline as an adjunct to opioids for postoperative orthopedic pain: a placebo-controlled trial. *Pain*. 1993; **52**: 325–30.

139. Reuben SS, Makari-Judson G, Lurie SD. Evaluation of efficacy of the perioperative administration of venlafaxine XR in the prevention of postmastectomy pain syndrome. *Journal of Pain and Symptom Management*. 2004; **27**: 133–9.

140. Bowsher D. The effects of pre-emptive treatment of postherpetic neuralgia with amitriptyline: a randomized, double-blind, placebo-controlled trial. *Journal of Pain and Symptom Management*. 1997; **13**: 327–31.

141. Scholz J, Steinfath M, Tonner PH. Postoperative nausea and vomiting. *Current Opinion in Anaesthesiology*. 1999; **12**: 657–61.

142. Baxendale BR, Vater M, Lavery KM. Dexamethasone reduces pain and swelling following extraction of third molar teeth. *Anaesthesia*. 1993; **48**: 961–4.

143. Schmelzeisen R, Frolich JC. Prevention of postoperative swelling and pain by dexamethasone after operative removal of impacted third molar teeth. *European Journal of Clinical Pharmacology*. 1993; **44**: 275–7.

144. Bisgaard T. Analgesic treatment after laparoscopic cholecystectomy: a critical assessment of the evidence. *Anesthesiology*. 2006; **104**: 835–46.

145. Aasboe V, Raeder JC, Groegaard B. Betamethasone reduces postoperative pain and nausea after ambulatory surgery. *Anesthesia and Analgesia*. 1998; **87**: 319–23.

146. Pappas AL, Sukhani R, Hotaling AJ *et al.* The effect of preoperative dexamethasone on the immediate and delayed postoperative morbidity in children undergoing adenotonsillectomy. *Anesthesia and Analgesia*. 1998; **87**: 57–61.

147. Afman CE, Welge JA, Steward DL. Steroids for post-tonsillectomy pain reduction: meta-analysis of randomized controlled trials. *Otolaryngology, Head and Neck Surgery*. 2006; **134**: 181–6.

148. Henzi I, Walder B, Tramer MR. Dexamethasone for the prevention of postoperative nausea and vomiting: a quantitative systematic review. *Anesthesia and Analgesia*. 2000; **90**: 186–94.

*149. Visser EJ. A review of calcitonin and its use in the treatment of acute pain. *Acute Pain*. 2005; **7**: 185–9.

150. Blau LA, Hoehns JD. Analgesic efficacy of calcitonin for vertebral fracture pain. *Annals of Pharmacotherapy*. 2003; **37**: 564–70.

151. Brown JP, Josse RG. 2002 clinical practice guidelines for the diagnosis and management of osteoporosis in Canada. *Canadian Medical Association Journal*. 2002; **167**: S1–34.

152. Halbert J, Crotty M, Cameron ID. Evidence for the optimal management of acute and chronic phantom pain: a systematic review. *Clinical Journal of Pain*. 2002; **18**: 84–92.

153. Kessel C, Worz R. Immediate response of phantom limb pain to calcitonin. *Pain*. 1987; **30**: 79–87.

154. Jaeger H, Maier C, Wawersik J. [Postoperative treatment of phantom pain and causalgias with calcitonin]. *Anaesthesist*. 1988; **37**: 71–6.

155. Simanski C, Lempa M, Koch G *et al.* [Therapy of phantom pain with salmon calcitonin and effect on postoperative patient satisfaction]. *Der Chirurg*. 1999; **70**: 674–81.

156. Jaeger H, Maier C. Calcitonin in phantom limb pain: a double-blind study. *Pain*. 1992; **48**: 21–7.

157. Gilbert CR, Hanson IR, Brown AB, Hingson RA. Intravenous use of xylocaine. *Current Research in Anesthesia and Analgesia*. 1951; **30**: 301–13.

*158. Boas RA, Covino BG, Shahnarian A. Analgesic responses to i.v. lignocaine. *British Journal of Anaesthesia*. 1982; **54**: 501–5.

159. Chabal C, Russell L, Burchiel K. The effect of intravenous lidocaine, tocainide and mexiletine on spontaneously active fibres originating in rat sciatic neuromas. *Pain*. 1989; **38**: 333–8.

160. Tanelian DL, Brose WG. Neuropathic pain can be relieved by drugs that are use-dependent sodium channel blockers: lidocaine, carbamazepine, and mexiletine. *Anesthesiology*. 1991; **74**: 949–51.

*161. Tremont-Lukats IW, Challapalli V, McNicol ED *et al.* Systemic administration of local anesthetics to relieve neuropathic pain: a systematic review and meta-analysis. *Anesthesia and Analgesia*. 2005; **101**: 1738–49.

162. Challapalli V, Tremont-Lukats IW, McNicol ED *et al.* Systemic administration of local anesthetic agents to relieve neuropathic pain. *Cochrane Database of Systematic Reviews*. 2005; **CD003345**.

*163. Herroeder S, Pecher S, Schonherr ME *et al.* Systemic lidocaine shortens length of hospital stay after colorectal surgery: a double-blinded, randomized, placebo-controlled trial. *Annals of Surgery*. 2007; **246**: 192–200.

164. Koppert W, Weigand M, Neumann F *et al.* Perioperative intravenous lidocaine has preventive effects on postoperative pain and morphine consumption after major abdominal surgery. *Anesthesia and Analgesia*. 2004; **98**: 1050–5.

165. Groudine SB, Fisher HA, Kaufman Jr RP *et al.* Intravenous lidocaine speeds the return of bowel function, decreases postoperative pain, and shortens hospital stay in patients undergoing radical retropubic prostatectomy. *Anesthesia and Analgesia*. 1998; **86**: 235–9.

166. Wasiak J, Cleland H. Lidocaine for pain relief in burn injured patients. *Cochrane Database of Systematic Reviews*. 2007; **CD005622**.

167. Brose WG, Cousins MJ. Subcutaneous lidocaine for treatment of neuropathic cancer pain. *Pain*. 1991; **45**: 145–8.

7

Clinical pharmacology: local anesthetics

JONATHAN McGHIE AND MICHAEL G SERPELL

KEY LEARNING POINTS

- Local anesthetics reversibly block nerve transmission.
- Na^+ channel blockade is their primary action.
- Physicochemical properties determine potency, onset, and duration.
- Cardiotoxicity, neurotoxicity, and anaphylaxis can occur.

- Dosing is based upon the drug used, the patient's co-morbidities and site of injection.
- Certain local anesthetic stereoisomers have better safety profiles.

INTRODUCTION

Local anesthetics (LA) are a class of chemicals that produce anesthesia (absence of sensation – pain, touch, temperature, proprioception) in a body part without loss of consciousness or impairment of central control of vital functions. They bind to Na^+ channels within nerves and will block the action potentials for nerve conduction in every type of nerve fiber. Therefore, afferent, efferent, and sympathetic fibers may all be blocked, when often it is only sensory block or analgesia that is needed. The necessary characteristics of LAs are that their action is reversible at clinically relevant concentrations. Cold, pressure, and other drugs can produce LA effects, e.g. phenothiazines, β-blockers and antihistamines, tricyclic antidepressants and anticonvulsants.[1] However, because the above have problems with poor penetration into nerve tissue and intolerable side effects, today's useful LAs are chemical descendants of the amino-ester cocaine.

HISTORY

Cocaine was the first LA to be used in clinical practice as a topical anesthetic for ophthalmic surgery in 1884 by Carl Koller.[2] It was used for centuries by Andean natives for its stimulatory and euphoric effects. It occurs in abundance in the leaves of the coca shrub (*Erythroxylon coca*) and was first isolated in 1860 by Albert Niemann. Although he noticed the numbing effect it had on the tongue, it was not until Sigmund Freud passed on this observation to Koller that medical use was made of this action in the form of topical anesthesia for eye surgery.[3] The first nerve to be blocked was the mandibular by Halsted and Hall in the same year and, thereafter, the use of LAs exploded. Crile first used the term "blocked" in 1897 and Cushing was the originator of regional anesthesia in 1901.

The toxicity and addictive properties of cocaine were disadvantageous and led to the search for synthetic substitutes. This resulted in the synthesis of procaine in 1905, the prototype of LA drugs for the next 50 years. However, it was the development and use of lidocaine by Lofgren in 1948 (the first amino-amide drug) that heralded the reign of the modern LAs. Lidocaine is still commonly used today and is the forefather of all the recent arrivals (**Table 7.1**).

CELLULAR ELECTROPHYSIOLOGY

Butterworth and Strichartz[4] present a more comprehensive account of the electrophysiology of cellular membrane potentials in their review. A nerve fiber or axon is a cylinder of axoplasm that is separated from the extracellular fluids by a semipermeable membrane. This membrane is a lipid bilayer that encases proteins, it is semipermeable because it is relatively impermeable to various ions, except at protein channels where selective ions can pass through.

The ionic composition of the axoplasm and extracellular fluids differ markedly. This state is produced and maintained by an electrogenic, energy requiring, membrane bound enzyme Na^+-K^+ ATPase, which pumps three Na^+ ions out of the cell for every two K^+ ions in. The electrical gradient that exists across the membrane is predicted by the Nernst equation.[5] At rest, the predicted membrane potential for K^+ ions alone gives a value of $-86\,mV$ which agrees closely with the measured normal resting potentials of cells (-50 to $-90\,mV$ with the interior of the cell negative to the exterior). This would imply that at rest the nerve cell behaves as a potassium electrode, thus changes in intra/extracellular K^+ would markedly alter the resting potential, whereas changes in Na^+ concentration have little effect.

An action potential (AP) is an event that is complete within 1–2 ms and consists of a depolarization phase followed by a repolarization phase. The depolarization phase is due to the influx of Na^+ ions through Na^+ channels. As the Na^+ channel closes spontaneously, the duration of the Na^+ influx is limited. Repolarization,

which accounts for 70 percent of the AP duration, is due to the efflux of K^+ ions through K^+ channels.

The AP produces electrical fields sufficient to initiate depolarization at a neighboring site and result in a self-propagating process that will continue along the entire length of the nerve fiber. After an AP, there is a refractory period that prevents the membrane from depolarizing again. This will prevent further depolarizations occurring in the wake following behind an AP until a fresh impulse arrives. The velocity of transmission is increased as the diameter of the unmyelinated axon increases.

Larger fibers (greater than 1 µm in diameter) are covered with a myelin sheath accounting for more than half the thickness of the fiber. The myelin is a bilayer lipid membrane extension from the Schwann cell that wraps around the axon several hundred times and which conserves current leakage and enhances electrical efficiency. The sheath is interrupted and deficient at intervals along the axon (nodes of Ranvier) and at these points the cell membrane is in closer contact with the extracellular fluid. Most of the Na^+ and K^+ channels are present at these nodes. This results in more rapid transmission as the AP jumps from node to node (saltatory conduction). The distance between nodes is proportional to the diameter of the axon; so larger diameter fibers have nodes further apart resulting in faster impulse transmission.

MECHANISM OF ACTION OF LOCAL ANESTHETICS

The primary effect of LAs involves altering Na^+ influx to decrease the rate of depolarization, prolong the refractory period, and slow the conduction velocity.[5] In subminimal concentrations, they will not prevent the development or transmission of an AP, but will decrease the frequency of impulses transmitted per second. When the minimum blocking concentration (C_m) of an LA is exposed to the nerve, complete conduction block is achieved primarily because the rate and degree of depolarization is sufficiently depressed that the threshold potential is never reached. There is also a concomitant but lesser decrease in the rate of repolarization. Initially, it was thought that LAs have little or no inhibitory effect on K^+ conductance and that a direct relationship between the rates of depolarization and repolarization existed.[6] However, recent evidence investigating the toxic side effects of LAs implicates distinct K^+ blockade in both cardiac and neurotoxicity.[7, 8, 9] Additionally, LAs can directly and indirectly affect Ca^{2+} stores via calcium receptors and muscarinic receptors.[10]

Site of action

Local anesthetics primarily act upon voltage-gated Na^+ channels ($Na_{(v)}$). The Na^+ channel is a complex of glycosylated proteins consisting of one α subunit and two β

Table 7.1 History of local anaesthetics.

Anesthetic	Date
Esters (aromatic end–ester chain–amine end)	
Cocaine	1884
Procaine	1905
Amides (aromatic end–amide chain–amine end)	
Lignocaine	1948
Prilocaine	1960
Bupivacaine	1963
Ropivacaine	1996
Levobupivacaine	1998

subunits (**Figure 7.1**).[11] The α subunit consists of four homologous domains (DI–IV), which each contain six transmembrane helices (S1–S6). The transmembrane pore of the Na^+ channel is created by the circular arrangement of the domains and lined by an additional helix between S5–S6 (P segment).[12, 13] The β subunits help to stabilize the channel and modify the ion gating.

There are at least ten isoforms of the α subunit and five genes coding the β subunit.[14] Importantly, they have differing gating properties and are expressed to different levels in the body; they can be distinguished by their affinity for tetrodotoxin.[15, 16] Certain isoforms are clustered to specific tissues, e.g. $Na_{(v)}1.2$ brain, $Na_{(v)}1.4$ skeletal muscle, and $Na_{(v)}1.5$ in cardiac muscle, suggesting the possibility for targeted therapeutic interventions if specific $Na_{(v)}$ blocking drugs can be synthesized.[17]

The internal hydrophobic residues on (S6) of domain IV are critical for LA binding and stabilization of the receptor in the inactivated state.[18] Mutagenic work with amino acids in the α subunit and computer models have confirmed that residues in S6–D4, and to a lesser degree on D1 and D3, contribute to the binding and positioning of the LA within the pore.[14, 19, 20]

While the neutral type of LA drugs such as benzocaine, n-butanol, and benzyl alcohol act within the nerve membrane, causing membrane expansion and a change in Na^+ channel configuration, most LAs exist in equilibrium between their nonionized tertiary amine base and their ionized quaternary amine cation.

$$B + H^+ \quad \Leftrightarrow \quad BH^+$$

Nonionized	Ionized
Base	Cation

Approximately 90 percent of the blocking action is due to its internal action of the cation and 10 percent is due to the base form.[21] Once the LA is internalized in the pore it prevents Na^+ entry by three mechanisms.[16] First, via steric interaction with amino acids on S6–D4 it occludes the pore and gating mechanism, initiating fast and slow inactivation. Second, the hydrophobic aromatic component excludes water, creating a low dielectric environment that interferes with Na^+ current. Finally, the quaternary or ionized end of the LA lies in the center of the pore, creating an electrostatic barrier to ion movement.

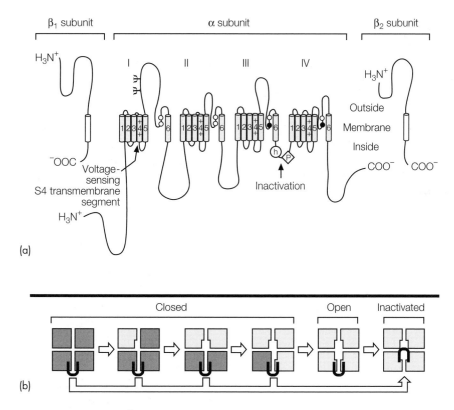

Figure 7.1 Structure and function of the Na^+ channel. (a) A two-dimensional representation of the α and β subunits of the Na^+ channel. (b) The four domains of the Na^+ channel α subunit are illustrated as a square array as viewed looking down on the membrane. Upon depolarization, each of the four domains undergoes a conformational change in sequence to an activated state. When all four domains have activated, the Na^+ channel can open. Within a few milliseconds after opening, the inactivation gate between domains III and IV closes over the intracellular mouth of the channel and occludes it, preventing further ion conductance. Adapted from Catterall W, Mackie K. Local Anaesthetics. In: Hardman JG, Limbird LL (eds). *Goodman and Gilman's the pharmacological basis of therapeutics*, 9th edn. New York: McGraw-Hill, 1996: 331–47, with permission.[7] © The McGraw-Hill Companies, Inc.

External sites on the Na$^+$ channel are acted upon by the naturally occurring biotoxins, saxitoxin (shellfish), and tetrodotoxin (pufferfish), which are the most potent Na$^+$ channel blockers known.[4, 5] Both toxins, in nanomolar concentrations, cause death by paralysis of the respiratory muscles. Although the toxins are chemically different from each other, their mechanism of action is indistinguishable. Some Na$^+$ channels are tetrodotoxin resistant, such as those on cardiac myocytes (1.5) and small sensory nerves (1.9).[22] Recent work suggests that the cardiac myocyte isoform may also have an external hydrophilic pathway for LA cation.[15]

Frequency- and voltage-dependent actions

A nerve which is repeatedly stimulated is much more sensitive to LAs than one that is resting because a higher frequency of stimulation produces a more positive membrane potential.[5] These frequency- and voltage-dependent effects occur because the LA molecule in its charged form gains access to its binding site within the pore only when the Na$^+$ channel is in an open state and because it binds more tightly to and stabilizes the inactivated state of the Na$^+$ channel, this is called the modulated-receptor hypothesis.[23] LAs exhibit these properties to differing extents. In general, small molecules with modest lipid solubility (i.e. lidocaine) bind and dissociate very rapidly. Therefore, a high frequency of stimulation is required so that drug binding during the action potential exceeds drug dissociation between action potentials. Frequency dependence appears only at high frequencies when these drugs will act as antiarrhythmics (for tachydysrhythmias). Conversely, large molecules with high lipid solubility (i.e. bupivacaine) dissociate slowly and frequency dependence occurs at lower rates of channel activation and so they can act as potent depressors of cardiac function at normal heart rates (i.e. more cardiotoxic).

Differential sensitivity

There is a differential block exhibited by fibers of varying size and frequency of discharge. Blockade of pain and sympathetic function usually appears first, followed by temperature, touch, deep pressure, and finally motor function (**Table 7.2**). From this it was deduced that the C_m was lower for smaller and unmyelinated fibers. For example, an Aδ fiber requires half the C_m compared with an Aα fiber. The theory to explain this for unmyelinated nerves was that the critical length over which an impulse could passively propagate (space constant) was shorter. For myelinated nerves, C_m had to be achieved at three nodes of Ranvier before conduction was blocked. The internodal distance is shorter in smaller myelinated nerves and so less LA is needed to block conduction than in larger myelinated ones. However, *in vitro* work failed to show that fiber diameter was the explanation.[24] Instead, it is suggested that with low concentrations of LA, it is the length of nerve exposed that matters. Partial inactivation of the nerve extends the decay of the AP along the axon, if the length is sufficiently long then conduction block will ultimately occur, this is called decremental blockade.[25, 26]

In vivo demonstration of differential block may be due to anatomical reasons.[27] LAs are injected as close to the target nerve as possible, but several factors affect delivery to the nerve membrane. The LA molecules, which are diluted by tissue fluid, must spread by mass movement to the nerve. Diffusion of the LA is dependent on the concentration gradient and the concentration achieved will depend on local distribution into nonneural tissue and systemic absorption. The myelin sheath also acts as a barrier for penetration into the nerve membrane. If these factors are sufficient to reduce the concentration to below C_m, conduction block will not occur. It is possible that a block can result in absence of pain (Aδ and C fibers blocked), whereas motor function and touch (Aα and Aβ fibers) are unaffected.

In addition, the frequency-dependence of LA action favors block of small sensory fibers as they generate APs of

Table 7.2 Susceptibility of nerve fibers to block.

Type	Function	Diameter (μm)	Velocity (m/s)	Sensitivity to block
Myelinated				
Aα	Motor, proprioception	12–20	70–120	+
Aβ	Touch, pressure	5–12	30–70	++
Aγ	Muscle spindles and tone	3–6	15–30	++
Aδ	Pain, temp, touch	2–5	12–30	+++
B	Pre-ganglionic autonomic	<3	3–15	++++
Unmyelinated				
C	Pain Post-ganglionic sympathetic	1	0.5–2	++++

longer duration (3 ms) at high frequencies, whereas motor fibers generate APs of shorter duration (<0.5 ms) at low frequencies.

Pattern of onset and offset: local disposition

The differential effects above explain why the onset and recovery of blockade in a peripheral nerve often occurs in a predictable order. Once at the nerve trunk, LA molecules diffuse inward toward the center of the nerve. The outer sections (mantle fibers) achieve higher concentrations with resultant blockade before the core fibers. This results in the more proximal fibers being blocked first, followed by the distal core fibers. However, this may vary amongst individuals and also in large mixed nerves, such as the brachial plexus, where motor fibers in the mantle of the nerve bundle are exposed to the LA drug first as they branch off before the sensory nerves.[28]

After equilibrium has been established between the surrounding tissues and the interior of the nerve, the process is reversed. The LA is removed mainly by systemic absorption from the exterior of the nerve. The core fibers retain a higher concentration and so take longer to recover.[28] Recovery is more dependent on lipid solubility.

Structure of local anesthetics

The structure of a typical LA consists of a hydrophilic amine joined to a hydrophobic aromatic domain by an intermediate ester or amide link (**Figure 7.2**). Either of these broad classes may be broken into four subunits that are common to both.[29] Additionally, most of these molecules have an asymmetric carbon and can therefore be further divided into two enantiomers (mirror images of the same chemical structure). This is clinically useful as each enantiomer, whilst having the same physiochemical properties, display different pharmacokinetic and pharmacodynamic properties and thus exhibits a unique anesthetic character and/or toxicity. The nomenclature for these molecules is based upon absolute descriptors (R and S), by arranging the atoms in a clockwise/anticlockwise fashion (**Figure 7.3**), and relative descriptors (+/−), according to their rotation of polarized light. The descriptors are not interchangable (i.e. both R^+ and S^+ can exist depending on the compound). Most of the commercially available LA agents are racemic mixtures, containing equal concentrations of the R and S enantiomers, but the two most recently developed LAs are both S(−) enantiomers.[31, 32][II] Stereoselectivity will be an important factor for all future LAs.[30]

Effect of pH

LAs are weak bases. The relative proportion between the base and cation is dependent on the pH of the solution

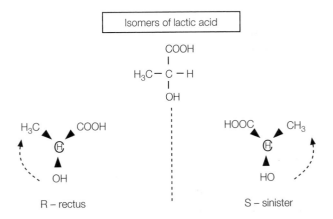

Figure 7.2 Structural formula for lidocaine divided into four important subunits. Subunit 1, The aromatic substituted benzene nucleus determines lipid solubility, which determines potency, duration, and toxicity. Subunit 2, Ester or amide linkage determines stability. Esters undergo spontaneous hydrolysis outside the body and so have a shorter bench life. They also have a higher incidence of allergic reactions. Amides are more stable and consequently have a longer bench life in the ampoule and can be resterilized more often. Subunit 3, The hydrocarbon chain connects the ester or amide group to the terminal amine. The longer or more substituted it is, the greater the lipid solubility. Subunit 4, The terminal tertiary amine group determines the hydrophilicity. Reprinted from Denson DD, Mazoit JX. Physiology and Pharmacology of Local Anaesthetics. In: Sinatra RS, Hord AH, Ginsbery B, Preble LM (eds). *Acute pain; mechanisms and management*. St Louis, MO: Mosby-Year Book, 1992: 124–39, with permission from Elsevier.[29]

Figure 7.3 Stereoisomers of lactic acid. Reprinted from Whiteside JB, Wildsmith JAW. Developments in local anaesthetic drugs. *British Journal of Anaesthesia* 2001; **87**: 27–35. © The Board of Management and Trustees of the British Journal of Anaesthesia. Reproduced by permission of Oxford University Press/British Journal of Anaesthesia.[30]

and the pKₐ of the specific agent and can be determined by the Henderson–Hasselbalch equation.[6] The pKₐ is defined as the pH at which 50 percent of the agent is in the unionized form.

$$pH = pK_a - \log(B)/(BN+)$$

Since the pKₐ is constant for any specific LA, the relative proportion of free base to cation is dependent on the pH of the solution. LAs are added to weak acids, usually hydrochlorides, in order to increase the cationic water-soluble form needed for injection. The cation is the form required for diffusing through body fluids to the nerve fiber (**Figure 7.4**). After injection, tissue buffering raises the pH and a percentage of the drug dissociates to become free base. The base form is the optimal form for penetrating the lipid membranes and getting inside the cell. It then becomes reionized, due to the acidic conditions within the cell, into the active form which blocks the Na^+ channel from the intracellular side.[33]

The clinical characteristics of an LA can be correlated with its pK_a value (**Figure 7.5**). Note that at body pH, lidocaine will be 35 percent unionized compared with 5–10 percent for bupivacaine.[12] There is, therefore, more lidocaine available in the appropriate form to enter the nerve cell. This partly explains why lidocaine has a faster onset of action than bupivacaine. The physicochemical properties of four commonly used amino-amides and their resulting clinical profiles are listed in **Table 7.3**.

Additives

A vasoconstrictor, usually epinephrine (adrenaline), is often added to LAs in clinical practice. The vasoconstriction reduces the rate of systemic absorption by up to one third,[34] which will increase the duration of block and will reduce the risk of toxicity. Vasoconstrictors should not be used for intravenous regional anesthesia or in regions that are poorly vascularized or supplied by end-arteries such as digits, as they may cause ischemia and tissue necrosis. Epinephrine is often used in a concentration of 1:200 000 (5 µg/mL); if intravascular, it may exhibit its own systemic effects and so should be used with caution in patients with cardiac disease.[35] Felypressin is often used in dentistry as an alternative as it has less systemic effect, but it is still a coronary vasoconstrictor.

Commercial LA solutions containing epinephrine are usually buffered to a lower pH than the standard solution in order to minimize oxidation of the additive. These acidic solutions are less effective at blocking nerves because there is less base available to diffuse into the cell.[36] Hence, if a vasoconstrictor is required, it is more logical to add a few drops of epinephrine concentrate to the LA solution just before injection.

Sodium pyrosulfite, sodium metabisulfite, methylhydroxybenzoate, and EDTA (ethylenediaminetetracetate) are widely used in the pharmaceutical industry as antioxidants and stabilizers. Some of them have been proven to be neurotoxic and so solutions containing these additives are not recommended for use with subarachnoid or epidural anesthesia.[27, 37]

Some drugs have to be prepared as the carbonated salt instead of the hydrochloride salt. This was shown by

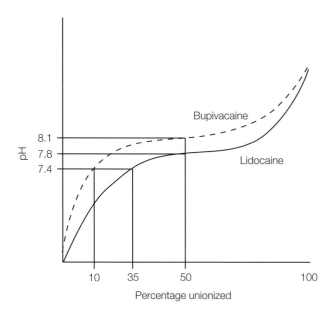

Figure 7.5 Graph of pH and pK_a of lidocaine and bupivacaine.

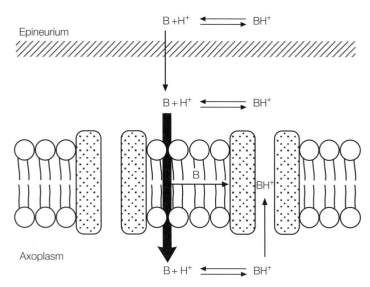

Figure 7.4 Penetration of local anesthetic in base form (B) into nerve axon.

Table 7.3 Physicochemical properties and resultant clinical profile of four commonly used amino-amide local anesthetics.

	Prilocaine	Lidocaine	Bupivacaine	Ropivacaine
Partition coefficient	50	110	560	230
Potency[a]	0.5	1	4	3
pK_a (latency)	7.7	7.8	8.1	8.2
Latency (minutes)	2–5	2–5	15–30	15–30
% protein binding	55	64	95	94
Duration[a]	1.5	1	2–4	2–4
Toxicity	Low	Medium	Medium	Medium
MSD mg/kg	6	3	2	3

[a]Lidocaine = 1.
MSD, maximum safe dose.

in vitro studies to hasten the onset of block as the carbon dioxide (CO_2) diffuses readily into the axoplasm and reduces the intracellular pH. This will promote ionization of the base form and result in ion trapping. The CO_2 also directly depresses the axon and may enhance diffusion of the LA into the cell.[38] *In vivo* work supports this effect, but it is only relevant for the slow onset blocks.[39][II]

Some authors advocate the alkalinization of LAs with sodium bicarbonate towards their pK_a in order to increase the proportion of free base form for more rapid penetration of the nerve and therefore onset of blockade. This process also produces CO_2, which can enhance the block as described above. Best results are seen with epidural blocks compared with brachial plexus or femoral/sciatic blocks.[40, 41][II] The amount of alkali that can be added is limited by the pH (causing precipitation of the LA into crystals).[42][III]

The addition of the enzyme hyaluronidase is used to enhance spread of the LA through the tissues. There is little clinical evidence to support this, except in ophthalmology.[43][III], [44, 45]

LA drugs can be mixed together in order to optimize the clinical profile. For instance, lidocaine and bupivacaine are often mixed with the aim of providing a solution that has a rapid onset, but long duration. Unfortunately, in clinical practice such a solution rarely performs as well as expected and it is possible that this failure is due to pharmacological interactions.[46]

High molecular weight dextrans have been used to try to prolong the duration of LA blocks, and these are more effective when used with epinephrine.[47][II]

The use of LAs with K^+ channel blocker drugs has shown promise in rat models and opens up new additive combinations for the future.[48][III]

CLINICAL PHARMACOKINETICS

The important factors determining the plasma concentrations of LA drugs are described below under Absorption and distribution, Metabolism and elimination, and Effect of age (**Figure 7.6**).[49]

Absorption and distribution

The dose of LA is the major factor over which the clinician has most control. Ideally, this should be kept to the lowest level that is clinically effective. The concept of maximum safe dose (MSD) of LAs based on the patient's weight is not supported by the pharmacokinetics, but may still be a useful concept.[50] Best practice is to dose according to the type of block needed and site administered and modify this up or down according to the patient's physique and medical condition.[51, 52]

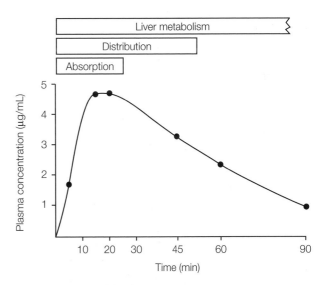

Figure 7.6 Factors affecting plasma concentration of a local anesthetic after injection. Reprinted from Arthur GR, Wildsmith JAW, Tucker GT. Pharmacology of local anaesthetic drugs. In: Wildsmith JAW, Armitage EN (eds). *Principles and practice of general anaesthesia*. Edinburgh: Churchill-Livingstone, 1993: 29–45, with permission from Elsevier.[1]

The vascularity of the tissue into which the LA is injected determines absorption. A tissue of high vascularity will give a more rapid rise and greater peak of systemic concentration. For example, the rate of absorption of LA without a vasoconstrictor from various anatomic locations follows this order:

mucosal > intercostal > caudal > lumbar epidural

> brachial plexus > subcutaneous

Accidental, direct intravenous (i.v.) injection results in a very rapid and high plasma concentration. Low concentrations of most LAs tend to produce slight vasoconstriction, but vasodilatation occurs with the doses used in most conventional blocks.[53][III] The use of epinephrine, by its vasoconstriction effects, allows the MSD dose of lidocaine to be increased by 50–100 percent.

Other important determinants of absorption are the partition coefficient and pK_a of the agent. If fat solubility is very high, then absorption into the blood will be low. Also, if the pK_a is high, there will be more of the ionized form and greater absorption.

LAs bind to two main proteins, α_1-acid glycoprotein, and albumin.[54][IV] The former binds avidly, but has a limited capacity above a plasma concentration of 10 μg/mL, whereas albumin has a low affinity but a large capacity. This results in a very high proportion of protein binding when there is a low concentration of LA. As the concentration of LA increases, all the binding sites on the α_1-acid glycoproteins become occupied and the proportion of protein binding decreases. When α_1-acid glycoprotein concentrations are increased, as occurs in cancer, protein binding is increased dramatically. This increase results in a decrease in total clearance and an accumulation of total plasma bupivacaine.[55][III] There is no increased risk of toxicity as this is related to the free proportion of drug in the plasma, which is in equilibrium with protein bound drug. Overall, protein binding has little effect.

The dose of LA absorbed is buffered by distribution throughout the rest of the body. Unless the drug is injected directly into an artery, it will have to pass through the lungs before entering the systemic circulation. The lungs are capable of a first-pass uptake of approximately 95 percent, which is then followed by a rapid release.[56] The lungs may also possibly metabolize large amounts of LA. However, these processes are limited so if the amount of drug is large or if it is absorbed rapidly, the lungs will be less able to prevent a toxic reaction. On reaching the systemic circulation, the LA is distributed preferentially to the vessel rich group of organs, such as the brain, heart, liver, and spleen, that have a high blood supply. The vessel-poor group, such as muscle and fat, equilibrate more slowly but the high lipid solubility of LAs means that large amounts are absorbed there temporarily and then leach back into the circulation.

Metabolism and elimination

Esters are hydrolyzed rapidly by plasma cholinesterase to carboxylic acid and alcohol. It is difficult to measure their concentrations in blood. Theoretically, an abnormal cholinesterase concentration could result in an increased risk of toxicity, but this situation rarely presents a clinical problem. Cocaine is metabolized by the liver.

Amides are metabolized in the liver by oxidative dealkylation. These enzymes have a high capacity or clearance by the liver (CL_H). Therefore, liver failure must be very severe before metabolism is delayed.[29, 52]

$$CL_H = Q_H \times E = Q_H \times (C_{HEPATIC\ ART} - C_{HEPATIC\ VEIN})/C_{HEPATIC\ ART}(C = conc^n)$$

Lidocaine and etidocaine both have high hepatic extraction ratios (E) near the value of 1, which means that their metabolism is perfusion limited (limited by hepatic blood flow, Q_H).

$$CL_H = Q_H$$

Bupivacaine and mepivacaine exhibit low E values, so their clearance depends more on intrinsic clearance and free drug concentration.

The metabolism of lidocaine is illustrated in **Figure 7.7**. It is dealkylated and then hydrolyzed before or after a second dealkylation. Hydroxylation of the ring also occurs. Most other amides undergo similar dealkylation and hydrolysis pathways.

Excretion of less active metabolites occurs via the kidneys. As very little of the parent drug is handled by the kidneys, renal failure has very little clinical effect with single administration, but in severe renal disease accumulation of amide metabolites may occur when using repeated blocks or continuous infusion techniques.[52]

Effect of age

It is important to remember the differences in anatomy, physiology, and metabolism between adults, children, and infants when using LAs. Central and peripheral nervous system maturation is not complete at birth. Myelination may not be completed until 8–12 years of age and so children show an increased sensitivity (lower C_m), particularly with A fibers.[57] Newborns have reduced concentrations of both albumin and α_1-acid glycoprotein (60 and 30 percent, respectively) compared with adults. Therefore, plasma LA concentrations are usually lower. However, the concentration of free drug in equilibrium will be the same so that tissue drug concentrations are similar.[58] Infants have a higher proportion of total and extracellular fluids. Thus, the volume of distribution of the hydrophilic LA drugs is much greater and these drugs

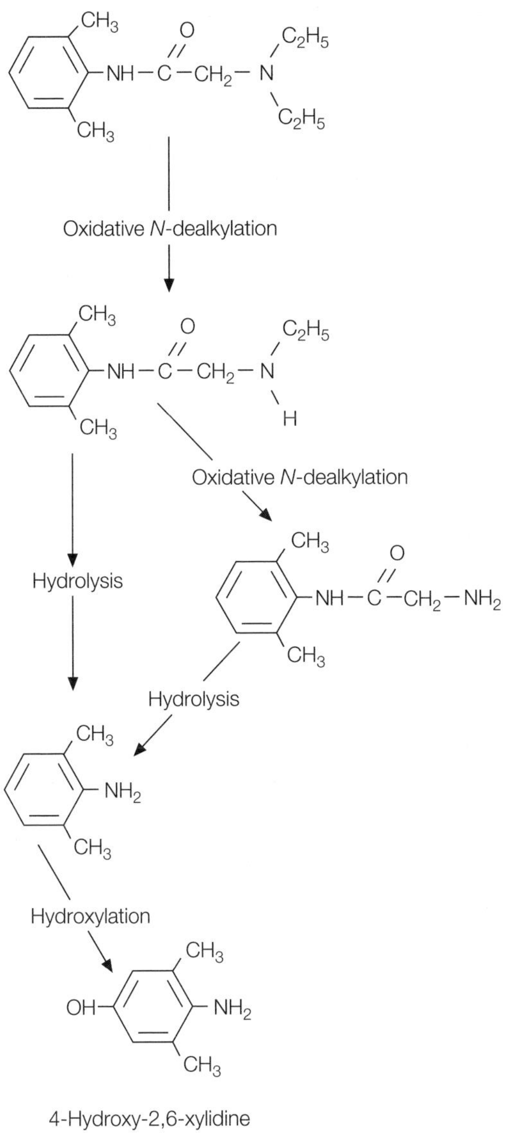

4-Hydroxy-2,6-xylidine

Figure 7.7 Metabolic pathway for lidocaine. Reprinted from Arthur GR, Wildsmith JAW, Tucker GT. Pharmacology of local anaesthetic drugs. In: Wildsmith JAW, Armitage EN (eds). *Principles and practice of general anaesthesia.* Edinburgh: Churchill-Livingstone, 1993: 29–45, with permission from Elsevier.[1]

distribute extensively in the body water. This will result in a lower systemic concentration compared with adults.[59] Drugs with low protein binding, such as lidocaine or mepivacaine, have historically been recommended;[60] however, the newer drugs, levobupivacaine and ropivacaine, are becoming the default standard for pediatric peripheral and central blockade.[61]

In infants and young children, the liver is immature and this impairs the metabolism of LAs. Weight and postnatal age are the most important variables affecting hepatic clearance.[62, 63][II] Ropivacaine is metabolized by CYP 1A2, which matures later than the CYP 3A4 cytochrome P_{450} responsible for bupivacaine clearance.[64] The

clearance of ropivacaine reaches its maximum by ≥5 years of age.[65]

Greater systemic absorption of LA from central blocks is suggested by the vascular and less fatty epidural space of children when compared to adults.[66][III] However, studies have found that the rate of absorption is slow and the peak concentration occurs at one hour for bupivacaine and up to two hours for ropivacaine.[61, 62] This means the peak plasma concentration of ropivacaine is lower than that of bupivacaine, offsetting the reduced clearance, providing a greater therapeutic safety margin for the newer drug.[64]

In pediatric clinical practice, there is little difference between levobupivacaine and ropivacaine for single-shot blocks, but when used in continuous infusions ropivacaine appears safer[61] (see also Chapter 27, Acute pain management in children).

In the elderly, there is an increased threshold but reduced tolerance to painful stimuli. These pharmacodynamic and anatomical changes in the nervous system, in addition to other organ co-morbidities, warrants a reduction in dose by up to 20 percent in those over 70 years of age[52] (see also Chapter 28, Acute pain management in the elderly patient).

COMPLICATIONS OF LOCAL ANESTHETICS

Local

The majority of complications are self-evident and are preventable with good technique and safe practice (**Table 7.4**); however, the neurotoxic potential of LAs remains an area for concern. In general, neurotoxicity is rare but the spinal cord and roots are more vulnerable as they have no protective covering.[36] Despite its longstanding safety record, lidocaine has been implicated with cauda equina syndrome when administered via an intrathecal catheter.[67] Often 5 percent hyperbaric lidocaine was used in excessive doses and the problem was attributed to maldistribution of the agent resulting in pooling of excessively high concentrations on unsheathed nerve roots.[68] A concentration and time-dependent phenomenon is proposed, causing raised intracellular calcium, leading to irreversible depolarization and cell death.[69] Experiments exposing crayfish nerves to 2 percent lidocaine for 15 minutes resulted in reversible nerve injury, but the same concentration for 30 minutes resulted in irreversible block of the action potential.[70] Strichartz has demonstrated that 2.5 percdent hyperbaric lidocaine or 5 percent isobaric lidocaine cause permanent neural dysfunction after exposure to isolated mammalian cauda nerves.[71] *In vitro* studies of the growth cone of developing chick dorsal root ganglia (DRG) neurons showed neuronal injury and cell death with clinically relevant concentrations of lidocaine, mepivacaine, bupivacaine, and

Table 7.4 Complications of local anesthetics.

Complication	
Local	
Pain	
Infection	
Tissue damage:	Direct nerve trauma or neurotoxicity
	Bleeding, hematoma, or vascular compromise due to epinephrine
	Neighboring structures – depends on actual block
Needle breakage	
Drug error	
Block failure:	Inactive drug
	Inadequate delivery to nerve, e.g. i.v. injection, anatomy
	Inadequate waiting time
Systemic	
Toxicity	
Allergic reactions	
Drug interactions	
Miscellaneous	

ropivacaine.[72][II] Despite the implications of these studies, with appropriate caution, intrathecal LAs continue to be used safely.[73][V], [74][IV]

The first cases of transient radicular irritation (TRI) after spinal anesthesia with lidocaine were reported in 1993.[75] This is a purely sensory phenomenon and prospective studies have shown an incidence of 10–37 percent.[76][IV] TRI has been unrecognized over the past 50 years despite an estimated 50 million spinal anesthetics being administered.[77][V] There are case reports of TRI occurring with bupivacaine, prilocaine, and mepivicaine, but it occurs most frequently with lidocaine.[78] The cause of TRI appears to be multifactorial and the LA is implicated, but the mechanism may even be a musculoskeletal one involving sciatic stretching and facet joint irritation.[79] [V], [80][IV] To date, lithotomy position, outpatient status, and obesity are implicated as important variables, but neither glucose (hyperbaric solutions), needle type or size, nor the dose of LA used have been shown to be related.[69] TRI occurs five times as often in lidocaine groups when compared with bupivacaine,[81][III] and its incidence is similar in patients exposed to 0.5, 1, and 2 percent lidocaine.[82][II]

Systemic complications

TOXICITY

Systemic toxicity is directly related to the amount of drug absorbed by the circulation and delivered to the particular organ involved. It can be due to the LA or the vasoconstrictor. The principal organ systems affected are the central nervous system (CNS) and the cardiovascular system (CVS). Disturbance of sarcolemma calcium release, Na^+/Ca^{2+} pumping, and cAMP inhibition lead to the cardiotoxic manifestations, with arrhythmias caused by conduction block due to the slow dissociation of the LA from the Na^+ channel.[8] Work on receptor affinities has established that (R)-bupivacaine, alone or in racemic mixture, is seven times more potent on cardiac K^+ channels[83] and 70 times more potent on neuronal K^+ channels[84, 85] when compared to levobupivacaine. These receptor affinity differences are thought to be important factors in the reduced neurotoxicity and cardiotoxicity seen with S-bupivacaine and ropivacaine.[7, 29] Both levobupivacaine and ropivacaine produce similar CNS and CVS symptoms when infused into healthy individuals.[86] [II] Intracoronary studies in animals show that ropivacaine and levobupivacaine have similar toxic effects, but both are considerably safer than racemic bupivacaine.[87] Additionally, ropivacaine exhibits less contractile depression in rabbit myocardium when compared to either levobupivacaine or racemic bupivacaine.[88][III] Current evidence supports the use of the newer LAs on the basis of their improved toxicity profile; however, incremental dosing and cautious usage are still recommended, particularly with large volume blocks.[89][IV]

Frequently in toxicity, a selective depression of the inhibitory pathways occurs, followed by the excitatory pathways.[36] This produces a clinical picture of initial stimulation followed by depression, such as occurs with alcohol (**Table 7.5**). The rapid administration of most LAs may produce convulsions or death with only transient signs of CNS stimulation. Animal studies[90][III] and human case reports[91][IV] of successful resuscitation

Table 7.5 Usual clinical presentation of local anesthetic toxicity.

Clinical presentation	
1. Central nervous system	Clinical picture of stimulation followed by depression
Stimulatory	
Auditory	Tinnitus, vertigo
Lips and tongue	Numb, tingling, metallic taste
Occular	Nystagmus
General	Tremor, restlessness
Inhibitory	
General	Drowsy, slurred speech, unconscious, convulsions
2. Cardiovascular system	Can present anywhere in range from (a) to (b)
(a) Moderate hypotension	Pallor, nausea, sweating, trembling
(b) Acute CVS collapse	Feeble or slow pulse, unconscious, cardiac arrest
3. Respiratory	Effects are secondary to central nervous system
Initial stimulation	Tachypnea, shallow respirations
Then depression	Apnea, hypoxia

Acidosis, hypercarbia, and hypoxia worsen toxicity symptoms.

Table 7.6 Treatment of toxicity reaction.

Treatment
1. Prevention: Repeat aspirations, inject slowly, do not exceed MSD, look for early symptoms and signs of toxicity. If toxicity occurs, stop injecting
2. Administer oxygen, maintain airway ± hand ventilation, performed early, will often prevent progression to convulsions
3. Treat convulsions, i.v. diazepam or sodium thiopental
4. Treat cardiac depression, i.v. fluids, inotropes, e.g. epinephrine, cardiopulmonary resuscitation
5. Give i.v. intralipid® if patient remains unresponsive.[92] Give 1 mL/kg stat, repeat up to twice more every 3–5 minutes, start infusion 0.25 mL/kg/min (do not exceed 8 mL/kg)

MSD, maximum safe dose.

following i.v. LA injection have established a role for intralipid administration in these circumstances. This lipophilic medium essential soaks up free bupivacaine and establishes an intravascular concentration gradient for the myocardial bupivacaine. Recommendations have been published[92][V] and the treatment of toxicity is described in **Table 7.6.** Careful use of this therapy must be employed as debate still remains about the dosage, timing, duration of effect, and possible pulmonary injury that intralipid may cause.[93][V], [94, 95, 96][IV] There is now a UK website (www.lipidrescue.org) with information on recent advances in use of lipid emulsion for toxicity. It contains sample protocols, case reports, recent research, and is a portal for clinicians to exchange ideas on the matter. A future development on this front may be the use of nanotechnology to more effectively soak up bupivacaine.[97] The smaller particle size is better at sequestering LA than intralipid, but further development and clinical trials are required to determine whether it also has a better safety profile.

ALLERGY

True allergic reactions to the LAs are extremely rare,[98] most are due to a preservative in the solution.[37] Reactions to the esters are relatively common, particularly with procaine as it is hydrolyzed to the allergenic constituent para-amino-benzoic acid. There is cross-sensitivity between this acid and methylparaben, a common preservative. Reactions present in a range from mild to fatal

and the onset is usually within five minutes, but may be delayed until 40 minutes. Even personnel handling the drug can experience allergic reactions, but these tend to be mild dermal ones. If a patient presents with a history of allergy to LAs, skin sensitivity testing or an i.v. challenge can be given using small doses.[98] However, people experienced in resuscitation, with necessary equipment on hand, should perform these tests.

Mild reactions present as a local erythema and weal at the injection site; there may be accompanying systemic flushing of the skin, especially in the upper trunk. Moderate reactions include generalized urticaria and weals, bronchospasm, and angioneurotic edema. Treatment of these may require antihistamines, steroids, and bronchodilators. Severe reactions result in full cardiorespiratory collapse and warrant the early use of epinephrine and adherence to anaphylactic treatment guidelines, as resuscitation may also be required.

DRUG INTERACTIONS

Drug interactions are theoretically possible, but rarely give rise to clinical problems. All LAs have a weak inhibitory effect at the neuromuscular junction and autonomic ganglia.[99] However, there is no clear evidence that this is a problem, even in myasthenic patients. The metabolism of esters by plasma cholinesterase may be prolonged when the enzyme is competitively blocked by anticholinesterases, amides,[100] and ecothiopate. LA drugs may be displaced from plasma-binding sites by various other drugs, but again this is of minimal clinical significance.[101]

Central nervous system depressants, such as anticonvulsants, antidepressants, and benzodiazepines, may mask the early CNS signs of toxicity so that the first manifestation could be cardiorespiratory collapse.

Drugs used to treat cardiovascular disease may contribute to the cardiac failure induced when toxic concentrations of LA drugs occur.

MISCELLANEOUS SYSTEMIC EFFECTS

LAs have myotoxic effects, causing reversible necrosis in a dose-related phenomenon, with bupivacaine implicated the most.[102] Indeed, the S-enantiomer appears to be most potent in this regard as it was associated with greater Ca^{2+} release when the enantiomers were compared.[103] [III] The damage is mediated through blockage of the Ca^{2+}-ATPase and the ryanodine (Ry1) receptor directly. Whilst it is rare for myotoxicity to be clinically significant, it may have implications for continuous peripheral nerve blocks and ophthalmic blocks.[102]

Effects of LA drugs include the reduction of the risk of thromboembolism by several mechanisms. They decrease platelet aggregation directly,[104] as well as reduce blood viscosity and improve blood flow from sympatholytic effects.[105][III]

LA drugs also directly relax vascular and bronchial smooth muscle, although low concentrations may initially produce contraction.[106] They depress bowel and uterine muscle contraction directly, though spinal and epidural administration cause sympathetic paralysis that can result in increased tone of gastrointestinal musculature.

Recent work highlights the potential anti-inflammatory affects of LAs.[107] They reduce the release and activity of proinflammatory mediators, impair leukocyte migration, and reduce neutrophil superoxide radicals. To date, there is no obvious increase in infection through the use of LAs and clinical evidence for therapeutic benefit is also lacking, but there is hope that by understanding the mechanisms involved, appropriate immunomodulating drugs may be formulated. It is hypothesized that these actions and those on the coagulation are mediated by interference with G-protein-coupled receptors and are independent of any Na^+ channel action.[108] This interference may also explain the delay wound healing that LAs can cause in cell culture and animal work, through impaired inflammatory migration and fibroblast granulation.[109] Again, there does not appear to be a cause for clinical concern and LAs continue to be used safely for wound infiltration.

Analgesic properties of systemically administered lidocaine are discussed in Chapter 6, Clinical pharmacology: other adjuvants.

DIFFERENTIAL DIAGNOSIS

If an adverse event occurs during or after a block, it should be assumed to be drug related until proven otherwise and toxicity and allergy in particular should be excluded. Common causes of collapse may also include syncope, myocardial infarction, stroke, epilepsy, and diabetes (hypoglycemia or ketoacidosis) and these should be considered if the event is unrelated to the drug. Patients are predisposed to fainting if they are nervous, exhausted, and hypoglycemic. Therefore, it is best to avoid prolonged fasting before the procedure.

COMMON LOCAL ANESTHETICS

The physicochemical properties of each LA drug can explain most of the characteristics seen when used in clinical practice (**Table 7.3** and **7.7**).

Amino-esters

Cocaine (1884) is unique as it is the only LA to produce vasoconstriction due to inhibition of norepinephrine reuptake. Currently, it is still used as a single agent that can provide both topical anesthesia and shrinkage of the oronasopharyngeal mucosa. Cocaine hydrochloride is used as a 1, 4, or 10 percent solution for topical use only. Its abuse potential (euphoric action from dopamine accumulation), makes it a controlled drug.[12, 36]

Procaine (1905) was the first synthetic LA. Due to its low potency, slow onset, and short duration of action, it is not useful for peripheral nerve or epidural blocks but can be for skin infiltration and the 10 percent solution can be used in spinal anesthesia. It is hydrolyzed to produce para-aminobenzoic acid that inhibits the action of sulfonamide antibiotics.

Tetracaine (1932) is significantly more potent and has a longer duration than procaine. It is metabolized more slowly and hence is more toxic. It is widely used for spinal anesthesia in the USA as a 1 percent solution or as anhydrous crystals that can be reconstituted into an isobaric, hypobaric, or hyperbaric solution. It is also incorporated into several topical preparations.

Chloroprocaine (1952) is a chlorinated derivative of procaine. It has a rapid onset, short duration, and reduced toxicity due to its short plasma half-life of 25 seconds. Reports of prolonged sensory and motor block after epidural or spinal use have decreased its popularity. Some preparations are associated with a higher incidence of muscle pain when given epidurally, possibly due to Ca^{2+} binding by the EDTA, which results in tetany.[110][II]

Amino amides

Lidocaine (1948) is the prototypical member of the amino-amide class of LAs.[12, 36] It produces anesthesia with a faster onset, longer duration, and more extensive spread and of greater intensity than an equal concentration of procaine. It comes in various preparations: 0.5 percent for infiltration, 1–2 percent for peripheral nerve block, 1.5–5 percent for spinal anesthesia, and 10 percent for topical anesthesia for the mucosa. Lidocaine is also a class I antiarrhythmic.

Table 7.7 Structure, physicochemical properties, and clinical profile of ester and amide local anesthetics.

Proper name/ formula	Equivalent concentration (%)[a]	Relative duration[a]	Toxicity	pK_a	Partition coefficient	Protein bound (%)
Esters						
Cocaine	1	0.5	Very high	8.7	?	?
Benzocaine	NA	2	Low	NA	132	?
Procaine	2	0.75	Low	8.9	3.1	5.8
Chloroprocaine	1	0.75	Low	9.1	17	?
Amethocaine	0.25	2	High	8.4	541	76
Amides						
Lidocaine	1	1	Medium	7.8	110	64
Mepivacaine	1	1	Medium	7.7	42	77

(Continued over)

Table 7.7 Structure, physicochemical properties, and clinical profile of ester and amide local anesthetics (continued).

Proper name/formula	Equivalent concentration (%)[a]	Relative duration[a]	Toxicity	pK_a	Partition coefficient	Protein bound (%)
Prilocaine	1	1.5	Low	7.7	50	55
Cinchocaine	0.25	2	High	7.9	?	?
Ropivacaine	0.25	2–4	Medium	8.1	230	94
Bupivacaine	0.25	2–4	Medium	8.1	560	95
Etidocaine	0.5	2–4	Medium	7.9	1853	94

[a] Lidocaine = 1.

NA, not applicable; ?, information not available.

Reprinted from Arthur GR, Wildsmith JAW, Tucker GT. Pharmacology of local anaesthetic drugs. In: Wildsmith JAW, Armitage EN (eds). *Principles and practice of general anaesthesia*. Edinburgh: Churchill–Livingston, 1993: 29–45, with permission from Elsevier.[1]

Mepivacaine (1957) has pharmacological properties similar to lidocaine with a duration of about 20 percent longer. It is, however, more toxic in the neonate because of ion trapping due to its lower pK_a.[111][IV] This has restricted its use in obstetric anesthesia by the epidural route, but lower doses have been used intrathecally, for cesarean section, without adverse effects.[112][II]

Prilocaine (1960) is also similar in clinical profile to lidocaine. However, it causes very little vasodilatation and so can be used without a vasoconstrictor if desired. It has a large volume of distribution that reduces its toxicity, making it a suitable agent for intravenous regional anesthesia. Prilocaine is metabolized to ortho- and nitro-toluidine, both of which can oxidize hemoglobin. Cyanosis is seen if greater than 15 percent of the circulating hemoglobin is in the methemoglobin form and this may occur if more than 8 mg/kg of prilocaine is administered. Oxygen liberation is reduced, as there is a shift in the dissociation curve to the left. If necessary, it can be reconverted to hemoglobin with reducing enzymes, such as methylene blue, in a dose of 1–2 mg/kg. Fetal hemoglobin is more sensitive to oxidant stresses, therefore, prilocaine is not suitable for obstetric or neonatal purposes. However, topical cream containing prilocaine (eutectic mixture of local anesthetics, EMLA) can be used safely in neonatal practice providing the number of applications is restricted.[113][II]

Etidocaine (1972) has a rapid onset of action similar to lidocaine, yet its duration is comparable to bupivacaine. It tends to produce preferential motor block, whilst this may be useful for surgical anesthesia it is not beneficial during labor or postoperative analgesia. Cardiac toxicity is similar to that of bupivacaine.

Articaine (1974)[114] is a common dental LA (as a 4 percent solution with epinephrine) as it has good tissue and bone penetration. It has a faster onset than lidocaine and less toxicity giving it a promising role in intravenous regional anesthesia (IVRA).

Bupivacaine (1963) is a potent agent with a long duration of action. It has a low therapeutic index, as little as 50 mg has caused ventricular fibrillation on accidental i.v. administration in a susceptible patient.[30] Bupivacaine depresses the maximal rate of increase of the cardiac action potential (V_{max}) more than any other LA; this is manifest by prolongation of the PR and QRS intervals resulting in reentrant phenomena and ventricular arrhythmia.[115] The enhanced cardiotoxicity may be due to its slower dissociation from the Na^+ channel, resulting in a prolonged block.[116] This toxicity involves a significant degree of stereospecificity, whereby the S isomer has significantly less cardiac depressant effect than the R.[117, 118] The incidence of arrhythmia is similar for both enantiomers, but the related mortality for equipotent doses of racemic bupivacaine versus S-bupivacaine is significantly different (50 percent for R versus 30 percent for S).[119] Bupivacaine may also act centrally to produce malignant ventricular arrhythmias.[120] Toxicity can occur without the usual early warning phase of CNS symptoms.

Levobupivacaine (1998)[121] is the S(−) isomer of bupivacaine. It has an improved safety profile and has the same speed of onset and duration as the racemic drug.[30, 117, 118]

Ropivacaine (1996) is the S(−) isomer of 1-propyl-2′,6′-pipecoloxylidide. Compared with racemic bupivacaine in equivalent doses, the sensory block is similar but the motor block is slower in onset, less intense, and shorter in duration.[31] It has less cardiotoxicity; the ratio of fatal doses in sheep was 1:2:9 for bupivacaine:ropivacaine:lidocaine.[122] This improved safety profile and differential block are desirable assets in regional anesthetic practice and its promise was further bolstered by an initial meta-analysis in obstetric analgesia that showed that its use compared to bupivacaine resulted in less instrumental deliveries and better neonatal outcome.[123][I] However, more rigorous studies have failed to replicate this finding,[124][II] and ropivacaine has been troubled by confusion surrounding its potency. Minimum local anesthetic concentrations (MLAC) studies calculated its potency ratio compared to bupivacaine at only 0.6 (levobupivacaine was 0.98).[125] This implied that the increased amount of ropivacaine required for equipotent dosing could negate the safety benefits. A recent review on the clinical use of ropivacaine concludes that in peripheral blocks its efficacy and dosing is similar to levobupivacaine and bupivacaine, while in central blocks the potency of ropivacaine is less and doses established from appropriate trials should be used.[124]

When the difference in potency is taken into account, most studies have found that ropivacaine versus levobupivacaine provides an almost identical block in onset and duration.[126, 127][II] There were no differences found between them in epidural randomized controlled trials (RCT) using low-dose infusions in postsurgical,[128][II] pediatric,[129][II] and labor[130][II] populations. A study of intrathecal bupivacaine (8 mg) versus ropivacaine (12 mg) versus levobupivacaine (8 mg), in an adult postsurgical hernia population, found comparable, satisfactory analgesia in all groups.[131][II] In this study, despite the higher dose of ropivacaine, the block still regressed significantly faster, but did not improve time to discharge. Similarly, in the epidural postsurgical study,[128] significantly more patients in the epidural ropivacaine group were mobilizing by day two. While faster block regression may be desirable clinically, it is yet to be determined whether it has a beneficial effect on overall outcome or length of hospital stay.

CLINICAL USES OF LOCAL ANESTHETICS

Indications and contraindications

The majority of LA blocks are performed to provide anesthesia during the operation and analgesia in the postoperative period. They can also be used in the diagnostic evaluation and therapeutic management of chronic pain. Contraindications are either absolute or relative and are listed in **Table 7.8**.

Types of anesthetic block

All of the aforementioned LAs can be used for peripheral nerve, plexus blocks, and infiltration according to clinical need. Topical anesthesia, ophthalmic, and IVRA deserve further discussion. Continuous neural blockade techniques are discussed in Chapter 12, Continuous peripheral neural blockade for acute pain, and epidural and spinal blockade in Chapter 13, Epidural and spinal analgesia.

Topical anesthesia

Some LAs are useful as topical agents on the skin or mucous membranes and can be effective in the symptomatic relief of dermatoses. Anesthesia is entirely superficial and does not extend to the submucosal structures. Topical administration is usually safe unless used in excessive doses or on raw inflamed areas. Commonly, tetracaine, lidocaine, and cocaine are used. The first two can achieve comparable vasoconstriction to cocaine by the addition of phenylephrine 0.005 percent; epinephrine applied topically has no effect due to poor membrane penetration. Benzocaine is used topically as it is poorly soluble in water. Its structure is similar to procaine, but lacks the terminal diethylamino group. It is therefore absorbed slowly, resulting in a sustained local action and low systemic toxicity, but methemoglobinemia has occurred.[12, 132][V]

Table 7.8 Contraindications to local anesthetic blocks.

Absolute	Relative
Unwilling patient	Severe tissue ischemia close to injection site
Local sepsis	Severe liver and renal disease
Coagulopathy	Epileptic
Drug allergy	Pregnancy
Absence of resuscitation equipment	Neuropathy
Block specific:	Drugs:
Fixed cardiac output (neuroaxial block)	Anticonvulsants
Contralateral pneumothorax (brachial plexus block)	Anticoagulants (aspirin, NSAIDs OK)
	Antidepressants
	Antihypertensives

EMLA is produced by mixing equal amounts of prilocaine 2.5 percent with lidocaine 2.5 percent. The eutectic property refers to the fact that when the crystal (solid) state of these two agents are mixed, the melting point is less than either compound alone, producing a liquid form. This is then mixed with oil to form an emulsion that is applied to the skin under an occlusive dressing and is able to penetrate to a maximum depth of 5 mm. It is useful for procedures such as venepuncture, skin graft harvesting, and treating burns. The topical use of EMLA and Ametop in children is discussed further in Chapter 27, Acute pain management in children.

Delivering local anesthetics to the dermis has also been achieved by microaerosol drug delivery technology. Devices using lidocaine particles with a helium propellant have been trialed in children to improve topical anesthesia for venepuncture.[133][II]

The use of an electric current to transfer polarized lidocaine transcutaneously, iontophoresis, is under investigation and may become a useful tool for topical anesthesia in the future.[45]

Ophthalmic anesthesia

Most LAs are either too irritating or ineffective when applied to the eye. Cocaine, though effective, has the disadvantage of producing mydriasis and corneal sloughing. The compounds used most frequently are tetracaine and proparacaine; the latter has the advantage of bearing little antigenic resemblance to the other benzoate LAs and is therefore useful in those patients sensitive to amino-esters.

Intravenous regional anesthesia (Bier's block)

This technique[134] consists of exsanguinating a limb, inflating a tourniquet above systolic blood pressure, and injecting LA i.v. into the ischemic limb. Most of the LA pools in the antecubital fossa and is distributed to the perivascular structures where it blocks the peripheral nerves travelling alongside the vessels. Additionally, the pressure and ischemic effects of the tourniquet contribute to the anesthesia. The tourniquet must remain inflated for at least 20 minutes to allow binding of the drug into the tissues. If there is a leak or premature release, toxic amounts of LA may enter the circulation. Prilocaine, lidocaine, and articaine are commonly used as they each have a short duration of action and a high therapeutic index. Low-dose levobupivacaine (0.125 percent) and adjuvants such as clonidine, nonsteroidal anti-inflammatory drugs (NSAID), opioids, and ketamine have also been used in an attempt to maximize the block. Only practitioners aware of the risks and familiar with the drugs involved should attempt this procedure.

FUTURE DIRECTIONS

Pain, where is thy sting?

René Fülöp-Miller[135]

Exciting developments lie ahead for LAs, as researchers and pharmaceutical companies try and develop the holy grail of an ultralong-acting LA. Two routes are being followed to achieve this aim:

1. LA drug modulation and development;
2. by the creation of new LA delivery systems.[136]

Drug alteration, by cyclizing and polarizing molecules so that they cannot readily diffuse out of cells, increases the duration of effect. For example, tetra-ethylammonium derivatives bind irreversibly to the channel proteins and their effects can last for several weeks until new channels are produced. Tonicaine, a charged lidocaine derivative, offers a greater duration of block than lidocaine itself,[137] [III] but can cause local skin toxicity when combined with epinephrine in skin infiltration. Phenylcarbamate esters of classic LA molecules can increase the duration of effect 100–300-fold.[138][III] Additionally, these molecules show exciting potential as their potency increases in acidic environments, making their use in inflamed tissue possible. Biotoxins (tetrodotoxin) have a narrow therapeutic index, which limits their clinical usage, but they still hold promise as they act synergistically with LAs to provide enhanced analgesia and preferentially block small fiber $Na^+(v)$ isoforms.[139, 140][II] Another promising drug is butyl amino-benzoate (BAB), an amino-ester with very low lipid solubility.[30] It appears to block only C and Aδ fibers, resulting in analgesia with minimal sensory and motor blockade and a highly selective differential effect. It can be suspended in polyethylene glycol and polysorbate-80 (butamben), which releases it very slowly, resulting in a prolonged duration. An effect on $K_v1.1$ and N- and T-type Ca^{2+} channels is proposed to explain its nontypical action.[141, 142] It has been successfully used for both cancer and noncancer pain.[143][V], [144][IV] Ultimately, it is hoped that further human clinical work on these drugs will lead to improved efficacy, safety, and wider therapeutic options.

Prolonged release preparations can be created by the addition of viscous substances such as peanut oil, dextrans, hyaluronic acid, and lipids to the LA mixture. Alternatively, slow release reservoirs in the form of gels,[145] polymers,[146] and bone acrylic cement[147][III] have been developed. While the gels can be used topically, polymers and cement mix are viscous and require wide-bore needles or open surgical placement. The addition of dexamethasone and TTX (tetrodotoxin) to synergistically enhance the duration of LA block offers a new way to develop these techniques.[140, 146]

The most promising form of slow release LA preparation is in the use of liposomes. These are lipid vesicles < 1-μ diameter, or microspheres, polymers of 10–150-μ diameter, that allow the encapsulation and controlled release of drugs, including LA agents. The advantages of reduced toxicity from lowered plasma peak concentrations[148] combined with a prolonged sensory effect are promising and they have been used successfully in animal[149, 150][III] and human models.[151][V], [152][IV] However, the hydrolysis of the liposomal phospholipids may produce toxic metabolites, peroxides, and free radicals, which have caused behavioral change and inflammation in animal models.[153] Additionally, myotoxicity and local inflammation occur and persist for up to a month after injection in rats.[140] Extremely high concentrations of LA in depot-formulation can also cause neurotoxicity, with lidocaine causing more damage than would be caused by absolute alcohol.[154][IV] While better *in vitro* techniques are being used to predict release rate and blood concentration,[155] further development and better human clinical trials are needed to optimize these delivery systems, maximize the LA effect and establish a safe dose range that minimizes side effects.[156][V]

REFERENCES

1. Arthur GR, Wildsmith JAW, Tucker GT. Pharmacology of local anaesthetic drugs. In: Wildsmith JAW, Armitage EN (eds). *Principles and practice of general anaesthesia.* Edinburgh: Churchill-Livingstone, 1993: 29–45.
2. Rushman GB, Davies NJH, Atkinson RS (eds). Regional anaesthesia. In: *A short history of anaesthesia: the first 150 years.* Oxford: Butterworth Heinemann, 1996: 137–53.
3. Galbis-Reig D. Sigmund Freud and Carl Koller: the controversy surrounding the discovery of local anaesthetics. *International Congress Series.* 2002; **1242**: 571–5.
4. Butterworth JF, Strichartz GR. The molecular mechanisms by which local anaesthetics produce impulse blockade: a review. *Anesthesiology.* 1990; **72**: 711–34.
5. Covino BG. Mechanism of impulse block. In: Wildsmith JAW, McClure JH (eds). *Conduction blockade for postoperative anaesthesia.* London: Arnold, 1991: 26–54.
6. Hille B. The common mode of action of three agents that decrease the transient charge in sodium permeability in nerves. *Nature.* 1966; **210**: 1220–2.
7. Kindler CH, Spencer Yost C. Two-pore domain potassium channels: new sites of local anaesthetic action and toxicity. *Regional Anaesthesia and Pain Medicine.* 2005; **30**: 260–74.
* 8. Mather LE, Chang D. Cardiotoxicity with modern local anaesthetics. *Drugs.* 2001; **61**: 333–42.
9. Nilsson J, Madeja M, Arhem P. Local anaesthetic block of Kv channels: Role of the S6 helix and the S5–S6 linker for

Bupivacaine action. *Molecular Pharmacology*. 2003; **63**: 1417–29.

10. Fang Xu, Garavito-Aguilar Z, Recio-Pinto E, Zhang J. Local anesthetics modulate neuronal calcium signaling through multiple sites of action. *Anesthesiology*. 2003; **98**: 1139–46.

11. Catterall W, Mackie K. Local anaesthetics. In: Hardman JG, Limbird LL (eds). *Goodman and Gilman's the pharmacological basis of therapeutics*, 9th edn. New York: McGraw-Hill, 1996: 331–47.

12. Catterall WA. Structure and function of voltage-sensitive ion channels. *Science*. 1988; **242**: 50–61.

13. Amir R, Argoff CE, Bennett GJ *et al.* The role of sodium channels in chronic inflammatory and neuropathic pain. *Journal of Pain*. 2006; **7**: S1–29.

14. Chevrier P, Vijayaragavan K, Chahine M. Differential modulation of Nav1.7 and Nav1.8 peripheral nerve sodium channels by the local anesthetic lidocaine. *British Journal of Pharmacology*. 2004; **142**: 576–84.

∗ 15. Fozzard HA, Lee PJ, Lipkind GM. Mechanism of local anesthetic drug action on voltage gated sodium channels. *Current Pharmaceutical Design*. 2005; **11**: 2671–86.

16. Lipkind GM, Fozzard HA. Molecular modeling of local anesthetic drug binding by voltage gated sodium channels. *Molecular Pharmacology*. 2005; **68**: 1611–22.

∗ 17. Attal N, Bouhassira D. Translating basic research on sodium channels in human neuropathic pain. *Journal of Pain*. 2006; **7**: S31–7.

18. French RJ, Zamponi GW, Sierralta IE. Molecular and kinetic determinants of local anaesthetic action on sodium channels. *Toxicology Letters*. 1998; **100–01**: 247–54.

19. Nau C, Wang GK. Interactions of local anaesthetics with voltage gated Na^+ channels. *Journal of Membrane Biology*. 2004; **201**: 1–8.

20. Bai C, Glaaser IW, Sawanobori T, Sunami A. Involvement of local anesthetic binding sites on IVS6 of sodium channels in fast and slow inactivation. *Neuroscience Letters*. 2003; **337**: 41–5.

21. Narahashi T, Frazier DT. Site of action and active form of local anesthetics. *Neuroscience Research Program Bulletin*. 1971; **4**: 65–99.

22. Rang HP, Bevan SJ, Dray A. Nociceptive peripheral neurons: Cellular properties. In: Wall PD, Melzack R (eds). *Textbook of pain*. London: Churchill-Livingstone, 1994: 57–78.

23. Hille B. Local anaesthetics: hydrophilic and hydrophobic pathways for the drug–receptor reaction. *Journal of General Physiology*. 1977; **69**: 497–515.

24. Fink BR, Cairns AM. Lack of size-related differential sensitivity to equilibrium conduction block among mammalian myelinated fibers with lidocaine. *Anaesthesia and Analgesia*. 1987; **66**: 948–53.

25. Fink BR. Mechanisms of differential axial blockade in epidural and subarachnoid anaesthesia. *Anesthesiology*. 1989; **68**: 948–53.

26. Fink BR. Labat Lecture. Toward the mathematization of spinal anaesthesia. *Regional Anaesthesia*. 1992; **17**: 263–73.

27. Gissen AJ, Covino BG, Gregus J. Differential sensitivity of fast and slow fibers in mammalian nerve. II. Margin of safety for nerve transmission. *Anaesthesia and Analgesia*. 1982; **61**: 561–9.

28. DeJong RH. Dynamics of nerve block. In: *Local anaesthetics*. St Louis, MO: Mosby-Year Book, 1994: 230–49.

29. Denson DD, Mazoit JX. Physiology and pharmacology of local anaesthetics. In: Sinatra RS, Hord AH, Ginsbery B, Preble LM (eds). *Acute pain; mechanisms and management*. St Louis, MO: Mosby-Year Book, 1992: 124–39.

∗ 30. Whiteside JB, Wildsmith JAW. Developments in local anaesthetic drugs. *British Journal of Anaesthesia*. 2001; **87**: 27–35.

31. McClure JH. Ropivacaine. *British Journal of Anaesthesia*. 1996; **76**: 300–07.

32. Lyons G, Columb M, Wilson RC, Johnson RV. Epidural pain relief in labour: potencies of levobupivacaine and racemic bupivacaine. *British Journal of Anaesthesia*. 1998; **81**: 899–901.

33. Ragsdale DR, McPhee JC, Scheuer T, Catterall WA. Molecular determinants of state-dependent block of Na^+ channels by local anaesthetics. *Science*. 1994; **265**: 1724–8.

∗ 34. Cox B, Durieux ME, Marcus MA. Toxicity of local anaesthetics. *Best Practice and Research Clinical Anaesthesiology*. 2003; **17**: 111–36.

35. Kennedy WF, Bonica JJ, Ward RJ *et al.* Cardiorespiratory effects of epinephrine when used in regional anaesthesia. *Acta Anaesthesiologica Scandinavica*. 1966; **23**: 320–33.

36. Covino BG. Clinical pharmacology of local anesthetic agents. In: Cousins MJ, Bridenbaugh PO (eds). *Neural blockade in clinical anaesthesia and management of pain*, 2nd edn. Philadelphia: JB Lippincott, 1988: 111–44.

37. Reichert MG, Butterworth J. Local anesthetic additives to increase stability and prevent organism growth. *Techniques in Regional Anaesthesia and Pain Management*. 2004; **8**: 106–09.

38. Catchlove RFH. The influence of CO_2 and pH on local anesthetic action. *Journal of Pharmacology and Experimental Therapeutics*. 1972; **181**: 298–309.

39. McClure JH, Scott DB. Comparison of bupivacaine hydrochloride and carbonated bupivacaine in brachial plexus block by interscalene technique. *British Journal of Anaesthesia*. 1981; **53**: 523–6.

40. Capogna G, Celleno D, Laudano D, Giunta F. Alkalinization of local anaesthetics; Which block, which local anesthetic? *Regional Anaesthesia*. 1995; **20**: 369–77.

41. Swann DG, Armstrong PJ, Douglas E *et al.* The alkalinisation of bupivacaine for intercostal nerve blockade. *Anaesthesia*. 1991; **46**: 174–6.

42. Ikuta PT, Raza SM, Durrani Z *et al.* pH adjustment schedule for the amide local anaesthetics. *Regional Anaesthesia*. 1989; **14**: 229–35.

43. Keeler JF, Simpson KH, Ellis FR, Kay SP. Effect of addition of hyaluronidase to bupivacaine during axillary brachial plexus block. *British Journal of Anaesthesia*. 1992; **68**: 68–71.

44. Nicoll JMV, Trueren B, Acharya PA et al. Retrobulbar anaesthesia: the role of hyaluronidase. Anaesthesia and Analgesia. 1986; 65: 1324–8.

45. Rosenberg PH. Additives to increase tissue spread of local anesthetics. Techniques in Regional Anaesthesia and Pain Management. 2004; 8: 114–8.

46. Covino BG. Pharmacology of local anaesthetic agents. British Journal of Anaesthesia. 1986; 58: 701–16.

47. Simpson PJ, Hughes DR, Long DH. Prolonged local analgesia for inguinal herniorrhaphy with bupivacaine and dextran. Annals of the Royal College of Surgeons of England. 1982; 64: 243–6.

48. Smith FL, Lindsay RJ. Enhancement of bupivacaine local anaesthesia with the potassium channel blocker ibutilide. European Journal of Pain. 2007; 11: 551–6.

49. Tucker GT, Mather LE. Properties, absorption, and disposition of local anesthetic agents. In: Cousins MJ, Bridenbaugh PO (eds). Neural blockade in clinical anaesthesia and management of pain, 2nd edn. Philadelphia: JB Lippincott, 1988: 47–110.

50. Reynolds F. Maximum recommend doses of local anaesthetics: a constant cause of confusion. Regional Anaesthesia and Pain Medicine. 2005; 30: 314–6.

51. Scott DB. Maximum recommended doses of local anaesthetic drugs British Journal of Anaesthesia. 1989; 63: 373–4 (editorial).

* 52. Rosenberg PH, Veering B, Urmey WF. Maximum recommended doses of local anaesthetics: A multifactorial concept. Regional Anaesthesia and Pain Medicine. 2004; 29: 564–75.

53. Newton DJ, McLeod GA, Khan F, Belch JJF. Vasoactive characteristics of bupivicaine and levobupivacaine with and without adjuvant epinephrine in peripheral human skin. British Journal of Anaesthesia. 2005; 94: 662–7.

54. Denson DD, Coyle DE, Thompson GA, Myers JA. The role of alpha1 acid glycoprotein and albumin in human serum binding of bupivacaine. Clinical Pharmacology Therapeutics. 1984; 35: 409–16.

55. Denson DD, Raj PP, Saldahna F et al. Continuous perineural infusion of bupivacaine for prolonged analgesia: pharmacokinetic considerations. International Journal of Clinical Pharmacology, Toxicology and Therapeutics. 1983; 21: 591–7.

56. Post C. Studies on the pharmacokinetic function of the lung with special reference to lidocaine. Acta Pharmacologica et Toxicologica. 1979; 44: 1–53.

57. Benzon HT, Strichartz GR, Gissen AJ et al. Developmental neurophysiology of mammalian peripheral nerves and age-related differential sensitivity to local anesthetic. British Journal of Anaesthesia. 1988; 61: 754–60.

58. Morishima HO, Santos AC, Pedersen H et al. Effect of lidocaine on the asphyxial responses in mature fetal lamb. Anesthesiology. 1987; 66: 501–07.

59. Ecoffey C, Desparmet J, Maury M et al. Bupivacaine in children: pharmacokinetics following caudal anaesthesia. Anesthesiology. 1985; 63: 447–8.

60. Morselli PL, Franco-Morselli R, Bossi L. Clinical pharmacokinetics in newborns and infants: age-related differences and therapeutic implications. Clinical Pharmacokinetics. 1980; 5: 485–527.

61. Dalens B. Some current controversies in paediatric regional anaesthesia. Current Opinion in Anaesthesiology. 2006; 19: 301–08.

62. McCann ME, Sethna NF, Mazoit JX et al. The pharmacokinetics of epidural ropivacaine in infants and young children. Anesthesia and Analgesia. 2001; 93: 893–7.

63. Chalkiadis GA, Anderson BJ. Age and size are the major covariates for prediction of levobupivacaine clearance in children. Paediatric Anaesthesia. 2006; 16: 275–82.

* 64. Mazoit JX, Dalens BJ. Ropivaciane in infants and children. Current Opinion in Anaesthesiology. 2003; 16: 305–07.

65. De Negri P, Ivani G, Tirri T, Del Piano AC. New local anesthetics for paediatric anaesthesia. Current Opinion in Anaesthesiology. 2005; 18: 289–92.

66. Eyers RL, Kidd J, Oppenheim R, Brown TCK. Local anesthetic plasma levels in children. Anaesthesia and Intensive Care. 1978; 6: 243–7.

67. Rigler ML, Drasner K, Krejcie TC. Cauda equina syndrome after continuous spinal anaesthesia. Anaesthesia and Analgesia. 1991; 72: 275–81.

68. Drasner K. Models for local anesthetic toxicity from continuous spinal anaesthesia. Regional Anaesthesia. 1993; 18: 434–8.

69. Hampl KF, Schneider MC, Drasner K. Toxicity of spinal local anaesthetics. Current Opinion in Anaesthesiology. 1999; 12: 559–64.

70. Kanai T, Katsuki H, Takasaki M. Graded, irreversible changes in crayfish giant axon as manifestations of lidocaine neurotoxicity in vitro. Anaesthesia and Analgesia. 1998; 86: 569–73.

71. Meissner K, Holst D, Mädler S, Strichartz GR. Potential neurotoxicity of lidocaine and bupivacaine for continuous spinal anaesthesia. The International Monitor 16th Annual ESRA Congress, London, 1997; 9: 8 (abstract issue).

* 72. Radwan IA, Saito S, Goto F. The neurotoxicity of local anaesthetics on growing neurons: a comparative study of lidocaine, bupivacaine, mepivacaine and ropivacaine. Anaesthesia and Analgesia. 2002; 94: 319–24.

73. Thompson GE. Continuous spinal anaesthesia: an ASRA perspective. Regional Anaesthesia. 1993; 18: 387–9.

74. Standl T, Eckert S, Schulte am Esch J. Microcatheter continuous spinal anaesthesia in the post-operative period: a prospective study of its effectiveness and complications. European Journal of Anaesthesiology. 1995; 12: 273–9.

75. Schneider M, Ettlin T, Kaufmann M et al. Transient neurologic toxicity after hyperbaric subarachnoid anaesthesia with 5% lidocaine. Anaesthesia and Analgesia. 1993; 76: 1154–7.

76. Panadero A, Monedero P, Fernandez-Liesa JI et al. Repeated transient neurological symptoms after spinal

anaesthesia with hyperbaric 5% lidocaine. *British Journal of Anaesthesia*. 1998; **81**: 471–2.

77. Dahlgren N. Transient radicular irritation after spinal anaesthesia *Acta Anaesthesiologica Scandinavica*. 1996; **40**: 864–5 (letter).

* 78. Pollock JE. Neurotoxicity of intrathecal local anaesthetics and transient neurological symptoms. *Best Practice and Research Clinical Anaesthesiology*. 2003; **17**: 471–84.

79. Neal JM, Pollock JE. Can scapegoats stand on shifting sands? *Regional Anaesthesia and Pain Medicine*. 1998; **23**: 533–7.

80. Aguilar JL, Pelaez R. Transient neurological syndrome does it really exist? *Current Opinion in Anaesthesiology*. 2004; **17**: 423–6.

81. Freedman JM, Li DK, Drasner K *et al*. Transient neurological symptoms after spinal anaesthesia: an epidemiological study of 1,863 patients. *Anesthesiology*. 1998; **89**: 633–41.

82. Pollock JE, Liu SS, Neal JM, Stephenson CA. Dilution of spinal lidocaine does not alter the incidence of transient neurological symptoms. *Anesthesiology*. 1999; **90**: 445–50.

83. Valenzuela C, Delpon E, Tamkun MM *et al*. Stereoselective block of human cardiac potassium channel (Kv1.5) by bupivacaine enantiomers. *Biophysical Journal*. 1995; **69**: 418–27.

84. Lee-son S, Wang GK, Concus A *et al*. Stereoselective inhibition of neuronal sodium channels by local anaesthetics: evidence for two sites of action? *Anesthesiology*. 1992; **77**: 324–35.

85. Nau C, Vogel W, Hempelmann G *et al*. Stereoselectivity of bupivacaine in local anesthetic-sensitive ion channels of peripheral nerve. *Anesthesiology*. 1999; **91**: 786–95.

86. Stewart J, Kellet N, Castro D. The CNS and CVS effects of levobupivacaine and ropivacaine in healthy volunteers. *Anaesthesia and Analgesia*. 2003; **97**: 412–6.

87. Veering BT. Complications and local anesthetic toxicity in regional anaesthesia. *Current Opinion in Anaesthesiology*. 2003; **16**: 455–9.

* 88. Royse CF, Royse AG. The myocardial and vascular effects of bupivacaine, levobupivacaine and ropivacaine using pressure volume loops. *Anaesthesia and Analgesia*. 2005; **101**: 679–87.

89. Mulroy MF. Local anesthetics: helpful science, but don't forget the basic safety steps. *Regional Anesthesia and Pain Medicine*. 2005; **30**: 513–5.

90. Weinberg GL, Ripper R, Murphy P *et al*. Lipid infusion accelerates removal of bupivacaine and recovery from bupivacaine toxicity in the isolated rat heart. *Regional Anesthesia and Pain Medicine*. 2006; **31**: 296–303.

91. Litz RJ, Popp M, Stehr SN, Koch T. Successful resuscitation of a patient with ropivacaine induced asystole after axillary plexus block using lipid infusion. *Anaesthesia*. 2006; **61**: 800–01.

* 92. Picard J, Meek T. Lipid emulsion to treat overdose of local anaesthetic: the gift of the glob. *Anaesthesia*. 2006; **61**: 107–09.

* 93. Weinberg GL. Current concepts in resuscitation of patients with local anesthetic cardiac toxicity. *Regional Anaesthesia and Pain Medicine*. 2002; **27**: 568–75.

94. Weinberg GL. In defence of lipid resuscitation *Anaesthesia*. 2006; **61**: 807–21 (letter).

95. Greensmith JE, Murray WB. Complications of regional anaesthesia. *Current Opinion in Anaesthesiology*. 2006; **19**: 531–7.

96. Moore N, Kirkton C, Bane J. Lipid emulsion to treat overdose of local anesthetic. *Anaesthesia*. 2006; **61**: 605–16.

97. Renehan EM, Enneking K, Varshney M *et al*. Scavenging nanoparticles: An emerging treatment for local anesthetic toxicity. *Regional Anaesthesia and Pain Medicine*. 2005; **30**: 380–4.

98. Raj PP, Winnie AP. Immediate reaction to local anaesthetic. In: Orkin FK, Coopperman LH (eds). *Complications in anesthesiology*. Philadelphia, PA: JB Lippincott, 1983.

99. Charnet P, Labarca C, Leonard RJ *et al*. An open-channel blocker interacts with adjacent turns of the alpha-helices in the nicotinic acetylcholine receptor. *Neuron*. 1990; **4**: 87–95.

100. Zsigmond EK, Kothary SP, Flynn KB. In vitro inhibitory effect of amide-type local analgesics on normal and atypical human plasma cholinesterases. *Regional Anaesthesia*. 1978; **3/4**: 7–9.

101. McNamara PJ, Slaughter RL, Pieper JA *et al*. Factors influencing serum protein binding of lidocaine in humans. *Anaesthesia and Analgesia*. 1981; **60**: 395–400.

*102. Zink W, Graf BM. Local anaesthetic myotoxicity. *Regional Anaesthesia and Pain Medicine*. 2004; **29**: 333–40.

103. Ibarra CA, Ichihara Y, Hikita M *et al*. Effect of bupivacaine enantiomers on Ca^{2+} release from sarcoplasmic reticulum in skeletal muscle. *European Journal of Pharmacology*. 2005; **512**: 77–83.

104. Borg T, Modig J. Potential antithrombotic effects of local anaesthetics due to their inhibition of platelet function. *Acta Anaesthesiologica Scandinavica*. 1985; **29**: 739–42.

105. Henny CP, Odoom JA, ten Cate H *et al*. Effects of extradural bupivacaine on the haemostatic system. *British Journal of Anaesthesia*. 1986; **58**: 301–5.

106. Covino BG. Toxicity and systemic effects of local anesthetic agents. In: Strichartz GR (ed.). *Local anaesthetics. Handbook of experimental pharmacology*. Berlin: Springer-Verlag, 1987: 187–212.

107. Swanton BJ, Shorten GD. Anti-inflammatory effects of local anesthetic agents. *International Anesthesiology Clinics*. 2003; **41**: 1–19.

108. Hollmann MW, DiFazio CA, Durieux ME. Ca-signalling G-protein-coupled receptors: A new site of local anesthetic action? *Regional Anaesthesia and Pain Medicine*. 2001; **26**: 565–71.

109. Brower MC, Johnson ME. Adverse effects of local anesthetic infiltration on wound healing. *Regional Anaesthesia and Pain Medicine*. 2003; **28**: 233–40.

110. Stevens RA, Urmey WF, Urquhart BL, Kao TC. Back pain after epidural anaesthesia with chloroprocaine. *Anesthesiology*. 1993; **78**: 492–7.

111. Brown WU, Bell GC, Alper MH. Acidosis, local anesthetics and the newborn. *Obstetrics and Gynecology*. 1976; **48**: 27–30.

112. Meninger D, Byhahn C, Kessler P *et al.* Intrathecal fentanyl, sufentanil or placebo combined with hyperbaric mepivacaine 2% for parturients undergoing elective cesarean delivery. *Anaesthesia and Analgesia*. 2003; **96**: 852–8.

113. Taddio A, Ohlsson A, Einarson TR *et al.* A systematic review of lidocaine-prilocaine cream (EMLA) in the treatment of acute pain in neonates. *Pediatrics*. 1998; **101**: E1.

114. Vree TB, Gielen MJM. Clinical pharmacology and the use of articaine for local and regional anaesthesia. *Best Practice and Research in Clinical Anaesthesiology*. 2005; **19**: 293–308.

115. Kasten GW. High serum bupivacaine concentrations produce rhythm disturbances similar to torsades de points in anesthetised dogs. *Regional Anaesthesia*. 1986; **11**: 20–5.

116. Clarkson CW, Hondeghem LM. Mechanism for bupivacaine depression of cardiac conduction: fast block of sodium channels during the action potential with slow recovery from block during diastole. *Anesthesiology*. 1985; **62**: 396–405.

117. Aberg G. Toxicological and local anaesthetic effects of optically active isomers of two local anaesthetic compounds. *Acta Pharmacologica et Toxicologica*. 1972; **31**: 273–86.

118. Vanhoutte F, Vereecke J, Verbeke N, Carmeliet E. Stereo-selective effects of enantiomers of bupivacaine on the electrophysiological properties of the guinea pig papillary muscle. *British Journal of Pharmacology*. 1991; **103**: 1275–81.

119. Groban L, Deal DD, Vernon JC *et al.* Cardiac resuscitation after incremental overdosage with lidocaine, bupivicaine, levobupivicaine and ropivicaine in anesthetised dogs. *Anaesthesia and Analgesia*. 2001; **92**: 37–43.

120. Thomas RD, Behbehani MM, Coyle DE, Denson DD. Cardiovascular toxicity of local anaesthetics: an alternative hypothesis. *Anaesthesia and Analgesia*. 1986; **65**: 444–50.

121. Foster RH, Markham A. Levobupivacaine: a review. *Drugs*. 2000; **59**: 551–79.

122. Nancarrow C, Rutten AJ, Runciman WG *et al.* Myocardial and cerebral drug concentrations and the mechanisms of death after fatal intravenous doses of lidocaine, bupivacaine, and ropivacaine in the sheep. *Anaesthesia and Analgesia*. 1989; **69**: 276–83.

123. Writer WD, Stienstra R, Eddleston JM *et al.* Neonatal outcome and mode of delivery after epidural analgesia for labour with ropivacaine and bupivacaine: a prospective meta-analysis. *British Journal of Anaesthesia*. 1998; **81**: 713–7.

*124. Simpson D, Curran MP, Oldfield V, Keating GM. Ropivacaine: A review of its use in regional anaesthesia and acute pain management. *Drugs*. 2005; **65**: 2675–717.

125. Lyons G, Reynolds F. Toxicity and safety of epidural local anaesthetics. *International Journal of Obstetric Anaesthesia*. 2001; **10**: 259–62.

126. McClellan KJ, Faulds D. Ropivacaine: an update of its use in regional anaesthesia. *Drugs*. 2000; **60**: 1065–93.

127. Casati A, Borghi B, Fanelli G *et al.* Interscalene brachial plexus anaesthesia and analgesia for open shoulder surgery: A randomized, double blinded comparison between levobupivacaine and ropivacaine. *Anaesthesia and Analgesia*. 2003; **96**: 253–9.

128. Senard M, Kaba A, Jacquemin MJ *et al.* Epidural levobupivacaine 0.1% or Roopivacaine 0.1% combined with morphine provides comparable analgesia after abdominal surgery. *Anaesthesia and Analgesia*. 2004; **98**: 389–94.

129. De Negri P, Ivani G, Tirri T *et al.* A comparison of epidural bupivacaine, levobupivacaine and ropivacaine on postoperative analgesia and motor blockade. *Anaesthesia and Analgesia*. 2004; **99**: 45–8.

130. Lee BB, Ngan Kee W *et al.* Epidural infusion of ropivacaine and bupivacaine for labour analgesia: A randomized, double blind study of obstetric outcome. *Anaesthesia and Analgesia*. 2004; **98**: 1145–52.

131. Casati A, Moizo E, Marchetti C, Vinciguerra F. A prospective, randomized, double blind comparison of unilateral spinal anaesthesia with hyperbaric bupivacaine, ropivacaine or levobupivacaine for inguinal herniorrhaphy. *Anaesthesia and Analgesia*. 2004; **99**: 1387–92.

132. Mofenson HC, Caraccio TR, Miller H, Greensher J. Lidocaine toxicity from topical mucosal application. *Clinical Pediatrics*. 1983; **22**: 190–2.

133. Wolf AR, Stoddart PA, Murphy PJ, Sasada M. Rapid skin anaesthesia using high velocity lignocaine particles: a prospective placebo controlled trial. *Archives of Disease in Childhood*. 2002; **86**: 309–12.

134. Marchant AE, McConachie I. Intravenous regional anaesthesia. *Current Anaesthesia and Critical Care*. 2003; **14**: 32–7.

135. Fülöp-Miller R. *The story of anaesthesia: triumph over pain*. New York: The Literary Guild of America, 1936: 391.

136. Kuzma PJ, Kline MD, Calkins MD, Staats PS. Progress in the development of ultra-long-acting local anaesthetics. *Regional Anaesthesia*. 1997; **22**: 543–51.

137. Khan MA, Gerner P, Sudoh Y, Wang GK. Use of charged lidocaine derivative, tonicaine, for prolonged infiltration anaesthesia. *Regional Anaesthesia and Pain Medicine*. 2002; **27**: 173–9.

*138. Vegh V, Cizmarik J, Hahnenkamp K. Is there a place for local anesthetics structurally different from classical amide or ester local anesthetics? *Current Opinion in Anaesthesiology*. 2006; **19**: 509–15.

139. Rang HP, Urban L. New molecules in analgesia. *British Journal of Anaesthesia*. 1995; **75**: 534–48.

140. Kohane DS, Smith SE, Louis DN *et al.* Prolonged duration local anaesthesia from tetrodotoxin enhanced local anesthetic microspheres. *Pain.* 2003; **104**: 415–21.

141. Beekwilder JP, Winkelman DLB, van Kempen G *et al.* The block of total and n-type calcium conductance in mouse sensory neurons by the local anesthetic n-butyl-p-aminobenzoate. *Anaesthesia and Analgesia.* 2005; **100**: 1674–9.

142. Beekwilder JP, van Kempen G, van den Berg RJ, Ypey DL. The local anesthetic butamben inhibits and accelerates low voltage activated t-type currents in small sensory neurons. *Anaesthesia and Analgesia.* 2006; **102**: 141–5.

143. Shulman M. Treatment of cancer pain with epidural butyl-amino-benzoate suspension. *Regional Anaesthesia and Pain Management.* 1987; **12**: 1–4.

144. Shulman M, Lubenow TR, Nath HA *et al.* Nerve blocks with 5% butamben suspension for the treatment of chronic pain syndromes. *Regional Anaesthesia and Pain Medicine.* 1998; **23**: 395–401.

145. Shin SC, Cho CW, Yang K. Development of lidocaine gels for enhanced local anesthetic action. *International Journal of Pharmaceutics.* 2004; **287**: 73–8.

146. Castillo J, Curley J, Hotz J *et al.* Glucocorticoids prolong rat sciatic nerve blockade in vivo from bupivacaine microspheres. *Anesthesiology.* 1996; **85**: 1157–66.

147. Bond DM, Rudan J, Kobus SM, Adams MA. Depot local anesthetic polymethylacrylate bone cement. *Clinical Orthopaedics and Related Research.* 2004; **418**: 242–5.

148. Grant GJ, Bansinath M. Liposomal delivery systems for local anaesthetics. *Regional Anaesthesia and Pain Medicine.* 2001; **26**: 61–3.

∗149. Grant SA. The holy grail: long-acting local anaesthetics and liposomes. *Best Practice and Research. Clinical Anaesthesiology.* 2002; **16**: 345–52.

150. Yu HY, Sun P, Hou WY. Prolonged local anesthetic effect of bupivacaine liposomes in rats. *International Journal of Pharmaceutics.* 1998; **176**: 133–6.

151. Lafont ND, Legros FJ, Boogaerts JG. Use of liposome-associated bupivacaine in a cancer pain syndrome. *Anaesthesia.* 1996; **51**: 578–9.

152. Boogaerts JG, Lafont ND, Declercq AG *et al.* Epidural administration of liposome-associated bupivaicaine for the management of postsurgical pain: a first study. *Journal of Clinical Anesthesia.* 1994; **6**: 315–20.

∗153. Rose JS, Neal JM, Kopacz DJ. Extended duration analgesia: update on microspheres and liposomes. *Regional Anaesthesia and Pain Medicine.* 2005; **30**: 275–85.

154. Dyhre H, Soderberg L, Bjorkman S, Carlsson C. Local anesthetics in lipid-depot formulations. Neurotoxicity in relation to duration of analgesia in a rat model. *Regional Anaesthesia and Pain Medicine.* 2006; **31**: 401–08.

155. Soderberg L, Dyhre H, Roth B, Bjorkman S. The inverted cup – a novel in vitro release technique for drugs in lipid formulations. *Journal of Controlled Release.* 2006; **113**: 80–8.

156. Duncan L, Wildsmith JAW. Liposomal local anaesthetics *British Journal of Anaesthesia.* 1995; **75**: 260–1 (editorial).

8

Assessment, measurement, and history

DAVID A SCOTT AND WENDY M McDONALD

KEY LEARNING POINTS

- Patients with acute pain must be reassessed at frequent intervals, with decisions regarding clinical interventions being based on clearly described criteria.
- Acute pain assessment involves a careful pain history including past experiences and treatments and the characteristics of the current pain.
- The patient's self-reporting of pain intensity is a key guide to management and should be documented wherever possible using appropriate tools and scales.

- Assessment and reporting of functional capacity is critical to titrating analgesia to maximize patient recovery.
- A number of tools are available to facilitate pain assessment in those who cannot communicate verbally or who are cognitively impaired.
- Monitoring for side effects and complications of analgesic interventions is necessary to ensure the provision of pain relief is both effective and safe.

INTRODUCTION

Assessment of pain in patients with acute pain is often undertaken quickly, with a view to rapid titration of analgesia and removal of the problem. Unfortunately, because of the nature of acute pain, the reality is that underassessment leads to inadequate pain management and contributes to poor outcomes.

As with chronic pain, the assessment of acute pain should include an appropriate pain history, including the evaluation of pain intensity, location, character, and recent changes. The functional impact of the pain should also be assessed. All of this must be undertaken within the context of the patient's situation, i.e. history of the acute pain event, history of past and ongoing long-term pain experiences, and full knowledge of current analgesic and medical history. Ideally, in a perioperative setting there would be an opportunity beforehand to discuss the pain

history with the patient, consider a pain management plan, advise on appropriate expectations, and also to discuss pain measurement tools and the importance of communicating pain experiences openly with his or her clinical carers. In many other environments this is simply not achievable, such as acute severe trauma in the Accident and Emergency Department or with patients with poor communication ability, including dementia.

ASSESSMENT

Reliable and accurate assessment of acute pain is necessary to ensure safe and effective pain management. **Table 8.1** summarizes the key objectives for acute pain assessment. The International Association for the Study of Pain (IASP) definition of pain emphasizes that it is a subjective experience, that it can be affected profoundly by other

Table 8.1 Key objectives of pain assessment.

Key objectives

1. Identification of the patient's *clinical context*
    history of acute pain event
    pain history
    current and recent past analgesic strategies
2. Measurement of the current level of pain *intensity, location, and character*
    to enable *prioritization*
        triage (Emergency Departments)
        alter review frequency (ward-based care)
        consultation by senior/more skilled clinicians
    to identify *inconsistencies*
        has something been missed?
        has a new problem emerged?
    to decide on a *treatment* strategy
        appropriate to type of pain
        ongoing – plus or minus modifications
        new interventions
3. Measurement of current *functional impact* of the pain (or its treatment)
    effect on immediate quality of life (sleep, nausea, etc.)
    ability to engage in rehabilitation therapies
4. Evaluation of *safety parameters*
    pharmacological side effects or toxicity, e.g.
        opioids: nausea, sedation, respiratory depression
        NSAIDs: GI discomfort, renal function
        local anesthetics: inappropriate motor or sensory block
    physical injury, e.g.
        intravenous, subcutaneous, or epidural infusion site inflammation
        neuraxial block and potential complications (hematoma, abscess)
5. *Plan* for next steps including further assessments
6. *Communication* of findings
    with patient
    in clinical record – documentation of current findings
        as a record of assessment
        to provide an indication of change of condition
        a source of information regarding the quality of care

GI, gastrointestinal; NSAID, nonsteroidal anti-inflammatory drugs.

factors in the environment such as anxiety and depression, and that its expression is related to the social and cultural background of the individual. In addition, it is now well recognized that acute pain, like chronic pain, is not uni-dimensional and may not be effectively categorized by one measurable index. Many scales have been developed to attempt to record the perceived level of pain (pain intensity scores) or to assess the degree of pain relief (analgesia scores). A number of these have direct application in a tightly controlled research environment, whilst others have less reliability or are less complex but are simpler to apply and hence more useful on a day-to-day basis.

In acute pain management, assessment must be undertaken at appropriate frequent intervals. At these times, evaluation of pain intensity, functional impact, and side effects of treatment must be undertaken and recorded using tools and scales that are consistent, valid, and reliable. There is evidence that more frequent assessment leads to improved pain management.[1] While it is always hoped that pain scores would remain at satisfactory levels or improve, deterioration in any of these is not auto-matically a signal for increasing or modifying analgesic therapy. In particular, a significant unexpected increase in pain may be due to the onset of a new clinical condition (e.g. perforated viscus or compartment syndrome) and should be evaluated accordingly. Likewise, aggressive pain management without appropriate clinical safety mon-itoring may lead to increased adverse outcomes.[2]

HISTORY

The pain history is necessary in order to place the pain measurements into context and therefore to prioritize and guide appropriate therapy. In chronic pain management, the pain history forms part of the complete biopsychosocial assessment of the patient in a multidisciplinary environment. Complex and long-standing issues need to be evaluated in a considered fashion in order to develop a long-term strategy for effective management. In acute pain, the clinical situation is often clearly defined and the expectations are for a relatively rapid recovery from the initiating condition. Nonetheless, although in some circumstances clinical priorities may dictate a need for a rapid initial intervention (e.g. in the Accident and Emergency Department), an exploration of the patient's pain history, both acute and chronic, is important to provide both effective and safe pain relief.

The key elements of the pain history in patients with acute pain are:

1. establish communication and rapport with the patient;
2. understand the context of the current condition;
3. learn the location, character, and intensity of the pain being experienced;
4. establish the functional impact of the pain on the patient's activity;
5. identify all current drug therapies and the indications for their use;
6. identify drug adverse reactions or allergies that might affect analgesic options;
7. determine underlying chronic pain issues and treatments;
8. learn about previous relevant acute pain episodes and how they responded to treatment.

Items 1–6 are essential for safe management of acute pain conditions. Items 7 and 8 are important in maximizing the effectiveness of treatment and also in interpreting pain intensity measurements.

Communication with patients experiencing acute pain may be difficult, especially in the early stages of treatment if adequate pain control has not been achieved. Patients may be agitated and distressed and impatient for an effective intervention to occur. However, a considerable amount can be gained by concise and relevant questioning and listening to what the patient says. Knowledge of the patient's cultural, social, and medical background aids the establishment of a relationship of trust and commitment, which is an important initial step in therapy.

It is essential to determine the context of the acute pain condition. In some cases this will be immediately obvious, such as an acutely fractured limb secondary to trauma, or a postoperative patient, but in others there may be much to reveal such as a patient with a long-standing inflammatory bowel condition with an acute abdomen requiring laparotomy. In either case, there will be many factors that need to be considered, including emotional status, cultural factors, and practical considerations such as cognitive state and medicolegal consent issues.

When reviewing patients during treatment for acute pain, it is important to remember that the patient's current condition may well have altered since the last visit, even if it were only a few hours previously. Recent mobilization, changes in drug therapy, side effects of drug treatment (e.g. nausea), the effects of altered sleep patterns, and even relationships with carers may all impact on the current situation.

The pain description is a core component of the history. The patient's pain needs to be described in a comprehensive and efficient manner. In acute pain, as in chronic pain, it is the subjective interpretation of the pain by the patient that provides the most information. Typically, acute pain assessment has focused on unidimensional pain scores without further description; however, whenever possible a detailed description of the patient's pain should be made including the following characteristics, remembering that there are often multiple sites or sensations of pain:

- site:
  - where the pain is located – site of injury, surgical wound, frontal headache;
- intensity:
  - the subjective pain rating (see measurement below);
  - reported both at rest and with movement/activity;
- nature:
  - descriptive characteristics of the pain (it is important to differentiate nociceptive from neuropathic pain, both of which may often present at the same time, see below);
- radiation:
  - visceral radiation patterns, e.g. cardiac, renal;
  - neurological distribution, e.g. sciatica;
  - referred patterns, e.g. diaphragmatic irritation;
- modifying factors:
  - aggravating or relieving factors:
    - activities, posture, etc.
  - temporal factors:
    - change over time
    - cyclical exacerbations (including, of course, "colicky" patterns typical of spasm of a hollow viscus;
    - periodic changes;
- associated symptoms:
  - nausea/vomiting;
  - syncope/dizziness;
  - neurological symptoms, e.g. visual changes with migraine;
- emotional impact of the pain, e.g. distress.

The process of eliciting the above characteristics need not be complex and time-consuming. For example, patients following knee joint replacement surgery often have significant pain, but there may be multiple components. The knee itself may be acutely painful secondary to surgical resection and manipulation, there may be muscle spasm and pain in the thigh as a reflex response to joint irritation or due to muscle injury from the leg tourniquet, and there may be radiating pains or burning discomfort in the lower leg due to nerve injury during surgery. The therapeutic strategies and expected time course for resolution of each of these components differs significantly, and management of any one element will lead to incomplete treatment.

Pain intensity is measured and recorded using one or more scales/tools as detailed below under Measurement. At different times, the measurement tool may change because of the circumstances of the patient (sedation/ cognitive state/dexterity, etc.). For example, in the postoperative period, the residual effects of anesthesia medications may make it more appropriate to use verbal scales until the patient is settled back in the ward.

Pain intensity should be assessed both at rest and with movement relevant to the patient's condition. Both values should be recorded. These measures give an indication of the subjective component of the pain, but they do not enable the clinician to determine the impact that the pain is having on limiting physical activity. For this to be done, a functional activity assessment must be made (see below under Functional assessment).

It is becoming increasingly apparent that acute pain comprises both nociceptive components (somatic and visceral) and neuropathic components. Neuropathic pain may be manifest in the immediate postoperative period[3, 4] and provides one explanation for the limited opioid responsiveness in some conditions. Phantom sensations, including pain, have been identified to be present within a few days following amputation in up to 75 percent of patients.[5] Descriptive characteristics useful for differentiating nociceptive from neuropathic pain are listed in **Table 8.2**.

The functional impact of the patient's pain can be assessed by history and, if possible, direct observation. Pain management can only be considered to be fully effective if it both relieves the patient's suffering and enables appropriate physical function. Without being able to undertake relevant activities, which in most cases involve rehabilitation, recovery from an underlying injury will most likely be impaired. Further information regarding scoring functional impact as a Functional Activity Scale (FAS) score is provided below (see Functional Activity Scale). The activity to be used for assessing the FAS score must be determined on an individual basis – coughing may be an appropriate activity target following abdominal surgery, whereas tolerance of physiotherapy and joint mobilization may be appropriate following knee surgery, or the ability to tolerate a lighted room for migraine headaches. Pain also impacts on other aspects of function, such as the ability to sleep, which should be assessed.

It is important to be aware of the chronic use of analgesics as part of a pain history as the presence of opioid tolerance requires modification of analgesic strategies in acute pain. Specific treatments, such as buprenorphine patches or naltrexone in substance abuse disorders, also need to be considered (see Chapter 30, The opioid-tolerant patient, including those with a substance abuse disorder).

Finally it should be re-emphasized that the emotional status of the patient (e.g. depression, anxiety, anger, distress) has a significant impact on their reaction to pain and their response to clinical intervention.[6]

MEASUREMENT

Appropriate measurement of acute pain at the bedside or in the clinic, both before and following interventions, is

Table 8.2 Characteristics of nociceptive and neuropathic pain.

Nociceptive		Neuropathic
Somatic	**Visceral**	
Well localized ± tenderness	Poorly localized ± referred radiation pattern	Often located in a somatic region rather than precisely to a site of injury
Sharp/stinging/hot	Dull/cramping/colicky	Burning/shooting/stabbing
Autonomic symptoms – sympathetic predominate	Autonomic symptoms – vagal predominates	Poorly identified triggers
		Poor response to opioid therapy
		Abnormal sensations in the affected region (dysesthesias)
		Burning, allodynia
		Evidence of neurological dysfunction
		Numbness, hypoesthesia
		Associated with other phenomena, such as phantom sensations or pain

the most important first step in providing effective acute pain relief. A wide range of acute pain measurement tools has been developed for both routine clinical use and research use. There are vastly different clinical and patient factors which make it necessary to have a choice of measurement tools available. Apart from personal preferences, language, past experience, and education level often influences a patient's choice of a pain-reporting tool.

There is frequently no pre-education of surgical patients or admission-time education of hospital inpatients about methods available to enable effective communication of pain intensity. Patients are rarely given the opportunity to choose the pain-reporting tool that best suits their needs and communication abilities. The tool used to measure pain could change during a patient's stay, depending on their clinical circumstances (e.g. time in postanesthesia care unit (PACU)). Having pre-education would facilitate such changes.

As has been mentioned, the measurement of pain intensity is only one component of measuring acute pain and must be done with the patient moving (or deep breathing/coughing, etc.) as well as at rest, and in conjunction with a functional assessment in order to gain an accurate impression of the adequacy of analgesia.

Pain intensity scales

Pain intensity is the subjective component of the perception of pain by the patient. It is an important parameter because ultimately from the patient's perspective this is what counts. It is this parameter that is referred to by the American Pain Society as the "fifth vital sign." Important as it is, it should be remembered that it is nonetheless only one component of the complete pain assessment (**Table 8.1**). As noted above, different measurement tools suit different patients and clinical circumstances. Ultimately, it is helpful to reduce the value recorded by all tools to a reporting value that is easily transcribed and able to be used by different clinicians over time to assess absolute levels and also change in pain intensity over time. Thus, most tools should be converted to a 0 to 10 (i.e. 11-point) scale. Any scale that is non-ranked is not clinically useful for long-term management.

VERBAL DESCRIPTOR SCALES

Forms of verbal rating scales (description of pain intensity) are tools that can be applied when others fail or when cognition is impaired, provided that communication is not compromised. The variability of interpretation of the specific verbal descriptors weakens the overall reliability.

The verbal descriptor scale (VDS) is also called the verbal rating scale (VRS) or graphic rating scale (GRS). It includes a series of word descriptors of pain intensity in ascending order, the pain intensity score of the McGill Pain Questionnaire (MPQ) being the most frequently used form which have been updated from time to time.[7] The VRS has been validated in 1997 by Paice and Cohen,[8] and a five words format in 1971 by Melzack.[9]

Examples of scales include the four-level VRS-4[10] (0, no pain; 1, mild pain; 2, moderate pain; 3, severe pain) and the five-level scale[11] (mild, discomforting, distressing, horrible, excruciating). The latter scale was thought to be too open-ended and so defined end points were added by Aitken in 1969 ("no pain" and "unendurable.")[12] This version therefore has a seven-point scale.

Advantages of VDS

- Descriptor scales are used to measure the sensory dimension of pain. Except for the (MPQ), they have seldom been examined for reliability or validity but show strong correlations between visual analog scale (VAS) and VDS in studies over 20 years.
- Simple VDSs have been used to measure pain intensity, as well as "expectation" of relief and actual pain relief.[13]
- Descriptive terms added to measurement scales are thought to increase the likelihood of recording the same degree of severity in the same position on the scale.[12] Although this may improve the reliability, it also narrows the range available and may introduce bias depending on the subject's interpretation of the descriptors.
- VDS techniques successfully quantify sensory intensity and affective aspects of pain, and VDS provides a more sensitive tool for separating intensity and unpleasantness than nondescriptive scales.[14]

Disadvantages of VDS scales

- The literature suggests variability in use of verbal descriptors is associated with affective distress, especially in cancer pain, and therefore variability in reports of pain intensity may be due to the use of different descriptors, different tools and a lack of standardization in measurement.[13] This also applies across population groups.[15]
- VDSs have a limited number of possible responses and the scale is noncontinuous, so that the use of nonparametric statistical analysis is required, potentially making this scale weaker in research than the VAS.[16]
- The VRS is consistently regarded as being simple to apply and scale measurements correlate somewhat with other tools, such as the VAS. The choice of words is important, and the pain intensity scale of the MPQ appears to be the most widely used English language version. In particular, it is the most effective scale in elderly patients with cognitive impairment – possibly due to the retention of long-term verbal associations. Even in English-speaking patients, word

choice is very variable, however.[17] Translation into other languages has been carried out, but many of these versions have not been as extensively validated.

In emergency medicine, triage scales, such as the Manchester Triage Scale and the Australasian Triage Scale, incorporate categorical or numeric descriptors of pain as part of their overall patient assessment.[18] These scales highlight the need to take into consideration both subjective and objective data. The purpose of the triage assessment is to prioritize patients for care, based on a combination of past history, physiological factors, pain, and other acute clinical conditions. Pain assessment is an important component, but it must be taken into consideration as part of the entire patient presentation. All triage systems require appropriate education and training by those applying the criteria for them to be reproducible.

NUMERICAL RATING SCALE

The numerical rating scale (NRS) is one of the most widely used pain rating scales in clinical practice settings.[19] The NRS can be administered verbally as a 0–10 (or 0–5) scale or visually with both words and numbers along a vertical or horizontal line. Patients are asked to choose a number that relates to their pain intensity: 0 represents no pain and 10 the worst possible pain.[20] The NRS competes with the VAS as the gold standard of pain intensity measurement.[21]

The verbal NRS (NRS or VNRS) is typically administered using a phrase such as: "On a scale of 0 to 10, with 0 being no pain at all and 10 being the worst pain you could imagine, where would you rate the pain you are experiencing right now?" NRSs are also known as NRS-11 (patients rate from 11 points 0–10) and NRS-100 (patients rating from 0–100).[22]

The most straightforward visual representation of the NRS is not unlike a VAS, except that there are tick-marks and numbers registering the units that the scale is divided into (**Figure 8.1**). A hybrid scale using a vertical visual NRS along with faces can be used for patient populations who have difficulty with horizontal scales.[12]

The point box scale (PS-11) is a simple variant where the patient points to a selection of 11 numerals[23] displayed in a line of boxes (**Figure 8.2**). There is also a 21-point box scale (PS-21). Patients point to the number which represents their pain level or alternatively place an X on the appropriate number. The use of visual alternatives was highlighted in the Department of Veterans Affairs Project "Pain as the 5th Vital Sign Toolkit" as

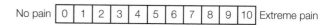

No pain | 0 | 1 | 2 | 3 | 4 | 5 | 6 | 7 | 8 | 9 | 10 | Extreme pain

Figure 8.2 Point-box variant of numerical rating scale, useful for pointing to with finger.

being important in accommodating the specific requirements of particular patients. Such patient groups included the hearing-impaired and dysphasic patients or settings of care where oral responses are limited.[24]

Advantages of NRS

- Overall, the NRS correlates well with conventional VAS[25] and Faces Scales,[12] and correlation with coughing has been shown to be better than at rest.[26]
- The NRS has been validated as a verbal alternative or complementary to the VAS[27] and categorical scales,[25] especially in more acutely ill patients.[8]
- The verbal form of the NRS may be used without instrumentation (visual aids).
- Sensitivity is improved by spacing equal numeric increments.[28]
- The NRS is straightforward and quick to use, and therefore encourages frequent assessment of pain.[26]
- The verbal NRS was completed by more postoperative patients (99.5 percent) than the VAS (85.5 percent) during nighttime assessment in an orthopedic ward.[29]
- The results are simple to record.[12]
- It is valid for use in assessment of acute, cancer of chronic nonmalignant pain, and in varied clinical settings.

Disadvantages of NRS

- It is a unidimensional assessment tool. Supplemental scales are required to assess other dimensions, e.g. pain distress.[20]
- In postoperative patients, the NRS-11 correlated poorly with orthopedic pain or rest pain scores, despite better correlation in other surgical groups with activity.[26]
- Some patients have difficulty visualizing their pain in numerical terms and cannot complete pain assessments this way.
- NRSs are not useful for patients who are confused. Alternative methods of assessing pain in these populations must be employed.
- Verbal explanation and cues should be standardized to ensure reliable scores are obtained.
- In the Accident and Emergency Department, verbal NRSs (0–10) are commonly used in triage and following treatment interventions. Simple VDSs are used when this is not possible ("no pain" … "it hurts a lot"). Behavioral assessment using observed parameters (including physiological factors) are also used to assess severity of pain.[18]

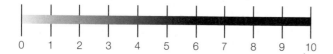

0   1   2   3   4   5   6   7   8   9   10

Figure 8.1 Linear representation of a numerical rating scale.

Clinical correlates of the actual numerical score are similar to the VAS, with 0–3 constituting mild pain, 4–6 moderate pain, and 7–10 severe pain on an NRS-11 scale.[30] The Department of Veterans Affairs project indicated that scores between 1 and 4 were indicative of a mild level of pain intensity, 5 and 6 a moderate level, and 7 or greater reflective of severe pain.[24] Like the VAS, it is widely accepted that a level over 3 (out of 10) is a threshold of clinical relevance. Thus a value of 4 or more is often used to guide clinical nursing judgment as to the need for further intervention or documentation that a patient's goals for analgesia have been achieved.[26]

The NRS is a versatile and well-validated tool. However, it exists in many variants and the implications from testing with one variant may not necessarily flow on to others. The NRS-11 (0–10 scale) is most widely used in one form or another, especially in clinical practice investigations. As a research tool, its metrics have not been as fully characterized as the VAS, but in clinical use the thresholds (e.g. mild, moderate, and severe) are consistent with those for VAS. Caution is advised with interpreting some of the literature as a number of study populations have been patients with chronic or subacute pain. The NRS has some limitations in those with communication difficulties, the elderly, and cognitively impaired, and indeed in some postoperative categories of patient. However, these limitations have not been consistently found by all authors and the use of the NRS as an acute pain assessment tool is recommended.

VISUAL ANALOG SCALE

VAS scores are reliable, validated, and produce a "standardized" numerical pain rating that is widely understood. Although VAS scores are not applicable in some patient circumstances, appropriate patient education may improve their utility. The VAS is a horizontal line, typically 100 mm in length, anchored by textual descriptors and/or pictures at each end (**Figure 8.3**). An end point descriptor such as "no pain" (a score of 0) is marked at the left end, and "worst pain imaginable" or "worst possible pain" (a score of 10 or 100) is marked at the right end. The patient is asked to indicate a point along the line at the position which they feel represents their perception of their current state or state they are rating (if for example they were asked to rate their overall pain over the last six hours). The VAS score out of 10 or 100 is

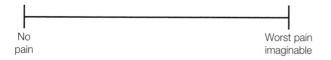

No pain   Worst pain imaginable

Figure 8.3 Horizontal visual analog scale. May be drawn on paper or used with a sliding indicator on a handheld ruler. Redrawn from McCaffrey M, Pasero C. *Pain: clinical manual.* St Louis, MO: Mosby Inc., 1999: 62. © 1999, Mosby, Inc.[20]

determined by measuring the distance in centimeters or millimeters from the left end of the line to the point that the patient indicates.[31]

The VAS may be applied using pen and paper (the subject places a line on a 10-cm printed scale), using a handheld ruler with a slider that can be positioned between the anchor points, or by pointing a finger at a printed line (which is less precise).

The design of the VAS is important. Descriptors should only be used for the anchor points. The choice of verbal descriptors needs to be meaningful, unambiguous, and culturally appropriate (e.g. "worst pain" might mean "worst pain today" to one patient or "worst pain ever" to another; "severe pain" might mean "worst possible pain" to one patient and "bad but not agonizing" to another). The line itself should not have numbers marked below it nor should it have tick marks at points along its length – these tend to act as focal points and limit the range that patients might feel free to use. The orientation of the line (horizontal or vertical) does not appear to have a significant impact on the use of the tool.[32]

Advantages of VAS

- This scale is of value for current pain intensity, as well as looking at change within individuals.
- The VAS is a validated ratio measure of chronic and experimental pain,[33] but more importantly from a clinical acute pain perspective, changes in the VAS score represent a proportionate change in magnitude of pain perception, especially for mild to moderate pain.[34] As such, it may be reasonable to analyze pooled VAS data using parametric statistics (see below under Outcomes and research). It has also been shown that the VAS is a linear scale in subjects with severe acute pain. Changes in the VAS score therefore represent a relative change in magnitude of pain intensity. Overall, these studies support the linearity of the VAS over a wide range of acute pain intensity.[35]
- The VAS scale is well described in research and has been shown to be valid and reliable,[36, 37, 38, 39] and a sensitive clinical measure of pain that is amenable to statistical analysis.[40]
- This scale is simple to use and the wording can be written in many different languages.
- It can also be adapted to measure other subjective variables, such as patient satisfaction, mood, distress, pain relief, and nausea.[41]
- The VAS is systematically more powerful and sensitive than the VRS-4 in acute pain populations and is approximately equal to the NRS-11.[10] Other investigations found that the VAS correlated well with the NRS-11, although it was not always numerically equivalent.[42]
- VAS showed significant positive correlation with NRSs and faces pain scale (FPS). Previous studies have shown reliability, validity and clinical sensitivity of VAS as a measure of intensity of subjective pain.[12]

Disadvantages of VAS

- The VAS is a unidimensional measure of pain intensity and cannot adequately represent all aspects of pain perception.
- Some studies have questioned the validity of VAS scores when used to measure retrospective pain scores or assess treatment efficacy.[37, 43]
- Some patients have difficulty conceptualizing pain as a straight-line continuum.
- The ability to use the VAS has been reported to be affected by personality, mood, age, and culture.[40] Hence, as a research tool, it is often recommended that anxiety scores be measured simultaneously.
- VAS scales may be difficult to use in situations of severe pain or immediately following anesthesia.[44] Nonetheless, in one study of 60 patients, residual anesthesia, blurred vision, and nausea limited VAS use in only four patients in the postoperative PACU period.[42]
- Although VAS is a validated measure of pain, its administration requires additional nursing resources that may reduce compliance. The use of complex measurement tools that preserve scientific validity at the expense of comprehensive compliance do not necessarily serve patients' needs.[26]
- VAS scores may be not numerically interchangeable with the NRS-11 in all circumstances. In one acute pain study, linear relationships were noted in labor and in postoperative patients during coughing (thoracic and abdominal incisions), but no such correlations noted for the same patients during rest or for postoperative orthopedic patients.[26]
- Modifications to pain assessment rulers for VAS scores (e.g. by pharmaceutical companies) have in some instances created confusion, e.g. by adding colors to the scales. As yet, no research is available to prove or disprove the effectiveness of color in measuring pain intensity.[40]

The VAS pain score has been used extensively in research projects investigating acute pain, including acute postoperative pain. In this setting, once a series of VAS scores are obtained (either as pain scores or pain relief ratings), they may be analyzed by a number of techniques that assess area under the curve (AUC) over time with further analyses following interventions, etc. As a result of research validation of the VAS score and its conceptual simplicity, it has been applied in clinical settings as well. The VAS score is subjective, validated, and correlates well with other indices of pain measurement. It is usable in a wide range of clinical environments, although there are clearly circumstances where it fails. Such situations are the cognitively impaired, those with visual impairment (although tactile modifications may be employed) or impaired motor skills, those who are moderately sedated (as in PACU), and those in very severe pain with agitation.

The VAS scale provides a numerical rating, with a score out of 10 being most useful clinically because it translates to other indices (e.g. NRS). It has been shown to provide a relatively linear index from mild to severe pain. From studies involving pain relief, requests for analgesia, and verbal descriptors, it is reasonable to categorize a rating of 3/10 or less as mild pain, often not being associated with requests for further analgesia, and 8/10 or more as severe pain requiring prompt intervention.

One of the reasons VAS scores work well in research is that there is often a high level of motivation and bedside support to obtain the readings. In day-to-day clinical practice, this may not always be achievable. For VAS scores to be reliably used in routine practice, patients would have to be introduced to the methodology early in their stay or even before their admission (e.g. in the pre-admission process or Accident and Emergency Department waiting area). In some circumstances, repeated explanation regarding VAS use may be required in the postoperative period as well.

PICTORIAL FACE SCALES

Pictorial scales such as the FPS – a row of face pictures indicating increasing pain intensity – are well accepted in pediatric pain assessment and have been used successfully in adults. Debate still exists regarding anchor expressions and the attribution of "nonpain" characteristics to the cartoons. The data resolution is crude but useable, especially within the one patient.

The FPS was first developed by Wong and Baker and is recommended for people aged three years and older.[45, 46] An explanation is given to the patient that each face is a person who feels happy because he has no pain (or hurt) or sad because he has some or a great deal of pain. The patient is then asked to choose the face that best describes how they feel.[47] There are typically six (but occasionally seven faces) in the scale (**Figure 8.4**), which enables easy translation to a numerical rating.

Although numbers may be printed under the faces, they are to be used for transcription to the medical chart and should not be shown to the patient. Variants exist with other facial cartoons or even real photographs of facial expressions as in the Oucher Scale.[49] These photographic scales also come in versions appropriate to the age and ethnicity of the children being assessed. Overall, the ranking amongst scales is similar.[47] Concern has been raised regarding the affective contribution of a smiling face at the "no pain" end of the scale.[50] The scale was originally developed by asking children to draw their impression of facial expressions from no pain to worst pain and a smiling face was most frequently drawn as the "no pain" anchor. This has been replicated with adults.[47] The Faces Pain Scale-Revised (FPS-R) (**Figure 8.5**), adapted from Bieri et al.[51] has a neutral rather than happy

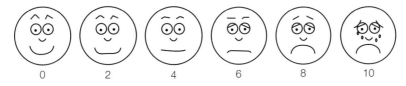

Figure 8.4 Modified Wong–Baker FACES Pain Rating Scale. The numbers beneath the faces were changed from 0–5 to a 0–10 scale so that the recording of pain intensity is consistently on a 0–10 scale. Modified from Wong DL. *Whaley and Wong's essentials of pediatric nursing*, 5th edn. St Louis, MO: Mosby Inc., 1997: 1215–16.[48]

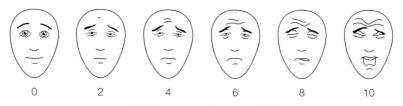

Numbers are not shown to child

Figure 8.5 Faces Pain Scale-Revised. This version has less "emotive" low and no-pain images. Instructions: "These faces show how much something can hurt. This face (point to the leftmost face) shows no pain. The faces show more and more pain (point to each face from left to right) up to this one (point to rightmost face) – it shows very much pain. Point to the face that shows how much you hurt right now." Note: The full-size version of the Faces Pain Scale (FPS-R), together with instructions for administration (available in 33 languages), are freely available for noncommercial clinical and research use from www.painsourcebook.ca. Redrawn with permission from Hicks CL, von Baeyer CL, Spafford PA *et al*. The Faces Pain Scale-Revised: toward a common metric in pediatric pain measurement. *Pain*. 2001; **93**: 173–83. Scale adapted from Bieri D, Reeve RA, Champion GD *et al*. The Faces Pain Scale for the self-assessment of the severity of pain experienced by children: development, initial validation, and preliminary investigation for ratio scale properties. *Pain*. 1990; **41**: 139–50. © 2001 International Association for the Study of Pain.[51, 52]

no-pain anchor, and no tears at the upper anchor. These scales too have been validated in adults.[52]

Advantages of faces scales

- Face scales are validated and reliable in children.[45, 51]
- They are useful in adults, especially those with cognitive disabilities or communication difficulties.[53]
- They are simple to administer.
- They are able to be converted to a numerical value for charting.

Disadvantages of faces scales

- Although notionally unidimensional, the use of facial images adds the possibility of confounding with emotional interpretations.
- "The … scales with 'faces' may have different degrees of sensitivity, and although reported to be valid and reliable for measuring pain, may create a 'picture' of what one experiencing pain should look like, a value that has potential of being psychosocially, or culturally biased."[40]
- Although ranked categories, the differences between faces may not be linear in terms of pain intensity.
- Thresholds for intervention have not been described.
- A physical tool is required to present to the patient.

Overall, the FPS is a useful tool for patients, including adults, unable to use alternative ranking systems (see also Chapter 38, Pain assessment in children in the *Practice and Procedures* volume of this series).

PAIN DRAWINGS

This method of pain assessment is used to identify the distribution of pain and the characteristics of the pain syndromes experienced.[54] The patient is asked to mark the areas where he/she feels pain on a line drawing of a person. Shading is used for identifying qualities of pain, i.e. stabbing, pins and needles, cramping, numbness, etc.[23] This tool is used extensively for chronic pain conditions, including back pain location and diagnosis. Recent developments have used computers in the production and analysis of pain drawings.[31]

An intensive care unit (ICU)-based study reported that patients were still able to communicate extensive information about pain even when intubated. The patients in the study were able to use a body outline diagram to locate the painful areas and a word list to communicate their sensations and emotions.[55]

Advantages

- Patients can map multiple pain locations and can describe radiation characteristics.
- Extra notations can incorporate the character of the pain (aching, stabbing, etc.).
- Pain drawings may be an aid to nonverbal communication.
- The potential for multidimensional pain assessment exists.

Disadvantages

- Pain drawings do not measure intensity.
- They are not very useful for diffuse pain (e.g. headache, pelvic pain).
- They take time to complete.
- They require education, visual acuity, and dexterity (unless just pointing).
- They need physical tools.

Overall, graphical representations of pain are well suited to the assessment of chronic pain conditions. They also have a role in pain assessment of acute pain on admission (e.g. via the Accident and Emergency Department) or initial assessment (e.g. in a Pre-admission Clinic), providing the patient is able to concentrate and is not too distressed. Apart from specific situations of nonverbal communication, the use of pictographic representations of pain is less practical for routine hospital use in acute care.

MCGILL PAIN QUESTIONNAIRE

The MPQ was developed in 1975 by Melzack primarily for the assessment of chronic pain conditions. It comprises three major measures: (1) a pain rating index (PRI) (numerical score assigned to descriptions); (2) a count of the total number of words chosen; and (3) the present pain intensity (modified single dimension five-point verbal descriptive scale).

The major strengths of the MPQ are the PRIs, which are also an area of controversy. There are three dimensions: evaluative, affective, and sensory. The subclasses of the PRI have been found to be a reliable and valid measure of pain in diverse conditions.[9, 31, 56]

Advantages

- Where there is a need to measure the multidimensional aspects of pain, the MPQ is regarded as a "gold standard" by many authors.[57]
- MPQ has been used in a variety of clinical settings, including dentistry, postoperative pain and complications, low back pain evaluation, and obstetric pain. Over time, the MPQ has shown validity and reliability in the evaluation of acute and chronic pain.
- A major modification occurred when Melzack introduced the short form MPQ (SF-MPQ) in 1987.[9] This has proved to be advantageous, as it is simpler and easier to use yet it correlates with the full MPQ. The SF-MPQ has been translated into a variety of languages.

Disadvantages

- The questionnaire is often long and tedious to administer the abbreviated version simplifies the task without losing the multidimensional assessment.

- The MPQ often requires completion with the help of a research assistant and can take up to 15 minutes to complete.[57]
- The need for concentration, assistance, and time make it unsuitable for routine ward use, even in short form.

The MPQ and the brief pain inventory (BPI) are well-validated multilanguage tools for assessing chronic pain and its impact. The Fifth Vital Sign project includes two components that are similar to the SF-MPQ – the present pain intensity and the VAS scales. Other elements of this multidimensional scale are not included.

BEHAVIORAL ASSESSMENT TOOLS AND SCALES

Patients unable to interact to communicate effectively may be assessed using behavioral pain scores. The relationship between behavioral tools and pain intensity ratings has not been established for many reasons, although work in ICU patients suggests that validation can be undertaken. There is no clear threshold score to indicate pain severity; instead the observations that may be indicative of pain are used to determine what warrants further investigation, treatment, and monitoring. Behavioral assessments may be unreliable indices of severity, but this does not mean that signs should not be considered.

There are many circumstances when meaningful self-reporting of acute pain is not feasible and behavioral tools have a role, including:

- patients under the influence of residual sedatives or general anesthetic agents;
- the absence of adequate verbal skills (neonates, children younger than three years);
- those who cannot respond verbally or participate in using conventional tools;
- patients with severe cognitive impairment;
- some geriatric patients (regression of linguistic ability);
- patients who are intubated and sedated (e.g. in ICU);
- patients who are too sick to respond purposefully.

In many of these situations, pain severity can only be estimated by observation of patients' behavioral and physiological responses to pain or pain relief. Observation over time is also useful.

Physiological responses to pain are numerous and are reflected in many bodily systems including respiratory (tachypnea), cardiovascular (tachycardia, hypertension, vasoconstriction), gastrointestinal (abdominal rigidity, guarding), urinary (frequency), neuroendocrine (sweating, pupillary dilation, hyperglycemia), and of course nonspecific behavioral (posturing, crying, moaning, etc.).[23] Unfortunately, many of these features are not specific to acute pain and clinical assessment needs to consider a number of factors before conclusions are drawn. Nonetheless, observation is a key area of clinical assessment and is used in critical areas such as Emergency Department triage and PACU to assist with management. It is not well codified for clinical use on hospital wards.

Direct observation

The most common method for determining the behavioral component of a patient's pain is by direct observation. One example is the Checklist for Interpersonal Pain Behavior (CHIP),[58] although this is intended for chronic pain sufferers. This system can be used with adults and children and focuses on rates of occurrence of painful episodes and frequency of response to various activities. Particular attention should be given to the known affected region.[31] Modified versions of the Face, Legs, Activity, Cry, Consolability (FLACC) scale have been developed that have criteria and descriptors that are more appropriate for adult patients (**Figure 8.6**) (see also under Pain assessment in pediatrics and Pain assessment in dementia).[59] These provide reliable systems for grading pain intensity objectively.

Advantages

- Behavioral assessments can be used in patients who cannot self-report pain verbally or with selected tools.
- These tools can be applied to adults and children.
- Where subjective tools are inappropriate, systems exist that enable a "score" to be documented, enabling change over time in an individual to be assessed.

Disadvantages

- The relationship between behavioral tools and pain intensity rating has not been established. There is, therefore, no clear threshold score to indicate pain severity, therefore behavioral assessments may be unreliable indices of severity, but this does not mean that signs should not be considered.[60]
- Pain itself, being a subjective phenomenon, cannot be observed – it can only be inferred from observed actions. Thus, because ratings are judgments, rater (observer) bias may come into play and can be influenced by many factors including sex, age, weight, and race. The use of multiple raters may alleviate this problem, but is often impractical in an acute clinical setting.[31]
- Tools such as scoring charts or guides need to be available for reliable assessments and evaluation over time.

Behavioral measures of pain in children and adolescents have recently been systematically reviewed.[61]

PAIN ASSESSMENT IN PEDIATRICS

It is recognized that pain can be felt at all ages, even in neonates. It is therefore the responsibility of clinicians to ensure that appropriate steps are undertaken to prevent painful stimuli in all children and to respond to signs or reports of pain appropriately. The assessment of pain in children has recently been described in an evidence-based guideline,[62] and a systematic review,[61] and is also discussed in more detail in Chapter 27, Acute pain management in children and Chapter 38, Pain assessment in children in the *Practice and Procedures* volume of this series.

It is important that pain assessment in pediatrics is appropriate to the age and developmental level of the child. The opinions of parents and carers should also be valued. Generalized behavioral responses are characteristic of younger children and infants, but physiological changes (heart rate, blood pressure, etc.) may not be as useful, especially in the neonate. For neonates, composite behavioral and physiological indexes have been developed such as the CRIES scale[63] for postoperative pain, or the Neonatal Facial Coding Scale in procedural pain.[64] These have both been validated to some extent. In older infants and children, the FLACC index,[65] which includes a consolability response, is one of a number of useful scales. The response to analgesia in children who cannot verbalize also provides a guide to the cause of their distress.

Self-reporting of pain is useful in children from an early age, and quantifiable scales are usable from the age of three to four years and above. These sometimes help in separating emotional distress from that due to pain. Although VAS scores can be used by older children, the pictorial scales such as the FPS[52] or Wong–Baker Faces Scale[45] are well described and validated. As noted above, there are varying opinions regarding the influence of the character of the faces at the anchor points. However, both tools facilitate communication of pain to carers and thus achieve the primary objective of optimizing pain relief.

There are many scales available for pain assessment in children.[66] In the absence of demonstrated superiority of any one tool, it is important for a single institution to adopt a consistent multidimensional approach to pain measurement and reporting that facilitates communication amongst carers, while at the same time being flexible enough to cope with the needs of children over a wide range of ages and abilities.

PAIN ASSESSMENT IN DEMENTIA

In response to the challenge of finding an effective pain assessment tool for patients with advanced dementia the Geriatric Research Education Clinical Centre (GRECC) at the Bedford Veterans' Administration Hospital sought to develop an assessment tool that would be simple, usable,

Behavioral pain assessment scale				
(For patients unable to provide a self-report of pain: scored 0–10 clinical observation)				
Face	0 Face muscles relaxed	1 Facial muscle tension, frown, grimace	2 Frequent to constant frown, clenched jaw	Face score:
Restlessness	0 Quiet, relaxed appearance, normal movement	1 Occasional restless movement, shifting position	2 Frequent restless movement may include extremities or head	Restlessness score:
Muscle tone*	0 Normal muscle tone, relaxed	1 Increased tone, fexion of fingers and toes	2 Rigid tone	Muscle tone score:
Vocalization**	0 No abnormal sounds	1 Occasional moans, cries, whimpers or grunts	2 Frequent or continuous moans, cries, whimpers or grunts	Vocalization score:
Consolability	0 Content, relaxed	1 Reassured by touch or talk. Distractible	2 Difficult to comfort by touch or talk	Consolability score:
Behavioral Pain Assessment Scale total (0 to 10)				/10

*Assess muscle tone in patients with spinal cord lesion or injury at a level above the lesion or injury. Assess patients with hemiplegia on the unaffected side. **This item cannot be measured in patients with artificial airways.

How to use the pain assessment behavioral scale:
- Observe behaviors and mark appropriate number for each category.
- Total the numbers in the Pain Assessment Behavioral Score column.
- Zero = no evidence of pain. Mild pain = 1–3. Moderate pain = 4–5. Severe uncontrolled pain is ≥ 6.

Considerations:
- Use the standard Pain Scale whenever possible to obtain the patient's self-report of pain. Self-report is the best indicator of the presence and intensity of pain.
- Use this scale for patients who are unable to provide a self-report of pain.
- In addition, a "Proxy pain evalution" from family, friends, or clinicians close to the patient may be helpful to evaluate pain based on previous knowledge of patient response
- When in doubt, provide an analgesic. "If there is reason to suspect pain, an analgesic trial can be diagnostic as well as therapeutic". (AHCPR Acute Pain Management Guidelines Panel)

Figure 8.6 Behavioral assessment scale. This modified version of the Face, Legs, Activity, Cry, Consolability (FLACC) scale is useful for adults and children.[59]

reliable, and valid.[67] This group developed a pain assessment tool known as "PAINAD." It is based on elements from three other pain assessment tool areas. Including the 0 to 10 VAS used for pain assessment in Alzheimer's disease,[68] the FLACC pediatric scale,[65] and the Discomfort Scale for Dementia of the Alzheimer Type (DS-DAT).[69] The DS-DAT, however, has some limitations including time-consuming observation periods, a requirement for extensive training, and a cumbersome scoring schema. Literature describing and defining pain behaviors was also taken into consideration.

The PAINAD scale consists of five items:

1. breathing independent of vocalization;
2. negative vocalization;
3. facial expression;
4. body language;
5. consolability.

Each of the elements is scored 0 to 2 giving a total score of 0 to10. The PAINAD contributes to other projects in the field of assessment of pain in dementia and some components, such as the modified FLACC scale, may be used for adults in other circumstances.

An alternative tool developed for the assessment of pain in dementia is the Abbey pain scale.[70] This was initially evaluated in 24 residential care facilities in four Australian states using patients with moderate to advanced dementia pre- and postanalgesic interventions. The tool comprises six items (vocalization, facial expression, change in body language, behavioral change, physiological change, physical change) each graded from 0 to 3 points (0, absent to 3, severe). These are then added to arrive at a total score ranging from 0 to 18 and graded as: 0–2, no pain; 3–7, mild pain; 8–13, moderate pain; 14 and above, severe pain. Pain assessment in dementia and more generally in elderly patients is also covered in Chapter 28, Acute pain management in the elderly patient.

Advantages

- The Abbey scale has been shown to be valid and reliable in clinical trials.
- It correlates with analgesic therapy.
- It is claimed to be rapid to administer, taking less than one minute.
- It enables tracking of measures over time.

Disadvantages

- Wider clinical experience is still lacking, especially in nondemented patients.
- The scale is 0–18 rather than 0–10, although validation across scales has not yet been undertaken.
- A scoring aid or chart is required.

SURROGATES

In order to assist behavioral assessment, other resources may be useful, such as surrogates who may include family members or carers and asking questions, such as "Is this behavior usual for him/her?" or "Could these behaviors be a signal for pain?" Surrogates have been found to be moderately successful 50 percent of the time in a study of critically ill sedated patients.[71]

RESPONSE TO THERAPY

An additional approach in noncommunicative patients, once other causes are ruled out, is to consider a time-limited trial of mild analgesic. Once given, careful observation needs to be undertaken for changes in behavior and movement consistent with alleviation of pain.[72, 73]

Functional assessment

The functional impact of pain on patients must not be overlooked. As mentioned earlier, analgesia should be titrated to achieve both decreased pain intensity and the ability to undertake appropriate functional activity. This will enable analgesia to optimize recovery. Most tools for measuring the functional impact of pain are based on chronic pain assessment and therefore are not routinely applicable to the acute pain environment.

BRIEF PAIN INVENTORY

The BPI[74] may be utilized for an overall assessment necessary for patients with acute pain to determine functional difficulties which may be related to pain.[12, 75] This includes the impact of pain on general activity, relationships with other people and sleep patterns. The BPI is an assessment tool for cancer patients developed by the Pain Research Group of the WHO Collaborating Centre for Symptom Evaluation and Cancer Care. The tool measures the intensity of pain in patient's life and has been used as an outcome measure in advanced cancer patients.[76] The initial version of the BPI was called the Wisconsin Brief Pain Questionnaire (WBPQ).[77]

Advantages

The BPI assessment takes 15 minutes to complete. It is not intended for use with all patients in pain – one of the recommendations is that an overall assessment may be necessary for patients with acute pain that is not easily controlled with customary pain treatments.

Validity has been assessed by correlating pain ratings both with pain medication usage and with interference rating on the quality-of-life indicators. Acceptable correlation coefficients were obtained.[78] Data from patients with cancer at four primary sites and from patients with rheumatoid arthritis suggest that the BPI is sufficiently reliable and valid for research purposes.

Where a clinical researcher wishes to measure the emotional aspects of pain, the Short Pain Inventory (short version of BPI) has been claimed to be the better instrument when compared with the MPQ.[57]

As well as measuring the current impact of pain, the BPI has a quality improvement aspect. It measures satisfaction with caregiver responsiveness to pain, as well as satisfaction with the intervention used.[79]

Disadvantages

Twycross et al.[76] concluded after a study of 111 patients with advanced cancer that the BPI is not brief enough for routine clinical use, and the short form of the BPI (BPI-SF) is too limited.

The BPI takes less time to administer than tools such as the MPQ, but in both cases the respondent must be alert. A useful aspect of these tools for acute pain assessment in a clinical setting are the multilanguage descriptors, especially of the BPI. It also reinforces the concept that it is the functional impact of the pain, as well as its perceived intensity that is important to assess.

FUNCTIONAL ACTIVITY SCALE

A recently introduced tool for the assessment of the functional impact of acute pain was developed as part of a government-sponsored initiative in Australia.[80] The functional activity scale (FAS) score is a simple three-level ranked categorical score designed to be applied at the point of care. Its fundamental purpose is to assess whether the patient can undertake appropriate activity at their current level of pain control and to act as a trigger for intervention should this not be the case. This is different, but related to, pain intensity scoring with movement. It comprises both objective and subjective components in that the clinician asks the patient if they are able to perform the activity and if possible gains the pain intensity score at the time. The patient is then asked to perform the activity, or is taken through the activity in the case of structured physiotherapy (joint mobilization) or nurse-assisted care (e.g. ambulation, turned in bed). The ability to complete the activity is then assessed using the FAS as follows:

A. No limitation: The patient is able to undertake the activity without limitation due to pain (pain intensity score typically 0–3).
B. Mild limitation: The patient is largely able to undertake the activity, but experiences moderate to severe pain (pain intensity score typically 4–10).
C. Significant limitation: The patient is unable to complete the activity due to pain (or pain treatment related side effects) (independent of pain intensity scores).

A FAS score of A represents optimal pain control. A FAS score of B represents an adequate functional outcome, but further pain relief is required for comfort. A FAS score of C represents inadequate pain control or unacceptable complications of pain control (motor block from neuraxial analgesia, nausea, or sedation from opioids, etc.). The score of A needs to be determined relative to the patient's preacute baseline function (which may already have limitations, e.g. due to severe arthritis).

Advantages

- It is simple to use.
- It incorporates an evaluation of what patients can do, in addition to what they feel.
- It may be applied to the evaluation of any acute pain condition.
- Change over time can be assessed.
- It provides a trigger for advanced intervention.

Disadvantages

- Education is required to enable consistent use.
- It has not yet been validated in large clinical trials (although there exists no gold standard for reference).

- Care must be used in determining the acceptable baseline level of functional ability.
- Residual sedation or spinal motor blockade in the immediate postsurgical period should not be graded as no active intervention is required at this time because the expectation is for progressive resolution.
- It is not a linear scale, therefore it must be reported using proportions in each grade or nonparametric techniques.

Overall, it is well recognized that functional capacity must be optimized if recovery is to be facilitated in patients with acute pain. The combination of careful patient questioning with the use of selected tools to measure pain intensity and functional capacity will help achieve these outcomes provided that there are appropriate guidelines for intervention should pain relief be demonstrated to be inadequate.

OUTCOMES AND RESEARCH

Research

The assessment of pain and pain relief is often the focus of clinical research projects. In these circumstances, a baseline pain rating is usually followed by repeated assessments at specified time points over a period of time. The tools that are used need to be appropriate to the outcome being measured. The many important issues of research trial design, implementation, and analysis are beyond the scope of this chapter; however, a few characteristics relating to pain assessment will be discussed.

Pain measurement tools need to be well validated (i.e. they measure what you think you are measuring), reliable (they will produce similar results on retesting or with other assessors), and are graded or ranked (providing a hierarchy of responses). The tool employed should be appropriate to the patient population and the outcomes clinically relevant, e.g. reductions in VAS scores by 30 to 35 percent have been considered meaningful in a clinical sense in a number of studies.[81] A change of this magnitude is also necessary because the random variation in scores needs to be allowed for. In the immediate postoperative period, the variation of VAS scores was ± 20 percent, indicating that in an individual a change greater than this would be needed to imply improvement (or deterioration), although from a study population point of view, a smaller change could still achieve statistical significance and may usefully be described as providing an indication of direction of change.

In order to make overall comparisons of analgesic interventions as a change from baseline, the individual pain intensity difference (PID) scores may be summed (summed pain intensity difference, SPID) or if pain relief is being assessed (PAR) the area under the curve of pain relief scores over time may be calculated (TOTPAR).[25]

Further outcome scores include the combined pain relief and intensity difference (PRID) and the sum (SPRID). The time epoch used varies depending on the intervention and protocol, but is typically from 6 to 24 hours (hence SPID-6, etc.). These scores can be expressed as absolute values or compared to the maximum possible scores because the scales used have floor and ceiling values.

A common criticism of integrating pain scores over time is that the analysis will be flawed if the scoring system is not proportionate over the scale (e.g. linear). Some studies have established that VAS scores are suitable for such analyses because they are linearly related to verbal descriptor rankings and pain relief criteria.[35] Overall, nonparametric statistical analysis is more appropriate for categorical scales (e.g. VDSs) and provides a more robust assessment.

Another difficulty with integration of scores over time is that information regarding peaks, troughs, and duration of effect is lost. In some circumstances, it may be more useful to describe how many patients reported pain scores over certain intensity, or how many achieved over a 50 percent reduction in intensity or for how long. When analgesics are administered before or during anesthesia, a useful criterion is the time to the first/next analgesic request (TFA), which can be analyzed using parametric statistics.

A frequent tool for 'measuring' the analgesic efficacy of an intervention is to assess the change in dose requirements of another analgesic used as a "rescue" medication. Ideally, with appropriate rescue analgesia, pain scores for patients in all study groups should be similar, which is appealing from an ethical point of view. Patient controlled analgesia (PCA) is commonly used in this way, although by the nature of its design patients must experience some degree of pain to trigger a request for analgesia. The reduction in opioid requirements over time epochs may then be calculated and compared with simple parametric statistical analysis. Caution should be used with interpretation of such results, however, as a small reduction in opioid requirements may not be clinically relevant even though it was statistically significant. An alternative approach is to determine the proportion of patients who required no supplemental opioid during the study period.

Meta-analysis

As a consequence of the issues of variability in inter- and intraindividual pain measurements noted above, clinical trials assessing analgesic outcomes need to enroll large numbers of subjects to ensure that they are sufficiently powered to avoid the error of a false-negative conclusion, i.e. failing to find a difference when one truly existed. Alternatively, if a treatment effect is large (i.e. benefiting a large proportion of subjects or making a large change in pain scores in individuals) then the trial population size

may not need to be so great. Unfortunately, most interventions do not have a large effect in comparison with a control group and therefore many published investigations are too small to draw reliable conclusions.

Meta-analysis is a statistical tool that combines the results of a number of smaller studies into one single assessment. This is particularly useful in clinical pain investigations for the reasons outlined above. For a meta-analysis to be meaningful, it has to have a rigorous design and the trials to be included must be selected carefully.[82] There must be a clearly stated research question, an unbiased and detailed literature review and an appropriate analytic methodology (e.g. random effects versus fixed effects models). The trials selected must be of similar design, meet clear criteria, be of high quality, and have definable end points or outcomes. Failings in these areas can make a meta-analysis come to biased or flawed conclusions. When used appropriately, however, meta-analysis is a powerful tool and provides valuable information.

The results of meta-analysis may be expressed in a number of ways. Often, the treatment effect of individual trials is expressed as an odds ratio with its 95 percent confidence interval (CI). For a given trial, if the 95 percent CI crosses unity, then the outcome is not statistically significant. When multiple trial outcomes are appropriately combined, the resultant odds ratio and 95 percent CI is more powerful and is used to express the outcome in terms of significance (crossing unity) and treatment effect or relative risk. Another technique is to describe the numbers needed to treat (NNT). This is based on the reciprocal of the absolute risk reduction and provides an indication of the effectiveness of an intervention if a successful analgesic outcome can be clearly defined and measured as a dichotomous variable for an individual (e.g. at least 50 percent pain relief).[25] The NNT describes the number of patients needed to be given the treatment for one to have a successful outcome.

Systematic reviews are similar to meta-analyses in terms of the quality of literature reviewed and the level of critical evaluation. Statistical analyses are also applied. The Cochrane Collaboration provides a high-quality source of ongoing systematic reviews in a wide range of clinical areas, including pain medicine (www.cochrane.org).

Satisfaction scoring

Satisfaction scores should be used with caution and only as a supplement to other pain outcome measures. In a study of 391 day-surgery patients, change in pain intensity scores were compared with treatment evaluations for perceived effectiveness and found that these correlated poorly.[83] In the "worst pain" group, 42 percent of patients rated their treatment as effective! This was despite the use of an assessor who was identified as being independent of the treatment team to avoid the potential for bias in patient reporting.

Satisfaction may be measured using ranked categorical scales (completely dissatisfied to completely satisfied) or a VAS with similar anchor words. Unlike pain-intensity scoring, there is no evidence that such scales are linear and so they should be described and analyzed using nonparametric statistics.[84]

Satisfaction scores are most frequently used in the context of a retrospective appraisal, e.g. "How satisfied were you with the quality of your pain management over the last day/hospital stay, etc.?" The reliance on recall, compounded with whatever the current state of the patient's satisfaction is, adds to the imprecision of the measurement.

The rating an individual gives regarding their level of satisfaction with pain management may relate to a number of factors and thus further add to creating an inaccurate representation of the quality of pain management. Emotional state, interpersonal relationships (including those with the clinical carers), "signature" events (e.g. a bad diagnosis, surgical complications, size of the hospital account), and the passage of time may all contribute to how "satisfaction" is scored. Patients may rate satisfaction highly even in the presence of moderate to severe pain.[84, 85] The evaluation of patient satisfaction is also discussed in Chapter 15, Psychological therapies – adults, and specifically in relation to PCA in Chapter 11, Patient-controlled analgesia.

Side effects of treatment and adverse outcomes

Provision of safe and effective acute pain management involves regular evaluation of the patient in order to detect and limit any side effects or complications. These assessments should be documented. All patients receiving parenteral opioids, by any route, should have frequent assessment for sedation as this almost always precedes respiratory depression.[2] The greatest weakness of sedation scoring is for patients who are assumed to be asleep and who are therefore not disturbed by clinical staff. At these times, patients should be noted to rouse slightly when clinical observations are made, e.g. pulse or blood pressure, and if they do not do so then the stimulus should be increased until they respond.

Patients receiving neuraxial infusions (i.e. epidural or subarachnoid) need regular assessment of motor and sensory block. Any unexpected increase in motor block needs to be investigated because delay in decompression of epidural hematoma or abscess leads to poor recovery of function.

OVERVIEW

A thorough assessment of the patient with acute pain is important because it will improve understanding of the patient's problems and guide therapy. Acute pain assessment needs more than just a unidimensional pain intensity rating. The character, location, and history of the pain are important to determine, as well as contributing factors, including patient anxiety and distress. The functional limitations imposed by the patient's pain should also be assessed.

The particular tool used to assess acute pain intensity is less important than the process of regular assessment and review. Nonetheless, tools used should enable consistent recording of a pain score over time in order to facilitate response to treatment and progress of the condition. Ideally, patients should be educated in pain reporting and select a tool that is reflective of their needs. Consistency of tools used within an institution will aid communication and thus improve treatment.

Underlying all assessment of pain is a need to ensure that observations for safety are also performed. In particular, inappropriate changes in sedation level need to be managed before respiratory depression occurs, and neurological changes in the presence of neuraxial analgesia need to be acted on promptly. By combining frequent evaluation of acute pain with appropriate responses and monitoring, safe and effective pain management can be provided.

REFERENCES

1. Gould TH, Crosby DL, Harmer M et al. Policy for controlling pain after surgery: effect of sequential changes in management. British Medical Journal. 1992; 305: 1187–93.

* 2. Vila Jr H, Smith RA, Augustyniak MJ et al. The efficacy and safety of pain management before and after implementation of hospital-wide pain management standards: is patient safety compromised by treatment based solely on numerical pain ratings? Anesthesia and Analgesia. 2005; 101: 474–80.

3. Hayes C, Browne S, Lantry G et al. Neuropathic pain in the acute pain service: a prospective survey. Acute Pain. 2002; 4: 45–8.

4. Hayes C, Molloy AR. Neuropathic pain in the perioperative period. International Anesthesiology Clinics. 1997; 35: 67–81.

5. Nikolajsen L, Ilkjaer S, Kroner K et al. The influence of preamputation pain on postamputation stump and phantom pain. Pain. 1997; 72: 393–405.

6. Edwards D, Gatchel R, Adams L, Stowell AW. Emotional distress and medication use in two acute pain populations: jaw and low back. Pain Practice. 2006; 6: 242–53.

7. Towery S, Fernandez E. Reclassification and rescaling of McGill Pain Questionnaire verbal descriptors of pain sensation: a replication. Clinical Journal of Pain. 1996; 12: 270–6.

8. Paice JA, Cohen FL. Validity of a verbally administered numeric rating scale to measure cancer pain intensity. *Cancer Nursing.* 1997; **20**: 88–93.

9. Melzack R. The Short Form McGill Pain Questionnaire. *Pain.* 1987; **30**: 191–7.

10. Breivik EK, Bjornsson GA, Skovlund E. A comparison of pain rating scales by sampling from clinical trial data. *Clinical Journal of Pain.* 2000; **16**: 22–8.

11. Melzack R, Torgerson WS. On the language of pain. *Anesthesiology.* 1971; **34**: 50–9.

∗ 12. Jaywant SS, Pai AV. A comparative study of pain measurement in acute burn patients. *Indian Journal of Occupational Therapy.* 2003; **35**: 13–17.

13. Dalton JA, Toomey T, Workman MR. Pain relief for cancer patients. *Cancer Nursing.* 1988; **11**: 322–8.

14. Duncan GH, Bushnell MC, Lavigne GJ. Comparison of verbal and visual analogue scales for measuring the intensity and unpleasantness of experimental pain. *Pain.* 1989; **37**: 295–303.

15. Tammaro S, Berggren U, Bergenholtz G. Representation of verbal pain descriptors on a visual analogue scale by dental patients and dental students. *European Journal of Oral Sciences.* 1997; **105**: 207–12.

16. Ohnhaus EE, Adler R. Methodological problems in the measurement of pain: a comparison between the verbal rating scale and the visual analogue scale. *Pain.* 1975; **1**: 379–84.

17. Closs SJ, Briggs M. Patients' verbal descriptions of pain and discomfort following orthopaedic surgery. *International Journal of Nursing Studies.* 2002; **39**: 563–72.

18. Bible D. Pain assessment at nurse triage: a literature review. *Emergency Nurse.* 2006; **14**: 26–9.

19. Puntillo KA, Neighbor ML. Two methods of assessing pain intensity in English-speaking and Spanish-speaking emergency department patients. *Journal of Emergency Nursing.* 1997; **23**: 597–601.

20. McCaffery M, Pasero C. *Pain: clinical manual.* St Louis, MO: Mosby, 1999.

21. Panel APMG. *Acute pain management: operative or medical procedures and trauma.* Rockville, MD: US Department of Health and Human Services, 1992.

22. Jensen MP, Karoly P, Braver S. The measurement of clinical pain intensity: a comparison of six methods. *Pain.* 1986; **27**: 117–26.

∗ 23. Ho K, Spence J, Murphy MF. Review of pain-measurement tools. *Annals of Emergency Medicine.* 1996; **27**: 427–32.

24. VHA. Pain as the 5th vital sign: take 5. 2000. Available from: www.va.gov/OAA/pocketcard/pain.

25. Moore A, Edwards J, Barden J, McQuay H. *An evidence-based guide to treatments.* Bandolier's little book of pain. Oxford: Oxford University Press, 2003.

26. Hartrick CT, Kovan JP, Shapiro S. The numeric rating scale for clinical pain measurement: a ratio measure? *Pain Practice.* 2003; **3**: 310–6.

27. Jensen MP, Karoly P. Pain-specific beliefs, perceived symptom severity, and adjustment to chronic pain. *Clinical Journal of Pain.* 1992; **8**: 123–30.

28. Downie WW, Leatham PA, Rhind VM *et al.* Studies with pain rating scales. *Annals of Rheumatic Diseases.* 1978; **37**: 378–81.

29. Briggs M, Closs JS. A descriptive study of the use of visual analogue scales and verbal rating scales for the assessment of postoperative pain in orthopedic patients. *Journal of Pain and Symptom Management.* 1999; **18**: 438–46.

30. Serlin RC, Mendoza TR, Nakamura Y *et al.* When is cancer mild, moderate or severe? Grading pain severity by its interference with function. *Pain.* 1995; **61**: 277–84.

31. Prithvi Raj P. *Pain medicine: a comprehensive review.* St Louis, MO: Mosby-Year Book, 1996.

32. Breivik EK, Skoglund LA. Comparison of present pain intensity assessments on horizontally and vertically oriented visual analogue scales. *Methods and Findings in Experimental and Clinical Pharmacology.* 1998; **20**: 719–24.

33. Price DD, McGrath PA, Rafii A, Buckingham B. The validation of visual analogue scales as ratio scale measures for chronic and experimental pain. *Pain.* 1983; **17**: 45–56.

34. Myles PS, Troedel S, Boquest M, Reeves M. The pain visual analog scale: is it linear or nonlinear? *Anesthesia and Analgesia.* 1999; **89**: 1517–20.

∗ 35. Myles PS, Urquhart N. The linearity of the visual analogue scale in patients with severe acute pain. *Anaesthesia and Intensive Care.* 2005; **33**: 54–8.

36. Ahles TA, Blanchard EB, Ruckdeschel JC. The multidimensional nature of cancer-related pain. *Pain.* 1983; **17**: 277–88.

37. Carlsson AM. Assessment of chronic pain. I. Aspects of the reliability and validity of the visual analogue scale. *Pain.* 1983; **16**: 87–101.

38. Chapman CR, Casey KL, Dubner R *et al.* Pain measurement: an overview. *Pain.* 1985; **22**: 1–31.

39. Stewart M. Measurement of clinical pain. In: Jacox A (ed.). *Pain: a sourcebook for nurses and other health professionals.* Boston: Little Brown, 1977: 107–37.

40. Dalton JA, McNaull F. A call for standardizing the clinical rating of pain intensity using a 0 to 10 rating scale. *Cancer Nursing.* 1998; **21**: 46–9.

41. MacIntyre PE, Ready LB, Atkins JR, Wild L. *Acute pain management: a practical guide.* London: WB Saunders, 1996.

∗ 42. DeLoach LJ, Higgins MS, Caplan AB, Stiff JL. The visual analog scale in the immediate postoperative period: intrasubject variability and correlation with a numeric scale. *Anesthesia and Analgesia.* 1998; **86**: 102–6.

43. Lui W, Aitkenhead AR. Comparison of contemporaneous and retrospective assessment of postoperative pain using the visual analogue scale. *British Journal of Anaesthesia.* 1991; **67**: 768–71.

44. Aubrun F, Paqueron X, Langeron O et al. What pain scales do nurses use in the postanaesthesia care unit? *European Journal of Anaesthesiology*. 2003; **20**: 745–9.

45. Wong DL, Baker CM. Pain in children: comparison of assessment scales. *The Oklahoma Nurse*. 1988; **33**: 8.

46. Wong D, Baker C. *Reference manual for the Wong-Baker Faces Pain Rating Scale*. Tulsa: Wong and Baker, 1995.

47. Wong DL, Baker CM. Smiling faces as anchor for pain intensity scales. *Pain*. 2001; **89**: 295–300.

48. Wong DL. *Whaley and Wong's essentials of pediatric nursing*, 5th edn. St Louis, MO: Mosby Inc., 1997: 1215–6.

49. Beyer JE, Denyes MJ, Villarruel AM. The creation, validation, and continuing development of the Oucher: a measure of pain intensity in children. *Journal of Pediatric Nursing*. 1992; **7**: 335–46.

50. Chambers CT, Craig KD. An intrusive impact of anchors in children's faces pain scales. *Pain*. 1998; **78**: 27–37.

51. Bieri D, Reeve RA, Champion GD et al. The Faces Pain Scale for the self-assessment of the severity of pain experienced by children: development, initial validation, and preliminary investigation for ratio scale properties. *Pain*. 1990; **41**: 139–50.

* 52. Hicks CL, von Baeyer CL, Spafford PA et al. The Faces Pain Scale-Revised: toward a common metric in pediatric pain measurement. *Pain*. 2001; **93**: 173–83.

53. Frank AJ, Moll JM, Hort JF. A comparison of three ways of measuring pain. *Rheumatology and Rehabilitation*. 1982; **21**: 211–7.

54. Margolis RB, Tait RC, Krause SJ. A rating system for use with pain drawings. *Pain*. 1986; **24**: 57–65.

55. Puntillo KA. Dimensions of procedural pain and its analgesic management in critically ill surgical patients. *American Journal of Critical Care*. 1994; **3**: 116–22.

56. Prieter EJ, Geisinger KF. Factor-analytic studies of the McGill Pain Questionnaire. In: Melzack R (ed.). *Pain measurement and assessment*. New York: Raven Press, 1983.

57. Kilminster SG, Mould GP. Comparison of internal reliability and validity of the McGill Pain Questionnaire and the Short Pain Inventory. *International Journal of Pharmaceutical Medicine*. 2002; **16**: 87–95.

58. Keefe FJ. Behavioral assessment and treatment of chronic pain: current status and future directions. *Journal of Consulting and Clinical Psychology*. 1982; **50**: 896–911.

59. Erdek MA, Pronovost PJ. Improving assessment and treatment of pain in the critically ill. *International Journal for Quality in Health Care*. 2004; **16**: 59–64.

60. Briggs M. Principles of acute pain assessment. *Nursing Standard*. 1995; **9**: 23–7.

61. von Baeyer CL, Spagrud LJ. Systematic review of observational (behavioral) measures of pain for children and adolescents aged 3 to 18 years. *Pain*. 2007; **127**: 140–50.

62. Royal College of Nursing. Clinical practice guidelines. The recognition and assessment of acute pain in children. Available from: www2.rcn.org.uk/cyp/resources/a-z_of_resources/pain_management.

63. Krechel SW, Bildner J. CRIES: a new neonatal postoperative pain measurement score. Initial testing of validity and reliability. *Paediatric Anaesthesia*. 1995; **5**: 53–61.

64. Grunau RE, Holsti L, Haley DW et al. Neonatal procedural pain exposure predicts lower cortisol and behavioral reactivity in preterm infants in the NICU. *Pain*. 2005; **113**: 293–300.

65. Merkel SI, Voepel-Lewis T, Shayevitz JR, Malviya S. The FLACC: a behavioral scale for scoring postoperative pain in young children. *Pediatric Nursing*. 1997; **23**: 293–7.

66. Franck LS, Greenberg CS, Stevens B. Pain assessment in infants and children. *Pediatric Clinics of North America*. 2000; **47**: 487–512.

67. Lane P, Kuntupis M, MacDonald S et al. A pain assessment tool for people with advanced Alzheimer's and other progressive dementias. *Home Healthcare Nurse*. 2003; **21**: 32–7.

68. Scherder EJ, Bouma A. Visual analogue scales for pain assessment in Alzheimer's disease. *Gerontology*. 2000; **46**: 47–53.

69. Hurley AC, Volicer BJ, Hanrahan PA et al. Assessment of discomfort in advanced Alzheimer patients. *Research in Nursing and Health*. 1992; **15**: 369–77.

70. Abbey J, Piller N, De Bellis A et al. The Abbey pain scale: a 1-minute numerical indicator for people with end-stage dementia. *International Journal of Palliative Nursing*. 2004; **10**: 6–13.

* 71. Payen JF, Bru O, Bosson JL et al. Assessing pain in critically ill sedated patients by using a behavioral pain scale. *Critical Care Medicine*. 2001; **29**: 2258–63.

72. Kovach CR, Weissman DE, Griffie J et al. Assessment and treatment of discomfort for people with late-stage dementia. *Journal of Pain and Symptom Management*. 1999; **18**: 412–9.

73. Weiner DK, Hanlon JT. Pain in nursing home residents: management strategies. *Drugs and Aging*. 2001; **18**: 13–29.

74. Cleeland CS, Ryan KM. Pain assessment: global use of the Brief Pain Inventory. *Annals of the Academy of Medicine, Singapore*. 1994; **23**: 129–38.

75. Carr DB, Jacox AK, Chapman CR. *Acute pain management: operative or medical procedures and trauma: clinical practice guideline*, vol. 92. Rockville, MD: Agency for Health Care Policy and Reseach, US Department of Human Service, 1992.

76. Twycross R, Harcourt J, Bergl S. A survey of pain in patients with advanced cancer. *Journal of Pain and Symptom Management*. 1996; **12**: 273–82.

77. Daut RL, Cleeland CS. The prevalence and severity of pain in cancer. *Cancer*. 1982; **50**: 1913–8.

78. Daut RL, Cleeland CS, Flanery RC. Development of the Wisconsin Brief Pain Questionnaire to assess pain in cancer and other diseases. *Pain*. 1983; **17**: 197–210.

79. Janken JK, Dufault MA. Improving the quality of pain assessment through research utilization. *Online Journal of Knowledge Synthesis for Nursing.* 2002; **9**: 2C.

80. VQC. Acute Pain Management Performance Assessment Toolkit. Victorian Quality Council. Accessed February 2008. http://www.health.vic.gov.au/qualitycouncil/activities/acute.htm

* 81. Cepeda MS, Africano JM, Polo R *et al.* What decline in pain intensity is meaningful to patients with acute pain? *Pain.* 2003; **105**: 151–7.

82. Naylor CD. Meta-analysis and the meta-epidemiology of clinical research. *British Medical Journal.* 1997; **315**: 617–9.

83. Mamie C, Morabia A, Bernstein M *et al.* Treatment efficacy is not an index of pain intensity. *Canadian Journal of Anaesthesia.* 2000; **47**: 1166–70.

84. Miaskowski C, Nichols R, Brody R, Synold T. Assessment of patient satisfaction utilizing the American Pain Society's Quality Assurance Standards on acute and cancer-related pain. *Journal of Pain and Symptom Management.* 1994; **9**: 5–11.

* 85. Svensson I, Sjostrom B, Haljamae H. Influence of expectations and actual pain experiences on satisfaction with postoperative pain management. *European Journal of Pain.* 2001; **5**: 125–33.

9

Preventive analgesia and beyond: current status, evidence, and future directions

JOEL KATZ AND HANCE CLARKE

KEY LEARNING POINTS

- *What is preemptive analgesia?* The classic definition of preemptive analgesia requires two groups of patients to receive identical treatment before or after incision or surgery. The only difference between the two groups is the timing of administration of the pharmacological agent relative to incision. The constraint to include a postincision or postsurgical treatment group is methodologically appealing, because in the presence of a positive result, it provides a window of time within which the observed effect occurred, and thus points to possible mechanisms underlying the effect: the classic view assumes that the intraoperative nociceptive barrage contributes to a greater extent to postoperative pain than does the postoperative nociceptive barrage. However, this view is too restrictive and narrow in part because we know that sensitization is induced by factors other than the peripheral nociceptive barrage associated with incision and subsequent noxious intraoperative events.

- *What is preventive analgesia?* A broader approach to the prevention of postoperative pain has evolved that aims to minimize the deleterious immediate and long-term effects of noxious perioperative afferent input. The focus of preventive analgesia is not on the relative timing of analgesic or anesthetic interventions, but on attenuating the impact of the peripheral nociceptive barrage associated with noxious preoperative, intraoperative, and/or postoperative events/stimuli. These stimuli induce peripheral and central sensitization which increase postoperative pain intensity and analgesic requirements. Preventing sensitization will reduce pain and analgesic requirements. Preventive analgesia is demonstrated when postoperative pain and/or analgesic use are reduced beyond the clinical duration of action of the target agent which we have defined as 5.5 half-lives of the target agent. This requirement ensures that the observed effects are not analgesic effects.

- *What does the recent preemptive analgesia literature tell us?* The results of the present literature review indicate that the proportion of significant preemptive effects (0.63) is not significantly different from the proportion of negative preemptive effects (0.37) across the different classes of drugs studied ($p = 0.36$). This is understandable when one considers that both preincisional and postincisional (or postsurgical) noxious inputs contribute to postoperative sensitization, pain, and analgesic consumption. The most likely conclusion, therefore, is that for a certain proportion of studies of preemptive analgesia, the postincision or postsurgical administration condition is as beneficial in reducing central sensitization as is the preoperative condition, but these benefits go undetected when the comparison is made between the two groups. The lack of a control group in studies of preemptive analgesia is a serious limitation that confounds interpretation of the results and has contributed to the premature and erroneous conclusion that there is no clinical benefit to preoperative nociceptive blockade.

- *What does the recent preventive analgesia literature tell us?* In contrast to the results for preemptive analgesia, the proportion of significant preventive effects (0.72) is significantly greater than the proportion of negative effects (0.28) across the different classes of drugs studied ($p = 0.03$). Overall, administration of these agents appears to reduce pain, analgesic consumption, or both at a point in time that exceeds 5.5 half-lives of the target agent. Since these extended effects are observed after the clinical actions of the agents have worn off, they are not analgesic effects. Rather, these effects appear to be due to the reduction in perioperative peripheral and central sensitization associated with preventive analgesia. The benefits of preventive analgesia are clinically relevant and include reduced pain and/or analgesic consumption that extend beyond the duration of action of the target drug.

- *What other important factors do we need to measure perioperatively?* Measures of postoperative pain and analgesic use are important, but given the prominent role played by psychosocial factors in the experience of preoperative, acute postoperative, and chronic postsurgical pain, relevant psychological, emotional, and physical variables should be routinely assessed before and after surgery. Assessment of these additional domains of functioning may help to shed light on the predictors of severe acute postoperative pain, the processes involved in recovery from surgery, and the risk factors for developing chronic postsurgical pain.

BACKGROUND LITERATURE

Acute postoperative pain management has been dominated by an outdated concept of pain. Pain is viewed as the end product of a passive system that faithfully transmits a peripheral "pain" signal from receptor to a "pain centre" in the brain.[1] This view has resulted in a strategy for managing postoperative pain that is inadequate, in part, because it treats the patient only after the pain is well established. Patients arrive in the post-anesthetic care unit after surgery, often in extreme pain, where they then receive multiple doses of opioids in an effort to bring the pain down to a tolerable level. However, basic science and clinical data show that brief, noxious inputs or frank injury due to C-fiber activation (e.g. cutting tissue, nerve, and bone) induce long-lasting changes in central neural function that persist well after the offending stimulus has been removed or the injury has healed.[2, 3] This view of pain, involving a dynamic interplay between peripheral and central mechanisms, is inconsistent with the outdated notion that pain results from transmission of impulses along a straight-through pathway from the site of injury to the brain.[1]

The practice of treating pain only after it has become well entrenched is slowly being supplanted by a preventive approach that aims to block transmission of the primary afferent injury barrage before, during, and after surgery.[4, 5, 6, 7] The idea behind this approach is not simply that it reduces nociception and stress during surgery – although these are obviously worthwhile goals. The hypothesis is that the transmission of noxious afferent input from the periphery (e.g. arising from preoperative pain, incision, noxious intraoperative events, postoperative inflammation, and ectopia) to the spinal cord induces a prolonged state of central neural sensitization or hyperexcitability that amplifies subsequent input from the wound and leads to heightened postoperative pain and a greater requirement for postoperative analgesics. By interrupting the transmission of the peripheral nociceptive barrage to the spinal cord at various points in time throughout the perioperative period, a preventive approach aims to block the induction of central sensitization, resulting in reduced pain intensity and lower analgesic requirements. The goal of this chapter is to critically review the recent literature on preemptive and preventive analgesia. The first section provides a description of the perioperative targets of a preventive analgesic approach. This is followed by a brief review of the factors that have been shown to predict the development of acute and chronic postsurgical pain. Next, the history and recent progress in preemptive analgesia are presented with emphasis on the confusion and lack of clarity that characterizes the field. Under Controversy and confusion about preemptive analgesia, we attempt to clear up the confusion by highlighting clinical trial designs and examples from the literature that distinguish preventive analgesia from preemptive analgesia. This is followed by a quantitative review of the preemptive and preventive analgesia literatures (see below under Preventive analgesia), organized according to class of drug administered. Outcomes are described in terms of the presence or absence or a preemptive or preventive effect and a detailed tabular summary is presented of all studies that met our criteria for inclusion in the review. The chapter concludes with recommendations for future research.

TARGETS OF A PREVENTIVE APPROACH TO ACUTE PAIN MANAGEMENT

The perioperative period can be divided into three distinct phases: preoperative, intraoperative, and postoperative (**Figure 9.1**). Specific factors within these phases contribute to the development of acute postoperative pain. These factors include: (1) preoperative noxious inputs and pain; (2) C-fiber injury barrage arising from the cutting of skin, muscle, nerve and bone, wound retraction, etc.; and (3) postoperative peripheral nociceptive activity, including that arising from the inflammatory response and ectopic neural activity in the case of postsurgical nerve injury. Each of these factors can contribute to peripheral and central sensitization and each is a legitimate target for a preventive approach. The relative contribution of these three factors to acute postoperative pain is dependent on the surgical procedure, extent and nature of tissue damage, duration of surgery, timing of treatments relative to incision, pharmacokinetics of the agent(s) used preoperatively, presence or absence of additional analgesia intraoperatively, nature of postoperative analgesia, and a host of other variables. Minimizing the negative impact of as many of these factors as possible in the three phases will increase the likelihood of preventing the induction and maintenance of peripheral and central sensitization. Preventing sensitization will reduce pain and analgesic requirements.

Figure 9.1 depicts the eight possible treatment combinations of administering or not administering analgesics across the three perioperative phases (preoperative, intraoperative, and postoperative). The preoperative period encompasses interventions that begin days before surgery and up to those administered just minutes before skin incision. The intraoperative period includes interventions started immediately after incision to those initiated just prior to the end of surgery (i.e. skin closure). The postoperative period includes interventions started immediately after the end of surgery and may extend for days or weeks thereafter. Within each phase there is potential for extensive variability in the timing of administration of analgesic agents. While this potential is greatest in the pre- and postoperative phases (e.g. ranging from minutes to days or weeks) even within the intraoperative period, evidence shows that there are considerable interstudy differences in timing of the postincisional intervention (e.g. ranging from minutes to hours).

PREDICTORS OF ACUTE AND CHRONIC POSTSURGICAL PAIN

The ability to predict who will develop severe acute postoperative pain and who will go on to develop chronic postsurgical pain is at the heart of efforts to understand

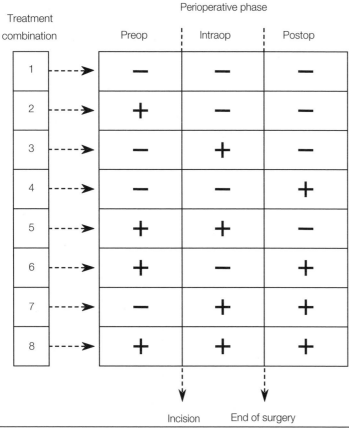

Figure 9.1 Schematic representation showing the administration (+) or non-administration (−) of analgesic agents across the three perioperative phases of surgery (preop, preoperative; intraop, intraoperative; postop, postoperative). The administration or nonadministration of analgesics during the three phases yields eight different treatment combinations and 28 possible two-group designs to evaluate the efficacy of preemptive and preventive analgesia. The classic preemptive analgesia design requires two groups of patients to receive identical treatment before or after incision or surgery (treatment combination 2 versus 3 and 2 versus 4). This represents only one of many possible hypotheses concerning the effects of blocking noxious perioperative inputs on postoperative pain and analgesic consumption.

the role played by the various factors within the three perioperative phases depicted in **Figure 9.1**. One of the most robust findings to emerge from the postoperative pain and anesthesia literatures is that current pain predicts future pain.[8, 9, 10, 11] This appears to be true across surgery types and regardless of time frame. Preoperative pain intensity or pain duration is a risk factor for development of severe early acute postoperative pain,[12] acute pain days,[13, 14, 15, 16, 17] and weeks[18] after surgery, as well as long-term postsurgical pain.[14, 15, 18, 19, 20, 21, 22] Preoperative pain ratings in response to the cold pressor task,[23] suprathreshold heat pain stimuli,[24] and a first-degree burn injury[25] also predict acute postoperative pain intensity days after surgery. Severity of acute postoperative pain not only predicts pain after discharge,[18, 26] but it is also a risk factor for development of chronic postsurgical pain.[27, 28, 29, 30, 31, 32]

No other factor is as consistently related to the development of future pain problems as is current pain. Younger age,[12, 18] female gender,[12, 18] anxiety,[12, 19] and various other psychological variables[8, 33, 34, 35, 36] predict postoperative pain in some studies, but not with the consistency or magnitude with which pain predicts pain. What must be determined is the aspect(s) of pain that is predictive. Is it something about the pain *per se* (e.g. intensity, quality, duration) or the individuals who report the pain (e.g. response bias, psychological vulnerability, genetic predisposition)? Will reducing surgery-induced sensitization alter the course of acute pain and lead to a decreased incidence of long-term pain problems? What factors are responsible for the transition of acute postoperative pain to chronic, intractable, pathological pain? We do not have answers to these important questions but one of the factors that has been linked to increased pain and analgesic consumption in the short and long term is the perioperative peripheral nociceptive injury barrage associated with surgery. The remainder of this chapter will focus on an evidence-based presentation of the literature that examines the efficacy of preemptive and preventive interventions aimed at reducing surgically induced sensitization.

HISTORY AND RECENT PROGRESS IN PREEMPTIVE ANALGESIA

The idea that acute postoperative pain might be intensified by a state of central neural hyperexcitability induced during surgery was first proposed by Crile (see Katz[37]) and later by Wall[38] who suggested that "preemptive preoperative analgesia" would block the induction of central neural sensitization brought about by incision and thus reduce acute postoperative pain intensity. Since its introduction into the pain and anesthesia literatures, this concept has been refined, based in part on confirmatory and contradictory evidence from clinical studies, new developments in basic science, and critical thought. The suggestion that surgical incision triggered central

sensitization[38] has been expanded to include the sensitizing effects of preoperative noxious inputs and pain, other noxious intraoperative stimuli, as well as postoperative peripheral and central inflammatory mediators and ectopic neural activity.

It is now well documented that while general anesthesia may attenuate transmission of afferent injury barrage from the periphery to the spinal cord and brain, it does not block it.[39] Moreover, systemic opioids may not provide a sufficiently dense blockade of spinal nociceptive neurons to prevent central sensitization.[40] The clinical significance of these findings for patients who receive general anesthesia during surgery is that although they are unconscious, the processes leading to sensitization of dorsal horn neurons are largely unaffected by general anesthesia or routine doses of opioids. This sets the stage for heightened postoperative pain and an increased requirement for analgesics.

CONTROVERSY AND CONFUSION ABOUT PREEMPTIVE ANALGESIA

Debate over the appropriate definition of preemptive analgesia[5, 6, 41, 42, 43, 44, 45, 46, 47] has spawned a variety of different terms, including anoci-association,[48] preemptive preoperative analgesia,[38] preemptive analgesia,[49] preventive analgesia,[4, 6] balanced periemptive analgesia,[50] broad versus narrow preemptive analgesia,[51] and protective analgesia.[52] Substantial confusion has developed over the benefits and meaning of preemptive analgesia.

Two general approaches have dominated the literature.[53] The classic view of preemptive analgesia[49] requires two groups of patients to receive identical treatment before or after incision or surgery (treatment combination 2 versus 3 and 2 versus 4 in **Figure 9.1**). Accordingly, the only difference between the two groups is the timing of administration of the pharmacological agent relative to incision with one group receiving the target agent before surgery, and the other, after incision or surgery (see **Figures 9.2** and **9.3** depicting studies by Katz *et al.*[54] and Dierking *et al.*[55] who used these designs, respectively). The constraint to include a postincision or postsurgical treatment group is methodologically appealing because in the presence of a positive result, it provides a window of time within which the observed effect occurred and thus points to possible mechanisms underlying the effect. However, this view of preemptive analgesia is too restrictive and narrow[5, 6, 56] in part because we do not know the relative extent to which pre-, intra-, and postoperative peripheral nociceptive inputs contribute to central sensitization and postoperative pain.

The narrow conceptualization of preemptive analgesia in conjunction with the classic pre- versus postsurgery design assumes that the intraoperative nociceptive barrage contributes to a greater extent to postoperative pain than does the postoperative nociceptive barrage. However, the

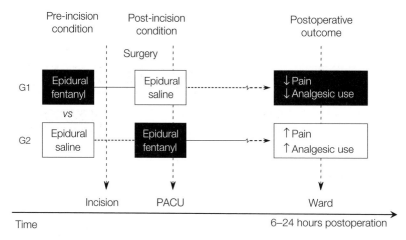

Figure 9.2 Experimental design and expected postoperative outcome for studies of preemptive analgesia in which a preincisional intervention is compared with the very same intervention initiated after incision, but before the end of surgery (treatment combination 2 versus 3 in **Figure 9.1**). This design was used in the study by Katz et al.[54][II] in which the two groups of patients undergoing lateral thoracotomy received epidural fentanyl or saline before, and epidural saline or fentanyl 15 minutes after, incision, respectively. Pain ratings in the group that received preincisional epidural fentanyl were significantly lower six hours after surgery and morphine consumption was significantly lower between 12 and 24 hours after surgery.

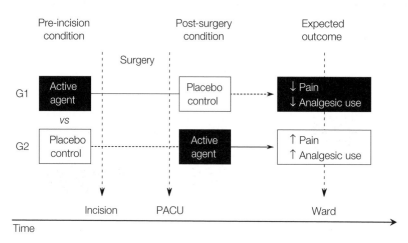

Figure 9.3 Experimental design and expected postoperative outcome for studies of preemptive analgesia in which a preincision intervention is compared with the very same intervention initiated after surgery (treatment combination 2 versus 4 in **Figure 9.1**). According to the classic view of preemptive analgesia, the expected outcome is based on the assumption that the intraoperative nociceptive barrage contributes to a greater extent to postoperative pain and analgesic use than do postoperative noxious inputs. This design was used in the study by Dierking et al.[55] who compared a lidocaine inguinal field block administered 15 minutes before hernia repair with the same treatment administered immediately after surgery. Significant differences in pain or analgesic use were not found between the pre- and postsurgical treatment groups raising the possibility that a preventive effect went undetected due to lack of a control group (see **Figures 9.4** and **9.5**).

design does not allow for other equally plausible alternatives. For certain surgical procedures, central sensitization may be induced to an equal extent by incision and intraoperative trauma on the one hand (i.e. in the postsurgical treatment group) and postoperative inflammatory inputs and/or ectopia on the other (i.e. in the preoperative treatment group) which would lead to nonsignificant intergroup differences in pain and analgesic consumption.[57, 58]

Two-group studies that fail to find significant differences in postoperative pain or analgesic consumption between groups treated before or after incision or surgery are inherently flawed because of the absence of an appropriate control group (e.g. treatment combination 1 or 8, or both in **Figure 9.1**). The negative results may point to the relative efficacy in reducing central sensitization of postincisional or postsurgical blockade and not the inefficacy of preoperative blockade (for examples, see **Figures 9.4** and **9.5** depicting studies Katz et al.[57, 58] and Gordon et al.[59]). Recent studies[57, 58] have highlighted the critical importance of a standard treatment control group. Inclusion of such as group has made it possible to

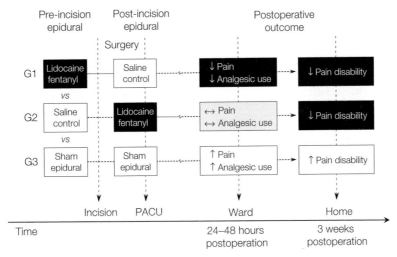

Figure 9.4 Experimental design (treatment combination 1 versus 2 versus 3 in **Figure 9.1**) used by Katz et al.[57, 58][II] to address the design flaw inherent in two-group studies of preemptive analgesia (**Figure 9.2**). In females undergoing abdominal gynecological surgery by laparotomy, preincisional (G1) but not postincisional (G2) administration of epidural lidocaine and fentanyl was associated with a significantly lower rate of morphine use, lower cumulative morphine consumption, and reduced hyperalgesia compared with a sham epidural condition (G3).[58][II] Three-week follow up showed that pain disability ratings were significantly lower in the two groups that received the epidural when compared with the standard treatment group.[57][II] Results highlight the importance of including a standard treatment control group to avoid the problems of interpretation that arise when two-group studies of preemptive analgesia (pre- versus postincision) fail to find the anticipated effects.

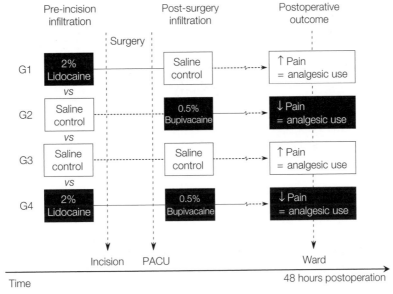

Figure 9.5 Experimental design used by Gordon et al.[59][II] to assess the relative effects on late postoperative pain of blocking, or not blocking, noxious intraoperative and/or postoperative inputs (treatment combination 1 versus 2 versus 4 versus 6 in **Figure 9.1**). Patients were randomly assigned in a double-blinded manner to receive a local anesthetic (lidocaine or bupivacaine) or saline before and/or at the end of third molar extraction surgery. Preventive analgesia is demonstrated by the finding that 48 hours after surgery, pain intensity was significantly less in the groups whose postoperative pain was blocked by bupivacaine (G2, G4) compared with preoperative administration of lidocaine (G1) or the saline control group (G3). The results suggest that for third molar extraction surgery, the peripheral nociceptive barrage in the hours following surgery contributes to a greater extent to central sensitization and late postoperative pain than does the intraoperative nociceptive barrage since local anesthetic blockade after surgery was more efficacious than preoperative blockade.

demonstrate reductions in acute postoperative pain and morphine consumption,[58] as well as pain disability three weeks after surgery[57] that would otherwise have gone undetected using the classic, two-group design.

The near exclusive focus in the literature on the narrow view of preemptive analgesia has had the unintended effect of diverting attention away from other clinically significant findings because they do not conform to what has become the accepted definition of preemptive analgesia.[4] For example, certain studies[60, 61] evaluate the effects of altering the timing of administration of various analgesic agents in a manner similar to that described above for the classic two-group preemptive analgesia design, except that the intent is not to compare pre-versus postincisional or postsurgical treatments. Rather, as illustrated in **Figure 9.6**, both groups may receive the target intervention preoperatively, differing only in how long before surgery the treatment is given.[61] Such a study evaluates the effect on postoperative pain and analgesic consumption of blocking versus not blocking preoperative pain in the context of intraoperative and postoperative epidural blockade and demonstrates that relief of preoperative pain is associated with reduced analgesic use 48 hours after surgery.[61] Finally, other reports[59] have demonstrated that for certain types of surgery, blocking the peripheral nociceptive barrage in the hours after surgery decreases pain at later time periods, whereas blocking the intraoperative nociceptive barrage does not (**Figure 9.5**). Taken together, these shortcomings of the classic view of preemptive analgesia, and its associated design, indicate that an expanded conceptualization and explication of the rationale for, and effects of, blockade across the three perioperative phases is required to move us beyond the current state of confusion that pervades the field of preemptive analgesia.

PREVENTIVE ANALGESIA

A more encompassing approach, termed preventive analgesia,[4, 6] has evolved with the aim of minimizing sensitization induced by noxious perioperative stimuli including those arising preoperatively, intraoperatively,

and postoperatively. A preventive analgesic effect is demonstrated when postoperative pain and/or analgesic consumption is reduced relative to another treatment, and/or a placebo treatment or no treatment as long as the effect is observed at a point in time that exceeds the clinical duration of action of the target agent (e.g. treatment combination 1 versus 2, 1 versus 5, or 1 versus 8 in **Figure 9.1**). The requirement that the reduced pain and/or analgesic consumption be observed after the duration of action of the target agent ensures that the preventive effect is not simply an analgesic effect. As we have previously pointed out,[4, 5, 56][I] such a design does not provide information about the factors underlying the effect or the time frame within which the effect occurred due the absence of a post-treatment condition (see **Figures 9.7** and **9.8** for illustrations of studies by Tverskoy et al.[62][II] and Reuben et al.,[63][II] respectively, who used these designs).

Demonstration of a preventive effect does not require that an intervention be initiated before surgery; the timing of treatment may be during the procedure (e.g. treatment combination 1 versus 3 in **Figure 9.1**) or even after surgery (e.g. treatment combination 1 versus 4 in **Figure 9.1**). For example, a preventive effect is present if postoperative administration of a target analgesic agent, but not a placebo, results in reduced postoperative pain or analgesic consumption after the effects of the target agent have worn off (for a case in point see **Figure 9.9** depicting the study by Reuben et al.[64][II]). In fact, any two or more treatment combinations in **Figure 9.1** can produce preventive effects. The focus of preventive analgesia is not on the relative timing of analgesic or anesthetic interventions, but on attenuating the impact of noxious perioperative stimuli that induce peripheral and central sensitization and that increase postoperative pain intensity and

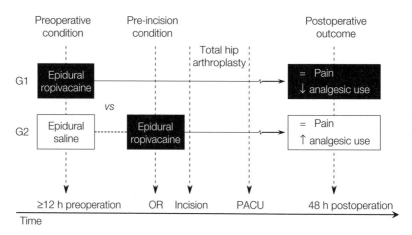

Figure 9.6 Two-group experimental design used by Klasen et al.[61][II] comparing the administration of an active agent at different times before surgery in order to examine the effect on postoperative pain and analgesic consumption of blocking versus not blocking preoperative pain in the context of intraoperative and postoperative epidural blockade (treatment combination 8 versus 8 in **Figure 9.1**). This study[61][II] demonstrates that relief of preoperative pain by epidural ropivacaine for at least 12 hours before surgery followed by intraoperative epidural ropivacaine (G1) is associated with reduced patient-controlled epidural analgesia (PCEA) ropivacaine consumption 48 hours after surgery compared with preoperative epidural saline and intraoperative epidural ropivacaine (G2).

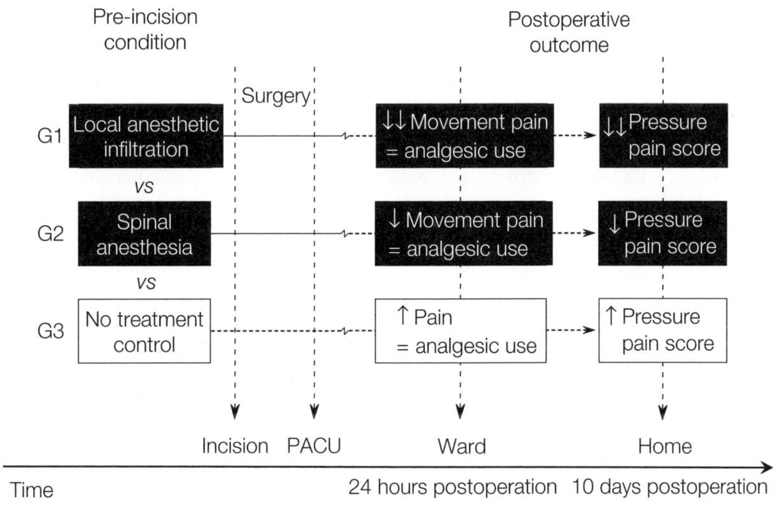

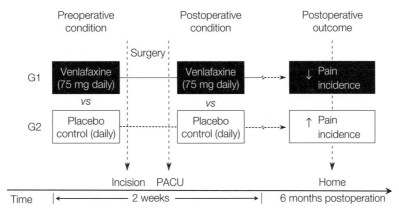

Figure 9.7 Experimental design comparing two different preoperative interventions with a no treatment control condition (treatment combination 1 versus 2 versus 2 in **Figure 9.1**). This design was used by Tverskoy et al.[62][II] in the very first prospective study of preventive analgesia. Patients undergoing inguinal herniorraphy were randomly assigned to receive one of three types of anesthesia: general plus preoperative local anesthetic infiltration (G1), spinal (G2), or general (G3). While anesthesia (infiltration or spinal) significantly decreased movement-associated pain intensity at 24 hours after surgery compared with the control group, the infiltration group reported the least pain overall. This pattern of pain scores was still apparent ten days after surgery in response to mechanical pressure applied to the wound.

Figure 9.8 Experimental design comparing a preoperative plus postsurgical intervention with a placebo control condition (treatment combination 1 versus 8 in **Figure 9.1**). Preventive analgesia is demonstrated if the preoperative plus postsurgical intervention condition shows less pain and/or analgesic consumption than the placebo control group beyond the clinical duration of action of the target analgesic. This design was used by Reuben et al.[63][II] who randomly assigned females to receive venlafaxine (75 mg daily) or placebo (daily) for a two-week period beginning the night before radical mastectomy. Six-month follow up showed that the incidence of chest wall pain, arm pain, and axilla pain was significantly lower in the venlafaxine group than the placebo group.

analgesic requirements. A preventive analgesic effect involves demonstrating reduced pain and/or analgesic use beyond the clinical duration of action of the target agent.

RATIONALE FOR PRESENT REVIEW

Recent evidence-based reviews of randomized, double-blind studies reported in the literature on preemptive[4, 47, 52, 65, 66][I] and preventive[4, 47, 67][I] analgesia suggest that there are clinically significant benefits associated with

both approaches to postoperative pain prevention, although the positive evidence is more abundant for the latter than the former. The more equivocal results for preemptive analgesia likely reflect the fact that intra-operative and postoperative noxious inputs contribute to central sensitization, thus diminishing the magnitude of the effect when pre- and posttreated groups are compared. The aim of the present review is to critically evaluate the recent literature on preemptive and preventive analgesia and to compare and contrast the results from both approaches.

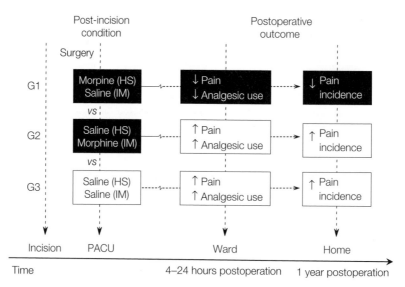

Figure 9.9 Experimental design comparing two postincision analgesic interventions with a placebo or no treatment control condition (treatment combination 1 versus 4 versus 4 in **Figure 9.1**). Preventive analgesia is demonstrated if the postincision condition shows less pain and/or analgesic consumption than the control group beyond the clinical duration of action of the target analgesic. This design was used by Reuben *et al.*[64][II] who showed that morphine, but not saline, administered into the iliac bone graft harvest site (HS) during cervical spinal fusion surgery reduced short-term pain and analgesic consumption, as well as the incidence of chronic donor site pain one year after surgery when compared with a group that received intramuscular morphine and a placebo control group that received saline. The study illustrates that preventive analgesia can be achieved even when the analgesic intervention is started after incision and bone graft harvest (i.e. in the context of an unchecked peripheral nociceptive injury barrage during surgery).

SEARCH STRATEGIES AND CRITERIA FOR INCLUDING STUDIES

A PubMed database search was conducted from January 2001 to September 2006. Search strategies were limited to English language and studies using human subjects. Each of the following key words was searched: pre-emptive analgesia, preemptive analgesia, preempts, pre-operative, preoperative, postoperative, pre-incision, preincision, post-incision, postincision. A second search was conducted using the same time period and the same limits. The terms searched were as follows: (gabapentin *or* NSAIDs *or* (NSAIDs and preoperative) *or* (NSAIDs and postoperative) *or* NMDA *or* (NMDA and preoperative) or (NMDA and postoperative) or opioids or (opioid and preemptive) or (opioid and preoperative) or (opioid and postoperative) or local anesthetics or (local anesthetics and preemptive) or (local anesthetics and preoperative) or (local anesthetics and postoperative)).

The above search strategies yielded 333 publications which were retrieved and reviewed by both authors. All clinical trials were evaluated according to the following inclusion criteria for entry into the present review: (1) randomized; (2) double-blind assessments of pain and analgesic use; (3) report of pain using a reliable and valid measure; (4) report of analgesic consumption; (5) absence of design flaws, methodological problems, or confounds that render interpretation of the results ambiguous. Trials that fit the above definition of preventive analgesia were

considered not relevant and were not considered further if they did not report measures of postoperative pain and analgesic consumption at a point in time that equaled or exceeded 5.5 half-lives of the target agent. This criterion was included to ensure that the observed effects are not simply analgesic effects. We excluded clinical trials that involved third molar extraction and those evaluating neuraxial opioids due to controversy over half-life data.[68] **Table 9.1** lists the half-lives of the drugs used for the present chapter.

Of the 333 publications, 61 clinical trials were identified that met the above inclusion and exclusion criteria. **Table 9.2** contains the 34 studies that were excluded from review, showing which one or more of the five inclusion criteria were not met. The 61 studies were evaluated and scored for methodological quality by both authors using the Jadad quality index scale.[72] The scale uses a six point (0–5) rating system (in which lower quality articles receive lower scores) to assess the likelihood of bias in pain research reports based on descriptions of randomization, blinding, and withdrawals. A data extraction process was performed on the articles that met inclusion criteria. The following items were collected: publication details, sample size, surgical procedure, nature and timing of interventions, target agent, route and dose of target agent, nature and time after surgery of preemptive or preventive effect.

Table 9.3 shows the various experimental designs (depicted in **Figure 9.1**) and the frequency with which

Table 9.1 Half-lives of drugs and source of half-live information used in studies of preventive analgesia.

Drug/source of information	Half-life	Criterion value of 5.5 half-lives
Local anesthetics		
Bupivacaine[69]	i.v.: 3.5 hours	i.v.: 19.25 hours
	epidural: 2–5 hours	epidural: 27.5 hours
	PNB: 4–12 hours	PNB: 66 hours
	Infilt: 2–8 hours	Infilt: 44 hours
Lidocaine[69]	i.v.: 1.6 hours	i.v.: 8.8 hours
	epidural: 1–3 hours	epidural: 16.5 hours
	PNB: 1–3 hours	PNB: 16.5 hours
	Infilt: 1–4 hours	Infilt: 22 hours
Mexiletine[70]	10–12 hours	66 hours
Ropivacaine[69]	i.v.: 1.9 hours	i.v.: 10.45 hours
	epidural: 2–6 hours	epidural: 33 hours
	PNB: 5–8 hours	PNB: 44 hours
	Infilt: 2–6 hours	Infilt: 33 hours
Nonsteroidal anti-inflammatory drugs		
Celecoxib[71]	6–12 hours	66 hours
Flurbiprofen[71]	6 hours	33 hours
Ibuprofen[71]	2–4 hours	22 hours
Ketoprofen[71]	2 hours	11 hours
Ketorolac[71]	4–6 hours	33 hours
Piroxicam[71]	45–50 hours	11.4 days
Potassium diclofenac[69]	1.5 hours	8.25 hours
Rofecoxib	17 hours	93.5 hours
Tenoxicam[69]	60 hours	13.75 days
NMDA receptor antagonists		
Dextromethorphan[69]	1.2–3.9 hours	21.45 hours
Ketamine[70]	2.5–3 hours	16.5 hours
Magnesium[70]	8 hours	44 hours
Opioids		
Fentanyl[70]	3–4 hours	22 hours
Morphine[70]	4 hours	22 hours
Pethidine[70]	3 hours	16.5 hours
Remifentanil[70]	8–20 minutes	1.8 hours
Sufentanil[70]	3–4 hours	22 hours
Other analgesic and nonanalgesic agents		
Paracetamol (acetaminophen)[70]	4 hours	22 hours
Clonidine[70]	6–20 hours	4.6 days
Dexmedetomidine[70]	2 hours	11 hours
Gabapentin[69]	6–7 hours	38.5 hours
Nitroglycerin[70]	1–4 minutes	1.5 hours
Promethazine[70]	9–16 hours	3.6 days
Venlafaxine[70]	11 hours	60.5 hours

i.m., intramuscular; Infilt, infiltration; i.v., intravenous; NMDA, N-methyl-D-aspartate; p.o., per os; PNB, peripheral nerve block.
Also shown is the criterion value of 5.5 half lives used to determine inclusion of studies evaluating preventive analgesia (i.e. with a no treatment or placebo control group). Only studies that reported a measure of pain and analgesic consumption beyond the criterion value were eligible for inclusion in the present review as assessing preventive effects. This requirement was not in place for studies of preemptive analgesia (i.e. in which treatment control groups received the same intervention but at different times).

Table 9.2 Studies excluded from review in the present chapter for failing to meet one or more of the following criteria: randomized (R), double-blind assessments (DB), report of pain using a reliable and valid measure (P), report of analgesic consumption (A), and absence of methodological problem, design flaw, or confound that renders interpretation of the results ambiguous (MF).

Author	Year	Drug class	Criterion not met
Lee et al.[73]	2001	LA	R
Senturk et al.[31]	2002	LA	DB
Yegin et al.[74]	2003	LA	DB
Senagore et al.[75]	2003	LA	DB
Cerfolio et al.[76]	2003	LA	A
Korhonen et al.[77]	2004	LA	DB
Karakaya et al.[78]	2004	LA	DB
Lee-Elliott et al.[79]	2004	LA	DB
Batra et al.[80]	2005	LA	DB
Sundarathiti et al.[81]	2005	LA	DB
Abramov et al.[82]	2005	LA	MF
Herbland et al.[83]	2006	LA	A
Seet et al.[84]	2006	LA	DB
Yukawa et al.[85]	2005	Multimodal	DB
Busch et al.[86]	2006	Multimodal	DB
Subramaniam et al.[87]	2001	NMDA antagonist	P
Papaziogas et al.[88]	2001	NMDA antagonist	A
Weinbroum et al.[89]	2001	NMDA antagonist	R
Weinbroum et al.[90]	2002	NMDA antagonist	MF
Weinbroum[91]	2002	NMDA antagonist	R
Weinbroum et al.[92]	2003	NMDA antagonist	MF
O'Flaherty and Lin[93]	2003	NMDA antagonist	A, P
Hayes et al.[94]	2004	NMDA antagonist	A
Bolcal et al.[95]	2005	NMDA antagonist	DB
Carney et al.[96]	2001	NSAID	R
Mallory et al.[97]	2002	NSAID	R, DB
Wnek et al.[98]	2004	NSAID	DB
Nikanne et al.[99]	2005	NSAID	A
Canbay et al.[100]	2006	NSAID	A
Louizos et al.[101]	2006	NSAID	DB
Wordliczek et al.[102]	2002	Opioid	DB
Machida et al.[103]	2004	Opioid	DB
Bellissant et al.[104]	2004	Opioid	P
De Pietri et al.[105]	2006	Opioid	DB

LA, local anesthetic; NSAID, nonsteroidal anti-inflammatory drug; NMDA, N-methyl-D-aspartate.

they were used across the 61 studies for each class of analgesic and anesthetic agent. For each design, the table also shows whether the effect being evaluated is preemptive or preventive as defined above. The enormous variability in timing of treatment is evident from the fact that 23 different designs have been implemented. **Table 9.4** summarizes the outcomes of the studies reviewed below according to the target agent administered, including gabapentin, local anesthetics, opioids, nonsteroidal anti-inflammatory drugs (NSAID), N-methyl-D-aspartate

(NMDA) receptor antagonists, multimodal therapy (three or more target agents), and other, traditionally, non-analgesic/anesthetic agents. Positive studies are defined as those that report a significant preemptive or preventive effect (i.e. reduced pain or analgesic consumption, or both). Negative studies are defined as those for which the treatment and control groups did not differ significantly in terms of pain or analgesic consumption. Also listed in the table is the frequency of studies reporting effects opposite to that predicted (e.g. in a study of preemptive analgesia, the postsurgical treatment group demonstrated significantly less pain and/or used fewer analgesics than the preincisional treatment group).

LITERATURE REVIEW

Gabapentin

Gabapentin is a structural analogue of γ-aminobutyric acid (GABA) and was introduced into clinical practice as an anticonvulsant drug. Its main binding site is believed to be the alpha-2-delta subunit of voltage-dependent calcium channels, but its full mechanism of action is not well understood.[106] Other postulated mechanisms of action have been proposed, such as selectively activating $GABA_B$ receptors, selectively enhancing the NMDA current at GABAergic interneurons, or blocking α-amino-3-hydroxy-5-methylisoxazole-4-propionic acid (AMPA) receptor-mediated transmission in the spinal cord.[106] More recently, gabapentin has been shown to increase tonic inhibitory conductance in mammalian hippocampal neurons.[107] Thus, a combination of peripheral and central effects likely mediate the clinical effects of this drug.

Gabapentin has been demonstrated to be effective in the treatment of neuropathic pain, diabetic neuropathy, postherpetic neuralgia, and reflex sympathetic dystrophy.[108] Gabapentin has been described as an anti-hyperalgesic drug that selectively affects the nociceptive process involving central sensitization.[108] In volunteers, oral gabapentin profoundly suppressed established cutaneous hyperalgesia after heat-capsaicin sensitization and was able to prevent the development of cutaneous sensitization.[109]

Over the past six years, there have been 20 clinical trials examining the effects of gabapentin on postoperative pain.[110, 111, 112, 113, 114, 115, 116, 117, 118, 119, 120, 121, 122, 123, 124, 125, 126, 127, 128, 129] All but two of these studies[114, 123] have found that gabapentin significantly reduces pain, as well as the amount of postoperative opioid required (16–67 percent).

Table 9.5 shows the six studies that were found to have examined designs assessing preemptive and preventive analgesic effects of perioperative gabapentin. The Jadad et al.[72] quality index scores of the six articles ranged from four to five with a mean $\pm$ S.D. of 4.3 ± 0.52. Of the six

Table 9.3 Variety and frequency of experimental designs used to evaluate the preemptive and/or preventive effects of different classes of analgesic agents.

Design number	Treatment combinations in Figure 9.1	Preemptive and/or preventive	Gabapentin	Local anesthetics	Opioids	NSAIDs	NMDA antagonists	Multimodal	Other	Total No. of studies
1	1, 2	PV	1	–	1	1	5	1	3	12
2	1, 2, 3	PE and PV	1	2	–	–	1	–	–	4
3	1, 2, 3, 5	PE and PV	–	1	–	–	–	–	–	1
4	1, 2, 4	PE and PV	–	–	–	3	1	–	1	5
5	1, 2, 5	PE and PV	–	–	–	–	1	–	–	1
6	1, 3, 3, 3	PE and PV	–	–	1	–	–	–	–	1
7	1, 3, 5	PE and PV	–	–	–	–	1	–	–	1
8	1, 4	PV	–	1	–	1	–	–	–	2
9	1, 4, 4	PV	–	1	–	–	–	–	–	1
10	1, 4, 6	PE and PV	–	–	–	1	–	–	–	1
11	1, 5	PV	–	1	–	–	3	–	–	4
12	1, 8	PV	2	2	–	2	1	1	–	8
13	1, 8, 8	PV	1	–	–	–	–	–	–	1
14	1, 8, 8, 8	PV	1	–	–	–	–	–	–	1
15	2, 2	PE	–	–	–	1	–	–	–	1
16	2, 3	PE	–	–	–	2	–	–	–	2
17	2, 4	PE	–	2	2	2	–	2	–	8
18	2, 4, 5	PE and PV	–	–	–	–	1	–	–	1
19	2, 4, 6	PE and PV	–	–	–	1	–	–	–	1
20	3, 4	PE	–	–	1	–	–	–	–	1
21	4, 4, 4	PV	–	–	–	–	–	1	–	1
22	4, 8	PE	–	2	–	–	–	–	–	2
23	8, 8	PE	–	1	–	–	–	–	–	1
Total			6	13	5	14	14	5	4	61

NSAIDs, nonsteroidal anti-inflammatory drugs; NMDA, *N*-methyl-ᴅ-aspartate; PE, preemptive; PV, preventive.
Each design (column 1) is defined in terms of specific treatment combinations (column 2) depicted in **Figure 9.1**. Each design is also described as evaluating preemptive and/or preventive effects (column 3).

Table 9.4 Summary of studies according to target agent administered showing total number of studies, number (%) with positive and negative preemptive and preventive effects.

Agent(s)	No. studies	Preemptive effects		Preventive effects		Opposite effects (%)	Total No. effects (%)
		Positive (%)	Negative (%)	Positive (%)	Negative (%)		
Gabapentin	6	0 (0)	1 (16.7)	4 (66.6)	1 (16.7)	0 (0)	6 (100)
Local anesthetics	13	3 (20)	3 (20)	6 (40)	1 (6.7)	2 (13.3)	15 (100)
Opioids	5	3 (60)	1 (20)	0 (0)	1 (20)	0 (0)	5 (100)
NSAIDs	14	7 (43.8)	3 (18.8)	4 (25)	2 (12.4)	0 (0)	16 (100)
NMDA antagonists	14	2 (11.8)	1 (5.9)	9 (53)	4 (23.4)	1 (5.9)	17 (100)
Multimodal	5	1 (16.7)	1 (16.7)	2 (33.3)	2 (33.3)	0 (0)	6 (100)
Other	4	1 (25)	0 (0)	3 (75)	0 (42.9)	0 (0)	4 (100)
Total[a]	61	17[b] (24.6)	10 (14.5)	28[c] (40.6)	11 (15.9)	3 (4.4)	69 (100)

Also shown is the number (%) of studies reporting effects opposite to that predicted and the total number of effects. The total number of effects exceeds the number of studies because some studies were designed to evaluate both preemptive and preventive effects. See text for definition of preemptive and preventive effects.
[a] $p = 0.02$ for *z*-test comparison of proportion of total positive preemptive plus preventive effects (0.64) versus proportion of total negative preemptive plus preventive effects (0.31).
[b] $p = 0.36$ for *z*-test comparison of proportion of total positive preemptive effects ($17/27 = 0.63$) versus proportion of total negative preemptive effects ($10/27 = 0.37$).
[c] $p = 0.03$ for *z*-test comparison of proportion of total positive preventive effects ($28/39 = 0.72$) versus proportion of total negative preventive effects ($11/39 = 0.28$).
NSAIDs, nonsteroidal anti-inflammatory drugs; NMDA, *N*-methyl-ᴅ-aspartate.

Table 9.5 Studies examining the preemptive and preventive effects of perioperative gabapentin.

Author	Surgical procedure (No. patients)	Treatment combinations (Figure 9.1)	Group: first intervention drug/ second intervention drug	Route and dose	Timing of first intervention	Timing of second intervention	Quality score	Nature and time after surgery of preventive and/or preemptive analgesic effects
Menigaux et al.[117]	Arthroscopic anterior cruciate ligament repair (40)	1, 2	GA plus: G1: GABA/na G2: PLA/na	p.o. 1200 mg	1–2 h preop	NA	4	[a]Preventive effect – yes VAS pain: no inter-group differences beyond t1/2 = 5.5 lives Cumulative i.v. PCA morphine consumption: G1 < G2 at 48 h [a]First/maximal and passive/active flexion on post-op day 2: G1 < G2
Fassoulaki et al.[114]	Abdominal hysterectomy (60)	1, 8	GA plus: G1: GABA/GABA G2: PLA/PLA	400 mg p.o.	18 h preoperation and every 6 h (3 doses) until surgery	Continues on same schedule until 5 days postoperatively	4	[a]Preventive effect – yes One month follow up: [a]Pain incidence: G1 < G2 Analgesic use: G1 = G2
Turan et al.[129]	Abdominal hysterectomy (100)	1, 8, 8	GA plus: G1: PLA/PLA G2: ROF+PLA/ ROF+ PLA G3: GABA+PLA/ GABA+PLA G4: ROF+GABA/ ROF+GABA	ROF p.o. 50 mg GABA p.o. 1.2 g	1 h preoperatively	9 a.m. on the first and second postoperative days	5	Preventive effect – no 3-month follow up No intergroup differences in pain incidence

(Continued over)

Study	Surgery (n)	Group	Groups	Drug/dose	Timing		Outcome[a]
Turan et al.[127]	Elective lower limb surgery (40)	1, 8	GA plus: G1: PLA/PLA G2: GABA/GABA	1.2 g p.o.	9 a.m. on the first and second postoperative days	5	Preventive effect – yes VRS-R pain: no inter-group differences beyond $t_5 = 5.5$ lives PCEA requirements: G2 < G1 at 48–72 h PARACET usage: G2 < G1
Pandey et al.[122]	Open donor nephrectomy (60)	1, 2, 3	GA plus: G1: GABA/PLA G2: PLA/GABA G3: PLA/PLA	GABA p.o. 600 mg GABA 600 mg NG	2 h preoperatively Immediately after surgical incision	4	Preventive effect – na Preemptive effect – no VAS-R: G1 = G2 < G3 at 0, 6, 12, 18, and 24 h Fentanyl use: G1 < G3 = G2
Fassoulaki et al.[113]	Breast cancer surgery (75)	1, 8, 8	GA plus: G1: MEXIL+PLA/ MEXIL+PLA G2: GABA+PLA/ GABA+PLA G3: PLA+PLA/PLA+ PLA	MEXIL p.o. 200 mg TID postoperatively GABA p.o. 400 mg TID postoperatively	One dosage the evening before the operation TID for 10 days postoperatively	4	Preventive effect – yes 3 month follow up chronic pain characteristics: Neuropathic/burning pain: G1 = G2 < G3 Analgesic use: no intergroup differences

[a] Nature and time after surgery of preventive analgesic effects.

G, group; GA, general anesthesia; GABA, gabapentin; i.v., intravenous; MEXIL, mexiletine; na, not applicable; NG, nasogastric; PARACET, paracetamol; PCEA, patient-controlled epidural analgesia; PLA, placebo; p.o., per os; ROF, rofecoxib; TID, three times daily; VAS-R/M, visual analog scale pain score at rest/on movement.

studies identified, only one fits the classification of a preemptive design.[122] The other five studies[113, 114, 117, 127, 129] provided data to assess the preventive effects of gabapentin beyond the 5.5 half-lives (40 hours) after the final administration of the drug. Four of the five studies (80 percent) demonstrated impressive preventive effects in favor of the gabapentin treated versus placebo control group. Perioperative gabapentin administration was associated with a significant decrease in postoperative opioid consumption,[117, 127][II] a reduction in the incidence of pain at the surgical incision site one month after surgery,[114][II] and a reduction in neuropathic pain three months after surgery.[113][II]

Only one study[122][II] evaluated the preemptive effects of gabapentin. Pandey and colleagues[122][II] compared preincisional versus immediate postincisional administration of gabapentin (600 mg) with a placebo control group (treatment combination 1 versus 2 versus 3 in **Figure 9.1**) in open donor nephrectomy patients. The results showed that patients in the pre- and postincision groups had significantly lower pain and used less fentanyl than those in the control group. The absence of a preemptive effect likely is due to the fact that the gabapentin was given too early after incision in the postincisional group.

The optimal dose of gabapentin for perioperative use has not been established, but a recent meta-analysis[130] and systematic review[131] suggest that doses between 600 and 1200 mg have robust opioid-sparing and pain-relieving effects in the acute postoperative period. The preventive effects of gabapentin are quite promising. For example, the study by Menigaux et al.[117] demonstrated the effectiveness of gabapentin in decreasing anxiety scores and improving early functional recovery after anterior cruciate ligament knee surgery. Patients treated with one preoperative dose of 1200 mg of gabapentin had significantly improved range of motion on active and passive knee flexion on postoperative day two in comparison to placebo-treated patients.

Although only six studies have examined the preemptive or preventive effects of gabapentin in the perioperative period, the perioperative pain-reducing and opioid-sparing effects of gabapentin beyond the acute perioperative period are quite promising; including the possibility that pain incidence may be reduced up to three months after surgery. Future studies are needed to clarify the optimal dosing and timing of gabapentin in the perioperative period.

Local anesthetics

Table 9.6 describes the 13 studies that were found to have examined designs assessing preemptive and preventive analgesic effects using local anesthetic agents. Surgical procedures included major gynecologic surgery by laparotomy,[57, 58, 132] major abdominal surgery,[133] thoracic surgery,[134] median sternotomy,[135] laparoscopic surgery,[136] laparoscopic cholecystecomy,[137] appendectomy,[138] total hip replacement,[61] total knee arthroplasty,[139] knee arthroscopy,[140, 141] and craniotomy.[142] Routes of administration included epidural[58, 61, 132, 134] intravenous (i.v.),[133, 135] subcutaneous (s.c.),[136, 137, 138, 142] intra-articular (i.a.),[140, 141] and a combination of intramuscular (i.m.), s.c., and i.a.[139]

Although only two[58, 134] of the 13 studies were designed to assess the effects of co-administration of a local anesthetic and an opioid, all but two studies[61, 139] administered opioids at induction of general anesthesia and/or during surgery, so that it is not possible to attribute effects solely to the target local anesthetic agent.

As shown in **Table 9.4**, of the 15 effects that were tested (in the 13 trials), 37.5 percent (3/8) showed significant preemptive effects, approximately 87 percent (6/7) showed significant preventive effects, and 25 percent (2/8) showed preemptive effects that were opposite in direction to the hypothesized effect, in that the postincisional group showed reduced pain compared with the preincisional group. Of note is the study by Katz et al.,[58][II] who found that short-term beneficial effects of preventive epidural analgesia (whether administered before or after incision) translated into less pain disability at three weeks but not six months after surgery.[57]

Opioid analgesics

The effect of preinjury treatment with opioids on preventing spinal postinjury hyperexcitability is well documented.[143] Early studies by Woolf and Wall[144] showed that the amount of morphine required to prevent the development of this spinal hyperexcitability was ten-fold less than the amount required to reverse it after it was well established. More recent animal studies have also shown that the application of mu-opiate receptor agonists preempt development of hyperalgesia and allodynia following inflammation, surgery, or nerve injury.[145, 146]

However, the efficacy of opioid pretreatment in decreasing central sensitization and thus reducing pain is somewhat more equivocal in human trials. Several studies have demonstrated that preoperative opioid administration reduces postoperative pain and consumption of analgesics when compared with postoperative administration[147] or a placebo control,[148] the latter effect occurring beyond the clinical duration of action of the target opioid. However, others have failed to demonstrate preemptive effects.[149] A growing body of evidence over the past ten years has also suggested that under certain conditions opioids may induce some forms of central sensitization and facilitate development of hyperalgesia.[150] Despite the mixed picture of opioids with respect to their hyperalgesic and analgesic actions, they continue to have a major role in perioperative pain management.

Table 9.7 shows the five studies that were found to have examined designs assessing preemptive and

Table 9.6 Studies examining the preemptive and preventive effects of local anesthetics ($\pm$ opioid) as the target treatment.

Author	Procedure (No. patients)	Treatment combinations (Figure 9.1)	Group: First intervention drug/second intervention drug	Route and dose	Timing of first intervention	Timing of second intervention	Quality score	Nature and time after surgery of preventive and/or preemptive analgesic effects
Katz et al.[58] and Katz and Cohen[57]	Major gynecologic surgery by laparotomy (141)	1, 2, 3	GA plus: G1: LID+FENT/ SAL G2: SAL/ LID+FENT G3: SAL/SAL	Epidural 12 mL LID 2 Epidural FENT 4 µg/kg	After placement of epidural catheter before incision	40 min post-incision	5	[a]Preventive effect – yes [b]Preemptive effect – yes VAS-R: No inter group differences, [a]VAS-M: G1<G3 at 24 h Hourly PCA Morphine: [b]G1<G2=G3 for day 1; [a,b]G1<G2<G3 for day 2 Von Frey pain threshold at 24 h: [a]G1>G3 at 24 h 3-week follow-up: Pain Disability Index: [a]G1=G2<G3 No differences analgesic use 6 month follow-up: No differences in pain incidence, intensity, disability or analgesic use
Neustein et al.[134]	Thoracic surgery (32)	4, 8	GA plus: G1: BUP+FENT/ BUP+FENT/ BUP+FENT G2: SAL/SAL/ BUP+FENT	Epidural 20 mg BUP and 100 µg FENT followed by an intra-operative infusion of BUP 0.1 and FENT 10 µg/mL at 6 mL per h reduced to 2 mL per h in PACU	After induction but pre-incision followed by intra op infusions	Postoperative infusion started in PACU (G1, G2)	3	[b]Preemptive effect – no VAS pain: G1<G2 at 0–6 h (exact time of effect not known) PCEA: no differences in median epidural infusion rate (Continued over)

Table 9.6 Studies examining the preemptive and preventive effects of local anesthetics (± opioid) as the target treatment (continued).

Author	Procedure (No. patients)	Treatment combinations (Figure 9.1)	Group: First intervention drug/ second intervention drug	Route and dose	Timing of first intervention	Timing of second intervention	Quality score	Nature and time after surgery of preventive and/or preemptive analgesic effects
Vendittoli et al.[139]	Total knee arthroplasty (42)	1, 8	Spinal BUP plus: G1: Nad/Nad/Nad G2: ROP/ROP/ROP	i.m. (deep tissues) 275 mg s.c. 125 mg i.a. 150 mg	i.m. before prosthesis implantation	s.c. before wound closure and i.a. on first day postoperation	4	[a]Preventive effect – yes [a]VAS pain at 2 days: G2<G1 Analgesic use: G2<G1 up to 48 h Active assisted knee flexion day 1–5: No inter group differences
Koppert et al.[133]	Major abdominal surgery (40)	1, 8	GA plus: G1: SAL/na G2: LID/na	i.v. LID bolus 1.5 mg/kg followed by i.v. LID infusion 1.5 mg/kg/h	Bolus after intubation; infusion started 30 min before surgical incision and maintained until 60 min post op	na	5	[a]Preventive effect – yes VRS-R: No differences post-op at any time VRS-MAUC: [a]G2<G1 24–48 h and 48–72 h PCA morphine: [a]G2<G1 at 36–48, 48–60 and 60–72 h Cumulative PCA morphine: G2<G1
Lohsiriwat et al.[138]	Appendectomy (123)	1, 5	GA plus: G1: SAL/na G2: BUP/na	s.c. 10 mL 0.5	5 min before incision and just after incision of skin and s.c. tissue	na	3	[a]Preventive effect – yes [a]VAS-M: G2<G1 at 48 h Total morphine consumption: G2<G1 at 48 h
Lam et al.[136]	Laparoscopy (144)	1, 2, 3	GA plus: G1: LID/SAL G2: SAL/LID G3: SAL/SAL	s.c. 10 mL 1 LID	Before incision	Before closure	5	[b]Preemptive effect – opposite [a]Preventive effect – yes Pain levels: [a]G2<G3 at 24 h [b]G2<G1 at 24 h No differences in analgesic consumption prior to discharge

(Continued over)

Study	Surgery (n)	Groups	Drug and dose	Timing (first)	Timing (second)	Quality	Outcome
Burmeister et al.[132]	Major gynecological surgery (30)	4, 8	GA plus: G1: PLA/ROP, G2: ROP/ROP	Epidural bolus 10 mL 0.375 followed by epidural infusion 6 mL/h	Bolus before induction; infusion until end of skin closure	At end of skin closure; continuously until 24 hours postoperatively	4	Preemptive effect – no
Nguyen et al.[142]	Craniotomy (30)	1, 4	GA plus: G1: na/ROP, G2: na/PLA	s.c. 20 mL 0.75	na	At skin closure	4	Preventive effects – no
Louizos et al.[137]	Laparoscopic cholecystectomy (108)	1, 2, 3, 5	GA plus: G1: SAL/SAL, G2: L-BUP/SAL, G3: SAL/L-BUP, G4: L-BUP/L-BUP	s.c. 20 mL 0.25 L-BUP, i.p. 20 mL 0.25 L-BUP	Before incision	Before skin closure	4	Preventive effect – na; bPreemptive effect – opposite; bIncidence of right shoulder pain: G3 < G2
Fagan et al.[141]	Knee arthroscopy (40)	2, 4	GA plus: G1: BUP+EPI/PLA, G2: PLA/BUP+EPI	i.a. 15 mL 0.5	15 min preoperation	After surgery	5	Preemptive effect – no
Tuncer et al.[140]	Arthroscopic knee surgery (40)	2, 4	i.v. sedation plus: G1: BUP/SAL, G2: SAL/BUP	i.a. BUP 20 mL 0.25	30 min before incision	Immediately after skin closure	3	bPreemptive effect – yes; bVAS-R/M: G1 < G2 at 1, 2, 4 and 6 h
Klasen et al.[61]	Total hip replacement (42)	8c, 8	i.v. sedation plus: G1: ROP/ROP, G2: SAL/ROP	Epidural: ROP 0.2 at 5 mL/h	Continuously starting 12 h preoperation up until arrival in OR	Pre-incision 1 ROP to achieve sensory blockade to T8 and throughout surgery	4	bPreemptive effect – yes; bVAS pain: No intergroup differences post-operation; bTotal PCEA ROP consumption at 48 h: G1 < G2
White et al.[135]	Median sternotomy (36)	1, 4, 4	GA plus: G1: na/PLA, G2: na/BUP 0.25, G3: na/BUP 0.5	i.v. infusion 4 mL/h	na	Continuously from end of surgery until 48 h post-operation	3	aPreventive effect – yes; aVAS Pain: G3 < G1 at 72 h; Mean i.v. PCA morphine usage: G3 < G1 at 72 h; aHospital stay: G3 < G1

AUC, area under the curve; FENT, fentanyl; G, group; GA, general anesthesia; i.a., intraarticular; i.p., intraperitoneal; i.v., intravenous; L-BUP, levo-bupivacaine; LID, lidocaine; na, not applicable; OR, operating room; PACU, postanesthetic care unit; PCEA, patient controlled epidural analgesia; PLA, placebo; ROP, ropivacaine; SAL, saline; s.c., subcutaneous.

aNature and time after surgery of preventive analgesic effects.

bNature and time after surgery of preemptive analgesic effects.

cThe classification of this study as evaluating preemptive analgesia is not entirely accurate. While it does evaluate the effect of altering the timing of administration, it does not do so before versus after incision.

Table 9.7 Studies examining the preemptive and preventive effects opioids as the target treatment.

Author	Procedure (No. of patients)	Treatment combinations (Figure 9.1)	Group: First intervention drug/ second intervention drug	Route and dose	Timing of first intervention	Timing of second intervention	Quality Score	Nature and time after surgery of preventive and/or preemptive analgesic effects
Reuben et al.[155]	Arthroscopic knee surgery (40)	2, 4	IV sedation plus IA BUP plus: G1: MORPH/Nad G2: Nad/MORPH	MORPH i.a. 3 mg	30 min preoperation	At end of surgery	3	Preemptive – yes VAS-R/M: G1 = G2 at 1, 2 and 24 h 24 h analgesic consumption: G1 < G2
McCarty et al.[153]	Anterior cruciate ligament reconstruction (62)	1, 2	GA plus post-operation femoral nerve block: G1: PLA/na G2: MORPH/na	5 mg i.a.	After induction but pre-incision	na	3	Preventive effect – no
Mavioglu et al.[152]	Total abdominal hysterectomy (64)	3, 4[a]	GA plus: G1: PETH/Nad G2: Nad/PETH	0.5 mg/kg i.v.+bolus doses of 10 mg	During closure of fascia	In PACU	4	Preemptive – yes VAS-R: G1 < G2 at 0, 15, 30, 60 and 120 min PETH use: G1 < G2 at 0–15, 15–30, 30–60 and 60–120 min (Continued over)

Study		Surgery (N)	Intervention groups (GA plus)	Drug	First/second intervention	Third intervention	Preventive/Preemptive effect
Munoz et al.[154]	1, 3, 3, 3[a]	Laparoscopic cholecystectomy (120)	G1: SAL/SAL/SAL G2: SAL/SAL/MORPH G3: SAL/MORPH/SAL G4: MORPH/SAL/SAL	MORPH i.v.150 µg/kg	First intervention: >40 min from end of surgery Second intervention: 20–40 min from end of surgery	Third intervention <20 min from end of surgery — 4	Preventive effect – na Preemptive effect – no
Akural et al.[151]	2, 4	Abdominal hysterectomy (41)	G1: SUFENT/SAL G2: SAL/SUFENT	Epidural 50 µg	20 min pre-anesthesia	20 min after closure of peritoneum — 3	Preemptive effect – yes NRS pain-R/M: no inter group differences postop to 1 month PCEA SUFENT consumption: G1<G2 at 8–16 h Touch detection threshold AUC for 4 days: G1<G2 Pain threshold AUC for 4 days: G1<G2

AUC, area under the curve; BUP, bupivacaine; G, group; GA, general anesthesia; i.a., inta-articular; i.v, intravenous; min, minutes; MORPH, morphine; na, not applicable; NRS pain – R/M, numeric rating scale for pain at rest/on movement; Nad, nothing administered; PACU, postanesthetic care unit; PCEA, patient controlled epidural analgesia; PETH, pethidine; PLA, placebo; SAL, saline; SUFENT, sufentanil; VAS-R/M, visual analog scale pain score at rest/movement.

[a]The classification of this study as evaluating preemptive analgesia is not entirely accurate. While it does evaluate the effect of altering the timing of administration, it does not do so before versus after incision.

preventive analgesic effects of opioids in the perioperative period.[151, 152, 153, 154, 155] The Jadad et al.[72] quality index scores of the five articles ranged from three to four with a mean ± S.D. of 3.4 ± 0.55. Routes of administration included were i.a. (morphine), i.v. (pethidine [meperidine], morphine) and epidural (sufentanil, treatment combination 2 versus 4 in **Figure 9.1**). The relatively few studies examining the preventive effects of opioids (i.e. five) was due to our exclusion of all trials involving neuraxial opioids since there is a lack of a consensus on half-life values of opioids delivered by the epidural and spinal routes.[68] The five trials included in **Table 9.7** studied the effects of opioids in the following four surgical populations: total abdominal hysterectomy,[151, 152] laparoscopic cholecystectomy,[154] anterior cruciate ligament repair,[153] and arthroscopic meniscectomy.[155]

Of the five studies, four used preemptive designs (three positive[151, 152, 155][II] and one negative[154]), while only one[153] met the criteria for a preventive trial. Reuben et al.[155][II] (treatment combination 2 versus 4 in **Figure 9.1**) demonstrated that preoperative i.a. injection of morphine was superior to postoperative injection in decreasing pain scores and morphine consumption following arthroscopic knee surgery. Akural et al.[151][II] (treatment combination 2 versus 4 in **Figure 9.1**) demonstrated that preoperative epidural sufentanil was superior to epidural sufentanil administration near the end of surgery. Postoperative pain was significantly lower in the pre- versus postincisional group for up to four days after surgery.[151][II] The only negative preemptive study[154] used a clinically nonrelevant design (treatment combination 1 versus 3 versus 3 versus 3 in **Figure 9.1**) and evaluated the effects on postoperative pain and analgesic consumption of i.v. morphine administered at three time points during laparoscopic cholecystectomy versus a saline control. The sole preventive study[153] we identified compared the effects of preincisional i.a. morphine compared to placebo in patients undergoing anterior cruciate ligament reconstruction. The authors did not find evidence of an effect of i.a. morphine on pain or analgesic consumption, but this not surprising since all patients received postoperative femoral nerve blocks with at least 20 mL of 0.5 percent bupivacaine. Thus, the only plausible conclusion is that i.a. morphine provides no additional benefit when combined with effective postoperative femoral nerve blocks.

Opioids continue to have a significant role in perioperative pain management despite significant adverse effects such as nausea, vomiting, sedation, pruritus, constipation, urinary retention, and respiratory depression.[156] The problem of accurately identifying the half-life of neuraxially administered opioids[68] essentially limited our review of these agents to studies using preemptive designs. Longer follow-up times after surgery (e.g. weeks or months) would obviate the problem of determining an accurate half-life of epidural and spinal opioids. More research is needed to clarify the role of opioids in preemptive/preventive analgesia.

NSAIDs

The analgesic effects of NSAIDs have been attributed to their anti-inflammatory actions in inhibiting the synthesis of prostaglandins.[157] Prostaglandin (PG) synthesis is essential for the generation of inflammatory pain and this depends not only on prostaglandin production at the site of inflammation, but also on the actions of prostaglandins synthesized within the central nervous system (CNS). Prostaglandins derive from arachidonic acid liberated from phospholipids in the cell membrane by the action of phospholipase A_2 (PLA_2) enzymes.[158] Cyclooxygenase (COX) catalyzes the first two reactions of the PG pathway. The identification of two COX isoforms, COX-1 and COX-2, led to intense efforts to characterize the relative contribution of each isoform to prostaglandin production in specific situations.[158]

Marked increases in PLA_2 and COX-2 expression occur at the site of peripheral inflammation. Prostaglandins themselves do not produce pain, but sensitize receptors at the site of injury to a variety of neurochemicals (e.g. bradykinin, serotonin, substance P, calcitonin gene-related peptide).[157] Recent evidence has also demonstrated that peripheral inflammation induces a widespread increase in COX-2 and prostaglandin synthase expression in neurons and nonneuronal cells in the spinal cord.[159] An elevation of COX-2 also occurs at many levels in the brain, mainly in the endothelial cells of the brain vasculature.

Samad et al.[158] proposed two signaling systems through which peripheral injury and its inflammatory sequelae are relayed to the CNS. The first is the traditional, electrically mediated transmission system, in which neural activity in sensitized nerve fibers innervating inflamed tissue signals the location of injury, as well as the onset, duration, and nature of any stimuli applied to this tissue. The second is a nonneuronally mediated system in which a humoral signaling molecule (or molecules), originating in inflamed tissue, acts via the bloodstream to produce a widespread induction of COX-2 in the CNS. Following peripheral injury, there is an immediate (within minutes) and delayed (within hours) spinal release of PGE_2, the former produced by COX-1 and/or COX-2, and the latter by COX-2.[157, 160] This suggests that acute postoperative pain may not be as sensitive to COX-2 inhibitors as the pain experienced some time later.[158] The net effect of both the peripheral and central actions of NSAIDs would be to prevent or attenuate development of a hyperexcitable state in spinal cord dorsal horn neurons. In terms of the patient's experience of pain after surgery, this would translate into less intense pain and a reduced requirement for postoperative analgesics. Based on data from basic science and clinical research, NSAIDs may preempt different components of postoperative pain (e.g. central and peripheral sensitization) by more than one mechanism, and prolonged blockade of inflammation by NSAIDs throughout the perioperative period and beyond has demonstrated a decrease in the development of chronic pain.

Table 9.8 shows the 14 studies that were found to have examined the preemptive and preventive effects of NSAID administration in the perioperative period. The Jadad *et al.*[72] quality index scores of the 14 articles ranged from two to five with a mean ± S.D. of 3.8 ± 0.89. Routes of administration include oral, rectal, and i.v. A variety of NSAIDs were used which differ in the extent of their anti-inflammatory activity, analgesic effects, antipyretic actions, and pharmacokinetics.

Of the 14 studies identified, ten fit the classification of a preemptive design.[60, 161, 162, 163, 164, 166, 168, 169, 170, 172] Two of the 14 studies also examined effects beyond 5.5 half-lives of the target drug, one demonstrating a positive,[170][II] and the other, a negative[169] preventive effect. The other four studies used designs that assessed the preventive effects of NSAID interventions.[165, 167, 171, 173]

Of the six studies that reported preventive effects, four (66.7 percent) reported positive findings, and of these, both Buvanendran *et al.*[167][II] and Rueben *et al.*[161][II] demonstrated significant long-term benefits at one month and one year after surgery, respectively. Buvanendran *et al.*[167] found that a two-week perioperative regimen of rofecoxib in total knee arthroplasty patients improved range of motion in comparison to controls at a one month follow up. Reuben *et al.*[161][II] administered celecoxib or placebo, to patients scheduled for spinal fusion, for five days beginning one hour before surgery. The incidence of chronic donor-site pain was significantly lower in the celecoxib group (four of 40 patients, or 10 percent) compared with the placebo group (12 of 40 patients, or 30 percent) at one year after surgery. Celecoxib-treated patients had a 74 percent lower risk for developing chronic pain than the placebo-treated patients at one year.

COX-2 selective inhibitors were originally marketed as safer alternatives to nonselective nonsteroidal anti-inflammatory drugs. Recent studies demonstrating a link to long-term use and cardiac and renal morbidity[174, 175] have culminated in the withdrawal of rofecoxib and valdecoxib from the marketplace. Although the evidence suggests a fairly consistent cardiovascular risk rate with rofecoxib, the evidence for cardiovascular risk with celecoxib is equivocal.[176] It is important to note that the long-term cardiovascular risk associated with COX-2 inhibitors, which resulted in the withdrawal of rofecoxib, was demonstrated in patients taking the medication for more than two years. The analgesic and opioid-sparing effects associated with COX-2 inhibition were demonstrated with short-term use (eight days at most).[161, 165, 167]

In summary, the results of the present review suggest that perioperative NSAID use is associated with clinically significant preemptive and preventive effects with a success rate approaching 70 percent. Long-term benefits at one month and one year after surgery were associated with COX-2-selective NSAID (rofecoxib/celecoxib) administration. Given their long half-life (**Table 9.1**), the anti-inflammatory properties of these agents continued to

be active for some time after surgery, even when administered as a single preoperative dose.[161] This may contribute to a longstanding block of the inflammatory response and a reduction in peripheral sensitization. Prolonged central effects of NSAIDs may also contribute to the prevention of central sensitization significantly attenuating the development of hyperexcitability in spinal cord dorsal horn neurons. Further research is required to confirm and extend the initial promising short- and long-term benefits of preventive COX-2 inhibition.

NMDA receptor antagonists

A variety of agents that have an antagonistic action at the NMDA receptor are clinically available, including amantadine, dextromethorphan, ketamine, ketobemidone, memantine, and methadone. At the present time, preventive or preemptive analgesic effects have been investigated using ketamine or dextromethorphan, but not the other NMDA antagonists. Although ketamine hydrochloride[177] and dextromethorphan[178] act on a variety of receptor systems, their NMDA channel-blocking properties quickly became the focus of intense research once this receptor–ion channel complex was discovered to play a critical role in the induction and maintenance of central sensitization and pathological pain.[179, 180] The mechanism proposed to underlie the reduced opioid consumption and pain in studies of preemptive analgesia is the prevention (or reversal) of NMDA-mediated sensitization of spinal cord dorsal horn neurons.[4, 51] The NMDA channel blockers dextromethorphan and ketamine are of particular interest, therefore, in testing the hypothesis that perioperative administration will lead to reduced pain and analgesic consumption using preventive and preemptive designs.

Table 9.9 shows the 14 studies that were found to have examined designs assessing preemptive and preventive analgesic effects of ketamine ($n = 10$) or dextromethorphan ($n = 4$). The Jadad *et al.*[72] quality index scores of the 14 articles ranged from three to four with a mean ± S.D. of 4.4 ± 0.64. The most frequent designs have compared preoperative administration of dextromethorphan or ketamine with a placebo or an active agent (i.e. evaluation of preventive effects). The next most commonly used designs compare preoperative administration of dextromethorphan or ketamine with the same agent administered either intraoperatively, postoperatively, or both preoperatively and postoperatively (**Table 9.3**).

KETAMINE

The preemptive and preventive use of ketamine has been studied on a variety of surgical procedures including lower abdominal surgery,[193] total knee arthroplasty,[182, 187] gynecological laparotomy[183] and laparoscopy,[184] gastrectomy,[185] major ear, nose, and throat surgery,[186] tonsillectomy,[194]

Table 9.8 Studies examining the preemptive and preventive effects of NSAIDs.

Author	Procedure (No. of patients)	Treatment combinations (Figure 9.1)	Group: first intervention drug/ second intervention drug	Route and dose	Timing of first intervention	Timing of second intervention	Quality Score	Nature and time after surgery of preventive and/or preemptive analgesic effects
Reuben et al.[161]	Arthroscopic knee surgery (60)	1, 2, 4	Sedation i.v. plus IA BUP plus: G1: ROF/PLA G2: PLA/ROF G3: PLA/PLA	50 mg p.o.	1 h preoperation	15 min after surgery	4	Preventive effect – na Preemptive effect – yes Verbal Analogue Pain at rest: G1=G2<G3 at 2+24 h Verbal Analogue Pain at movement: G1<G2<G3 at 1, 2+24 h 24 h consumption of PARACET/OXYCOD: G1<G2=G3
Kokki and Salonen[162]	Pediatric tonsillectomy (109)	1, 4, 6	GA plus: G1: KETOP /SAL/ KETOP G2: SAL/KETOP/ KETOP G3: SAL/SAL/SAL	Bolus i.v. 0.5 mg/kg Infusion i.v. 3 mg/kg/h	Bolus 5 min after induction but before surgery	PACU bolus followed by 24 h infusion	4	Preventive effect – na Preemptive effect – no
Gramke et al.[163]	Laparoscopic bilateral inguinal hernia repair (52)	2, 4	GA plus: G1: PIROXI/PLA G2: PLA/PIROXI	Sublingual 40 mg	2 h preoperation	10 min postoperation	3	Preemptive effect – yes VAS-R: G1<G2 at 6 and 20 h Cumulative i.v. PCA tramadol:
Norman et al.[164]	Ankle fracture surgery (48)	2, 3	GA plus: G1: KETOR/PLA G2: PLA/KETOR	30 mg i.v.	After induction, while the leg was being prepared	Immediately after tourniquet inflation (<15 min after intervention 1)	5	Preemptive effect – yes VAS-R: G1<G2 at 2 and 4 h PCA morphine: No inter group differences *(Continued over)*

Study		Surgery (n)	Intervention	Dose	Timing 1	Timing 2		Outcomes
Reuben et al.[165]	1, 8	Spinal fusion (80)	GA plus infiltration of proposed incision sites with BUP plus: G1: CELECOX/CELECOX G2: PLA/PLA	400 mg preoperation p.o., 200 BID postoperation	1 h preoperation	Every 12 h postoperation until 5th day	3	Preventive effect – yes One year follow up: Chronic donor site pain: G1<G2 G1 patients had a 74 lower risk for chronic pain than G2
Boccara et al.[166]	2, 4	Laparoscopic cholecystectomy (104)	GA plus: G1: KETOP/PLA G2: PLA/KETOP G3: PARACET/PLA G4: PLA/PARACET	KETOP 100 mg i.v. PARACET 2 g i.v.	Before induction	After surgery	4	Preventive effect – na Preemptive effect – yes VAS Pain: G1<G2=G3=G4 at 0, 1, 2, 3, 10 and 12 h No of pain-free patients during 24 h: G1<G2=G3=G4 No. of patients with severe pain (VAS ≥50): G1<G2=G3 Cumulative nalbuphine consumption at 24 h: G1=G2
Buvanendran et al.[167]	1, 8	Total knee arthroplasty (70)	Sedation (i.v.) plus spinal BUP preop plus epidural post-op plus: G1: ROF/ROF G2: PLA/PLA	50 mg per day p.o.	24 h and 1–2 h preoperation	Once daily for 5 days then 25 mg/day for 8 more days	5	Preventive effect – yes One-month follow-up: Range of motion of affected knee: G1>G2

(Continued over)

Table 9.8 Studies examining the preemptive and preventive effects of NSAIDs (continued).

Author	Procedure (No. of patients)	Treatment combinations (Figure 9.1)	Group: first intervention drug/ second intervention drug	Route and dose	Timing of first intervention	Timing of second intervention	Quality Score	Nature and time after surgery of preventive and/or preemptive analgesic effects
Priya et al.[168]	Breast surgery (50)	2, 3	GA plus: G1: KETOP/SAL G2: SAL/KETOP	100 mg i.v.	30 min before incision	Immediately after incision	4	Preemptive effect – yes VAS pain: G1<G2 at all time points until 10 h No. of patients requiring rescue analgesia: G1<G2 at 2, 4, 6, 8 and 10 h
Norris et al.[169]	Ambulatory knee arthroscopy (127)	2, 6, 4	GA plus: G1: DICLOF/PLA G2: DICLOF/ DICLOF G3: PLA/DICLOF	50 mg p.o.	1 h preoperation	30 min postoperation	4	Preventive effect – no Preemptive effect – no Functional Score: No differences at 0, 1, 2 and 3 days VAS pain: No differences at 1, 2 and 3 days
Nakayama et al.[170]	Abdominal hysterectomy (45)	1, 2, 4	GA plus epidural BUP post-op plus: G1: SAL/SAL G2: FLURBIP/SAL G3: SAL/FLURBIP	1 mg/kg i.v.	30 min preoperation	At end of surgery	3	Preventive effect – yes Preemptive effect – yes VAS-R: G2<G1=G3 at 15 and 24 h VAS-C: G2<G1=G3 at 24, 48 and 72 h N of diclofenac in 24 h: G2=G3<G1
Bugter et al.[171]	Total hip surgery (50)	1, 2	Sedation (i.v.) plus spinal anesthesia plus: G1: IBU/na G2: PLA/na	600 mg p.o.	TID for 2 weeks until surgery	na	2	Preventive effect – no

(Continued over)

Study	Surgery (n)		Intervention	Dose	After induction but preincision	In the PACU / After	n	Results
Salonen et al.[172]	Tonsillectomy (106)	1, 2, 4	GA plus postoperative KETOP infusion 3 mg/kg for 24 h plus: G1: KETOP/SAL G2: SAL/KETOP G3: SAL/SAL	0.5 mg/kg i.v. bolus	After induction but preincision	In the PACU	5	Preventive effect – na Preemptive effect – no
Lim et al.[173]	Cesarean section (48)	1, 4	Spinal anesthesia plus: G1: na/DICLOF G2: na/na	100 mg p.r.	na	After Cesarean section	3	Preventive effect – yes VAS-M: no inter group differences post-operation PCEA consumption: G1<G2 at 12–18 h Total PCEA consumption: G1<G2 at 24 h
O'Hanlon et al.[60]	Ambulatory breast biopsy (73)	2, 2[a]	GA plus wound infiltration with BUP at end of procedure plus: G1: TENOX/Nad G2: NadTENOX	20 mg i.v.	30 min preoperation	At induction of anesthesia	4	Preemptive effect – yes VAS pain: G1<G2 at 30, 60, 120 and 240 min No. of patients requiring additional analgesia: G1<G2 Demerol and DICLOF usage for first 4 h: G1<G2

BID, twice daily; BUP, bupivacaine; CELECOX, celecoxib; DICLOF, diclofenac; G, group; GA, general anesthesia; IA, intaarticular; IBU, ibuprofen; IV, intravenous; KETOP, ketoprofen; KETOR, ketorolac; min, minutes; na, not applicable; Nad, nothing administered; OXYCOD, oxycodone; PACU, postanesthetic care unit; PARACET, paracetamol (acetaminophen); PCA, patient controlled analgesia; PCEA, patient controlled epidural analgesia; PIROXI, piroxicam; PLA, placebo; p.o., per os; p.r., per rectum; ROF, rofecoxib; SAL, saline; TENOX, tenoxicam; TID, three times daily; VAS-C, visual analog scale pain score when coughing; VAS-R/M, visual analog scale pain score at rest/movement.

[a]The classification of this study as evaluating preemptive analgesia is not entirely accurate. While it does evaluate the effect of altering the timing of administration, it does not do so before versus after incision.

Table 9.9 Studies examining the preemptive and preventive effects of the NMDA receptor antagonists ketamine and dextromethorphan.

Author	Procedure (No. of patients)	Treatment Combinations (Figure 9.1)	Group: First intervention drug/ second intervention drug	Route and dose	Timing of first intervention	Timing of second intervention	Quality score	Nature and time after surgery of preventive and/or preemptive analgesic effects
Helmy and Bali[181]	Upper-abdominal surgery (60)	1, 2, 3	GA plus: G1: DEXTRO/SAL G2: SAL/DEXTRO G3: SAL/SAL	120 mg i.m.	30 min before incision	30 min before end of surgery	4	Preventive effect – na Preemptive – yes VAS-R/M: G1 < G2 = G3 at 6 h Total i.v. PCA pethidine (meperidine) consumption: G1 < G2 = G3
Himmelseher et al.[182]	Total knee arthroplasty (37)	1, 2	Lumbar epidural ROP plus: G1: SAL/na G2: KETAM/na	Epidural 0.25 mg/kg	10 min before incision	na	5	Preventive effect – yes VAS-R/M: G2 < G1 at 24 and 48 h Cumulative PCEA ROP:
Bilgin et al.[183]	Gynecologic laparotomy surgery (45)	2, 4, 5	GA plus: G1: KETAM/SAL/ SAL G2: KETAM/KETAM /SAL G3: SAL/SAL/ KETAM	Bolus i.v. 0.5 mg/kg Infusion i.v. 600 µg/kg/ h (G2)	Before induction of anesthesia followed by infusion	Third intervention after wound closure (G3)	4	Preventive effect – yes Preemptive effect – opposite VAS-R: G2 = G3 < G1 at 0–24 h VAS-C: G2 = G3 < G1 at 24 h i.v. PCA morphine: G1 = G2 = G3 at 0–24 h
Kwok et al.[184]	Gynecologic laparoscopic surgery (135)	1, 2, 4	GA plus: G1: KETAM/SAL G2: SAL/KETAM G3: SAL/SAL	0.15 mg/kg i.v.	Immediately before induction of anesthesia	After wound closure	5	Preventive effect – no Preemptive effect – yes VAS pain: G1 < G2 = G3 at 0 to 6 h Cumulative i.m. morphine: G1 < G2 = G3

(Continued over)

Study		Groups	Dose	Timing		Score	Outcomes
Xie et al.[185]	1, 2	Gastrectomy (45)	GA plus PCEA post op plus: G1: KETAM/na G2: KETAM/na G3: SAL/na	G1: 0.5 mg/kg i.v. G2: Epidural 0.5 mg/kg	15 min before incision	na	4	Preventive effect – yes VAS-R: G1 <G3 at 24 h G2 <G3 at 24, 36 and 48 h G2 <G1 at 24, 36 and 48 h Cumulative PCEA morphine at 48 h: G2 <G1 <G3
Ganne et al.[186]	1, 5	Major ear, nose, and throat surgery (62)	GA plus: G1: KETAM/na G2: SAL/na	Bolus i.v. 0.15 mg/kg followed by i.v. infusion 2 µg/kg	Bolus just before induction followed by continuous infusion during anesthesia	na	5	Preventive effect – no
Adam et al.[187]	1, 8	Total knee arthroplasty (40)	GA plus: G1: KETAM/KETAM/ KETAM G2: SAL/SAL/SAL	Bolus i.v. 0.05 mL/kg followed by intraoperation Infusion i.v. 3 µg/kg/ min then reduced to 1.5 µg/kg/min for 48 h	Just after induction of anesthesia Maintained at second level from initial bolus until emergence from anesthesia, then reduced until 48 h postoperation	5	Preventive effect – yes Maximal active knee flexion at days 6 and 7: G1 >G2 Maximal active knee flexion at 6 weeks and 3 months: G1 = G2
Katz et al.[188]	1, 3, 5	Radical prostatectomy (143)	GA plus: G1: KETAM/SAL G2: SAL/KETAM G3: SAL/SAL	Bolus i.v. 0.2 mg/kg followed by i.v. infusion 0.0025 mg/kg/min	Bolus 10 min before incision followed by infusion for 70 min intraoperation Bolus 70 min after incision followed by infusion until the end of surgery	5	Preventive effect – no Preemptive effect – no VAS-R/M: no inter group differences at any time Von Frey thresholds: no inter group differences at any time Cumulative i.v. PCA morphine consumption at 72 h: G1 = G2 = G3 (but G1 vs G2 and G1 vs G3; p = 0.08) (Continued over)

Table 9.9 Studies examining the preemptive and preventive effects of the NMDA receptor antagonists ketamine and dextromethorphan (continued).

Author	Procedure (No. of patients)	Treatment Combinations (Figure 9.1)	Group: First intervention drug/ second intervention drug	Route and dose	Timing of first intervention	Timing of second intervention	Quality score	Nature and time after surgery of preventive and/or preemptive analgesic effects
								Hourly PCA consumption: G1 < G2 = G3 from 48 h to 72 h 2 week follow-up: VAS- R: G1 = G2 = G3
Ozyalcin et al.[189]	Thoracotomy (60)	1, 2	GA plus: G1: KETAM+SAL/ na G2: SAL+KETAM/ na G3: SAL+SAL/na	(G1) 1 mg/kg i.m. Epidural (G2) 1 mg/kg	15 min preoperation	na	5	Preventive effect – yes At 48 h: pinprick hyperalgesia: G2 < G1 = G3 Pressure hyperalgesia: G1 = G2 < G3 Brush allodynia: G2 < G1 < G3 Cumulative PCEA morphine at 48 h: G2 < G1 < G3 Cumulative PCEA morphine BUP: G2 < G1 = G3 15 day follow up Brush allodynia: G2 < G1 < G3 Pinprick hyperalgesia: G2 < G1 = G3 Pressure hyperalgesia: G2 < G3 30 day follow-up Brush allodynia: G2 < G1 < G3 (Continued over)

Study	Surgery (n)		Groups	Drug/dose	Timing	Duration		Results
Yeh et al.[190]	Colonic surgery (90)	1, 5	GA plus thoracic epidural plus: G1: PLA/SAL; G2: PLA/LID; G3: DEXTRO/LID	DEXTRO i.m. 20 mg; Epidural 2 LID (8-10 mL/h)	30 min preincision	Intraoperatively until end of surgery	3	Pin-prick hyperalgesia: G2<G1<G3; Pressure hyperalgesia No intergroup differences; Preventive effect – yes; VAS-C: G1=G2>G3 at 24h; Cum PCEA volume at 48h and 72h: G1>G2>G3
Wu et al.[191]	Laparoscopic cholecystectomy (100)	1, 2, 5	GA plus: G1: PLA+PLA/na; G2: DEXTRO+PLA/na; G3: PLA+LID/na	DEXTRO i.m. 40 mg; LID i.v. 3 mg/kg/h until end of surgery	30 min preincision	na	4	Preventive effect – yes; VAS-C: G4<G2<G1=G3 at24h; Cumulative i.m. pethidine at 48 h: G4<G3=G2<G1
Weinbroum et al.[192]	Lower body surgery (60)	1, 2	Epidural LID plus: G1: PLA/na; G2: DEXTRO/na; G3: DEXTRO/na	DEXTRO p.o. 60 mg (G2); DEXTRO p.o. 90 mg (G3)	90 min preoperation	na	4	Preventive effect – yes; 3-day follow-up VAS Pain: G2=G3<G1; Analgesic use: G2=G3<G1
Kafali et al.[193]	Lower abdominal surgery (60)	1, 2	GA plus: G1: SAL/na; G2: KETAM/na	150 µg/kg i.v.	Before incision	na	4	Preventive effect – yes; VAS pain: G2<G1 at 48 h; Cumulative i.v. PCA Morphine to 48 h: G2<G1; i.v. PCA morphine: G2<G1 at 24–48 h
Van Elstraete et al.[194]	Tonsillectomy (40)	1, 5	GA plus: G1: KETAM/KETAM; G2: SAL/SAL	0.5 mg/kg i.v. bolus followed by i.v. infusion 2 µg/kg/min	At induction of anesthesia before incision	Infusion continued until end of surgery	5	Preventive effect – no

BUP, bupivacaine; DEXTRO, dextromethorphan; G, group; GA, general anesthesia; i.m., intramuscular; i.v., intravenous; KETAM, ketamine; LID, lidocaine; Na, not applicable; PCA, patient controlled analgesia; PCEA, patient controlled epidural analgesia; PLA, placebo; ROP, ropivacaine; SAL, saline; VAS-C, visual analog scale pain score when coughing; VAS-R/M, visual analog scale pain score at rest/movement.

radical prostatectomy,[188] and thoracotomy.[189] There is usually no rationale given for the patient population studied, in spite of the fact that important differences clearly exist among the various surgical procedures that may have a bearing on the outcome of the results (e.g. duration of procedure relative to that of the target agent, extent (deep versus superficial) and nature (nerve, muscle, viscera) of tissue damage and inflammation).

Ketamine has been administered by via the i.m.,[189] i.v.,[183, 184, 185, 186, 187, 188, 193, 194] and epidural[182, 185, 189] routes. Two studies compared the route of administration, including 1.0 mg/kg ketamine i.m. or epidurally[189] and 0.5 mg/kg ketamine i.v. or epidurally.[185] In both studies,[185, 189][II] preventive effects were observed for epidural ketamine compared with the other route.

Intravenous ketamine has been administered as a single bolus dose,[184, 185, 193] or as a bolus dose followed by a continuous infusion[183, 186, 187, 188, 194] for the duration of the surgical procedure. Intravenous bolus doses of ketamine have ranged from 0.15 to 0.5 mg/kg with infusions ranging from 2–10 µg/kg/minute.

The three studies of epidural ketamine[182, 185, 189][II] administered a single, preoperative bolus dose (0.25–1.0 mg/kg) without infusion. All three showed significant preventive effects; 48 hours after surgery, pain intensity and postoperative analgesic consumption were significantly lower in the ketamine-treated patients compared with the placebo control condition.[182, 185, 189][II] In one study,[189][II] patients were followed up 15 and 30 days after surgery. At both follow-up assessments, brush-evoked allodynia and pin-prick hyperalgesia were still significantly less pronounced in the epidural ketamine group compared with the i.m. ketamine and saline control groups. The pattern of intergroup differences for pressure hyperalgesia at the wound was the same for the 15-day follow up, but the differences were no longer significant 30 days after surgery.

The surgical procedures were performed under general anesthesia in all but one of the studies, the exception being a positive preventive study of patients undergoing total knee arthroplasty with epidural ropivacaine.[182][II]

Of the ten studies evaluating ketamine, significant preventive effects were observed in seven studies.[182, 183, 184, 185, 187, 189, 193][II] One study[183] showed a preemptive effect that was opposite to what had been predicted in that the group receiving i.v. ketamine after wound closure reported significantly lower pain scores at rest and after coughing up to 24 hours after surgery compared with the preincisional group. As noted above, these results may point to the relative greater efficacy in reducing central sensitization of postsurgical i.v. ketamine versus preoperative blockade.

DEXTROMETHORPHAN

Surgical procedures for the four studies using dextromethorphan include upper abdominal surgery,[181] colonic surgery,[190] laparoscopic cholecystectomy,[191] and lower body surgery.[192] For all studies, dextromethorphan was administered by the i.m. route as a single bolus dose ranging between 20 and 120 mg, either before surgery,[89, 190, 191] or before versus during surgery.[181] Intramuscular dextromethorphan resulted in a preventive effect in three[89, 190, 191][II] of the four studies; pain intensity was significantly lower between 24 hours[190, 191][II] and three days[89][II] after a single bolus dose of i.m. dextromethorphan. The one study[181] that did not find a preventive effect did, however, show a short-term preemptive effect in that total patient-controlled analgesia (PCA) opioid consumption, as well as pain at rest and after movement six hours after surgery, were significantly lower in the group that received dextromethorphan 30 minutes before surgery versus 30 minutes before the end of surgery.

Taken together, the results of the studies that have examined administration of ketamine or dextromethorphan have proved quite successful in that approximately 65 percent (11/17) of the effects reported supported the efficacy of preemptive or preventive analgesia. As shown in **Table 9.3**, almost 69 percent (9/13) of the effects evaluating only preventive analgesia show that preoperative ketamine or dextromethorphan administration results in significantly lower pain intensity and/or reduced analgesic requirements after the duration of action of the NMDA antagonists have worn off (i.e. after more than 5.5 half-lives). These results are very similar to those reported by McCartney et al.[67][I] in a recent qualitative review of the preventive analgesia literature from 1966 to 2003. They found that among the clinically available NMDA receptor antagonists, dextromethorphan (67 percent (8/12) of studies) and ketamine (58 percent (14/24) of studies) showed the greatest number of significant preemptive or preventive effects. Their data show that 16 of the 30 studies (53 percent) evaluating preventive analgesia only (i.e. excluding preemptive analgesia) showed evidence of a reduction in pain, analgesic consumption, or both beyond the clinical duration of action of the drug concerned. The similarity in outcome between the present review and that of McCartney et al.[67][I] is unlikely to be due to the two-year (2001–2003) overlap in the literature reported since, of the 36[67][I] and 24 (present review) studies covered, only three[181, 182, 192] were common to both reviews.

The preponderance of positive studies of ketamine and dextromethorphan may be due not only to the ability of these agents to block the neural processes underlying central sensitization,[177] but in a related vein, to their ability to attenuate the development of acute opioid tolerance[7, 195] and reverse opioid-induced facilitation of nociceptive processing.[196, 197] Since opioids were administered (as premedication or during surgery) in all but three[89, 182, 183] of the studies, preoperative administration of ketamine or dextromethorphan may also have prevented acute opioid tolerance, opioid-facilitated activation of NMDA processes, and opioid-induced hyperalgesia relative to the control group leading to a reduction in postoperative opioid requirements and postoperative pain intensity in the preoperatively treated groups.

Multimodal analgesic therapy

The rationale for a preoperative multimodal approach to postoperative pain management is to capitalize on the combined actions of a variety of classes of analgesic and anesthetic agents at different receptor sites in reducing peripheral and central sensitization.[198, 199] For the purpose of the present review, we have defined a multimodal regimen as involving administration of three or more agents in combination. Expectations of the therapeutic benefits associated with multimodal regimens include improved efficacy, lower doses, and fewer adverse effects.[200]

Table 9.10 describes the five studies[115, 201, 202, 203, 204] that evaluated the effects of multimodal, combination therapy on pain and analgesic consumption using preemptive or preventive designs. The Jadad et al.[72] quality index scores of the five articles ranged from two to five with a mean ± S.D. of 4.2 ± 1.3. Surgical procedures include breast cancer surgery,[115] arthroscopic knee surgery,[201, 203] nephrectomy,[202] and tonsillectomy.[204] Of the five studies, two[201, 202] evaluated preemptive effects using the classic design (treatment combination 2 versus 4 in **Figure 9.1**) and one[201][II] showed significant effects in favor of the preoperative treatment. Two[115, 204][II] of the remaining three studies[115, 203, 204] that evaluated preventive effects found significant benefits that long outlasted the clinical duration of action of the target agents. In a triple-dummy, placebo-controlled study by Fassoulaki et al.,[115] [II] patients undergoing breast cancer surgery received placebo or preoperative gabapentin and transdermal eutectic mixture of local anesthetics (EMLA) followed by intraoperative ropivacaine irrigation of the brachial plexus and several intercostal spaces. After surgery, patients continued to receive placebo or gabapentin every six hours for eight days in addition to transdermal EMLA daily for three days. Three months (but not six months) after surgery, patients in the multimodal treatment group had a lower incident of axilla pain, arm pain, chronic pain, and analgesic use compared with the placebo control patients. Naja et al.[204][II] compared the effects of no treatment with a preincisional tonsillar infiltration of a placebo solution or a solution containing lidocaine with epinephrine, bupivacaine, fentanyl, and clonidine in 90 pediatric patients undergoing tonsillectomy. Pain at rest, on jaw opening, and when eating soft foods were all significantly lower in the combination pharmacotherapy group for up to at least one week after tonsillectomy. These studies provide some of the strongest and most promising evidence of the therapeutic benefits of a (prolonged[115][II]) multimodal analgesic regimen.[204][II]

The study by Rosaeg et al.,[201] which compared a combination of local anesthesia, morphine, epinephrine, and ketorolac (treatment combination 2 versus 4 in **Figure 9.1**), was designed to look at long-term outcomes as well (i.e. preventive effects). The authors found that administration of their three-component analgesic drug combination resulted in lower pain scores in patients that received the intervention before versus after surgery. Pain scores and i.v. PCA morphine consumption were significantly lower during the initial stay in the postanesthesia care unit (PACU) (i.e. a positive preemptive effect). However, pain scores did not differ significantly between the groups on postoperative days one, three, and seven; thus there was no measurable long-term advantage associated with preemptive multimodal drug administration in arthroscopic knee surgery (i.e. a negative preventive effect).[201]

At first glance, the results describing the multimodal studies shown in **Table 9.10** seem equivocal. However, it is important to note the two studies[201, 203] that reported negative preventive effects and the one negative preemptive study[202] both lacked a placebo control group. Thus, the conclusion that these multimodal interventions do not exert a clinically relevant benefit may be incorrect. Until similar studies are conducted with the appropriate control condition(s), these conclusions are premature.

Other nonanalgesic agents

Table 9.11 describes the four studies that examined the preemptive and/or preventive analgesic effects of other, traditionally, nonanalgesic agents, including venlafaxine[63] [II] (a serotonin and norepinephrine reuptake inhibitor (SNRI)), promethazine[205][II] (a histamine$_1$ (H$_1$) receptor antagonist), nitroglycerine,[206][II] and dexmedetomidine[207] [II] (an alpha-2 agonist). All evaluated preventive effects with the exception of the study by Chia et al.,[205][II] in which both preemptive and preventive effects were examined (treatment combination 1 versus 2 versus 4 in **Figure 9.1**). Thus, of the five effects examined, there were three positive preventive effects,[63, 206, 207][II] one negative preventive effect[205] and one positive preemptive effect.[205][II]

The most interesting and promising of these studies, conducted by Reuben et al.[63][II] and depicted in **Figure 9.8**, involved administration of venlafaxine 75 mg or placebo capsules to women (n = 50 per group) the night before surgery and daily for two weeks after radical mastectomy. Six month follow-up assessment revealed that pain on movement, as well as the incidence of chest wall pain, arm pain, axilla pain, chronic pain, and analgesic use were all significantly lower in the venlafaxine group. Consistent with the results of a rat study,[208] the authors suggest that the lower incidence of chronic neuropathic pain six months after surgery may have been result of an SNRI-induced reduction of activity in adrenergic nociceptive pathways that contribute to central sensitization.[63]

Table 9.10 Studies examining the preemptive and preventive effects of multimodal analgesic regimens.

Author	Procedure (No. of patients)	Design	Group: First intervention drug/second intervention drug	Route and dose	Timing of first intervention	Timing of second intervention	Quality score	Nature and time after surgery of preventive and/or preemptive analgesic effects
Fassoulaki et al.[115]	Breast cancer surgery (50)	1, 8	GA plus: G1: PLA+PLACRM/ SAL/ PLA+PLACRM G2: GABA+EMLA/ROP/ GABA+EMLA	GABA p.o. 400 mg Irrigation ROP 10 mL Transdermal EMLA 20 g	GABA starting 6 pm preoperation and every 6 h thereafter EMLA – 5 min before surgery Intraop – ROP irrigation of brachial plexus, third, fourth, and fifth intercostal spaces	GABA – every 6 h until 8th day postoperation EMLA – sternal area, close to the wound, around the incision in the axilla daily for 3 days postoperation	5	Preventive effect – yes 3 month follow-up Incidence of: axilla pain: G2<G1; arm pain: G2<G1; chronic pain: G2<G1; analgesic use: G2<G1 6-month follow up no group differences in pain or analgesic use
Rosaeg et al.[201]	Arthroscopic knee ligament repair (40)	2, 4	GA plus: G1: ROP+MORPH+EPI +KETOR/Nad G2: Nad/ROP+MORPH +EPI+KETOR	Femoral nerve block ROP 20 mL 0.25 ROP i.a. 20 mL 0.25 MORPH i.a. 2 mg (plus EPI) KETOR i.v. 30 mg	15 min before skin incision	Immediately after completion of surgery	4	Preventive effect – no Preemptive effect – yes VRS Pain: G1<G2 at 0.5, 1, 1.5 and 2 h Cumulative i.v. PCA morphine usage: G1<G2 at 1, 2, 3, 4 and 5 h
Holthusen et al.[202]	Nephrectomy (30)	2, 4	GA plus: G1: MORPH+KETAM +CLON/Nad G2: Nad/MORPH +KETAM+CLON	150 µg/kg i.v. MORPH 150 µg/kg KETAM	15 min preoperation	Immediately after completion of surgery	2	Preemptive effect – no
Ng et al.[203]	Arthroscopic knee surgery (63)	4, 4, 4	LID infiltration plus: G1: na/BUP G2: na/ROP G3: na/ROP+MORPH +KETOR	BUP i.a. 150 mg ROP i.a. 150 mg ROP i.a. 150 mg MORPH 4 mg KETOR 30 mg	na	At end of surgery	5	Preventive effect – no

(Continued over)

| Naja et al.[204] | Pediatric tonsillectomy (90) | 1, 2 | GA plus: G1: LID+EPI+BUP+FENT +CLON/na G2: SAL/na G3: Nad/na | Preincisional infiltration (each tonsil 1.5 mL) mixture of LID+EPI, BUP, FENT and CLON | Before incision | na | 5 | Preventive effect – yes VAS-R: G1<G2=G3 at 1, 2, 3, 4, 7 and 8 days VAS-R: G1<G3 at 5, 6, 9 and 10 days VAS pain on jaw opening: G1<G2=G3 at 1, 2, 3, 4, 7, 8 and 10 days G1<G3 at 5 and 6 days G1<G2 at 9 days VAS pain when eating soft foods: G1<G2=G3 at 1, 2, 3, 4, 8 days No. of patients taking paracetemol (acetaminophen): G1<G2<G3 at 1, 2, 3, 4, 5 and 6 days No. of patients taking tramadol: G1<G2<G3 at 1, 2 and 3 days G1<G2=G3 at 4 and 5 days VAS-R: G1<G2=G3 at 1, 2, 3, 4, 7 and 8 days |

BUP, bupivacaine; CLON, clonidine; EMLA, eutectic mixture of local anesthetics; FENT, fentanyl; G, group; GA, general anesthesia; GABA, gabapentin; i.a., inta-articular; i.v., intravenous; KETAM, ketamine; KETOR, ketorolac; LID, lidocaine; MORPH, morphine; Nad, nothing administered; PCA, patient controlled analgesia; PLA, placebo; PLACRM, placebo cream; PO, per os; ROP, ropivacaine; VAS-R, visual analog scale pain score at rest; VRS, verbal rating scale.

Table 9.11 Studies examining the preemptive and preventive effects of other nonanalgesic agents.

Author	Procedure (No. of patients)	Treatment combinations (Figure 9.1)	Group: First intervention drug/second intervention drug	Route and Dose	Timing of first intervention	Timing of second intervention	Quality score	Nature and time after surgery of preventive and/or preemptive analgesic effects
Reuben et al.[63]	Radical mastectomy with axillary lymph node dissection (100)	1, 2	GA plus: G1: VENLAF/na G2: PLA/na	75 mg p.o.	Night before surgery and daily for 2 weeks postoperatively	na	5	Preventive effect – yes At 6 month follow up: Pain on movement: G1<G2 6 month incidence of: chest wall pain: G1<G2 arm pain: G1<G2 axilla pain: G1<G2 chronic pain: G1<G2 analgesic use: G1<G2
Chia et al.[205]	Total abdominal hysterectomy (90)	1, 2, 4	GA plus: G1: PROMETH/SAL G2: SAL/PROMETH G3: SAL/SAL	0.1 mg/kg i.v.	30 min preoperation	At end of surgery	4	Preventive effect – na Preemptive effect – yes VAS-R/M: No inter group differences to 24 h Cumulative PCA MORPH: G1<G2=G3 at 3, 6, 12 and 24 h
Unlegenc et al.[207]	Abdominal surgery (60)	1, 2	GA plus: G1: PLA/na G2: DEXMED/na	1 µg/kg i.v. for 10 min	10 min before anesthesia	na	4	Preventive effect – yes VAS pain: no inter group differences up to 24 h Cumulative PCA MORPH: G2<G1 at 24 h PCA morphine 12–24 h: G2<G1
Sen et al.[206]	Hand surgery (30)	1,2	Sedation i.v. plus: G1: LID/na G2: NITRO+LID/na	LID i.v. 2 3 mg/kg NITRO i.v. 200 µg	Immediately preoperation	na	4	Preventive effect – yes VAS for tourniquet pain: G2<G1 at 30 min intraoperation VAS pain: G2<G1 for 1st 4 h postoperation DICLOF consumption: G2<G1 PARACET consumption: G2<G1

DEXMED, dexmedetomidine; DICLOF, diclofenac; G, group; GA, general anesthesia; i.v., intravenous; LID, lidocaine; min, minute; MORPH, morphine; NITRO, nitroglycerin; PARACET, paracetamol (acetaminophen); PCA, patient-controlled analgesia; PLA, placebo; PROMETH, promethazine; SAL, saline; VAS-R/M, visual analog scale pain score at rest/on movement; VENLAF, venlafaxine.

RECOMMENDATIONS FOR FUTURE RESEARCH

Relationship between preexisting pain and timing of analgesic administration

We know very little about the effects of preexisting, preoperative pain on the subsequent development of acute and chronic postoperative pain. As it turns out, this important issue prompted the very first controlled study[209][III] of "preoperative preemptive analgesia"[38] which suggested that epidural anesthesia started before and continuing for the duration of surgery conferred protection from long-term phantom limb pain six months after surgery. These promising results were not supported by a subsequent randomized trial evaluating the long-term effects on phantom limb and stump pain of continuous epidural morphine and bupivacaine administered 18 hours before, during and for about one week after lower limb amputation.[15] The control group received epidural saline before and throughout surgical procedure followed by epidural morphine and bupivacaine postoperatively. There were no significant differences between the groups in pain incidence, intensity, or opioid consumption at any time up to 12 months after surgery.[15]

Other more recent studies in nonamputee populations have examined the same issue as it pertains to the development of acute, as opposed to chronic, postsurgical pain. The data suggest that in the presence of presurgical pain, preoperative administration of analgesics does not lead to the anticipated lessening of postoperative pain or analgesic consumption, perhaps because central sensitization has already been established. Postoperative pain and analgesic consumption were significantly reduced by pre- and intra-operative epidural morphine, but not saline, for patients who did not report presurgical pain.[210][II] However, among patients with presurgical pain, pre- and intraoperative epidural morphine was no more effective than saline.[210] This raises the important issue of what effect blocking preoperative pain would have on the intensity of acute postoperative pain. A recent study of patients undergoing total knee arthroplasty showed that relief of preoperative pain by epidural ropivacaine for at least 12 hours before surgery, followed by intraoperative epidural ropivacaine, reduced patient-controlled epidural analgesia (PCEA) ropivacaine consumption 48 hours after surgery compared with preoperative epidural saline and intraoperative epidural ropivacaine.[61][II] Based on these interesting and controversial findings, future studies should report presence (and duration) or absence of presurgical pain.

Offsetting the competing effects of opioid analgesia and opioid-induced tolerance and hyperalgesia

As noted above, recent basic science evidence points to the possibility that under certain circumstances,

preoperative administration of opioid analgesics may contribute to the establishment of acute opioid tolerance[195] and opioid-induced hyperalgesia.[197, 211] The mechanisms underlying the reduced pain and opioid consumption brought about by preemptive opioid analgesia, and the increased pain and opioid consumption underlying acute opioid tolerance and opioid-induced hyperalgesia, involve competing processes involving the NMDA receptor–ion channel complex. These findings have important implications for the conduct of clinical studies evaluating the timing of administration of opioid analgesics since the main outcome measures (pain and opioid consumption) will be directly affected by the mechanisms underlying these competing neural processes. The net effect of this competition is to attenuate (or even reverse) the desired preemptive and preventive effects. Coadministration of opioids and low-dose NMDA antagonists or low-dose opioid antagonists has been found to interfere with the development of acute opioid tolerance[7, 212] and opioid-induced hyperalgesia.[213] A mechanism-based approach to postoperative pain management involving coadministration of these agents would be expected to facilitate the preventive and preemptive analgesic effects of opioids in patients undergoing major surgery.

Recommendations to improve the quality of studies

MEASURES OF PAIN

The most appropriate pain measurement instruments are patient-rated pain scales that have demonstrated reliability and validity (e.g. visual analog scale (VAS), numeric rating scale, McGill pain questionnaire).[214] Measurement of pain with the patient in a resting position is reported by almost all studies. However, the measurement of hyperalgesia is important. The simplest and most clinically significant test of mechanical hyperalgesia is to have the patient perform a standardized movement after surgery (e.g. sitting up from a lying position, inspirational spirometry) and rate the intensity of the pain that ensues. More sophisticated measures of primary and secondary mechanical and thermal hyperalgesia include pressure algometry applied either on or near the wound dressing[215] or on the side of the body contralateral to the incision,[216] measurement of thresholds to electrical stimulation,[217] temperature,[89] and use of pinprick, brush,[189] and Von Frey filaments[58, 188] at a distance from the wound to determine the extent of secondary mechanical allodynia and hyperalgesia. Baseline (preoperative) measures are important as is testing at a control site (e.g. a noninjured body part) to rule out a generalized effect due to factors such as anxiety, anticipatory pain, or a response bias.

MEASURES OF ANALGESIC CONSUMPTION

The degree of pain a patient experiences in the post-operative setting is in part a function of postoperative analgesic consumption. Use of patient-controlled analgesia (either i.v. or epidural) as a modality for post-operative pain management has dominated the pre-emptive analgesia literature. This is largely because PCA/PCEA is now the gold standard for postoperative pain management at most institutions worldwide. Analgesic consumption is usually the primary outcome measure since patients self-administer the agent to achieve a relatively constant pain level. However, from the point of view of demonstrating preemptive analgesia, analgesic consumption is not the most ideal measure because the main hypothesis deals with pain and hyperalgesia. Allowing pain to fluctuate by holding constant the level of postoperative analgesics administered would be a more direct test of the hypothesis, but this is not always feasible or ethical given the evolving standards of pain management practice.

Cumulative analgesic consumption at the end of the study is a common measure, but report of a single value may not provide specific enough information to pinpoint exactly when the effect is observed. This point is not as important if a postincision control group is employed. However, it is especially relevant in studies that evaluate the preventive effect of a preoperative intervention (i.e. when comparing it to a placebo) since it is likely that the largest difference in PCA consumption between treated and untreated groups will occur around the time of peak effect of the target agent used preventively. Cumulative analgesic consumption at the end of the study may be misleading depending on the pattern of consumption over time. For example, if a difference in analgesic consumption occurs within the first few hours after surgery, when the effects of the analgesics used preventively are still active, then this is an analgesic effect. Unless cumulative analgesic consumption is reported at multiple times across the study period, an analgesic effect may be mis-interpreted as a preventive effect or a preventive effect may be missed. Likewise, report of a single value for cumulative analgesic consumption at the end of the study may result in failure to detect the presence of group differences at earlier time points. Another approach that circumvents this problem is to calculate analgesic consumption within intervals bounded by the times when pain is assessed.[54, 148, 218] This method has the advantage of specifying an interval within which an opioid-sparing effect has occurred.

SUMMARY AND CONCLUSIONS

Preoperative pain intensity is a risk factor for development of severe acute postoperative pain, as well as long-term postsurgical pain. Severity of acute postoperative pain predicts pain after discharge and also is a risk factor for chronic postsurgical pain. These findings have, in part, fueled recent preventive and preemptive efforts to reduce acute pain intensity and long-term pain problems by blocking noxious perioperative inputs.

Overall, across the classes of agents reviewed, the proportion of significant preventive and preemptive effects is significantly greater than the proportion of negative effects ($p = 0.02$, **Table 9.4**). The same is true for the proportion of positive versus negative preventive effects ($p = 0.03$, **Table 9.4**). Administration of these agents appears to reduce pain, analgesic consumption or both at a point in time that exceeds 5.5 half-lives of the target agent. Since these extended effects are observed after the clinical actions of the agents have worn off, they are not analgesic effects. Rather, these effects appear to be due to the reduction in perioperative peripheral and central sensitization in the treated patients. The greatest proportion of positive preventive effects were found for the NMDA antagonists ketamine and dextromethorphan for which significantly lower pain intensity and/or reduced analgesic requirements were found in approximately 69 percent of the effects tested. In spite of the heterogeneity in designs (**Figure 9.3**) across the 61 clinical trials (69 effects) evaluated, it appears that, in general, there is a benefit in terms of reduced pain and/or analgesic consumption that extends beyond the duration of action of the target drug.

The absence of a difference in the proportion of positive preemptive versus negative preemptive effects is understandable when one considers that both preincisional and postincisional (or postsurgical) noxious inputs contribute to postoperative sensitization.[4][I] The most likely conclusion is that for a certain proportion of studies of preemptive analgesia, the postincision or postsurgical administration condition is as beneficial in reducing central sensitization as is the preoperative condition but that these benefits go undetected when the comparison is made between the two groups. The lack of a control group in studies of preemptive analgesia is a serious limitation that confounds interpretation of the results and has contributed to the premature and erroneous conclusion that there is no clinical benefit to preoperative nociceptive blockade.

The continued use of incomplete designs that consist of preincisional and postincisional or postsurgical conditions without a standard treatment group or a complete blockade condition will hinder progress in our understanding of the benefits of preemptive analgesia. Adhering to the narrow definition of preemptive analgesia currently accepted by many in the field will perpetuate problems of interpretation and will not lead to the evolution and progress that is needed to move us beyond the current state of confusion. Inclusion of appropriate control conditions is essential if we are to advance our knowledge about the factors that contribute to acute postoperative pain and enhance our ability to detect clinical benefits associated with blockade of noxious perioperative inputs. Future work should focus on maximizing the prevention of surgically induced sensitization by ensuring as complete a blockade as possible of nociceptive transmission throughout the three phases of the perioperative period. Long-term follow-up studies are needed to assess the efficacy of the perioperative interventions and to ascertain the true incidence of chronic post-surgical pain.

Given the prominent role of psychosocial factors in chronic pain[219] and the recent recommendations for assessment of core measures and domains in clinical trials,[220] relevant psychological, emotional, and physical variables should be added to those routinely assessed before and after surgery. Assessment of additional domains of functioning may help to shed light on the predictors of severe acute postoperative pain, the processes involved in recovery from surgery, and the risk factors for developing chronic postsurgical pain.[57]

ACKNOWLEDGMENTS

Joel Katz is supported by a Canada Research Chair in Health Psychology at York University, Toronto, Canada. We would like to thank Maria Dzyuba and Eileen Halket for retrieving the articles reviewed in this chapter and Matthew Dubins for his help with data extraction and creation of the tables.

REFERENCES

1. Melzack R, Wall PD. *The challenge of pain*, 2nd edn. New York: Basic Books, 1988: 447.
2. Woolf CJ, Salter MW. Neuronal plasticity: increasing the gain in pain. *Science*. 2000; **288**: 1765–9.
* 3. Coderre TJ, Katz J. Peripheral and central hyperexcitability: differential signs and symptoms in persistent pain. *Behavioral and Brain Sciences*. 1997; **20**: 404–19; discussion 35-513.
* 4. Katz J, McCartney CJL. Current status of pre-emptive analgesia. *Current Opinion in Anaesthesiology*. 2002; **15**: 435–41.
5. Katz J. Pre-emptive analgesia: evidence, current status and future directions. *European Journal of Anaesthesiology* Supplement. 1995; **10**: 8–13.
6. Kissin I. Preemptive analgesia: Terminology and clinical relevance. *Anesthesia and Analgesia*. 1994; **79**: 809.
7. Kissin I, Bright CA, Bradley Jr EL. The effect of ketamine on opioid-induced acute tolerance: can It explain reduction of opioid consumption with ketamine-opioid analgesic combinations? *Anesthesia and Analgesia*. 2000; **91**: 1483–8.
8. Perkins FM, Kehlet H. Chronic pain as an outcome of surgery. A review of predictive factors. *Anesthesiology*. 2000; **93**: 1123–33.

9. Katz J. Pain begets pain – Predictors of long-term phantom limb pain and post-thoracotomy pain. *Pain Forum*. 1997; **6**: 140–4.
10. Dworkin RH. Which individuals with acute pain are most likely to develop a chronic pain syndrome? *Pain Forum*. 1997; **6**: 127–36.
* 11. Kehlet H, Jensen TS, Woolf CJ. Persistent postsurgical pain: risk factors and prevention. *Lancet*. 2006; **367**: 1618–25.
12. Kalkman CJ, Visser K, Moen J et al. Preoperative prediction of severe postoperative pain. *Pain*. 2003; **105**: 415–23.
13. Tasmuth T, Blomqvist C, Kalso E. Chronic post-treatment symptoms in patients with breast cancer operated in different surgical units. *European Journal of Surgical Oncology*. 1999; **25**: 38–43.
14. Jensen TS, Krebs B, Nielsen J, Rasmussen P. Immediate and long-term phantom limb pain in amputees: incidence, clinical characteristics and relationship to pre-amputation limb pain. *Pain*. 1985; **21**: 267–78.
15. Nikolajsen L, Ilkjaer S, Christensen JH et al. Randomised trial of epidural bupivacaine and morphine in prevention of stump and phantom pain in lower-limp amputation. *Lancet*. 1997; **350**: 1353–7.
16. Caumo W, Schmidt AP, Schneider CN et al. Preoperative predictors of moderate to intense acute postoperative pain in patients undergoing abdominal surgery. *Acta Anaesthesiologica Scandinavica*. 2002; **46**: 1265–71.
17. Scott LE, Clum GA, Peoples JB. Preoperative predictors of postoperative pain. *Pain*. 1983; **15**: 283–93.
18. Thomas T, Robinson C, Champion D et al. Prediction and assessment of the severity of post-operative pain and of satisfaction with management. *Pain*. 1998; **75**: 177–85.
19. Harden RN, Bruehl S, Stanos S et al. Prospective examination of pain-related and psychological predictors of CRPS-like phenomena following total knee arthroplasty: a preliminary study. *Pain*. 2003; **106**: 393–400.
20. Brander VA, Stulberg SD, Adams AD et al. Predicting total knee replacement pain: a prospective, observational study. *Clinical Orthopaedics and Related Research*. 2003: 27–36.
21. Liem MS, van Duyn EB, van der Graaf Y, van Vroonhoven TJ. Recurrences after conventional anterior and laparoscopic inguinal hernia repair: a randomized comparison. *Annals of Surgery*. 2003; **237**: 136–41.
22. Poobalan AS, Bruce J, King PM et al. Chronic pain and quality of life following open inguinal hernia repair. *British Journal of Surgery*. 2001; **88**: 1122–6.
23. Bisgaard T, Klarskov B, Rosenberg J, Kehlet H. Characteristics and prediction of early pain after laparoscopic cholecystectomy. *Pain*. 2001; **90**: 261–9.
24. Granot M, Lowenstein L, Yarnitsky D et al. Postcesarean section pain prediction by preoperative experimental pain assessment. *Anesthesiology*. 2003; **98**: 1422–6.
25. Werner MU, Duun P, Kehlet H. Prediction of postoperative pain by preoperative nociceptive responses to heat stimulation. *Anesthesiology*. 2004; **100**: 115–9; discussion 5A.

26. Beauregard L, Pomp A, Choiniere M. Severity and impact of pain after day-surgery. *Canadian Journal of Anaesthesia*. 1998; **45**: 304–11.

27. Lau H, Patil NG, Yuen WK, Lee F. Prevalence and severity of chronic groin pain after endoscopic totally extraperitoneal inguinal hernioplasty. *Surgical Endoscopy*. 2003; **17**: 1620–3.

28. Callesen T, Bech K, Kehlet H. Prospective study of chronic pain after groin hernia repair. *British Journal of Surgery*. 1999; **86**: 1528–31.

* 29. Katz J, Jackson M, Kavanagh BP, Sandler AN. Acute pain after thoracic surgery predicts long-term post-thoracotomy pain. *Clinical Journal of Pain*. 1996; **12**: 50–5.

* 30. Hayes C, Browne S, Lantry G, Burstal R. Neuropathic pain in the acute pain service: a prospective survey. *Acute Pain*. 2002; **4**: 45–8.

31. Senturk M, Ozcan PE, Talu GK *et al.* The effects of three different analgesia techniques on long-term postthoracotomy pain. *Anesthesia and Analgesia*. 2002; **94**: 11–5.

32. Tasmuth T, Kataja M, Blomqvist C *et al.* Treatment-related factors predisposing to chronic pain in patients with breast cancer – a multivariate approach. *Acta Oncologica*. 1997; **36**: 625–30.

33. Jorgensen T, Teglbjerg JS, Wille-Jorgensen P *et al.* Persisting pain after cholecystectomy. A prospective investigation. *Scandinavian Journal of Gastroenterology*. 1991; **26**: 124–8.

34. Borly L, Anderson IB, Bardram L *et al.* Preoperative prediction model of outcome after cholecystectomy for symptomatic gallstones. *Scandinavian Journal of Gastroenterology*. 1999; **34**: 1144–52.

35. Cohen L, Fouladi RT, Katz J. Preoperative coping strategies and distress predict postoperative pain and morphine consumption in women undergoing abdominal gynecologic surgery. *Journal of Psychosomatic Research*. 2005; **58**: 201–09.

36. Hanley MA, Jensen MP, Ehde DM *et al.* Psychosocial predictors of long-term adjustment to lower-limb amputation and phantom limb pain. *Disability and Rehabilitation*. 2004; **26**: 882–93.

37. Katz J. George Washington Crile, anoci-association, and pre-emptive analgesia. *Pain*. 1993; **53**: 243–5.

* 38. Wall PD. The prevention of post-operative pain. *Pain*. 1988; **33**: 289–90.

39. Rundshagen I, Kochs E, Schulte am Esch J. Surgical stimulation increases median nerve somatosensory evoked responses during isoflurane-nitrous oxide anaesthesia. *British Journal of Anaesthesia*. 1995; **75**: 598–602.

40. Abram SE, Yaksh TL. Morphine, but not inhalation anesthesia, blocks post-injury facilitation. The role of preemptive suppression of afferent transmission. *Anesthesiology*. 1993; **78**: 713–21.

* 41. Taylor BK, Brennan TJ. Preemptive analgesia: Moving beyond conventional strategies and confusing terminology. *Journal of Pain*. 2000; **1**: 77–84.

42. Futter M. Preventive not pre-emptive analgesia with piroxicam. *Canadian Journal of Anaesthesia*. 1997; **44**: 101–02.

* 43. Kissin I. Preemptive analgesia. Why its effect is not always obvious. *Anesthesiology*. 1996; **84**: 1015–9.

44. Yaksh TL, Abram SE. Preemptive analgesia: A popular misnomer, but a clinically relevant truth? *Psychological Science*. 1993; **2**: 116–21.

45. Penning JP. Pre-emptive analgesia: what does it mean to the clinical anaesthetist? *Canadian Journal of Anaesthesia*. 1996; **43**: 97–101.

46. Dionne R. Preemptive vs preventive analgesia: which approach improves clinical outcomes? *Compendium of Continuing Education in Dentistry*. 2000; **21**: 48, 51–4, 6.

47. Pogatzki-Zahn EM, Zahn PK. From preemptive to preventive analgesia. *Current Opinion in Anaesthesiology*. 2006; **19**: 551–5.

48. Crile GW. The kinetic theory of shock and its prevention through anoci-association (shockless operation). *Lancet*. 1913; **185**: 7–16.

49. McQuay HJ. Pre-emptive analgesia. *British Journal of Anaesthesia*. 1992; **69**: 1–3.

50. Amantea B, Gemelli A, Migliorini F, Tocci R. Preemptive analgesia or balanced periemptive analgesia? *Minerva Anestesiologica*. 1999; **65**: 19–37.

51. Kissin I. Preemptive analgesia. *Anesthesiology*. 2000; **93**: 1138–43.

52. Moiniche S, Kehlet H, Dahl JB. A qualitative and quantitative systematic review of preemptive analgesia for postoperative pain relief: the role of timing of analgesia. *Anesthesiology*. 2002; **96**: 725–41.

53. Kissin I. Preemptive analgesia at the crossroad. *Anesthesia and Analgesia*. 2005; **100**: 754–6.

* 54. Katz J, Kavanagh BP, Sandler AN *et al.* Preemptive analgesia. Clinical evidence of neuroplasticity contributing to postoperative pain. *Anesthesiology*. 1992; **77**: 439–46.

55. Dierking GW, Dahl JB, Kanstrup J *et al.* Effect of pre- vs postoperative inguinal field block on postoperative pain after herniorrhaphy. *British Journal of Anaesthesia*. 1992; **68**: 344–8.

56. Coderre TJ, Katz J, Vaccarino AL, Melzack R. Contribution of central neuroplasticity to pathological pain: review of clinical and experimental evidence. *Pain*. 1993; **52**: 259–85.

* 57. Katz J, Cohen L. Preventive analgesia is associated with reduced pain disability 3 weeks but not 6 months after major gynecologic surgery by laparotomy. *Anesthesiology*. 2004; **101**: 169–74.

58. Katz J, Cohen L, Schmid R *et al.* Postoperative morphine use and hyperalgesia are reduced by preoperative but not intraoperative epidural analgesia: implications for preemptive analgesia and the prevention of central sensitization. *Anesthesiology*. 2003; **98**: 1449–60.

* 59. Gordon SM, Brahim JS, Dubner R *et al.* Attenuation of pain in a randomized trial by suppression of peripheral nociceptive activity in the immediate postoperative period. *Anesthesia and Analgesia*. 2002; **95**: 1351–7.

60. O'Hanlon DM, Thambipillai T, Colbert ST *et al*. Timing of pre-emptive tenoxicam is important for postoperative analgesia. *Canadian Journal of Anaesthesia*. 2001; **48**: 162–6.

∗ 61. Klasen J, Haas M, Graf S *et al*. Impact on postoperative pain of long-lasting pre-emptive epidural analgesia before total hip replacement: a prospective, randomised, double-blind study. *Anaesthesia*. 2005; **60**: 118–23.

62. Tverskoy M, Cozacov C, Ayache M *et al*. Postoperative pain after inguinal herniorrhaphy with different types of anesthesia. *Anesthesia and Analgesia*. 1990; **70**: 29–35.

∗ 63. Reuben SS, Makari-Judson G, Lurie SD. Evaluation of efficacy of the perioperative administration of venlafaxine XR in the prevention of postmastectomy pain syndrome. *Journal of Pain and Symptom Management*. 2004; **27**: 133–9.

∗ 64. Reuben SS, Vieira P, Faruqi S *et al*. Local administration of morphine for analgesia after iliac bone graft harvest. *Anesthesiology*. 2001; **95**: 390–4.

65. Dahl JB, Mathiesen O, Moiniche S. 'Protective premedication': an option with gabapentin and related drugs? A review of gabapentin and pregabalin in the treatment of post-operative pain. *Acta Anaesthesiologica Scandinavica*. 2004; **48**: 1130–6.

66. Ong CK, Lirk P, Seymour RA, Jenkins BJ. The efficacy of preemptive analgesia for acute postoperative pain management: a meta-analysis. *Anesthesia and Analgesia*. 2005; **100**: 757–73.

∗ 67. McCartney CJ, Sinha A, Katz J. A qualitative systematic review of the role of N-methyl-D-aspartate receptor antagonists in preventive analgesia. *Anesthesia and Analgesia*. 2004; **98**: 1385–400.

68. George MJ. The site of action of epidurally administered opioids and its relevance to postoperative pain management. *Anaesthesia*. 2006; **61**: 659–64.

69. Evers A, Maze M. *Anesthetic pharmacology: physiologic principles and clinical practice*. Philadelphia, PA: Churchill Livingstone, 2004.

70. *Mosby's drug consult 2006*. St Louis, MO: Mosby, 2006.

71. Hardman JG, Limbird LE, Gilman AG. *Goodman & Gilman's the pharmacological basis of therapeutics*, 10th edn. New York: McGraw-Hill, 2001.

72. Jadad AR, Moore RA, Carroll D *et al*. Assessing the quality of reports of randomized clinical trials: is blinding necessary? *Controlled Clinical Trials*. 1996; **17**: 1–12.

73. Lee IO, Kim SH, Kong MH *et al*. Pain after laparoscopic cholecystectomy: the effect and timing of incisional and intraperitoneal bupivacaine. *Canadian Journal of Anaesthesia*. 2001; **48**: 545–50.

74. Yegin A, Erdogan A, Kayacan N, Karsli B. Early postoperative pain management after thoracic surgery; pre- and postoperative versus postoperative epidural analgesia: a randomised study. *European Journal of Cardiothoracic Surgery*. 2003; **24**: 420–4.

75. Senagore AJ, Delaney CP, Mekhail N *et al*. Randomized clinical trial comparing epidural anaesthesia and patient-controlled analgesia after laparoscopic segmental colectomy. *British Journal of Surgery*. 2003; **90**: 1195–9.

76. Cerfolio RJ, Bryant AS, Bass CS, Bartolucci AA. A prospective, double-blinded, randomized trial evaluating the use of preemptive analgesia of the skin before thoracotomy. *Annals of Thoracic Surgery*. 2003; **76**: 1055–8.

77. Korhonen AM, Valanne JV, Jokela RM *et al*. A comparison of selective spinal anesthesia with hyperbaric bupivacaine and general anesthesia with desflurane for outpatient knee arthroscopy. *Anesthesia and Analgesia*. 2004; **99**: 1668–73.

78. Karakaya D, Baris S, Ozkan F *et al*. Analgesic effects of interpleural bupivacaine with fentanyl for post-thoracotomy pain. *Journal of Cardiothoracic and Vascular Anesthesia*. 2004; **18**: 461–5.

79. Lee-Elliott CE, Dundas D, Patel U. Randomized trial of lidocaine vs lidocaine/bupivacaine periprostatic injection on longitudinal pain scores after prostate biopsy. *Journal of Urology*. 2004; **171**: 247–50.

80. Batra YK, Mahajan R, Bangalia SK *et al*. Bupivacaine/ketamine is superior to intra-articular ketamine analgesia following arthroscopic knee surgery. *Canadian Journal of Anaesthesia*. 2005; **52**: 832–6.

81. Sundarathiti P, Pasutharnchat K, Kongdan Y, Suranutkarin PE. Thoracic epidural anesthesia (TEA) with 0.2 ropivacaine in combination with ipsilateral brachial plexus block (BPB) for modified radical mastectomy (MRM). *Journal of the Medical Association of Thailand*. 2005; **88**: 513–20.

82. Abramov Y, Sand PK, Gandhi S *et al*. The effect of preemptive pudendal nerve blockade on pain after transvaginal pelvic reconstructive surgery. *Obstetrics and Gynecology*. 2005; **106**: 782–8.

83. Herbland A, Cantini O, Reynier P *et al*. The bilateral superficial cervical plexus block with 0.75 ropivacaine administered before or after surgery does not prevent postoperative pain after total thyroidectomy. *Regional Anesthesia and Pain Medicine*. 2006; **31**: 34–9.

84. Seet E, Leong WL, Yeo AS, Fook-Chong S. Effectiveness of 3-in-1 continuous femoral block of differing concentrations compared to patient controlled intravenous morphine for post total knee arthroplasty analgesia and knee rehabilitation. *Anaesthesia and Intensive Care*. 2006; **34**: 25–30.

85. Yukawa Y, Kato F, Ito K *et al*. A prospective randomized study of preemptive analgesia for postoperative pain in the patients undergoing posterior lumbar interbody fusion: continuous subcutaneous morphine, continuous epidural morphine, and diclofenac sodium. *Spine*. 2005; **30**: 2357–61.

86. Busch CA, Shore BJ, Bhandari R *et al*. Efficacy of periarticular multimodal drug injection in total knee arthroplasty. A randomized trial. *Journal of Bone and Joint Surgery*. 2006; **88**: 959–63.

87. Subramaniam B, Subramaniam K, Pawar DK, Sennaraj B. Preoperative epidural ketamine in combination with morphine does not have a clinically relevant intra- and

postoperative opioid-sparing effect. *Anesthesia and Analgesia*. 2001; **93**: 1321–6.

88. Papaziogas B, Argiriadou H, Papagiannopoulou P *et al*. Preincisional intravenous low-dose ketamine and local infiltration with ropivacaine reduces postoperative pain after laparoscopic cholecystectomy. *Surgical Endoscopy*. 2001; **15**: 1030–3.

89. Weinbroum AA, Gorodezky A, Niv D *et al*. Dextromethorphan attenuation of postoperative pain and primary and secondary thermal hyperalgesia. *Canadian Journal of Anaesthesia*. 2001; **48**: 167–74.

90. Weinbroum AA, Gorodetzky A, Nirkin A *et al*. Dextromethorphan for the reduction of immediate and late postoperative pain and morphine consumption in orthopedic oncology patients: a randomized, placebo-controlled, double-blind study. *Cancer*. 2002; **95**: 1164–70.

91. Weinbroum AA. Dextromethorphan reduces immediate and late postoperative analgesic requirements and improves patients' subjective scorings after epidural lidocaine and general anesthesia. *Anesthesia and Analgesia*. 2002; **94**: 1547–52.

92. Weinbroum AA, Bender B, Bickels J *et al*. Preoperative and postoperative dextromethorphan provides sustained reduction in postoperative pain and patient-controlled epidural analgesia requirement: a randomized, placebo-controlled, double-blind study in lower-body bone malignancy-operated patients. *Cancer*. 2003; **97**: 2334–40.

93. O'Flaherty JE, Lin CX. Does ketamine or magnesium affect posttonsillectomy pain in children? *Paediatric Anaesthesia*. 2003; **13**: 413–21.

94. Hayes C, Armstrong-Brown A, Burstal R. Perioperative intravenous ketamine infusion for the prevention of persistent post-amputation pain: a randomized, controlled trial. *Anaesthesia and Intensive Care*. 2004; **32**: 330–8.

95. Bolcal C, Iyem H, Sargin M *et al*. Comparison of magnesium sulfate with opioid and NSAIDs on postoperative pain management after coronary artery bypass surgery. *Journal of Cardiothoracic and Vascular Anesthesia*. 2005; **19**: 714–8.

96. Carney DE, Nicolette LA, Ratner MH *et al*. Ketorolac reduces postoperative narcotic requirements. *Journal of Pediatric Surgery*. 2001; **36**: 76–9.

97. Mallory TH, Lombardi Jr AV, Fada RA *et al*. Pain management for joint arthroplasty: preemptive analgesia. *Journal of Arthroplasty*. 2002; **17**: 129–33.

98. Wnek W, Zajaczkowska R, Wordliczek J *et al*. Influence of pre-operative ketoprofen administration (preemptive analgesia) on analgesic requirement and the level of prostaglandins in the early postoperative period. *Polish Journal of Pharmacology*. 2004; **56**: 547–52.

99. Nikanne E, Kokki H, Salo J, Linna TJ. Celecoxib and ketoprofen for pain management during tonsillectomy: a placebo-controlled clinical trial. *Otolaryngology – Head and Neck Surgery*. 2005; **132**: 287–94.

100. Canbay O, Karakas O, Celebi N *et al*. The preemptive use of diclofenac sodium in combination with ketamine and remifentanil does not enhance postoperative analgesia after laparoscopic gynecological procedures. *Saudi Medical Journal*. 2006; **27**: 642–5.

101. Louizos AA, Pandazi AB, Koraka CP *et al*. Preoperative administration of rofecoxib versus ketoprofen for pain relief after tonsillectomy. *Annals of Otology, Rhinology, and Laryngology*. 2006; **115**: 201–04.

102. Wordliczek J, Banach M, Garlicki J *et al*. Influence of pre- or intraoperational use of tramadol (preemptive or preventive analgesia) on tramadol requirement in the early postoperative period. *Polish Journal of Pharmacology*. 2002; **54**: 693–7.

103. Machida M, Imamura Y, Usui T, Asai T. Effects of preemptive analgesia using continuous subcutaneous morphine for postoperative pain in scoliosis surgery: a randomized study. *Journal of Pediatric Orthopedics*. 2004; **24**: 576–80.

104. Bellissant E, Estebe JP, Sebille V, Ecoffey C. Effect of preoperative oral sustained-release morphine sulfate on postoperative morphine requirements in elective spine surgery. *Fundamental and Clinical Pharmacology*. 2004; **18**: 709–14.

105. De Pietri L, Siniscalchi A, Reggiani A *et al*. The use of intrathecal morphine for postoperative pain relief after liver resection: a comparison with epidural analgesia. *Anesthesia and Analgesia*. 2006; **102**: 1157–63.

106. Cheng JK, Chiou LC. Mechanisms of the antinociceptive action of gabapentin. *Journal of Pharmacological Sciences*. 2006; **100**: 471–86.

107. Cheng VY, Bonin RP, Chiu MW *et al*. Gabapentin increases a tonic inhibitory conductance in hippocampal pyramidal neurons. *Anesthesiology*. 2006; **105**: 325–33.

108. Rose MA, Kam PC. Gabapentin: pharmacology and its use in pain management. *Anaesthesia*. 2002; **57**: 451–62.

109. Dirks J, Petersen KL, Rowbotham MC, Dahl JB. Gabapentin suppresses cutaneous hyperalgesia following heat-capsaicin sensitization. *Anesthesiology*. 2002; **97**: 102–07.

110. Al-Mujadi H, A-Refai AR, Katzarov MG *et al*. Preemptive gabapentin reduces postoperative pain and opioid demand following thyroid surgery. *Canadian Journal of Anaesthesia*. 2006; **53**: 268–73.

111. Dierking G, Duedahl TH, Rasmussen ML *et al*. Effects of gabapentin on postoperative morphine consumption and pain after abdominal hysterectomy: a randomized, double-blind trial. *Acta Anaesthesiologica Scandinavica*. 2004; **48**: 322–7.

112. Dirks J, Fredensborg BB, Christensen D *et al*. A randomized study of the effects of single-dose gabapentin versus placebo on postoperative pain and morphine consumption after mastectomy. *Anesthesiology*. 2002; **97**: 560–4.

113. Fassoulaki A, Patris K, Sarantopoulos C, Hogan Q. The analgesic effect of gabapentin and mexiletine after breast surgery for cancer. *Anesthesia and Analgesia*. 2002; **95**: 985–91.

114. Fassoulaki A, Stamatakis E, Petropoulos G *et al.* Gabapentin attenuates late but not acute pain after abdominal hysterectomy. *European Journal of Anaesthesiology.* 2006; **23**: 136–41.

*115. Fassoulaki A, Triga A, Melemeni A, Sarantopoulos C. Multimodal analgesia with gabapentin and local anesthetics prevents acute and chronic pain after breast surgery for cancer. *Anesthesia and Analgesia.* 2005; **101**: 1427–32.

116. Gilron I, Orr E, Tu D *et al.* A placebo-controlled randomized clinical trial of perioperative administration of gabapentin, rofecoxib and their combination for spontaneous and movement-evoked pain after abdominal hysterectomy. *Pain.* 2005; **113**: 191–200.

*117. Menigaux C, Adam F, Guignard B *et al.* Preoperative gabapentin decreases anxiety and improves early functional recovery from knee surgery. *Anesthesia and Analgesia.* 2005; **100**: 1394–9.

118. Mikkelsen S, Hilsted KL, Andersen PJ *et al.* The effect of gabapentin on post-operative pain following tonsillectomy in adults. *Acta Anaesthesiologica Scandinavica.* 2006; **50**: 809–15.

119. Pandey CK, Navkar DV, Giri PJ *et al.* Evaluation of the optimal preemptive dose of gabapentin for postoperative pain relief after lumbar diskectomy: a randomized, double-blind, placebo-controlled study. *Journal of Neurosurgical Anesthesiology.* 2005; **17**: 65–8.

120. Pandey CK, Priye S, Singh S *et al.* Preemptive use of gabapentin significantly decreases postoperative pain and rescue analgesic requirements in laparoscopic cholecystectomy. *Canadian Journal of Anaesthesia.* 2004; **51**: 358–63.

121. Pandey CK, Sahay S, Gupta D *et al.* Preemptive gabapentin decreases postoperative pain after lumbar discoidectomy. *Canadian Journal of Anaesthesia.* 2004; **51**: 986–9.

122. Pandey CK, Singhal V, Kumar M *et al.* Gabapentin provides effective postoperative analgesia whether administered pre-emptively or post-incision. *Canadian Journal of Anaesthesia.* 2005; **52**: 827–31.

123. Radhakrishnan M, Bithal PK, Chaturvedi A. Effect of preemptive gabapentin on postoperative pain relief and morphine consumption following lumbar laminectomy and discectomy: a randomized, double-blinded, placebo-controlled study. *Journal of Neurosurgical Anesthesiology.* 2005; **17**: 125–8.

124. Rorarius MG, Mennander S, Suominen P *et al.* Gabapentin for the prevention of postoperative pain after vaginal hysterectomy. *Pain.* 2004; **110**: 175–81.

125. Turan A, Karamanlioglu B, Memis D *et al.* Analgesic effects of gabapentin after spinal surgery. *Anesthesiology.* 2004; **100**: 935–8.

126. Turan A, Karamanlioglu B, Memis D *et al.* The analgesic effects of gabapentin after total abdominal hysterectomy. *Anesthesia and Analgesia.* 2004; **98**: 1370–3.

127. Turan A, Kaya G, Karamanlioglu B *et al.* Effect of oral gabapentin on postoperative epidural analgesia. *British Journal of Anaesthesia.* 2006; **96**: 242–6.

128. Turan A, Memis D, Karamanlioglu B *et al.* The analgesic effects of gabapentin in monitored anesthesia care for ear-nose-throat surgery. *Anesthesia and Analgesia.* 2004; **99**: 375–8.

129. Turan A, White PF, Karamanlioglu B *et al.* Gabapentin: an alternative to the cyclooxygenase-2 inhibitors for perioperative pain management. *Anesthesia and Analgesia.* 2006; **102**: 175–81.

130. Seib RK, Paul JE. Preoperative gabapentin for postoperative analgesia: a meta-analysis. *Canadian Journal of Anaesthesia.* 2006; **53**: 461–9.

131. Ho KY, Gan TJ, Habib AS. Gabapentin and postoperative pain – a systematic review of randomized controlled trials. *Pain.* 2006; **126**: 91–101.

132. Burmeister MA, Gottschalk A, Freitag M *et al.* Pre- and intraoperative epidural ropivacaine have no early preemptive analgesic effect in major gynecological tumour surgery. *Canadian Journal of Anaesthesia.* 2003; **50**: 568–73.

133. Koppert W, Weigand M, Neumann F *et al.* Perioperative intravenous lidocaine has preventive effects on postoperative pain and morphine consumption after major abdominal surgery. *Anesthesia and Analgesia.* 2004; **98**: 1050–5.

134. Neustein SM, Kreitzer JM, Krellenstein D *et al.* Preemptive epidural analgesia for thoracic surgery. *Mount Sinai Journal of Medicine.* 2002; **69**: 101–04.

135. White PF, Rawal S, Latham P *et al.* Use of a continuous local anesthetic infusion for pain management after median sternotomy. *Anesthesiology.* 2003; **99**: 918–23.

136. Lam KW, Pun TC, Ng EH, Wong KS. Efficacy of preemptive analgesia for wound pain after laparoscopic operations in infertile women: a randomised, double-blind and placebo control study. *BJOG.* 2004; **111**: 340–4.

137. Louizos AA, Hadzilia SJ, Leandros E *et al.* Postoperative pain relief after laparoscopic cholecystectomy: a placebo-controlled double-blind randomized trial of preincisional infiltration and intraperitoneal instillation of levobupivacaine 0.25. *Surgical Endoscopy.* 2005; **19**: 1503–06.

138. Lohsiriwat V, Lert-akyamanee N, Rushatamukayanunt W. Efficacy of pre-incisional bupivacaine infiltration on postoperative pain relief after appendectomy: prospective double-blind randomized trial. *World Journal of Surgery.* 2004; **28**: 947–50.

139. Vendittoli PA, Makinen P, Drolet P *et al.* A multimodal analgesia protocol for total knee arthroplasty. A randomized, controlled study. *Journal of Bone and Joint Surgery.* 2006; **88**: 282–9.

140. Tuncer B, Babacan CA, Arslan M. The pre-emptive analgesic effect of intra-articular bupivacaine in arthroscopic knee surgery. *Acta Anaesthesiologica Scandinavica.* 2005; **49**: 1373–7.

141. Fagan DJ, Martin W, Smith A. A randomized, double-blind trial of pre-emptive local anesthesia in day-case knee arthroscopy. *Arthroscopy.* 2003; **19**: 50–3.

142. Nguyen A, Girard F, Boudreault D et al. Scalp nerve blocks decrease the severity of pain after craniotomy. Anesthesia and Analgesia. 2001; 93: 1272–6.

143. Stubhaug A. Can opioids prevent post-operative chronic pain? European Journal of Pain. 2005; 9: 153–6.

144. Woolf CJ, Wall PD. Morphine-sensitive and morphine-insensitive actions of C-fibre input on the rat spinal cord. Neuroscience Letters. 1986; 64: 221–5.

145. Kouya PF, Xu XJ. Buprenorphine reduces central sensitization after repetitive C-fiber stimulation in rats. Neuroscience Letters. 2004; 359: 127–9.

146. Gonzalez MI, Field MJ, Bramwell S et al. Ovariohysterectomy in the rat: a model of surgical pain for evaluation of pre-emptive analgesia? Pain. 2000; 88: 79–88.

147. Aida S, Yamakura T, Baba H et al. Preemptive analgesia by intravenous low-dose ketamine and epidural morphine in gastrectomy: a randomized double-blind study. Anesthesiology. 2000; 92: 1624–30.

148. Katz J, Clairoux M, Redahan C et al. High dose alfentanil pre-empts pain after abdominal hysterectomy. Pain. 1996; 68: 109–18.

149. Motamed C, Mazoit X, Ghanouchi K et al. Preemptive intravenous morphine-6-glucuronide is ineffective for postoperative pain relief. Anesthesiology. 2000; 92: 355–60.

150. Ruscheweyh R, Sandkuhler J. Opioids and central sensitisation: II. Induction and reversal of hyperalgesia. European Journal of Pain. 2005; 9: 149–52.

151. Akural EI, Salomaki TE, Tekay AH et al. Pre-emptive effect of epidural sufentanil in abdominal hysterectomy. British Journal of Anaesthesia. 2002; 88: 803–08.

152. Mavioglu O, Ozkardesler S, Tasdogen A et al. Effect of analgesia administration timing on early post-operative period characteristics: a randomized, double-blind, controlled study. Journal of International Medical Research. 2005; 33: 483–9.

153. McCarty EC, Spindler KP, Tingstad E et al. Does intraarticular morphine improve pain control with femoral nerve block after anterior cruciate ligament reconstruction? American Journal of Sports Medicine. 2001; 29: 327–32.

154. Munoz HR, Guerrero ME, Brandes V, Cortinez LI. Effect of timing of morphine administration during remifentanil-based anaesthesia on early recovery from anaesthesia and postoperative pain. British Journal of Anaesthesia. 2002; 88: 814–8.

155. Reuben SS, Sklar J, El-Mansouri M. The preemptive analgesic effect of intraarticular bupivacaine and morphine after ambulatory arthroscopic knee surgery. Anesthesia and Analgesia. 2001; 92: 923–6.

156. Strassels SA, McNicol E, Suleman R. Postoperative pain management: a practical review, part 2. American Journal of Health-System Pharmacy. 2005; 62: 2019–25.

157. Yaksh TL, Dirig DM, Malmberg AB. Mechanism of action of nonsteroidal anti-inflammatory drugs. Cancer Investigation. 1998; 16: 509–27.

*158. Samad TA, Sapirstein A, Woolf CJ. Prostanoids and pain: unraveling mechanisms and revealing therapeutic targets. Trends in Molecular Medicine. 2002; 8: 390–6.

159. Samad TA, Moore KA, Sapirstein A et al. Interleukin-1beta-mediated induction of Cox-2 in the CNS contributes to inflammatory pain hypersensitivity. Nature. 2001; 410: 471–5.

160. Tegeder I, Niederberger E, Vetter G et al. Effects of selective COX-1 and -2 inhibition on formalin-evoked nociceptive behaviour and prostaglandin E(2) release in the spinal cord. Journal of Neurochemistry. 2001; 79: 777–86.

161. Reuben SS, Bhopatkar S, Maciolek H et al. The preemptive analgesic effect of rofecoxib after ambulatory arthroscopic knee surgery. Anesthesia and Analgesia. 2002; 94: 55–9.

162. Kokki H, Salonen A. Comparison of pre- and postoperative administration of ketoprofen for analgesia after tonsillectomy in children. Paediatric Anaesthesia. 2002; 12: 162–7.

163. Gramke HF, Petry JJ, Durieux ME et al. Sublingual piroxicam for postoperative analgesia: preoperative versus postoperative administration: a randomized, double-blind study. Anesthesia and Analgesia. 2006; 102: 755–8.

164. Norman PH, Daley MD, Lindsey RW. Preemptive analgesic effects of ketorolac in ankle fracture surgery. Anesthesiology. 2001; 94: 599–603.

*165. Reuben SS, Ekman EF, Raghunathan K et al. The effect of cyclooxygenase-2 inhibition on acute and chronic donor-site pain after spinal-fusion surgery. Regional Anesthesia and Pain Medicine. 2006; 31: 6–13.

166. Boccara G, Chaumeron A, Pouzeratte Y, Mann C. The preoperative administration of ketoprofen improves analgesia after laparoscopic cholecystectomy in comparison with propacetamol or postoperative ketoprofen. British Journal of Anaesthesia. 2005; 94: 347–51.

167. Buvanendran A, Kroin JS, Tuman KJ et al. Effects of perioperative administration of a selective cyclooxygenase 2 inhibitor on pain management and recovery of function after knee replacement: a randomized controlled trial. Journal of the American Medical Association. 2003; 290: 2411–8.

168. Priya V, Divatia JV, Sareen R, Upadhye S. Efficacy of intravenous ketoprofen for pre-emptive analgesia. Journal of Postgraduate Medicine. 2002; 48: 109–12.

169. Norris A, Un V, Chung F et al. When should diclofenac be given in ambulatory surgery: preoperatively or postoperatively? Journal of Clinical Anesthesia. 2001; 13: 11–15.

170. Nakayama M, Ichinose H, Yamamoto S et al. Perioperative intravenous flurbiprofen reduces postoperative pain after abdominal hysterectomy. Canadian Journal of Anaesthesia. 2001; 48: 234–7.

171. Bugter ML, Dirksen R, Jhamandas K et al. Prior ibuprofen exposure does not augment opioid drug potency or modify

opioid requirements for pain inhibition in total hip surgery. *Canadian Journal of Anaesthesia.* 2003; **50**: 445–9.

172. Salonen A, Kokki H, Tuovinen K. I.v. ketoprofen for analgesia after tonsillectomy: comparison of pre- and post-operative administration. *British Journal of Anaesthesia.* 2001; **86**: 377–81.

173. Lim NL, Lo WK, Chong JL, Pan AX. Single dose diclofenac suppository reduces post-Cesarean PCEA requirements. *Canadian Journal of Anaesthesia.* 2001; **48**: 383–6.

174. Graham DJ, Campen D, Hui R et al. Risk of acute myocardial infarction and sudden cardiac death in patients treated with cyclo-oxygenase 2 selective and non-selective non-steroidal anti-inflammatory drugs: nested case–control study. *Lancet.* 2005; **365**: 475–81.

175. Levesque LE, Brophy JM, Zhang B. The risk for myocardial infarction with cyclooxygenase-2 inhibitors: a population study of elderly adults. *Annals of Internal Medicine.* 2005; **142**: 481–9.

176. Brophy JM. Celecoxib and cardiovascular risks. *Expert Opinion on Drug Safety.* 2005; **4**: 1005–15.

*177. Schmid RL, Sandler AN, Katz J. Use and efficacy of low-dose ketamine in the management of acute postoperative pain: a review of current techniques and outcomes. *Pain.* 1999; **82**: 111–25.

178. Weinbroum AA, Rudick V, Paret G, Ben-Abraham R. The role of dextromethorphan in pain control. *Canadian Journal of Anaesthesia.* 2000; **47**: 585–96.

179. Woolf CJ, Thompson SWN. The induction and maintenance of central sensitization is dependent on *N*-methyl-D-aspartic acid receptor activation: Implications for the treatment of post-injury pain hypersensitivity states. *Pain.* 1991; **44**: 293–9.

180. Wilcox GL. Excitatory neurotransmitters and pain. In: Bond MR, Charlton JE, Woolf CJ (eds). *Proceedings of the VIth World Congress on Pain.* Amsterdam: Elsevier Science Publishers BV, 1991: 97–117.

181. Helmy SA, Bali A. The effect of the preemptive use of the NMDA receptor antagonist dextromethorphan on postoperative analgesic requirements. *Anesthesia and Analgesia.* 2001; **92**: 739–44.

182. Himmelseher S, Ziegler-Pithamitsis D, Argiriadou H et al. Small-dose S(+)-ketamine reduces postoperative pain when applied with ropivacaine in epidural anesthesia for total knee arthroplasty. *Anesthesia and Analgesia.* 2001; **92**: 1290–5.

183. Bilgin H, Ozcan B, Bilgin T et al. The influence of timing of systemic ketamine administration on postoperative morphine consumption. *Journal of Clinical Anaesthesia.* 2005; **17**: 592–7.

184. Kwok RF, Lim J, Chan MT et al. Preoperative ketamine improves postoperative analgesia after gynecologic laparoscopic surgery. *Anesthesia and Analgesia.* 2004; **98**: 1044–9.

185. Xie H, Wang X, Liu G, Wang G. Analgesic effects and pharmacokinetics of a low dose of ketamine preoperatively administered epidurally or intravenously. *Clinical Journal of Pain.* 2003; **19**: 317–22.

186. Ganne O, Abisseror M, Menault P et al. Low-dose ketamine failed to spare morphine after a remifentanil-based anaesthesia for ear, nose and throat surgery. *European Journal of Anaesthesiology.* 2005; **22**: 426–30.

187. Adam F, Chauvin M, Du Manoir B et al. Small-dose ketamine infusion improves postoperative analgesia and rehabilitation after total knee arthroplasty. *Anesthesia and Analgesia.* 2005; **100**: 475–80.

188. Katz J, Schmid R, Snijdelaar DG et al. Pre-emptive analgesia using intravenous fentanyl plus low-dose ketamine for radical prostatectomy under general anesthesia does not produce short-term or long-term reductions in pain or analgesic use. *Pain.* 2004; **110**: 707–18.

189. Ozyalcin NS, Yucel A, Camlica H et al. Effect of pre-emptive ketamine on sensory changes and postoperative pain after thoracotomy: comparison of epidural and intramuscular routes. *British Journal of Anaesthesia.* 2004; **93**: 356–61.

190. Yeh CC, Jao SW, Huh BK et al. Preincisional dextromethorphan combined with thoracic epidural anesthesia and analgesia improves postoperative pain and bowel function in patients undergoing colonic surgery. *Anesthesia and Analgesia.* 2005; **100**: 1384–9.

191. Wu CT, Borel CO, Lee MS et al. The interaction effect of perioperative cotreatment with dextromethorphan and intravenous lidocaine on pain relief and recovery of bowel function after laparoscopic cholecystectomy. *Anesthesia and Analgesia.* 2005; **100**: 448–53.

192. Weinbroum AA, Lalayev G, Yashar T et al. Combined pre-incisional oral dextromethorphan and epidural lidocaine for postoperative pain reduction and morphine sparing: a randomised double-blind study on day-surgery patients. *Anaesthesia.* 2001; **56**: 616–22.

193. Kafali H, Aldemir B, Kaygusuz K et al. Small-dose ketamine decreases postoperative morphine requirements. *European Journal of Anaesthesiology.* 2004; **21**: 916–7.

194. Van Elstraete AC, Lebrun T, Sandefo I, Polin B. Ketamine does not decrease postoperative pain after remifentanil-based anaesthesia for tonsillectomy in adults. *Acta Anaesthesiologica Scandinavica.* 2004; **48**: 756–60.

195. Mao J, Price DD, Mayer DJ. Mechanisms of hyperalgesia and morphine tolerance: a current view of their possible interactions. *Pain.* 1995; **62**: 259–74.

196. Celerier E, Laulin J, Larcher A et al. Evidence for opiate-activated NMDA processes masking opiate analgesia in rats. *Brain Research.* 1999; **847**: 18–25.

197. Celerier E, Rivat C, Jun Y et al. Long-lasting hyperalgesia induced by fentanyl in rats: preventive effect of ketamine. *Anesthesiology.* 2000; **92**: 465–72.

198. Dickenson AH. Plasticity: implications for opioid and other pharmacological interventions in specific pain states. *Behavioral and Brain Sciences.* 1997; **20**: 392–403; discussion 35–513.

199. Dickenson AH, Sullivan AF. Combination therapy in analgesia: Seeking synergy. *Current Opinion in Anaesthesiology.* 1993; **6**: 86–9.

200. Gilron I, Max MB. Combination pharmacotherapy for neuropathic pain: current evidence and future directions. *Expert Review of Neurotherapeutics.* 2005; **5**: 823–30.

201. Rosaeg OP, Krepski B, Cicutti N *et al.* Effect of preemptive multimodal analgesia for arthroscopic knee ligament repair. *Regional Anesthesia and Pain Medicine.* 2001; **26**: 125–30.

202. Holthusen H, Backhaus P, Boeminghaus F *et al.* Preemptive analgesia: no relevant advantage of preoperative compared with postoperative intravenous administration of morphine, ketamine, and clonidine in patients undergoing transperitoneal tumor nephrectomy. *Regional Anesthesia and Pain Medicine.* 2002; **27**: 249–53.

203. Ng HP, Nordstrom U, Axelsson K *et al.* Efficacy of intra-articular bupivacaine, ropivacaine, or a combination of ropivacaine, morphine, and ketorolac on postoperative pain relief after ambulatory arthroscopic knee surgery: a randomized double-blind study. *Regional Anesthesia and Pain Medicine.* 2006; **31**: 26–33.

204. Naja MZ, El-Rajab M, Kabalan W *et al.* Pre-incisional infiltration for pediatric tonsillectomy: a randomized double-blind clinical trial. *International Journal of Pediatric Otorhinolaryngology.* 2005; **69**: 1333–41.

205. Chia YY, Lo Y, Liu K *et al.* The effect of promethazine on postoperative pain: a comparison of preoperative, postoperative, and placebo administration in patients following total abdominal hysterectomy. *Acta Anaesthesiologica Scandinavica.* 2004; **48**: 625–30.

206. Sen S, Ugur B, Aydin ON *et al.* The analgesic effect of nitroglycerin added to lidocaine on intravenous regional anesthesia. *Anesthesia and Analgesia.* 2006; **102**: 916–20.

207. Unlugenc H, Gunduz M, Guler T *et al.* The effect of pre-anaesthetic administration of intravenous dexmedetomidine on postoperative pain in patients receiving patient-controlled morphine. *European Journal of Anaesthesiology.* 2005; **22**: 386–91.

208. Lang E, Hord AH, Denson D. Venlafaxine hydrochloride (Effexor) relieves thermal hyperalgesia in rats with an experimental mononeuropathy. *Pain.* 1996; **68**: 151–5.

209. Bach S, Noreng MF, Tjellden NU. Phantom limb pain in amputees during the first 12 months following limb amputation, after preoperative lumbar epidural blockade. *Pain.* 1988; **33**: 297–301.

210. Aida S, Fujihara H, Taga K *et al.* Involvement of presurgical pain in preemptive analgesia for orthopedic surgery: a randomized double blind study. *Pain.* 2000; **84**: 169–73.

211. Eisenach JC. Preemptive hyperalgesia, not analgesia? *Anesthesiology.* 2000; **92**: 308–09.

212. Crain SM, Shen KF. Antagonists of excitatory opioid receptor functions enhance morphine's analgesic potency and attenuate opioid tolerance/dependence liability. *Pain.* 2000; **84**: 121–31.

213. Li X, Angst MS, Clark JD. Opioid-induced hyperalgesia and incisional pain. *Anesthesia and Analgesia.* 2001; **93**: 204–09.

214. Katz J, Melzack R. Measurement of pain. *Surgical Clinics of North America.* 1999; **79**: 231–52.

215. Tverskoy M, Oz Y, Isakson A *et al.* Preemptive effect of fentanyl and ketamine on postoperative pain and wound hyperalgesia. *Anesthesia and Analgesia.* 1994; **78**: 205–09.

216. Kavanagh BP, Katz J, Sandler AN *et al.* Multimodal analgesia before thoracic surgery does not reduce postoperative pain. *British Journal of Anaesthesia.* 1994; **73**: 184–9.

217. Wilder-Smith OH, Tassonyi E, Senly C *et al.* Surgical pain is followed not only by spinal sensitization but also by supraspinal antinociception (published erratum appears in *British Journal of Anaesthesia.* 1996; **77**: 566–7). *British Journal of Anaesthesia.* 1996; **76**: 816–21.

218. Katz J, Clairoux M, Kavanagh BP *et al.* Pre-emptive lumbar epidural anaesthesia reduces postoperative pain and patient-controlled morphine consumption after lower abdominal surgery. *Pain.* 1994; **59**: 395–403.

219. Turk DC. Cognitive-behavioral approach to the treatment of chronic pain patients. *Regional Anesthesia and Pain Medicine.* 2003; **28**: 573–9.

*220. Dworkin RH, Turk DC, Farrar JT *et al.* Core outcome measures for chronic pain clinical trials: IMMPACT recommendations. *Pain.* 2005; **113**: 9–19.

PART II

MANAGEMENT – TECHNIQUES

Routes of administration

JEREMY CASHMAN

KEY LEARNING POINTS

- Nonsteroidal anti-inflammatory drugs (NSAID) given rectally or by injection do not perform better or faster than the same dose of the same drug given by mouth.
- Topical NSAIDs are effective for acute pain of musculoskeletal origin.
- Opioids by injection are effective in the treatment of moderate-to-severe acute postoperative pain (intramuscular≡subcutaneous ≤ intravenous/intravenous patient-controlled analgesia (PCA)).
- Epidural opioid administration is superior to parenteral routes of opioid administration.
- Transdermal iontophoretic opioid administration may be as effective as opioids by injection.
- Other new formulations and systems of drug delivery also show promise.

INTRODUCTION

Since antiquity, man has used the extracts of plant products to produce medicaments which have then been ingested. The Ebers Papyrus (circa 1552BC) provides evidence of the medicinal use of the dried powdered extract of unripe capsules of the poppy head (opium), in ancient Egyptian prescriptions. Salicylic acid, a constituent of several plants, has an equally long history of use as a medicament. The Ebers Papyrus recommended the application of a decoction of dried leaves of myrtle to the abdomen and back to expel rheumatic pains from the womb. Hippocrates in the fifth century BC recommended the use of willow bark for pain in childbirth and for fever, whilst Theophrastus at the beginning of the third century BC provides the first authentic reference to the use of opium. Throughout Roman times and the Middle Ages, topically applied willow bark was used for its healing effects and to relieve mild to moderate pain. Thomas Sydenham introduced tincture of opium (laudanum) into England in the latter part of the fifteenth century, but it is Sir Christopher Wren who is credited in 1665 with the first intravenous injection of laudanum into a dog using a bladder attached to a sharpened quill. In 1763 Rev. Edward Stone reported to the Royal Society on the successful use of extract of the bark of the willow *Salix alba vulgaris* in the treatment of fever. At the time, Stone remarked on the extreme bitter taste. The techniques of intranasal and inhalation administration of dried plant extracts followed the discovery of tobacco. Although the routes of administration of drugs continued to evolve up until the end of the twentieth century, more recently attention has focused on developing new formulations and mechanisms for enhancing drug delivery. This trend has continued (even since the first edition of this book), such that there are now a wide variety of routes and formulations available for administration of analgesic drugs. Indeed the Food and Drug Administration (FDA) recognizes 111 distinct routes for drug administration (www.fda.gov/cder/dsm/DRG/drg00301). However, only a proportion of these routes are appropriate for systemic analgesic drug administration (**Table 10.1**). Furthermore, some routes (e.g. dermal, intranasal, inhalational) can be used for both systemic administration as well as topical effect. This chapter will consider the available routes for systemic (as opposed to topical) administration of analgesic drugs before presenting the evidence for advantage of one route of administration over another for both nonopioid and for opioid analgesic drugs.

ORAL

The oral route is the most commonly used route of administration and is the route of choice so long as the gastrointestinal tract is intact and the patient is able to take fluids by mouth. However, the delay between drug administration and onset of effect is at least 20 minutes and often much longer. Differences in rates of absorption depend on whether tablets, capsules, suspension, enteric coating, or slow-, sustained-, or controlled-release preparations are used. In addition, absorption into the portal circulation can result in significant presystemic metabolism resulting in markedly reduced bioavailability of

Table 10.1 Routes of systemic drug administration.

Route of administration		
Enteral	Oral	
	Rectal	
Parenteral (by injection)	Intramuscular	
	Subcutaneous	
	Intravenous	
Parenteral (other than by injection)	Transdermal	
	Transmucosal	Buccal
		Sublingual
		Intranasal
	Inhalational	
Neuraxial	Perineural	
	Epidural	
	Intrathecal	
Other	Intra-articular	
	Intrawound	

the drug. Thus, oral dosing regimens may need to be modified to take account of drug loss due to first-pass hepatic metabolism. It is also preferable that drug metabolites should be inactive and noncumulative.

Nonopioid analgesics

Nonsteroidal anti-inflammatory drugs (NSAID) as a group are insoluble acidic compounds. The time to peak plasma concentration (t_{max}) after oral administration in humans has been determined for a number of NSAIDs (**Table 10.2**). However, it has been noted for many NSAIDs that peak analgesia is delayed after maximum plasma concentration (C_{max}). The speed of absorption of ibuprofen can be increased using arginine and lysine salts. Both are nonessential amino acids which improve the rate of absorption of NSAIDs by enhancing transfer across gastric and enteric mucosa. A similar acceleration of absorption is achieved by linking the NSAID to β-cyclodextrin (e.g. piroxicam).[1][V] The t_{max} for a standard oral formulation of ibuprofen to produce maximum plasma concentration is approximately 1–1.5 hours after oral administration. Ibuprofen arginine is absorbed much more rapidly, with peak plasma concentration occurring within 15–20 minutes,[2][IV] while C_{max} for ibuprofen lysine occurs in 45 minutes.[3][III] An equivalent dose of ibuprofen arginine results in approximately 30 percent higher C_{max} than an identical dose of the standard formulation. The relative bioavailability of the two preparations is similar, as are the mean values for elimination half-life, total area under the concentration–time curve (AUC), apparent volume of distribution (V_d), and clearance (CL).[2][IV] Another formulation of ibuprofen (liquid filled capsule; ibuprofen liquigel) has a kinetic profile similar to ibuprofen suspension, with both a higher C_{max} and an earlier t_{max} than any solid tablet and onset of pain relief in under 25 minutes.[4][II] Similarly, an effervescent solution of paracetamol (acetaminophen) halves the time to onset of pain relief compared with tablet formulation following dental surgery.[5][II]

In surgical patients, oral ibuprofen arginine has a similar efficacy profile to intramuscular ketorolac, both being superior to placebo,[6][II] whilst in postcesarian section pain, the time to maximum analgesia of ibuprofen arginine is similar to intramuscular ketorolac.[7][II] Feldene "melt," a matrix of freeze-dried piroxicam in a fast dissolving excipient, rapidly dissolves in saliva and is swallowed as a solution. In a double-blind, randomized, double-dummy study, Feldene "melt" provided equivalent analgesia to rectal diclofenac when given 1 hour before surgery.[8][II] Speed of absorption is also increased using a single isomer compared with a racemic mixture of the same NSAID. Median values for t_{max} are shorter (30 versus 75 minutes) and for C_{max} are higher and less variable with dexketoprofen trometamol than for racemic ketoprofen.[9][III] At least one clinical study has confirmed

Table 10.2 Pharmacokinetic data of various nonopioids.

Drug	Bioavailability (%)		Time to peak plasma concentration t_{max} (h)	Half-life (h)
	Oral	Rectal		
Paracetamol	60–70	30–40	0.4–0.9	~3
Celecoxib	~40		2.0–4.0	9–11
Diclofenac	50–60	~65	2.0–3.0	2–3
Flurbiprofen	>95		1.5–3.0	3–6
Ibuprofen	>95		0.5–1.5	2–5
Indometacin	100	80	1.0–2.0	4–8
Ketoprofen	~100		0.3	2–4
Ketorolac	80		0.5–1.0	4–6
Naproxen	95		1.0–2.0	10–20
Piroxicam	~100		2.0	40–80
Tenoxicam	100	80	1.0–4.0	44–100

Adapted from published data.

a rapid onset of analgesic action of dexketoprofen. Following removal of impacted third molars, the time to reduce pain by at least 50 percent was shorter in patients treated with oral dexketoprofen trometamol than in patients who had received oral ibuprofen (mean 0.9 versus 2.1 hours).[10][II] There are a limited number of trials of the few coxibs that are licensed for postoperative pain relief. A Cochrane review has concluded that single-dose oral celecoxib is at least as effective as paracetamol for relieving postoperative pain, despite finding only two trials of celecoxib that met their inclusion criteria.[11][I] A subsequent larger systematic review of 22 trials (2246 patients) concluded that preoperative oral coxibs (mainly celecoxib and rofecoxib) were effective in reducing postoperative pain, but were unable to draw any conclusions from three trials comparing coxibs with traditional NSAIDs.[12][I]

Opioid analgesics

There are several formulations of oral morphine. For simplicity, these can be considered as morphine in solution, immediate-release morphine tablets, and controlled-release morphine tablets. After ingestion, oral morphine undergoes significant first-pass metabolism. Peak plasma concentrations occur within one hour of morphine in solution and immediate-release tablets, while controlled-release morphine tablets produce delayed peak plasma concentrations at two to four hours, but long-lasting (up to 24 hours depending on the formulation) analgesia. Furthermore, a systematic review found no difference in dose-corrected C_{max} or t_{max} between morphine in solution and immediate-release morphine tablets or between different morphine salts, and little difference between the various controlled-release morphine formulations.[13][I] The potency ratio of oral to parenteral morphine is 1:6 for acute pain, but 1:2 to 1:3 for nonacute pain (**Table 10.3**).

Table 10.3 Potency of oral morphine relative to other routes of administration.

Oral to	Morphine potency ratio
Rectal	1:1
Subcutaneous	1:2
Intravenous	1:3–1:6

There are reports of the satisfactory[14, 15][III] and unsatisfactory[16][II] use of oral morphine preparations in the early treatment of postoperative pain. Nevertheless, oral morphine administered regularly is superior to intramuscular morphine administered on-demand,[17][II] but the tendency for oral preparations to delay gastric emptying would seem to be a significant disadvantage.[15][II] A number of other oral opioids can be used for postoperative pain relief, including dihydrocodeine, oxycodone, and oxymorphone. A Cochrane review found that a single dose of oral dihydrocodeine was inferior to ibuprofen and does not provide adequate postoperative pain relief.[18][I] In contrast, a single dose of oral oxycodone is of comparable efficacy to intramuscular morphine, albeit at the expense of a high incidence of adverse effects.[19][I] Immediate-release oral oxymorphone is also effective for postsurgical pain with a safety profile similar to oxycodone.[20][I] In an early meta-analysis, oral tramadol was found to have an analgesic efficacy comparable with simple combination analgesics (tramadol 100 mg NNT 4.8),[21][I] but a subsequent review suggested that the overall analgesic efficacy of oral tramadol was similar to equianalgesic doses of morphine.[22][IV]

Controlled-release preparations have been used for postoperative pain relief. There are conflicting reports of the effectiveness of controlled-release oxycodone (usually administered preoperatively) in the early treatment of postoperative pain. However, a direct comparison of controlled-release oxycodone with standard oxycodone following joint arthroplasty surgery revealed that the controlled-release formulation did not provide better pain control than the immediate release formulation administered regularly.[23][IV] Nevertheless, both controlled-release oxycodone[24, 25][II] and controlled-release oxymorphone[26] [IV] significantly reduce postoperative intravenous (i.v.)-patient-controlled analgesia (PCA) opioid consumption, whilst conversion from i.v.-PCA to regular controlled-release oxycodone can provide adequate pain control for up to seven days postoperatively.[27][IV]

RECTAL

Rectal administration results in absorption directly into the systemic circulation, with resultant greater drug bioavailability. Correct placement of the suppository is important; too high inside the rectum results in absorption into the superior rectal vein (which drains into the portal system) rather than middle and inferior rectal veins, resulting in greater first-pass metabolism. Similarly, the formulation of the suppository affects the rapidity of absorption: hydrophilic formulations result in much more efficient and rapid absorption than fatty suppositories.[28, 29][IV] Hydrogels are biologically inert and hydrophilic, expanding to two to four times their original volume on hydration.

Nonopioid analgesics

Rectal administration is associated with a slow onset of effect which may be influenced by patient factors, as well as formulation. The bioavailability of rectally administered paracetamol is only 30–40 percent, whilst the time to peak plasma concentration is two to four hours.[30][III] There are no major pharmacokinetic differences between infants <1 year and adults after rectal administration of ibuprofen apart from a faster absorption.[31][III] In a single-dose crossover study comparing rectal with oral administration of a diclofenac–codeine combination, the AUC was similar but C_{max} following rectal administration was 50 percent of that following oral administration, whilst t_{max} was prolonged.[32][IV] A liquid gel suppository is associated with enhanced rectal bioavailability of ibuprofen, higher initial plasma concentration and AUC, than a solid suppository.[33][III] The pharmacokinetics of rectal ketoprofen are unaffected by whether a fatty or gelatin-capsulated formulation is used, but surgery may markedly influence absorption. Thus C_{max} was decreased, t_{max} was prolonged, and the absorption rate constant was significantly lower with rectal ketoprofen in surgical patients than in healthy controls.[34][III] Furthermore, the bioavailability of diclofenac suppositories is decreased by insertion into a colostomy due to an increased first-pass effect. Consequently, the dose of diclofenac suppository

should be increased with intrastomal insertion.[35] However, there seems to be no significant difference between rectal and parenteral, or for that matter oral, administration of NSAIDs[36][I] or of paracetamol[37][I] for postoperative pain relief. In renal colic, NSAIDs are as effective as opioids,[38][I] but although rectal administration is inferior to intravenous administration,[36][I] it is associated with fewer side effects than either intravenous administration[39][II] or opioids.[37][I]

A reduction in adverse gastric effects is the perceived advantage of NSAIDs as a suppository, but although rectal administration of NSAIDs can reduce adverse gastric effects, there is marked variation between NSAIDs in the extent to which gastric mucosal damage is systemically or topically mediated. In the case of naproxen, damage is almost entirely topically mediated and use of a suppository formulation is not associated with gastric mucosal damage.[40][III] Nevertheless, rectal NSAID administration is not without its own problems. Proctitis has been reported with rectal indometacin (indomethacin) administration in postoperative orthopedic patients.[41][II]

Opioid analgesics

In general, rectal opioid dosing roughly equates to oral opioid dosing. Morphine suppositories have similar bioavailability and duration of effect as oral morphine with a potency ratio relative to oral morphine of 1:1. Morphine is presented commonly as a hydrogel suppository. Morphine hydrogel suppositories can provide sustained analgesia over a long period of time. In a volunteer study, morphine hydrogel suppository had 53 percent bioavailability, whilst C_{max} was achieved in 30–60 minutes.[42][III] In contrast, rectal administration of codeine results in rapid absorption and identical plasma concentration profile to that following oral administration.[43][IV] In a comparison of morphine hydrogel suppository, morphine-in-solution suppository, and intravenous morphine in children, morphine hydrogel suppository was associated with greater bioavailability than morphine-in-solution suppository. Significant first-pass metabolism occurred.[44][III] Oxycodone suppositories have a similar bioavailability to that of morphine, but provide sustained analgesia over a longer period of time (8–12 hours).[45][IV] Morphine suppository inserted into a colostomy results in much greater variability in absorption than with the rectal route and is not recommended.[46][III]

INTRAMUSCULAR AND SUBCUTANEOUS

The intramuscular route is popular for analgesic drug administration, but absorption can be erratic and repeat needling is often necessary. This latter problem can be avoided by use of an indwelling cannnula, e.g. into the deltoid muscle. Results are variable with respect to speed of onset, intensity, and duration of analgesia. Injection into a well-perfused muscle results in faster onset and greater peak plasma levels than injection into a less well-perfused muscle or indeed adipose tissue. There has also been a resurgence of interest in subcutaneous administration of opioid analgesics in acute and nonacute pain management. Aqueous, nonirritating solutions are preferred. Analgesic solutions should be concentrated to ensure small volume. Nevertheless, the infusion site should be changed regularly (every four days or so). Absorption can be unpredictable. In general, subcutaneous and intramuscular drug administration regimens can be used interchangeably.

Nonopioid analgesics

As few NSAIDs can be given intramuscularly, there are limited data comparing intramuscularly administered NSAIDs with NSAIDs given by other routes. Oral ketorolac 10 mg is at least as effective as intramuscular ketorolac 30 mg.[47][I] Furthermore, intramuscular ketorolac 60 mg is comparable with parecoxib 40 mg which is equally effective whether administered intramuscularly or intravenously.[48][II] Preoperative intramuscular lornoxicam is more effective than intramuscular ketoprofen in reducing postoperative pain.[49][II]

Opioid analgesics

Traditionally, opioids have been given intramuscularly. The precise muscle chosen is not important as long as it is of sufficiently large bulk. Thus, morphine absorption is similar from the gluteal and deltoid muscles.[50][III] The subcutaneous route is generally less painful than the intramuscular one, although it may not be practical in many patients, e.g. in patients with generalized edema. Intermittent injections of morphine or diamorphine subcutaneously seem to be as effective as the intravenous or intramuscular routes with greater patient acceptance.[51][III], [52][IV], [53][II] An early study by Rutter and colleagues suggested that the intravenous route of opioid administration was superior to the intramuscular one.[54][III] The efficacy of injected morphine relative to that provided by oral analgesics in patients with moderate to severe postoperative pain has been examined in a systematic review of randomized trials.[55][I] The authors considered randomized controlled trials of the use of opioids in the management of postoperative pain. They were unable to find any suitable studies of subcutaneous administration and were able to find only one intravenous study. It was only in the case of 10-mg intramuscular morphine that sufficient numbers of patients were studied to allow a pooling of results. A single intramuscular dose of

morphine had a number needed to treat (NNT) of 2.9 for at least 50 percent pain relief compared with placebo. By comparison, a similar NNT of 2.7 for 400 mg ibuprofen has been reported by the same authors.

INTRAVENOUS

The intravenous route of analgesic drug administration is the "gold standard" against which all other routes of administration are compared. This is because of the rapidity of onset of action associated with intravenous drug administration and because it avoids uncertainty of drug absorption. However, the plasma concentration of drug following bolus dosing declines rapidly, resulting in short-lived analgesia; this problem can be overcome by using a continuous infusion.

Nonopioid analgesics

A number of NSAIDs are available for parenteral administration. Despite the more rapid absorption rate and shorter time to C_{max} associated with parenteral compared with oral administration, there is a delay in the time to maximum pharmacological effect relative to the time to peak plasma concentration. It has been shown, using radiolabeled ketorolac, that the time to peak plasma concentration after intravenous administration is achieved in less than five minutes and more slowly after intramuscular (45 minutes) and oral (30 minutes) administration.[56][III] Parenteral dexketoprofen is associated with similar values.[57][III] However, the time to peak plasma concentration correlates poorly with onset of analgesia, which does not reach a peak until 30 minutes after i.v. administration. This delay in effect has also been noted with ibuprofen[2][IV] and aspirin.[58][IV] Furthermore, serum ibuprofen concentration shows poor correlation with clinical analgesia over time.[59][III] The evidence for an advantage of injected or rectal over oral administration of NSAIDs has been examined in a systematic review of randomized controlled trials.[36][I] The authors considered randomized controlled trials of the use of NSAIDs in the management of postoperative pain. Only five trials satisfied the authors' strict criteria for internal sensitivity and validity. In comparisons of just two drugs, diclofenac and ketorolac, across routes, they found no evidence of the superiority of one route over another. Subsequently published studies of diclofenac,[60, 61, 62][II] ketorolac,[63, 64][II] dipyrone,[65][II] and indometacin,[66, 67][II] have not contradicted these findings. A systematic review of oral valdecoxib and intravenous parecoxib for acute postoperative pain has also found no evidence of the superiority of one route over the other.[68][I] Similarly, a study comparing oral versus intravenous paracetamol following dental extraction found no difference in pain intensity between the two routes, although onset of analgesia was faster with intravenous para-cetamol.[69][II]

Opioid analgesics

The concept has been promoted that for every opioid there is a minimum effective analgesic concentration (MEAC) which can be expected to provide freedom from severe pain in at least 95 percent of cases.[70][III] Therefore, intravenous infusion regimens should aim to achieve and maintain this concentration, usually by means of a bolus loading dose followed by an infusion rate set to equal elimination rate. Unfortunately, there is great inter-individual variability, with MEAC varying four-fold in patients recovering from surgery.[71][III] Although MEAC has not achieved widespread acceptance, a recent study has found evidence to support the concept of a therapeutic window for fentanyl.[72][III]

In practice, it is simpler to titrate to effect rather than to a predetermined plasma concentration. Intravenous opioid bolus dose titration is a simple and effective technique used to obtain pain relief, particularly in the postanesthesia care unit (PACU) or recovery ward. A predetermined dose of opioid is administered intravenously at fixed time intervals until pain is relieved, this is then followed by subcutaneous opioid administration after a further time interval.[73][IV]

Patient-controlled analgesia

Patient-controlled analgesia is a further development of intravenous analgesic delivery. PCA refers to the on-demand, intermittent, self-administration of an analgesic drug (predominantly opioid, but other classes of drugs can be used) by a patient. The traditional route of drug delivery has been intravenous (i.v.-PCA), but the sub-cutaneous (s.c.-PCA), epidural (patient-controlled epidural analgesia; PCEA), and intranasal (i.n.-PCA) routes can also be used. The quality of analgesia is normally good and allows for wide interpatient variation. The basic variables of PCA are demand (bolus) dose, lockout interval (length of the time between patient demands), background infusion rate (if used), and hourly or four-hourly limit.

Intravenous PCA is more effective than conventional administration of opioid analgesics with no increase in opioid-related side effects,[74][I], [75][1I1], [76][III] whilst subcutaneous PCA is as effective as intravenous PCA,[77] [II] but see Chapter 11, Patient-controlled analgesia, for a more detailed analysis.

TRANSDERMAL

Transdermal drug delivery allows for slow but controlled release of drug with avoidance of first-pass metabolism. Unfortunately, the skin provides an impermeable barrier to most molecules, although highly lipid-soluble drugs can penetrate into and beyond the stratum corneum by passive diffusion. Uptake from skin capillaries provides the basis for systemic efficacy, but skin blood flow can virtually cease with extreme vasoconstriction and can increase by up to ten-fold with vasodilatation. Drug delivery rate with the earlier patches was dependent on a rate-controlling membrane, such that the area of the applied patch determined the dose. However, with the newer transdermal therapeutic matrix systems there is no drug reservoir or rate-controlling membrane as the opioid is dissolved in the adhesive matrix itself. Washin and washout of drug after patch removal tends to be slow, probably because the skin acts as a depot for the drug. Various physical methods have been developed to over-come some of these obstacles, including microporation, liposome encapsulation, needleless high pressure gas jet injectors, ultrasound sonophoresis, pulsed magnetic fields, and iontophoresis.[78] The technique of iontophor-esis has proved particularly useful in overcoming some of the problems inherent in transdermal drug administra-tion. In this method of transdermal administration, electrically charged molecules of ionized drug are pro-pelled through the skin by an external electrical field (electrorepulsion). Further increase in transdermal drug permeation can be achieved by combining iontophoresis with chemical enhancers and sonophoresis.[79]

Nonopioid analgesics

Transdermal penetration varies considerably among NSAIDs. An *in vitro* study using human skin has inves-tigated the transdermal absorption of a series of NSAIDs.[80] The authors found that diclofenac had the highest *in vitro* transdermal penetration whilst ketoprofen had the highest flux, but ketorolac provided plasma concentrations at steady state that were closest to ther-apeutic concentration. These findings suggest that ketor-olac might be suitable for formulation as a transdermal delivery system. For other NSAIDs, the formation of an eutectic mixture with a permeation enhancer may markedly increase transdermal permeation. Feasibility studies conducted on a membrane-controlled transder-mal drug delivery system indicate that oleic acid provides the maximum enhancement of permeation of ketoprofen across an artificial membrane.[81] An increase in ketoprofen loading also increased permeation. An *in vitro* investiga-tion of permeation of ibuprofen–terpene mixtures across human epidermal membranes showed a significant increase in transdermal penetration and a greater than 12-fold increase in flux compared with an aqueous solution of ibuprofen.[82] The profile of distribution of ibuprofen within the tissues differs with transdermal or oral administration.[83][IV] Oral administration is associated with higher concentrations of ibuprofen in plasma and synovial fluid than transdermal application.

Conversely, higher concentrations of ibuprofen are found in the subcutaneous tissue and muscle directly beneath the site of application. This might explain the advantage of transdermal over oral administration of ibuprofen in the management of pain of muscular origin.[84][III]

An early review considered that topical NSAIDs were of uncertain value in the treatment of soft-tissue injuries and called for more convincing evidence.[85][IV] A recent systematic review of the evidence that topical NSAIDs are effective and safe for soft-tissue injuries, strains, sprains, and minor trauma (but not postoperative pain) has come to the same conclusions as an earlier review.[86, 87][I] The authors reviewed studies which were either placebo-controlled or compared different topical NSAIDs, formulations, or routes of administration. Only three trials in their sample compared topical with oral NSAIDs, one of which included a placebo control. In acute painful conditions, topical NSAIDs are significantly better than placebo over a period of one week. The number needed to treat was 3.9. Pooling data for each drug indicated that, of the drugs studied, ketoprofen, felbinac, ibuprofen, and piroxicam were significantly superior to placebo. However, none of the three studies comparing topical with oral NSAID showed significant benefit of topical over oral NSAID. Local or systemic effects were rare. The same group has conducted a systematic review of the evidence that topical rubefacients containing salicylates are effective and safe for acute (soft-tissue injuries, strains, sprains, and minor trauma) pain. They identified only three eligible trials. Based on this limited information, they concluded that such preparations were significantly better than placebo (NNT, 2.1) and adverse events were rare.[88][I]

Opioid analgesics

Highly lipophilic opioids are ideally suited to transdermal delivery. Thus, the transdermal fentanyl patch system provides sustained delivery of fentanyl at a constant rate for up to 72 hours, varying between 25 and 100 μg/hour depending on the patch. Unfortunately, there is a considerable delay between patch application and minimum concentration for effective analgesia (>12 hours) and t_{max} (>17 hours).[89][III] The delay in achieving an adequate blood fentanyl concentration may be due to depot accumulation of the drug within the skin under the patch before the drug diffuses into the systemic circulation.[89][III] Two systems of transdermal fentanyl delivery are currently available; the original "transdermal reservoir" system and a new "drug-in-adhesive matrix" system. The two systems are comparable with respect to bioequivalence and patient tolerability.[90][III] Buprenorphine is also available as a drug-in-adhesive matrix delivery system, but in a comparative study with fentanyl the system was associated with greater skin irritation than the fentanyl matrix system.[91][III] Clinical studies of transdermal fentanyl in the management of acute,

nonstable pain, such as postoperative pain, have revealed wide variability in clinical effect. In some clinical trials, transdermal patches were applied up to eight hours before surgery in an attempt to circumvent the slow washin of fentanyl. Unfortunately, the therapeutic benefits of transdermal fentanyl are largely outweighed by the risks.[92][II] Hypoventilation is the most serious adverse respiratory event, being especially common in opioid-naive patients when there is no opportunity for dose titration. Consequently, transdermal fentanyl administration is not recommended for postoperative pain relief,[93, 94][II] although subsequent studies of transdermal fentanyl for postoperative pain sought to avoid additional opioid administration by utilizing intramuscular ketorolac.[95][III], [96][II]

Studies of iontophoretically delivered opioids have been encouraging. Unlike passive transdermal fentanyl delivery, absorption of fentanyl (and of sufentanil) is rapid with no evidence of a skin depot.[97] A fentanyl HCl patient-controlled transdermal system (PCTS) for iontophoretic analgesia was granted market authorization by the European Union in January 2006; in North America, FDA approval was granted in May 2006. In a crossover study of healthy subjects, the system was shown to have a similar pharmacokinetic profile to intravenous fentanyl infusion.[98][IV] Furthermore, in a study of 636 patients, the efficacy of fentanyl HCl PCTS was therapeutically equivalent to a standard regimen of morphine i.v.-PCA.[99][II] The incidences of opioid-related adverse events were similar in both groups, but erythema after system removal occurred in more than half of patients and took up to four weeks to resolve.[99][II]

TRANSMUCOSAL

Buccal, sublingual, and intranasal routes of administration provide direct drug entry into the systemic circulation with avoidance of the problems of presystemic metabolism. These routes are also unaffected by the delay in gastric emptying that occurs during the perioperative period, which can limit the usefulness of orally administered analgesic drugs. In addition to lipophilicity, unionized drugs of low molecular weight have higher transmucosal permeability. Furthermore, drug bioavailability by these routes will depend on the proportion of drug swallowed. Mucoadhesive microparticulate drug delivery systems have been developed to improve residence time on buccal, sublingual, and intranasal mucosa, as well as drug dissolution rate.

Buccal and sublingual

NONOPIOID ANALGESICS

A buccal formulation of aspirin was associated with buccal ulceration and is no longer available. In contrast, piroxicam loaded into microparticles shows promise as a mucoadhesive sublingual drug delivery sytem.[100]

OPIOID ANALGESICS

Lipophilic opioid drugs exhibit better sublingual absorption than hydrophilic opioid drugs. Buprenorphine and fentanyl are well absorbed at the pH level found in the mouth. For these lipophilic opioids, a contact time of 2.5 minutes is sufficient to achieve extensive absorption. For morphine, a very much more prolonged contact time (six hours) is necessary before buccal bioavailability becomes equivalent to that of the intramuscular route.[101][IV] The time to maximum plasma concentration following buccal administration is longer than with oral administration, but C_{max} is the same.[102][IV] In another study, buccal morphine bioavailability was <20 percent and C_{max} was reached at six hours.[103][IV] Changing the formulation may help. A new bioadhesive buccal morphine tablet can be retained in place for up to six hours to provide sustained analgesia.[104][IV] Alternatively, sodium glycocholate may be useful as a permeation-enhancing agent.[105] Studies of buccal morphine have been confined to its use as a premedicant rather than in the treatment of postoperative pain. In one study, buccal morphine (30 mg) resulted in a lower C_{max}, worse absorption, and worse analgesia than intramuscular morphine (10 mg).[106][IV] In an early volunteer study, the pharmacokinetics and bioavailability of a new aerosolized sublingual morphine were the same as oral morphine, but there was a suggestion that analgesia was more rapid in onset.[107][IV] Currently, there is no evidence of any clinical advantage over oral morphine of the buccal, sublingual, or even nebulized sublingual routes for morphine administration. However, the sublingual and transdermal routes of administration of other more lipid-soluble opioids may constitute a useful alternative to morphine. Oral transmucosal fentanyl citrate (OTFC) lollipops in doses up to 20 µg/kg are useful for premedication in children and for procedure pain. Plasma concentrations rapidly reach levels associated with analgesia and peak within 25 minutes.[108][II], [109][II], [110][III] Rapid consumption is desirable as delay results in decreased absorption. Although experience is limited, OTFC is unlikely to be of great use in postoperative pain.[111][II] Fentanyl effervescent buccal tablet (FEB) may be a promising alternative, having a significantly faster t_{max} and greater C_{max} than OTFC.[112][IV]

Intranasal

Intranasal drug delivery takes advantage of the significant systemic absorption that occurs throughout the nasal mucosa. However, drug-metabolizing enzymes are present in the nasal mucosa that may create a pseudo-first-pass effect,[113] although the significance of this effect is not known.[114]

OPIOID ANALGESICS

A number of opioids are available for intranasal administration, but most experience has been with butorphanol. Butorphanol undergoes significant presystemic hepatic metabolism, resulting in a low oral bioavailability of 5–17 percent. This compares with a bioavailability of approximately 70 percent when administered intranasally. Intravenous, intramuscular, and intranasal administration results in similar plasma concentration-time curves. Onset of analgesia occurs within 15 minutes, with peak concentrations reached 30–60 minutes after intranasal administration.[115][IV] **Table 10.4** outlines the pharmacokinetics of other intranasally administered opioids. The pharmacokinetics of intranasal butorphanol are unaffected by inflammation of nasal passages, as in allergic rhinitis. In contrast, nasal vasoconstriction significantly decreases C_{max} and extends t_{max}, but AUC and absolute bioavailability are not affected.[115][IV] In a single-dose study, intranasal butorphanol provided similar analgesia to intramuscular pethidine (meperidine) in postoperative patients with moderate to severe pain.[116] [II] In a multiple dose study, intranasal butorphanol provided similar analgesia to intravenous butorphanol in postcesarian section pain. Intravenous butorphanol resulted in a more rapid onset of action (5 versus 15 minutes), but intranasal butorphanol was associated with a significantly longer duration of analgesia.[117][II] Intranasal diamorphine, although associated with fewer side effects, is less effective than i.v.-PCA diamorphine in the early postoperative period,[118][II] whilst intranasal pethidine is superior to subcutaneous pethidine with a similar incidence of nausea and vomiting.[119][IV] Intranasal fentanyl provides similar analgesia to intravenous fentanyl in children[120][II] and in adults.[121][II], [122] [III], [123][IV] with rapid (<5 minutes) onset.[123][IV] However, as a result of stinging associated with the intranasal spray, patients tend to prefer the intravenous over the intranasal route of administration.[123][IV] Intranasal sufentanil also provides effective postoperative analgesia.[124][IV]

Table 10.4 Pharmacokinetics of intranasal opioids.[114]

Drug	Bioavailability (%)	Time to peak plasma concentration t_{max} (min)
Alfentanil	65	9
Buprenorphine	48	30
Butorphanol	71	49
Fentanyl	71	5
Hydromorphone	55	20
Oxycodone	46	25
Sufentanil	78	10

Adapted from published data.

INHALATIONAL

The lungs provide a large potential area for absorption of analgesic drugs. However, unless nebulization results in the correct droplet size, very little drug will reach the alveoli. NSAIDs have not been administered by this route and there is limited experience of nebulized opioids administered as an aerosol.

Opioid analgesics

Aerosolized morphine results in dose-dependent analgesic blood concentrations of morphine within five minutes. In a comparison of inhaled morphine with intramuscular morphine, Chrubasik and colleagues found that the maximum serum morphine concentration following inhaled morphine was six times lower than that following intramuscular morphine.[125][IV] Another study compared systemic absorption of nebulized morphine with oral morphine in healthy subjects.[126][II] The bioavailability of inhaled morphine was 5 percent (i.e. only one-twentieth of the nebulized dose reached the lungs), where it was rapidly absorbed, with the result that C_{max} was reached sooner than with the oral route. These authors concluded that it was a rapid but inefficient method of administering morphine. Morphine bioavailability with a new aerosol delivery system was increased to 59 percent, of which 43 percent was absorbed instantaneously with an onset to effect time similar to intravenous administration.[127][IV] A fixed metered dose of aerosolized fentanyl has been compared with the same dose administered by intravenous injection in volunteers. The pharmacokinetics of fentanyl by the pulmonary route were similar to intravenous administration. The bioavailability was 100 percent, having exceeded 50 percent within five minutes. Side effects were similar.[128][IV]

PERINEURAL

In contrast to all of the preceding routes of drug administration, analgesic drugs may be delivered by direct neuraxial administration to peripheral and spinal (encompassing epidural and intrathecal) nerves. There is now extensive clinical experience with direct neuraxial administration of opioid analgesics for postoperative pain management.

Opioid analgesics

The evidence that opioids injected, with or without local anesthetic, close to nerve trunks or nerve endings may have an analgesic effect has been examined by Picard and colleagues.[129][I] The authors considered randomized controlled clinical trials in which an opioid, with the specific exception of pethidine, was injected into the brachial plexus, Bier block, or perineural or other sites. The authors concluded that the trials provided no evidence for a clinically relevant peripheral analgesic efficacy of opioids in acute pain.

EPIDURAL

Drug administration into the epidural space must pass through the dura and into the intradural space in order to reach the spinal cord. There is some drug loss because of absorption into the systemic circulation and some loss because of absorption into the extradural fat, where it acts as a depot. The concentration of opioid in cerebrospinal fluid (CSF) required for analgesia is very low. In addition to high lipid solubility, the molecular weight, molecular size, drug concentration, and receptor binding affinity of opioids are also important characteristics. Opioids may be administered as intermittent injection, continuous infusion, or even as PCEA. As Chapter 13, Epidural and spinal analgesia, provides a comprehensive analysis of the epidural route of analgesic administration, only a brief review follows.

Opioid analgesics

The lipophilicity, site of injection, and mode of injection (bolus, infusion, or PCEA) all influence the efficacy of epidurally administered opioids. Onset of analgesia is most rapid with lipophilic opioids,[130][III] whilst bolus dose administration provides analgesia that is superior to the same dose given parenterally.[131][I] Administering opioids by the epidural route provides analgesia that is superior to i.v.-PCA,[132, 133, 134, 135][II] and epidural opioid infusions are superior to the same drug given as a continuous intravenous infusion.[136][I] Furthermore, PCEA opioid administration is superior to i.v.-PCA.[137, 138, 139][II] Also, compared with systemically administered opioids, epidural opioids are associated with a reduced overall incidence of pulmonary complications.[140][I] Finally, extended-release epidural morphine (EREM) is a liposomal morphine preparation that has been recently granted FDA approval. There have been few trials of EREM, but in a comparison with standard epidural morphine, EREM provided better and more prolonged analgesia in postcesarian section patients.[141][II]

INTRATHECAL

A more detailed analysis of intrathecal analgesic administration can be found in Chapter 13, Epidural and spinal analgesia.

Nonopioid analgesics

Numerous animal studies attest to the efficacy of intrathecally administered NSAIDs. However, only one case
series has shown that an intrathecally administered
NSAID (lysine acetylsalicylate) can relieve intractable pain
in humans.[142][III] So far, no clinical trials have been
conducted.

Opioid analgesics

Direct injection of opioid into the CSF is associated with
potent segmental analgesia using much smaller doses of
opioid. The dose employed is commonly one-fifth of that
required for epidural analgesia. Onset is also faster than
the epidural route. Lipid solubility is important in determining the extent and duration of analgesia. Thus,
intrathecal fentanyl provide short-acting, intense analgesia, whereas morphine provides more prolonged analgesia.[143][II], [144][II], [145][III] Furthermore, intrathecal
morphine provides superior postoperative pain relief
compared with i.v. patient-controlled morphine analgesia
alone.[144][II] Although single-bolus dosing is usual,
indwelling subarachnoid catheters for continuous infusion
are available in some countries. Combining intrathecal
bolus dosing with a continuous epidural catheter infusion
technique (combined spinal epidural (CSE)) offers many
potential advantages over continuous epidural analgesia
or intrathecal analgesia methods alone.[146][IV]

OTHER

Other routes of analgesic drug administration include
intra-articular and intrawound injection. Morphine has
even been reported to have a systemic effect following
topical application to the eye in an animal model.[147]

Intra–articular

NONOPIOID ANALGESICS

Intra-articular injection of NSAIDs may be useful in the
treatment of acute, painful, local inflammatory processes,
rather than postoperative pain. In a study of periarticular
injection, tenoxicam 20 mg was effective in alleviating the
pain of rotator cuff tendinitis.[148][II] A systematic review of
intra-articular NSAID administration has confirmed the
effectiveness of this route for postoperative analgesia.[149][I]

OPIOID ANALGESICS

The demonstration of endogenous opioid ligands in
inflamed synovium has led to the application of exogenous opioids directly into the joint capsule. The low

lipid solubility of morphine combined with the relatively
low blood flow to the articular region results in prolonged
analgesia (up to three days) associated with this route of
administration. The evidence that intra-articular injection
of morphine can reduce postoperative pain has been
examined in a systematic review of randomized controlled trials.[150][I] The authors considered 36 randomized
controlled trials of intra-articular morphine. Because of
the perceived prolonged analgesic effect by this route, they
sought evidence of efficacy in both early (up to six hours
after intra-articular injection) and late (6–24-hour) periods. All of the studies comparing morphine with saline
that included an index of internal sensitivity demonstrated efficacy of intra-articular morphine. Evidence for a
prolonged analgesic effect was more compelling than an
early effect. However, comparison of intra-articular with
parenteral morphine was less compelling. There were no
adverse effects attributable to intra-articular morphine.
Subsequent studies by De Andres and colleagues[151][II]
and Kanbak and colleagues[152][III] support these conclusions, whereas Wrench and colleagues found no evidence
of peripherally mediated opioid analgesic effect.[153][II]

Intrawound

Studies of wound infiltration with NSAIDs in postoperative pain are inconclusive. A systematic review
found that no more than two out of five studies comparing intrawound NSAIDs with systemic administration
showed a significant analgesic effect.[149][I]

SUMMARY

The choice of routes of administration and formulations
of analgesic drugs is bewildering.

Of the many different routes of administration, the
oral route is effective, the simplest to use, and usually
the least expensive. Nevertheless, alternative routes of
administration may be necessary for patients who are
unable to take drugs orally. The intravenous route has the
advantages of a rapid onset of action and ease of titration,
although other parenteral and neuraxial routes are also
effective. Furthermore, many of the new formulations and
systems of drug delivery that have been developed show
promise, but have yet to become universally adopted.
Delayed release formulations (oral, parenteral, or transdermal) are best not used, at least intially, for the sole
management of acute postoperative pain.

NSAIDs and opioid, alone or in combination, remain
important components of any analgesic regimen. There is
no evidence, with the exception of paracetamol, that
NSAIDs given rectally or by injection perform better or
faster than the same dose of the same drug given by
mouth, although topical NSAIDs are effective for acute
pain of musculoskeletal origin. Intravenous paracetamol

is associated with faster onset of analgesia than the oral route, but there is no difference in pain relief between the two routes. Opioids by injection are effective in the treatment of moderate-to-severe acute postoperative pain (intramuscular≡subcutaneous ≤ intravenous/i.v.-PCA). Epidural opioid administration, with or without a background infusion, is superior to parenteral routes of opioid administration. Finally transdermal opioid administration may be as effective as opioids by injection and offers the prospect of effective needle-free pain control in the future.

Thus, when immediate relief of severe pain is required, intravenous injection, usually of an opioid, is the obvious choice.[154][IV], [155][I] Otherwise, with the exception of the epidural route of opioid administration, as long as the patient can swallow, there is no evidence for the superiority of one route over another.

REFERENCES

1. Wenz G. An overview of host–guest chemistry and its application to nonsteroidal anti-inflammatory drugs. *Clinical Drug Investigation.* 2000; **19** (Suppl. 2): 21–5.
2. Ceppi Monti N, Gazzaniga A, Gianesello V *et al.* Activity and pharmacokinetics of a new oral dosage form of soluble ibuprofen. *Arzneimittel-Forschung.* 1992; **42**: 556–9.
3. Martin W, Koselowske G, Töberich H *et al.* Pharmacokinetics and absolute bioavailability of ibuprofen after oral administration of ibuprofen lysine in man. *Biopharmaceutics and Drug Disposition.* 1990; **11**: 265–78.
4. Olson NZ, Otero AM, Marrero I *et al.* Onset of analgesia for liquigel ibuprofen 400 mg, acetaminophen 1000 mg, ketoprofen 25 mg, and placebo in the treatment of postoperative dental pain. *Journal of Clinical Pharmacology.* 2001; **41**: 1238–47.
5. Moller PL, Norholt SE, Ganry HE *et al.* Time to onset of analgesia and analgesic efficacy of effervescent acetaminophen 1000 mg compared to tablet acetaminophen 1000 mg in postoperative dental pain: a single-dose, double-blind, randomized, placebo-controlled study. *Journal of Clinical Pharmacology.* 2001; **40**: 370–8.
6. Laveneziana D, Riva A, Bonazzi M *et al.* Comparative efficacy of oral ibuprofen arginine and intramuscular ketorolac in patients with postoperative pain. *Clinical Drug Investigation.* 1996; **11** (Suppl. 1): 8–14.
7. Pagnoni B, Vignali M, Colella S *et al.* Comparative efficacy of oral ibuprofen arginine and intramuscular ketorolac in post caesarian section pain. *Clinical Drug Investigation.* 1996; **11** (Suppl. 1): 15–21.
8. Wakeling HG, Barry PC, Butler PJ. Postoperative analgesia in dental day case surgery: a comparison between Feldene "Melt" (piroxicam) and diclofenac suppositories. *Anaesthesia.* 1996; **51**: 784–6.
9. Evans AM. Enantioselective pharmacodynamics and pharmacokinetics of chiral non-steroidal antiinflammatory drugs. *European Journal of Clinical Pharmacology.* 1992; **42**: 237–56.
10. Gay C, Planas E, Donado M *et al.* Analgesic effect of low doses of dexketoprofen in the dental pain model: a randomised, double-blind, placebo-controlled study. *Clinical Drug Investigation.* 1996; **11**: 320–30.
11. Barden J, Edwards JE, McQuay HJ, Moore RA. Single dose oral celecoxib for postoperative pain. *Cochrane Database of Systematic Reviews.* 2003; **CD004233**.
12. Straube S, Derry S, McQuay HJ, Moore RA. Effect of preoperative Cox-II-selective NSAIDs (coxibs) on postoperative outcomes: a systematic review of randomised studies. *Acta Anaesthesiologica Scandinavica.* 2005; **49**: 601–13.
13. Collins SL, Faura CC, Moore RA, McQuay HJ. Peak plasma concentrations after oral morphine: a systematic review. *Journal of Pain and Symptom Management.* 1998; **16**: 388–402.
14. Derbyshire DR, Bell A, Parry PA, Smith G. Morphine sulphate slow release: comparison with i.m. morphine for postoperative analgesia. *British Journal of Anaesthesia.* 1985; **57**: 858–65.
15. Lew JK, Mobley KA, Achola KJ *et al.* Postoperative absorption of controlled-release morphine sulphate: a study in patients given no parenteral opioids. *British Journal of Anaesthesia.* 1989; **44**: 101–3.
16. Hanks GW, Rose NM, Aherne GW *et al.* Controlled release morphine tablets: a double-blind trial in dental surgery patients. *British Journal of Anaesthesia.* 1981; **53**: 1259–64.
17. McCormack JP, Warriner CB, Levine M, Glick N. A comparison of regularly dose oral morphine and on-demand intramuscular morphine in the treatment of postsurgical pain. *Canadian Journal of Anaesthesia.* 1993; **40**: 819–24.
18. Edwards JE, McQuay HJ, Moore RA. Single dose dihydrocodeine for acute postoperative pain. *Cochrane Database of Systematic Reviews.* 2000; **CD002760**.
19. Edwards JE, Moore RA, McQuay HJ. Single dose oxycodone and oxycodone plus paracetamol (acetaminophen) for acute postoperative pain. *Cochrane Database of Systematic Reviews.* 2000; **CD002763**.
20. Gimbel J, Ahdieh H. The efficacy and safety of oral immediate-release oxymorphone for poststurgical pain. *Anesthesia and Analgesia.* 2004; **99**: 1472–7.
21. Moore RA, McQuay HJ. Single-patient data meta-analysis of 3453 postoperative patients: oral tramadol versus placebo, codeine and combination analgesics. *Pain.* 1997; **69**: 287–94.
22. Scott LJ, Perry CM. Tramadol. A review of its use in perioperative pain. *Drugs.* 2000; **60**: 139–76.
23. Kerpsack JM, Fankhauser RA. The use of controlled-release versus scheduled oxycodone in the immediate postoperative period following total joint arthroplasty. *Orthopedics.* 2005; **28**: 491–4.

24. Reuben SS, Connelly HR, Maciolek H. Preoperative administration of controlled-release oxycodone for the management of pain after ambulatory laparoscopic tubal ligation surgery. *Journal of Clinical Anesthesia*. 2002; **14**: 223–7.

25. Kampe S, Warm M, Kaufman J et al. Clinical efficacy of controlled-release oxycodone 20 mg administered in a 12-hour dosing schedule on the management of postoperative pain after breast surgery for cancer. *Current Medical Research and Opinion*. 2005; **20**: 199–202.

26. Ahdieh H, Ma T, Babul N, Lee D. Efficacy of oxymorphone extended release in postsurgical pain: a randomized clinical trial in knee arthroplasty. *Journal of Clinical Pharmacology*. 2004; **44**: 767–7.

27. Ginsberg R, Sinatra RS, Adler LJ et al. Conversion to oral controlled-release oxycodone from intravenous opioid analgesic in the postoperative setting. *Pain Medicine*. 2003; **4**: 31–8.

28. Morgan DJ, McCormick Y, Cosolo W et al. Prolonged release of morphine alkaloid from a lipophilic suppository base *in vitro* and *in vivo*. *International Journal of Clinical Pharmacology, Therapy, and Toxicology*. 1992; **30**: 576–81.

29. Takatori T, Yamamoto K, Yamaguchi T et al. Design of controlled-release morphine suppositories containing polyglycerol ester of fatty acid. *Biological and Pharmaceutical Bulletin*. 2005; **28**: 1480–4.

30. Stocker ME, Montgomery JE. Serum paracetamol concentrations in adult volunteers following rectal administration. *British Journal of Anaesthesia*. 2001; **87**: 638–40.

31. Kyllonen M, Olkkola KT, Seppala T, Ryhanen P. Perioperative pharmacokinetics of ibuprofen enantiomers after rectal administration. *Paediatric Anaesthesia*. 2005; **15**: 566–73.

32. Hanses A, Spahn-Lanqquth H, Meiss F, Mutschler E. Pharmacokinetics and drug input characteristics of a diclofenac–codeine phosphate combination following oral and rectal administration. *Arzneimittel-Forschung*. 1996; **46**: 57–63.

33. Yong CS, Oh YK, Jung SH et al. Preparation of ibuprofen-loaded liquid suppository using eutectic mixture system with menthol. *European Journal of Pharmaceutical Sciences*. 2004; **23**: 347–53.

34. Kanamoto I, Nagakawa T, Horikoshi I et al. Pharmacokinetics of two rectal dosage forms of ketoprofen in patients after anal surgery. *Journal of Pharmacobio-dynamics*. 1988; **11**: 141–5.

35. Nagasawa K, Nakanishi H, Matsuda T et al. Pharmacokinetics of diclofenac after its intrarectal and intracolostomal administration to rabbits with rectal resection or colostoma construction. *Biopharmaceutics and Drug Disposition*. 2001; **22**: 31–9.

* 36. Tramèr MR, Williams JE, Carroll D et al. Comparing analgesic efficacy of non-steroidal anti-inflammatory drugs given by different routes in acute and chronic pain: a qualitative systematic review. *Acta Anaesthesiologica Scandinavica*. 1998; **42**: 71–9.

* 37. Romsing J, Moiniche S, Dahl JB. Rectal and parenteral paracetamol, and paracetamol in combination with NSAIDs, for postoperative pain. *British Journal of Anaesthesia*. 2002; **88**: 215–26.

38. Holdgate A, Pollock T. Nonsteroidal anti-inflammatory drugs (NSAIDs) versus opioids for acute renal colic. *Cochrane Database of Systematic Reviews*. 2005; **CD004137**.

39. Lee C, Gnanasegaram D, Maloba M. Best evidence topic report. Rectal or intravenous non-steroidal anti-inflammatory drugs in acute renal colic. *Emergency Medicine Journal*. 2005; **22**: 653–4.

40. Lipscomb GR, Rees WD. Gastric mucosal injury and adaptation to oral and rectal administration of naproxen. *Alimentary Pharmacology and Therapeutics*. 1996; **10**: 133–8.

41. Twiston-Davies CW, Goodwin MI, Baxter PJ. Rectal indomethacin for postoperative pain in orthopaedic surgery: a double-blind study. *Journal of Bone and Joint Surgery*. 1990; **72**: 510–1.

42. Jonsson T, Christensen CB, Jordening H, Frolund C. The bioavailability of rectally administered morphine. *Pharmacology and Toxicology*. 1988; **62**: 203–5.

43. Moolenaar F, Grasmeijer G, Visser J, Meijer DK. Rectal versus oral absorption of codeine phosphate in man. *Biopharmaceutics and Drug Disposition*. 1983; **4**: 195–9.

44. Lundeberg S, Beck O, Olsson GL, Boreos L. Rectal administration of morphine in children: pharmacokinetic evaluation after a single-dose. *Acta Anaesthesiologica Scandinavica*. 1996; **40**: 445–51.

45. Lugo RA, Kern SE. The pharmacokinetics of oxycodone. *Journal of Pain and Palliative Care Pharmacotherapy*. 2004; **18**: 17–30.

46. Hojsted J, Rubeck-Petersen K, Rask H et al. Comparative bioavailability of a morphine suppository given rectally and in a colostomy. *European Journal of Clinical Pharmacology*. 1990; **39**: 49–50.

47. Smith LOA, Carroll D, Edwards JE et al. Single dose ketorolac and pethidine in acute postoperative pain: systematic review with meta-analysis. *British Journal of Anaesthesia*. 2000; **84**: 48–58.

48. Daniels SE, Grossman EH, Kuss ME et al. A double-blind, randomized comparison of intramuscularly and intravenously administered parecoxib sodium versus ketorolac and placebo in a post-oral surgery pain model. *Clinical Therapeutics*. 2001; **23**: 1018–31.

49. Karaman S, Gunusen I, Uyar M, Firat V. The effect of pre-operative lornoxicam and ketoprofen application on the morphine consumption of post-operative patient-controlled analgesia. *Journal of International Medical Research*. 2006; **34**: 168–75.

50. Kirkpatrick T, Henderson PD, Nimmo WS. Plasma morphine concentrations after intramuscular injection into the deltoid or gluteal muscles. *Anaesthesia*. 1988; **43**: 293–5.

51. Semple TJ, Upton RN, Macintyre PE et al. Morphine blood concentration in elderly postoperative patients following

administration via an indwelling subcutaneous cannula. *Anaesthesia.* 1997; **52**: 318–23.

52. Semple D, Aldridge LA, Doyle E. Comparison of i.v. and s.c. diamorphine infusions for the treatment of acute pain in children. *British Journal of Anaesthesia.* 1996; **76**: 310–2.

53. Cooper IM. Morphine for postoperative analgesia: a comparison of intramuscular and subcutaneous routes of administration. *Anaesthesia and Intensive Care.* 1996; **24**: 574–8.

54. Rutter PC, Murphy F, Dudley HAF. Morphine: controlled trial of different methods of administration for postoperative pain relief. *British Medical Journal.* 1980; **280**: 12–13.

* 55. McQuay HJ, Carroll D, Moore RA. Injected morphine in postoperative pain; a quantitative systematic review. *Journal of Pain and Symptom Management.* 1999; **17**: 164–74.

56. Greenwald RA. Ketorolac: an innovative non-steroidal analgesic drug. *Drugs Today.* 1992; **28**: 41–6.

57. Valles J, Artigas R, Crea A. Clinical pharmacokinetics of parenteral dexketoprofen trometamol in healthy subjects. *Methods and Findings in Experimental and Clinical Pharmacology.* 2006; **28** (Suppl. A): 7–12.

58. Levy G. Clinical pharmacokinetics of salicylates: a reassessment. *British Journal of Clinical Pharmacology.* 1980; **10**: S285–90.

59. Laska EM, Sunshine A, Marrero I *et al.* The correlation between blood levels of ibuprofen and clinical analgesic response. *Journal of Clinical Pharmacy and Therapeutics.* 1986; **40**: 1–7.

60. Campbell WI, Kendrick R, Patterson C. Intravenous diclofenac sodium: does its administration before operation suppress postoperative pain? *Anaesthesia.* 1990; **45**: 763–6.

61. Hyrkas T, Ylipaavalniemi P, Oikarinen VJ, Hampf G. Postoperative pain prevention by a single-dose formulation of diclofenac producing a steady plasma concentration. *Journal of Oral and Maxillofacial Surgery.* 1992; **50**: 124–7.

62. Jakobsson J, Rane K, Davidson S. Intramuscular NSAIDs reduce postoperative pain after minor outpatient anaesthesia. *European Journal of Anaesthesiology.* 1996; **13**: 67–71.

63. Parke TJ, Millett S, Old S *et al.* Ketorolac for early postoperative analgesia. *Journal of Clinical Anesthesia.* 1995; **7**: 465–9.

64. Ben-David B, Baune-Goldstein U, Goldik Z, Gaitini L. Is preoperative ketorolac a useful adjunct to regional anaesthesia for inguinal herniorrhaphy? *Acta Anaesthesiologica Scandinavica.* 1996; **40**: 358–63.

65. Muriel-Villoria C, Zungri-Telo E, Diaz-Curiel M *et al.* Comparison of the onset and duration of the analgesic effect of dipyrone, 1 or 2 g, by the intramuscular or intravenous route, in acute renal colic. *European Journal of Clinical Pharmacology.* 1995; **48**: 103–7.

66. Nelson CE, Nylander C, Olsson AM *et al.* Rectal v. intravenous administration of indomethacin in the treatment of renal colic. *Acta Chirurgica Scandinavica.* 1988; **154**: 253–5.

67. Nissen I, Birke H, Olsen JB *et al.* Treatment of ureteric colic: intravenous versus rectal administration of indomethacin. *British Journal of Urology.* 1990; **65**: 576–9.

68. Barden J, Edwards JE, McQuay HJ, Moore RA. Oral valdecoxib and injected parecoxib for acute postoperative pain: a quantitative systematic review. *BMC Anesthesiology.* 2003; **3**: 1.

69. Moller PL, Sindet-Petersen S, Petersen CT *et al.* Onset of paracetamol analgesia: comparison of oral and intramuscular routes after third molar surgery. *British Journal of Anaesthesia.* 2005; **94**: 642–8.

70. Austin KL, Stapleton JV, Mather LE. Relationship between blood meperidine concentrations and analgesic response: a preliminary report. *Anesthesiology.* 1980; **53**: 460–6.

71. Austin KL, Stapleton JV, Mather LE. Multiple intramuscular injections: a major source of variability of analgesic response to meperidine. *Pain.* 1980; **83**: 47–62.

72. Woodhouse A, Mather LE. The minimum effective concentration of opioids: a revisitation with patient controlled analgesia fentanyl. *Regional Anesthesia and Pain Medicine.* 2000; **25**: 259–67.

73. Aubrun F, Monsel S, Langeron O *et al.* Postoperative titration of intravenous morphine. *European Journal of Anaesthesiology.* 2001; **18**: 159–61.

* 74. Walder B, Schafer M, Henzi I, Tramer M. Efficacy and safety of patient-controlled opioid analgesia for acute postoperative pain. *Acta Anaesthesiologica Scandinavica.* 2001; **45**: 795–804.

* 75. Dolin SJ, Cashman JN, Bland JM. Effectiveness of acute postoperative pain management: I. Evidence from published data. *British Journal of Anaesthesia.* 2002; **89**: 409–23.

* 76. Cashman JN, Dolin SJ. Respiratory and haemodynamic effects of acute postoperative pain management: evidence from published data. *British Journal of Anaesthesia.* 2004; **93**: 212–23.

77. Urquhart ML, Klapp K, White PF. Patient-controlled analgesia: a comparison of intravenous versus subcutaneous hydromorphone. *Anesthesiology.* 1988; **69**: 428–32.

* 78. Nanda A, Nanda S, Ghilzai NM. Current developments using emerging transdermal technologies in physical enhancement methods. *Current Drug Delivery.* 2006; **3**: 233–42.

* 79. Batheja O, Thakur R, Michniak B. Transdermal iontophoresis. *Expert Opinion on Drug Delivery.* 2006; **3**: 127–38.

80. Cordero JA, Alarcon L, Escribano E *et al.* A comparative study of the transdermal penetration of a series of nonsteroidal antiinflammatory drugs. *Journal of Pharmaceutical Sciences.* 1997; **86**: 503–8.

81. Singh SK, Durrani MJ, Reddy IK, Khan MA. Effect of permeation enhancers on the release of ketoprofen

through transdermal drug delivery systems. *Die Pharmazie.* 1996; **51**: 741–4.

82. Stott PW, Williams AC, Barry BW. Transdermal delivery from eutectic systems: enhanced permeation of a model drug, ibuprofen. *Journal of Controlled Release.* 1998; **50**: 297–308.

83. Dominkus M, Nicolakis M, Kotz R *et al.* Comparison of tissue and plasma levels of ibuprofen after oral and topical administration. *Arzneimittel-Forschung.* 1996; **46**: 1138–43.

84. Svensson P, House L, Arendt-Nielsen L. Effect of systemic versus topical nonsteroidal anti-inflammatory drugs on post exercise jaw-muscle soreness: a placebo controlled study. *Journal of Orofacial Pain.* 1997; **11**: 353–62.

85. Anonymous. More topical NSAIDs: worth the rub? *Drug and Therapeutics Bulletin.* 1990; **28**: 27–8.

86. Mason L, Moore RA, Edwards JE *et al.* Topical NSAIDS for acute pain: a meta-analysis. *BMC Family Practice.* 2004; **5**: 10.

87. Moore RA, Tramèr MR, Carroll D *et al.* Quantitative systematic review of topically applied non-steroidal anti-inflammatory drugs. *British Medical Journal.* 1998; **316**: 333–8.

88. Mason L, Moore RA, Edwards JE *et al.* Systematic review of efficacy of topical rubefacients containing salicylates for the treatment of acute and chronic pain. *British Medical Journal.* 2004; **328**: 995.

89. Gourlay GK, Kowalski SR, Plummer JL *et al.* The transdermal administration of fentanyl in the treatment of postoperative pain: pharmacokinetics and pharmacodynamic effects. *Pain.* 1989; **37**: 193–202.

90. Sathyan G, Guo C, Sivakumar K *et al.* Evaluation of two transdermal fentanyl systems following single and repeat applications. *Current Medical Research and Opinion.* 2005; **21**: 1961–8.

91. Schmid-Grendelmeier P, Pokorny R, Gasser UE, Richarz U. A comparison of the skin irritation potential of transdermal fentanyl versus transdermal buprenorphine in middle-aged to elderly healthy volunteers. *Current Medical Research and Opinion.* 2006; **22**: 501–9.

92. Sandler AN, Baxter AD, Katz J *et al.* A double-blind, placebo-controlled trial of transdermal fentanyl after abdominal hysterectomy: analgesic, respiratory and pharmacokinetic effects. *Anesthesiology.* 1994; **81**: 1169–80.

93. Jeal W, Benfield P. Transdermal fentanyl: a review of its pharmacological properties and therapeutic efficacy in pain control. *Drugs.* 1997; **53**: 109–38.

94. Sandler A. Transdermal fentanyl: acute analgesic clinical studies. *Journal of Pain and Symptom Management.* 1992; **7**: S27–35.

* 95. Lehmann LJ, DeSio JM, Radvany T, Bikhazi GB. Transdermal fentanyl in postoperative pain. *Regional Anesthesia.* 1997; **22**: 24–8.

96. Reinhart DJ, Goldberg ME, Roth JV *et al.* Transdermal fentanyl system plus im ketorolac for the treatment of

postoperative pain. *Canadian Journal of Anaesthesia.* 1997; **44**: 377–84.

97. Thysman S, Préat V. *In vivo* iontophoresis of fentanyl and sufentanil in rats: pharmacokinetics and acute antinociceptive effects. *Anesthesia and Analgesia.* 1993; **77**: 61–6.

* 98. Sathyan G, Jaskowiak J, Evashenk M, Gupta S. Characterisation of the pharmacokinetics of fentanyl HCl patient-controlled transdermal system (PCTS): effect of current magnitude and multiple-day dosing and comparison with IV fentanyl administration. *Clinical Pharmacokinetics.* 2005; **44** (Suppl. 1): 7–15.

99. Viscusi ER, Reynolds L, Chung F *et al.* Patient-controlled transdermal fentanyl hydrochloride vs intravenous morphine pump for postoperative pain. *Journal of the American Medical Association.* 2004; **291**: 1333–41.

100. Cilurzo F, Selmin F, Mingetti P *et al.* Fast-dissolving mucoadhesive microparticulate delivery system containing piroxicam. *European Journal of Pharmaceutical Sciences.* 2005; **24**: 355–61.

101. Weinberg DS, Inturrisi CE, Reidenberg B *et al.* Sublingual absorption of selected opioid analgesics. *Journal of Clinical Pharmacy and Therapeutics.* 1988; **44**: 335–42.

102. Fisher AP, Fung C, Hanna M. Absorption of buccal morphine: a comparison with slow-release morphine sulphate. *Anaesthesia.* 1988; **43**: 552–3.

103. Hoskin PJ, Hanks GW, Aherne GW *et al.* The bioavailability and pharmacokinetics of morphine after intravenous, oral and buccal administration in healthy volunteers. *British Journal of Clinical Pharmacology.* 1989; **27**: 499–505.

104. Beyssac E, Touaref F, Meyer M *et al.* Bioavailability of morphine after administration of a new bioadhesive buccal tablet. *Biopharmaceutics and Drug Disposition.* 1998; **19**: 401–5.

105. Senel S, Duchene D, Hincal AA *et al.* *In vitro* studies on enhancing effect of sodium glycocholate on transbuccal permeation of morphine hydrochloride. *Journal of Controlled Release.* 1998; **51**: 107–13.

106. Simpson KH, Tring IC, Ellis FR. An investigation of premedication with morphine given by the buccal or intramuscular route. *British Journal of Clinical Pharmacology.* 1989; **27**: 377–80.

107. Watson NW, Taylor KM, Joel SP *et al.* A pharmacokinetic study of sublingual aerosolized morphine in healthy volunteers. *Journal of Pharmacy and Pharmacology.* 1996; **48**: 1256–9.

108. Schechter NL, Weisman SJ, Rosenblum M *et al.* The use of oral transmucosal fentanyl citrate for painful procedures in children. *Pediatrics.* 1995; **95**: 335–9.

109. Goldstein-Dresner MC, Davis PJ, Kretchman E *et al.* Double-blind comparison of oral transmucosal fentanyl citrate with oral meperidine, diazepam and atropine as preanesthetic medication in children with congenital heart disease. *Anesthesiology.* 1991; **74**: 28–33.

110. Lind GH, Marcus MA, Mears SL *et al.* Oral transmucosal fentanyl citrate for analgesia and sedation in the

emergency department. *Annals of Emergency Medicine*. 1991; **20**: 1117–20.

111. Ashburn MA, Lind GH, Gillie MH *et al*. Oral transmucosal fentanyl citrate (OTFC) for the treatment of postoperative pain. *Anesthesia and Analgesia*. 1993; **76**: 377–81.

112. Darwish M, Tempero K, Kirby M, Thompson J. Relative bioavailability of the fentanyl effervescent buccal tablet (FEBT) 1,080 pg versus oral transmucosal fentanyl citrate 1,600 pg and dose proportionality of FEBT 270 to 1,300 microg: a single-dose, randomized, open-label, three-period study in healthy adult volunteers. *Clinical Therapeutics*. 2006; **28**: 715–24.

113. Sarkar MA. Drug metabolism in the nasal mucosa. *Pharmaceutical Research*. 1992; **9**: 1–9.

∗114. Dale O, Hjortkjaer R, Kharasch ED. Nasal administration of opioids for pain management in adults. *Acta Anaesthesiologica Scandinavica*. 2002; **46**: 759–70.

115. Gillis JC, Benfield P, Goa KL. Transnasal butorphanol: a review of its pharmacodynamic and pharmacokinetic properties, and therapeutic potential in acute pain management. *Drugs*. 1995; **50**: 157–75.

116. Schwesinger WH, Reynolds JC, Harshaw DH *et al*. Transnasal butorphanol and intramuscular meperidine in the treatment of postoperative pain. *Advances in Therapy*. 1992; **9**: 123–9.

117. Abboud TK, Zhu J, Gangolly J *et al*. Transnasal butorphanol: a new method for pain relief of postcesarian section pain. *Acta Anaesthesiologica Scandinavica*. 1991; **35**: 14–18.

118. Ward M, Minto G, Alexander-Williams JM. A comparison of patient-controlled analgesia administered by the intravenous or intranasal route during the early postoperative period. *Anaesthesia*. 2002; **57**: 48–52.

119. Striebel HW, Bonillo B, Schwagmeier R *et al*. Self-administered nasal meperidine for postoperative pain management. *Canadian Journal of Anaesthesia*. 1995; **42**: 287–91.

120. Manjushree R, Lahiri A, Ghosh BR *et al*. Intranasal fentanyl provided adequate postoperative analgesia in paediatric patients. *Canadian Journal of Anaesthesia*. 2002; **49**: 190–3.

121. Toussaint S, Maidl J, Schwagmeier R, Striebel HW. Patient-controlled intranasal analgesia: effective alternative to PCA for postoperative pain relief. *Canadian Journal of Anaesthesia*. 2000; **47**: 299–302.

122. Striebel HW, Oelmann T, Spies C *et al*. Patient-controlled intranasal analgesia: a method for non-invasive postoperative pain management. *Anesthesia and Analgesia*. 1996; **83**: 548–51.

123. Paech MJ, Lim CB, Banks SL *et al*. A formulation of nasal spray for postoperative analgesia: a pilot study. *Anaesthesia*. 2003; **58**: 740–4.

124. Mathieu N, Cnudde N, Engelman E, Barvais L. Intranasal sufentanil is effective for postoperative analgesia in adults. *Canadian Journal of Anaesthesia*. 2006; **53**: 60–6.

125. Chrubasik J, Wüst H, Friedrich G, Geller E. Absorption and bioavailability of nebulized morphine. *British Journal of Anaesthesia*. 1988; **61**: 228–30.

126. Masood AR, Thomas SH. Systemic absorption of nebulized morphine compared with oral morphine in healthy subjects. *British Journal of Clinical Pharmacology*. 1996; **41**: 250–2.

127. Dershwitz M, Walsh JL, Morishige RJ *et al*. Pharmacokinetics and pharmacodynamics of inhaled versus intravenous morphine in healthy volunteers. *Anesthesiology*. 2000; **93**: 619–28.

128. Mather LE, Woodhouse A, Ward ME *et al*. Pulmonary administration of aerosolized fentanyl: pharmacokinetic analysis of systemic delivery. *British Journal of Clinical Pharmacology*. 1998; **46**: 37–43.

∗129. Picard PR, Tramèr MR, McQuay HJ, Moore RA. Analgesic efficacy of peripheral opioids (all except intra-articular): a qualitative systematic review of randomized controlled trials. *Pain*. 1997; **72**: 309–18.

∗130. Sandler AN. Epidural opiate analgesia for acute pain relief. *Canadian Journal of Anaesthesia*. 1990; **37** (Suppl.): Sxxxiii–ix.

131. Nishimori M, Ballantyne JC, Lows JHS. Epidural pain relief versus systemic opioid-based pain relief for abdominal aortic surgery. *Cochrane Database of Systematic Reviews*. 2006; **CD005059**.

132. Eriksson-Mjoberg M, Svensson JO, Almkvist O, Olund A. Extradural morphine gives better pain relief than patient-controlled i.v. morphine after hysterectomy. *British Journal of Anaesthesia*. 1997; **78**: 10–16.

133. Boylan JF, Katz J, Kavanagh BP *et al*. Epidural bupivacaine-morphine analgesia versus patient controlled analgesia following aortic abdominal surgery: analgesic, respiratory, and myocardial effects. *Anesthesiology*. 1998; **89**: 585–93.

134. Motamed C, Spencer A, Farhat F *et al*. Postoperative hypoxaemia: continuous extradural bupivacaine and morphine vs patient-controlled analgesia with morphine. *British Journal of Anaesthesia*. 1998; **80**: 742–7.

135. Welchew EA, Breen DP. Patient-controlled on-demand fentanyl: a comparison of patient-controlled on demand fentanyl delivered epidurally or intravenously. *Anaesthesia*. 1991; **46**: 438–41.

136. Werawatganon T, Charuluxanun S. Patient controlled intravenous opioid analgesia versus continuous epidural analgesia for pain after intra-abdominal surgery. *Cochrane Database of Systematic Reviews*. 2005; **CD004088**.

137. Grant RP, Dolman JF, Harper JA *et al*. Patient-controlled lumbar epidural fentanyl compared with patient controlled intravenous fentanyl for post-thoracotomy pain. *Canadian Journal of Anaesthesia*. 1992; **39**: 214–9.

138. Paech MJ, Moore JS, Evans SF. Meperidine for patient controlled analgesia after cesarian section: intravenous versus epidural administration. *Anesthesiology*. 1994; **80**: 1268–76.

139. Ngan Kee WD, Lam KK, Chen PP, Gin T. Comparison of patient-controlled epidural analgesia with patient controlled intravenous analgesia using pethidine or

fentanyl. *Anaesthesia and Intensive Care.* 1997; **25**: 126–32.

*140. Ballantyne JC, Carr DB, de Ferranti S *et al.* The comparative effects of postoperative analgesic therapies on pulmonary outcome: cumulative meta-analyses of randomized, controlled trials. *Anesthesia and Analgesia.* 1998; **86**: 598–612.

141. Carvalho B, Riley E, Cohen SE *et al.* Single-dose, sustained-release epidural morphine in the management of postoperative pain after elective cesarian section. Results of a multicenter randomized controlled study. *Anesthesia and Analgesia.* 2005; **100**: 1150–8.

142. Devoghel J-C. Small intrathecal doses of lysineacetylsalicylate relieve intractable pain in man. *Journal of International Medical Research.* 1983; **11**: 90–1.

143. Niemi L, Pitkanen MT, Tuominen MK, Rosenberg PH. Comparison of intrathecal fentanyl infusion with intrathecal morphine infusion or bolus for postoperative pain relief after hip arthroplasty. *Anesthesia and Analgesia.* 1993; **77**: 126–30.

144. Liu N, Kuhlman G, Dalibon N *et al.* A randomized, double-blinded comparison of intrathecal morphine, sufentanil and their combination versus IV morphine patient-controlled analgesia for postthoracotomy pain. *Anesthesia and Analgesia.* 2001; **92**: 31–6.

145. Fleron MH, Weiskopf RB, Bertrand M *et al.* A comparison of intrathecal opioid and intravenous analgesia for the incidence of cardiovascular, respiratory, and renal complications after abdominal aortic surgery. *Anesthesia and Analgesia.* 2003; **97**: 2–12.

*146. Rawal N, van Zundert A, Holmstrom B, Crowhurst JA. Combined spinal-epidural technique. *Regional Anesthesia.* 1997; **22**: 406–23.

147. Chast F. Systemic morphine pharmacokinetics after ocular administration. *Journal of Pharmaceutical Sciences.* 1990; **80**: 911–7.

148. Itzkowitch D, Ginsberg F, Leon M, Appelboom T. Periarticular injection of tenoxicam for painful shoulders: a double-blind, placebo controlled trial. *Clinical Rheumatology.* 1996; **15**: 604–9.

*149. Römsing J, Moiniche S, Ostergaard D, Dahl JB. Local infiltration with NSAIDs for postoperative analgesia: evidence for a peripheral analgesic action. *Acta Anaesthesiologica Scandinavica.* 2000; **44**: 672–83.

*150. Kalso E, Tramèr MR, Carroll D *et al.* Pain relief from intra-articular morphine after knee surgery: a qualitative systematic review. *Pain.* 1997; **71**: 127–34.

151. De Andres J, Valia JC, Barrera L, Colimina R. Intra-articular analgesia after arthroscopic knee surgery: comparison of three different regimens. *European Journal of Anaesthesiology.* 1998; **15**: 10–15.

152. Kanbak M, Akpolat N, Ocal T *et al.* Intra-articular morphine administration provides pain relief after knee arthroscopy. *European Journal of Anaesthesiology.* 1997; **14**: 153–6.

153. Wrench IJ, Taylor P, Hobbs PJ. Lack of efficacy of intra-articular opioids for analgesia after day-case arthroscopy. *Anaesthesia.* 1996; **51**: 920–2.

*154. Shang AB, Gan TJ. Optimising postoperative pain management in the ambulatory patient. *Drugs.* 2003; **63**: 855–67.

*155. McQuay H, Moore A (eds). *An evidence-based resource for pain relief.* Oxford: Oxford University Press, 1998.

11

Patient-controlled analgesia

PAMELA E MACINTYRE AND JULIA COLDREY

KEY LEARNING POINTS

- The concept of patient-controlled analgesia (PCA) commonly refers to methods of pain relief which use electronic or disposable devices and allow patients to self-administer analgesic drugs. However, it could/should apply to any analgesic technique used in the acute pain setting.
- PCA results in better pain relief than traditional (simple) methods of opioid analgesia, although the magnitude of the difference may be small.
- PCA is neither a "one size fits all" nor a "set and forget" therapy. By making appropriate alterations to the bolus dose, PCA can be tailored to suit the individual patient.
- Individual titration of the loading dose is usually required for each patient prior to starting PCA. If the

loading dose is omitted, patients are unlikely to obtain good analgesia from PCA alone.
- The routine use of a background infusion with PCA in opioid-naive patients does not improve pain relief or sleep, but does increase the risk of respiratory depression.
- The level of knowledge that nursing and medical staff have about PCA may also influence the effectiveness and safety of PCA.
- As with other methods of opioid administration, the best early clinical indicator of respiratory depression resulting from PCA opioids is increasing sedation.
- There is little difference in efficacy between the opioids used with PCA.

INTRODUCTION

The concept of patient control over the timing of administration of analgesic drugs, as well as the dose taken (albeit usually within a suggested dose range), has been standard practice for many hundreds of years and remains the common practice for analgesic medications taken outside the hospital setting. In contrast, the idea that patients may be "allowed" some control over the

timing and dose of analgesics needed for management of pain in the hospital setting is relatively recent.

While the idea of patient control could apply to any analgesic technique, the term patient-controlled analgesia (PCA) more commonly refers to methods of pain relief which use electronic or disposable devices and allow patients to self-administer analgesic drugs. This chapter will review the use of PCA and systemically administered medications: discussion of PCA regimens used for peripheral nerve, epidural, and other regional analgesia is included in Chapter 12, Continuous peripheral neural blockade for acute pain and Chapter 13, Epidural and spinal analgesia.

In 1968, Sechzer[1] investigated the analgesic response to small intravenous (i.v.) doses of opioid given by a dedicated bedside attendant to postsurgical patients able to choose the timing of administration of additional doses according to the pain perceived. Later, in 1971, he described a machine that allowed patients to self-administer 1 mL bolus doses of either morphine or pethidine (meperidine) as needed.[2] He concluded that his analgesic-demand system provided improved analgesia compared with fixed-dose nurse-administered regimens. Interestingly, the bolus doses delivered by his machine were considerably smaller than those used today (just 0.2 or 0.5 mg morphine and 2.0 or 5.0 mg pethidine). He also noted that analgesic requirements varied considerably between patients.

Early PCA systems were the Demand Dropmaster,[3] Demanalg,[4] and Cardiff Palliator.[5] Only the latter system, which was able to deliver drugs at a variety of rates and had adjustable parameters that were very similar to modern-day machines, was available commercially.

Subsequent development of PCA machines has seen: the ability to run continuous infusions in addition to delivery of bolus doses; increases in security and data output capacity; introduction of error reduction programs; and a choice of mains or battery power. In addition, a variety of disposable delivery systems is now available.

TYPES OF PCA EQUIPMENT

It is not possible in a chapter such as this to cover in detail all the PCA devices available. The basic principles and features of the various PCA systems are therefore covered as generic groups.

Programmable PCA pumps

The earliest forms of PCA pumps were electronic. While the basic principles involved have changed little over the years, the introduction of sophisticated microprocessors has meant that they are now more compact, more reliable, and more flexible in use. All require disposable items, e.g. generic or dedicated syringes or cartridges, and tubing, to be used for each patient. Antisiphon valves to prevent siphoning of drug from the drug reservoir and antireflux valves to prevent backflow of drug into the intravenous infusion line should also be incorporated into the system.

The major advantage of these types of pumps is their flexibility of use. Adjustments can be made to the dose delivered and lockout intervals, background infusions can

be added, and accurate assessments can be made of the total dose of drug delivered. In some, the rate of delivery of the bolus dose can also be changed. In addition, access to the syringe (or other drug reservoir) and the microprocessor program is only possible using a key or access code.

Disposable PCA devices

A variety of disposable PCA devices is now available although, as yet, most are not widely used. They have the major advantage of being portable and so do not hinder patient mobility, and may not require i.v. access. However, these devices do not allow much flexibility in use. In some, both the drug administered and bolus dose delivered are fixed; in others the drug and drug concentration may be varied, but the volume of the bolus dose cannot be changed. There are also security issues as the drug reservoirs for these devices are more readily accessible.

Parenteral PCA devices

Many disposable PCA devices are based on the same physical principle, that is the volume of pressurized fluid delivered (dependent upon spring or elastomer technology) is determined by mechanical restrictions within the flow path; the speed of filling of the bolus dose reservoir determines the "lockout" interval.[6]

In a review of disposable infusion pumps, Skryabina and Dunn[6] summarized both advantages and disadvantages. Advantages include: small size and weight; freedom from an external power source; elimination of programming errors; and simplicity of use. Disadvantages include: an inability to alter the volume of the bolus dose delivered, add a background infusions, or to accurately determine the amount of drug the patient has received; the possibility of inaccurate flow rates; and long-term costs.

Disposable pumps may also be used in conjunction with patient-controlled epidural and other regional or nerve block analgesia (see Chapter 12, Continuous peripheral neural blockade for acute pain and Chapter 13, Epidural and spinal analgesia).

Transmucosal PCA devices

Metered-dose, patient-controlled intranasal analgesia (PCINA) devices are available that allow the intranasal administration of a fixed dose of opioid. The drugs must be administered in small volumes to avoid significant run-off into the pharynx. It has been suggested that the maximum volume given into each nostril should not exceed 150 μL.[7]

Intranasal PCA devices were initially developed that delivered spray doses of a reasonable dose but large volume (e.g. 25 µg fentanyl/0.5 mL[8, 9][II] or smaller volume, but with smaller doses than commonly used with i.v. PCA (e.g. 9 µg fentanyl/180 µL[10][V]). Using a specially formulated solution of 300 µg/mL fentanyl, Paech et al. developed a device that enables fentanyl doses of 54 µg to be delivered in just 180 µL.[11][II]

Transdermal PCA devices

An iontophoretic transdermal PCA fentanyl system is now available. It uses a low-intensity electric current to drive the drug from the reservoir through the skin and into the systemic circulation.[12] Following activation, the battery-generated electric current passes through the drug-containing anode hydrogel (reservoir) ionizing the fentanyl, which, as a positively charged molecule, is then repelled from the positively charged anode (electrostatic repulsion) and transported across the skin.[13]

The credit-card sized IONSYS[TM] device, which is applied to the chest or upper outer arm, delivers a fixed dose of 40 µg fentanyl over a ten-minute period following a patient demand.[12, 14] The device allows delivery of up to six doses each hour, up to a maximum of 80 doses in 24 hours.[13, 14] It must be replaced every 24 hours, is not yet available in all countries, and is designed for in-hospital use only.

In contrast to the passive transdermal fentanyl systems commonly used for the treatment of cancer and chronic pain (they are contraindicated for use in the management of acute pain), when it may take 24 hours or longer for peak blood concentrations to be seen, time to peak concentration of fentanyl using the IONSYS[TM] device is about 40 minutes.[13]

ADJUSTABLE PCA PARAMETERS

The comments below apply to electronic microprocessor-controlled PCA pumps and not the disposable PCA systems. As already noted above, the electronic PCA pumps allow flexibility in use through variations in programmed parameter settings. It is necessary to specify the required parameter settings as part of the PCA "prescription" and this should be done in a way that aims to maximize both the efficacy and safety of the technique. It is therefore important to have some appreciation of the role of these variable parameters and the rationale for choosing a particular setting.

Bolus dose

The bolus dose is the amount of analgesic drug the patient receives after a successful demand. Its size can influence the success or otherwise of PCA. If the dose is too small, the patient may be unable to achieve adequate analgesia; if the dose is too large, there may be excessive side effects, reducing the safety of the technique and/or discouraging the patient from using the machine.

The optimal bolus dose is one that provides consistent, satisfactory analgesia without producing excessive or dangerous side effects. In clinical practice, relatively standard i.v. bolus doses such as morphine 1 mg, fentanyl 10–20 µg, tramadol 10 mg, hydromorphone 0.2 mg and pethidine 10 mg are commonly prescribed. If this dose is not "optimal," and as long it is not too small, the patient will be able to compensate to some degree by changing their demand rate.[15]

In other patients, the size of the bolus dose will need to be increased or decreased according to subsequent reports of pain or the onset of any side effects. As Etches said,[16] PCA is neither a "one size fits all" nor a "set and forget" therapy. By making appropriate alterations to the bolus dose, PCA can be tailored to suit the individual patient. In selecting the size of the initial bolus dose, factors such as age and previous opioid use must also be taken into account.

Relatively few studies have attempted to determine the optimal dose. In one, patients were prescribed 0.5, 1, or 2 mg morphine. Most patients who self-administered 0.5 mg were unable to achieve good pain relief, while patients who received 2 mg with every demand had a high incidence of respiratory depression.[15][II] The conclusion was that 1 mg was the optimal dose of morphine.

Different doses of fentanyl have also been investigated. Three different demand doses (20, 40, and 60 µg) delivered over ten minutes were compared in patients after major surgery. Based on efficacy and incidence of adverse effects, it was concluded that 40 µg was the optimal dose.[17][II]

Four different demand doses of fentanyl (10, 20, 30, and 40 µg) were assessed for the management of pain during burns dressings changes. Pain relief was significantly better with the 30 and 40 µg doses; no patient became sedated or experienced nausea and vomiting.[18][II]

In a further attempt to obtain an optimal PCA dose, a handpiece was designed by Love and colleagues[19][II] that allowed patients to choose between 0.5, 1, or 1.5 mg bolus doses of morphine. When the effectiveness of this system was compared with a standard PCA machine, there were no differences noted in analgesia, total morphine doses, patient satisfaction, or nausea and vomiting.

Lockout interval

Little work has been carried out to investigate the "ideal" lockout interval; that is, the time following the end of the delivery of one dose during which the machine will not administer another dose despite further demands by the patient.

So that the risk of side effects from the drug being administered is minimized, the lockout interval should ideally reflect the time necessary for the patient to appreciate the effect of one bolus dose before another is delivered, and would therefore be related to the drug used. In practice, however, lockout intervals of five to ten minutes are commonly prescribed for i.v. PCA, regardless of the drug, and despite the fact that the full effect of i.v. morphine (most commonly used in PCA) may not be seen for 15 minutes or more.[20] One study that looked at the effects of varying the lockout interval from 7 to 11 minutes for morphine and five to eight minutes for fentanyl, was unable to show any differences in analgesia, anxiety, or side effects.[20][II]

The route of administration will influence the rate of uptake of a drug. If PCA is used to deliver opioids via a route other than i.v., longer lockout intervals are commonly used.

Loading dose

The loading dose is the amount of drug required to achieve an initial level of analgesia, the minimum effective analgesic concentration (MEAC). It can be administered by presetting the PCA pump and allowing automatic administration. However, a set dose is unlikely to be effective for all patients. There are enormous interpatient differences in loading dose requirements and the total dose that will be necessary is impossible to predict. Individual titration of the loading dose by the anesthesiologist or nurse is usually required for each patient before starting PCA. If the loading dose is omitted, patients are unlikely to obtain good analgesia from PCA alone, because even if the demand button is pressed as often as permitted by the program, the MEAC may not be achieved.

Background infusion

It had been hoped that the addition of a background infusion would improve pain relief, particularly at night, by reducing the frequency of demands required to maintain an analgesic blood concentration. The risk is that opioid will continue to be delivered, regardless of whether it is needed by the patient and regardless of the sedation level of the patient.

Most studies investigating the effect of background infusions have concluded that this practice neither improves the effectiveness of analgesia[21][II] nor sleep[22][II] and does not reduce the number of demands made.[22][II] It does, however, result in higher opioid consumption[21][II], [22][II], [23][II] and an increased risk of respiratory depression.[24][V]

Guler et al.[25][II] did show that addition of a background infusion improved analgesia, but the lockout interval used was 15 minutes with a bolus dose of 0.015 mg/kg (i.e. about 1 mg in an average 70-kg patient), so PCA alone might not have been effective anyway.

For the reasons noted above, the routine use of background infusions in adults is usually not recommended. However, their relative safety may be improved if a patient's opioid requirements are already known.[26] For example, it may be suitable in patients who are opioid-tolerant, when it can be used to replace the patient's normal maintenance opioids.

Dose limit

In most pumps, it is possible to program a dose limit (commonly hourly or four-hourly), that allows only a predetermined total amount of drug to be administered within a given time. While those who use a dose limit do so to improve the safety of PCA, there is no reliable method of determining how much opioid a patient will require for analgesia, far less how much will result in dangerous side effects. To date, there is no good evidence to show that the inclusion of a dose limit has resulted in a decrease in side effects related to PCA.[27] Indeed, for PCA to be used effectively in all patients, a wide range of opioid doses may be required.

PREPARATION FOR PCA

Patient education

To enable patients to use PCA to its maximum potential, they should be given instructions about the technique before use, preferably before surgery. Several studies have shown that providing patients with written information[28] [II], [29][II] or information on CD[30][III] significantly improves their knowledge and understanding of PCA compared with verbal instruction alone.

Current literature gives conflicting results with regard to the effect of preoperative education on patient satisfaction and opioid consumption. The use of a multimedia CD educational package in a group of patients, scheduled to have a total knee replacement, showed improved pain relief,[30][III] but other studies using written[28][II], [29][II], [31] [I] or verbal[29, 32][III] information have not replicated these findings. One study found that the use of structured preoperative patient education decreased the amount of opioid consumed and thus may reduce the severity of any unwanted effects;[33][II] more recent work has failed to find a similar correlation.[28][II], [29][II], [30][III], [32][III]

A lack of patient education, on the other hand, has been associated with patient concerns about the use of opioids. Early work by Chumbley and colleagues,[34] found that 22 percent of patients said they feared addiction to the drugs used in PCA and 30 percent feared that they could overdose. This may have been related to a lack of patient education about PCA as 43 percent of patients did not receive any preoperative education and 24 percent received no instruction at any time during the study.[34][V] However, in subsequent work,[28][II], [29][II] they found that although the patients receiving structured information had better knowledge levels, there was no difference between patient groups with regard to postoperative anxiety levels, including fear of addiction and overdose.

Staff education

Education of all staff involved in the use of PCA is important if the technique is to be used safely and effectively.

The level of knowledge that nursing and medical staff have about PCA may also influence the effectiveness of PCA. Introduction of an acute pain service (APS) nurse, whose role included staff and patient education, led to a 50 percent reduction in moderate to severe pain with PCA, a marked improvement in patient satisfaction and significantly fewer side effects.[35][III]

Similarly, when PCA was supervised by an APS compared with the primary clinic a year earlier, patients used significantly more opioids but the incidence of side effects was almost halved; PCA bolus doses were altered more often to suit the individual patient.[36][III]

Nursing staff need to be educated regarding the importance of the patient having control of the PCA machine in order to achieve maximal individual benefit.[37][V] There is evidence that nursing staff approve of patients who use the PCA sparingly, which may not provide all patients with adequate analgesia.[37][V] Conversely, those patients who use more than expected via the PCA may be censured for abusing it.[28][V], [37][V]

Standard orders and nursing procedure protocols

Institutions may vary with regard to responsibility for the setting up and programming of the PCA machine. This responsibility may lie with the anesthesiologist, a member of the APS, or ward nursing staff. Standardized orders (often preprinted) and procedure protocols for PCA need to be available, as they play a key role in ensuring the ongoing safe management of the technique and allow appropriate alterations to be made to these orders so that maximum analgesia can be obtained with minimum possible side effects.

In order to standardize care and ensure safe practice, it is suggested that each institution develop its own standard orders and nursing procedure protocols (for more details see Chapter 24, Intravenous and subcutaneous patient-controlled analgesia and Chapter 47, Organization and role of acute pain services, both in the *Practice and procedures* volume of this series).

Monitoring requirements

Traditionally, in patients receiving opioids, respiratory rate has been monitored and used as an indicator of respiratory depression. A normal respiratory rate may coexist with marked rises in blood carbon dioxide levels and a decrease in respiratory rate has been found to be a late and unreliable sign of respiratory depression.[26] Vila et al.[38][III] described their results before and after the hospital-wide introduction of pain management standards. Only three of 29 patients reported to have respiratory depression exhibited a fall in respiratory rate, compared with 27 of the 29 who experienced a decrease in conscious state.[38][III] Thus, the best early clinical indicator of respiratory depression is increasing sedation, which can be monitored using a simple sedation score.

Regular monitoring of oxygen saturation levels is also recommended. It should be noted however, that oxygen saturation readings may be unreliable indicators of an underlying problem if the patient is receiving supplemental oxygen, as is standard with for many patients receiving parenteral opioids.[26]

PSYCHOLOGICAL FACTORS ASSOCIATED WITH PCA

Patient-controlled analgesia allows patients to self-administer pain-relieving medication, giving them a significant measure of control over an important aspect of their care, at a time when they have very little control over other aspects of their life. Patients are able to balance the degree of pain relief achieved against the severity of any side effects that may occur.

Egan and Ready[39] found that postoperative patients expressed a high degree of satisfaction with the pain relief afforded by PCA. Characteristics of the method that patients have found particularly satisfying were: PCA worked quickly,[39][V] personal control over pain relief,[39] not having to wait for injections,[34][V], [40][V] and not having to bother nurses.[34][V], [37][V], [40][V]

A significant association has also been noted between perceived control and higher satisfaction with lower pain ratings.[34][V], [41][V] In contrast, others have failed to show any perceived benefit from having control.[42][V] In fact, some patients found the element of control disturbing, as it meant that they were also responsible for the production of unpleasant side effects. These authors questioned whether the patient is really in control or is heavily influenced by medical and nursing staff, for whom PCA has certain advantages.[42]

A recent study looked at the correlation between a number of psychological factors and postoperative pain reports, as well as analgesic consumption.[43][III] Emotional support and religious-based coping showed a positive correlation with postoperative morphine consumption; preoperative self-distraction coping correlated positively with pain while in hospital; and preoperative distress, religious-based coping, behavioral disengagement, and emotional support coping positively predicted pain levels four weeks after surgery.[43]

Patient anxiety may also affect how well PCA is used. High levels of anxiety are significantly related to higher pain scores and analgesic requirements in patients using PCA,[44][V], [45][V], [46][V], [47][V] and may be associated with more frequent unsuccessful demands (i.e. demands during the lockout period).[45][V], [48][V]

In adolescents, those expecting high levels of postoperative pain generally experienced more pain in the postoperative period indicating a degree of self-fulfilling prophecy.[49, 50]

Lastly, PCA, or rather the unavailability of it, can have a detrimental effect on the patient's psychology,[51] leading to a "let down" when a machine is not available. This may be overcome by providing alternative analgesia according to the PCA principle (providing patients with rapid analgesia titrated to individual requirements);[52][V] however, this requires more nursing time than conventional PCA.

EFFICACY OF PCA

Analgesic efficacy

A meta-analysis[53][I] published in 1993 reported that significantly better analgesia was provided by PCA compared with intramuscular (i.m.) opioid analgesia; a more recent systematic review has supported these earlier findings.[54][I] In both studies, the magnitude of the difference in analgesia was small (5.9[53] and 8.0[54] on a pain scale of 0–100). A third meta-analysis by Walder et al.[55] found no difference in pain scores and that analgesia with PCA was only better if all pain outcomes (pain relief, pain intensity, and need for rescue analgesia) were considered.

Not all authors have found improved analgesia with PCA.[56][II], [57][II], [58][II], [59][II], [60][II] Of these studies in which no difference was found in analgesia, four[56, 58, 59, 60] examined pain relief in settings where there are high nurse:patient ratios. In these settings, it may be easier to provide any analgesia when required and with minimal delay, i.e. they follow the "PCA principle."[52][V] In general wards, where there are fewer nurses, PCA may facilitate more immediate drug delivery. A more recent meta-analysis of the use of PCA versus nurse-administered analgesia following cardiac surgery[61][I] found no difference in analgesia at 24 hours, but significantly better analgesia with PCA at 48 hours which would support the assertions above, as nursing attention is likely to be higher in the first 24 hours after surgery.

The results of Ballantyne et al.,[53] Walder et al.,[55] and Hudcova et al.[54] are probably a little unexpected given the continuing popularity of i.v.-PCA. It is possible, under

study conditions when greater attention is paid to the technique by investigators and staff alike, that conventional opioid analgesia is more effective. It is also possible that the way in which PCA was used did not adequately allow for interpatient variations (e.g. fixed program parameters) and significantly limited the flexibility of the technique.[62] Information obtained from published cohort studies, case-controlled studies and audit reports as well as randomized-controlled trials[63] suggests that i.v.-PCA may be appreciably more effective than intermittent i.m. opioid analgesia in a real-life clinical setting. Patients given i.m. analgesia were more than twice as likely to experience moderate-to-severe pain and severe pain as those given PCA. These authors also reviewed the incidence of side effects with these techniques (see below under Problems related to the PCA opioid).

PCA analgesia has been found to be less effective for pain than continuous epidural analgesia (CEA) and patient-controlled epidural analgesia (PCEA) in a Cochrane review,[64][I] and another meta-analysis.[65] When a hydrophilic opioid alone was used for epidural analgesia, it failed to confer any advantage over PCA.[65, 66]

Patient satisfaction

Patient satisfaction is significantly higher with PCA than i.m. opioid analgesia.[53][I], [54][I], [55][I] Others have found higher satisfaction with i.v. PCA compared with epidural morphine PCA,[66][II] possibly due to a faster onset of analgesia with the i.v. route.

There may be a correlation between satisfaction and lower pain ratings,[41, 48][V] although some patients report high levels of satisfaction and high pain scores.[34][V], [35][III], [46][V] It would appear that the evaluation of satisfaction is complex. Satisfaction scores may reflect satisfaction with overall treatment or a reluctance to criticize treatment.[34][V], [37][V] Preoperative expectations for analgesia also appear to have an effect on postoperative satisfaction.[66][II]

In addition to patient preference, there is a definite preference for PCA by nurses, not just because it reduces their workload,[67][II] but also because it helps the nurses to distance themselves from the patient's pain and suffering by making the patient responsible for their own analgesia.[37]

Opioid consumption

Ballantyne and colleagues[53][I] reported a nonsignificant trend towards lower opioid use with PCA. However, two more recent systematic reviews of PCA versus conventional opioid analgesia published in 2005[54][I], [61][I] found that opioid consumption was higher in the PCA group.

The same reviews[53, 54, 61] also concluded that there was no difference in the incidence of opioid-related side effects from the use of PCA compared with conventional opioid analgesia, meaning that total opioid dose may be relatively unimportant.

Different opioids used with parenteral PCA

Several different opioids have been used with parenteral PCA, including morphine, fentanyl, pethidine, oxycodone, tramadol, sufentanil, alfentanil, piritramide, nalbuphine, and remifentanil.

The comparative efficacy of these opioids has been studied by a number of authors in double-blinded randomized control trials.[68][II], [69][II], [70][II], [71][II], [72][II], [73][II], [74][II], [75][II], [76][II], [77][II], [78][II], [79][II], [80][II], [81][II], [82][II] On the whole, they have found little difference in efficacy between the opioids studied. This is probably a real finding, although it is possible that differences between the opioids may have been masked by flaws in the calculation of equianalgesic doses.

Three of the five studies that compared pethidine with other opioids,[70][II], [78][II], [79][II] found that analgesia, when moving or coughing, was significantly worse with pethidine. This result, combined with the high incidence of adverse drug reactions,[83][V], [84][III] including norpethidine (normeperidine) toxicity and serotonergic syndrome,[85][V], [86][V], [87][V] means that pethidine should not be used routinely for intravenous PCA.[85, 88]

Individual patients may gain benefit from one opioid over another. This was shown by Woodhouse et al.,[73][II] in a three way cross-over double-blinded randomized control trial comparing morphine, fentanyl, and pethidine. Overall analgesia was equivalent for all drugs; however, subjectively some patients found that they were better able to tolerate one or more of the opioids than the others.

The use of remifentanil PCA has increased, including for applications other than obstetric analgesia.[76][II], [77][II], [89][V], [90][V] It offers potential advantages for analgesia due to its very rapid onset/offset of action and lack of accumulation with repeated dosing. Studies have found that it provides at least equivalent analgesia to morphine[76][II], [77][II] and fentanyl[77][II] and may be associated with fewer side effects.[77][II]

Genetic polymorphism at the μ-opioid receptor may influence the efficacy of PCA opioid in the individual patient. Polymorphism of the μ-opioid receptor at the 118 nucleotide position, encoding for a GG homozygote, has been associated with increased PCA morphine requirements in the postoperative period.[91][III], [92][III] A number of other polymorphisms at genes encoding for morphine metabolism and transport across the blood--brain barrier have also been found to have an influence on the clinical efficacy of morphine.[93][III] Patients who have absent activity of the CYP2D6 enzyme have been found to have a poorer response to tramadol compared with those with normal enzyme activity.[94][III] The literature is yet to

report on the influence of phamacogenetics on other opioids commonly used in PCA; however, there may be similar differences.

Cost comparisons

A review[95] of seven studies that compared costs related to PCA and i.m. analgesia concluded that, while PCA may provide superior analgesia and patient satisfaction, it does so at a greater cost. Other authors have reported similar results.[55, 96, 97]

A decrease in average length of stay (ALOS) in hospital would also have important cost implications. However, neither systematic reviews[53][I], [54][I], [55][I], [61][I] nor other studies,[57, 67] have been able to show that PCA is associated with a decreased ALOS.

PCA has been found to be three times more cost-effective than epidural analgesia, for each pain-free day, after major abdominal surgery.[98][V]

Efficacy via other non-i.v. routes

Other routes can also be used for PCA. The subcutaneous (s.c.),[99][II], [100][II] oral,[101][II] intranasal,[7][V], [102][II], [103][III], [104][II] and transdermal[105][II], [106][II] routes have all be shown to provide effective analgesia.

Compared with i.v. PCA, s.c. PCA may result in higher opioid use.[99][II], [100][II], [107][II] Studies of efficacy have not provided consistent results as both significantly better pain relief[99][II] and no difference in analgesic efficacy[100][II], [107][II] have been reported. Similarly, some authors found no difference in the incidence of nausea and vomiting,[99, 100] whereas others found an increase in nausea and vomiting with s.c. PCA.[107]

The intranasal route has also been used for PCA (PCINA) with general acceptance of the method by patients and nurses. Toussaint et al.[102] found that fentanyl PCINA is equally effective as intravenous fentanyl PCA; similar results have been noted by Paech et al. using a formulation that allows the delivery of larger bolus doses of fentanyl (see Transmucosal PCA devices).[11] Bioavailability of fentanyl via the intranasal route is 0.7, so doses need to be adjusted accordingly.[7, 104] Other drugs that have been administered by PCINA include diamorphine[104] and pethidine.[108] Equivalent efficacy for intranasal diamorphine compared with i.v. was not found in a study by Ward et al.;[104] PCINA pethidine was more effective than s.c. pethidine injections.[108]

Transdermal administration of fentanyl via PCA has emerged in the literature over recent years. The technique is described earlier. Unlike fentanyl patches used for chronic pain management, there is no reservoir of drug left in the skin once the device is removed.[109]

Transdermal fentanyl PCA has been shown to be more effective than placebo for pain relief after major surgery, when the end point was withdrawal from the study due to inadequate analgesia.[105][II], [106][II] A study by Viscusi et al.[110][II] found that transdermal fentanyl PCA (40 μg bolus dose) was as effective as intravenous morphine PCA (1 mg bolus) following major surgery, using patient satisfaction with the technique as the primary end point. Side effects were similar between the two groups. The transdermal fentanyl system is currently only commercially available with a 40 μg bolus dose and a maximum delivery rate of six bolus doses per hour, which may limit its use due to an inability to tailor a regimen for each patient.

Efficacy of other drugs added to PCA opioid regimens

Many drugs have been added to opioids in PCA over the past several years in an attempt to either reduce side effects, improve analgesia, or both.

KETAMINE

A Cochrane review by Bell et al.[111][I] found that the use of low-dose ketamine (that is, subanesthetic doses) in addition to PCA morphine (run as a separate infusion or added to PCA morphine) reduced morphine requirements in the first 24 hours after surgery, as well as the incidence of postoperative nausea and vomiting. There was considerable variation in the doses of ketamine used in the included trials and so no comment could be made regarding the best dose regimen.

Just six of the studies included in this meta-analysis involved the addition of ketamine to the PCA morphine solution.[112][II], [113][II], [114][II], [115][II], [116][II], [117][II] Morphine consumption was reduced in three[113, 115, 117] and pain scores were lower in four of these studies.[113, 114, 115, 117] The amount of ketamine added to PCA morphine varied from 0.5 to 2 mg per bolus dose.

NALOXONE

Naloxone in varying doses has been added to PCA morphine (1 mg/mL). "Ultra-low" doses of naloxone (0.6 μg to 1 mg morphine) added to PCA morphine led to a lower incidence of nausea (not vomiting) and pruritus, but no change in pain relief or morphine requirements.[118][II] However, use of "low" doses (6 μg added to 1 mg morphine) led to increased pain and a clinically insignificant increase in morphine requirements.[119][II]

Naloxone added to PCA morphine (0.8 mg naloxone to 60 mg morphine) did not alter pain relief compared with PCA morphine alone.[120][II]

OTHER DRUGS

Clonidine[121][II] significantly reduces the incidence of nausea and vomiting without an increase in sedation,

and leads to lower pain scores up to 12 hours and higher patient satisfaction.

Magnesium[117][II], [122][II] added to morphine was opioid-sparing and led to better pain relief; added to tramadol it was opioid-sparing but only provided better pain relief for the first two hours.

Ketorolac[123][II] added to PCA morphine was opioid-sparing; there was no difference in pain relief or adverse effects, although the times to first bowel movement and first ambulation were earlier.

Lidocaine[124][II], when added to morphine, shows no advantage in terms of pain relief, opioid use, or nausea, vomiting and pruritus, but the addition of lidocaine leads to higher sedation scores.

STEP-DOWN ANALGESIA

Patients using higher doses of PCA morphine (average and for the 24 hours before stopping PCA) were more likely to want to restart PCA. However, there is no information on the doses of i.m. analgesic (morphine or pethidine) ordered or given, or whether the doses were based on the last 24-hour PCA requirements.[125][V] It has been suggested that doses of opioid prescribed to follow PCA (whether i.m. or oral) be based on the PCA requirements in the 24-hours prior to ceasing.[26]

Use of a controlled-release oxycodone preparation to follow PCA morphine and based on a conversion factor of 1:1.2 morphine:oxycodone provided effective pain relief after cessation of PCA.[126][V]

PCA IN SPECIFIC PATIENT GROUPS

Although PCA allows significant flexibility and variations in opioid use, enabling a wide variety of patients to achieve effective analgesia, additional considerations may be required if some specific patient groups are to obtain safe and effective pain relief using this technique. These groups include pediatric, elderly, and opioid-tolerant patients, and those with obstructive sleep apnea (OSA).

Considerations for three of these groups are discussed in the relevant chapters: pediatric patients (Chapter 27, Acute pain management in children); elderly patients (Chapter 28, Acute pain management in the elderly patient); opioid-tolerant patients (Chapter 30, The opioid-tolerant patient, including those with a substance abuse disorder).

Patients with obstructive sleep apnea syndrome

Concerns about the potential risks associated with administration of opioids in patients with OSA have led to suggestions that nonopioid or opioid-sparing acute pain management techniques should be used where possible.[127, 128] Some of these concerns arise from case reports related to respiratory depression associated with the use of PCA in OSA patients.[129, 130, 131, 132]

However, other factors in these reports could have led to an increased risk of respiratory depression, even in patients who do not have OSA. These included use of background infusions and concurrent administration of sedatives. More importantly, in all cases, it seemed that there was an overreliance on the use of respiratory rate as an indicator of respiratory depression, as vital signs were reported to be normal. The significance of increasing sedation (noted with these patients) as the better clinical indicator of early respiratory depression (see under Monitoring requirements) was missed.

In all patients given opioids, it is wise to reduce the dose should the patient become sedated, and at a stage where they are still easy to rouse but have difficulty staying awake, not once they become unconscious.[26] Proper monitoring and appropriate alteration of opioid dose is especially important as many patients with undiagnosed OSA will be given opioids. The prevalence of OSA in the adult population is known to be high; up to 20 percent of adults have at least mild OSA and 7 percent have moderate to severe OSA; and up to 75 percent of patients who could benefit from treatment remain undiagnosed.[133] Therefore, the chance of unknowingly giving opioids to a patient with OSA is significant.

Morbid obesity is significantly associated with OSA.[133] The use of PCA (without a background infusion) in these patients has been investigated and reported to be a safe and reasonably effective method of providing analgesia,[134] [II], [135][V], [136][III] although the number of patients in these studies was small.

COMPLICATIONS OF PCA

A number of complications related to the use of PCA have been reported. In general, they can be divided into operator or patient-related errors, and problems due to the equipment or the opioid used.

Of the 5377 PCA-related errors reported from September 1998 to August 2003 and examined by the United States Pharmacopeia (USP), the most common were improper dose/quantity 38.9 percent, unauthorized drug 18.4 percent, omission error 17.6 percent, and prescribing error 9.2 percent. Other errors included wrong administration technique, wrong drug preparation, wrong patient, and wrong route.[137]

A prospective study of 4000 patients given PCA postoperatively found nine cases of respiratory depression. These were associated with drug interactions, continuous (background) infusions, nurse- or physician-controlled analgesia, and inappropriate use of PCA by patients.[138]

In a similar-sized prospective survey of 3785 patients, use of PCA was associated with 14 critical events: eight programming errors (all associated with the setting of a continuous infusion); three family members activating PCA; one patient tampering; and three errors in clinical judgment.[139]

Other examples of reported problems are given below.

Operator errors

PROGRAMMING ERRORS

Misprogramming of PCA pumps is thought to account for around 30 percent of PCA errors, be twice as likely to result in injury or death than errors involving general-purpose infusion pumps, and lead to more harm than errors in other types of medication administration.[140]

Vicente et al.[141] sought to obtain an evidence-based estimate of the risk of death from programming errors associated with one type of PCA. They searched Food and Drug Administration (FDA) and other databases and, based on a denominator of 22,000,000 (for use between 1988 and 2000) provided by the device manufacturer, concluded that mortality from programming errors was low (1 in 33,000 to 1 in 338,000); this equated to between 65 and 667 deaths.[141] Interestingly, the case that prompted the review was of a young woman who, after a cassette containing the wrong concentration of drug was placed in the PCA machine, was noted to be unrousable and snoring. However, nothing was done at that time as the nurse "considered the vital signs to be normal" (respiratory rate was 20 breaths/minute) – another reminder of the danger of using respiratory rate to monitor for respiratory depression. Other errors found during the review were all related to incorrect programming of the concentration.[141]

Other reports of incorrect drug concentrations leading to the inadvertent delivery of high doses of opioid (with fatal results)[142, 143] have led to suggestions that drug concentrations should be standardized within institutions.[140]

Oversedation and respiratory depression has also followed the programming of an incorrect bolus dose size,[144, 145] incorrect background infusions,[146] and background infusions when none were prescribed.[139, 146]

Some PCA pump manufacturers have introduced dose error reduction systems in response to such problems. These systems use internal software to guide manual programming by checking programmed doses against preset limits and alerting the programmer to inappropriate dose or continuous infusion settings.[140] Preset dosing protocols can also be used, so that "standard" settings can be programmed for each of the opioids administered.[140]

In addition to programming errors, incorrect checking procedures may also lead to the "wrong" drug being placed in the PCA pump. In one case the first sign of a problem was when the nurses observed that a patient using PCA was a little "twitchy." The drug being delivered was mixture of bupivacaine and fentanyl intended for an epidural infusion in another patient.[147]

Integrated barcode readers, available in some pumps, will identify the drug and drug concentration being used; in some cases the appropriate dosing protocol will be selected automatically.[140]

INAPPROPRIATE PATIENT SELECTION

Patient suitability for PCA requires more than just an assessment of factors such as a patient's understanding of the technique, age, cognitive ability, and willingness to be in control of their own pain relief. The presence of concurrent patient diseases also needs to be taken into account before PCA is prescribed. For example, renal impairment may reduce excretion of the metabolites of morphine, leading to respiratory depression,[148] and pethidine leading to norpethidine toxicity.[149]

The potential problems associated with the use of PCA in morbidly obese patients or patients with sleep apnea have already been described.

INAPPROPRIATE USE OF CONCURRENT MEDICATIONS

Inadequate knowledge about the risks of PCA and prescribing by more than one team, have led to reports of oversedation and respiratory depression due to inappropriate prescriptions of supplementary opioids (by other routes) or sedatives, including benzodiazepines and antihistamines.[129, 139, 150, 151, 152]

Patient-related errors

FAILURE TO UNDERSTAND PCA

Most patients manage PCA well after just some initial education, but others may need reminding about its method of use. Confusion between the nurse call and PCA demand button has been reported.[150, 153]

The design of the patient button has also been given as a reason for an inability to use PCA adequately. Some PCA machines have small buttons and are not easy for elderly or disabled patients to use. Some workers have produced purpose-built buttons to overcome particular disabilities so the machine can be activated by foot,[154] or attached plastic tubing to the machine in place of the handset, allowing activation by the patient blowing into the tube.[155, 156]

PCA BY PROXY

Unauthorized activation of the demand button by nurses[157, 158] or family or visitors[24, 139, 157, 159, 160, 161] has led to respiratory depression.

TAMPERING WITH PCA MACHINES

Access to the syringe (or other drug reservoir) and the microprocessor program in electronic PCA pumps should only be possible using a key or access code. Therefore, "successful" tampering would usually leave obvious signs of damage to the pump casing. However, this may not always be the case. Access to the syringe without a key is possible in one of the current models of PCA machine.[162]

Problems related to equipment

In general, modern PCA pumps have a high degree of reliability. However, problems continue to be reported, as well as problems related to the disposable items required for each patient.

"RUN-AWAY" PUMP

Early reports of "run-away" pumps, where the machine has unexpectedly changed the program and delivered an unprescribed dose of drug (e.g. when the mains electricity leads became loose or disconnected),[151] were attributed to derangements in the software used to control the syringe driver mechanism. While the number of reports has decreased following changes made to the pump design, they continue to occur, including a report of spontaneous triggering made in 1998,[163] and another, made in 2001, of a frayed wire in the demand apparatus leading to triggering as a result of an electrical short circuit.[164]

INCORRECT USE OF, OR FAILURE TO USE, ANTIREFLUX VALVES

Since the early days of PCA, it has been recognized that retrograde flow of opioid along the intravenous line is a potential hazard. In 1979, a one-way antireflux valve was developed to prevent this.[165]

The routine use of antireflux valves has been recommended for many years,[166] but as late as 1998 there was a report of a respiratory arrest resulting from a failure to incorporate such a valve in the PCA system.[167] Respiratory depression has also resulted from a wrongly connected Y-piece.[151] If PCA is to run with an intravenous infusion, antireflux valves must be used and they should be an integral part of the infusion system.

INCORRECT PLACEMENT OF, OR DAMAGE TO, SYRINGE/ CARTRIDGE

For the PCA pump to function properly, the syringe or cassette must be correctly placed into the syringe carriage. If this is not done, there is a risk that the contents of the syringe may empty by gravity (siphon) into the patient.

Uncontrolled siphoning of syringe contents has been reported when the syringe plunger was not engaged in its carriage,[168] a damaged drive mechanism failed to retain the syringe plunger,[169] and with improper cassette attachment.[170] Cracked glass PCA syringes may also allow uncontrolled siphoning.[171, 172]

Care should also be taken when syringes are changed. Failure to cross-clamp the line from the syringe when changing resulted in the inadvertent giving of a large bolus dose of sufentanil, rendering the patient apneic within one to two minutes.[144]

Occurrences such as those detailed above have led to advice that the machine should always be placed level with or below the patient, or, better still, that an anti-siphon valve be included in the infusion system.[172, 173, 174]

Problems related to the PCA opioid

Whenever opioids are given to patients, some opioid-related side effects are to be expected. In general, the risk of side effects from opioids administered by PCA is similar to the risks related to traditional methods of systemic opioid administration (i.v., i.m., or s.c.).[54][I], [55][I]

A review of randomized-controlled trials reporting postoperative opioid-related adverse effects concluded that the incidences with PCA were respiratory depression 1.8 percent, gastrointestinal (mainly nausea and vomiting) 37.1 percent, and pruritus 14.7 percent. This compared with 2.4, 28.2, and 17.5 percent, respectively, for i.v./i.m. opioids combined.[175][IV]

A later review of published cohort studies, case-controlled studies, and audit reports, as well as randomized-controlled trials, found reasonably similar incidences associated with the use of PCA: respiratory depression 1.2 to 11.5 percent (depending whether respiratory rate or oxygen saturation were used as indicators), nausea 32 percent, vomiting 20.7 percent, and pruritus 13.8 percent.[176][V], [177][V]

RESPIRATORY DEPRESSION

The true incidence of respiratory depression associated with PCA is almost impossible to determine from published studies because of the variety of definitions used, including respiratory rate, hypercarbia, low oxygen saturation, and use of naloxone. Most commonly, when reporting incidences of opioid-related side effects, authors use a decrease in respiratory rate as an indicator of respiratory depression. However, as noted earlier in this chapter, this may be a late and unreliable sign of respiratory depression (the better early clinical indicator being increasing sedation).[26, 38] The converse is also true in that respiratory depression can be present in a patient with a "normal" respiratory rate.

As noted above, Cashman and Dolin[176] found an incidence of PCA-related respiratory depression of 1.2–11.5 percent (depending on definition used). The incidence of sedation, reported by the same authors in a later paper looking at other opioid-related side effects, was found to be just over 5 percent.[177] However, the methods and definitions used by the various authors of the studies included in the survey also varied considerably.

Shapiro et al.[178][V] audited 700 patients who received PCA for postoperative pain relief looking for the incidence of respiratory depression defined as a respiratory rate of <10 breaths/minute and/or a sedation score of 2 (defined as "asleep but easily roused"). They reported that 13 patients (1.86 percent) developed respiratory depression; all had respiratory rates of <10 breaths/minute and 11 also had sedation scores of 2.

Factors that may increase the incidence of respiratory depression with PCA include: the use of concurrent (background) infusions; concurrent administration of sedatives or additional opioids; use in the elderly patient; or if the patient becomes hypovolemic.[16, 24, 139, 157]

Concurrent administration of nonsteroidal anti-inflammatory drugs (NSAID) significantly reduces PCA opioid requirements and the incidence of opioid-related nausea and vomiting, and sedation.[179][I]

NAUSEA AND VOMITING

Two meta-analysis have shown that there is no difference in the incidence of nausea and vomiting[54][I], [55][I] with PCA compared with conventional methods of opioid delivery.

However, in the review by Dolin and Cashman[177] referred to earlier, the incidences of nausea and vomiting with PCA were 32 and 20.7 percent, respectively. The incidence of nausea was higher with PCA than following i.m./s.c. opioid analgesia (17 percent), but there was no difference in the incidence of vomiting.[177] However, some of these differences may be related to opioid dose. The much higher number of patients reporting moderate-to-severe or severe pain with i.m. analgesia[63] would suggest that lower opioid doses were used.

There is a known correlation between the risk of nausea and vomiting and increasing opioid dose.[179][V], [180][V] Significant opioid-sparing effects and reductions in the incidence of nausea and vomiting are seen if patients using PCA morphine are also given concurrent NSAIDs.[179][I] In contrast, paracetamol (acetaminophen) given to patients with PCA morphine results in significant opioid-sparing, but no decrease in morphine-related adverse effects.[181]

The risk of nausea and vomiting can be also be reduced by administration of antiemetic drugs. In this chapter, discussion will include only those studies where antiemetics have been added to the PCA opioid solution and not those where the drugs were administered separately.

The addition of droperidol to morphine PCA significantly reduces the incidence of nausea and vomiting,[182][I], [183][I] and may lead to lower total morphine use.[183][I] Tramer and Walder[182][I] calculated that the number needed to treat (NNT) was 2.7 for nausea and 3.1 for vomiting. They found no evidence of a dose-response for effectiveness of droperidol, but the risk of side effects was dose-dependent. Minor adverse effects were more likely if the patients received total doses of more than 4 mg/day; extrapyramidal side effects were not seen.[182][I]

Culebras et al.[184][II] investigated the effectiveness of three different doses of droperidol (5, 15, and 50 μg) added to 1 mg morphine in PCA and did show dose-responsiveness. The effect on nausea and vomiting was significantly related to the dose given: 5 μg had no effect, 15 μg was effective against nausea but not vomiting, and 50 μg was effective against both nausea and vomiting. The antinausea efficacy was more than 40 percent greater with the largest dose and also suggests that droperidol is more effective for the treatment of nausea than vomiting.[184] In contrast to the NNTs reported by Tramer et al.,[182] these results translate to NNTs of 3.7 for nausea and 8.3 and for vomiting; the higher dose, however, increased the risk of sedation.[184][II]

Gan and others[185][II] compared the addition of droperidol to PCA morphine with droperidol given separately and found both regimens to be equally effective.

The success of the 5HT$_3$ antagonists in controlling nausea and vomiting associated with PCA remains unclear. Cherian and Smith[186][II] compared prophylactic ondansetron given both as a bolus at the end of surgery and mixed with morphine in the PCA solution with plain PCA morphine; there was no significant difference in the incidence of nausea and vomiting. Tramer and Walder[182][II] included studies using antiemetics other than droperidol in their analysis and concluded that 5HT$_3$ receptor antagonist drugs (e.g. ondansetron) showed antivomiting, but not antinausea, effects.

Addition of some other antiemetics added to PCA has also been studied. In summary, the results are:

- promethazine reduced the incidence of nausea and vomiting when mixed with morphine for PCA;[187][II]
- diphenhydramine added to PCA morphine in a ratio of 4.8:1 (but not 1.2:1) reduced the incidence of nausea, severe nausea, and vomiting, without increasing side effects such as sedation and dry mouth;[188][II]
- cyclizine added to PCA morphine in a ratio of 2:1 gave low and comparable incidences of severe nausea and vomiting compared with droperidol 50 μg added to 1 mg PCA morphine.[189][II]

Other drugs have also been added to PCA solutions in an attempt to reduce emetic side effects. These include:

- propofol combined with PCA morphine showed no benefit;[190][II]

- nalmefene added to the PCA solution reduced the incidence of nausea and vomiting, but did not reduce analgesia;[191][II]
- naloxone added to PCA morphine (0.8 mg naloxone to 60 mg morphine) did not reduce the incidence of nausea and vomiting compared with PCA morphine alone.[120][II]

The practice of adding antiemetics to PCA is, however, still controversial, as the risk of side effects may increase with increased use of PCA. The NNT for droperidol of 2.7 for nausea and 3.1 for vomiting calculated by Tramer and Walder[182][I] means that that if 100 patients are treated in this manner, 30 will benefit. Cost–benefit and risk–benefit therefore need to be considered.

PRURITUS

The incidence of pruritus is significantly higher in patients given PCA compared with those receiving systemic opioids by other routes.[54][I] Dolin and Cashman[177][V] also found that the incidence of pruritus was higher with PCA (13.8 percent) compared with i.m./s.c. opioids (3.1 percent).

The mechanism of opioid-related pruritus is not fully understood. The role of histamine remains unclear as pruritus may occur after the administration of opioids that do not release histamine. The fact that drugs such as naloxone (a μ-receptor antagonist) can reverse opioid-related pruritus suggests that there may be a μ-receptor-mediated mechanism.[192]

In a systematic review, Kjellberg and Tramer[192][I] concluded that naloxone, naltrexone, nalbuphine, and droperidol were effective in the prevention of opioid-induced pruritus, but that there was a lack of evidence for any beneficial effect with propofol, i.v. ondansetron, epidural clonidine, and epinephrine, or i.m. hydroxyzine.

When droperidol was added to PCA morphine in three different dose regimens (5, 15, and 50 μg added to 1 mg morphine), the two larger doses reduced the incidence of pruritus (NNT 10).[184] However, naloxone added to PCA morphine (0.8 mg naloxone to 60 mg morphine) did not reduce the incidence compared with PCA morphine alone.[120]

Urinary retention

There is no difference in the incidence of urinary retention in patients given PCA compared with other methods of systemic opioid administration.[177][III], [54][I]

NORPETHIDINE TOXICITY

After reviewing records of patients receiving PCA pethidine and assessing the presence of signs and symptoms of central nervous system (CNS) excitation (suggesting norpethidine toxicity), Simopulos et al.[86] recommended that no more than 600 mg pethidine should be given each day and for no more than three days. However, because pethidine offers no benefit in terms of analgesic effect or incidence of adverse effects compared with other opioids used in PCA, it has been recommended that the use of pethidine should be discouraged.[85, 88]

Masking of postoperative and other complications

Obviously, if sufficient analgesic is given (or taken), it may be possible to mask other disease processes or postoperative complications. There have been reports of PCA "masking" signs of urinary retention,[193] compartment syndrome,[194, 195] pulmonary embolus[196] and myocardial infarction.[197]

The concerns expressed in reports such as these relate to the fact that a patient with PCA can increase their opioid use to cover any "new" pain. However, assessment of pain and opioid use should be regular and frequent. Any unexpected change in opioid use, or the site, severity, or character of the pain, warrants careful diagnosis as it may signal the development of a new medical or surgical diagnosis.

REFERENCES

∗ 1. Sechzer PH. Objective measurement of pain. *Anesthesiology.* 1968; **29**: 209–10.

2. Sechzer PH. Studies in pain with the analgesic-demand system. *Anesthesia and Analgesia.* 1971; **50**: 1–10.

3. Forrest Jr WH, Smethurst PW, Kienitz ME. Self-administration of intravenous analgesics. *Anesthesiology.* 1970; **33**: 363–5.

4. Keeri-Szanto M. Apparatus for demand analgesia. *Canadian Anaesthetists' Society Journal.* 1971; **18**: 581–2.

5. Evans JM, Rosen M, MacCarthy J, Hogg MI. Apparatus for patient-controlled administration of intravenous narcotics during labour. *Lancet.* 1976; **1**: 17–18.

∗ 6. Skryabina EA, Dunn TS. Disposable infusion pumps. *American Journal of Health-System Pharmacy.* 2006; **63**: 1260–8.

∗ 7. Dale O, Hjortkjaer R, Kharasch ED. Nasal administration of opioids for pain management in adults. *Acta Anaesthesiologica Scandinavica.* 2002; **46**: 759–70.

8. Striebel HW, Olmann T, Spies C, Brummer G. Patient-controlled intranasal analgesia (PCINA) for the management of postoperative pain: a pilot study. *Journal of Clinical Anesthesia.* 1996; **8**: 4–8.

9. Striebel HW, Pommerening J, Rieger A. Intranasal fentanyl titration for postoperative pain management in an unselected population. *Anaesthesia.* 1993; **48**: 753–7.

10. O'Neil G, Paech M, Wood F. Preliminary clinical use of a patient-controlled intranasal analgesia (PCINA) device. *Anaesthesia and Intensive Care.* 1997; **25**: 408–12.

11. Paech MJ, Lim CB, Banks SL et al. A new formulation of nasal fentanyl spray for postoperative analgesia: a pilot study. *Anaesthesia.* 2003; **58**: 740–4.

12. Banga AK. Iontophoretic topical and transdermal drug delivery. *Drug Delivery Report.* 2005; Autumn/Winter: 51–3.

13. Chelly JE. An iontophoretic, fentanyl HCl patient-controlled transdermal system for acute postoperative pain management. *Expert Opinion on Pharmacotherapy.* 2005; **6**: 1205–14.

14. Koo PJ. Postoperative pain management with a patient-controlled transdermal delivery system for fentanyl. *American Journal of Health-System Pharmacy.* 2005; **62**: 1171–6.

15. Owen H, Plummer JL, Armstrong I et al. Variables of patient-controlled analgesia. 1. Bolus size. *Anaesthesia.* 1989; **44**: 7–10.

16. Etches RC. Patient-controlled analgesia. *Surgical Clinics of North America.* 1999; **79**: 297–312.

17. Camu F, Van Aken H, Bovill JG. Postoperative analgesic effects of three demand-dose sizes of fentanyl administered by patient-controlled analgesia. *Anesthesia and Analgesia.* 1998; **87**: 890–5.

18. Prakash S, Fatima T, Pawar M. Patient-controlled analgesia with fentanyl for burn dressing changes. *Anesthesia and Analgesia.* 2004; **99**: 552–5.

19. Love DR, Owen H, Ilsley AH et al. A comparison of variable-dose patient-controlled analgesia with fixed-dose patient-controlled analgesia. *Anesthesia and Analgesia.* 1996; **83**: 1060–4.

20. Ginsberg B, Gil KM, Muir M et al. The influence of lockout intervals and drug selection on patient-controlled analgesia following gynecological surgery. *Pain.* 1995; **62**: 95–100.

21. Dal D, Kanbak M, Caglar M, Aypar U. A background infusion of morphine does not enhance postoperative analgesia after cardiac surgery. *Canadian Journal of Anaesthesia.* 2003; **50**: 476–9.

22. Parker RK, Holtmann B, White PF. Effects of a nighttime opioid infusion with PCA therapy on patient comfort and analgesic requirements after abdominal hysterectomy. *Anesthesiology.* 1992; **76**: 362–7.

23. Owen H, Szekely SM, Plummer JL et al. Variables of patient-controlled analgesia. 2. Concurrent infusion. *Anaesthesia.* 1989; **44**: 11–13.

24. Sidebotham D, Dijkhuizen MR, Schug SA. The safety and utilization of patient-controlled analgesia. *Journal of Pain and Symptom Management.* 1997; **14**: 202–9.

25. Guler T, Unlugenc H, Gundogan Z et al. A background infusion of morphine enhances patient-controlled analgesia after cardiac surgery. *Canadian Journal of Anaesthesia.* 2004; **51**: 718–22.

26. Macintyre PE, Schug SA. *Acute pain management: a practical guide*, 3rd edn. London: Elsevier, 2007.

✱ 27. Macintyre PE. Safety and efficacy of patient-controlled analgesia. *British Journal of Anaesthesia*. 2001; **87**: 36–46.

28. Chumbley GM, Hall GM, Salmon P. Patient-controlled analgesia: what information does the patient want? *Journal of Advanced Nursing*. 2002; **39**: 459–71.

29. Chumbley GM, Ward L, Hall GM, Salmon P. Pre-operative information and patient-controlled analgesia: much ado about nothing. *Anaesthesia*. 2004; **59**: 354–8.

30. Chen HH, Yeh ML, Yang HJ. Testing the impact of a multimedia video CD of patient-controlled analgesia on pain knowledge and pain relief in patients receiving surgery. *International Journal of Medical Informatics*. 2005; **74**: 437–45.

✱ 31. McDonald S, Hetrick S, Green S. Pre-operative education for hip or knee replacement. *Cochrane Database of Systematic Reviews*. 2004; **CD003526**.

32. Griffin MJ, Brennan L, McShane AJ. Preoperative education and outcome of patient controlled analgesia. *Canadian Journal of Anaesthesia*. 1998; **45**: 943–8.

33. Lam KK, Chan MT, Chen PP, Kee WD. Structured preoperative patient education for patient-controlled analgesia. *Journal of Clinical Anesthesia*. 2001; **13**: 465–9.

34. Chumbley GM, Hall GM, Salmon P. Patient-controlled analgesia: an assessment by 200 patients. *Anaesthesia*. 1998; **53**: 216–21.

35. Coleman SA, Booker-Milburn J. Audit of postoperative pain control. Influence of a dedicated acute pain nurse. *Anaesthesia*. 1996; **51**: 1093–6.

36. Stacey BR, Rudy TE, Nelhaus D. Management of patient-controlled analgesia: a comparison of primary surgeons and a dedicated pain service. *Anesthesia and Analgesia*. 1997; **85**: 130–4.

37. Salmon P, Hall GM. PCA: patient-controlled analgesia or politically correct analgesia? *British Journal of Anaesthesia*. 2001; **87**: 815–18.

✱ 38. Vila Jr H, Smith RA, Augustyniak MJ *et al*. The efficacy and safety of pain management before and after implementation of hospital-wide pain management standards: is patient safety compromised by treatment based solely on numerical pain ratings? *Anesthesia and Analgesia*. 2005; **101**: 474–80.

39. Egan KJ, Ready LB. Patient satisfaction with intravenous PCA or epidural morphine. *Canadian Journal of Anaesthesia*. 1994; **41**: 6–11.

40. Kluger MT, Owen H. Patients' expectations of patient-controlled analgesia. *Anaesthesia*. 1990; **45**: 1072–4.

41. Pellino TA, Ward SE. Perceived control mediates the relationship between pain severity and patient satisfaction. *Journal of Pain and Symptom Management*. 1998; **15**: 110–16.

42. Taylor NM, Hall GM, Salmon P. Patients' experiences of patient-controlled analgesia. *Anaesthesia*. 1996; **51**: 525–8.

43. Cohen L, Fouladi RT, Katz J. Preoperative coping strategies and distress predict postoperative pain and morphine consumption in women undergoing abdominal gynecologic surgery. *Journal of Psychosomatic Research*. 2005; **58**: 201–9.

44. Thomas V, Heath M, Rose D, Flory P. Psychological characteristics and the effectiveness of patient-controlled analgesia. *British Journal of Anaesthesia*. 1995; **74**: 271–6.

45. Gil KM, Ginsberg B, Muir M *et al*. Patient-controlled analgesia in postoperative pain: the relation of psychological factors to pain and analgesic use. *Clinical Journal of Pain*. 1990; **6**: 137–42.

46. Perry F, Parker RK, White PF, Clifford PA. Role of psychological factors in postoperative pain control and recovery with patient-controlled analgesia. *Clinical Journal of Pain*. 1994; **10**: 57–63; discussion 82–5.

47. Ozalp G, Sarioglu R, Tuncel G *et al*. Preoperative emotional states in patients with breast cancer and postoperative pain. *Acta Anaesthesiologica Scandinavica*. 2003; **47**: 26–9.

48. Jamison RN, Taft K, O'Hara JP, Ferrante FM. Psychosocial and pharmacologic predictors of satisfaction with intravenous patient-controlled analgesia. *Anesthesia and Analgesia*. 1993; **77**: 121–5.

49. Logan DE, Rose JB. Gender differences in post-operative pain and patient controlled analgesia use among adolescent surgical patients. *Pain*. 2004; **109**: 481–7.

50. Logan DE, Rose JB. Is postoperative pain a self-fulfilling prophecy? Expectancy effects on postoperative pain and patient-controlled analgesia use among adolescent surgical patients. *Journal of Pediatric Psychology*. 2005; **30**: 187–96.

51. Riley RH. Patient-controlled analgesia "letdown". *Medical Journal of Australia*. 1991; **155**: 648.

52. Lehmann KA. Recent developments in patient-controlled analgesia. *Journal of Pain and Symptom Management*. 2005; **29**: S72–89.

✱ 53. Ballantyne JC, Carr DB, Chalmers TC *et al*. Postoperative patient-controlled analgesia: meta-analyses of initial randomized control trials. *Journal of Clinical Anesthesia*. 1993; **5**: 182–93.

✱ 54. Hudcova J, McNicol E, Quah C *et al*. Patient controlled intravenous opioid analgesia versus conventional opioid analgesia for postoperative pain control; a quantitative systematic review. *Acute Pain*. 2005; **7**: 115–32.

✱ 55. Walder B, Schafer M, Henzi I, Tramer MR. Efficacy and safety of patient-controlled opioid analgesia for acute postoperative pain. A quantitative systematic review. *Acta Anaesthesiologica Scandinavica*. 2001; **45**: 795–804.

56. Evans E, Turley N, Robinson N, Clancy M. Randomised controlled trial of patient controlled analgesia compared with nurse delivered analgesia in an emergency department. *Emergency Medicine Journal*. 2005; **22**: 25–9.

57. Choiniere M, Rittenhouse BE, Perreault S *et al*. Efficacy and costs of patient-controlled analgesia versus regularly administered intramuscular opioid therapy. *Anesthesiology*. 1998; **89**: 1377–88.

58. Munro AJ, Long GT, Sleigh JW. Nurse-administered subcutaneous morphine is a satisfactory alternative to intravenous patient-controlled analgesia morphine after cardiac surgery. *Anesthesia and Analgesia*. 1998; **87**: 11–15.

59. Tsang J, Brush B. Patient-controlled analgesia in postoperative cardiac surgery. *Anaesthesia and Intensive Care*. 1999; **27**: 464–70.

60. Myles PS, Buckland MR, Cannon GB *et al*. Comparison of patient-controlled analgesia and nurse-controlled infusion analgesia after cardiac surgery. *Anaesthesia and Intensive Care*. 1994; **22**: 672–8.

∗ 61. Bainbridge D, Martin JE, Cheng DC. Patient-controlled versus nurse-controlled analgesia after cardiac surgery – a meta-analysis. *Canadian Journal of Anaesthesia*. 2006; **53**: 492–9.

∗ 62. Macintyre PE. Intravenous patient-controlled analgesia: one size does not fit all. *Anesthesiology Clinics of North America*. 2005; **23**: 109–23.

∗ 63. Dolin SJ, Cashman JN, Bland JM. Effectiveness of acute postoperative pain management: I. Evidence from published data. *British Journal of Anaesthesia*. 2002; **89**: 409–23.

∗ 64. Werawatganon T, Charuluxanun S. Patient controlled intravenous opioid analgesia versus continuous epidural analgesia for pain after intra-abdominal surgery. *Cochrane Database of Systematic Reviews*. 2005; **CD004088**.

∗ 65. Wu CL, Cohen SR, Richman JM.*et al*. Efficacy of postoperative patient-controlled and continuous infusion epidural analgesia versus intravenous patient-controlled analgesia with opioids: a meta-analysis. *Anesthesiology*. 2005; **103**: 1079–88; quiz 109–10.

66. Lebovits AH, Zenetos P, O'Neill DK *et al*. Satisfaction with epidural and intravenous patient-controlled analgesia. *Pain Medicine*. 2001; **2**: 280–6.

67. Colwell Jr CW, Morris BA. Patient-controlled analgesia compared with intramuscular injection of analgesics for the management of pain after an orthopaedic procedure. *Journal of Bone and Joint Surgery*. 1995; **77**: 726–33.

∗ 68. Rapp SE, Egan KJ, Ross BK *et al*. A multidimensional comparison of morphine and hydromorphone patient-controlled analgesia. *Anesthesia and Analgesia*. 1996; **82**: 1043–8.

69. Pang WW, Mok MS, Lin CH *et al*. Comparison of patient-controlled analgesia (PCA) with tramadol or morphine. *Canadian Journal of Anaesthesia*. 1999; **46**: 1030–5.

70. Plummer JL, Owen H, Ilsley AH, Inglis S. Morphine patient-controlled analgesia is superior to meperidine patient-controlled analgesia for postoperative pain. *Anesthesia and Analgesia*. 1997; **84**: 794–9.

71. Sinatra R, Chung KS, Silverman DG *et al*. An evaluation of morphine and oxymorphone administered via patient-controlled analgesia (PCA) or PCA plus basal infusion in postcesarean-delivery patients. *Anesthesiology*. 1989; **71**: 502–7.

72. Stanley G, Appadu B, Mead M, Rowbotham DJ. Dose requirements, efficacy and side effects of morphine and pethidine delivered by patient-controlled analgesia after gynaecological surgery. *British Journal of Anaesthesia*. 1996; **76**: 484–6.

73. Woodhouse A, Hobbes AF, Mather LE, Gibson M. A comparison of morphine, pethidine and fentanyl in the postsurgical patient-controlled analgesia environment. *Pain*. 1996; **64**: 115–21.

74. Woodhouse A, Ward ME, Mather LE. Intra-subject variability in post-operative patient-controlled analgesia (PCA): is the patient equally satisfied with morphine, pethidine and fentanyl? *Pain*. 1999; **80**: 545–53.

75. Howell PR, Gambling DR, Pavy T *et al*. Patient-controlled analgesia following caesarean section under general anaesthesia: a comparison of fentanyl with morphine. *Canadian Journal of Anaesthesia*. 1995; **42**: 41–5.

76. Kucukemre F, Kunt N, Kaygusuz K *et al*. Remifentanil compared with morphine for postoperative patient-controlled analgesia after major abdominal surgery: a randomized controlled trial. *European Journal of Anaesthesiology*. 2005; **22**: 378–85.

77. Gurbet A, Goren S, Sahin S *et al*. Comparison of analgesic effects of morphine, fentanyl, and remifentanil with intravenous patient-controlled analgesia after cardiac surgery. *Journal of Cardiothoracic and Vascular Anesthesia*. 2004; **18**: 755–8.

78. Bahar M, Rosen M, Vickers MD. Self-administered nalbuphine, morphine and pethidine. Comparison, by intravenous route, following cholecystectomy. *Anaesthesia*. 1985; **40**: 529–32.

79. Sinatra RS, Lodge K, Sibert K *et al*. A comparison of morphine, meperidine, and oxymorphone as utilized in patient-controlled analgesia following cesarean delivery. *Anesthesiology*. 1989; **70**: 585–90.

80. Dopfmer UR, Schenk MR, Kuscic S *et al*. A randomized controlled double-blind trial comparing piritramide and morphine for analgesia after hysterectomy. *European Journal of Anaesthesiology*. 2001; **18**: 389–93.

81. Erolcay H, Yuceyar L. Intravenous patient-controlled analgesia after thoracotomy: a comparison of morphine with tramadol. *European Journal of Anaesthesiology*. 2003; **20**: 141–6.

82. Silvasti M, Tarkkila P, Tuominen M *et al*. Efficacy and side effects of tramadol versus oxycodone for patient-controlled analgesia after maxillofacial surgery. *European Journal of Anaesthesiology*. 1999; **16**: 834–9.

83. Seifert CF, Kennedy S. Meperidine is alive and well in the new millennium: evaluation of meperidine usage patterns and frequency of adverse drug reactions. *Pharmacotherapy*. 2004; **24**: 776–83.

84. Silverman ME, Shih RD, Allegra J. Morphine induces less nausea than meperidine when administered parenterally. *Journal of Emergency Medicine*. 2004; **27**: 241–3.

∗ 85. Latta KS, Ginsberg B, Barkin RL. Meperidine: a critical review. *American Journal of Therapeutics*. 2002; **9**: 53–68.

86. Simopoulos TT, Smith HS, Peeters-Asdourian C, Stevens DS. Use of meperidine in patient-controlled analgesia and

the development of a normeperidine toxic reaction. *Archives of Surgery.* 2002; **137**: 84–8.

87. Stone PA, Macintyre PE, Jarvis DA. Norpethidine toxicity and patient controlled analgesia. *British Journal of Anaesthesia.* 1993; **71**: 738–40.

* 88. Australian and New Zealand College of Anaesthetists. *Acute pain management: scientific evidence*, 2nd edn. Melbourne: ANZCA, 2005 (www.anzca.edu.au/publications/acutepain).

89. Krishnan K, Elliot SC, Berridge JC, Mallick A. Remifentanil patient-controlled analgesia following cardiac surgery. *Acta Anaesthesiologica Scandinavica.* 2005; **49**: 876–9.

90. Dill-Russell PC, Ng L, Ravalia A. Use of a remifentanil PCA for a patient with multiple rib fractures. *Canadian Journal of Anaesthesia.* 2002; **49**: 757.

91. Chou WY, Yang LC, Lu HF *et al.* Association of mu-opioid receptor gene polymorphism (A118G) with variations in morphine consumption for analgesia after total knee arthroplasty. *Acta Anaesthesiologica Scandinavica.* 2006; **50**: 787–92.

92. Chou WY, Wang CH, Liu PH *et al.* Human opioid receptor A118G polymorphism affects intravenous patient-controlled analgesia morphine consumption after total abdominal hysterectomy. *Anesthesiology.* 2006; **105**: 334–7.

93. Klepstad P, Dale O, Skorpen F *et al.* Genetic variability and clinical efficacy of morphine. *Acta Anaesthesiologica Scandinavica.* 2005; **49**: 902–8.

94. Stamer UM, Lehnen K, Hothker F *et al.* Impact of CYP2D6 genotype on postoperative tramadol analgesia. *Pain.* 2003; **105**: 231–8.

95. Jacox A, Carr DB, Mahrenholz DM, Ferrell BM. Cost considerations in patient-controlled analgesia. *Pharmacoeconomics.* 1997; **12**: 109–20.

96. D'Haese J, Vanlersberghe C, Umbrain V, Camu F. Pharmaco-economic evaluation of a disposable patient-controlled analgesia device and intramuscular analgesia in surgical patients. *European Journal of Anaesthesiology.* 1998; **15**: 297–303.

97. Chang AM, Ip WY, Cheung TH. Patient-controlled analgesia versus conventional intramuscular injection: a cost effectiveness analysis. *Journal of Advanced Nursing.* 2004; **46**: 531–41.

98. Bartha E, Carlsson P, Kalman S. Evaluation of costs and effects of epidural analgesia and patient-controlled intravenous analgesia after major abdominal surgery. *British Journal of Anaesthesia.* 2006; **96**: 111–17.

99. Dawson L, Brockbank K, Carr EC, Barrett RF. Improving patients' postoperative sleep: a randomized control study comparing subcutaneous with intravenous patient-controlled analgesia. *Journal of Advanced Nursing.* 1999; **30**: 875–81.

100. Urquhart ML, Klapp K, White PF. Patient-controlled analgesia: a comparison of intravenous versus subcutaneous hydromorphone. *Anesthesiology.* 1988; **69**: 428–32.

101. Striebel HW, Scheitza W, Philippi W *et al.* Quantifying oral analgesic consumption using a novel method and comparison with patient-controlled intravenous analgesic consumption. *Anesthesia and Analgesia.* 1998; **86**: 1051–3.

102. Toussaint S, Maidl J, Schwagmeier R, Striebel HW. Patient-controlled intranasal analgesia: effective alternative to intravenous PCA for postoperative pain relief. *Canadian Journal of Anaesthesia.* 2000; **47**: 299–302.

103. Hallett A, O'Higgins F, Francis V, Cook TM. Patient-controlled intranasal diamorphine for postoperative pain: an acceptability study. *Anaesthesia.* 2000; **55**: 532–9.

104. Ward M, Minto G, Alexander-Williams JM. A comparison of patient-controlled analgesia administered by the intravenous or intranasal route during the early postoperative period. *Anaesthesia.* 2002; **57**: 48–52.

105. Chelly JE, Grass J, Houseman TW *et al.* The safety and efficacy of a fentanyl patient-controlled transdermal system for acute postoperative analgesia: a multicenter, placebo-controlled trial. *Anesthesia and Analgesia.* 2004; **98**: 427–33.

106. Viscusi ER, Reynolds L, Tait S *et al.* An iontophoretic fentanyl patient-activated analgesic delivery system for postoperative pain: a double-blind, placebo-controlled trial. *Anesthesia and Analgesia.* 2006; **102**: 188–94.

107. White PF. Subcutaneous-PCA: an alternative to IV-PCA for postoperative pain management. *Clinical Journal of Pain.* 1990; **6**: 297–300.

108. Striebel HW, Bonillo B, Schwagmeier R *et al.* Self-administered intranasal meperidine for postoperative pain management. *Canadian Journal of Anaesthesia.* 1995; **42**: 287–91.

109. Sathyan G, Jaskowiak J, Evashenk M, Gupta S. Characterisation of the pharmacokinetics of the fentanyl HCl patient-controlled transdermal system (PCTS): effect of current magnitude and multiple-day dosing and comparison with IV fentanyl administration. *Clinical Pharmacokinetics.* 2005; **44** (Suppl. 1): 7–15.

110. Viscusi ER, Reynolds L, Chung F *et al.* Patient-controlled transdermal fentanyl hydrochloride vs intravenous morphine pump for postoperative pain: a randomized controlled trial. *Journal of the American Medical Association.* 2004; **291**: 1333–41.

* 111. Bell RF, Dahl JB, Moore RA, Kalso E. Perioperative ketamine for acute postoperative pain. *Cochrane Database of Systematic Reviews.* 2006; **CD004603**.

112. Hercock T, Gillham MJ, Sleigh JW, Jones SF. The addition of ketamine to patient controlled morphine analgesia does not improve quality of analgesia after total abdominal hysterectomy. *Acute Pain.* 1999; **2**: 68–72.

113. Snijdelaar DG, Cornelisse HB, Schmid RL, Katz J. A randomised, controlled study of peri-operative low dose s(+)-ketamine in combination with postoperative patient-controlled s(+)-ketamine and morphine after radical prostatectomy. *Anaesthesia.* 2004; **59**: 222–8.

114. Burstal R, Danjoux G, Hayes C, Lantry G. PCA ketamine and morphine after abdominal hysterectomy. *Anaesthesia and Intensive Care.* 2001; **29**: 246–51.

115. Javery KB, Ussery TW, Steger HG, Colclough GW. Comparison of morphine and morphine with ketamine for postoperative analgesia. *Canadian Journal of Anaesthesia*. 1996; **43**: 212–15.

116. Murdoch CJ, Crooks BA, Miller CD. Effect of the addition of ketamine to morphine in patient-controlled analgesia. *Anaesthesia*. 2002; **57**: 484–8.

117. Unlugenc H, Ozalevli M, Guler T, Isik G. Postoperative pain management with intravenous patient-controlled morphine: comparison of the effect of adding magnesium or ketamine. *European Journal of Anaesthesiology*. 2003; **20**: 416–21.

118. Cepeda MS, Alvarez H, Morales O, Carr DB. Addition of ultralow dose naloxone to postoperative morphine PCA: unchanged analgesia and opioid requirement but decreased incidence of opioid side effects. *Pain*. 2004; **107**: 41–6.

119. Cepeda MS, Africano JM, Manrique AM et al. The combination of low dose of naloxone and morphine in PCA does not decrease opioid requirements in the postoperative period. *Pain*. 2002; **96**: 73–9.

120. Sartain JB, Barry JJ, Richardson CA, Branagan HC. Effect of combining naloxone and morphine for intravenous patient-controlled analgesia. *Anesthesiology*. 2003; **99**: 148–51.

121. Jeffs SA, Hall JE, Morris S. Comparison of morphine alone with morphine plus clonidine for postoperative patient-controlled analgesia. *British Journal of Anaesthesia*. 2002; **89**: 424–7.

122. Unlugenc H, Gunduz M, Ozalevli M, Akman H. A comparative study on the analgesic effect of tramadol, tramadol plus magnesium, and tramadol plus ketamine for postoperative pain management after major abdominal surgery. *Acta Anaesthesiologica Scandinavica*. 2002; **46**: 1025–30.

123. Chen JY, Wu GJ, Mok MS et al. Effect of adding ketorolac to intravenous morphine patient-controlled analgesia on bowel function in colorectal surgery patients – a prospective, randomized, double-blind study. *Acta Anaesthesiologica Scandinavica*. 2005; **49**: 546–51.

124. Cepeda MS, Delgado M, Ponce M et al. Equivalent outcomes during postoperative patient-controlled intravenous analgesia with lidocaine plus morphine versus morphine alone. *Anesthesia and Analgesia*. 1996; **83**: 102–6.

125. Chen PP, Chui PT, Ma M, Gin T. A prospective survey of patients after cessation of patient-controlled analgesia. *Anesthesia and Analgesia*. 2001; **92**: 224–7.

126. Ginsberg B, Sinatra RS, Adler LJ et al. Conversion to oral controlled-release oxycodone from intravenous opioid analgesic in the postoperative setting. *Pain Medicine*. 2003; **4**: 31–8.

127. Benumof JL. Obesity, sleep apnea, the airway and anesthesia. *Current Opinion in Anaesthesiology*. 2004; **17**: 21–30.

128. Loadsman JA, Hillman DR. Anaesthesia and sleep apnoea. *British Journal of Anaesthesia*. 2001; **86**: 254–66.

129. Etches RC. Respiratory depression associated with patient-controlled analgesia: a review of eight cases. *Canadian Journal of Anaesthesia*. 1994; **41**: 125–32.

130. VanDercar DH, Martinez AP, De Lisser EA. Sleep apnea syndromes: a potential contraindication for patient-controlled analgesia. *Anesthesiology*. 1991; **74**: 623–4.

131. Parikh SN, Stuchin SA, Maca C et al. Sleep apnea syndrome in patients undergoing total joint arthroplasty. *Journal of Arthroplasty*. 2002; **17**: 635–42.

132. Lofsky A. Sleep apnea and narcotic postoperative pain medication: morbidity and mortality risk. *Anesthesia Patient Safety Foundation Newsletter*. 2002; **17**: 24.

133. Young T, Skatrud J, Peppard PE. Risk factors for obstructive sleep apnea in adults. *Journal of the American Medical Association*. 2004; **291**: 2013–16.

134. Choi YK, Brolin RE, Wagner BK et al. Efficacy and safety of patient-controlled analgesia for morbidly obese patients following gastric bypass surgery. *Obesity Surgery*. 2000; **10**: 154–9.

135. Kyzer S, Ramadan E, Gersch M, Chaimoff C. Patient-controlled analgesia following vertical gastroplasty: a comparison with intramuscular narcotics. *Obesity Surgery*. 1995; **5**: 18–21.

136. Charghi R, Backman S, Christou N et al. Patient controlled i.v. analgesia is an acceptable pain management strategy in morbidly obese patients undergoing gastric bypass surgery. A retrospective comparison with epidural analgesia. *Canadian Journal of Anaesthesia*. 2003; **50**: 672–8.

*137. USP. Patient-controlled analgesia pumps USP quality review; cited November 2006. Available from: www.usp.org/patientSafety/newsletters/qualityReview/qr812004-09-01.html.

138. Looi-Lyons LC, Chung FF, Chan VW, McQuestion M. Respiratory depression: an adverse outcome during patient controlled analgesia therapy. *Journal of Clinical Anesthesia*. 1996; **8**: 151–6.

139. Ashburn MA, Love G, Pace NL. Respiratory-related critical events with intravenous patient-controlled analgesia. *Clinical Journal of Pain*. 1994; **10**: 52–6.

140. ECRI. Patient-controlled analgesic infusion pumps. *Health Devices*. 2006; **35**: 5–35.

*141. Vicente KJ, Kada-Bekhaled K, Hillel G et al. Programming errors contribute to death from patient-controlled analgesia: case report and estimate of probability. *Canadian Journal of Anaesthesia*. 2003; **50**: 328–32.

142. ECRI. Abbott PCA Plus II patient-controlled analgesic pumps prone to misprogramming resulting in narcotic overinfusions. *Health Devices*. 1997; **26**: 389–91.

143. ECRI. Medication safety: PCA pump programming errors continue to cause fatal overinfusions. *Health Devices*. 2002; **31**: 342–6.

144. White PF. Mishaps with patient-controlled analgesia. *Anesthesiology*. 1987; **66**: 81–3.

145. White PF, Parker RK. Is the risk of using a "basal" infusion with patient-controlled analgesia therapy justified? *Anesthesiology*. 1992; **76**: 489.

146. Heath ML. Safety of patient controlled analgesia. *Anaesthesia*. 1995; **50**: 573.

147. Wright DG. 'That chap on the PCAS is a bit twitchy today'. *Anaesthesia*. 1993; **48**: 354.

148. Richtsmeier Jr AJ, Barnes SD, Barkin RL. Ventilatory arrest with morphine patient-controlled analgesia in a child with renal failure. *American Journal of Therapeutics*. 1997; **4**: 255–7.

149. Geller RJ. Meperidine in patient-controlled analgesia: a near-fatal mishap. *Anesthesia and Analgesia*. 1993; **76**: 655–7.

150. Tsui SL, Irwin MG, Wong CM *et al*. An audit of the safety of an acute pain service. *Anaesthesia*. 1997; **52**: 1042–7.

151. Notcutt WG, Morgan RJ. Introducing patient-controlled analgesia for postoperative pain control into a district general hospital. *Anaesthesia*. 1990; **45**: 401–6.

152. Lotsch J, Skarke C, Tegeder I, Geisslinger G. Drug interactions with patient-controlled analgesia. *Clinical Pharmacokinetics*. 2002; **41**: 31–57.

153. Farmer M, Harper NJ. Unexpected problems with patient controlled analgesia. *British Medical Journal*. 1992; **304**: 574.

154. Dawson P, Ashworth M. A footplate for conventional PCA demand buttons. *Anaesthesia and Intensive Care*. 1990; **18**: 585–6.

155. Southall L, Macintyre PE, Semple TG. PCA demand buttons. *Anaesthesia and Intensive Care*. 1990; **18**: 268.

156. Jastrzab G, Khor KE. Use of breath-activated patient controlled analgesia for acute pain management in a patient with quadriplegia. *Spinal Cord*. 1999; **37**: 221–3.

157. Fleming BM, Coombs DW. A survey of complications documented in a quality-control analysis of patient-controlled analgesia in the postoperative patient. *Journal of Pain and Symptom Management*. 1992; **7**: 463–9.

158. Wheatley RG, Madej TH, Jackson IJ, Hunter D. The first year's experience of an acute pain service. *British Journal of Anaesthesia*. 1991; **67**: 353–9.

159. Chisakuta AM. Nurse-call button on a patient-controlled analgesia pump? *Anaesthesia*. 1993; **48**: 90.

160. Lam FY. Patient-controlled analgesia by proxy. *British Journal of Anaesthesia*. 1993; **70**: 113.

161. Wakerlin G, Larson Jr CP. Spouse-controlled analgesia. *Anesthesia and Analgesia*. 1990; **70**: 119.

162. Peady C. Unauthorised access to the contents of a Graseby 3300 PCA pump. *Anaesthesia*. 2007; **62**: 98–9; discussion 9.

163. Christie L, Cranfield KA. A dangerous fault with a PCA pump. *Anaesthesia*. 1998; **53**: 827.

164. Doyle DJ, Vicente KJ. Electrical short circuit as a possible cause of death in patients on PCA machines: report on an opiate overdose and a possible preventive remedy. *Anesthesiology*. 2001; **94**: 940.

165. Rosen M, Williams B. The Valved-Y-Cardiff connector (V.Y.C. Con). *Anaesthesia*. 1979; **34**: 882–4.

166. Kluger MT, Owen H. Antireflux valves in patient-controlled analgesia. *Anaesthesia*. 1990; **45**: 1057–61.

167. Paterson JG. Intravenous obstruction and PCA machines. *Canadian Journal of Anaesthesia*. 1998; **45**: 284.

168. Grover ER, Heath ML. Patient-controlled analgesia. A serious incident. *Anaesthesia*. 1992; **47**: 402–4.

169. Kwan A. Overdose of morphine during PCA. *Anaesthesia*. 1995; **50**: 919.

170. ECRI. Improper cassette attachment allows gravity free-flow from SIMS-Deltec CADD-series pumps. *Health Devices*. 1995; **24**: 84–6.

171. Thomas DW, Owen H. Patient-controlled analgesia – the need for caution. A case report and review of adverse incidents. *Anaesthesia*. 1988; **43**: 770–2.

172. ECRI. Overinfusion caused by gravity free-flow from a damaged prefilled glass syringe. *Health Devices*. 1996; **25**: 476–7.

173. Harmer M. Overdosage during patient controlled analgesia. Follow manufacturers' instructions. *British Medical Journal*. 1994; **309**: 1583.

174. Notcutt WG, Kaldas R. Patient-controlled analgesia – a serious incident. *Anaesthesia*. 1992; **47**: 1008.

175. Wheeler M, Oderda GM, Ashburn MA, Lipman AG. Adverse events associated with postoperative opioid analgesia: a systematic review. *Journal of Pain*. 2002; **3**: 159–80.

*176. Cashman JN, Dolin SJ. Respiratory and haemodynamic effects of acute postoperative pain management: evidence from published data. *British Journal of Anaesthesia*. 2004; **93**: 212–23.

*177. Dolin SJ, Cashman JN. Tolerability of acute postoperative pain management: nausea, vomiting, sedation, pruritis, and urinary retention. Evidence from published data. *British Journal of Anaesthesia*. 2005; **95**: 584–91.

178. Shapiro A, Zohar E, Zaslansky R *et al*. The frequency and timing of respiratory depression in 1524 postoperative patients treated with systemic or neuraxial morphine. *Journal of Clinical Anesthesia*. 2005; **17**: 537–42.

*179. Marret E, Kurdi O, Zufferey P, Bonnet F. Effects of nonsteroidal antiinflammatory drugs on patient-controlled analgesia morphine side effects: meta-analysis of randomized controlled trials. *Anesthesiology*. 2005; **102**: 1249–60.

180. Roberts GW, Bekker TB, Carlsen HH *et al*. Postoperative nausea and vomiting are strongly influenced by postoperative opioid use in a dose-related manner. *Anesthesia and Analgesia*. 2005; **101**: 1343–8.

*181. Remy C, Marret E, Bonnet F. Effects of acetaminophen on morphine side-effects and consumption after major surgery: meta-analysis of randomized controlled trials. *British Journal of Anaesthesia*. 2005; **94**: 505–13.

*182. Tramer MR, Walder B. Efficacy and adverse effects of prophylactic antiemetics during patient-controlled analgesia therapy: a quantitative systematic review. *Anesthesia and Analgesia*. 1999; **88**: 1354–61.

183. Lo Y, Chia YY, Liu K, Ko NH. Morphine sparing with droperidol in patient-controlled analgesia. *Journal of Clinical Anesthesia*. 2005; **17**: 271–5.

184. Culebras X, Corpataux JB, Gaggero G, Tramer MR. The antiemetic efficacy of droperidol added to morphine

patient-controlled analgesia: a randomized, controlled, multicenter dose-finding study. *Anesthesia and Analgesia.* 2003; **97**: 816–21.

185. Gan TJ, Alexander R, Fennelly M, Rubin AP. Comparison of different methods of administering droperidol in patient-controlled analgesia in the prevention of postoperative nausea and vomiting. *Anesthesia and Analgesia.* 1995; **80**: 81–5.

186. Cherian VT, Smith I. Prophylactic ondansetron does not improve patient satisfaction in women using PCA after Caesarean section. *British Journal of Anaesthesia.* 2001; **87**: 502–4.

187. Silverman DG, Freilich J, Sevarino FB *et al.* Influence of promethazine on symptom-therapy scores for nausea during patient-controlled analgesia with morphine. *Anesthesia and Analgesia.* 1992; **74**: 735–8.

188. Lin TF, Yeh YC, Yen YH *et al.* Antiemetic and analgesic-sparing effects of diphenhydramine added to morphine intravenous patient-controlled analgesia. *British Journal of Anaesthesia.* 2005; **94**: 835–9.

189. Laffey JG, Boylan JF. Cyclizine and droperidol have comparable efficacy and side effects during patient-controlled analgesia. *Irish Journal of Medical Science.* 2002; **171**: 141–4.

190. Bree SE, West MJ, Taylor PA, Kestin IG. Combining propofol with morphine in patient-controlled analgesia to prevent postoperative nausea and vomiting. *British Journal of Anaesthesia.* 1998; **80**: 152–4.

191. Joshi GP, Duffy L, Chehade J *et al.* Effects of prophylactic nalmefene on the incidence of morphine-related side effects in patients receiving intravenous patient-controlled analgesia. *Anesthesiology.* 1999; **90**: 1007–11.

*192. Kjellberg F, Tramer MR. Pharmacological control of opioid-induced pruritus: a quantitative systematic review of randomized trials. *European Journal of Anaesthesiology.* 2001; **18**: 346–57.

193. Hodsman NB, Kenny GN, McArdle CS. Patient controlled analgesia and urinary retention. *British Journal of Surgery.* 1988; **75**: 212.

194. Harrington P, Bunola J, Jennings AJ *et al.* Acute compartment syndrome masked by intravenous morphine from a patient-controlled analgesia pump. *Injury.* 2000; **31**: 387–9.

195. Richards H, Langston A, Kulkarni R, Downes EM. Does patient controlled analgesia delay the diagnosis of compartment syndrome following intramedullary nailing of the tibia? *Injury.* 2004; **35**: 296–8.

196. Meyer GS, Eagle KA. Patient-controlled analgesia masking pulmonary embolus in a postoperative patient. *Critical Care Medicine.* 1992; **20**: 1619–21.

197. Finger MJ, McLeod DG. Postoperative myocardial infarction after radical cystoprostatectomy masked by patient-controlled analgesia. *Urology.* 1995; **45**: 155–7.

12

Continuous peripheral neural blockade for acute pain

KIM E RUSSON AND WILLIAM HARROP-GRIFFITHS

KEY LEARNING POINTS

- Continuous neural blockade usually supplements a multimodal approach to acute pain management; rarely does it completely replace it.
- Although the knowledge and skills of the physician are critical for successful continuous neural blockade, the knowledge and skills of an appropriately trained multidisciplinary team are also vitally important for its safe and successful use in acute pain management.
- There is an increasing body of evidence that supports the use of continuous neural blockade and shows that, compared with opioid analgesia alone, continuous neural blockade results in better pain relief and fewer side effects.
- Compared with central neuraxial blockade, pain relief with continuous neural blockade may be as effective

with fewer side effects, although there may be a higher risk of neurological complications.
- Continuous nerve blocks are more expensive and difficult to perform and maintain than single-injection blocks. It is therefore critically important to assess the benefits that the patient will gain from their use and the risks to which the patients will be exposed.
- The development of sustained-release formulations of local anesthetic drugs may provide an alternative to continuous peripheral neural blockade in the future. However, these drugs are not yet in clinical use. Administration of a fixed dose may also limit the ability to titrate to effect (or adverse effects) for individual patients.

INTRODUCTION

The use of continuous peripheral nerve blocks (CPNB) was first described by Ansbro in 1946.[1] The only local anesthetic available to him, procaine, was short-acting: unfortunately, the surgeons with whom he worked were long-acting. By inserting a needle near the brachial plexus and fixing it to the skin, he

was able to top up the initial block and match the duration of anesthesia to that of the surgery. In the 60 years since then, surgeons have become a little faster and local anesthetic drugs have become longer-acting, and there have been key advances in the needles and catheters available and techniques to assist with their placement, as well as developments in infusion pump technology.

The pain experienced after surgery often outlasts the duration of action of single-shot peripheral nerve blocks. Continuous peripheral neural blockade therefore seeks to extend the duration of local analgesia from the hours of the single-shot block to many hours or even days, enabling the duration of analgesia to better match the likely duration of significant pain.

Currently, CPNB is most often used for postoperative analgesia and the treatment of other acutely painful conditions. Pain is a multimodal experience and it is important to note that CPNB should be used as part of a multimodal analgesic technique. Some general principles of initiating and managing CPNB can be proposed.

- The operator should be an experienced and successful single-shot blocker, and should be assisted by someone who is familiar with both the technique and the equipment.
- Suitable monitoring regimens and appropriate resuscitation equipment must be available during the insertion of the catheter and initiation of the regional block; monitoring requirements during CPNB (using repeated bolus doses and/or continuous infusions) may vary according to patient location (in hospital ward or at home).
- There needs to be a multidisciplinary team, the members of which are familiar with the principles of the use of CPNB, the catheters, and infusion pumps, and have received the appropriate training. They should be aware of the goals of the treatment, of its potential complications, and of the initial actions needed should complications occur. The team will include the operating room, recovery and ward staff, physiotherapists, and, where appropriate, patients and their carers in the community, as well as their general practitioners.
- If CPNB is used for analgesia after discharge from hospital, appropriate patient selection and education are essential and adequate follow up is crucial. There should be a 24-hour point of contact available to advise on problems should they occur; this is ideally an anesthesiologist familiar with the technique.

A number of reviews have confirmed that CPNB provides safe and effective postoperative analgesia in both elective and emergency situations, and can be used for patients of all ages in hospital or at home.[2, 3, 4, 5]

In general, and in comparison with systemic opioid analgesia, CPNB is associated with better pain relief and a lower incidence of opioid-related side effects, regardless of the site of catheter insertion.[6][I] In comparison with single-shot blocks, reports published to date do not suggest a higher complication rate with CPNB.[7] However, as it is possible that the risks might be greater than those of the single-shot block on which they are based, it is important to assess whether the benefits that may accrue to the patient with the use of CPNB outweigh the additional time, expertise, expense, and possible risks. More detail about complications associated with CPNB is given below under Complications.

There are many different types of CPNB that can be used in clinical practice and the more common ones are under Equipment below. Examples of indications for their use are listed in **Table 12.1**.

COMMON TYPES OF CPNB

Upper limb

AXILLARY BRACHIAL PLEXUS BLOCKS

The first description of continuous brachial plexus blockade in the modern era was provided by Selander.[8] In this paper, he describes the successful placement of an intravenous cannula into the axillary brachial plexus sheath.

Since then, many investigators have confirmed that axillary catheters can provide effective anesthesia and analgesia during and after hand, forearm, and elbow surgery.[9, 10, 11, 12] Success of this technique may be affected by the dose regimens used and the provision of additional analgesia. For example, Salonen et al.[13][II] found that after elective hand surgery, continuous axillary infusions of 0.1 or 0.2 percent ropivacaine was no better than a saline infusion and all groups needed additional analgesia. However, both continuous infusion and repeated bolus dose regimens using 0.25 percent bupivacaine have resulted in good pain relief with no difference between the techniques for pain scores, degree of motor block, or opioid requirements, although plasma bupivacaine levels were higher in the patients given the continuous infusions.[14][II] Similarly, both 0.125 percent bupivacaine and 0.125 percent ropivacaine, given as patient-controlled bolus doses of 10 mL at home, provided equal and effective pain relief.[9][II]

As well as improving pain relief, continuous axillary blocks have been used to increase vascular flow in patients after digital reimplantation surgery.[15]

The naive original notion that the three nerves in greatest proximity to the axillary artery (median, ulnar, and radial nerves) can be blocked equally by a catheter placed in the notional axillary sheath[16] is proving not to be correct.[17] Many of those who use this technique identify and then place the catheter by the nerve that primarily supplies the part of the arm that is the target of the surgery. In attempts to reduce the risk of infection and limit catheter movement and therefore the chance of dislodgement, some anesthesiologists also tunnel the catheter away from the apex of the axilla in order to

Table 12.1 Catheter locations and examples of indications.

Block technique	Examples of indications for each catheter technique
Upper limb	
Interscalene block (anterior or posterior approach)	Shoulder replacement, hemi-arthroplasty
	Open rotator cuff repair
	Capsular release and manipulation for frozen shoulder
	Acromioclavicular joint reconstruction
	Surgery for proximal humeral fractures
Supraclavicular or subclavian perivascular block	Shoulder procedures
	Elbow replacement or arthrolysis
	Elbow fracture dislocation
	Forearm and hand fractures
	Hand surgery
Infraclavicular block (vertical or other more lateral approaches), axillary block	Elbow replacement or arthrolysis
	Elbow fracture dislocation
	Forearm and hand fractures
	Hand surgery
Lower limb	
Proximal sciatic nerve block	Hip arthroplasty
	Knee arthroplasty
	Cruciate ligament repair
	Above or below knee amputation
	Foot and ankle surgery
Popliteal fossa sciatic nerve	Foot and ankle surgery
Psoas compartment/lumbar plexus block	Femoral fractures and surgery
	Hip arthroplasty
	Knee arthroplasty
	Cruciate ligament repair
Femoral nerve block	Femoral fractures and surgery
	Knee arthroplasty
	Cruciate ligament repair
Fascia iliaca block	Femoral fractures and surgery
	Skin graft harvesting
	Knee arthroplasty
	Cruciate ligament repair
Saphenous nerve block	Foot or ankle surgery involving the medial side
	Varicose vein surgery on the long saphenous nerve
Trunk blocks	
Intercostal blocks	Rib fractures
	Open cholecystectomy
Thoracic paravertebral blocks	Rib fractures
	Breast surgery
	Thoracic and abdominal surgery

allow it to emerge from a cleaner and less mobile piece of skin.

PERICLAVIULAR BRACHIAL PLEXUS BLOCKS

The periclavicular area offers advantages as a site for the placement of brachial plexus catheters. In contrast to the axilla, the skin in this area is clean and relatively immobile. The increasing popularity of a variety of infraclavicular blocks has coincided with the increasing use of these approaches for plexus catheterization.

Infraclavicular catheters have been used for pain relief after elbow, forearm, and hand surgery, including after the patient has been discharged home.[18][II], [19][II], [20][II] Ilfeld et al.[18][II] compared the use of an infraclavicular brachial plexus ropivacaine infusion with a saline infusion in patients discharged home after surgery of the upper extremity; patients receiving the ropivacaine infusion had less pain, fewer sleep disturbances, used less opioid, had fewer opioid-related side effects, and were more satisfied.

The vertical infraclavicular block was first described by Mehrkens and Geiger[21] and has become a popular approach for catheter insertion in some hospitals. Compared with axillary plexus blocks, this approach is associated with more rapid block onset and a higher success rate.[22][II]

The possibility of using the subclavian perivascular approach originally described by Winnie and Collins[23] for continuous techniques was first mooted by the great man himself.[16] Although there exist proponents of this approach and the technique is used by some as the basis of a continuous technique, it has not achieved widespread popularity.

INTERSCALENE BRACHIAL PLEXUS BLOCKS

Shoulder operations can be extremely painful, and early and effective rehabilitation is important in improving postoperative outcome.[24] With pain as a significant feature and placing substantial limitations on rehabilitation, it is perhaps not surprising that the subject of local anesthetic infusions via interscalene catheters made a relatively early appearance in the literature on CPNB[25, 26] or that their use for pain relief after major shoulder surgery, has become widespread.[5, 27, 28, 29, 30, 31]

A growing body of evidence now confirms that, in general, continuous interscalene brachial plexus blockade can provide analgesia that is superior to intravenous opioids.[6][I] For example, patient-controlled (set to deliver a continuous infusion and allow delivery of bolus doses)[27][II], [31][II] and continuous infusion-only interscalene analgesia[30][II] improved pain relief and patient satisfaction and reduced opioid-related side effects compared with i.v. opioid patient-controlled analgesia (PCA)[27][II], [31][II] and oral opioid analgesia.[30][II] Continuous interscalene analgesia also provided better pain relief and reduced opioid requirements following shoulder surgery compared with single-injection interscalene blockade[32][II] and local anesthetic infusions into the glenohumeral joint or subacromial bursa,[33][II] although the incidence of minor side effects may be increased.[33][II]

There have been reports of successful interscalene brachial plexus catheterization by the posterior approach to this part of the brachial plexus using the techniques described by Pippa et al.[34] and Boezaart et al.[35] Although this approach has been criticized,[36] it has been shown to be relatively safe and effective when used as a single-shot block,[37][V] or continuous infusion after painful shoulder surgery.[38][V]

As a footnote, it is worth mentioning that the skin over the most popular entry point for access to the interscalene brachial plexus – the lateral approach or Winnie technique[39] – is also relatively mobile. For this reason, some anesthesiologists who use this technique tunnel the catheter to more immobile skin.[40, 41]

Discussion about the complications that might be associated with this block are covered below under Complications.

Lower limb

It is arguable that whereas the available published evidence indicates that continuous regional analgesia of the upper limb consistently offers better pain relief and outcome compared with opioid analgesia, the data for the lower limb are perhaps not as convincing.

One of the great appeals of CPNB for pain relief after lower limb surgery is the avoidance of many of the side effects and complications associated with the regional anesthetic and analgesic alternatives: spinal and epidural blockade. The use of CPNB avoids the possibility of significant sympathetic block and limits blockade to a specific extremity while making analgesia virtually limitless.[42]

PSOAS COMPARTMENT BLOCKS

Psoas compartment blocks, also called lumbar plexus blocks, were first described by Chayen et al. in 1976.[43] By blocking the three primary components of the lumbar plexus (femoral nerve, obturator nerve, and the lateral cutaneous nerve of the thigh), this block can provide analgesia for hip, thigh, and knee surgery. If combined with a sciatic nerve block, it can provide analgesia for virtually the whole lower limb.

The traditional landmarks for the block have been refined on a number of occasions[44, 45] with the aim of maximizing the success rate and minimizing the incidence of complications, most notably accidental epidural and spinal injection of large volumes of local anesthetic drug. Prolongation of this block can readily be achieved by insertion of a catheter, and the relatively immobile skin over the insertion site of the block is associated with a low incidence of accidental dislodgement.[46]

Continuous psoas compartment blocks have been shown to provide more effective analgesia than i.v. opioid PCA after surgery for acetabular fractures,[47][III] or hip fractures,[48][II] total knee joint replacement,[49][II] and total hip replacement.[44][II] In patients having partial hip replacement surgery, there was no difference in pain relief or patient satisfaction between continuous psoas compartment blocks and epidural analgesia, although patients in the epidural group had greater motor blockade and significantly more complications, and delayed ambulation.[50][II]

As mentioned above, complications of this block have included accidental placement of attempted psoas compartment catheters into the subarachnoid or epidural spaces.[51, 52, 53]

FEMORAL NERVE AND FASCIA ILIACA BLOCKS

The traditional anterior femoral nerve block remains popular for analgesia after knee surgery. It can also provide effective pain relief after lower limb vascular surgery and skin grafting.[54, 55]

After total knee arthroplasty, there is conflicting evidence whether continuous femoral nerve infusions provide better analgesia than single-shot femoral blocks with both better pain relief[56][II] and no difference[57][II] reported. However, compared with i.v. PCA opioids, most studies show that continuous femoral nerve infusions lead to better pain relief at rest and with movement, [49][II], [58][II], [59][II] better postoperative knee flexion,[58] [II], [59][II] and earlier discharge;[58][II], [59][II] although this may not always be the case.[60][II] Pain relief, knee flexion, and length of stay were similar to epidural analgesia, although side effects were more common with the latter technique.[58][II], [59][II], [60][II], [61][II]

Although it has been shown that continuous femoral nerve blocks can improve analgesia after total knee replacement, the knee is also innervated by the sciatic nerve and, on occasion, the obturator nerve. It has been suggested that fully effective analgesia of the knee may therefore require the blockade of both femoral and sciatic nerves,[62] although another study showed that combined sciatic and femoral nerve blockade did not improve analgesia compared with femoral block alone.[63]

Similarly, in a study that compared combined continuous femoral–sciatic nerve blocks with epidural analgesia for pain relief after total knee replacement, pain on mobilization was well controlled in both groups and there were no differences in the length of hospital stay or rehabilitation indices; there was a greater incidence of motor blockade in the combined femoral/sciatic nerve block group, but a lower incidence of other side effects compared with those given epidural analgesia.[64][II]

Similar results have also been reported after total hip replacement. Continuous three-in-one blocks provided pain relief that was comparable to i.v. morphine and epidural analgesia; the incidence of nausea, vomiting, pruritus, and sedation was reduced compared with i.v. morphine and there was a reduced incidence of urinary retention and hypotension compared with epidural analgesia.[65]

The original description of the three-in-one block claimed that local anesthetic injected into the femoral sheath just below the level of the inguinal ligament would spread proximally to provide blockade of the femoral, obturator, and lateral cutaneous nerves of the thigh.[66] The increasing realization that blockade of the latter two

nerves of this trio is produced by lateral rather than proximal spread of the local anesthetic has supported the use of subfascial blocks, such as the fascia iliaca block. Successful reports of the use of fascia iliaca catheters exist for both adults and children who undergo knee surgery.[67, 68, 69] Continuous fascia iliaca blocks result in opioid-sparing and improved range of motion during the immediate postoperative period.[68][II] Morau et al.[69][II] showed that it may be faster to place a fascia iliaca catheter compared with a three-in-one catheter, but that there was no difference in pain relief or opioid requirements.

While the use of continuous local anesthetic infusions via femoral nerve catheters can provide safe and reliable analgesia after anterior cruciate ligament repair, there is no evidence of better pain relief or fewer side effects compared with PCA opioid analgesia.[70][III] However, pain relief is better than intra-articular local anesthesia following this type of surgery.[71][II], [72][II] Clear demonstrations that outcome in terms of decreases in significant morbidity, or even mortality, with any form of pain relief are unlikely to ever be forthcoming in this relatively minor procedure on fit people.

SCIATIC NERVE BLOCK

The sciatic nerve is the largest peripheral nerve in the body and is easy to block. Although Labat's original posterior approach has much to commend it and little to criticize,[73] it has not prevented the development of an increasing number of allegedly novel approaches to this nerve. Blockade of the sciatic nerve can be achieved at any place along its course, the exact location of blockade affecting the distribution of analgesia.[46] Proximal blockade of the nerve will provide effective analgesia after knee, shin, ankle, and foot surgery; popliteal sciatic nerve blockade will provide effective foot and ankle analgesia,[46] and can be used for postoperative pain relief at home.[74]

As with most blocks that can be performed using a single-shot approach, insertion of a catheter is also possible. However, the depth of the nerve at the Labat approach and the right-angle that the needle makes with the nerve can make this far from simple. Smith et al.[75] was the first to describe the use of a Tuohy needle for this approach, a technique that has since been used by others.[76, 77] The subgluteal approach appears to be increasing in popularity, perhaps in part because it is possible to alter the direction of the needle so that it approaches the nerve at an angle that is more conducive to easy catheterization. Insertion of a catheter by the anterior approach is also possible.[78]

The use of a peripheral nerve catheter sited at the level of the popliteal fossa to block the sciatic nerve has been well described, and many studies report its success for analgesia after foot and ankle surgery, with few side effects.[46] After lower extremity surgery[74][II] and foot surgery[79][II], [80][II] continuous popliteal sciatic nerve blockade has been shown to result in better pain relief, [74][II], [79][II], [80][II], [81][II] lower opioid requirements, [74][II], [80][II] fewer side effects,[74][II] greater patient satisfaction,[74][II], [80][II] improved sleep,[74][II], [81][II] and earlier patient discharge,[80][II] compared with opioid analgesia alone. Most authorities report the use of a posterior approach, but the successful use of a lateral approach has also been described.[82, 83] Continuous popliteal sciatic nerve infusions have been effectively and safely used in patients who are discharged home with the catheter in place.[74, 80]

RECOMMENDATIONS FOR CPNB AFTER HIP AND KNEE SURGERY

The European PROSPECT group (PROcedure-SPECific postoperative pain managemenT)[84] has recommended femoral nerve block for analgesia after hip arthroplasty, largely based on its efficacy for analgesia after hip fracture surgery.[85][II] The group concluded that femoral nerve blockade is preferred to neuraxial blockade or parenteral opioids, in part because of the lower incidence of side effects (see above under Femoral nerve and fascia iliaca blocks), they suggest use of a continuous infusion rather than a single-shot block, and note that while psoas compartment blocks are more effective, there is a greater potential for more serious complications.[84][II]

More recently, the same group assessed the evidence for pain relief after total knee arthroplasty.[84][V] While they again recommended femoral nerve block based on efficacy of analgesia, they found that the available data did not allow them to say that a continuous block was preferable to a single-shot block (they note one study published after the cut-off date for their literature search suggested that continuous blockade was more effective); they did not recommend psoas compartment blocks because femoral nerve blocks are equally effective with fewer complications.[84][V]

Trunk

CONTINUOUS PARAVERTEBRAL BLOCKADE

Paravertebral blockade as an analgesic technique resided in the doldrums until it was revived by a report by Eason and Wyatt in 1979.[86] Publications by groups in the UK, USA, the Middle East, and Scandinavia then led to a revival in interest in this technique.[87, 88, 89, 90] Although indications for paravertebral blockade are relatively few in number, they can prove useful in a number of situations. Continuous paravertebral blockade has now been described for major unilateral breast surgery,[91] bilateral breast surgery,[92] outpatient breast surgery,[93] rib fractures,[94, 95] shoulder surgery,[96, 97] after minimally invasive

direct coronary artery bypass surgery,[98] after major vascular surgery,[99] and in the treatment of postherpetic neuralgia.[100]

Continuous paravertebral blockade has been shown to be superior to systemic opioid administration as part of a multimodal analgesia technique after thoracotomy.[101] [III] The comparison between postthoracotomy analgesia provided by paravertebral blockade and epidural blockade has attracted a great deal of academic interest. A recent meta-analysis identified ten qualifying, randomized prospective trials that compared these two techniques in patients undergoing thoracotomy.[102][I] After meta-analysis of the results from 520 patients, the majority of whom underwent continuous epidural or paravertebral blockade as opposed to single-shot techniques, the authors concluded that the analgesia provided by paravertebral and epidural blockade was equivalent. However, the use of paravertebral blockade was associated with a significantly lower incidence of pulmonary complications, urinary retention, nausea, vomiting, hypotension, and failed blocks. They concluded that paravertebral blockade has a better side effect profile than epidural blockade in this context and that its use can be recommended for major thoracic surgery. Other comparisons of continuous paravertebral blockade and epidural analgesia after thoracotomy for lung resection[103][II] and minimally invasive direct coronary artery bypass surgery[98][II] also concluded that there was no difference in pain relief, but that continuous paravertebral blockade may be associated with fewer adverse hemodynamic effects.[103][II]

INTERPLEURAL BLOCKADE

Interpleural blockade – the result of the administration of local anesthetic drugs between the parietal and visceral layers of the pleura – is termed by some as "intrapleural blockade." It has a shorter history than paravertebral blockade, having first been presented in 1984 and published in 1986;[104, 105] it has been the subject of a recent two-part review by Dravid and Paul.[106, 107] It has similar applications to paravertebral blockade and has been used for pain relief after upper abdominal surgery,[108] breast surgery,[109] renal surgery,[110] and thoracotomy.[111]

It is this last application about which debate has occurred on the subject of its efficacy. Studies have produced conflicting results, with some concluding that continuous interpleural analgesia is more effective than pain relief using opioids alone,[112][II], [113][II] and others concluding that it is not.[114][II], [115][II] It is possible that the variable results achieved with this technique after thoracotomy may be related to the presence of a chest drain, which would be expected to drain the local anesthetic away from the pleura.[112] Alternatively, the local anesthetic drugs may bind to blood proteins in effusions or suffer an uneven distribution within the postsurgical pleural cavity.[112] Diaphragmatic irritation and scapular retraction may be other reasons why interpleural block alone may not be completely effective after a thoracotomy.

Richardson et al.[116][II] performed a prospective, double-blind trial comparing interpleural with paravertebral block after thoracotomy. Compared with interpleural block, they found that paravertebral blockade was associated with similar pain scores and PCA opioid use, but fewer side effects and better preservation of lung function.

After thoracotomy for minimally invasive direct coronary artery bypass surgery, interpleural analgesia resulted in better pain relief than thoracic epidural analgesia for only the first 12 hours, but the incidence of complications was lower.[117][II]

INTERCOSTAL BLOCKS

Continuous intercostal blocks have also been used in acute pain management. However, analgesia after thoracotomy is not as effective as continuous epidural analgesia.[118][II]

CONTRAINDICATIONS

The contraindications to single-shot or continuous peripheral nerve blocks are well known, but bear repetition. Although it is popular to divide them into absolute and relative contraindications, the authors prefer not to create an artificial division, preferring to rank them starting with those factors most likely to prevent an anesthesiologist from performing the block.

Patient refusal

Obviously, nerve blocks should not be performed in a patient who is capable of consent and who refuses even after careful explanation of its risks and benefits – in many countries to do so would constitute common assault. In addition, not all patients may be willing or able to accept the responsibility that accompanies ambulatory use of CPNB techniques.

Allergy to local anesthetic drugs

Reports of alleged allergy are common but true allergy is rare.[119, 120] A common report of local anesthetic allergy often involves the systemic injection of a catecholamine vasoconstrictor in the dentist's chair.[121]

Disorders of coagulation

Treatment with anticoagulant drugs or the existence of a significant coagulopathy is considered by many to be a contraindication to central neuraxial blocks, although there exists ongoing debate about the extent of the coagulation derangement that would constitute an absolute contraindication. The American Society of Regional Anesthesia has published useful guidance on this which has been highlighted in a paper by Horlocker et al.[122]

The situation with regard to peripheral nerve blocks is perhaps not so clear cut. Although few significant problems have been reported in patients with a coagulopathy undergoing CPNB, the literature is not devoid of such reports.

One case report details the use of an axillary brachial plexus catheter in a hemophiliac patient with no adverse effects.[123] Another paper reports on three patients who had undergone total knee arthroplasty with femoral and sciatic nerve catheters being placed to provide postoperative analgesia; all patients were receiving enoxaparin.[124] In all three patients, some bleeding was noticed before catheter removal and in one of these massive thigh swelling occurred after catheter removal. Another report of a patient receiving low molecular weight heparin therapy in the presence of a lumber plexus catheter described the development of a sciatic nerve palsy after surgery.[125] Although the peripheral nerve catheter was initially suspected to be the cause of the complication, it was found to have resulted from a periarticular hematoma compressing the sciatic nerve. These case reports highlight the need for close postoperative supervision of the patient.

Little can be concluded from sporadic case reports of the safety or complications related to the use of CPNB in coagulopathic patients. In the absence, and likely continuing absence, of definitive data, the opinions of experts must be relied upon. The decision of whether to perform a block in patients with a pathological coagulopathy, being given anticoagulant drugs, or who are likely to be given anticoagulant or thromboprophylactic drugs after surgery, is one that cannot be definitively guided by the available literature. It is a decision that must be taken on an individual patient basis, taking into account the following factors:

- the likely benefits to the patient of the block (e.g. it may be that few would criticize an expert if they were to perform a sciatic nerve block by the posterior approach in an elderly, infirm, and anticoagulated patient with tight aortic stenosis and severe chronic obstructive pulmonary disease, in order to avoid general anesthesia or neuraxial blockade; this may not be the case if the anticoagulated patient were younger and fitter);
- the proximity of the block technique to major blood vessels and the likely incidence of arterial puncture;
- the experience, expertise and confidence of the anesthesiologst;
- the extent or likely extent of the coagulopathy.

Infection

LOCAL INFECTION

Few anesthesiologists would choose to pass their block needles through an overtly infected area of skin or into a part of the body in which sepsis is suspected. This is particularly true of catheter-based continuous techniques.

SYSTEMIC INFECTION

The literature contains articles on the risk of infectious complications after regional anesthesia in febrile or immunocompromised patients; some of these articles offer advice on clinical management, while admitting that this advice is often expert opinion at best.[126, 127] Although the focus of Wedel and Horlocker's article[126] on regional anesthesia in the febrile or infected patient is spinal and epidural blockade, presumably because they are associated with a higher incidence of infectious complications, such as meningitis or epidural abscess, the recommendations they make at the end of the paper can be paraphrased in the context of continuous peripheral nerve blocks:

- the decision to perform a peripheral nerve block must be made on an individual basis considering the anesthetic alternatives, the benefits of regional anesthesia and analgesia, and the risk of central nervous system (CNS) infection (which may theoretically occur in any bacteremic patient);
- consideration should be given to the removal of catheters in the presence of local erythema and/or discharge; there are no convincing data to suggest that concomitant infection at remote sites or the absence of antibiotic therapy are risk factors for infection.

Given the likely (or assumed) lower incidence of infectious complications associated with peripheral nerve blocks, or at least their likely lower risk of grave implications, experts may take slightly more license in the performance of CPNB in febrile patients. However, they may be more reluctant to perform such a block in a patient with significant, untreated systemic sepsis and even more so to pass their block needle or catheter through frankly infected skin. However, in some circumstances it may be believed that a septic patient may derive particular benefit from the avoidance of a general anesthetic and the decision to perform a nerve block will remain a matter for consideration on an individual patient basis.

Preexisting neurological problems

Some neurologists in the past may have advised against the use of peripheral nerve blocks in patients with degenerative neurological disorders, most commonly multiple sclerosis. While there are no published data to support the view that the use of either single-shot or continuous peripheral nerve blocks can lead to a deterioration in these diseases, if the performance of the peripheral nerve block coincides with an acute deterioration in the neurological disorder, the anesthesiologist is likely to be apportioned blame for the deterioration. In such cases, the decision to use CPNB will depend on an assessment of the risk and benefit for each patient and whether the technique is thought to offer particular clinical advantage to the patient.

Block-specific contraindications

There exist absolute and relative contraindications to particular peripheral nerve blocks and therefore to their associated, derived continuous techniques. These are more correctly considered in texts on single-shot blocks. However, as an example, Urmey et al.[128] demonstrated with ultrasound imaging that the performance of a successful interscalene brachial plexus block is associated with a 100 percent incidence ipsilateral hemidiaphragmatic paralysis, proposing this was due to the inevitable block of the phrenic nerve during interscalene block. Although few patients become subjectively or objectively breathless as a result, there have been reports of dyspnea and desaturation in association with this phenomenon.[129, 130] This effect of a single-shot interscalene brachial plexus block is sustained during continuous interscalene analgesia by infusion of local anesthetic drugs.[131] Therefore, any patient who might be compromised by hemidiaphragmatic paralysis, such as in the presence of significant lung disease, should undergo neither the single-shot nor the continuous technique. The incidence of phrenic nerve block as one descends the brachial plexus decreases such that it is thought to be 0 percent for the axillary brachial plexus block, although a low incidence has been claimed for just one relatively high brachial plexus block – the bent needle technique described by Cornish.[132] Bilateral interscalene blocks are to be avoided for fear of precipitating ventilatory failure even in healthy patients.

EQUIPMENT

Catheterization kits

There are now a number of different catheterization kits available. Catheterization equipment can be divided broadly into catheter-through-needle or cannula-over-needle-catheter-through-cannula designs. The latter formerly dominated the market; the former is now prevalent. The needles used are almost always insulated and designed to be used with a peripheral nerve stimulator.

The tips of the needle can be faceted, pencil-point, or Tuohy-tipped. The ability of the Tuohy tip to direct the catheter at an angle to the shaft of the needle is thought to aid catheterization in approaches in which the needle does not pass parallel to the nerve or nerve sheath. Denny et al.[133] describe early experiences with a Tuohy system, arguing that the design facilitates plexus sheath catheterization. The catheter can be a plain plastic tube or a stimulating catheter – one which can be connected to a peripheral nerve stimulator so as to allow the position of its tip to be identified if it is within reasonable proximity to a nerve that has provides innervation to a muscle.[134, 135] The stimulating catheters are more expensive than their nonstimulating counterparts and can be stiffer and therefore more difficult to place. While their ability to provide confirmation of correct placement both before initial injection and during postoperative use has been seen as an advantage,[136][III], [137][III] evidence of benefit compared with conventional catheters is mixed.[138][III]

In one study, stimulating catheters used for interscalene plexus blocks led to faster onset of the block and improved postoperative analgesia in patients undergoing shoulder surgery compared with conventional catheters.[139][II] However, in another study comparing stimulating and conventional interscalene catheters, although onset of motor block was faster in the stimulating catheter group, there was no difference in pain relief.[140][II] Results for continuous femoral nerve block are also mixed with one comparison of stimulating catheters versus nonstimulating catheters for anterior cruciate ligament reconstruction showing faster onset block, but no difference in pain relief,[141][II] while another group reported no difference in onset time of sensory and motor block or postoperative pain.[138][III] When comparisons were made for continuous posterior popliteal sciatic nerve blocks used for elective foot surgery, a significantly shorter onset time of both sensory and motor block was reported when stimulating catheters were used compared with nonstimulating catheters, but again there was no difference in quality of pain relief at rest and with movement between the two groups.[136][II]

If a stimulating catheter is to be used to aid placement, the anesthesiologist must be careful not to inject local anesthetic down the introducing needle before inserting the catheter – this will make nerve stimulation impossible. However, injection of some fluid is thought to aid catheter passage; the use of saline or dextrose for this purpose is both rational and effective.[134]

Ultrasound imaging is being increasingly used to guide needle placement in regional anesthesia,[142] and in the insertion of peripheral nerve catheters.[143] With skill and experience, it is possible to visualize the tip of a catheter and to thereby confirm its proximity to a target nerve. During injection down the catheter, it is possible to see the local anesthetic spreading around the catheter. Anesthesiologists are starting to use ultrasound contrast (agitated local anesthetic solutions that contain myriad small air bubbles that show well on ultrasound) to identify the spread of local anesthetic with some certainty.[142]

Pumps

An increasing number of infusion pumps for continuous regional analgesia are being brought into the market to match the increasing interest in this form of treatment. The pumps can be elastomeric or electronic; they can infuse at fixed rates or variable rates; and they can have the facility for patient-controlled bolus injections. Different pumps will suit different environments and different applications. In general, those pumps designed for epidural infusion are reasonably well suited to continuous neural blockade as they are designed to infuse against the relatively high resistance of a long, thin catheter.

Elastomeric pumps are usually used in patients who will be discharged with CPNB in place. These pumps have a (small) choice of infusion rates ± patient-controlled bolus doses, are robust and simple to use.

In a review of portable infusion pumps (three electronic and three elastomeric) used for continuous regional analgesia, it was noted that infusion rate accuracy differed significantly among the pumps; elastomeric pump infusion rates increased with an increase in temperature; and battery life was a limiting factor in one of the electronic pumps.[144] Another review of portable, bolus-capable infusion pumps used for patient-controlled continuous regional analgesia also showed this variation, suggesting that flow-rate accuracy and consistency, infusion profile, and temperature sensitivity should be taken into consideration when choosing a portable infusion pump for local anesthetic administration.[145]

DRUGS

Local anesthetics

CHOICE OF DRUG

Any local anesthetic can be used, but there are few who use the perhaps more logical choice of the shorter-acting agents lidocaine and prilocaine. Tachyphylaxis has been reported with the former[146] and the latter is known to be associated with occasional cyanosis caused by methemoglobinemia.[147] It is perhaps for these reasons that these drugs have not been favored. Bupivacaine,[31, 80, 148, 149] levobupivacaine,[150, 151] and ropivacaine[20, 149, 150, 152, 153, 154] have all been used for CPNB, but in general there are insufficient data available to suggest an optimal local anesthetic solution. It has been argued that ropivacaine should be favored as it has the capacity to be motor-sparing so that more movement is retained for a set degree of sensory block. Indeed, the late Andrea Casati preferred ropivacaine to lidocaine for this reason.[155][III] However, the evidence for this difference in CPNB is limited and mixed.

For example, 0.2 percent ropivicaine provided the same degree of pain relief when used in interscalene CPNB after shoulder surgery when compared with 0.15 percent bupivicaine,[149][II] or 0.125 percent levobupivicaine,[151][II] but a greater degree of motor block was observed following the bupivicaine[149][II] and no difference[151][II] noted with levobupivicaine. A similar study using double the concentrations of these drugs (0.25 percent levobupivacaine and 0.25 and 0.4 percent ropivacaine) showed that pain relief and motor block for an interscalene catheter infusion were similar after both 0.25 percent levobupivacaine and 0.4 percent ropivicaine and better than 0.25 percent ropivicaine.[156][II] In a study of popliteal catheter infusions, Casati et al.[150][II] also showed that 0.125 percent levobupivacaine was roughly equivalent to 0.2 percent ropivacaine, both in terms of analgesia and motor block sparing effect.

The term "analgesic gap" has been used for the period of inadequate analgesia that often occurs after the offset of the initial block associated with catheter placement, but before the subsequent local anesthetic infusion has taken full effect.[5, 157] This may be particularly difficult to manage if the patient is discharged after day-care surgery with a catheter and infusion system in place. It is important that regular oral analgesia is commenced prior to the block wearing off and that additional analgesia is readily available and used at first sign of discomfort.

DOSE REGIMENS

Anesthesiologists have used a number of different infusion strategies which range from simple continuous fixed infusion rates,[13, 20, 148, 154] through to patient-controlled intermittent bolus doses only,[20, 148, 152] and a combination of the two.[20, 148, 149, 152, 153] In general, the optimum local anesthetic regimen for CPNB appears to be a combination of continuous infusion plus patient-controlled bolus doses.[20][II], [148, 152][II] In their review article of CPNB, Grossi and Allegri[2] also concluded that the best infusion regimen was a combination of a preset basal infusion together with intermittent bolus dose administration for almost all CPNB in adults.

There is no good evidence as yet for the optimal infusion rate, size of bolus dose, or lockout interval, although infusion rates of 5–10 mL per hour, bolus doses of 2–5 mL per hour and lockout intervals of 20–60 minutes have been used successfully.[158] However, there will always be variation between patients, and infusion regimens should be adjusted to provide the desired effect.

TOXICITY

The continuous infusion of local anesthetic drugs creates the possibility that plasma levels may increase over time, such that toxic levels are eventually achieved. Although there have been no reports of cardiovascular collapse due to high plasma levels of local anesthetic, there have been reports of minor subjective sensations likely to be associated with high plasma levels.[26] Plasma ropivacaine levels after an interscalene block with ropivacaine 7.5 mg/mL 30 mL followed by infusions of ropivacaine 2 mg/mL 9 mL per hour in patients with a mean weight of 75 kg were well below thresholds for CNS toxicity and this dosing regimen would therefore appear to have a wide safety margin.[154] [III] Peak plasma levels may be lower with patient-controlled bolus doses than continuous infusions.[159][II] Although there are, as yet, no reports of local anesthetic toxicity resulting from infusion pump malfunction, this remains a potential hazard.

Local anesthetic toxicity due to accidental intravascular injection or rapid absorption is a known complication of all peripheral nerve blocks, and was associated with cardiac arrest (1.4 per 10,000) or seizures (7.5 per 10,000) in a prospective survey of over 21,000 cases.[160]

Adjuvant drugs

Most drugs added to local anesthetic solutions as adjuvants are added in order to prolong the duration of a single-shot block or to speed its onset. When using continuous regional analgesia, these considerations are not valid – the onset need not be rapid and the block can be prolonged with the simple expedient of not turning the pump off. The addition of adrenaline (epinephrine) has its advocates as an indicator that can be used for the first injection down a catheter to exclude intravascular positioning. Its addition to lidocaine for single-shot blocks prolongs duration and intensity.[161, 162, 163] However, there is little logic in its use for CPNB.

Clonidine is an alpha-2 adrenoceptor agonist – for more details on its pharmacology see Chapter 6, Clinical pharmacology: other adjuvants. There is some evidence that the addition of clonidine prolongs the duration of single-injection blocks,[164][II] [165][I] albeit at the cost of a slight increase in patient sedation.[164][II] However, there seems to be little benefit in terms of better pain relief when it is added to local anesthetic solutions use for CPNB,[19][II], [166][II], [167][III] and it may delay recovery of motor function.[166][II] Klein and Nielsen[168] have recently supported the view that although adjvants can prolong the duration of single-shot local anesthetic blocks, significant and flexible prolongation is only really possible with ongoing infusions.

POSTOPERATIVE CARE

The approach to the care of a patient with a peripheral nerve catheter needs to be multidisciplinary. The patient and their carers, whether in hospital on a ward or in the patient's home, need to be familiar with the catheter and pump, and know how to manage block failure and to recognize and treat local anesthetic toxicity. This requires an ongoing education program for all those who will be caring for the patient, and involves the patient, patient's family or carer, hospital nurses, community nurses, physiotherapists, and medical staff. Information sheets and guidelines are a useful resource and patient should be given written advice, including on the care of a numb limb.

There should be provision for a "plan B" for patients in hospital and those discharged home. Repeating blocks and the use of opioid analgesics are practicable for inpatients, but blocks cannot be repeated for patients at home. Plans for readmission should be devised and put in place if necessary. All must be aware of the early symptoms and signs of local anesthetic toxicity and arrangements should be made for the disposal of the catheter and infusion equipment in the home setting.

There have been many successful reports of outpatient management of CPNB.[5, 168, 169] Success in this respect appears to depend upon good communication and organization, along with careful choice of surgical procedure and patient. However, successful outpatient management of continuous neural blockade is not a universal experience. Readers are encouraged to read a series of three publications by Greengrass's group. The title of the first paper boldly declared, "Continuous interscalene brachial plexus blockade provides good analgesia at home after major shoulder surgery."[170] Later experience led them to entitle their next report of the program, "The difficulties of ambulatory interscalene and intra-articular infusions for rotator cuff surgery."[157] Their experiences are summarized in a more recent review that is well worth reading.[171]

COMPLICATIONS

Continuous neural blockade techniques carry with them all the general and block-specific complications of the single-shot block techniques upon which they are based.

Neurological

The possibility of producing permanent nerve damage rightly preoccupies many anesthesiologists. The subject is very well covered by three seminal papers that address this topic for single-shot blocks.[160][III], [172][III], [173][II]

The survey by Auroy et al.[160] of regional anesthesia in France in 1997 suggested that the incidence of neurological problems following peripheral nerve block (PNB) was 3.8:10,000 (0.4 percent) cases. Over double the number of PNBs (43,946) were included in their second survey in 2002[172] – compared with 1997 (21,278) – and the authors reported 12 (0.02 percent) patients with transient neuropathy and one with a permanent neuropathy, suggesting a rate of 1:43,946 (0.002 percent) for permanent neurological problems following PNB.

Brull et al.[173] reviewed 32 studies investigating the risk of complications after central neuraxial blockade and PNB over ten years. On analysis of the 16 papers (65,092 cases) that involved PNB, they found a 3:100 (3 percent) rate of neuropathy; there was only one report of permanent neurological injury. Of the common PNB techniques, they reported that the rate of neuropathy after interscalene brachial plexus block, axillary brachial plexus block, and femoral nerve block was 2.84, 1.48, and 0.34 percent, respectively.

The literature on the neurological complications associated with CPNB is not extensive but would suggest that there is no difference in the risks between single-shot blocks compared with CPNB. Borgeat's group[7] prospectively followed 520 patients for nine months after an interscalene block (single-shot or continuous infusion) for shoulder surgery and showed that 17 percent of the single-shot group and 11 percent of the continuous infusion group complained of neurological symptoms postoperatively. Only one of the 520 patients (0.2 percent) incurred a permanent neurological injury; unfortunately, this paper does not specify from which group this patient came.[7] Results from another later review by Borgeat's group[174] also concluded that there was no difference.

It may be that because most catheters for CPNB are placed by anesthesiologists who are already very experienced in single-shot block techniques, it is predictable that there appears to be little difference in the incidence of nerve damage between series of single-shot blocks and catheters. However, large, randomized prospective studies would be necessary to prove the lack of a difference conclusively. It is unlikely that such studies will be performed.

In a one-year prospective survey of CPNB after orthopedic surgery, Capdevila et al.[175][III] reported three nerve injuries (0.21 percent), all associated with femoral nerve catheters but resolving completely within 36 hours to ten weeks.[175] The study by Bergman et al.[176] of 368 patients (405 axillary nerve catheters) reported that four patients (1.0 percent) had new neurological deficits of which two were attributed to the surgery. Swenson et al.[143] also reported on complications associated with CPNB; two patients of the 620 included in their study had transient neurological problems that resolved within six weeks. The recent study by Wiegel et al.[177] of almost 1400 orthopedic patients with anterior sciatic, femoral, or interscalene brachial plexus CPNB found that 0.8 percent of patients had transient symptoms and that one patient (0.07 percent) suffered a permanent neurological injury.

So to summarize, a reasonable incidence of transient neurological symptoms following a peripheral nerve catheter to quote to patients would be 1–11 percent with the rate of permanent problems less than 1 percent. However, there have and will be further case reports of neurological irritation or damage.[178, 179]

Catheter-related

Just as accidental misplacement of a single-shot block is not only possible but occasionally inevitable, catheters can be misplaced. Amongst those reported to be associated with CPNB are accidental catheterization of the epidural space during an attempt at interscalene brachial plexus[180, 181] and psoas compartment[175] blocks, unintentional vertebral artery catheterization (which resulted in local anesthetic toxicity) during an interscalene approach,[182] and the placement of a planned lumbar plexus catheter into the subarachnoid space.[183] There are also reports of catheters knotting or breaking, which sometimes requires surgical assistance for catheter extrication.[176, 177, 184, 185] Catheter kinking, obstruction, and accidental removal are so common so as not to warrant individual publication.

Correctly placed catheters can also give rise to block-related complications. In one such report, use of a correctly placed interscalene brachial plexus catheter for analgesia at home after painful shoulder surgery resulted in chest pain, dyspnea, and lower lobe lung collapse, probably secondary to phrenic nerve palsy associated with this block.[186] Another report of respiratory distress following use of an interscalene brachial plexus catheter was probably due to the same reason.[187]

Reports of the migration of peripheral nerve catheters also exist.[188, 189] In both these reports, the authors claim that a catheter originally placed correctly in the interscalene brachial plexus sheath migrated thence to the pleural space. The latter of these two reports provoked publication of a letter querying whether this purported migration was in fact an original misplacement.[190]

Reports of signs of local anesthetic toxicity more than 24 hours after initiation of a continuous neural blockade[176] may also suggest catheter migration into a blood vessel, but more importantly, it highlights the need for the patient and carer to be aware of the signs of local anesthetic toxicity and how to manage it.

Infection

Peripheral nerve catheters left in place can lead to infection. Although inflammation of the catheter insertion site and bacterial colonization are relatively common, cases of overt sepsis are rare. Adam et al.[191] reported a psoas abscess that complicated a femoral nerve catheter. The catheter had been in place in a fit 35-year-old patient for

some 96 hours when sepsis was noted. The organism was *Staphylococcus aureus*; the patient responded well to antibiotic therapy. Capdevila et al.[175] studied more than 1400 patients undergoing CPNB. They noted that only 3 percent of catheter insertion sites became inflamed, whereas it was possible to culture bacteria from 28.7 percent of the sites; the bacteria found most frequently were coagulase-negative staphylococcus (61 percent) and Gram-negative bacillus (22 percent). A psoas abscess developed in a diabetic patient after femoral catheter placement; this too responded to antibiotic therapy.

Other studies have also reported high colonization rates, but low infection rates.[192, 193] Wiegel et al.[177] noted inflammation at the interscalene, femoral, and sciatic, but only found infection (pustules) at femoral nerve sites.

These reports support the view that strict asepsis should be adopted for catheter insertion and catheter sites should be observed closely, while continuous neural blockade is performed with extra care and vigilance for femoral nerve catheters.

CONCLUDING THOUGHTS

Single-shot blocks are well established in clinical practice and have demonstrable benefits over and above the excellent analgesia that they provide. We believe that we know a great deal about the incidence of the serious complications of single-shot blocks, and we are therefore in a position to give our patients the information they need about the benefits and material risks involved for them to make an informed choice about their treatment. The risks of continuous catheter techniques are not yet as well defined and, arguably, neither are their benefits.

However, the authors would argue that the jury is still to provide its final verdict on this question, if it ever reaches a verdict. In the meantime, CPNB should be used when it is specifically indicated, i.e. in situations in which significant pain will persist for some considerable time. They should not be used simply because it is possible to do them. Continuous techniques will form an important weapon in the armamentarium wielded by those involved in acute pain management. However, the role of CPNB may not be as significant as is envisaged by the many enthusiasts who currently expound the technique. The development of sustained release formulations of local anesthetics[194] may ultimately obviate the need for CPNB, but these formulations are not yet being used in clinical practice.

Whatever the future of continuous regional analgesia, we would advise caution, care, and communication – with your colleagues and your patients!

ACKNOWLEDGMENTS

This chapter is adapted and expanded from Murphy DF. Nerve blocks for acute pain: principles. In: Rowbotham

DJ and Macintyre PE (eds). *Clinical Pain Management: Acute Pain*, 1ˢᵗ edn. London: Hodder Arnold, 2003: 267–74. The assistance of Dr Nicholas M Denny in sourcing some of the references is also acknowledged.

REFERENCES

1. Ansbro FP. Method of continuous brachial plexus block. *American Journal of Surgery*. 1946; **71**: 716–22.

2. Grossi P, Allegri M. Continuous peripheral nerve blocks: state of the art. *Current Opinion in Anaesthesiology*. 2005; **18**: 522–6.

3. Klein SM, Evans H, Steele SM *et al.* Peripheral nerve blocks for ambulatory surgery. *Anesthesia and Analgesia*. 2005; **101**: 1663–76.

4. Dadure C, Capdevila X. Perioperative analgesia with continuous peripheral nerve blocks in children. *Annales Françaises d'Anesthésie et de Réanimation*. 2007; **26**: 136–44.

5. Russon K, Sardesai AM, Denny NM *et al.* Postoperative shoulder surgery initiative (POSSI): an interim report of major shoulder surgery as a day case procedure. *British Journal of Anaesthesia*. 2006; **97**: 869–73.

∗ 6. Richman JM, Liu SS, Wu CL *et al.* Does continuous peripheral nerve block provide superior pain control to opioids? A meta-analysis. *Anesthesia and Analgesia*. 2006; **102**: 248–57.

7. Borgeat A, Ekatodramis G, Kalberer F, Benz C. Acute and nonacute complications associated with interscalene block and shoulder surgery: a prospective study. *Anesthesiology*. 2001; **95**: 875–80.

8. Selander D. Catheter technique in axillary plexus block. Presentation of a new method. *Acta Anaesthesiologica Scandinavica*. 1977; **21**: 324–9.

9. Rawal N, Allvin R, Axelsson K *et al.* Patient-controlled regional analgesia (PCRA) at home: controlled comparison between bupivacaine and ropivacaine brachial plexus analgesia. *Anesthesiology*. 2002; **96**: 1290–6.

10. Randalls B. Continuous brachial plexus blockade. A technique that uses an axillary catheter to allow successful skin grafting. *Anesthesiology*. 1990; **45**: 143–4.

11. De Andres JA, Bolinches R, Serrano MT *et al.* Continuous block of the brachial plexus with nerve stimulation. Intra and postoperative control in orthopaedic surgery of the arm. *Revista Española de Anestesiología y Reanimación*. 1989; **36**: 198–201.

12. Sada T, Kobayashi T, Murakami S. Continuous axillary brachial plexus block. *Canadian Anesthesiologsts' Society Journal*. 1983; **30**: 201–05.

13. Salonen MH, Haasio J, Bachmann M *et al.* Evaluation of efficacy and plasma concentrations of ropivacaine in continuous axillary brachial plexus block: high dose for surgical anesthesia and low dose for postoperative analgesia. *Regional Anesthesia and Pain Medicine*. 2000; **25**: 47–51.

14. Mezzatesta JP, Scott DA, Schweitzer SA, Selander DE. Continuous axillary brachial plexus block for postoperative pain relief. Intermittent bolus versus continuous infusion. *Regional Anesthesia*. 1997; **22**: 357–62.

15. Berger A, Tizian C, Zenz M. Continuous plexus blockade for improved circulation in microvascular surgery. *Annals of Plastic Surgery*. 1985; **14**: 16–19.

∗ 16. Winnie AP. *Plexus anaesthesia 1*. Fribourg: Mediglobe SA, 1990.

17. Cornish PB, Leaper CJ, Hahn JL. The "axillary tunnel": an anatomic reappraisal of the limits and dynamics of spread during brachial plexus blockade. *Anesthesia and Analgesia*. 2007; **104**: 1288–91.

18. Ilfeld BM, Morey TE, Enneking FK. Continuous infraclavicular brachial plexus block for postoperative pain control at home. A randomized, double-blinded, placebo-controlled study. *Anesthesiology*. 2002; **96**: 1297–304.

19. Ilfeld BM, Morey TE, Enneking FK. Continuous infraclavicular perineural infusion with clonidine and ropivacaine alone: a randomized, double blinded, controlled study. *Anesthesia and Analgesia*. 2003; **97**: 706–12.

20. Ilfeld BM, Morey TE, Enneking FK. Infraclavicular perineural local anesthetic infusion. A comparison of three dosing regimens for postoperative analgesia. *Anesthesiology*. 2004; **100**: 395–402.

21. Mehrkens HH, Geiger PK. Continuous brachial plexus blockade via the vertical infraclavicular approach. *Anaesthesia*. 1998; **53**(Suppl. 2): 19–20.

22. Heid FM, Jage J, Bauwe N *et al.* Efficacy of vertebral infraclavicular plexus block vs. modified axillary plexus block: a prospective randomized, observer blinded study. *Acta Anaesthesiologica Scandinavica*. 2005; **49**: 677–82.

23. Winnie AP, Collins VJ. The Subclavian Perivascular technique of brachial plexus anesthesia. *Anesthesiology*. 1964; **25**: 353–63.

24. Borgeat A, Ekatodramis G. Anaesthesia for shoulder surgery. *Best Practice and Research. Clinical Anaesthesiology*. 2002; **16**: 211–25.

25. Tuominen M, Pitkanen M, Rosenberg PH. Postoperative pain relief and bupivacaine plasma levels during continuous interscalene brachial plexus block. *Acta Anaesthesiologica Scandinavica*. 1987; **31**: 276–8.

26. Rosenberg PH, Pere P, Hekali R, Tuominen M. Plasma concentrations of bupivacaine and two of its metabolites during continuous interscalene brachial plexus block. *British Journal of Anaesthesia*. 1991; **66**: 25–30.

27. Borgeat A, Tewes E, Biasca N, Gerber C. Patient-controlled interscalene analgesia with ropivacaine after major shoulder surgery: PCIA vs PCA. *British Journal of Anaesthesia*. 1998; **81**: 603–05.

28. Lucas MA, Harrop-Griffiths AW. Interscalene patient-controlled analgesia. *Anaesthesia*. 1997; **52**: 263–4.

29. Borgeat A, Dullenkopf A, Ekatodramis G, Nagy L. Evaluation of the lateral modified approach for continuous interscalene block after shoulder surgery. *Anesthesiology*. 2003; **99**: 436–42.

30. Ilfeld BM, Morey TE, Wright TW et al. Continuous interscalene brachial plexus block for postoperative pain control at home: a randomized, double-blinded, placebo-controlled study. Anesthesia and Analgesia. 2003; 96: 1089–95.

31. Borgeat A, Schappi B, Biasca N, Gerber C. Patient-controlled analgesia after major shoulder surgery: patient-controlled interscalene analgesia versus patient-controlled analgesia. Anesthesiology. 1997; 87: 1343–7.

32. Klein SM, Grant SA, Greengrass RA et al. Interscalene brachial plexus block with a continuous catheter insertion system and a disposable infusion pump. Anesthesia and Analgesia. 2000; 91: 1473–8.

33. Delaunay L, Souron V, Lafosse L et al. Analgesia after arthroscopic rotator cuff repair: subacromial versus interscalene continuous infusion of ropivacaine. Regional Anesthesia and Pain Medicine. 2005; 30: 117–22.

34. Pippa P, Cominelli E, Marinelli C, Aito S. Brachial plexus block using the posterior approach. European Journal of Anaesthesiology. 1990; 7: 411–20.

35. Boezaart AP, Koorn R, Borene S, Edwards JN. Continuous brachial plexus block using the posterior approach. Regional Anesthesia and Pain Medicine. 2003; 28: 70–1.

36. Harrop-Griffiths W, Denny NM. The cat in the kitchen: problems with the Pippa technique. Anaesthesia. 2006; 61: 1028–30.

37. Sandefo I, Iohom G, Polin B et al. Clinical efficacy of the brachial plexus block via the posterior approach. Regional Anesthesia and Pain Medicine. 2005; 30: 238–42.

38. Boezaart AP, de Beer JF, du Toit C, van Rooyen K. A new technique of continuous interscalene nerve block. Canadian Journal of Anaesthesia. 1999; 46: 275–81.

39. Winnie AP. Interscalene brachial plexus block. Anesthesia and Analgesia. 1970; 49: 455–66.

40. Harrop-Griffiths W. Subcutaneous tunnelling of interscalene catheters. Canadian Journal of Anaesthesia. 2001; 48: 102–03.

41. Boezaart AP. Continuous interscalene block for ambulatory shoulder surgery. Best Practice and Research. Clinical Anaesthesiology. 2002; 16: 295–310.

42. Mulroy MF, McDonald SB. Regional anaesthesia for outpatient surgery. Anesthesiology Clinics of North America. 2003; 21: 289–303.

43. Chayen D, Nathan H, Chayen M. The psoas compartment block. Anesthesiology. 1976; 45: 95–9.

44. Capdevila X, Macaire P, Dadure C et al. Continuous psoas compartment block for postoperative analgesia after total hip arthroplasty: new landmarks, technical guidelines, and clinical evaluation. Anesthesia and Analgesia. 2002; 94: 1606–13.

45. Farny J, Drolet P, Girard M. Anatomy of the posterior approach to the lumbar plexus. Canadian Journal of Anaesthesia. 1994; 41: 480–5.

∗ 46. Enneking FK, Chan V, Horlocker TT et al. Lower extremity peripheral nerve blockade: essentials of our current understanding. Regional Anesthesia and Pain Medicine. 2005; 30: 4–35.

47. Chelly JE, Casati A, Al-Samsam T et al. Continuous lumbar plexus block for acute postoperative pain management after open reduction and internal fixation of acetabular fractures. Journal of Orthopaedic Trauma. 2003; 17: 362–7.

48. Chudinov A, Berkenstadt H, Salai M et al. Continuous psoas compartment block for anesthesia and perioperative analgesia in patients with hip fractures. Regional Anesthesia and Pain Medicine. 1999; 24: 563–8.

49. Kaloul I, Guay J, Cote C, Fallaha M. The posterior lumbar plexus (psoas compartment) block and the three-in-one femoral nerve block provide similar postoperative analgesia after total knee replacement. Canadian Journal of Anaesthesia. 2004; 51: 45–51.

50. Turker G, Uckunkaya N, Yavascaoglu B et al. Comparison of the catheter-technique psoas compartment block and the epidural block for analgesia in partial hip replacement surgery. Acta Anaesthesiologica Scandinavica. 2003; 47: 30–6.

51. Litz RJ, Vicent O, Wiessner D, Heller AR. Misplacement of a psoas compartment catheter in the subarachnoid space. Regional Anesthesia and Pain Medicine. 2004; 29: 60–4.

52. Stevens RD, Van Gessel E, Flory N et al. Lumbar plexus block reduces pain and blood loss associated with total hip arthroplasty. Anesthesiology. 2000; 93: 115–21.

53. Biboulet P, Morau D, Capdevila X et al. Postoperative analgesia after total-hip arthroplasty: Comparison of intravenous patient-controlled analgesia with morphine and single injection of femoral nerve or psoas compartment block. A prospective, randomized, double-blinded study. Regional Anesthesia and Pain Medicine. 2004; 29: 102–09.

54. Griffith JP, Whitely S, Gough MJ. Prospective randomized study of a new method of providing post-operative pain relief following femoropliteal bypass. British Journal of Surgery. 1996; 83: 1735–8.

55. Cuignet O, Pirson J, Boughrouph J, Duville D. The efficacy of continuous fascia iliaca compartment block for pain management in burn patients undergoing skin grafting procedures. Anesthesia and Analgesia. 2004; 98: 1077–81.

56. Salinas FV, Liu SS, Mulroy MF. The effect of single-injection femoral nerve block versus continuous femoral nerve block after total knee arthroplasty on hospital length of stay and long term functional recovery within an established clinical pathway. Anesthesia and Analgesia. 2006; 102: 1234–9.

57. Hirst GC, Lang SA, Yip RW et al. Femoral nerve block. Single injection versus continuous infusion for total knee arthroplasty. Regional Anesthesia. 1996; 21: 292–7.

58. Singelyn FJ, Deyaert M, Joris D et al. Effects of intravenous patient controlled analgesia with morphine, continuous epidural analgesia and continuous three-in-one block on post-operative pain and knee rehabilitation after unilateral total knee arthroplasty. Anesthesia and Analgesia. 1998; 87: 88–92.

59. Capdevila X, Barthelet Y, Biboulet P et al. Effects of perioperative analgesic technique on the surgical outcome

and duration of rehabilitation after major knee surgery. *Anesthesiology.* 1999; **91**: 8–15.

60. Singelyn FJ, Ferrant T, Malisse MF, Joris D. Effects of intravenous patient-controlled analgesia with morphine, continuous epidural analgesia, and continuous femoral nerve sheath block on rehabilitation after unilateral total-hip arthroplasty. *Regional Anesthesia and Pain Medicine.* 2005; **30**: 452–7.

61. Barrington MJ, Olive D, Low K *et al.* Continuous femoral nerve blockade or epidural analgesia after total knee replacement: a prospective randomized controlled trial. *Anesthesia and Analgesia.* 2005; **101**: 1824–9.

62. Ben-David B, Schmalenberger K, Chelly JE. Analgesia after total knee arthroplasty: is continuous sciatic blockade needed in addition to continuous femoral blockade? *Anesthesia and Analgesia.* 2004; **98**: 747–9.

63. Allen HW, Liu SS, Ware PD *et al.* Peripheral nerve blocks improve analgesia after total knee replacement surgery. *Anesthesia and Analgesia.* 1998; **87**: 93–7.

64. Zaric D, Boysen K, Christiansen B *et al.* A comparison of epidural analgesia and continuous femoral-sciatic nerve blocks after total knee replacement. *Anesthesia and Analgesia.* 2006; **102**: 1240–6.

65. Singelyn FJ, Gouverneur JM. Postoperative analgesia after total hip arthroplasty: i.v. PCA with morphine, patient-controlled epidural analgesia, or continuous "3-in-1" block?: a prospective evaluation by our acute pain service in more than 1,300 patients. *Journal of Clinical Anesthesia.* 1999; **11**: 550–4.

66. Winnie AP, Ramamurthy S, Durrani Z. The inguinal paravascular technique of lumbar plexus anesthesia: the "3-in-1 block". *Anesthesia and Analgesia.* 1973; **52**: 989–96.

67. Longo SR, Williams DP. Bilateral fascia iliaca catheters for postoperative pain control after bilateral total knee arthroplasty: a case report and description of a catheter technique. *Regional Anesthesia.* 1997; **22**: 372–7.

68. Ganapathy S, Wasserman R, MacDonald C *et al.* Modified continuous femoral three-in-one block for postoperative pain after total knee arthroplasty. *Anesthesia and Analgesia.* 1999; **89**: 1197–202.

69. Morau D, Lopez S, Capdevila X *et al.* Comparison of continuous 3-in-1 and fascia iliaca compartment blocks for postoperative analgesia: feasibility, catheter migration, distribution of sensory block, and analgesic efficacy. *Regional Anesthesia and Pain Medicine.* 2003; **28**: 309–14.

70. Tetzlaff JE, Andrish J, O'Hara Jr J *et al.* Effectiveness of bupivacaine administered via femoral nerve catheter for pain control after anterior cruciate ligament repair. *Journal of Clinical Anesthesia.* 1997; **9**: 542–5.

71. Dauri M, Polzoni M, Fabbi E *et al.* Comparison of epidural, continuous femoral block and intraarticular analgesia after anterior cruciate ligament reconstruction. *Acta Anaesthesiologica Scandinavica.* 2003; **47**: 20–5.

72. Iskandar H, Benard A, Ruel-Raymond J *et al.* Femoral block provides superior analgesia compared with intra-articular ropivacaine after anterior cruciate ligament reconstruction. *Regional Anesthesia and Pain Medicine.* 2003; **28**: 29–32.

73. Labat G. *Regional anesthesia. Its technique and clinical applications.* Philadelphia: WB Saunders, 1923.

74. Ilfeld BM, Morey T, Enneking FK *et al.* Continuous popliteal sciatic nerve block for postoperative pain control at home. *Anesthesiology.* 2002; **97**: 959–65.

75. Smith BE, Fischer HB, Scott PV. Continuous sciatic nerve block. *Anaesthesia.* 1984; **39**: 155–7.

76. Vaghadia H, Kapnoudhis P, Jenkins LC, Taylor D. Continuous lumbosacral block using a Tuohy needle and catheter technique. *Canadian Journal of Anaesthesia.* 1992; **39**: 75–8.

77. Morris GF, Lang SA. Continuous parasacral sciatic nerve block: two case reports. *Regional Anesthesia.* 1997; **22**: 469–72.

78. Wiegel M, Reske A, Olthoff D *et al.* Anterior sciatic nerve block – new landmarks and clinical experience. *Acta Anaesthesiologica Scandinavica.* 2005; **49**: 552–7.

79. Singelyn FJ, Aye F, Gouverneur JM. Continuous popliteal sciatic nerve block: an original technique to provide postoperative analgesia after foot surgery. *Anesthesia and Analgesia.* 1997; **84**: 383–6.

80. White PF, Issioui T, Skrivanek GD *et al.* The use of a continuous popliteal sciatic nerve block after surgery involving the foot and ankle: does it improve the quality of recovery? *Anesthesia and Analgesia.* 2003; **97**: 1303–09.

81. Zaric D, Boysen K, Christiansen J *et al.* Continuous popliteal sciatic nerve block for outpatient foot surgery – a randomized, controlled trial. *Acta Anaesthesiologica Scandinavica.* 2004; **48**: 337–41.

82. Chelly JE, Greger J, Casati A *et al.* Continuous lateral sciatic blocks for acute postoperative pain management after major ankle and foot surgery. *Foot and Ankle International.* 2002; **23**: 749–52.

83. Fournier R, Weber A, Gamulin Z. No differences between 20, 30, or 40 ml ropivacaine 0.5% in continuous lateral popliteal sciatic-nerve block. *Regional Anesthesia and Pain Medicine.* 2006; **31**: 455–9.

84. PROSPECT Working Group. Procedure specific postoperative pain management. Cited December 2007. Available from: www.postoppain.org/frameset.htm.

85. Fischer HBJ, Simanski CJP. A procedure-specific systematic review and consensus recommendations for analgesia after total hip replacement. *Anaesthesia.* 2005; **60**: 1189–202.

86. Eason MJ, Wyatt R. Paravertebral thoracic block – a reappraisal. *Anaesthesia.* 1979; **34**: 638–42.

87. Richardson J, Lonnqvist PA. Thoracic paravertebral block. *British Journal of Anaesthesia.* 1998; **81**: 230–8.

88. Weltz CR, Klein SM, Arbo JE, Greengrass RA. Paravertebral block anesthesia for inguinal hernia repair. *World Journal of Surgery.* 2003; **27**: 425–9.

89. Lonnqvist PA. Entering the paravertebral space age again? *Acta Anaesthesiologica Scandinavica.* 2001; **45**: 1–3.

90. Naja MZ, Ziade MF, Lonnqvist PA. General anaesthesia combined with bilateral paravertebral blockade (T5–6) vs. general anaesthesia for laparoscopic cholecystectomy: a prospective, randomized clinical trial. *European Journal of Anaesthesiology*. 2004; **21**: 489–95.

91. Klein SM, Bergh A, Steele SM *et al.* Thoracic paravertebral block for breast surgery. *Anesthesia and Analgesia*. 2000; **90**: 1402–5.

92. Buckenmaier 3rd CC, Steele SM, Nielsen KC *et al.* Bilateral continuous paravertebral catheters for reduction mammoplasty. *Acta Anaesthesiologica Scandinavica*. 2002; **46**: 1042–5.

93. Buckenmaier 3rd CC, Klein SM, Nielsen KC, Steele SM. Continuous paravertebral catheter and outpatient infusion for breast surgery. *Anesthesia and Analgesia*. 2003; **97**: 715–17.

94. Karmakar MK, Critchley LA, Ho AM *et al.* Continuous thoracic paravertebral infusion of bupivacaine for pain management in patients with multiple fractured ribs. *Chest*. 2003; **123**: 424–31.

95. Karmakar MK, Chui PT, Joynt GM, Ho AM. Thoracic paravertebral block for management of pain associated with multiple fractured ribs in patients with concomitant lumbar spinal trauma. *Regional Anesthesia and Pain Medicine*. 2001; **26**: 169–73.

96. Koorn R, Tenhundfeld Fear KM, Miller C, Boezaart A. The use of cervical paravertebral block as the sole anesthetic for shoulder surgery in a morbid patient: a case report. *Regional Anesthesia and Pain Medicine*. 2004; **29**: 227–9.

97. Boezaart AP, De Beer JF, Nell ML. Early experience with continuous cervical paravertebral block using a stimulating catheter. *Regional Anesthesia and Pain Medicine*. 2003; **28**: 406–13.

98. Dhole S, Mehta Y, Trehan N *et al.* Comparison of continuous thoracic epidural and paravertebral blocks for postoperative analgesia after minimally invasive direct coronary artery bypass surgery. *Journal of Cardiothoracic and Vascular Anesthesia*. 2001; **15**: 288–92.

99. Richardson J, Vowden P, Sabanathan S. Bilateral paravertebral analgesia for major abdominal vascular surgery: a preliminary report. *Anaesthesia*. 1995; **50**: 995–8.

100. Naja ZM, Maaliki H, Al-Tannir MA *et al.* Repetitive paravertebral nerve block using a catheter technique for pain relief in post-herpetic neuralgia. *British Journal of Anaesthesia*. 2006; **96**: 381–3.

101. Marret E, Bazelly B, Bonnet FJ *et al.* Paravertebral block with ropivacaine 0.5% versus systemic analgesia for pain relief after thoracotomy. *Annals of Thoracic Surgery*. 2005; **79**: 2109–13.

*102. Davies RG, Myles PS, Graham JM. A comparison of the analgesic efficacy and side-effects of paravertebral vs. epidural blockade for thoracotomy – a systematic review and meta-analysis of randomized trials. *British Journal of Anaesthesia*. 2006; **96**: 418–26.

103. Casati A, Alessandrini P, Nuzzi M *et al.* A prospective, randomized, blinded comparison between continuous thoracic paravertebral and epidural infusion of 0.2% ropivacaine after lung resection surgery. *European Journal of Anaesthesiology*. 2006; **23**: 999–1004.

104. Kvalheim L, Reiestad F. Interpleural catheter in the management of postoperative pain. *Anesthesiology*. 1984; **61**: A231.

105. Reiestad F, Strømskag KE. Interpleural catheter in the management of postoperative pain: a preliminary report. *Regional Anesthesia*. 1986; **11**: 89–91.

*106. Dravid RM, Paul RE. Interpleural block – part 1. *Anaesthesia*. 2007; **62**: 1039–49.

*107. Dravid RM, Paul RE. Interpleural block – part 2. *Anaesthesia*. 2007; **62**: 1143–53.

108. Laurito CE, Kirz LI, VadeBoncouer TR *et al.* Continuous infusion of interpleural bupivacaine maintains effective analgesia after cholecystectomy. *Anesthesia and Analgesia*. 1991; **72**: 516–21.

109. Higgins PC, Ravalia A. Interpleural anaesthesia for mastectomy. *Anaesthesia*. 2005; **60**: 1150–1.

110. van Kleef JW, Logeman A, Burm AG *et al.* Continuous interpleural infusion of bupivacaine for postoperative analgesia after surgery with flank incisions: a double-blind comparison of 0.25% and 0.5% solutions. *Anesthesia and Analgesia*. 1992; **75**: 268–74.

111. Covino BG. Interpleural regional analgesia. *Anesthesia and Analgesia*. 1988; **67**: 427–9.

112. Francois T, Blanloeil Y, Pillet F *et al.* Effect of interpleural administration of bupivacaine or lidocaine on pain and morphine requirement after oesophagectomy with thoracotomy: a randomized, double-blind and controlled study. *Anesthesia and Analgesia*. 1995; **80**: 718–23.

113. Mann U, Young GR, Williams JK *et al.* Intrapleural bupivacaine in the control of post-thoracotomy pain. *Annals of Thoracic Surgery*. 1992; **53**: 449–54.

114. Silomon M, Claus T, Hanno H *et al.* Interpleural analgesia does not influence post-thoracotomy pain. *Anesthesia and Analgesia*. 2000; **91**: 44–50.

115. Schneider RF, Villamena PC, Harvey J *et al.* Lack of efficacy of intrapleural bupivacaine for postoperative analgesia following thoracotomy. *Chest*. 1993; **103**: 414–16.

116. Richardson J, Sabanathan S, Goulden C *et al.* A prospective, randomised comparison of interpleural and paravertebral analgesia in thoracic surgery. *British Journal of Anaesthesia*. 1995; **75**: 405–08.

117. Mehta Y, Swaminathan M, Mishra Y, Trehan N. A comparative evaluation of intrapleural and thoracic epidural analgesia for postoperative pain relief after minimally invasive direct coronary artery bypass surgery. *Journal of Cardiothoracic and Vascular Anesthesia*. 1998; **12**: 162–5.

118. Debreceni G, Molnar Z, Szelig L, Molnar TF. Continuous epidural or intercostal analgesia following thoracotomy: a prospective randomized double-blind clinical trial. *Acta Anaesthesiologica Scandinavica*. 2003; **47**: 1091–5.

119. Boren E, Teuber SS, Naguwa SM, Gershwin ME. A critical review of local anesthetic sensitivity. *Clinical Reviews in Allergy and Immunology*. 2007; **32**: 119–28.

120. Eggleston ST, Lush LW. Understanding allergic reactions to local anesthetics. *Annals of Pharmacotherapy*. 1996; **30**: 851.

121. Finder RL, Moore PA. Adverse drug reactions to local anesthesia. *Dental Clinics of North America*. 2002; **46**: 747–57.

*122. Horlocker TT, Wedel DJ, Benzon H *et al*. Regional anesthesia in the anticoagulated patient: defining the risks (the second ASRA Consensus Conference on Neuraxial Anesthesia and Anticoagulation). *Regional Anesthesia and Pain Medicine*. 2003; **28**: 172–97.

123. Kang SB, Rumball KM, Ettinger RS. Continuous axillary brachial plexus analgesia in a patient with severe hemophilia. *Journal of Clinical Anesthesia*. 2003; **15**: 38–40.

124. Bickler P, Brandes J, Lee M *et al*. Bleeding complications from femoral and sciatic nerve catheters in patients receiving low molecular weight heparin. *Anesthesia and Analgesia*. 2006; **103**: 1036–7.

125. Ben-David B, Joshi R, Chelly JE. Sciatic nerve palsy after total hip arthroplasty in a patient receiving continuous lumbar plexus block. *Anesthesia and Analgesia*. 2003; **97**: 1180–2.

*126. Wedel DJ, Horlocker TT. Regional anesthesia in the febrile or infected patient. *Regional Anesthesia and Pain Medicine*. 2006; **31**: 324–33.

127. Horlocker TT, Wedel DJ. Regional anesthesia in the immunocompromised patient. *Regional Anesthesia and Pain Medicine*. 2006; **31**: 334–45.

*128. Urmey WF, Talts KH, Sharrock NE. One hundred percent incidence of hemidiaphragmatic paresis associated with interscalene brachial plexus anesthesia as diagnosed by ultrasonography. *Anesthesia and Analgesia*. 1991; **72**: 498–503.

129. Smith MP, Tetzlaff JE, Brems JJ. Asymptomatic profound oxyhemoglobin desaturation following interscalene block in a geriatric patient. *Regional Anesthesia and Pain Medicine*. 1998; **23**: 210–13.

130. Kayerker UM, Dick MM. Phrenic nerve paralysis following interscalene brachial plexus block. *Anesthesia and Analgesia*. 1983; **62**: 536–7.

131. Borgeat A, Perschak H, Bird P *et al*. Patient-controlled interscalene analgesia with ropivacaine 0.2% versus patient-controlled intravenous analgesia after major shoulder surgery: effects on diaphragmatic and respiratory function. *Anesthesiology*. 2000; **92**: 102–08.

132. Cornish PB. Supraclavicular regional anaesthesia revisited – the bent needle technique. *Anaesthesia and Intensive Care*. 2000; **28**: 676–9.

133. Denny NM, Barber N, Sildown DJ. Evaluation of an insulated Tuohy needle system for the placement of interscalene brachial plexus catheters. *Anaesthesia*. 2003; **58**: 554–7.

134. Pham-Dang C, Kick O, Collet T *et al*. Continuous peripheral nerve blocks with stimulating catheters. *Regional Anesthesia and Pain Medicine*. 2003; **28**: 83–8.

135. Boezaart AP, De Beer JF, Nell ML. Early experience with continuous cervical paravertebral block using a stimulating catheter. *Regional Anesthesia and Pain Medicine*. 2003; **28**: 406–13.

136. Casati A, Faneli G, Koscielniak-Nielson Z *et al*. Using stimulating catheters for continuous sciatic nerve block shortens onset time of surgical block and minimizes postoperative consumption of pain medication after hallux valgus repair as compared with conventional nonstimulating catheters. *Anesthesia and Analgesia*. 2005; **101**: 1192–7.

137. Stevens MF, Werdehausen R, Lipfert P *et al*. Does interscalene catheter placement with stimulating catheters improve postoperative pain or functional outcome after shoulder surgery? A prospective, randomized and double-blinded trial. *Anesthesia and Analgesia*. 2007; **104**: 442–7.

138. Morin AM, Eberhart LH, Behnke HK *et al*. Does femoral nerve catheter placement with stimulating catheters improve effective placement? A randomized, controlled, and observer blinded trial. *Anesthesia and Analgesia*. 2005; **100**: 1503–10.

139. Birnbaum J, Kip M, Spies CD *et al*. The effect of stimulating versus nonstimulating catheters for continuous interscalene plexus blocks in short-term pain management. *Journal of Clinical Anesthesia*. 2007; **19**: 434–9.

140. Stevens MF, Werdehausen R, Golla E *et al*. Does interscalene catheter placement with stimulating catheters improve postoperative pain or functional outcome after shoulder surgery? A prospective, randomized and double-blinded trial. *Anesthesia and Analgesia*. 2007; **104**: 442–7.

141. Dauri M, Sidiropoulou T, Fabbi E *et al*. Efficacy of continuous femoral nerve block with stimulating catheters versus nonstimulating catheters for anterior cruciate ligament reconstruction. *Regional Anesthesia and Pain Medicine*. 2007; **32**: 282–7.

142. Marhofer P, Greher M, Kapral S. Ultrasound guidance in regional anaesthesia. *British Journal of Anaesthesia*. 2005; **94**: 7–17.

143. Swenson JD, Bay N, Loose E *et al*. Outpatient management of continuous peripheral nerve catheters placed using ultrasound guidance: an experience in 620 patients. *Anesthesia and Analgesia*. 2006; **103**: 1436–43.

144. Ilfeld BM, Morey TE, Enneking FK. Portable infusion pumps used for continuous regional analgesia: delivery rate accuracy and consistency. *Regional Anesthesia and Pain Medicine*. 2003; **28**: 424–32.

145. Ilfeld BM, Morey TE, Enneking FK. Delivery rate accuracy of portable, bolus-capable infusion pumps used for patient-controlled continuous regional analgesia. *Regional Anesthesia and Pain Medicine*. 2003; **28**: 17–23.

146. Mogensen T, Simonsen L, Kehlet H *et al*. Tachyphylaxis associated with repeated epidural injections of lidocaine is not related to changes in distribution or the rate of

elimination from the epidural space. *Anesthesia and Analgesia.* 1989; **69**: 180–4.

147. Vasters FG, Eberhart LH, Morin AM *et al.* Risk factors for prilocaine-induced methaemoglobinaemia following peripheral regional anaesthesia. *European Journal of Anaesthesiology.* 2006; **23**: 760–5.

148. Singelyn FJ, Seguy S, Gouverneur JM. Interscalene brachial plexus analgesia after open shoulder surgery: continuous versus patient-controlled infusion. *Anesthesia and Analgesia.* 1999; **89**: 1216–20.

149. Borgeat A, Kalberer F, Jacob H *et al.* Patient-controlled interscalene analgesia with ropivacaine 0.2% versus bupivacaine 0.15% after major open shoulder surgery: the effects on hand motor function. *Anesthesia and Analgesia.* 2001; **92**: 218–23.

150. Casati A, Vinciguerra F, Rivoltini P *et al.* Levobupivacaine 0.2% or 0.125% for continuous sciatic nerve block: a prospective, randomized, double-blind comparison with 0.2% ropivicaine. *Anesthesia and Analgesia.* 2004; **99**: 919–23.

151. Casati A, Borghi B, Fanelli G *et al.* Interscalene brachial plexus anesthesia and analgesia for open shoulder surgery: a randomized, double-blinded comparison between levobupivacaine and ropivacaine. *Anesthesia and Analgesia.* 2003; **96**: 253–9.

152. Ilfeld BM, Thannikary LJ, Enneking FK *et al.* Popliteal sciatic perineural local anesthetic infusion: a comparison of three dosing regimens for postoperative analgesia. *Anesthesiology.* 2004; **101**: 970–7.

153. Ilfeld BM, Morey TE, Wright TW *et al.* Interscalene perineural ropivacaine infusion: a comparison of two dosing regimes for postoperative analgesia. *Regional Anesthesia.* 2004; **29**: 9–16.

154. Ekatodramis G, Borgeat A, Sjovall J *et al.* Continuous interscalene analgesia with ropivacaine 2 mg/ml after major shoulder surgery. *Anesthesiology.* 2003; **98**: 143–50.

155. Casati A, Vinciguerra F, Chelly JE *et al.* Lidocaine versus ropivacaine for continuous interscalene brachial plexus block after open shoulder surgery. *Acta Anaesthesiologica Scandinavica.* 2003; **47**: 355–60.

156. Borghi B, Facchini F, Agnoletti V *et al.* Pain relief and motor function during continuous interscalene analgesia after open shoulder surgery: a prospective, randomized, double-blind comparison between levobupivacaine 0.25%, and ropivacaine 0.25% or 0.4%. *European Journal of Anaesthesiology.* 2006; **23**: 1005–09.

157. Klein SM, Steele SM, Nielsen KC *et al.* The difficulties of ambulatory interscalene and intra-articular infusions for rotator cuff surgery: a preliminary report. *Canadian Journal of Anaesthesia.* 2003; **50**: 265–9.

158. Ilfeld B. Continuous peripheral nerve blocks: past, present and future. In: ASA (eds). *American Society of Anesthesiologists Annual Meeting Refresher Course Lectures.* Park Ridge, IL: American Society of Anesthesiologists, 2007: 238.

159. Duflo F, Sautou-Miranda V, Pouyau A *et al.* Efficacy and plasma levels of ropivacaine for children: controlled regional analgesia following lower limb surgery. *British Journal of Anaesthesia.* 2006; **97**: 250–4.

*160. Auroy Y, Narchi P, Messiah A *et al.* Serious complications related to regional anesthesia: results of a prospective survey in France. *Anesthesiology.* 1997; **87**: 479–86.

161. Covino BG. Pharmacology of local anesthetic agents. *British Journal of Anaesthesia.* 1986; **58**: 701–16.

162. Butterworth J, Strichartz GR. Molecular mechanisms of local anesthetics. A review. *Anesthesia and Analgesia.* 1990; **72**: 711–34.

163. Richards A, McConachie I. The pharmacology of local anesthetic drugs. *Current Anaesthesia and Critical Care.* 1995; **6**: 41–7.

164. Casati A, Magistris L, Torri G *et al.* Small-dose clonidine prolongs postoperative analgesia after sciatic-femoral block with 0.75% ropivacaine after foot surgery. *Anesthesia and Analgesia.* 2000; **91**: 388–92.

165. Murphy DB, McCartney CJ, Chan VW. Novel analgesic adjuncts for brachial plexus block: a systematic review. *Anesthesia and Analgesia.* 2000; **90**: 1122–8.

166. Casati A, Vinciguerra F, Chelly JE *et al.* Adding clonidine to induction bolus and postoperative infusion during continuous femoral nerve block delays recovery of motor function after total knee arthroplasty. *Anesthesia and Analgesia.* 2005; **100**: 866–72.

167. Ilfeld BM, Morey TE, Thannikary LJ *et al.* Clonidine added to a continuous interscalene ropivacaine perineural infusion to improve postoperative analgesia: a randomized, double-blind, controlled study. *Anesthesia and Analgesia.* 2005; **100**: 1172–8.

168. Klein SM, Nielsen KC. Brachial plexus blocks: infusions and other mechanisms to provide prolonged analgesia. *Current Opinion in Anaesthesiology.* 2003; **16**: 393–9.

169. Ilfeld BM, Enneking FK. Continuous peripheral nerve blocks at home: a review. *Anesthesia and Analgesia.* 2005; **100**: 1822–33.

170. Nielsen KC, Greengrass RA, Pietrobon R *et al.* Continuous interscalene brachial plexus blockade provides good analgesia at home after major shoulder surgery – report of four cases. *Canadian Journal of Anaesthesia.* 2003; **50**: 57–61.

*171. Greengrass RA, Nielsen KC. Management of peripheral nerve block catheters at home. *International Anesthesiology Clinics.* 2005; **43**: 79–87.

*172. Auroy Y, Benhamou D, Samii K *et al.* Major complications of regional anesthesia in France: The SOS Regional Anesthesia Hotline Service. *Anesthesiology.* 2002; **97**: 1274–80.

*173. Brull R, McCartney CJ, Chan VW, El-Beheiry H. Neurological complications after regional anesthesia: contemporary estimates of risk. *Anesthesia and Analgesia.* 2007; **104**: 965–74.

174. Borgeat A, Blumenthal S. Nerve injury and regional anaesthesia. *Current Opinion in Anaesthesiology.* 2004; **17**: 417–21.

*175. Capdevila X, Pirat P, Bringuier S *et al.* French Study Group on Continuous Peripheral Nerve Blocks. Continuous peripheral nerve blocks in hospital wards after orthopedic surgery: a multicenter prospective analysis of the quality of postoperative analgesia and complications in 1,416 patients. *Anesthesiology.* 2005; **103**: 1035–45.

176. Bergman BD, Hebl JR, Kent J, Horlocker TT. Neurologic complications of 405 consecutive continuous axillary catheters. *Anesthesia and Analgesia.* 2003; **96**: 247–52.

*177. Wiegel M, Gottschaldt U, Reske A. Complications and adverse effects associated with continuous peripheral nerve blocks in orthopedic patients. *Anaesthesia and Analgesia.* 2007; **104**: 1578–82.

178. Ozalp G, Canoler O, Kadiogullari N *et al.* Sciatic nerve palsy after total hip arthroplasty in a patient receiving psoas compartment block for patient-controlled regional analgesia. *Journal of Anesthesia.* 2006; **20**: 251–2.

179. Ribeiro FC, Georgousis H, Bertram R, Scheiber G. Plexus irritation caused by interscalene brachial plexus catheter for shoulder surgery. *Anesthesia and Analgesia.* 1996; **82**: 870–2.

180. Mahoudeau G, Gaertner E, Loewenthal A *et al.* Interscalenic block: accidental catheterization of the epidural space. *Annales Françaises d'Aanesthèsie et de Reanimation.* 1995; **14**: 438–41.

181. Cook LB. Unsuspected extradural catheterisation in an interscalene block. *British Journal of Anaesthesia.* 1991; **67**: 473–5.

182. Tuominen MK, Pere P, Rosenberg PH. Unintentional arterial catheterisation and bupivicaine toxicity associated with continuous interscalene brachial plexus block. *Anesthesiology.* 1991; **75**: 356–8.

183. Litz RJ, Vicent O, Wiessner D, Heller AR. Misplacement of a psoas compartment catheter in the subarachnoid space. *Regional Anesthesia and Pain Medicine.* 2004; **29**: 60–4.

184. Hubner T, Gerber H. Knotting of a catheter in the plexus brachialis. A rare complication. *Anaesthesist.* 2003; **52**: 606–7.

185. Burgher AH, Hebl JR. Minimally invasive retrieval of knotted nonstimulating peripheral nerve catheters. *Regional Anesthesia and Pain Medicine.* 2007; **32**: 162–6.

186. Sardesai AM, Chakrabarti AJ, Denny NM. Lower lobe collapse during continuous interscalene brachial plexus local anesthesia at home. *Regional Anesthesia and Pain Medicine.* 2004; **29**: 65–8.

187. Bryan NA, Swenson JD, Greis PE, Burks RT. Indwelling interscalene catheter use in an outpatient setting for shoulder surgery: technique, efficacy, and complications. *Journal of Shoulder and Elbow Surgery.* 2007; **16**: 388–95.

188. Souron V, Reiland Y, De Traverse A. Interpleural migration of an interscalene catheter. *Anesthesia and Analgesia.* 2003; **97**: 1200–01.

189. Jenkins CR, Karmakar MK. An unusual complication of interscalene brachial plexus catheterization: delayed catheter migration. *British Journal of Anaesthesia.* 2005; **95**: 535–7.

190. Harrop-Griffiths W, Denny N. Migration of interscalene catheter – not proven. *British Journal of Anaesthesia.* 2006; **96**: 266.

191. Adam F, Jaziri S, Chauvin M. Psoas abscess complicating femoral nerve block catheter. *Anesthesiology.* 2003; **99**: 230–1.

192. Cuvillon P, Ripart J, Lalourcey L *et al.* The continuous femoral nerve block catheter for postoperative analgesia: bacterial colonization, infectious rate and adverse effects. *Anesthesia and Analgesia.* 2001; **93**: 1045–9.

193. Neuburger M, Buttner J, Blumenthal S *et al.* Inflammation and infection complications of 2285 perineural catheters: a prospective study. *Acta Anaesthesiologica Scandinavica.* 2007; **51**: 108–14.

194. Pedersen JL, Lilleso J, Hammer NA *et al.* Bupivacaine in microcapsules prolongs analgesia after subcutaneous infiltration in humans: a dose-finding study. *Anesthesia and Analgesia.* 2004; **99**: 912–18.

13

Epidural and spinal analgesia

SINA GRAPE AND STEPHAN A SCHUG

KEY LEARNING POINTS

- Neuraxial techniques are safe and provide better postoperative pain relief than parenteral opioids after a wide range of surgical interventions and across different patient populations.
- Co-administration of neuraxial local anesthetic agents and opioids enhances the quality of analgesia. New local anesthetic agents with improved safety profile and short-acting, highly potent opioids have been developed and licensed for neuraxial use.
- Different adjuvant drugs may have additional benefits in terms of analgesia and pharmacokinetic interaction with neuraxial local anesthetics and opioids.

- Specific indications exist for patient-controlled epidural analgesia, combined spinal–epidural analgesia and continuous spinal analgesia.
- In patients having neuraxial blockades, regular monitoring of analgesic efficacy and potential side effects is indispensable.
- Neuraxial analgesia appears to improve morbidity in specific settings, while its impact on mortality is not clear.
- Neuraxial techniques are associated with a high degree of patient satisfaction and procedure-related quality of life.

INTRODUCTION

Neuraxial analgesic techniques were first described in the late nineteenth and early twentieth century. The German surgeon August Bier reported the first intrathecal anesthesia in 1898,[1] while the first lumbar epidural probably dates back to 1921.[2] However, the safety and efficacy of neuraxial anesthesia and analgesia were only established in the 1970s.[3]

Over the following decades, significant progress was made in both surgical and anesthetic domains, enabling more and more complex procedures to be carried out in more and more fragile populations. In this context, neuraxial techniques cannot only produce reliable and flexible analgesia, but they also have been advocated as a method of attenuating detrimental physiologic responses in the perioperative period and improving postoperative outcome. This chapter presents a summary of the recent evidence about epidural and spinal analgesia, evolving indications in specific settings, and the impact of neuraxial techniques on different outcome variables.

NEURAXIAL ANALGESIA: INDICATIONS AND CONTRAINDICATIONS

There are no formal indications, but rather clinical situations where patient preference and physiology make a neuraxial block the technique of choice. Thoracic and abdominal, inguinal, urogenital, rectal, and lower extremity surgery, including ambulatory surgical procedures, are suited for neuraxial anesthesia and analgesia. While epidural techniques are indicated for major surgery where lasting postoperative analgesia is required, spinal techniques produce rapid anesthesia and analgesia for up to 24 hours and have advantages in ambulatory surgery.

Contraindications to neuraxial blockade are patient refusal, clotting defects, sepsis, poor or limited cardiac function, and severe hypovolemia. Relative contraindications are immunocompromise, preexisting neurologic deficits, or spinal deformities. That preexisting central nervous system (CNS) disorders should not be regarded as an absolute contraindication to neuraxial blockade has been confirmed recently, when a survey found no increased frequency of complications.[4] In contrast, clinicians should be aware that neuraxial blockade in patients with preexisting peripheral sensorimotor neuropathy or diabetic polyneuropathy may lead to worsening of neurologic function postoperatively; the incidence of such severe deterioration in a case series was 0.4 percent (95 percent confidence interval (CI), 0.1–1.3 percent).[5]

Regardless of formal indications or contraindications, the decision to perform a neuraxial block must be an individual one. Detailed physiological and pharmacological knowledge, as well as patient-informed consent prior to, meticulous technique during, and continuous follow up after performance of a neuraxial block are prerequisites for successful neuraxial analgesia.

MECHANISMS OF NEURAXIAL ANALGESIA

The precise sites of action and mechanisms of specific neuraxial drug effects are not known, but analgesia is likely to be mediated via extradural (radicular), subdural (spinal), and peripheral structures.[6] Pharmacokinetic studies have shown that an epidurally administered drug diffuses down its concentration gradient into the epidural fat, where it acts at the spinal nerves that traverse the epidural space. In addition, the drug diffuses through the spinal meninges, into the cerebrospinal fluid (CSF) and into the white matter of the spinal cord dorsal horn where its central effects are mediated. Spinal analgesics are given directly into the CSF and correspondingly traverse fewer structures. Finally, neuraxial drugs reach the plasma compartment via venous uptake.[7]

Neuraxially administered local anesthetic (LA) agents penetrate nerve axonal membranes and bind to sodium channels, thus reducing postsynaptic depolarization and nerve stimulus propagation. The effect is nonselective, involving both autonomic and somatic nerve fibers. In addition to sodium channels, multiple neurotransmitters are involved in nociceptive transmission in the dorsal horn of the spinal cord, such as tachykinins (for example, substance P), somatostatin, acetylcholine, γ-aminobutyric acid and N-methyl-D-aspartate (NMDA). Neuraxial administration of LA seems to decrease nociception by interference with these transmitters.

Clinically, a differential pattern of sensory and motor block can often be discerned with LA. Thinner C-fibers that convey pain and autonomic impulses are blocked first, followed by the preganglionic sympathetic B-fibers and finally the large A-fibers that transmit touch, pressure, and motor information.

The effects of neuraxial opioids are complex and are mediated by both peripheral and central mechanisms.[3, 8] At a spinal level, they bind to nonspecific presynaptic afferents to inhibit release of substance P. They also bind to specific μ (mu), κ (kappa), and δ (delta) receptors in the substantia gelatinosa of the dorsal horn where they decrease transmission of nociceptive inputs by hyperpolarization of postsynaptic neurones and inhibition of various neurotansmitter releases. After cephalad transport via the CSF, opioids exert an analgesic action on central μ, κ, and δ receptors. After intravascular absorption, opioids have systemic antinociceptive effects on peripheral μ receptors.

DRUGS USED FOR NEURAXIAL ANALGESIA

Local anesthetic agents

Almost every LA agent can be administered neuraxially. The first LA drugs to be used on a larger scale in the 1980s were of the ester type, such as procaine and tetracaine. These were then replaced by amino-amides (for example, lidocaine, bupivacaine) with an improved safety profile. When it was found that bupivacaine was associated with cardiac arrest and life-threatening arrhythmias, levobupivacaine and ropivacaine were introduced. These are S-enantiomers with similar anesthetic efficacy and reduced toxicity when compared to the racemic mixture.[9] While levobupivacaine is less cardiotoxic, ropivacaine also appears to cause less motor blockade. A meta-analysis of neuraxial ropivacaine in obstetric analgesia suggests clinical advantages, notably a differential block with improved motor function,[10] but the clinical relevance of this aspect continues to be debated.

Overall, neuraxial LA alone have never become widely used because of significant block failure and early regression of sensory block with lower doses and because of the unacceptable incidence of motor block and hypotension with larger doses.

Side effects of neuraxial local anesthetics

Serious complications can result from systemic absorption or inadvertent intravascular injection of LA in large doses, such as CNS toxicity (alterations of consciousness, seizures) or cardiovascular toxicity (arrhythmias, conduction abnormalities). These side effects will not be detailed further as this review is centered on complications resulting specifically from neuraxial administration of LA.

A review by Hodgson et al.[11] about the neurotoxicity of drugs given intrathecally found that all LA have the potential to be directly neurotoxic.[11] In usual concentrations, lidocaine and tetracaine seem to be more neurotoxic than bupivacaine. In animal experiments, neurotoxicity with lasting histopathologic and electrophysiologic changes and neurologic deficits occurred only when LA were given in high doses and concentrations within a restricted area.[12, 13] The exact mechanism of nerve injury induced by neuraxial LA remains undetermined, but may be related to electrolytic imbalances at the neuronal membrane. Despite these preclinical concerns, extensive epidural and spinal use of LA agents has attested to their relative safety in clinical doses.[14]

Another more recent concern with intrathecal LA in clinical doses are transient neurologic symptoms (TNS). Various types of paresthesias, as well as unilateral or bilateral pain in the lower extremity pain, were first reported in 1993 after the intrathecal use of 5 percent hyperbaric lidocaine.[15] Subsequent case series revealed an incidence of TNS between 4 and over 30 percent, depending on the type and concentration of LA, type of surgery, and patient position.[16, 17, 18] Average onset of TNS was 12 to 24 hours after surgery with a duration between six hours to four days and largely spontaneous resolution.[19] Proposed mechanism of TNS are disruption of the blood–nerve barrier by highly concentrated LA, decreased neural blood flow, and irritation of nerve cell membranes.[20] It is most likely not a manifestation of direct neurotoxicity, as neurological deficits are not part of the syndrome and all symptoms are fully reversible. In any patient presenting with neurologic symptoms, the exclusion of more sinister causes, such as nerve compression or infection, is mandatory.

Another concern, especially with spinal LA, are cardiovascular side effects. Blockade of sympathetic vasomotor fibers leads to a significant fall in peripheral vascular resistance by both arterial and venous dilation. If the block level is higher than T5, cardiac sympathetic outflow is affected, so that marked hypotension and bradycardia can occur. While hypotension is seen in over one-third of patients after spinal anesthesia, probably due to the sudden decrease in peripheral vascular resistance, the incidence is only between 0.7 and 6 percent with epidural LA.[21]

Motor blockade is the rule after intrathecal LA, but occurs rarely when low concentrations of local anesthetics are used to provide epidural analgesia. Patients under epidural analgesia with significant motor impairment should be followed up carefully, as this might be a symptom of beginning spinal cord compression.

Opioids

Neuraxial opioids produce intense analgesia without significant motor impairment. Morphine, fentanyl, and sufentanil are the most commonly used epidural and intrathecal opioids, and there is extensive clinical evidence attesting to their efficacy.

Hydrophilic opioids, such as morphine, penetrate neural tissue slowly, resulting in slower onset, delayed elimination and a longer duration of action. Furthermore, hydrophilic opioids have a widespread CSF distribution with the potential of significant cephalad migration.[22] Its prolonged analgesia (up to 24 hours) makes morphine suitable for single epidural or intrathecal bolus administration. However, respiratory depression limits the usefulness of intrathecal morphine doses over 300 µg and requires prolonged monitoring and some vigilance. Newer pharmacologic formulations of morphine were recently introduced into clinical practice, for example liposome-encapsulated morphine, which provides up to 48 hours of pain relief after total hip replacement surgery, but sedation and respiratory depression occurred frequently (4 percent of patients requiring naloxone) and requires careful monitoring and assessment for at least 48 hours.[23][II], [24][III]

As opposed to the preferential CSF distribution of hydrophilic opioids, lipophilic opioids tend to diffuse into perineural fat and are then released back into the epidural space. While fentanyl is the neuraxial opioid most often employed in Australia and in the USA, the fentanyl analog sufentanil is extensively used in Europe. Sufentanil is a µ receptor selective, highly lipophilic synthetic opioid five to ten times more potent than fentanyl.[25] Because of their good bioavailability at the spinal cord, fentanyl and sufentanil have a rapid onset of action. Analgesia tends to be segmentally restricted because of rapid uptake by neural and fatty tissue. The limited duration of lipophilic opioids aids in recovery after short procedures.

Side effects of neuraxial opioids

In contrast to LA, even in large doses neuraxial opioids do not seem to be neurotoxic,[26] and motor impairment is not an issue. However, opioids have several class-specific side effects, as well as complications specifically related to their epidural and spinal use.

The incidence of pruritus with intrathecal opioids varies from 30 to 100 percent and is higher than with epidural administration.[27][II] While the exact mechanism remains unclear, opioid-induced pruritus is probably not histamine-related, but rather due to activation of spinal μ receptors.[28] Reviews comparing the side effects of intravenous and epidural opioids concluded that epidural administration was associated with slightly more pruritus (16 versus 14 percent).[29, 30][I]

The treatment of opioid-related pruritus is difficult. 5-HT3 antagonists should be the first choice (for example odansetron 0.1 mg/kg i.v.).[28][V] Propofol has some efficacy (10 mg i.v., followed by a small continuous infusion), as well as opioid antagonists (for example, naloxone 1–2 μg/kg i.v. per hour, naltrexone 6–9 mg p.o.) or low doses of an agonist/antagonist (for example, nalbuphine 4 mg i.v.). There is no evidence in favor of the traditionally administered antihistamines.

Although intrathecal opioids distribute rapidly within the CSF and about 10 percent of the dose can reach the cisterna magna within 30 minutes after lumbar injection,[31] the overall incidence of respiratory depression with intrathecal opioids is less than 1 percent.[7][V] Respiratory depression after epidural injection is reported in 0.24–1.6 percent of patients.[21][V] As lipophilic opioids are highly potent with a rapid onset of action, they tend to cause early respiratory depression. In contrast, delayed respiratory depression is a concern with neuraxial morphine because of its high affinity to CSF with significant risk of late cephalad spread.

Urinary retention of up to 12 hours after neuraxial anesthesia is common; after epidural analgesia, urinary retention occurs in almost one-third of patients, compared to 15 percent with intramuscular opioids and 13 percent with intravenous patient-controlled opioids.[30][I] These figures may seem prohibitive. However, only patients after large surgical procedures are likely to require postoperative epidural analgesia, and urinary catheters are routinely inserted in these patients.

Nausea and vomiting are very distressing side effects of opioids and are probably mediated by direct stimulation of the chemoreceptor trigger zone. However, nausea and vomiting do not seem to be specifically related to neuraxial administration. In a recent review, the incidence was approximately 25 percent and was unaffected by route of administration (intravenous, intramuscular, or epidural).[30][I] Treatment of nausea and vomiting after neuraxial opioids follows the same principles as other types of opioid-induced nausea and vomiting.[32][V] It involves 5-HT3 antagonists, such as ondansetron (4–8 mg i.v.), dopamine (D_2), antagonists, such as droperidol (0.625–1.25 mg i.v.), and corticosteroids, such as dexamethasone (5–10 mg i.v.).

Another common side effect of opioids is sedation. While 4.6–6.4 percent of patients on intravenous patient-controlled analgesia (PCA) complained of excessive sedation, the incidence was only 0.9–1.4 percent with epidural opioids.[30][I] Administration of the smallest possible doses of neuraxial opioids, close clinical monitoring, as well as avoidance of additional intravenous sedatives are useful preventive measures.

Combination of local anesthetics and opioids

Various mixtures of neuraxial LA and opioids have been studied or are commonly used for both epidural and spinal analgesia; some are even commercially available in some countries. Compared with either component alone, such a combination achieves better analgesia with lower doses of each component.[21] This particularly reduces the hypotension and motor block seen with LA. However, one should always bear in mind that co-administration of LA agents and opioids not only combines the advantages, but also the potential side effects of each drug.

Systematic dose-finding studies with regard to optimal concentrations and combinations of LA-opioid mixtures have not been undertaken. Clinically, in terms of pain relief and side effects, differences between modern LA, such as levobupivacaine or ropivacaine, mixed with opioids, such as fentanyl or sufentanil, are probably minor. Typically, lipophilic opioids are chosen over hydrophilic ones for epidural administration in combination with local anesthetics. In contrast, hydrophilic opioids can have advantages in situations where catheter level and level of incision are incongruent. Probably the most often used epidural is combination bupivacaine 0.05–0.1 percent with 2–4 μg/mL of fentanyl. As co-administration of LA and opioids is routine practice, premixed solutions are available in many centers.

Other neuraxial drugs and adjuvants

EPINEPHRINE (ADRENALINE)

Epinephrine is a mixed α- and β-adrenergic receptor agonist. Its principal effect of interest in neuraxial use is the intense vasoconstriction it provokes. This markedly slows the systemic absorption of neuraxial LA and opioids, so that the sensory block is longer and more intense.[33][II] Addition of neuraxial epinephrine decreases the doses of LA and opioids used.[34][II] Epinephrine can be an adjunct to intrathecal, as well as epidural, analgesics; intrathecal doses are between 100 and 300 μg, and epidural doses are 0.5–3 μg/mL. Theoretical concerns have been raised about the detrimental effects of epinephrine on spinal cord blood flow, but these have been refuted in clinical studies.[35, 36]

Besides its vasoconstrictive effects, epinephrine may also have an analgesic effect of its own.[37] Indeed, several studies have shown that the addition of epinephrine to thoracic epidural analgesia (TEA) with fentanyl and bupivacaine improved analgesia.[38][II]

ALPHA-ADRENERGIC AGONISTS

Clonidine is an α_2-receptor agonist that was introduced for epidural use in the 1980s. It inhibits pain transmission by binding to pre- and postsynaptic receptors of nociceptive afferents, particularly in the dorsal horn of the spinal cord.[39] While having sympatholytic (antihypertensive) and sedative properties, the fact that clonidine is devoid of side effects such as respiratory depression, pruritus, and urinary retention makes it a potentially useful adjunct to neuraxial LA and opioid analgesia.

Several studies indicate that small doses of epidural clonidine (5–20 µg per hour) may improve analgesia, increase motor block, and reduce the dose of LA required, but the evidence is mostly weak and inconsistent.[40][II] Significant side effects, particularly hypotension and sedation, limit the use of clonidine in greater doses.

In 1998, Armand et al.[41][I] undertook a meta-analysis to analyze the efficacy of extradural clonidine to relieve postoperative pain. The authors found that meta-analysis was impossible due to serious methodological flaws in existing trials and due to lack of consistent study designs enabling direct comparison. They concluded that despite the frequent use of epidural clonidine, doses and indications remained widely a matter of personal habits and that no sound data for or against the use of epidural clonidine existed.

Dexmedetomidine is a more selective alpha$_2$-receptor agonist than clonidine. In a recent study, dexmedetomidine has been described as equipotent to clonidine and as effective for prolongation of bupivacaine spinal block.[42] [II] However, epidural dexmedetomidine is currently not in clinical use and further studies are needed to clarify its role.

KETAMINE

Ketamine, a phencyclidine derivative, had long been used as an anesthetic before it was discovered that it possessed significant analgesic properties in subanesthetic doses.[43] Among other target sites, ketamine acts as a noncompetitive antagonist at NMDA receptors where it is thought to play a role in blocking central sensitization, wind up, and pain memory. As ketamine is effective in both acute and chronic pain and has none of the side effects typically related to LA and opioids, it could be a very useful adjunct in neuraxial analgesia. Commercially available ketamine preparations contain potentially neurotoxic preservatives and should not be used for spinal or epidural analgesia, but preservative-free ketamine is well tolerated.

A systematic review assessed the effects of ketamine as adjuvant analgesic to various epidural regimens.[44][I] Eight trials were identified and five of these reported improved analgesia and opioid-sparing effects with no increase in ketamine-related adverse events, such as excessive salivation or psychomimetic effects.

Studies on intrathecal ketamine are scarce; in association with bupivacaine it does not appear to improve analgesia, but to increase side effects.[45]

More studies are warranted to identify the clinical applications of neuraxial ketamine.

NEOSTIGMINE BROMIDE

The acetylcholinesterase inhibitor neostigmine bromide reduces the breakdown of acetylcholine in the dorsal horn of the spinal cord. In animal experiments, it has been shown to potentiate muscarinic receptor-mediated analgesia, but human experience is limited. A multicenter study of intrathecal neostigmine after hysterectomy found that neostigmine reduced postoperative analgesic requirements, but this came at the price of increased and dose-dependent postoperative nausea and vomiting.[46][II] Epidural neostigmine is more promising and seems to have a LA-sparing effect, especially in labor analgesia with concurrent epidural clonidine.[47][II] Its routine use requires further evaluation.

MIDAZOLAM

Benzodiazepines act at GABA$_A$ receptors, which are thought to be involved in antinociception at a spinal level. Preservative-free midazolam for neuraxial use is presented in an aqueous solution buffered to pH 3.5. At physiologic pH, it becomes more lipophilic, which facilitates tissue penetration. Nishiyama et al.[48] reported improved pain control with a combination of epidural midazolam and LA compared to LA alone, but increased sedation occurred with midazolam. In another study, intrathecal midazolam potentiated the analgesic effect of intrathecal fentanyl.[49] A recent report by Yaksh et al.[50] reviewed the current data about neurotoxicity of neuraxial midazolam and concluded that, although there seems to be a degree of safety, further research is necessary and routine clinical use is currently not recommended.

TIMING AND TECHNIQUE

Timing and duration

Elective surgery can be defined as a "planned physical aggression." As the timing and extent of tissue injury are known, analgesic interventions can be given before, during, and after the noxious stimulation.

Over the last years, results of fundamental research and promising animal experiments have shaped the concept of preemptive analgesia, which means establishing an effective analgesic level before the actual noxious input arises.[51] Thus, central nervous perception of afferent nociceptive impulses could be blocked and acute pain, as well as central sensitization and pain memory, prevented. In order to provide preemptive analgesia, an analgesic intervention given before surgery must be shown to be more effective than the same analgesic intervention given after surgery. In this context, neuraxial regimens seem intuitively appealing because of their easy titrability and their combined peripheral and central actions. Various randomized controlled trials (RCT) of preemptive epidural analgesia have been conducted, but clinical benefit was marginal.[52] Currently, there does not seem to be a role for routine preemptive epidural analgesia.[51]

Even if neuraxial techniques are not used preemptively, it is reasonable that analgesia be titrated to an adequate level during the intraoperative and immediate postoperative period. The optimal duration of postoperative epidural analgesia is not clearly defined and decisions should be made on individual grounds (patient comorbidities, extent of surgery, postoperative rehabilitation program). Commonly, epidural analgesia is maintained for two to four days after major surgery until the patient can be switched to a step down regimen of other analgesics.

Level of insertion of epidural catheters

The location of epidural catheters affects analgesic efficacy.[53] Since it has become standard practice to insert an epidural catheter at the level of the incisional dermatome, a shift from lumbar to thoracic epidurals for major thoracoabdominal interventions has been observed. Although there are no randomized controlled trials comparing the efficacy of the same epidural drugs administered via a thoracic or a lumbar approach, numerous studies have demonstrated effective pain relief with thoracic epidural analgesia (TEA), especially dynamic pain relief after extensive thoracic surgery.[54][I]

Another advantage of TEA is that the sympathetic and sensory-motor innervation of the lower abdomen and the lower extremity remains intact. This translates into minimal motor blockade, less urinary retention, and less hypotension compared to lumbar epidurals. While there are theoretical concerns that the placement of a TEA may involve a greater risk of spinal cord injury, the current evidence does not support this view.[55]

Patient-controlled epidural analgesia and continuous epidural infusion

In the era of patient-oriented outcome variables and individualized pain management, giving patients control of their own analgesia is an important principle. Analogous to patient-controlled intravenous analgesia, patient-controlled epidural analgesia (PCEA) has been developed

and has become a standard modality of postoperative analgesia. In most cases, a continuous epidural infusion of LA and opioids is combined with patient-controlled bolus administration of the same mixture. To minimize side effects of repeated bolus doses, a lockout period – mostly 10–20 minutes – is defined before the patient can self-administer the next bolus. While this provides reliable background analgesia during periods of low activity and at night, the patient can manage his or her pain "on demand" according to his or her individual needs and activities. Dedicated color-coded PCEA pumps are available and should be used in order to avoid confusion with other intravenous drugs and infusions. Automatic lock of the PCEA pump after a certain time, and need of an access code to unlock and modify parameters, are useful features of safe epidural analgesia.

Combined spinal–epidural analgesia

For performance of combined spinal–epidural (CSE) analgesia, a needle-through-needle technique is commonly employed. First, the larger epidural needle (for example, an 18-gauge Tuohy needle) is placed in the lumbar epidural space. Then, the smaller spinal needle (for example, a 20- or 22-gauge pencil point needle) is put through the epidural needle until CSF is seen. A single shot spinal is then given through the spinal needle, which is subsequently taken out, and a lumbar epidural catheter is placed.

While the subarachnoid bolus produces immediate and dense analgesia, the epidural catheter can be used to top up the block during longer interventions and for postoperative analgesia. The small dural puncture makes significant intrathecal diffusion of epidurally administered drugs unlikely.

CSE analgesia is an option in prolonged surgery of the lower extremity and has also been incorporated into the practice of obstetrical anesthesia, both for labor analgesia and surgical anesthesia. While the intrathecal component has a rapid onset of action and offers a dense neuraxial blockade, the epidural catheter provides prolonged surgical anesthesia and postoperative analgesia as needed.

Continuous spinal analgesia

Continuous spinal analgesia (CSA) can be used for lower abdominal and lower extremity procedures. Placement of a catheter into the subarachnoid space produces rapid and reliable analgesia. By repeated injection of small doses of LA (for example, hyperbaric bupivacaine by steps in 2.5 mg), the block height can be titrated and analgesia can be extended as required. Especially in the elderly or in patients with significant cardiovascular compromise, it makes sense to avoid the cognitive dysfunction associated with general anesthesia on the one hand and the hemodynamic side effects associated with large intrathecal bolus administrations on the other. Orthopedic interventions, such as hip replacement surgery, are particularly suited for CSA.

Until the early 1990s, dedicated CSA microcatheters (<24 gauge) were available. After multiple case reports of cauda equina syndrome in 1992,[56, 57, 58] the Food and Drug Administration (FDA) issued a safety alert and banned these microcatheters. Subsequently it was found that the neurological complications most likely resulted from direct neurotoxicity when high concentrations of lidocaine were administered through these small needles. Currently, there is a prudent revival of interest in CSA with emphasis on meticulous insertion techniques and use of small doses and low concentrations of LA. A recent review concluded that CSA is a safe modality when patients are carefully selected and appropriately managed.[59] However, CSA catheters are still not available in most countries so that epidural catheters are often used for this purpose. A disadvantage of these catheters is the large dural leak they create and the subsequent risk of postdural puncture headache (see below under Postdural puncture headache). This means that CSA should preferably be used in patients over 75 years where the incidence of headache is very low.

COMPLICATIONS OF EPIDURAL AND SPINAL ANALGESIA

Spinal hematoma

Among the most dreaded and devastating adverse events associated with neuraxial techniques are bleeding complications with resultant permanent damage of the spinal cord. Fortunately, despite a rising number of patients on chronic or perioperative anticoagulant drugs, spinal hematomas remain very rare, and estimations of its incidence are difficult. In a large Finnish study based on 23,500 patient insurance claims from 1987 to 1993, the overall incidence was 0.005 percent, with 0.003 percent of spinal hematomas occurring after epidural and 0.004 percent after spinal anesthesia.[60] Another Swedish report summarizes severe neurological complications after central neuraxial blockades between 1990 and 1999.[61] Among 1,260,000 spinal blocks and 450,000 epidurals, spinal hematoma occurred in only 33 cases, 11 of which were associated with anticoagulation. However, the consequences of spinal and epidural hematoma in this review were severe. Only six patients made a full recovery and 27 suffered permanent neurological damage, such as paraparesis, cauda equina syndrome, and sensory deficits. A more recent review of 8120 patients with epidural catheters under the care of an acute pain service identified two epidural hematomas (incidence <0.05 percent) with no long-term neurological sequelae.[62]

Technical difficulties with block performance seem to be the single most important risk factor for spinal hematoma.[63] Therefore, indications for neuraxial blockade must be weighed carefully and abandoning the procedure should be considered in case of difficulties or "bloody taps."

Another risk factor for spinal–epidural hematoma is concurrent anticoagulation. In the late 1990s, after the introduction of low molecular weight heparin (LMWH) for routine thromboprophylaxis, a sharp rise in the incidence of spinal hematomas was observed.[64] This was mostly related to intraoperative or early postoperative administration of LMWH and a twice-daily, high-dose administration regimen, as practiced in the USA in contrast to the European once-daily administration.[65] Since then, there have been several consensus recommendations for safe practice of epidural and spinal blocks in anticoagulated patients. A summary of relevant guidelines according to the 2003 Second American Society of Regional Anesthesia and Pain Medicine Consensus Conference on Neuraxial Anesthesia and Anticoagulation will be given here.[66]

- Intraoperative systemic heparinization in patients under neuraxial blockade is safe. The same applies to low-dose unfractionated heparin (for example, 5000 IU/12 hours subcutaneously). Indwelling neuraxial catheters should be removed two to four hours after the last heparin dose; unfractionated heparin can be started two hours after removal.
- For patients on LMWH, at least 12 hours should elapse after a standard dose and 24 hours after higher doses before neuraxial blockade is considered. After surgery under neuraxial anesthesia, the first dose of LMWH should be administered after six to eight hours and then every 24 hours. Epidural catheters can be removed 12 hours after the last dose, and the next LMWH dose can be given two hours later.
- Oral anticoagulants should be stopped four to five days before a neuraxial block. The international normalized ratio (INR) must be closely monitored and should be less than 1.5 for catheter insertion and removal. Low-dose oral anticoagulants (for example warfarin 3–5 mg per day) started after catheter insertion seem safe.
- With regard to antiplatelet drugs, low-dose aspirin (for example, 100 mg per day) and nonsteroidal anti-inflammatory drugs (NSAIDs) do not appear to add a substantial risk, whereas neuraxial blocks should never be undertaken in patients on clopidogrel, GPIIb/IIIa antagonists, and direct thrombin inhibitors. However, as these anticoagulants have been introduced only recently, no formal studies and risk calculations exist.

Even with adherence to these guidelines, routine neurologic monitoring should be undertaken in every patient after neuraxial blockade, and more so in patients on any anticoagulant medication.

Infectious complications

Serious infectious complications related to neuraxial analgesia are very rare. A recent English survey of 8100 patients who had received epidural anesthesia between 2000 and 2005 identified six epidural abscesses and three cases of meningitis.[67] In another study which reviewed 17,372 epidurals, the overall incidence of infectious complications was 0.05 percent.[68] Risk factors, such as immunosuppression, diabetes, difficult insertion, or longer catheterization time (greater than three days), were present in 75 percent. No infections were seen when catheters were left in place for two days or less.[68] Similarly, a very recent review of 8120 patients with epidural catheters identified six epidural abscesses (incidence <0.1 percent) with no long-term neurological sequelae.[62]

Epidural analgesia in patients with localized infections is controversial. Septicemia is generally considered a contraindication. Although the data situation is not clear, expert advice is against the use of neuraxial blockade, other than single-shot spinal anesthesia in patients with untreated systemic infections.[69] However, Jakobsen et al.[70] undertook a retrospective study of 69 patients with localized skin infections who underwent repeated epidural catheterization and reported no infection. Immunocompromise should be regarded as a relative contraindication.[71]

Full sterile technique for performance of neuraxial blocks is mandatory. Moreover, careful follow up and a high index of suspicion for infectious complications and recognition of associated symptoms, such as erythema, severe back pain, and progressive neurologic deficit, are required. Early involvement of a neurologist and liberal use of imaging procedures, such as magnetic resonance, are indispensable when in doubt. In cases of confirmed spinal–epidural abcess or meningitis, the most frequent etiologic organism is *Staphylococcus aureus*, and timely administration of probabilistic antibiotics is important.[72] Surgical decompression must be realised as appropriate. The issue of infectious complications has been the topic of a recent practice advisory of the American Society of Regional Anesthesia and addressed in an accompanying editorial.[73]

Unfortunately, the outcome of patients with spinal or epidural abcess is bleak. Due to late recognition, the risk of persistent neurological deficit from an epidural abcess is almost 50 percent. In an analysis of the literature, Kindler et al.[74] found that this has not improved since the 1970s.

Postdural puncture headache

Postdural puncture headache (PDPH) is a common complication of spinal anesthesia and occurs in 2 to 3 percent.[75] The risk of accidental dural puncture with epidurals is estimated at 1 percent. Predictive factors for PDPH are younger patient age, possibly female sex (parturients), and size and type of needles.[76]

The pathophysiologic mechanism for PDPH is thought to be the dural defect induced by needle puncture with continuous transdural leakage of CSF. Headache occurs due to decreased CSF pressure, especially when the patient assumes an upright position because additional traction is then placed on the meninges.[76]

Smaller needles decrease the risk of PDPH, but are technically more difficult to handle. Noncutting (pencil point tip) needles are associated with fewer dural leaks. If PDPH has occurred, treatment by epidural blood patch provides effective tamponade of the CSF leak and increases subarachnoid pressure. Alternative, albeit less successful, options are hydration and intravenous administration of caffeine or intake of caffeinated beverages. Spontaneous improvement of PDPH occurs in ten days in over 90 percent of patients.[76]

EPIDURAL AND SPINAL ANALGESIA IN SPECIFIC SETTINGS

The use of neuraxial anesthesia and analgesia in obstetrics is the topic of Chapter 26, Pain in pregnancy, childbirth, and the puerperium and will not be discussed here.

Cardiac surgery

Cardiac surgery has several unique features that need to be considered before performing neuraxial analgesia. First, cardiac surgery is a highly invasive and stressful intervention that is carried out in a high-risk population. Second, intense postoperative pain can arise from sternotomy, thoracotomy, and chest tube insertion, and this can lead to chronic pain.[77] Third, intraoperative prolonged pulmonary collapse and postoperative atelectasis can cause significant pulmonary dysfunction. Fourth, a significant proportion of cardiac interventions is carried out under cardiopulmonary bypass. Significant platelet dysfunction or coagulopathy may arise from intraoperative anticoagulation. In addition, interventions, such as prosthetic heart valve surgery, warrant early long-term anticoagulation.

In this complex and unpredictable setting, it is difficult to evaluate the risks and benefits of neuraxial blockades for an individual patient. On the one hand, neuraxial analgesia seems attractive because it produces excellent analgesia and has the potential to attenuate the stress response and improve postoperative pulmonary dysfunction. On the other hand, a particular risk is associated with the use of epidural and spinal analgesia in anticoagulated patients. Several recent randomized controlled trials and meta-analyses have addressed this topic.

Intrathecal morphine given as a single-shot injection via a small needle provides effective postoperative analgesia up to 24 hours without the risk of spinal hematoma that might be associated with the use of large needles and the placement of indwelling catheters. Two reviews of intrathecal morphine in patients undergoing cardiac surgery found it to achieve good postoperative analgesia.[78, 79][I] However, no additional benefits were observed, in particular no impact on the perioperative stress response. Larger intrathecal doses of morphine may attenuate the stress response, but they cause an unacceptable delay of extubation.

Epidural techniques provide effective analgesia after cardiac surgery.[78, 79][I] Moreover, TEA has the potential to selectively block the cardiac sympathetic outflow (T1 to T5), which was found to attenuate stress-related increases in heart rate, blood pressure, inotropy, and myocardial oxygen consumption.[80] In a randomized controlled trial among patients with poor left ventricular function undergoing coronary artery bypass grafting, TEA was associated with improved cardiac index, reduced incidence of arrhythmias, and decreased inotropic requirements.[81] [III] While these advantages have been demonstrated, their clinical relevance is currently not clear.

In contrast, a recent randomized controlled trial designed to compare thoracic PCEA with intravenous PCA after elective cardiac surgery found no significant differences.[82][II] There was only a lower intraoperative consumption of anesthetics and a trend towards reduced incidence of confusion and pneumonia in patients receiving PCEA. In 2006, Chaney[79] published a review about intrathecal and epidural anesthesia and analgesia for cardiac surgery. They found that while TEA induced thoracic sympathectomy and attenuated the postoperative stress response, its impact on patient outcome remained unclear, and TEA seemed to offer no benefits other than analgesia. Similar results were found in a meta-analysis by Liu et al. which looked at the effects of perioperative neuraxial analgesia on outcome after coronary artery bypass surgery.[78][I] While TEA was associated with faster extubation, slightly decreased pulmonary complications, decreased cardiac dysrhythmias, and reduced pain scores, no differences in major morbidity or mortality were detected.

In conclusion, intrathecal and epidural analgesia for cardiac surgery remains controversial. The only proven benefit is good postoperative analgesia, but this can also be achieved by a combination of intravenous or oral opioid and nonopioid analgesics. The risks of neuraxial blockade in the fully anticoagulated or coagulopathic patient are substantial.

Thoracic surgery

Thoracic interventions probably come close to cardiac surgery in terms of invasiveness and perioperative risk. There is also a high level of intraoperative stress and

postoperative pain after thoracic interventions. In addition, intercostal nerve dysfunction may result from incision, retraction, trocar placement, or sutures.[83] Intense pain on respiration can cause postoperative hypoventilation and atelectasis in patients who often present significant pulmonary compromise at baseline, and such acute pain may predict chronic postthoracotomy pain.[84]

A meta-analysis by Ballantyne et al. concluded that TEA for thoracic surgery achieved good dynamic pain control, reduced pulmonary atelectasis, decreased the risk of infection, and increased oxygen saturation.[85][I] A more recent review found consistent evidence that TEA reduced perioperative pulmonary complications, especially in high-risk patients.[86][I]

In the future, less invasive surgical techniques, such as video-assisted thoracoscopy, are likely to be used more extensively. Whether the benefits of TEA will persist in this setting will be subject to reevaluation.

Apart from intravenous opioids, new analgesic techniques for thoracic surgery are emerging and compare favorably to epidurals. Davies et al. compared the efficacy of epidural and paravertebral blocks.[87][I] The latter were placed under direct vision by the thoracic surgeon. While both paravertebral and thoracic epidural blocks achieved good postoperative analgesia and dynamic pain control, the epidural group had significantly more adverse effects, such as block failure, hypotension, and urinary retention. Moreover, paravertebral blocks are less problematic with regard to anticoagulation.[88]

Vascular surgery and coagulation

It has long been known that major surgery is associated with a hypercoagulable state, which persists into the postoperative period so that patients are at risk of vaso-occlusive and thrombotic events. Some decades ago it was proven that the vasodilatation associated with neuraxial blockades reduced such events.[89, 90][II] A recent review, however, found minimal evidence that epidural analgesia affected the incidence of deep venous thrombosis or pulmonary embolism when state-of-the-art thromboprophylaxis was used.[86][I]

In a recent Cochrane review, epidural analgesia versus systemic opioids for abdominal aortic surgery was analyzed.[91][I] Epidural analgesia provided better pain relief at rest and dynamic pain relief for up to three postoperative days, and it reduced the duration of postoperative intubation by 20 percent. Epidural analgesia, in particular TEA, reduced overall cardiac complications, myocardial infarction, and gastric and renal complications. However, TEA had no impact on postoperative mortality.

Gastrointestinal surgery

Ileus is common after major abdominal surgery and can be associated with significant postoperative morbidity. In contrast, early enteral feeding reduces septic complications and improves wound healing.[92] The avoidance of parenteral opioids and the blockade of sympathetic afferents resulting from epidural analgesia can potentially reduce postoperative ileus.

A Cochrane review of randomized controlled trials revealed reduced gastrointestinal paralysis in patients after major abdominal surgery who had epidural analgesia as compared to systemic opioids.[29][I] High lumbar and thoracic epidurals were more effective than lower lumbar epidurals.[93] Another more recent review found consistent evidence that epidural analgesia hastened bowel recovery by 24–37 hours.[86][I] Continuous epidural analgesia was superior to PCA in relieving postoperative pain, but was associated with a higher incidence of pruritus.[29][I] Benefits with regard to improved analgesia and shortened duration of ileus have also been confirmed by a recent meta-analysis of RCTs in the setting of colorectal surgery; however, specific complications were also identified and length of hospital stay was not shortened.[94][I]

There was no evidence that epidural analgesia increases the risk of anastomotic leakage.[95][I]

Orthopedic surgery

After hip or knee replacement, epidurals provide better analgesia, especially dynamic pain relief, than parenteral opioids.[96][I] A review published in 1995 found less deep venous thrombosis in patients undergoing total hip replacement or knee arthroplasty under epidural than general anesthesia.[86] However, as pointed out above, the preventive effect of epidural analgesia on thrombosis may be less relevant today. Another review found less postoperative delirium, reduced deep venous thrombosis, and less pneumonia with epidural analgesia for hip replacement surgery.[97]

A recent meta-analysis in patients undergoing total hip replacement and spinal fusion surgery found that neuraxial techniques led to reduced blood loss and a reduced number of patients transfused.[98][I]

PROSPECT is a group which provides systematic reviews of randomized controlled trials leading to consensus recommendations for analgesia at a dedicated website (www.postoppain.org),[99] e.g. after total hip replacement.[100][I] The authors recommend general anesthesia combined with a peripheral nerve block, such as femoral nerve block, as the first option, because this combination provides reliable analgesia and has a favorable risk–benefit profile. An alternative recommendation is a single-shot spinal anesthesia with LA and opioids, followed by postoperative intravenous and oral analgesics. Epidural analgesia is recommended only for patients at particular risk for cardiopulmonary events.

Similar recommendations have been made by this group for the treatment of pain after total knee joint replacement, where again the evidence is more in favor of peripheral nerve blocks, when benefits and risks are weighted.

SAFETY AND EFFICACY OF NEURAXIAL ANALGESIA

Postoperative pain may result in a variety of unfavorable short- and long-term outcomes, such as psychological distress, inability to perform physiotherapy, delayed return to normal function, and chronic pain.[101] Over the last decades, the importance of aggressive pain management has been recognized and different forms of neuraxial analgesia with variable combinations of LA agents, opioids, and other adjuvants have been developed for treatment of postoperative pain. Numerous randomized controlled trials and meta-analyses have attested to the safety of epidural and spinal analgesia when performed according to recognized guidelines. Serious adverse events and mortality are so rare that it is difficult to obtain reliable data on their incidence.

As far as the efficacy of neuraxial analgesia is concerned, a study of almost 6000 patients who received intrathecal morphine for analgesia after different surgical procedures reported effective analgesia for up to 24 hours.[102] In a survey of 1057 patients with postoperative PCEA, Wigfull et al.[103] reported that nearly 94 percent of patients had adequate analgesia with PCEA. Block et al. undertook a meta-analysis on the analgesic efficacy of epidural versus intravenous patient-controlled analgesia, which included 100 randomized controlled trials.[104][I] They found that the overall analgesia with epidurals was better than with parenteral opioids at all time points, across all patient populations, and after all types of surgery. Similarly, a meta-analysis by Wu et al. found that PCEA after different surgical interventions provided superior analgesia compared to intravenous PCA for overall pain, pain at rest, and pain with activity.[105][I]

OUTCOME AFTER SPINAL AND EPIDURAL ANALGESIA

Cost–effectiveness

Cost-related issues are important aspects of anesthetic decision-making in a time where healthcare resources are scarce. As demographic changes and financial restrictions are only recent developments, no comprehensive reviews of costs and benefits associated with neuraxial analgesia have been published. In addition, no consensus exists as to which costs should be measured, in which clinical settings, and at what points in time this should be done. Comparison of cost-effectiveness data is likely to be hampered by major differences in healthcare systems.

A cost evaluation of epidural versus intravenous PCA after major abdominal surgery in Sweden published in 1995 found that epidurals provided more effective pain control, but were three times more expensive.[106] The beneficial effect of better pain control was only seen in the immediate postoperative period, so that the authors judged epidural analgesia poorly cost-effective and not overall justified. In contrast, a German analysis of 6349 patients comparing postoperative PCEA, intravenous PCA, and brachial plexus blockade concluded that the higher initial costs of PCEA could be set off by better pain relief and earlier discharge from the intensive care unit.[107]

In conclusion, a detailed cost-effectiveness analysis of neuraxial analgesia remains to be performed. It is most likely that neuraxial techniques become cost-effective by utilizing their advantages to permit aggressive postoperative rehabilitation.[108] Earlier discharge from high dependency wards, decreased postoperative complications, and long-term benefits, such as reduction in morbidity, may then outweigh the higher initial costs of epidural analgesia, especially in high-risk patients.[109] In low- and intermediate-risk patients undergoing less invasive interventions, neuraxial analgesia may not be cost effective.

Morbidity and mortality

Numerous studies have proven that major surgery and perioperative pain are powerful activators of the neuroendocrine stress response. Manifestations of this stress response include hypercoagulability, immunosuppression, increased myocardial workload and oxygen consumption, widespread inflammation, and increased catabolism with hyperglycemia, muscle breakdown and poor wound healing. Epidural analgesia has the potential to block this detrimental pathophysiology by improving analgesia and by blocking sympathetic afferents.

Indeed, many studies undertaken in the 1980s and 1990s found that epidural analgesia attenuated the postoperative stress response and improved outcome.[110, 111] [II] In 1987, Yeager et al. reported such a significant improvement in morbidity and mortality in high-risk patients receiving epidural analgesia that their study was stopped early by the local ethics committee.[112][II] In 2001, Beattie et al. published a meta-analysis including 11 randomized controlled trials with 1173 patients from 1966 to 1988.[113][I] They found that epidural anesthesia and analgesia was associated with a 40 percent reduction of postoperative myocardial infarction.

Yet the most comprehensive meta-analysis in favor of neuraxial anesthesia is the CORTRA analysis by Rodgers et al. that was published in 2000.[114][I] This review included 141 randomized controlled trials from 1977 to 1995 with almost 9600 patients, with the majority of trials coming from the 1980s. The authors observed a 30 percent reduction in overall mortality (1.9 versus 2.8

percent) with intraoperative neuraxial blockade compared to general anesthesia.

After much discussion of these impressive data, several large multicenter trials were undertaken with less striking results. In a study with 1021 patients published in 2001, epidural anesthesia and analgesia did not improve overall morbidity and mortality.[115][II] The only benefit was seen in a subgroup of patients undergoing abdominal aortic procedures. The MASTER trial (2002) analyzed data from 915 patients undergoing major abdominal surgery under combined epidural and general anesthesia or under general anesthesia alone.[116][II] Postoperative analgesia was either via epidural catheters or via intravenous PCA. There was no benefit in terms of mortality and only a slightly improved morbidity in the epidural group. In 2007, Liu et al. carried out a systematic update of the evidence to assess the effect of postoperative analgesia on major postoperative complications.[86][I] They analyzed randomized controlled trials from 1996 to 2006 and found that there was insufficient evidence to confirm or deny the ability of postoperative analgesia to affect postoperative mortality or morbidity.

In conclusion, several randomized controlled trials and meta-analyses report reduced morbidity and even mortality with epidural anesthesia and analgesia, while others find no significant benefit apart from good pain relief. Several aspects may explain these seemingly contradictory results.

Methodological difficulties most certainly play a role. Comparison of various data sets from heterogeneous studies with different patient groups undergoing a variety of surgical procedures is not evident. It is equally difficult to differentiate which effects are due to general anesthesia and which are due to intraoperative or postoperative neuraxial analgesia.[117] In the postoperative period, it is difficult to establish the exact impact of neuraxial analgesia amidst a multitude of therapeutic measures and individual patient factors. Therefore, the changes in mortality observed in several studies may not have been brought about by analgesia alone, but by a combination of different factors, such as optimization of preoperative medical status, use of short-acting anesthetic drugs and the laryngeal mask, less invasive surgical technique, modern thromboprophylaxis, and accelerated recovery. A corroborating aspect to this argument is that results of studies and meta-analyses seem to be affected by their publication date.[118][I] While older studies tend to find significant benefits from neuraxial analgesia, this effect is much attenuated in recent publications.

Modern anesthesia may also be a victim of its own success in that serious morbidity and mortality have become too rare to be measured in clinical trials of ordinary sample size. This aspect was addressed by Wu et al. in 2004, who analyzed a random sample of American Medicare beneficiaries undergoing different types of major surgery from 1997 to 2001.[119] In their database of 12,780 patients, they found that epidural analgesia was associated with a significantly lower odds ratio of death at 7 and 30 days postoperatively.

In conclusion, the impact of neuraxial analgesia on mortality remains to be determined and is likely to be less important than in the past due to surgical and anesthesiologic advances. However, epidural techniques, in particular, are very useful as part of a multimodal approach to control postoperative pain and hasten recovery.[117]

Nontraditional outcome measures

Over the last few years, patient-centered outcome variables have been introduced as monitors of anesthetic care and are likely to supplement or replace the traditional outcome measures, morbidity and mortality.

While many authors agree that patient satisfaction is an important outcome measure, no validated and standardized tools exist for rating patient satisfaction with regard to neuraxial analgesia.[120] Satisfaction is a complex psychosocial construct, which is likely to be influenced by numerous factors other than analgesia, for example patient expectations, level of information, baseline physical and psychological status, communication, and interaction with healthcare providers.[121] While it seems inherently difficult to measure patient satisfaction, reproducibility and comparison of such data from different studies is highly problematic.

Nevertheless, several trials have addressed this complex issue. In a survey of 1057 patients receiving postoperative PCEA, Wigfull et al.[103] found that PCEA produced excellent analgesia and high patient satisfaction. Another study of almost 6000 patients who received intrathecal morphine for analgesia after a range of surgical procedures equally reported high patient satisfaction.[102] A systematic review found that, compared with systemic opioids, epidural analgesia was associated with higher patient satisfaction.[122][I] Indeed, in a prospective seven-year survey of nearly 6000 surgical patients, neuraxial analgesia was associated with a high degree of patient satisfaction (mean satisfaction score of 8.5 on a scale from 0 to 10).[102]

As far as measurements of health-related quality of life are concerned, these have not been carried out with regard to postoperative analgesia. "Analgesia-related quality of life" is not yet an issue in most clinical studies. However, if the goal after a surgical intervention is to get the patient "up and functioning" and back to his or her preoperative state as soon as possible, neuraxial techniques may play an important role because they provide better pain relief and contribute to early rehabilitation. In one study, Carli et al.[123] found that epidural analgesia enhanced postoperative quality of life. Another contribution of neuraxial analgesia to better quality of life may be the avoidance of chronic pain by aggressive management of early postoperative pain.[101]

RESEARCH AGENDA AND FUTURE DIRECTIONS

Despite many recent advances with insight into pain mechanisms, further basic and clinical research is needed in order to elucidate the phenomenon of acute pain and associated physiology, such as the pain-related stress response. Better knowledge of peripheral and central pain reception and modulation may lead to better use of existing neuraxial techniques and to the development of new epidural and spinal analgesics.

As far as practical conduct of neuraxial analgesia is concerned, safer techniques of insertion, such as ultrasound-guided techniques, need to be studied, and safe catheters for epidural and intrathecal use are needed.

Based on further randomized controlled trials and meta-analyses, it is likely that more procedure-specific guidelines for postoperative pain management will be developed and that indications and contraindications will be tailored to specific subgroups of patients.

Finally, systematic outcomes research with regard to neuraxial analgesia needs to be conducted, with special emphasis on nontraditional outcome measures, analgesia-related quality of life, and cost-effectiveness.

CONCLUSIONS

The last decades have witnessed important advances in all aspects of patient care. In parallel with the introduction of less invasive and individualized surgical methods, new techniques of postoperative pain relief have been added to the armamentarium of the anesthetist. Specific guidelines about indications, contraindications, and the technical performance of neuraxial procedures are available.

Standard intrathecal and epidural analgesia and their variations, such as combined spinal–epidural analgesia and continuous spinal analgesia, provide effective pain relief after various types of surgical procedures. Patient-controlled epidural analgesia is an important component of effective and individualized management of postoperative pain.

Appropriately administered neuraxial analgesia is a key component of multimodal rehabilitation programs after major surgery and has benefits in terms of patient satisfaction and health-related quality of life. Significantly decreased morbidity has been proven in selected patients. The exact impact of epidural and spinal analgesia on mortality remains to be determined.

REFERENCES

1. Bier A. Versuche über Cocainisierung des Rückenmarkes. *Deutsche Zeitschrift für Chirurgie*. 1898; **51**: 361–9.
2. Brill S, Gurman GM, Fisher A. A history of neuraxial administration of local analgesics and opioids. *European Journal of Anaesthesiology*. 2003; **20**: 682–9.

3. Bromage PR, Camporesi E, Chestnut D. Epidural narcotics for postoperative analgesia. *Anesthesia and Analgesia.* 1980; **59**: 473–80.

∗ 4. Hebl JR, Horlocker TT, Schroeder DR. Neuraxial anesthesia and analgesia in patients with preexisting central nervous system disorders. *Anesthesia and Analgesia.* 2006; **103**: 223–8.

5. Hebl JR, Kopp SL, Schroeder DR, Horlocker TT. Neurologic complications after neuraxial anesthesia or analgesia in patients with preexisting peripheral sensorimotor neuropathy or diabetic polyneuropathy. *Anesthesia and Analgesia.* 2006; **103**: 1294–9.

∗ 6. Schug SA, Saunders D, Kurowski I, Paech MJ. Neuraxial drug administration: a review of treatment options for anaesthesia and analgesia. *CNS Drugs.* 2006; **20**: 917–33.

∗ 7. Rathmell JP, Lair TR, Nauman B. The role of intrathecal drugs in the treatment of acute pain. *Anesthesia and Analgesia.* 2005; **101**: S30–43.

8. Bernards CM, Shen DD, Sterling ES *et al.* Epidural, cerebrospinal fluid, and plasma pharmacokinetics of epidural opioids (part 1): differences among opioids. *Anesthesiology.* 2003; **99**: 455–65.

9. Groban L. Central nervous system and cardiac effects from long-acting amide local anesthetic toxicity in the intact animal model. *Regional Anesthesia and Pain Medicine.* 2003; **28**: 3–11.

10. Writer WD, Stienstra R, Eddleston JM *et al.* Neonatal outcome and mode of delivery after epidural analgesia for labour with ropivacaine and bupivacaine: a prospective meta-analysis. *British Journal of Anaesthesia.* 1998; **81**: 713–17.

∗ 11. Hodgson PS, Neal JM, Pollock JE, Liu SS. The neurotoxicity of drugs given intrathecally (spinal). *Anesthesia and Analgesia.* 1999; **88**: 797–809.

12. Ready LB, Plumer MH, Haschke RH *et al.* Neurotoxicity of intrathecal local anesthetics in rabbits. *Anesthesiology.* 1985; **63**: 364–70.

13. Lambert LA, Lambert DH, Strichartz GR. Irreversible conduction block in isolated nerve by high concentration local anesthetics. *Anesthesiology.* 1994; **80**: 1082–93.

14. Horlocker T, McGregor D, Matsushige D *et al.* A retrospective review of 4767 consecutive spinal anesthetics: central nervous system complications. *Anesthesia and Analgesia.* 1997; **84**: 578–84.

15. Schneider M, Ettlin T, Kaufmann M *et al.* Transient neurologic toxicity after hyperbaric subarachnoid anesthesia with 5% lidocaine. *Anesthesia and Analgesia.* 1993; **76**: 1154–7.

16. Hampl KF, Heinzmann-Wiedmer S, Luginbuehl I *et al.* Transient neurologic symptoms after spinal anesthesia: a lower incidence with prilocaine and bupivacaine than with lidocaine. *Anesthesiology.* 1998; **88**: 629–33.

17. Philip J, Sharma SK, Gottumukkala VNR *et al.* Transient neurologic symptoms after spinal anesthesia with lidocainie in obstetric patients. *Anesthesia and Analgesia.* 2001; **92**: 405–09.

∗ 18. Pollock JE. Neurotoxicity of intrathecal local anaesthetics and transient neurological symptoms. *Best Practice and Research. Clinical Anaesthesiology.* 2003; **17**: 471–84.

19. Pollock JE. Transient neurologic symptoms: etiology, risk factors, and management. *Regional Anesthesia and Pain Medicine.* 2002; **27**: 581–6.

20. Kitagawa N, Oda M, Totoki T. Possible mechanism of irreversible nerve injury caused by local anesthetics: detergent properties of local anesthetics and membrane disruption. *Anesthesiology.* 2004; **100**: 962–7.

∗ 21. Wheatley RG, Schug SA, Watson D. Safety and efficacy of postoperative epidural analgesia. *British Journal of Anaesthesia.* 2001; **87**: 47–61.

22. Bernards CM. Understanding the physiology and pharmacology of epidural and intrathecal opioids. *Best Practice and Research. Clinical Anaesthesiology.* 2002; **16**: 489–505.

23. Viscusi ER. Emerging techniques in the management of acute pain: epidural analgesia. *Anesthesia and Analgesia.* 2005; **101**: S23–9.

24. Viscusi ER, Kopacz D, Hartrick C *et al.* Single-dose extended-release epidural morphine for pain following hip arthroplasty. *American Journal of Therapeutics.* 2006; **13**: 423–31.

25. Schug SA, Buerkle H, Moharib M, Cardwell HMD. New drugs for neuraxial blockade. *Current Opinion in Anaesthesiology.* 1999; **12**: 551–7.

26. Sabbe MB, Grafe MR, Mjanger E *et al.* Spinal delivery of sufentanil, alfentanil, and morphine in dogs. Physiologic and toxicologic investigations. *Anesthesiology.* 1994; **81**: 899–920.

27. Shah MK, Sia AT, Chong JL. The effect of the addition of ropivacaine or bupivacaine upon pruritus induced by intrathecal fentanyl in labour. *Anaesthesia.* 2000; **55**: 1008–13.

∗ 28. Szarvas S, Harmon D, Murphy D. Neuraxial opioid-induced pruritus: a review. *Journal of Clinical Anesthesia.* 2003; **15**: 234–9.

29. Werawatganon T, Charuluxanun S. Patient controlled intravenous opioid analgesia versus continuous epidural analgesia for pain after intra-abdominal surgery. *Cochrane Database of Systematic Reviews.* 2005; **CD004088**.

∗ 30. Dolin SJ, Cashman JN. Tolerability of acute postoperative pain management: nausea, vomiting, sedation, pruritis, and urinary retention. Evidence from published data. *British Journal of Anaesthesia.* 2005; **95**: 584–91.

31. Swenson JD, Lee TH, McJames S. The effect of prior dural puncture on cerebrospinal fluid sufentanil concentrations in sheep after the administration of epidural sufentanil. *Anesthesia and Analgesia.* 1998; **86**: 794–6.

∗ 32. Gan TJ, Meyer T, Apfel CC *et al.* Consensus guidelines for managing postoperative nausea and vomiting. *Anesthesia and Analgesia.* 2003; **97**: 62–71.

33. Niemi G, Breivik H. The minimally effective concentration of adrenaline in a low-concentration thoracic epidural analgesic infusion of bupivacaine, fentanyl and adrenaline after major surgery. A randomized, double-blind, dose-

finding study. *Acta Anaesthesiologica Scandinavica*. 2003; **47**: 439–50.

* 34. Niemi G. Advantages and disadvantages of adrenaline in regional anaesthesia. *Best Practice and Research. Clinical Anaesthesiology*. 2005; **19**: 229–45.

35. Porter SS, Albin MS, Watson WA *et al.* Spinal cord and cerebral blood flow responses to subarachnoid injection of local anesthetics with and without epinephrine. *Acta Anaesthesiologica Scandinavica*. 1985; **29**: 330–8.

36. Neal JM. Effects of epinephrine in local anesthetics on the central and peripheral nervous systems: neurotoxicity and neural blood flow. *Regional Anesthesia and Pain Medicine*. 2003; **28**: 124–34.

37. Curatolo M, Petersen-Felix S, Arendt-Nielsen L, Zbinden AM. Epidural epinephrine and clonidine: segmental analgesia and effects on different pain modalities. *Anesthesiology*. 1997; **87**: 785–94.

38. Sakaguchi Y, Sakura S, Shinzawa M, Saito Y. Does adrenaline improve epidural bupivacaine and fentanyl analgesia after abdominal surgery? *Anaesthesia and Intensive Care*. 2000; **28**: 522–6.

39. Tamsen A, Gordh T. Epidural clonidine produces analgesia. *Lancet*. 1984; **2**: 231–2.

40. Eisenach JC. Three novel spinal analgesics: clonidine, neostigmine, amitriptyline. *Regional Anesthesia*. 1996; **21**: 81–3.

41. Armand S, Langlade A, Boutros A *et al.* Meta-analysis of the efficacy of extradural clonidine to relieve postoperative pain: an impossible task. *British Journal of Anaesthesia*. 1998; **81**: 126–34.

42. Kanazi GE, Aouad MT, Jabbour-Khoury SI *et al.* Effect of low-dose dexmedetomidine or clonidine on the characteristics of bupivacaine spinal block. *Acta Anaesthesiologica Scandinavica*. 2006; **50**: 222–7.

43. Visser E, Schug SA. The role of ketamine in pain management. *Biomedicine and Pharmacotherapy*. 2006; **60**: 341–8.

44. Subramaniam K, Subramaniam B, Steinbrook RA. Ketamine as adjuvant analgesic to opioids: a quantitative and qualitative systematic review. *Anesthesia and Analgesia*. 2004; **99**: 482–95.

45. Kathirvel S, Sadhasivam S, Saxena A *et al.* Effects of intrathecal ketamine added to bupivacaine for spinal anaesthesia. *Anaesthesia*. 2000; **55**: 899–904.

46. Lauretti GR, Hood DD, Eisenach JC, Pfeifer BL. A multi-center study of intrathecal neostigmine for analgesia following vaginal hysterectomy. *Anesthesiology*. 1998; **89**: 913–18.

47. Roelants F, Lavand'homme PM, Mercier-Fuzier V. Epidural administration of neostigmine and clonidine to induce labor analgesia: evaluation of efficacy and local anesthetic-sparing effect. *Anesthesiology*. 2005; **102**: 1205–10.

48. Nishiyama T, Matsukawa T, Hanaoka K. Continuous epidural administration of midazolam and bupivacaine for postoperative analgesia. *Acta Anaesthesiologica Scandinavica*. 1999; **43**: 568–72.

49. Tucker AP, Mezzatesta J, Nadeson R, Goodchild CS. Intrathecal midazolam II: combination with intrathecal fentanyl for labor pain. *Anesthesia and Analgesia*. 2004; **98**: 1521–7.

50. Yaksh TL, Allen JW. The use of intrathecal midazolam in humans: a case study of process. *Anesthesia and Analgesia*. 2004; **98**: 1536–45.

* 51. Grape S, Tramer MR. Do we need preemptive analgesia for the treatment of postoperative pain? *Best Practice and Research. Clinical Anaesthesiology*. 2007; **21**: 51–63.

* 52. Pogatzki-Zahn EM, Zahn PK. From preemptive to preventive analgesia. *Current Opinion in Anaesthesiology*. 2006; **19**: 551–5.

53. Richman JM, Wu CL. Epidural analgesia for postoperative pain. *Anesthesiology Clinics of North America*. 2005; **23**: 125–40.

54. Liu S, Angel JM, Owens BD *et al.* Effects of epidural bupivacaine after thoracotomy. *Regional Anesthesia*. 1995; **20**: 303–10.

55. Tanaka K, Watanabe R, Harada T, Dan K. Extensive application of epidural anesthesia and analgesia in a university hospital: Incidence of complications related to technique. *Regional Anesthesia*. 1993; **18**: 34–8.

56. Schell RM, Brauer FS, Cole DJ, Applegate 2nd RL. Persistent sacral nerve root deficits after continuous spinal anaesthesia. *Canadian Journal of Anaesthesia*. 1991; **38**: 908–11.

57. Denny NM, Selander DE. Continuous spinal anaesthesia. *British Journal of Anaesthesia*. 1998; **81**: 590–7.

58. Rigler ML, Drasner K, Krejcie TC *et al.* Cauda equina syndrome after continuous spinal anesthesia. *Anesthesia and Analgesia*. 1991; **72**: 275–81.

59. Bevacqua BK. Continuous spinal anaesthesia: what's new and what's not. *Best Practice and Research. Clinical Anaesthesiology*. 2003; **17**: 393–406.

60. Aromaa U, Lahdensuu M, Cozanitis DA. Severe complications associated with epidural and spinal anaesthesias in Finland 1987–1993. A study based on patient insurance claims. *Acta Anaesthesiologica Scandinavica*. 1997; **41**: 445–52.

61. Moen V, Dahlgren N, Irestedt L. Severe neurological complications after central neuraxial blockades in Sweden 1990–1999. *Anesthesiology*. 2004; **101**: 950–09.

* 62. Cameron CM, Scott DA, McDonald WM, Davies MJ. A review of neuraxial epidural morbidity: experience of more than 8,000 cases at a single teaching hospital. *Anesthesiology*. 2007; **106**: 997–1002.

63. Renck H. Neurological complications of central nerve blocks. *Acta Anaesthesiologica Scandinavica*. 1995; **39**: 859–68.

64. Horlocker TT, Wedel DJ. Neuraxial block and low-molecular-weight heparin: balancing perioperative analgesia and thromboprophylaxis. *Regional Anesthesia and Pain Medicine*. 1998; **23**: 164–77.

65. Tryba M. European practice guidelines: thromboembolism prophylaxis and regional anesthesia. *Regional Anesthesia and Pain Medicine*. 1998; **23**: 178–82.

* 66. Horlocker TT, Wedel DJ, Benzon H *et al*. Regional anesthesia in the anticoagulated patient: defining the risks (the second ASRA Consensus Conference on Neuraxial Anesthesia and Anticoagulation). *Regional Anesthesia and Pain Medicine*. 2003; **28**: 172–97.

67. Christie IW, McCabe S. Major complications of epidural analgesia after surgery: results of a six-year survey. *Anaesthesia*. 2007; **62**: 335–41.

68. Wang LP, Hauerberg J, Schmidt JF. Incidence of spinal epidural abscess after epidural analgesia: a national 1-year survey. *Anesthesiology*. 1999; **91**: 1928–36.

69. Wedel DJ, Horlocker TT. Regional anesthesia in the febrile or infected patient. *Regional Anesthesia and Pain Medicine*. 2006; **31**: 324–33.

70. Jakobsen KB, Christensen MK, Carlsson PS. Extradural anaesthesia for repeated surgical treatment in the presence of infection. *British Journal of Anaesthesia*. 1995; **75**: 536–40.

71. Horlocker TT, Wedel DJ. Regional anesthesia in the immunocompromised patient. *Regional Anesthesia and Pain Medicine*. 2006; **31**: 334–45.

72. Simpson RS, Macintyre PE, Shaw D *et al*. Epidural catheter tip cultures: results of a 4-year audit and implications for clinical practice. *Regional Anesthesia and Pain Medicine*. 2000; **25**: 360–7.

* 73. Hebl JR, Neal JM. Infectious complications: a new practice advisory. *Regional Anesthesia and Pain Medicine*. 2006; **31**: 289–90.

74. Kindler CH, Seeberger MD, Staender SE. Epidural abscess complicating epidural anesthesia and analgesia. An analysis of the literature. *Acta Anaesthesiologica Scandinavica*. 1998; **42**: 614–20.

75. Horlocker TT. Complications of spinal and epidural anesthesia. *Anesthesiology Clinics of North America*. 2000; **18**: 461–85.

76. Candido KD, Stevens RA. Post-dural puncture headache: pathophysiology, prevention and treatment. *Best Practice and Research. Clinical Anaesthesiology*. 2003; **17**: 451–69.

77. Perkins FM, Kehlet H. Chronic pain as an outcome of surgery. A review of predictive factors. *Anesthesiology*. 2000; **93**: 1123–33.

* 78. Liu SS, Block BM, Wu CL. Effects of perioperative central neuraxial analgesia on outcome after coronary artery bypass surgery: a meta-analysis. *Anesthesiology*. 2004; **101**: 153–61.

79. Chaney MA. Intrathecal and epidural anesthesia and analgesia for cardiac surgery. *Anesthesia and Analgesia*. 2006; **102**: 45–64.

80. Veering BT, Cousins MJ. Cardiovascular and pulmonary effects of epidural anaesthesia. *Anaesthesia and Intensive Care*. 2000; **28**: 620–35.

81. Kilickan L, Solak M, Bayindir O. Thoracic epidural anesthesia preserves myocardial function during intraoperative and postoperative period in coronary artery bypass grafting operation. *Journal of Cardiovascular Surgery*. 2005; **46**: 559–67.

82. Hansdottir V, Philip J, Olsen MF *et al*. Thoracic epidural versus intravenous patient-controlled analgesia after cardiac surgery: a randomized controlled trial on length of hospital stay and patient-perceived quality of recovery. *Anesthesiology*. 2006; **104**: 142–51.

83. Ochroch EA, Gottschalk A, Augostides J *et al*. Long-term pain and activity during recovery from major thoracotomy using thoracic epidural analgesia. *Anesthesiology*. 2002; **97**: 1234–44.

84. Katz J, Jackson M, Kavanagh BP, Sandler AN. Acute pain after thoracic surgery predicts long-term post-thoracotomy pain. *Clinical Journal of Pain*. 1996; **12**: 50–5.

* 85. Ballantyne J, Carr D, deFerranti S *et al*. The comparative effects of postoperative analgesia therapies on pulmonary outcome: cumulative meta-analysis of randomized, controlled trials. *Anesthesia and Analgesia*. 1998; **86**: 598–612.

* 86. Liu SS, Wu CL. Effect of postoperative analgesia on major postoperative complications: a systematic update of the evidence. *Anesthesia and Analgesia*. 2007; **104**: 689–702.

* 87. Davies RG, Myles PS, Graham JM. A comparison of the analgesic efficacy and side-effects of paravertebral vs epidural blockade for thoracotomy – a systematic review and meta-analysis of randomized trials. *British Journal of Anaesthesia*. 2006; **96**: 418–26.

88. Ng A, Swanevelder J. Pain relief after thoracotomy: is epidural analgesia the optimal technique? *British Journal of Anaesthesia*. 2007; **98**: 159–62.

89. Modig J, Borg T, Karlstrom G *et al*. Thromboembolism after total hip replacement: role of epidural and general anesthesia. *Anesthesia and Analgesia*. 1983; **62**: 174–80.

90. Jorgensen L, Rasmussen L, Nielsen P *et al*. Antithrombotic efficacy of continuous extradural analgesia after knee replacement. *British Journal of Anaesthesia*. 1991; **66**: 8–12.

91. Nishimori M, Ballantyne JC, Low JH. Epidural pain relief versus systemic opioid-based pain relief for abdominal aortic surgery. *Cochrane Database of Systematic Reviews*. 2006; **CD005059**.

92. Kehlet H. Fast-track colonic surgery: status and perspectives. *Recent Results in Cancer Research*. 2005; **165**: 8–13.

93. Fotiadis RJ, Badvie S, Weston MD, Allen-Mersh TG. Epidural analgesia in gastrointestinal surgery. *British Journal of Surgery*. 2004; **91**: 828–41.

* 94. Marret E, Remy C, Bonnet F. Meta-analysis of epidural analgesia versus parenteral opioid analgesia after colorectal surgery. *British Journal of Surgery*. 2007; **94**: 665–73.

95. Holte K, Kehlet H. Epidural analgesia and risk of anastomotic leakage. *Regional Anesthesia and Pain Medicine*. 2001; **26**: 111–17.

* 96. Choi PT, Bhandari M, Scott J, Douketis J. Epidural analgesia for pain relief following hip or knee replacement. *Cochrane Database of Systematic Reviews*. 2003; **CD003071**.

* 97. Tziavrangos E, Schug SA. Regional anaesthesia and perioperative outcome. *Current Opinion in Anaesthesiology.* 2006; **19**: 521–5.

* 98. Guay J. The effect of neuraxial blocks on surgical blood loss and blood transfusion requirements: a meta-analysis. *Journal of Clinical Anesthesia.* 2006; **18**: 124–8.

99. Neugebauer EA, Wilkinson RC, Kehlet H, Schug SA. PROSPECT: a practical method for formulating evidence-based expert recommendations for the management of postoperative pain. *Surgical Endoscopy.* 2007; **21**: 1047–53.

*100. Fischer HB, Simanski CJ. A procedure-specific systematic review and consensus recommendations for analgesia after total hip replacement. *Anaesthesia.* 2005; **60**: 1189–202.

*101. Kehlet H, Jensen TS, Woolf CJ. Persistent postsurgical pain: risk factors and prevention. *Lancet.* 2006; **367**: 1618–25.

102. Gwirtz KH, Young JV, Byers RS *et al.* The safety and efficacy of intrathecal opioid analgesia for acute postoperative pain: Seven years' experience with 5969 surgical patients at Indiana University Hospital. *Anesthesia and Analgesia.* 1999; **88**: 599–604.

103. Wigfull J, Welchew E. Survey of 1057 patients receiving postoperative patient-controlled epidural analgesia. *Anaesthesia.* 2001; **56**: 70–5.

104. Block BM, Liu SS, Rowlingson AJ *et al.* Efficacy of postoperative epidural analgesia: a meta-analysis. *Journal of the American Medical Association.* 2003; **290**: 2455–63.

*105. Wu CL, Cohen SR, Richman JM *et al.* Efficacy of postoperative patient-controlled and continuous infusion epidural analgesia versus intravenous patient-controlled analgesia with opioids: a meta-analysis. *Anesthesiology.* 2005; **103**: 1079–88.

106. Bartha E, Carlsson P, Kalman S. Evaluation of costs and effects of epidural analgesia and patient-controlled intravenous analgesia after major abdominal surgery. *British Journal of Anaesthesia.* 2006; **96**: 111–17.

107. Brodner G, Mertes N, Buerkle H *et al.* Acute pain management: Analysis, implications and consequences after prospective experience with 6349 surgical patients. *European Journal of Anaesthesiology.* 2000; **17**: 566–75.

108. Kehlet H. Effect of postoperative pain treatment on outcome-current status and future strategies. *Langenbeck's Archives of Surgery.* 2004; **389**: 244–9.

109. Kehlet H, Dahl JB. Anaesthesia, surgery, and challenges in postoperative recovery. *Lancet.* 2003; **362**: 1921–8.

110. Blomberg S, Curelaru I, Emanuelsson H *et al.* Thoracic epidural anaesthesia in patients with unstable angina pectoris. *European Heart Journal.* 1989; **10**: 437–44.

111. Saada M, Catoire P, Bonnet F *et al.* Effect of thoracic epidural anesthesia combined with general anesthesia on segmental wall motion assessed by transesophageal echocardiography. *Anesthesia and Analgesia.* 1992; **75**: 329–35.

112. Yeager MP, Glass DD, Neff RK, Brinck-Johnsen T. Epidural anesthesia and analgesia in high-risk surgical patients. *Anesthesiology.* 1987; **66**: 729–36.

*113. Beattie WS, Badner NH, Choi P. Epidural analgesia reduces postoperative myocardial infarction: a meta-analysis. *Anesthesia and Analgesia.* 2001; **93**: 853–8.

*114. Rodgers A, Walker N, Schug S *et al.* Reduction of postoperative mortality and morbidity with epidural or spinal anaesthesia: results from overview of randomised trials. *British Medical Journal.* 2000; **321**: 1493.

*115. Park WY, Thompson JS, Lee KK. Effect of epidural anesthesia and analgesia on perioperative outcome: a randomized, controlled Veterans Affairs cooperative study. *Annals of Surgery.* 2001; **234**: 560–9; discussion 569–71.

*116. Rigg JR, Jamrozik K, Myles PS *et al.* Epidural anaesthesia and analgesia and outcome of major surgery: a randomised trial. *Lancet.* 2002; **359**: 1276–82.

117. Wu CL, Caldwell MD. Effect of post-operative analgesia on patient morbidity. *Best Practice and Research. Clinical Anaesthesiology.* 2002; **16**: 549–63.

118. Ballantyne JC, Kupelnick B, McPeek B, Lau J. Does the evidence support the use of spinal and epidural anesthesia for surgery? *Journal of Clinical Anesthesia.* 2005; **17**: 382–91.

119. Wu CL, Hurley RW, Anderson GF *et al.* Effect of postoperative epidural analgesia on morbidity and mortality following surgery in medicare patients. *Regional Anesthesia and Pain Medicine.* 2004; **29**: 525–33; discussion 15–19.

120. Wu CL, Fleisher LA. Outcomes research in regional anesthesia and analgesia. *Anesthesia and Analgesia.* 2000; **91**: 1232–42.

121. Schug SA. Patient satisfaction – politically correct fashion of the nineties or a valuable measure of outcome? *Regional Anesthesia and Pain Medicine.* 2001; **26**: 193–5.

122. Wu CL, Naqibuddin M, Fleisher LA. Measurement of patient satisfaction as an outcome of regional anesthesia and analgesia: a systematic review. *Regional Anesthesia and Pain Medicine.* 2001; **26**: 196–208.

*123. Carli F, Mayo N, Klubien K *et al.* Epidural analgesia enhances functional exercise capacity and health-related quality of life after colonic surgery: results of a randomized trial. *Anesthesiology.* 2002; **97**: 540–9.

14

Transcutaneous electrical nerve stimulation (TENS) and acupuncture for acute pain

MARK I JOHNSON, STEPHEN G OXBERRY, AND KAREN H SIMPSON

KEY LEARNING POINTS

- Acute pain states tend to be treated with drugs although the burden of side effects can be considerable, especially in the elderly population.
- Nonpharmacological analgesic strategies, especially techniques involving nerve stimulation, are often simple to use, cheap and have few serious adverse effects.
- Transcutaneous electrical nerve simulation (TENS) has a role in the management of acute pain in selected patients and physiological studies provide a rationale for its use.
- Clinical experience is encouraging although systematic reviews of randomized controlled trials reveal a lack of good quality evidence. Evidence is equivocal for TENS

- for postoperative pain, labor pain, dysmenorrhea, angina, and procedural pain.
- Acupuncture has become standard therapy in many pain and palliative care services for the management of acute pain, although optimal treatment protocols remain uncertain.
- For acute dental pain and acute low back pain (LBP), results of systematic reviews of acupuncture are considered positive by some and difficult to interpret by others. For minor trauma, labor pain, and dysmenorrhea, the evidence for acupuncture is promising, but better research is needed.

INTRODUCTION

Successful acute pain management depends on a logical, stepwise approach to diagnosis and if there is a treatable cause then this should be managed. Where the cause of pain cannot be removed entirely, then treatment can be directed at modifying the disease process, reducing factors that exacerbate the pain, and managing symptoms with drugs. However, the burden of side effects is often considerable, especially in the elderly population.

Nonpharmacological analgesic strategies have many potential advantages. Techniques involving nerve stimulation have been used to provide analgesia in various forms for many centuries – suggesting that they are worthy of closer scrutiny. These strategies are often simple to use, cheap, and have few serious adverse effects. Acupuncture has become standard therapy in many pain and palliative care services in the management of acute pain. Much work remains to be done on the choice of optimal treatment for acute pain problems and more robust data are needed on efficacy. There has been increasing interest from pain practitioners in the role of TENS in the management of acute pain. The evidence from clinical experience and case reports is encouraging, and studies investigating the physiological basis of observed clinical effects provide a rationale for its use. However, more data from well-conducted clinical trials in acute pain are needed to underpin its use.

TENS

Historical context

Electric fish were used by the ancient Egyptians in 2500BC to relieve pain and, in pre-Christian times, electric ray fish were used to treat headache, gout, and arthritis.[1] In the modern era, publication of the Gate Control Theory of pain reawakened interest in electrical stimulation.[2] Percutaneous electrical nerve stimulation was shown to relieve chronic neuropathic pain and spinal cord stimulation (SCS) to relieve certain types of chronic pain.[3, 4] Originally, TENS was used to select patients for SCS, but it was realized that TENS was effective in its own right. With improvements in solid-state electronic technology in the 1970s, small battery-operated TENS devices became readily available and were tried on many types of pain with varying success.[5]

Definition of treatment

During TENS, a portable pulse generator delivers electrical currents across the intact surface of the skin via conducting pads called electrodes (**Figure 14.1**). By strict definition, TENS is any technique that delivers electricity across the intact surface of the skin to activate underlying nerves. However, healthcare professionals use the term to describe

a "standard TENS device" (**Figure 14.2**, **Table 14.1**). Minor variations in standard TENS devices between manufacturers have limited impact on the physiological effects produced.[6] Recently, a variety of TENS-like devices have flooded the market, although claims of their effectiveness are often inflated.[6] The common types of TENS are conventional TENS, acupuncture-like TENS (AL-TENS), and intense TENS (**Table 14.2**[7, 8, 9, 10, 11, 12]). Conventional TENS should be used in the first instance, and is most commonly used in practice, and AL-TENS used in specific situations (see Ref. 13 for discussion of AL-TENS).

Mechanism of action

The intention of conventional TENS is to selectively activate large diameter nonnoxious afferents (A-beta) without activating smaller diameter nociceptive fibers (A-delta and C). This has been shown to reduce activity in central nociceptive transmission cells (**Figure 14.3**)[14, 15] and is recognized by a strong but nonnoxious electrical paresthesia under the electrodes. Postulated mechanisms of TENS vary with the intensity, frequency, and amplitude of the electrical stimulus.

LOW INTENSITY STIMULATION

- Peripheral mechanisms. Antidromic activation of nerve fibers increases the latencies of compound action potentials and early somatosensory evoked potentials (SEP) in healthy subjects; this suggests that TENS could produce a "busy line-effect" on large afferent fibers.[16, 17] The conduction velocity and amplitude of A-alpha, A-beta, and A-delta components of the compound action potential recorded from isolated nerves in the cat are reduced, respectively, as the amplitude of TENS is increased.[18]

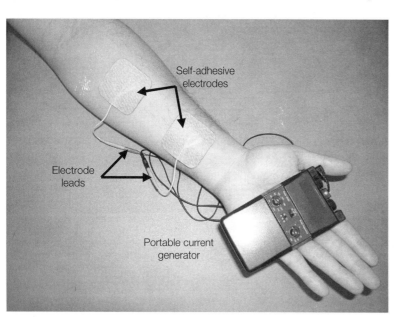

Figure 14.1 Transcutaneous electrical nerve stimulation.

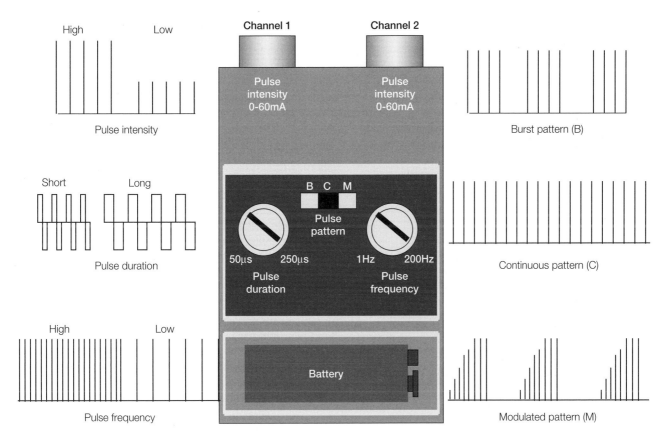

Figure 14.2 Schematic view of TENS controls on a "standard TENS device."

Table 14.1 Features of a typical TENS device.

Features	
Dimensions	6 × 5 × 2 cm (small device)
	12 × 9 × 4 cm (large device)
Weight	50–250 g
Channel (electrodes)	1(2) or 2(4)
Batteries	Usually 9 volt or rechargeable
Pulse amplitude (adjustable)	1–50 mA into a 1 kΩ load usually constant current output
Pulse waveform (usually preset)	Monophasic
	Biphasic (symmetrical or asymmetrical)
Pulse duration (usually adjustable)	50–500 μs
Pulse frequency (usually adjustable)	1–200 pulses per second
Pulse pattern (selection of preset options)	Continuous (burst, random frequency, modulated amplitude, modulated frequency, modulated pulse duration)
Additional features	Timer

Adapted from Johnson.[6, 7]

- Segmental mechanisms. Animal studies show that TENS segmentally inhibits central transmission of nociceptive information in the dorsal horn.[14, 15, 19, 20] This effect is maximal when TENS is applied to somatic receptive fields and is rapid in onset/offset.[21, 22, 23] Studies in animals also show that TENS reduces inflammation-induced sensitization of dorsal horn neurons in anesthetized rats.[14]

HIGH INTENSITY STIMULATION

- Spinal cord segmental mechanisms. In animal studies, high intensity stimulation of A-delta afferent activity produces long-term depression (LTD) of central nociceptor cells lasting up to two hours after stimulation.[24, 25] Although postulated as a mechanism underlying TENS, it is difficult to attain sufficient

Table 14.2 Common TENS techniques.

	Intention	Patient experience	Electrode location	TENS characteristics	Analgesic profile	Duration of treatment
Conventional TENS	Selective activation of large diameter nonnoxious afferents	Strong comfortable electrical paresthesia with minimal muscle activity	Dermatomal Site of pain	High frequency – 10–200 pulses per second Low amplitude – nonnoxious intensity Pulse duration – 100–200 µs Pulse pattern – continuous	Rapid onset and offset within 30 min	Continuously when in pain
AL-TENS	Indirect activation of small diameter muscle afferents through muscle twitches	Strong comfortable muscle contractions (twitches)	Myotomal over muscles or motor nerves	Low frequency bursts of pulses – 1–5 bursts of 100 pulses per second 'High' amplitude-nonnoxious intensity to generate muscle contractions Pulse duration – 100–200 µs Pulse pattern – burst	Rapid onset but delayed offset of over 1 h	~30 min per session
Intense TENS	Activation of small diameter noxious afferents	Electrical paresthesia that is uncomfortable but tolerable with post-stimulation hypoesthesia	Main nerve bundle from origin of pain	High frequency – 50–200 pulses per second High amplitude-noxious intensity Pulse duration > 500 µs Pulse pattern – continuous	Rapid onset and delayed offset over 1 h	~15 min per session

Adapted from Johnson.[6, 7]

intensity with TENS electrodes to stimulate A-delta fibers, and patients may find high intensity stimuli painful. LTD has been demonstrated in human volunteers following a low frequency, high intensity conditioning stimulus, which is delivered by punctate electrodes and initially evokes pain.[26] Longer post-stimulation analgesia may be obtained by administering conventional TENS in the first instance, followed by a brief period of intense TENS.[20]

- Extra-segmental mechanisms. Antinociceptive effects from TENS-induced A-delta activity are reduced by

spinal transection, suggesting that segmental spinal inputs activate a spinobulbar loop of ascending fibers to the brain stem and then descending pain inhibitory pathways.[27, 28, 29] Small diameter muscle afferent activity induced by AL-TENS is also believed to activate descending pain inhibitory pathways.[30]

NEUROPHARMACOLOGY OF TENS

Effects of TENS stimulation on neurotransmitter systems involved in nociception have been investigated in animal

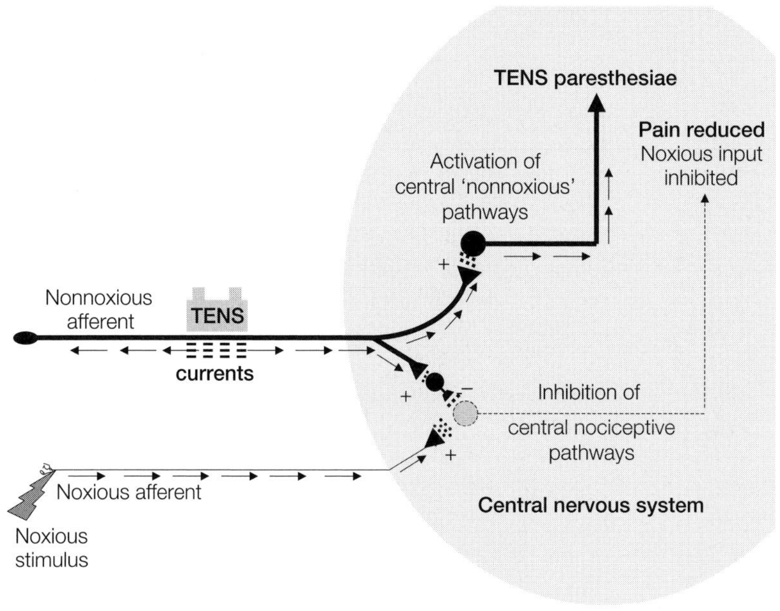

Figure 14.3 Simplified mechanism of action for conventional TENS. Current amplitude is titrated to cause selective activation of large diameter (Aβ) afferents. This leads to inhibition of ongoing central nociceptive transmission and increased activity in dorsal columns. This results in a sensation of TENS paresthesia and a reduction in pain sensation. Arrows indicate direction of nerve impulses. +, excitatory; –, inhibitory.

studies, but the contribution of these mechanisms have not been evaluated in clinical trials.

- Evidence suggests that TENS mediates opioid release throughout the central nervous system[31, 32] and that opioid tolerance may develop with repeated use of TENS.[33] Originally, it was suggested that AL-TENS, but not conventional TENS, was mediated by endorphins.[34, 35] Recent research suggests that the effects of low frequency TENS are diminished in morphine tolerant rats[36] and are mediated via mu opioid receptors. High frequency TENS effects may be mediated by delta opioid receptors, with kappa receptors having no involvement.[31, 37]
- Gamma-aminobutyric acid (GABA) may have a role in TENS[38] although LTD generated by low frequency stimulation of A delta fibers was not influenced by bicuculline, a $GABA_A$ receptor antagonist, but was abolished by D-2-amino-5-phosphonovaleric acid, an N-methyl-D-aspartate (NMDA) receptor antagonist, suggesting a role for glutamate.[20, 24] High-frequency, but not low-frequency, TENS reduces aspartate and glutamate release in the spinal cord dorsal horn.[39]
- High and low frequency TENS cause activation of spinal muscarinic receptors[40] and peripheral alpha-2A adrenergic receptors.[41] TENS effects are enhanced by systemic clonidine.[42]
- $5\text{-}HT_2$ and $5\text{-}HT_3$ receptors have been implicated in the effects of low frequency, but not high frequency TENS.[43]

Indications

TENS is used for symptomatic relief of pain. Most often it is used for nonmalignant chronic pain irrespective of origin, although any type of pain may respond to TENS.[44] Theoretically, pains that are widespread, deep seated, and/or severe are less likely to respond. TENS has been used for many acute pains including postoperative pain, labor pain, dysmenorrhea, angina, and procedural pain. TENS is inexpensive, easy to use, noninvasive, and has few adverse effects.[8, 9] TENS can be used in conjunction with other treatments and long-term use has been shown to reduce medication and physical therapy costs.[45]

GIVING A PATIENT A TRIAL OF TENS FOR THE FIRST TIME

Patients should administer TENS for themselves, following appropriate instruction by a healthcare professional. New TENS patients should be given a supervised trial to ensure that TENS does not aggravate pain, to determine whether the patient is likely to respond to TENS, and to check that the patient is competent in TENS technique. To maintain the patient's confidence, it is necessary to troubleshoot problems arising from poor response using early reviews of progress. In most circumstances, TENS is generated within, or close to, the site of pain.

Conventional TENS techniques should be used in the first instance (see **Table 14.2**). Patients should be instructed to administer TENS in 30-minute sessions for the first few times until they have familiarized themselves with the equipment. They should then be encouraged to use TENS as much as they like, and to experiment with stimulator settings, so that they achieve the most comfortable pulse frequency, pattern, and duration of stimulation. Patients should not use TENS in the shower or bath, but they can use TENS at bedtime providing the device has a timer so that it automatically switches off.

Determinants of TENS outcome

ELECTRICAL CHARACTERISTICS OF TENS

The characteristics of TENS currents include pulse amplitude, frequency, pattern, and duration. For conventional TENS, patients are instructed to alter the intensity (i.e. amplitude, 1–50 mA) of currents to achieve strong but comfortable electrical paresthesiae without muscle contraction in the area of pain. Patients are encouraged to experiment with other TENS settings to find what is comfortable and effective for them, as individual preferences vary.[7, 44, 46] Hypothetically, high frequency pulses (~10–200 pulses per second, pps) with pulse durations between 50–500 μs are optimal for differential recruitment of fiber type. However, research about the effect of TENS settings, such as pulse frequency, pattern, and duration, is conflicting, confusing, and generally of very poor quality. Studies comparing the effect of pulse frequencies (usually high ~100 pps and low ~2 pps) and pulse patterns either fail to standardize other TENS settings or are underpowered.[47]

ELECTRODE POSITIONS

Electrodes must be positioned on healthy innervated skin where sensation is intact. For most types of pain TENS electrodes are placed around the site of pain so that paresthesiae can be directed into the painful area (**Figure 14.4**). Alternatively, electrodes can be positioned along the main nerves proximal to the site of pain, at spinal segments related to the origin of pain or at contralateral dermatomes when there is diminished skin sensation or it is not possible to deliver currents within the site of pain (e.g. amputation, skin lesion). If allodynia and/or hyperalgesia exist, electrodes should be positioned along the main nerves well proximal to the site of pain in the first instance, because TENS may aggravate the pain. Dual channel devices with four electrodes should be used for pains covering large areas or for pains that change their location and quality over time. Accurate placement of electrodes can be time-consuming and is achieved by a process of informed trial and error.

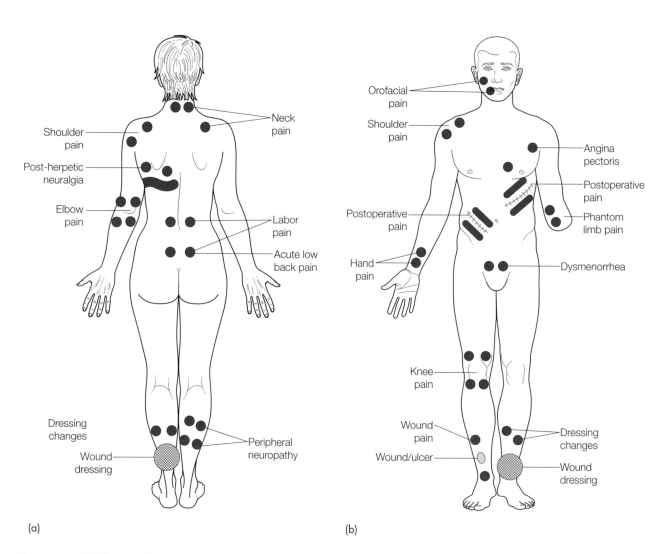

(a)

(b)

Figure 14.4 TENS electrode placement for common conditions: (a) anterior aspect; (b) posterior aspect.

TIMING AND DOSAGE

There is a lack of good quality evidence to support the belief that different TENS techniques have different analgesic profiles. Studies show that TENS analgesia is maximal when the stimulator is switched on[44, 48] and that long-term users administer TENS throughout the day to achieve adequate analgesia.[44, 45, 49] Regimens of 20 minutes of conventional TENS at daily, weekly, or monthly intervals are likely to be ineffective for persistent pains.[44, 46, 48, 50, 51, 52] Patients can leave electrodes *in situ* and use TENS intermittently providing they attend to skin care underneath the electrodes. Reports of poststimulation analgesia vary widely and are confounded by natural fluctuations in symptoms and the patient's expectation of treatment duration. Evidence suggests that TENS effects declines over time (see Table 92-1 in Ref.[11] for a summary of studies) and may be partly overcome by changing TENS settings, electrode placement, or temporarily withdrawing TENS treatment so that an objective assessment of the contribution of TENS to pain relief can be made.

CONTRAINDICATIONS AND PRECAUTIONS

TENS usually performs favorably in evaluations of risk when compared with other available treatments, including medication. There are few contraindications and adverse events with TENS, but the following should be noted:

- TENS manufacturers list cardiac pacemakers, pregnancy, and epilepsy as contraindications to its use because it may be difficult to exclude TENS as a potential cause of a problem in these patients. TENS may be used in some of these situations following consultation with the appropriate specialist, and providing electrodes are not applied locally and the patient's progress is carefully monitored.
- Electrodes should not be applied to damaged, inflamed, infected, or frail skin (e.g. open wounds, eczema). Hypoallergenic electrodes may be tolerated in patients who develop contact dermatitis.
- Pain may be aggravated in areas of allodynia and/or hyperalgesia, although this is not always the case.
- Avoid TENS over the anterior neck (as it may cause laryngeal spasm or hypotension), over the eyes, or placed in a transthoracic orientation.
- Nausea, light headedness, and fainting may occur in patients with a history of autonomic reactions to tactile allodynia, and caution or avoidance while operating hazardous equipment is suggested.
- TENS may not be acceptable to all patients due to an unpleasant sensation or aggravation of pain; fear of electrical equipment; inability to understand the instructions; inadequate manual dexterity to operate the controls.

CLINICAL EFFECTIVENESS OF TENS

Opinion is divided about the effectiveness of TENS for acute pain because clinical research findings do not always match clinical experience. Blinded controlled trials are difficult to conduct and systematic reviews (**Table 14.3**) often report that the evidence for TENS is inconclusive because of methodological shortcomings in randomized controlled trials (RCTs). Sometimes these shortcomings underestimate TENS effects because of inappropriate TENS technique which leads to inadequate dosing and inappropriate use and timing of outcome measures.[55]

Clinical trials suggest that TENS is useful for a wide range of acute pains. These include orofacial dental pain,[60, 61, 62, 63] pain caused by renal colic in emergency care,[64] acute LBP during emergency transport,[65] acute neck pain not due to whiplash,[59, 66] acute traumatic pain,[67] pain associated with multiple rib fractures,[68, 69] and acute hand infections.[70] However, a health technology assessment on TENS for acute pain in general, reported that TENS was more effective than controls in 22/39 RCTs, suggesting that available evidence was inconclusive.[53]

Acute postoperative pain

Systematic reviews have reported that in 12/20 RCTs[53] and 15/17 RCTs,[54][I] TENS did not produce significant postoperative pain relief when compared to controls. This conclusion has been challenged[55][I] as pain relief was taken as the primary outcome measure and patients had access to additional analgesic drugs, and therefore patients in both sham and TENS groups could titrate analgesic consumption to achieve similar levels of pain relief. This subsequent meta-analysis of 21 RCTs reported that TENS reduced analgesic consumption by 26.5 percent (range −6 to +51 percent) compared to sham.[55] A subgroup analysis of appropriate TENS techniques (i.e. 11 RCTs (964 patients) using a strong, subnoxious electrical stimulation at the site of pain) against inappropriate TENS technique (ten RCTs) revealed an outcome in favor of adequate TENS; this demonstrated the importance of using appropriate outcome measures and adequate TENS techniques in RCTs and meta-analyses.

Labor pain

There is widespread use of TENS as an adjunct during childbirth and many women are satisfied with its effect.[71] TENS is applied using a dual channel stimulator over thoracolumbar and sacral vertebrae. Systematic reviews have found TENS to be no better than control in 7/9 RCTs,[53] 5/8 RCTs,[56][I] and 7/10 RCTs,[57][I] although these reviews suffer from similar shortcomings to those regarding acute postoperative pain. Interestingly, two

Table 14.3 Systematic reviews of TENS for acute pain.

Reference and context	Condition	Data set (RCTs/patient numbers)	Outcome (trial vote count and/or meta-analysis)	Systematic review authors' conclusion	Our judgment	Comment
Reeve et al.[53]	Acute pain (postoperative pain, labor pain, dysmenorrhea, dental, back, cervical, orofacial)	39 RCTs 34 were 'grade 1' (suitable) quality	Pain relief and/or mobility: TENS > comparison in 22/39 RCTs and 19/34 grade 1 RCTs	Evidence inconclusive – RCT methodology weak	Evidence inconclusive	Comparisons included active and inactive interventions
Reeve et al.[53] (subgroup analysis performed post hoc by Johnson)	Postoperative pain	20 RCTs	Pain relief and/or functional outcomes (e.g. ventilation): TENS > comparison in 12/20 RCTs	Evidence inconclusive – RCT methodology weak	Evidence inconclusive	Comparisons included active and inactive interventions. Patients allowed free access to analgesic medication
Carroll et al.[54]	Postoperative pain	17 RCTs (786 patients)	Pain relief and/or analgesic sparing: TENS > comparison in 2/17 RCTs and TENS > sham in 0/14 RCTs	Evidence of no effect	Evidence inconclusive – shortcomings in RCTs/review	Comparisons included active and inactive interventions. Patients allowed free access to analgesic medication
Bjordal et al.[55]	Postoperative analgesic consumption with subgroup analysis on appropriateness of TENS intervention	21 RCTs (964 patients)	Only 11/21 RCTs met criteria for 'adequate TENS' Reducing analgesic consumption: TENS > sham (WMD = 35.5%) "Adequate" TENS > "Inadequate" TENS	Evidence of effect-analgesic sparing	Evidence of effect-analgesic sparing	Review reveals impact of applying TENS inappropriately on RCT and review outcome
Reeve et al.[53]	Labor pain	Nine were of suitable quality (grade 1)	Pain relief, analgesic sparing, and/or mobility: TENS > comparison in 3/9 'grade 1' RCTs	Evidence inconclusive – RCT methodology weak	Evidence inconclusive	Comparisons included active and inactive interventions. Patients allowed free access to analgesic medication

(Continued over)

Study	Condition	Sample	Pain relief:	Evidence of no effect	Evidence inconclusive – potential shortcomings in RCTs/review	Comments
Carroll et al.[56]	Labor pain	8 RCTs (712 women)	TENS > comparison in 1/8 RCTs TENS vs sham: Odds ratio = 1.89 (1 RCT) Analgesic sparing: TENS > comparison in 3/8 RCTs TENS > sham in 2/5RCTs: Odds ratio 0.57; NNT = 14; relative risk = 0.88 (4 RCTs)	Evidence of no effect		Comparisons included active and inactive interventions. Patients allowed free access to analgesic medication Positive outcome RCT used transcranial TENS
Carroll et al.[57] (update of Carroll et al.[56])	Labor pain	10 RCTs (877 women)	Pain relief: TENS > comparison in 0/10 RCTs Additional analgesics: TENS > comparison in 3/10 RCTs	Evidence of no effect	Evidence inconclusive – potential shortcomings in RCTs/review	Additional RCTs strengthen original conclusion
Proctor et al.[58]	Primary dysmenorrhea	7 RCTs (213 patients)	Pain relief HF TENS versus sham: Odds ratio = 7.2 (2 RCTs); WMD = 45 (1 RCT) Pain relief LF TENS versus sham: Odds ratio = 1.3 (2 RCTs); WMD = 24.1 (1 RCT)	Evidence of effect for HF TENS only	Evidence inconclusive	Comparisons used small samples
Vernon et al.[59]	Acute neck pain (not due to whiplash injury)	1 RCT (30 patients)	Pain relief: TENS > comparison group (1 RCT)	Evidence of effect	Evidence inconclusive	Comparisons used small sample

Adapted from Johnson.[7]

RCTs found that women favored TENS over sham at the end of childbirth, when women were relaxed yet still under double-blind conditions.[72, 73][II] It seems unreasonable to dismiss the use of TENS for labor pain without better quality evidence.

Dysmenorrhea

TENS on acupuncture points and over the thoracic spine has been reported to relieve symptoms in primary dysmenorrhea.[74, 75, 76] A Cochrane review of seven RCTs (213 patients) reported that high frequency, but not low frequency, TENS was superior to sham at reducing pain associated with primary dysmenorrhea.[58][I] There is clearly a role for TENS as an adjuvant to nonsteroidal anti-inflammatory drugs (NSAIDs) in severe cases[77] and as sole therapy in those women who are intolerant of NSAIDs.

Angina pectoris

TENS may be used when an angina attack occurs or is anticipated. It may benefit patients not responding satisfactorily to medical or surgical treatment, in patients waiting for surgery, and for those intolerant of nitrates.[78] Electrodes are sited on the anterior chest wall so that the stimulation paresthesia covers the area of radiation of the pain. Evidence suggests that TENS reduces the number and severity of angina episodes[78, 79][II] increases exercise capacity,[80, 81][II] improves tolerance to pacing,[79, 82, 83][II] decreases ST segment depression,[79, 81][III] improves myocardial lactate metabolism,[82, 83][II] and reduces myocardial oxygen consumption.[78, 79, 80, 81, 82, 83, 84][II]

Procedural pain

TENS has been used to manage the pain of dressing changes,[85][III] lithotripsy,[86, 87][II] distension shoulder arthrography,[88][II] cervical laser treatment,[89][II] venepuncture,[90][II], [91][III] and prior to injection of local anesthetic. Evidence for the use of TENS for electronic dental anesthesia (EDA) is equivocal, although it is well tolerated and preferred to injections by adults and children.[92, 93, 94, 95, 96][II] During dental hygiene procedures (scaling and root treatments) in patients with hypersensitive teeth, active EDA resulted in significantly reduced pain scores compared with inactive EDA.[97]

ACUPUNCTURE

Historical context

According to the principles of traditional Chinese medicine (TCM), disease alters the balance of the vital energies of life (Yin and Yang). Acupuncture is used to redress this imbalance in energy channels called meridians. It also affects internal organs such as the liver, kidney, and bladder; the TCM concept of these organs is somewhat different to the western understanding of their physiology. Acupuncture points are named and numbered to correspond to this Chinese concept of the various organs, e.g. liver or large intestine. Some knowledge of the Chinese point notation can help in the understanding of Chinese point selection. A large part of the world still practices TCM, including the use of tongue and pulse diagnosis; this can be very confusing for western health care professionals. Different styles of acupuncture and different theories about its putative method of action have added to this confusion. Chinese medicine is based on a holistic model and western medicine is founded on linear causality and reductionism. Chinese Taoism has distaste for explanatory theories and would rather observe nature's phenomena – if a needle in the hand cured toothache, that was enough – the Chinese did not care why! This basic dichotomy largely explains the rejection of acupuncture by the West until relatively recently. References to the use of acupuncture began to appear in the English medical literature about 150 years ago. Interest declined over the early part of the last century and has only reemerged in the past 40 years. The majority of western practitioners now adopt a different approach to acupuncture that involves diagnosis and treatment according to orthodox medicine.

Definition of treatment

Acupuncture involves inserting fine needles through the skin at particular points on the body. Needle placement varies with the disease being treated and the treatment philosophy being used. In western medicine it is claimed that acupuncture points are related to specific (neural) pathways and that needles stimulate underlying nerve and muscle tissue. Practitioners achieve additional (stronger) stimulation by "twirling" the inserted needle or by passing mild electrical currents through pairs of needles using a portable electrical stimulator (electroacupuncture, EA). Acupuncture can also be used in conjunction with heat, moxibustion (burning herbs on the end of the needle to heat the tip), and acupressure.

Indications

Clinical experience suggests that acupuncture reduces nociceptive and musculoskeletal pain, but may be less effective for neuropathic pain. Acupuncture can be combined with drug therapy or TENS.

Rationale and mechanism of action

At present, evidence to support the existence of meridians is weak and practitioners adopting a western approach to acupuncture usually subscribe to a neuro-physiological explanation for acupuncture analgesia. Needling during acupuncture activates high-threshold receptors and/or their afferents (A-delta and C).[98] This generates segmental and extrasegmental modulation of nociceptive inputs.[8] Activation of descending pain inhibitory pathways, release of endogenous opioids, and/or positive feedback neural circuitry in the mesolimbic region of the brain may account for the prolonged poststimulation effects often seen following needling.[99] Acupuncture also influences autonomic nervous system activity. Studies have found improvements in microcirculation, perhaps via axonal reflexes and the release of vasoactive substances such as calcitonin gene-related peptide and substance P. Acupuncture points have been shown to correspond to nerve bundles, nerves emerging from deep to superficial planes, motor points, myofascial trigger points, and perivascular plexuses.[100, 101] The relevance of these findings has been challenged.[102] However, when pain thresholds were measured before and after electroacupuncture of Hegu acupuncture points of the hand and nonacupuncture points in volunteers, the pain threshold increased significantly in all tested sites after electroacupuncture. Interestingly, the analgesic effect was predominant in those points lying along the acupuncture meridians, suggesting that point selection may be important for analgesia with acupuncture.[103]

Animal models may elucidate some mechanisms of acupuncture analgesia. For example, EA treatment in inflammatory pain models in mice prolonged paw withdrawal latency (a surrogate for analgesia) after single and multiple treatments when compared to sham acupuncture.[104] Another inflammatory pain model in mice demonstrated suppression of peripheral inflammation with EA, but not with traditional acupuncture; this suppression did not occur in the presence of peripheral (but not central) opioid inhibition.[105] The analgesic effect of EA in inflammatory pain models could be mediated via muscarinic cholinergic receptors or serotonin receptors, e.g. $5HT_{1a}$ and $5HT_3$.[106] Similarly, relief from cold allodynia in rat models of neuropathic pain appears to be mediated via the $5HT_{1a}$ and $5HT_3$ spinal serotonergic receptors, as well as via spinal alpha$_2$-adrenergic receptors.[107] EA may also affect the progress of experimental inflammatory pain by modulating the expression of NMDA receptors in primary sensory neurons.[108]

The use of functional imaging may be important in elucidating the mechanisms of acupuncture in humans.[98, 109, 110]

Principles underlying clinical techniques

Formal training is required for any healthcare professional to administer acupuncture (www.medical-acupuncture.co.uk).

POINT SELECTION AND NEEDLING TECHNIQUE

The site and depth of needle insertion is believed to be critical to the outcome and is determined by the practitioner on an individual basis. Optimal point selection is usually achieved through a process of trial and observation; the use of simple "cookbook"-type point selection is probably less effective than individualized treatments. Sometimes acupuncture points are selected according to physiological and anatomical principles, e.g. based on dermatomes, myotomes, and sclerotomes. Some practitioners select points based on principles of TCM diagnosis. Stronger stimulation techniques (e.g. EA and heat) are often used if distant acupuncture points away from the main site of pain are chosen.

NOCICEPTIVE PAIN AND MUSCULOSKELETAL PROBLEMS

Trigger points are often used for pains of musculoskeletal origin. These tender points are manipulated by inserting needles with or without injection of other substances, such as local anesthetics.[111] Dry needling is considered to be effective in the treatment of myofascial trigger point pain by deactivating the trigger point. Often these points can be relieved with superficial needling, occasionally deeper penetration of the needle is required particularly if nerve root compression is implicated.[112] It is important following successful needling that the correction of the underlying musculoskeletal abnormality is addressed.

NEUROPATHIC PAIN

Needles should be inserted into innervated regions with functioning nerves to achieve an effect; stimulation of hypo- or hyperesthetic areas should be avoided. In situations where there is definite nerve damage, needles are usually placed proximal to the damage or on the opposite side of the body. When hyperalgesia and/or mechanical allodynia are present, practitioners stimulate above and below affected segments or on contralateral "mirror" points. Needling areas of skin with compromised circulation or lymphedema should be avoided.

TIMING, DOSAGE, AND DE QI

Pain relief after acupuncture may be immediate or delayed in onset. Some patients may experience a transient increase in pain called an "aggravation." Analgesia often outlasts the period of needle insertion and may persist for several days or weeks. A cumulative increase in pain relief with subsequent acupuncture treatments usually occurs in those who respond.

A typical course of acupuncture consists of 6–12 treatments given once per week; this may be followed up by "top up" sessions thereafter; it would be unusual to treat more than twice per week. Fine disposable steel needles that are between 0.2–0.3 mm in diameter are commonly used. Needles may be placed briefly or left *in situ* for up to 30 minutes. Sensations of heaviness, soreness, dull aches, referred pain, numbness, and/or paresthesia may occur; these sensations are known as de qi. Some practitioners use intradermal needling, e.g. in fibromyalgia. Tapping the needle onto bone is sometimes practiced; this is called "periosteal pecking." Small studs may be left in the ear so that the patient can apply repeated stimulation. Some Japanese acupuncture techniques involved embedding tiny needles subcutaneously and leaving them in permanently.

The acupuncture needle sensation known as de qi has been difficult to describe and words such as dull, aching, and spreading are often used. Previously, there has been little agreement on which words are acceptable as descriptors for de qi. Recently, a group of international experts rated a scale of 25 possible sensations associated with acupuncture in two categories: those predominantly associated with de qi and those with acute pain at the site of needling.[113] Seven sensations were considered to be associated with de qi: aching, dull, heavy, numb, radiating, spreading, and tingling. Nine sensations were associated with acute pain at the site of needling: burning, hot, hurting, pinching, pricking, sharp, shocking, stinging, and tender. It is important for trials of acupuncture to have a standardized measure or description of the sensation experienced so that similar trials can be compared and that the technique of acupuncture used can be monitored for variation in needling sensation.[113]

Contraindications and precautions

Acupuncture generally has few side effects when administered by trained personnel. In an analysis of adverse events due to acupuncture in 391 patients, tiredness (8.2 percent), drowsiness (2.8 percent), and aggravation of pre-existing symptoms (2.8 percent) were the most common adverse events reported.[114] Localized problems due to needle insertion, needle withdrawal, or bleeding at needle sites were relatively uncommon in this study. More serious adverse events are rare, but can include death, pneumothorax, cardiac injury, spinal lesions, or infections.[115, 116, 117, 118, 119] Relative contraindications include bleeding disorders, anticoagulant medication, placing needles close to a pregnant uterus, and patients with a needle phobia. Care needs to be taken with those at particular risk of infection, e.g. those with diabetes, immune suppression, or endocarditis risk. Ear studs or other more permanent needles pose the most risk in this situation. EA is contraindicated for patients with cardiac pacemakers. Pain due to the needling, tiredness after therapy, and bleeding at the site of needling are common, but usually of minor consequence. Some patients may feel disorientated after treatment and driving capabilities may be compromised; they should be warned about this.

Occasionally patients may feel nauseated and/or faint after treatment.

CLINICAL EFFECTIVENESS OF ACUPUNCTURE

The methodological rigor of clinical trials on acupuncture has generally been poor. Standards for Reporting Interventions in Controlled Trials of Acupuncture (STRICTA) have been developed in line with the Consolidated Standards for Reporting Trials (CONSORT) and these should improve critical appraisal, analysis, and replication of future trials.[120, 121, 122] Common problems have been noted in acupuncture trials:[123]

- inadequate sample size;
- sample size calculations not performed;
- lack of appropriate randomization;
- difficulty in standardization of acupuncture technique;
- inherent difficulty in blinding or inappropriate sham techniques for both patient and assessor;
- appropriate control group not identified;
- inadequate follow up or description of drop-outs;
- incomplete presentation of data and statistics;
- endpoints not described;
- lack of generalizability of results;
- funding sources not appropriately acknowledged.

Important criteria in the design, implementation, and writing up of controlled clinical acupuncture trials have been described by Birch.[123]

Acute LBP

To date, all systematic reviews on the effectiveness of acupuncture for acute LBP have concluded that there is insufficient good quality evidence to make a firm judgment (**Table 14.4**). Van Tulder et al.[129][I] conducted a Cochrane Review of 11 RCTs of acupuncture for LBP, but found that no study evaluated acupuncture for acute LBP, and concluded that there was a need for more high-quality RCTs. An updated Cochrane Review including 35 RCTs for nonspecific LBP and low back myofascial pain syndrome was conducted by Furlan et al.[124][I] Three trials of acupuncture for acute LBP were included but, as these had small sample sizes and low quality methodology, it was not possible to draw conclusions about the effectiveness of acupuncture in acute LBP. Manheimer et al.[125][I] performed a meta-analysis on the effectiveness of acupuncture for acute and chronic LBP that included 33 RCTs. Acupuncture was significantly better than sham treatment or no additional treatment for short-term relief of chronic pain, but no more effective than other active therapies. Four RCTs on acute LBP were included in the review, but were excluded from the meta-analysis because

Table 14.4 Systematic reviews of acupuncture for acute pain.

Reference and context	Condition	Data set (RCTs/patient numbers)	Outcome (trial vote count and/or meta-analysis)	Systematic review authors' conclusion	Our judgment	Comment
Furlan et al.[124]	Acute LBP	Three RCTs (163 participants)	No evidence of effect (needle acupuncture versus sham 2/3 RCTs)	Unable to draw conclusion due to small sample sizes and study quality	Evidence in acute back pain inconclusive	No difference between acupuncture and analgesics in two RCTs
Manheimer et al.[125]	Acute LBP	Four RCTs (130 participants – 65 on treatment)	Pain relief; Acupuncture > sham or TENS (RCT 2/4)	Unable to draw conclusion due to small sample sizes	Evidence in acute back pain inconclusive	
Lee and Ernst[126]	Labor pain	Three RCTs (496 patients)	Reduction in analgesia required in needle acupuncture vs usual care (2/3 RCTs)	Promising role of acupuncture as an adjunct to conventional pain control in labor	More evidence required but may have an adjunctive role	Reasonable quality of available trials
Proctor et al.[58]	Dysmenorrhea	One RCT (48 patients)	Pain relief; Needle acupuncture > sham acupuncture (OR 9.5 95% CI 1.7–51.8)	Insufficient evidence to recommend	More evidence required	Acupuncture and TENS also compared in one trial
White[127]	Dysmenorrhea	Two blinded RCTs, two unblinded RCTs (133 participants)	Pain relief: Traditional acupuncture > nonpoint acupuncture or usual care (2/2 RCTs) Acupressure > sham acupressure or usual care (2/2 RCTs)	Acupuncture and acupressure may be promising	Evidence inconclusive	Unable to perform meta-analysis due to study heterogeneity
Ernst and Pittler[128]	Acute dental pain	11 RCTs (464 participants)	Pain relief: Postop needle acupuncture > sham acupuncture (5/7 RCTs). Postop electroacupuncture = conventional analgesics (1 RCT) Preop electroacupuncture = needle or sham acupuncture (2/2 RCTs)	Acupuncture can alleviate dental pain – future studies should identify optimal technique	Methodological quality of included trials quite low. Postop needle acupuncture may have promise	Unable to perform meta-analysis due to heterogeneity of study methods and outcomes

of heterogeneity; this meant that there was insufficient data to draw conclusions about the short-term effectiveness of acupuncture for acute pain.

Postoperative pain

To date, there have been no systematic reviews of acupuncture and postoperative pain. Usichenko et al.[130][II] conducted an RCT of auricular acupuncture for pain relief after total hip arthroplasty. They concluded that acupuncture could be used to reduce postoperative analgesic requirements, but that it had no effect on pain scores. The trial did not account for differences in mobilization after surgery that could be a confounding factor. In a similar study by Usichenko et al.,[131][II] 20 patients randomly received a true auricular acupuncture or sham before ambulatory knee arthroscopy; permanent press ear needles were retained in situ for one day after surgery. There was no difference in pain intensity and other parameters between the groups. As in the hip trial, postoperative analgesic requirement was reduced after acupuncture, but this is a poor surrogate for analgesic efficacy. Gilbertson et al.[132][II] demonstrated that acupuncture was superior to sham acupuncture for pain relief, analgesic consumption, and patient satisfaction following arthroscopic acromioplasty in 40 patients. However, Gupta et al.[133][II] could not demonstrate any such benefit from acupuncture when given under anaesthesia in an RCT of 42 patients undergoing knee arthroplasty. Sim et al.[134][II] showed that preoperative EA reduced intraoperative alfentanil consumption, though this effect may is nonspecific. EA had a morphine sparing effect during the early postoperative period; but this is a poor measure of analgesic efficacy as it is influenced by so many other factors. A number of trials have explored the use of EA in intra- and postoperative pain states with a variety of control groups; outcomes have been inconclusive.[134, 135, 136, 137][III] A study involving the use of acupressure following open abdominal surgery showed no benefit of acupressure versus sham acupressure on postoperative analgesic consumption or pain scores.[138][II]

Labor pain

Lee and Ernst[126][I] performed a systematic review on acupuncture for labor pain that included three RCTs. They concluded that there was insufficient evidence to make a judgment about acupuncture in this setting, although early data were promising. Acupuncture was compared with standard care in two RCTs and sham acupuncture in one RCT. Nesheim et al.[139][II] found that women receiving acupuncture requested opioids on fewer occasions than women receiving standard care; however, there was no difference in the dose of pethidine given between the groups. Ramnero et al.[140][II] demonstrated that women receiving acupuncture requested less epidural analgesia than those who did not have acupuncture; there were no differences in pain relief or requests for other analgesics between the groups. Skilnand et al.[141][II] found that pain relief after acupuncture was superior to that after sham acupuncture (superficial needling of non-acupuncture points). Nesheim and Kinge[142][V] conducted an observational study on laboring women; they concluded that those having acupuncture had reduced use of epidural analgesia compared with those not using acupuncture. An RCT by Lee et al.[143][II] compared acupressure versus sham-acupressure in 75 women; they demonstrated a significant reduction in labor pain at all time points and shortened delivery time in the true acupressure group compared with the sham group.

Dysmenorrhea

Proctor et al.[58][I] conducted a Cochrane Review on the effectiveness of TENS and acupuncture for primary dysmenorrhea. They found only one small trial of acupuncture on its own, but it was methodologically sound. The findings were promising; acupuncture was superior to sham acupuncture and no treatment control groups for pain relief. However, the reviewers concluded that there was insufficient evidence to make definitive judgments about acupuncture. White[127][I] conducted a systematic review of controlled trials of acupuncture or acupressure for gynecological conditions (four studies). He concluded that acupuncture and acupressure appeared promising for dysmenorrhea. An RCT of 216 high school students demonstrated similar analgesic efficacy between acupressure and ibuprofen in the management of primary dysmenorrhea.[144][II]

Angina pectoris

Richter et al.[145][III] demonstrated a significant reduction in angina attacks (10.6 to 6.1 with acupuncture) compared with a tablet placebo in a cross-over study of 21 patients who were using optimal medical therapy. However, a trial including 49 patients with less severe angina demonstrated no significant difference between genuine or sham acupuncture; although there was a 50 percent median reduction in angina attacks in both groups.[146][II] A similar study of 26 patients demonstrated an improvement in cardiac work as an outcome with genuine but not sham acupuncture.[147][II] There is currently little evidence to support the use of acupuncture in angina, although a cost–benefit analysis of this treatment has shown beneficial results.[148][V]

Acute dental pain

Ernst and Pittler[128][I] performed a systematic review on the effectiveness of acupuncture in treating acute dental pain. Sixteen controlled clinical trials were included and the reviewers concluded that acupuncture alleviated dental pain. Lao et al.[149][II] performed a small RCT in patients with acute dental pain following oral surgery that demonstrated a reduction in analgesic use in those treated with acupuncture versus placebo, but no effect on overall total pain scores.

Trauma

The use of acupuncture for minor acute trauma is an attractive idea, but there are few large well-designed studies. In a study of prehospital care in 38 patients with acute hip fracture, patients were randomized to receive bilateral auricular acupressure at three ear points for hip pain or bilateral auricular acupressure at sham points. Patients in the true intervention groups had less pain and anxiety and lower heart rates on arrival at the hospital than did patients in the sham control group.[150][II] Paramedics who are trained in acupressure treated 60 minor trauma patients in a double-blind randomized trial with three groups (true points, sham-points, and no acupressure). There was significantly less pain, anxiety, heart rate, and a greater satisfaction in the "true points" group.[151][II] However, both of these studies do have some fundamental methodological problems, e.g. heterogeneity, sample/group size, appropriate controls, and selection of comparators.

SUMMARY AND CONCLUSION

Acupuncture and TENS are generally well-tolerated treatments advocated by enthusiasts and dismissed by skeptics. They have the benefit of being utilized in conjunction with, and without detriment to, existing analgesic therapies. The potential analgesic benefits of both acupuncture and TENS have been compromised by previous methodological problems and poor quality trials. One of the major difficulties in designing the trials has been the identification of an appropriate control or sham control group. In some conditions the evidence of efficacy is sufficient to draw conclusions, e.g. acupuncture is effective for acute dental pain. For minor trauma, labor pain, and dysmenorrhea, the evidence for acupuncture is promising, but better research is needed. For acute LBP the results are considered positive by some and difficult to interpret by others.

TENS has a role in the management of acute pain in selected patients. Equivocal evidence exists for use of TENS in angina and procedural pain. It may have more of a role in the management of dysmenorrhea or acute labor pain. Future studies should not only be more methodologically robust, but should also utilize appropriate techniques by trained professionals.

ACKNOWLEDGMENTS

This chapter is adapted and expanded from Lynch L and Simpson KH. Transcutaneous electrical nerve stimulation and acute pain. In: Rowbotham DJ and Macintyre PE (eds). *Clinical Pain Management: Acute Pain*, 1st edn. London: Hodder Arnold, 2003: 275–84.

REFERENCES

1. Gildenberg PL. History of electrical neuromodulation for chronic pain. *Pain Medicine.* 2006; **7** (Suppl. 1): S7–13.
2. Melzack R, Wall P. Pain mechanisms: A new theory. *Science.* 1965; **150**: 971–9.
3. Wall PD, Sweet WH. Temporary abolition of pain in man. *Science.* 1967; **155**: 108–09.
4. Shealy CN, Mortimer JT, Reswick JB. Electrical inhibition of pain by stimulation of the dorsal columns: preliminary clinical report. *Anesthesia and Analgesia.* 1967; **46**: 489–91.
5. Long DM. Cutaneous afferent stimulation for relief of chronic pain. *Clinical Neurosurgery.* 1974; **21**: 257–68.
6. Johnson M. Transcutaneous electrical nerve stimulation (TENS) and TENS-like devices. Do they provide pain relief? *Pain Reviews.* 2001; **8**: 121–8.
* 7. Johnson MI. Transcutaneous electrical nerve stimulation. In: Watson T (ed.). *Electrotherapy: evidence-based Practice.* Edinburgh: Churchill Livingstone, 2008.
8. Barlas P, Lundeberg T. Transcutaneous electrical nerve stimulation and acupuncture. In: McMahon S, Koltzenburg M (eds). *Melzack and Wall's textbook of pain.* Philadelphia: Elsevier Churchill Livingstone, 2006: 583–90.
9. Walsh D. *TENS. Clinical applications and related theory,* 1st edn. New York: Churchill Livingstone, 1997.
10. Mannheimer J, Lampe G. *Clinical transcutaneous electrical nerve stimulation.* Philadelphia: FA Davis Company, 1988.
11. Sjölund B, Eriksson M, Loeser J. Transcutaneous and implanted electric stimulation of peripheral nerves. In: Bonica J (ed.). *The management of pain.* Philadelphia: Lea & Febiger, 1990: 1852–61.
12. Woolf C, Thompson J. Segmental afferent fibre-induced analgesia: transcutaneous electrical nerve stimulation (TENS) and vibration. In: Wall P, Melzack R (eds). *Textbook of pain.* Edinburgh: Churchill Livingstone, 1994: 1191–208.
13. Johnson M. The analgesic effects and clinical use of acupuncture-like TENS (AL-TENS). *Physical Therapy Reviews.* 1998; **3**: 73–93.
14. Ma YT, Sluka KA. Reduction in inflammation-induced sensitization of dorsal horn neurons by transcutaneous electrical nerve stimulation in anesthetized rats. *Experimental Brain Research.* 2001; **137**: 94–102.
15. Garrison DW, Foreman RD. Effects of transcutaneous electrical nerve stimulation (TENS) on spontaneous and

noxiously evoked dorsal horn cell activity in cats with transected spinal cords. *Neuroscience Letters.* 1996; **216**: 125–8.

16. Walsh DM, Lowe AS, McCormack K *et al.* Transcutaneous electrical nerve stimulation: effect on peripheral nerve conduction, mechanical pain threshold, and tactile threshold in humans. *Archives of Physical Medicine and Rehabilitation.* 1998; **79**: 1051–8.

17. Nardone A, Schieppati M. Influences of transcutaneous electrical stimulation of cutaneous and mixed nerves on subcortical and cortical somatosensory evoked potentials. *Electroencephalography and Clinical Neurophysiology.* 1989; **74**: 24–35.

18. Ignelzi RJ, Nyquist JK. Direct effect of electrical stimulation on peripheral nerve evoked activity: implications in pain relief. *Journal of Neurosurgery.* 1976; **45**: 159–65.

19. Garrison DW, Foreman RD. Decreased activity of spontaneous and noxiously evoked dorsal horn cells during transcutaneous electrical nerve stimulation (TENS). *Pain.* 1994; **58**: 309–15.

20. Sandkuhler J. Long-lasting analgesia following TENS and acupuncture: Spinal mechanisms beyond gate control. In: Devor M, Rowbotham MC, Wiesenfeld-Hallin Z (eds). *The 9th World Congress on Pain: Progress in Pain Research and Management.* Vol. 16. Austria: IASP Press, 2000: 359–69.

21. Woolf CJ, Mitchell D, Barrett GD. Antinociceptive effect of peripheral segmental electrical stimulation in the rat. *Pain.* 1980; **8**: 237–52.

22. Woolf C, Thompson S, King A. Prolonged primary afferent induced alterations in dorsal horn neurones, an intracellular analysis in vivo and in vitro. *Journal of Physiology.* 1988; **83**: 255–66.

23. Sjolund BH. Peripheral nerve stimulation suppression of C-fiber-evoked flexion reflex in rats. Part 1: Parameters of continuous stimulation. *Journal of Neurosurgery.* 1985; **63**: 612–6.

24. Sandkuhler J, Chen JG, Cheng G, Randic M. Low-frequency stimulation of afferent A delta-fibers induces long-term depression at primary afferent synapses with substantia gelatinosa neurons in the rat. *Journal of Neuroscience.* 1997; **17**: 6483–91.

25. Macefield G, Burke D. Long-lasting depression of central synaptic transmission following prolonged high-frequency stimulation of cutaneous afferents: a mechanism for post-vibratory hypaesthesia. *Electroencephalography and Clinical Neurophysiology.* 1991; **78**: 150–8.

26. Klein T, Magerl W, Hopf HC *et al.* Perceptual correlates of nociceptive long-term potentiation and long-term depression in humans. *Journal of Neuroscience.* 2004; **24**: 964–71.

27. Chung JM. Antinociceptive effects of peripheral nerve stimulation. *Progress in Clinical and Biological Research.* 1985; **176**: 147–61.

28. Chung JM, Fang ZR, Hori Y *et al.* Prolonged inhibition of primate spinothalamic tract cells by peripheral nerve stimulation. *Pain.* 1984; **19**: 259–75.

29. Chung JM, Lee KH, Hori Y *et al.* Factors influencing peripheral nerve stimulation produced inhibition of primate spinothalamic tract cells. *Pain.* 1984; **19**: 277–93.

30. Sjolund B. Peripheral nerve stimulation suppression of C-fiber-evoked flexion reflex in rats. Part 2: Parameters of low-rate train stimulation of skin and muscle afferent nerves. *Journal of Neurosurgery.* 1988; **68**: 279–83.

31. Kalra A, Urban MO, Sluka KA. Blockade of opioid receptors in rostral ventral medulla prevents antihyperalgesia produced by transcutaneous electrical nerve stimulation (TENS). *Journal of Pharmacology and Experimental Therapeutics.* 2001; **298**: 257–63.

32. Ainsworth L, Budelier K, Clinesmith M *et al.* Transcutaneous electrical nerve stimulation (TENS) reduces chronic hyperalgesia induced by muscle inflammation. *Pain.* 2006; **120**: 182–7.

33. Chandran P, Sluka KA. Development of opioid tolerance with repeated transcutaneous electrical nerve stimulation administration. *Pain.* 2003; **102**: 195–201.

34. Sjolund B, Terenius L, Eriksson M. Increased cerebrospinal fluid levels of endorphins after electro-acupuncture. *Acta Physiologica Scandinavica.* 1977; **100**: 382–4.

35. Eriksson MB, Sjolund BH, Nielzen S. Long term results of peripheral conditioning stimulation as an analgesic measure in chronic pain. *Pain.* 1979; **6**: 335–47.

36. Sluka KA, Judge MA, McColley MM *et al.* Low frequency TENS is less effective than high frequency TENS at reducing inflammation-induced hyperalgesia in morphine-tolerant rats. *Eur J Pain.* 2000; **4**: 185–93.

37. Sluka KA, Deacon M, Stibal A *et al.* Spinal blockade of opioid receptors prevents the analgesia produced by TENS in arthritic rats. *Journal of Pharmacology and Experimental Therapeutics.* 1999; **289**: 840–6.

38. Duggan AW, Foong FW. Bicuculline and spinal inhibition produced by dorsal column stimulation in the cat. *Pain.* 1985; **22**: 249–59.

39. Sluka KA, Vance CG, Lisi TL. High-frequency, but not low-frequency, transcutaneous electrical nerve stimulation reduces aspartate and glutamate release in the spinal cord dorsal horn. *Journal of Neurochemistry.* 2005; **95**: 1794–801.

40. Radhakrishnan R, Sluka KA. Spinal muscarinic receptors are activated during low or high frequency TENS-induced antihyperalgesia in rats. *Neuropharmacology.* 2003; **45**: 1111–9.

41. King EW, Audette K, Athman GA *et al.* Transcutaneous electrical nerve stimulation activates peripherally located alpha-2A adrenergic receptors. *Pain.* 2005; **115**: 364–73.

42. Sluka KA, Chandran P. Enhanced reduction in hyperalgesia by combined administration of clonidine and TENS. *Pain.* 2002; **100**: 183–90.

43. Radhakrishnan R, King EW, Dickman JK *et al.* Spinal 5-HT(2) and 5-HT(3) receptors mediate low, but not high, frequency TENS-induced antihyperalgesia in rats. *Pain.* 2003; **105**: 205–13.

44. Johnson MI, Ashton CH, Thompson JW. An in-depth study of long-term users of transcutaneous electrical nerve

stimulation (TENS). Implications for clinical use of TENS. *Pain.* 1991; **44**: 221–9.

45. Chabal C, Fishbain DA, Weaver M, Heine LW. Long-term transcutaneous electrical nerve stimulation (TENS) use: impact on medication utilization and physical therapy costs. *Clinical Journal of Pain.* 1998; **14**: 66–73.

46. Johnson MI, Ashton CH, Thompson JW. The consistency of pulse frequencies and pulse patterns of transcutaneous electrical nerve stimulation (TENS) used by chronic pain patients. *Pain.* 1991; **44**: 231–4.

47. Chen C, Tabasam G, Johnson M. Does the pulse frequency of transcutaneous electrical nerve stimulation (TENS) influence hypoalgesia? A systematic review of studies using experimental pain and healthy human participants. *Physiotherapy.* 2008; **94**: 11–20.

48. Johnson MI, Tabasam G. An investigation into the analgesic effects of interferential currents and transcutaneous electrical nerve stimulation on experimentally induced ischemic pain in otherwise pain-free volunteers. *Physical Therapy.* 2003; **83**: 208–23.

49. Nash T, Williams J, Machin D. TENS: does the type of stimulus really matter? *The Pain Clinic.* 1990; **3**: 161–8.

50. Johnson MI, Ashton CH, Bousfield DR, Thompson JW. Analgesic effects of different pulse patterns of transcutaneous electrical nerve stimulation on cold-induced pain in normal subjects. *Journal of Psychosomatic Research.* 1991; **35**: 313–21.

51. Johnson MI, Ashton CH, Bousfield DR, Thompson JW. Analgesic effects of different frequencies of transcutaneous electrical nerve stimulation on cold-induced pain in normal subjects. *Pain.* 1989; **39**: 231–6.

52. Johnson M, Tabasam G. A double blind placebo controlled investigation into the analgesic effects of interferential currents (IFC) and transcutaneous electrical nerve stimulation (TENS) on cold induced pain in healthy subjects. *Physiotherapy Theory and Practice.* 1999; **15**: 217–33.

53. Reeve J, Menon D, Corabian P. Transcutaneous electrical nerve stimulation (TENS): a technology assessment. *International Journal of Technology Assessment in Health Care.* 1996; **12**: 299–324.

* 54. Carroll D, Tramer M, McQuay H *et al.* Randomization is important in studies with pain outcomes: systematic review of transcutaneous electrical nerve stimulation in acute postoperative pain. *British Journal of Anaesthesia.* 1996; **77**: 798–803.

* 55. Bjordal JM, Johnson MI, Ljunggreen AE. Transcutaneous electrical nerve stimulation (TENS) can reduce postoperative analgesic consumption. A meta-analysis with assessment of optimal treatment parameters for postoperative pain. *European Journal of Pain.* 2003; **7**: 181–8.

56. Carroll D, Tramer M, McQuay H *et al.* Transcutaneous electrical nerve stimulation in labour pain: a systematic review. *British Journal of Obstetrics and Gynaecology.* 1997; **104**: 169–75.

* 57. Carroll D, Moore A, Tramer M, McQuay H. Transcutaneous electrical nerve stimulation does not relieve in labour pain: updated systematic review. *Contemporary Reviews in Obstetrics and Gynecology.* 1997; September: 195–205.

* 58. Proctor ML, Smith CA, Farquhar CM, Stones RW. Transcutaneous electrical nerve stimulation and acupuncture for primary dysmenorrhoea. *Cochrane Database of Systematic Reviews.* 2003; **CD002123**.

59. Vernon HT, Humphreys BK, Hagino CA. A systematic review of conservative treatments for acute neck pain not due to whiplash. *Journal of Manipulative and Physiological Therapeutics.* 2005; **28**: 443–8.

60. Hansson P, Ekblom A. Transcutaneous electrical nerve stimulation (TENS) as compared to placebo TENS for the relief of acute oro-facial pain. *Pain.* 1983; **15**: 157–65.

61. Hansson P, Ekblom A. Afferent stimulation induced pain relief in acute oro-facial pain and its failure to induce sufficient pain reduction in dental and oral surgery. *Pain.* 1984; **20**: 273–8.

62. Hansson P, Ekblom A, Thomsson M, Fjellner B. Influence of naloxone on relief of acute oro-facial pain by transcutaneous electrical nerve stimulation (TENS) or vibration. *Pain.* 1986; **24**: 323–9.

63. Ekblom A, Hansson P. Extrasegmental transcutaneous electrical nerve stimulation and mechanical vibratory stimulation as compared to placebo for the relief of acute oro-facial pain. *Pain.* 1985; **23**: 223–9.

64. Mora B, Giorni E, Dobrovits M *et al.* Transcutaneous electrical nerve stimulation: an effective treatment for pain caused by renal colic in emergency care. *Journal of Urology.* 2006; **175**: 1737–41; discussion 41.

65. Bertalanffy A, Kober A, Bertalanffy P *et al.* Transcutaneous electrical nerve stimulation reduces acute low back pain during emergency transport. *Academic Emergency Medicine.* 2005; **12**: 607–11.

66. Nordemar R, Thorner C. Treatment of acute cervical pain – a comparative group study. *Pain.* 1981; **10**: 93–101.

67. Ordog GJ. Transcutaneous electrical nerve stimulation versus oral analgesic: a randomized double-blind controlled study in acute traumatic pain. *American Journal of Emergency Medicine.* 1987; **5**: 6–10.

68. Sloan J, Muwanga C, Waters E *et al.* Multiple rib fractures: transcutaneous nerve stimulation versus conventional analgesia. *Journal of Trauma.* 1986; **26**: 1120–2.

69. Myers RA, Woolf CJ, Mitchell D. Management of acute traumatic pain by peripheral transcutaneous electrical stimulation. *South African Medical Journal.* 1977; **52**: 309–12.

70. Quinton DN, Sloan JP, Theakstone J. Transcutaneous electrical nerve stimulation in acute hand infections. *Journal of Hand Surgery. British Volume.* 1987; **12**: 267–8.

71. Johnson MI. Transcutaneous electrical nerve stimulation (TENS) in the management of labour pain: the experience of over ten thousand women. *British Journal of Midwifery.* 1997; **5**: 400–05.

72. Harrison R, Woods T, Shore M *et al.* Pain relief in labour using transcutaneous electrical nerve stimulation (TENS).

A TENS/TENS placebo controlled study in two parity groups. *British Journal of Obstetrics and Gynaecology.* 1986; **93**: 739–46.

73. Thomas IL, Tyle V, Webster J, Neilson A. An evaluation of transcutaneous electrical nerve stimulation for pain relief in labour. *Australian and New Zealand Journal of Obstetrics and Gynaecology.* 1988; **28**: 182–9.

74. Milsom I, Hedner N, Mannheimer C. A comparative study of the effect of high-intensity transcutaneous nerve stimulation and oral naproxen on intrauterine pressure and menstrual pain in patients with primary dysmenorrhea. *American Journal of Obstetrics and Gynecology.* 1994; **170**: 123–9.

75. Neighbors L, Clelland J, Jackson J *et al.* Transcutaneous electrical nerve stimulation for pain relief in primary dysmenorrhea. *Clinical Journal of Pain.* 1987; **3**: 17–22.

76. Kaplan B, Peled Y, Pardo J *et al.* Transcutaneous electrical nerve stimulation (TENS) as a relief for dysmenorrhea. *Clinical and Experimental Obstetrics and Gynecology.* 1994; **21**: 87–90.

77. Dawood MY, Ramos J. Transcutaneous electrical nerve stimulation (TENS) for the treatment of primary dysmenorrhea: a randomized crossover comparison with placebo TENS and ibuprofen. *Obstetrics and Gynecology.* 1990; **75**: 656–60.

78. Börjesson M, Eriksson P, Dellborg M *et al.* Transcutaneous electrical nerve stimulation in unstable angina pectoris. *Coronary Artery Disease.* 1997; **8**: 543–50.

79. Mannheimer C, Carlsson CA, Emanuelsson H *et al.* The effects of transcutaneous electrical nerve stimulation in patients with severe angina pectoris. *Circulation.* 1985; **71**: 308–16.

80. Murray S, Collins PD, James MA. An investigation into the 'carry over' effect of neurostimulation in the treatment of angina pectoris. *International Journal of Clinical Practice.* 2004; **58**: 669–74.

81. Mannheimer C, Carlsson C, Ericson K *et al.* Transcutaneous electrical nerve stimulation in severe angina pectoris. *European Heart Journal.* 1982; **3**: 297–302.

82. Mannheimer C, Emanuelsson H, Waagstein F. The effect of transcutaneous electrical nerve stimulation (TENS) on catecholamine metabolism during pacing-induced angina pectoris and the influence of naloxone. *Pain.* 1990; **41**: 27–34.

83. Mannheimer C, Emanuelsson H, Waagstein F, Wilhelmsson C. Influence of naloxone on the effects of high frequency transcutaneous electrical nerve stimulation in angina pectoris induced by atrial pacing. *British Heart Journal.* 1989; **62**: 36–42.

84. Jessurun GA, Tio RA, De Jongste MJ *et al.* Coronary blood flow dynamics during transcutaneous electrical nerve stimulation for stable angina pectoris associated with severe narrowing of one major coronary artery. *American Journal of Cardiology.* 1998; **82**: 921–6.

85. Merkel SI, Gutstein HB, Malviya S. Use of transcutaneous electrical nerve stimulation in a young child with pain from open perineal lesions. *Journal of Pain and Symptom Management.* 1999; **18**: 376–81.

86. Rawat B, Genz A, Fache JS *et al.* Effectiveness of transcutaneous electrical nerve stimulation (TENS) for analgesia during biliary lithotripsy. *Investigative Radiology.* 1991; **26**: 866–9.

87. Kararmaz A, Kaya S, Karaman H, Turhanoglu S. Effect of the frequency of transcutaneous electrical nerve stimulation on analgesia during extracorporeal shock wave lithotripsy. *Urological Research.* 2004; **32**: 411–5.

88. Morgan B, Jones AR, Mulcahy KA *et al.* Transcutaneous electric nerve stimulation (TENS) during distension shoulder arthrography: a controlled trial. *Pain.* 1996; **64**: 265–7.

89. Crompton AC, Johnson N, Dudek U *et al.* Is transcutaneous electrical nerve stimulation of any value during cervical laser treatment? *British Journal of Obstetrics and Gynaecology.* 1992; **99**: 492–4.

90. Coyne P, MacMurren M, Izzo T, Kramer T. Transcutaneous electrical nerve stimulator for procedural pain associated with intravenous needlesticks. *Journal of Intravenous Nursing.* 1995; **18**: 263–70.

91. Lander J, Fowler-Kerry S. TENS for children's procedural pain. *Pain.* 1993; **52**: 209–16.

92. Meechan J, Winter R. A comparison of topical anaesthesia and electronic nerve stimulation for reducing the pain of intra-oral injections. *British Dental Journal.* 1996; **181**: 333–5.

93. Meechan JG, Gowans AJ, Welbury RR. The use of patient-controlled transcutaneous electronic nerve stimulation (TENS) to decrease the discomfort of regional anaesthesia in dentistry: a randomised controlled clinical trial. *Journal of Dentistry.* 1998; **26**: 417–20.

94. Schafer E, Finkensiep H, Kaup M. Effect of transcutaneous electrical nerve stimulation on pain perception threshold of human teeth: a double-blind, placebo-controlled study. *Clinical Oral Investigations.* 2000; **4**: 81–6.

95. Modaresi A, Lindsay S, Gould A, Smith P. A partial double-blind, placebo-controlled study of electronic dental anaesthesia in children. *International Journal of Paediatric Dentistry.* 1996; **6**: 245–51.

96. Cho SY, Drummond BK, Anderson MH, Williams S. Effectiveness of electronic dental anesthesia for restorative care in children. *Pediatric Dentistry.* 1998; **20**: 105–11.

97. Bruzek D, Geistfeld N. Clinical study to evaluate the use of electronic anesthesia during dental hygiene procedures. *Northwest Dentistry.* 1996; **75**: 21–6.

98. Leung A, Khadivi B, Duann JR *et al.* The effect of Ting point (tendinomuscular meridians) electroacupuncture on thermal pain: a model for studying the neuronal mechanism of acupuncture analgesia. *Journal of Alternive and Complementary Medicine.* 2005; **11**: 653–61.

99. Han JS. Recent progress in the study of acupuncture mechanisms. *Zhen Ci Yan Jiu.* 1988; **13**: 36–42, 35.

100. Kao MJ, Hsieh YL, Kuo FJ, Hong CZ. Electrophysiological assessment of acupuncture points. *American Journal of Physical Medicine and Rehabilitation*. 2006; **85**: 443–8.

101. Melzack R, Stillwell DM, Fox EJ. Trigger points and acupuncture points for pain: correlations and implications. *Pain*. 1977; **3**: 3–23.

102. Birch S. Trigger point–acupuncture point correlations revisited. *Journal of Alternative and Complementary Medicine*. 2003; **9**: 91–103.

103. Farber PL, Tachibana A, Campiglia HM. Increased pain threshold following electroacupuncture: analgesia is induced mainly in meridian acupuncture points. *Acupuncture and Electro-therapeutics Research*. 1997; **22**: 109–17.

104. Li WM, Cui KM, Li N et al. Analgesic effect of electroacupuncture on complete Freund's adjuvant-induced inflammatory pain in mice: a model of antipain treatment by acupuncture in mice. *Japanese Journal of Physiology*. 2005; **55**: 339–44.

105. Kim HW, Roh DH, Yoon SY et al. The anti-inflammatory effects of low- and high-frequency electroacupuncture are mediated by peripheral opioids in a mouse air pouch inflammation model. *Journal of Alternative and Complementary Medicine*. 2006; **12**: 39–44.

106. Baek YH, Choi DY, Yang HI, Park DS. Analgesic effect of electroacupuncture on inflammatory pain in the rat model of collagen-induced arthritis: mediation by cholinergic and serotonergic receptors. *Brain Research*. 2005; **1057**: 181–5.

107. Kim SK, Park JH, Bae SJ et al. Effects of electroacupuncture on cold allodynia in a rat model of neuropathic pain: mediation by spinal adrenergic and serotonergic receptors. *Experimental Neurology*. 2005; **195**: 430–6.

108. Wang L, Zhang Y, Dai J et al. Electroacupuncture (EA) modulates the expression of NMDA receptors in primary sensory neurons in relation to hyperalgesia in rats. *Brain Research*. 2006; **1120**: 46–53.

109. Biella G, Sotgiu ML, Pellegata G et al. Acupuncture produces central activations in pain regions. *Neuroimage*. 2001; **14**: 60–6.

110. Chen AC, Liu FJ, Wang L, Arendt-Nielsen L. Mode and site of acupuncture modulation in the human brain: 3D (124-ch) EEG power spectrum mapping and source imaging. *Neuroimage*. 2006; **29**: 1080–91.

111. Baldry P. Superficial versus deep dry needling. *Acupuncture in Medicine*. 2002; **20**: 78–81.

112. Baldry P. Management of myofascial trigger point pain. *Acupuncture in Medicine*. 2002; **20**: 2–10.

113. MacPherson H, Asghar A. Acupuncture needle sensations associated with De Qi: a classification based on experts' ratings. *Journal of Alternative and Complementary Medicine*. 2006; **12**: 633–7.

114. Yamashita H, Tsukayama H, Hori N et al. Incidence of adverse reactions associated with acupuncture. *Journal of Alternative and Complementary Medicine*. 2000; **6**: 345–50.

115. Yamashita H, Tsukayama H, White AR et al. Systematic review of adverse events following acupuncture: the Japanese literature. *Complementary Therapies in Medicine*. 2001; **9**: 98–104.

*116. Ernst E, White AR. Prospective studies of the safety of acupuncture: a systematic review. *American Journal of Medicine*. 2001; **110**: 481–5.

117. Ernst G, Strzyz H, Hagmeister H. Incidence of adverse effects during acupuncture therapy – a multicentre survey. *Complementary Therapies in Medicine*. 2003; **11**: 93–7.

118. Ernst E, White A. Life-threatening adverse reactions after acupuncture? A systematic review. *Pain*. 1997; **71**: 123–6.

119. Ernst E. Acupuncture – a critical analysis. *Journal of Internal Medicine*. 2006; **259**: 125–37.

120. MacPherson H, White A, Cummings M et al. Standards for Reporting Interventions in Controlled Trials of Acupuncture: the STRICTA recommendations. *Journal of Alternative and Complementary Medicine*. 2002; **8**: 85–9.

121. MacPherson H, White A, Cummings M et al. Standards for reporting interventions in controlled trials of acupuncture: the STRICTA recommendations. *Complementary Therapies in Medicine*. 2001; **9**: 246–9.

*122. MacPherson H, White A, Cummings M et al. Standards for reporting interventions in controlled trials of acupuncture: The STRICTA recommendations. STandards for Reporting Interventions in Controlled Trails of Acupuncture. *Acupuncture in Medicine*. 2002; **20**: 22–5.

123. Birch S. Clinical research on acupuncture. Part 2. Controlled clinical trials, an overview of their methods. *Journal of Alternative and Complementary Medicine*. 2004; **10**: 481–98.

*124. Furlan AD, van Tulder M, Cherkin D et al. Acupuncture and dry-needling for low back pain: an updated systematic review within the framework of the Cochrane collaboration. *Spine*. 2005; **30**: 944–63.

*125. Manheimer E, White A, Berman B et al. Meta-analysis: acupuncture for low back pain. *Annals of Internal Medicine*. 2005; **142**: 651–63.

*126. Lee H, Ernst E. Acupuncture for labor pain management: A systematic review. *American Journal of Obstetric Gynecology*. 2004; **191**: 1573–9.

127. White AR. A review of controlled trials of acupuncture for women's reproductive health care. *Journal of Family Planning and Reproductive Health Care*. 2003; **29**: 233–6.

*128. Ernst E, Pittler MH. The effectiveness of acupuncture in treating acute dental pain: a systematic review. *British Dental Journal*. 1998; **184**: 443–7.

129. van Tulder MW, Cherkin DC, Berman B et al. The effectiveness of acupuncture in the management of acute and chronic low back pain. A systematic review within the framework of the Cochrane Collaboration Back Review Group. *Spine*. 1999; **24**: 1113–23.

130. Usichenko TI, Dinse M, Hermsen M et al. Auricular acupuncture for pain relief after total hip arthroplasty – a randomized controlled study. *Pain*. 2005; **114**: 320–7.

131. Usichenko TI, Hermsen M, Witstruck T *et al.* Auricular acupuncture for pain relief after ambulatory knee arthroscopy – A pilot study. *Evidence-based Complementary and Alternative Medicine.* 2005; **2**: 185–9.

132. Gilbertson B, Wenner K, Russell LC. Acupuncture and arthroscopic acromioplasty. *Journal of Orthopaedic Research.* 2003; **21**: 752–8.

133. Gupta S, Francis JD, Tillu AB *et al.* The effect of pre-emptive acupuncture treatment on analgesic requirements after day-case knee arthroscopy. *Anaesthesia.* 1999; **54**: 1204–7.

134. Sim CK, Xu PC, Pua HL *et al.* Effects of electroacupuncture on intraoperative and postoperative analgesic requirement. *Acupuncture in Medicine.* 2002; **20**: 56–65.

135. Christensen PA, Noreng M, Andersen PE, Nielsen JW. Electroacupuncture and postoperative pain. *British Journal of Anaesthesia.* 1989; **62**: 258–62.

136. Wang B, Tang J, White PF *et al.* Effect of the intensity of transcutaneous acupoint electrical stimulation on the postoperative analgesic requirement. *Anesthesia and Analgesia.* 1997; **85**: 406–13.

137. Christensen PA, Rotne M, Vedelsdal R *et al.* Electroacupuncture in anaesthesia for hysterectomy. *British Journal of Anaesthesia.* 1993; **71**: 835–8.

138. Sakurai M, Suleman MI, Morioka N *et al.* Minute sphere acupressure does not reduce postoperative pain or morphine consumption. *Anesthesia and Analgesia.* 2003; **96**: 493–7.

139. Nesheim BI, Kinge R, Berg B *et al.* Acupuncture during labor can reduce the use of meperidine: a controlled clinical study. *Clinical Journal of Pain.* 2003; **19**: 187–91.

140. Ramnero A, Hanson U, Kihlgren M. Acupuncture treatment during labour – a randomised controlled trial. *BJOG.* 2002; **109**: 637–44.

141. Skilnand E, Fossen D, Heiberg E. Acupuncture in the management of pain in labor. *Acta Obstetricia et Gynecologica Scandinavica.* 2002; **81**: 943–8.

142. Nesheim BI, Kinge R. Performance of acupuncture as labor analgesia in the clinical setting. *Acta Obstetricia et Gynecologica Scandinavica.* 2006; **85**: 441–3.

143. Lee MK, Chang SB, Kang DH. Effects of SP6 acupressure on labor pain and length of delivery time in women during labor. *Journal of Alternative and Complementary Medicine.* 2004; **10**: 959–65.

144. Pouresmail Z, Ibrahimzadeh R. Effects of acupressure and ibuprofen on the severity of primary dysmenorrhea. *Journal of Traditional Chinese Medicine.* 2002; **22**: 205–10.

145. Richter A, Herlitz J, Hjalmarson A. Effect of acupuncture in patients with angina pectoris. *European Heart Journal.* 1991; **12**: 175–8.

146. Ballegaard S, Pedersen F, Pietersen A *et al.* Effects of acupuncture in moderate, stable angina pectoris: a controlled study. *Journal of Internal Medicine.* 1990; **227**: 25–30.

147. Ballegaard S, Jensen G, Pedersen F, Nissen VH. Acupuncture in severe, stable angina pectoris: a randomized trial. *Acta Medica Scandinavica.* 1986; **220**: 307–13.

148. Ballegaard S, Johannessen A, Karpatschof B, Nyboe J. Addition of acupuncture and self-care education in the treatment of patients with severe angina pectoris may be cost beneficial: an open, prospective study. *Journal of Alternative and Complementary Medicine.* 1999; **5**: 405–13.

149. Lao L, Bergman S, Hamilton GR *et al.* Evaluation of acupuncture for pain control after oral surgery: a placebo-controlled trial. *Archives of Otolaryngology – Head and Neck Surgery.* 1999; **125**: 567–72.

150. Barker R, Kober A, Hoerauf K *et al.* Out-of-hospital auricular acupressure in elder patients with hip fracture: a randomized double-blinded trial. *Academic Emergency Medicine.* 2006; **13**: 19–23.

151. Kober A, Scheck T, Greher M *et al.* Prehospital analgesia with acupressure in victims of minor trauma: a prospective, randomized, double-blinded trial. *Anesthesia and Analgesia.* 2002; **95**: 723–7.

15

Psychological therapies – adults

H CLARE DANIEL

KEY LEARNING POINTS

- Psychological factors play an important role in all pain processing. These factors include mood, fear-avoidance, catastrophizing, perceived threat, beliefs and meanings, expectations and previous pain experience.
- Although medical interventions reduce acute pain intensity, they do not provide the complete solution.
- Using a broad definition, psychological interventions include the provision of information, education of healthcare providers, attentional techniques, relaxation, hypnosis, and cognitive-behavioral therapy (CBT).

- Evidence for the majority of these interventions for postoperative pain is mixed. The evidence for cognitive behavioral interventions for people with acute pain who are at risk of developing long-term problems is promising.
- Further research is required to help clinicians ascertain which interventions are appropriate for which population and at what time point.

INTRODUCTION

There is increasing emphasis on the need to reduce the occurrence and intensity of acute pain because:

- unrelieved acute pain can result in psychological and physiological effects;[1]
- acute pain is a factor in the development of persistent pain.[2]

For many years, the medical model of pain assumed a direct relationship between physical pathology and pain and neglected the influence of psychological factors. Treatments often continue to follow this assumption, seeking to identify the cause and eliminate pain by improving pathology or blocking pain pathways. As conventional medical treatments do not eradicate all acute pain, the focus needs to shift to multimodal rehabilitation techniques, which include psychological interventions. This chapter will focus on psychological interventions for two prevalent types of acute pain:

1. patients with postoperative pain;
2. patients with acute pain who are at risk of developing persistent pain and chronic problems.

The literature's interpretation of what constitutes a psychological intervention for acute pain ranges from the provision of basic information to complex cognitive-behavioral interventions provided by a range of healthcare providers (HCPs) with varying levels of training. For the purpose of this chapter, a broad range of interventions will be discussed and will include education for HCPs.

BACKGROUND

Moderate to severe pain continues to be a problem in medical and surgical hospital settings.[3, 4] It is thought to be experienced by 50–80 percent of people following surgery and trauma,[5, 6] and between 0.05 and 1.5 percent of people at one year postsurgery.[7] These statistics need to be improved because inadequate postoperative pain management may

- decrease patient satisfaction with the perioperative experience;[8]
- decrease psychological and physical quality of life in the immediate postoperative period;[4, 9]
- increase the risk of the development of chronic postoperative pain, defined as pain of at least two months duration following surgery,[10, 11] which accounts for up to 25 percent of referrals to chronic pain services.[12, 13, 14]

When considering the need to reduce the prevalence of postoperative pain, the current healthcare climate and the implications on resources cannot be ignored. For example, the drive to decrease the length of hospital stay and increase the numbers of day-cases means that the relief of acute pain is essential if targets are to be met and primary care and hospital visits following discharge are to be minimized.[15, 16, 17]

With regards to acute pain caused by musculoskeletal problems, the reported lifetime prevalence of at least one episode of low back pain (LBP) varies but has been stated as ranging from 49 to 70 percent.[18] The majority of the working population has at least one episode of work absenteeism due to LBP during their career.[19, 20, 21] Whilst most episodes of acute LBP resolve within one month, for some the pain will persist and reoccur. Reports of short-term recovery in primary care populations vary from 21 to 90 percent depending on the selection criteria and outcomes used in the studies,[22] but it is estimated that 3–10 percent develop long-term disability.[23]

Since the publication of various recommendations,[24, 25, 26, 27] acute pain services have gradually increased in number. These documents propose that acute pain should be managed by an interdisciplinary team. However, they rarely refer to the provision of psychological interventions, their focus being on medical and nursing interventions. It remains unusual for a clinical psychologist to be a member of an acute pain team. In 2004, only ten (4.9 percent) of the 227 UK National Health Service acute pain teams employed a psychologist.[28]

To understand the role of psychological interventions for acute pain, clinicians must move away from the artificial dualistic model of pain and develop an understanding of the role of psychosocial factors involved in pain perception.

An early explanation of pain physiology by Descartes in the seventeenth century proposed that

- a direct, unbroken pathway exists between peripheral pain receptors and specific brain centers;
- pain is always a result of damage;
- the intensity of pain is proportional to the amount of damage sustained;
- pain perception is purely a physiological process.

This model is now known to be too simplistic and has been surpassed by the gate control theory,[29] which itself has been refined since its inception.[30] As psychophysical and functional magnetic resonance imaging (fMRI) research has developed, so too has our understanding of (1) the neural correlates of the pain experience and (2) the role of psychological processes in the subjective experience of pain.[31] fMRI results suggest that reports of pain intensity do not correlate with stimulus intensity but with the degree of cortical activation in several brain regions that are not only important in pain processing but also cognitive processes.[32] Pain should not be viewed as either organic or psychological in origin as both physical and psychological factors play an important role in all pain perception. Considering only nociception and somatic factors when formulating people's experience of pain is inadequate. Using only psychological factors to explain pain is often unhelpful and distressing for the patient. Engel[33] developed the biopsychosocial model that highlights the dynamic interaction between biological, psychological, behavioral, and social factors during an episode of illness. This model has been applied to pain[34, 35] and has placed psychological and social factors firmly in the realm of pain research and practice.[36]

PSYCHOLOGICAL FACTORS INVOLVED IN PAIN PROCESSING

The psychological factors that are involved in pain processing include:

- mood (for example, anxiety and depression);
- catastrophizing (**Box 15.1**);
- fear-avoidance (**Box 15.2**);
- attention and perceived level of threat;
- thought content (for example, attitudes, beliefs, and meanings);
- expectations;
- previous pain experience.

Box 15.1 Catastrophizing

Catastrophizing describes extreme negative appraisals of internal and external stimuli and situations. It has been defined in relation to pain as "an exaggerated negative mental set brought to bear during actual or anticipated pain experience".[37] The pain literature suggests that catastrophizing consists of three dimensions: rumination about pain; magnification of the threat value of a painful stimulus; and perceived helplessness about ones' ability to control pain.[37, 38] An example of catastrophic thinking is: "I've heard that people can be in excruciating pain after an operation like this. I'm not very good at coping with pain. It'll be horrible and I know that something will go wrong."

These will be discussed in relation to postoperative pain and acute pain that is at risk of developing into chronic problems.

Psychological factors and postoperative pain

There are significant variations in reports of postoperative pain intensity, duration, and quality of the recovery period, even following the same procedure. This has led to work addressing the influence of cognitive and emotional factors on postoperative pain.[43, 44][III] However, results

Box 15.2 Fear-avoidance

The fear-avoidance model aids understanding about the development and maintenance of long-term disability in the presence of persistent pain.[39] The model highlights the interaction between psychological and physical processes. It proposes that the presence of pain can elicit beliefs and cognitions associated with a fear of movement and/or damage/injury. This results in avoidance of activity, the maintenance and exacerbation of fear[40, 41] and, in the long term, disuse, disability, and mood changes. Catastrophizing (Box 15.1) about pain is thought to be a salient feature in this process. In the absence of catastrophizing, people confront situations and engage in activities that are more likely to promote recovery. Fear-avoidance beliefs, for example, "physical activity might harm my back" and "I cannot do my normal work until my pain is treated"[42] predict disability in daily or occupational activity, treatment outcome, and return to work.[42]

vary due to the use of prospective or retrospective assessments; different types of analyses; or poor methodology such as omission of the numbers investigated, the follow-up measures used, and the time of follow up.[10] The available evidence suggests that the psychological factors associated with postoperative pain are not universally applicable to all surgical procedures or types of surgery[45] and have yet to be validated in predicting the risk of postsurgical pain in an individual patient.[11] In addition, it is not only the patient's experience that influences postoperative pain intensity. For example, a study focusing on elective cesarean sections reported that the fear experiences of the birth partner were significantly associated with the mother's level of postoperative pain.[46]

MOOD

Anxiety is commonly addressed in studies that attempt to understand the association between postoperative pain and psychological factors.[43] The available literature appears to support a positive association between preoperative anxiety and pain[45, 47, 48, 49, 50, 51, 52] and postoperative anxiety and pain[51, 53] in the first hour and up to a year postoperatively. There is also evidence that anxiety is a predictive factor in the amount of analgesia required.[54] However, significant positive relationships have not been reported in all studies[55] and methodological problems exist in many.[43] One difficulty when drawing conclusions from the available studies is that some address state (current) anxiety and some trait (dispositional) anxiety (**Box 15.3**) and many use different measures of anxiety.

In an attempt to make consistent comparisons across studies, a review[43] of the associations between preoperative anxiety and postoperative variables only included studies that assessed state and trait anxiety using the State-Trait Anxiety Inventory.[56] Of the 27 studies that met the review's inclusion criteria, 12 reported on the association between preoperative anxiety and postoperative pain. The effect sizes that could be calculated from the reviewed studies for state anxiety ranged from

Box 15.3 State and trait anxiety

- State anxiety is a transitory, unpleasant emotional arousal characterized by subjective feelings of tension and apprehension. A cognitive appraisal of threat is a prerequisite for the experience of this emotion.
- Trait anxiety is a stable feature of personality. Individuals scoring high on trait anxiety are more likely to anticipate and perceive situations as threatening and respond with state anxiety.

0.18 to 0.41. Only two effect sizes could be calculated for trait anxiety, these were 0.37 and 0.38. Despite inconsistencies between the studies' findings, the review tentatively concluded that preoperative state and trait anxiety both positively correlate with postoperative pain. The authors attributed the inconsistencies to variations between the studies (for example, type of surgery and the gender ratios and age range of the participants) and methodological problems (for example, differences in statistical analysis and no controlling for levels of preoperative pain).

The literature that attempts to understand adults' anxiety when facing surgery is surprisingly sparse. Anxiety about perioperative risks and problems is thought to be associated with worse than expected postoperative pain experience.[8]

Studies report minimal positive or no effects of preoperative anxiolytics on postoperative pain and analgesic requirements.[57, 58, 59] However, there is some evidence to the contrary[60] which may be mediated by the type and severity of surgery.[57]

Anxiety does not exist in isolation and its effect on postoperative pain may be mediated by other psychological variables such as coping style, cognitive style, and other aspects of mood. The association between postoperative pain and **depression** has received less attention than anxiety. The studies available suggest that preoperative depression is associated with higher postoperative pain intensity,[48, 61] morphine requirements, and requests for patient-controlled analgesia (PCA).[62] Even mild depression is a predictor of moderate to intense postoperative pain.[48]

CATASTROPHIZING

Research findings have consistently suggested that catastrophizing (**Box 15.1**) is associated with heightened pain experience across a range of diverse patient groups.[37]

Catastrophizing prior to surgery has been shown to be associated with greater postoperative pain intensity[38][III], [44][III] and may mediate the effect of anxiety on postoperative pain.[38][III] One study made a distinction between postoperative pain at rest and during activity, suggesting that people classified as "high" or "low" catastrophizers did not differ on reported pain intensity at rest following an operation. However, the high catastrophizers reported more pain during activity.[44][III] This may have a detrimental impact on postoperative rehabilitation. An association between postoperative catastrophizing and increased pain intensity has also been reported.[63][III]

Reports of the association between catastrophizing and the use of postoperative analgesia are varied: an increased use of analgesia has been found following breast surgery[63][III] but not following anterior cruciate ligament repair.[44][III]

THREAT VALUE

Perception of threat is a significant factor in pain perception.[64] If an event occurring in the presence of pain is perceived to be a greater threat than the pain, attention is likely to be removed from the pain and towards the threatening event. Thus the pain becomes less salient and disruptive. If the pain is caused by a stimulus that is perceived to be threatening, attention is likely to be focused towards the pain and attention on current tasks, activities, and events is disrupted.[65] Anticipation of pain results in a similar response.[66]

Perceived threat is thought to activate pain schemata (**Box 15.4**) that represent the sensory, spatial, temporal, and affective properties of the pain experience[67] and influence attention to pain. For example, a study reported that although people classified as high or low catastrophizers attended to pain to a similar degree, the high catastrophizers had more difficulty disengaging from the pain.[68] The authors postulated that the perceived threat activated the pain schemata. This may have elicited a negative state and increased the accessibility of schema-congruent information and interfered with the processing of schema-incongruent information (**Box 15.4**). This resulted in a difficulty disengaging from the pain-congruent information. This selective processing bias towards threat stimuli that is congruent with current concerns has been shown to be a predictive factor in postoperative pain.[43]

The extent to which the pain is perceived as personally threatening is thought to influence which pain-related schemata are activated. If attention is on the sensory aspects of the pain, the sensory schema overrides the affective schema and the pain is reduced. If the pain is perceived as threatening, the affective schema is activated and the pain intensity experienced increases.[69]

Box 15.4 Pain schemata, congruent and incongruent information

- **Schemata (plural)** are mental representations that mediate perceptions and guide responses. They can be revised by new information. Someone's pain schemata will contain beliefs, thoughts, and images about pain that have evolved through their experience.
- **Schema (singular) congruent information** is information that is compatible with someone's schema, in this context, someone's representations of pain.
- **Schema incongruent information** is information that is incompatible with someone's schema.

BELIEFS AND MEANINGS

Patients' beliefs and meanings

Beliefs and meanings influence the perception of and responses to pain.[8, 70, 71] They may be about, for example, the cause and consequences of the pain, expectations of pain intensity, or a treatment or diagnosis. Beliefs and meanings are shaped by factors such as past experiences of pain, family and cultural beliefs, and experiences with HCPs.

Different people hold different beliefs and meanings and these will influence their reports of their pain experience, including pain intensity. For example, it has been suggested that patients who have abdominal surgery to treat cancer are less likely to report moderate to intense postoperative pain than those who have abdominal surgery for a problem with a benign etiology.[48] The authors suggest that this may be because the patients with cancer viewed the pain as necessary if their heath was to improve. Conversely, if a patient believes that experiencing pain indicates postoperative complications or that their situation is graver than they thought, they may report greater pain intensity.

Patient beliefs can result in a reluctance to report pain even if severe pain is being experienced. Such beliefs may be about:

- clinicians being too busy to help;[72]
- having to show they can tolerate pain;[73, 74]
- concerns about addiction to analgesia.[75]

Fears of addiction and concerns about potential overdose and side effects have been reported to reduce the use of PCA in one-quarter of patients.[76] Most patients used the PCA as soon as they experienced pain or had to move, but over one-third waited until they could not tolerate the pain. Nearly half used the PCA only when told to do so by someone else, and many limited their use of analgesia because they were trying to balance analgesic effects against side effects and feared administering a possibly harmful drug[76] (see Chapter 11, Patient-controlled analgesia).

Patients' beliefs about how much knowledge they should have about their condition and the extent of their involvement in their health care can affect their pain management. For example, it has been proposed that those who seek information report less severe pain.[47] Patients adopt three general strategies for managing postoperative pain:[77]

- Passive recipient – Patients do not involve themselves in decision making about their pain management and refer this process to HCPs. This passivity can be reinforced by their context, such as the language used by HCPs.[78]
- Problem solving – Patients actively increase their knowledge about analgesia.

- Active negotiation – Patients ensure that they are involved in decision making regarding their pain management.

Adoption of a passive recipient role (60 percent of patients) was associated with poorer pain management and an increased likelihood of receiving nonopioid analgesia; whereas patients using problem solving and active negotiation (23 and 17 percent, respectively) were more likely to receive opioid analgeisia.[77]

Healthcare providers' beliefs and meanings

Studies have reported that HCPs' knowledge, beliefs, perceptions, attitudes, and behaviors also influence patient reports of postoperative pain and the quality of their pain management.[79] Examples associated with postoperative pain and inadequate postoperative analgesia include

- HCPs viewing adequate rather than absolute pain relief as a goal of postoperative analgesia;[79]
- a lack of agreement between the hospital team about treatment goals;[75]
- an underestimation by HCPs of postoperative pain intensity[80] and beliefs about how well patients are coping with their pain;[81]
- inadequate assessment and documentation of pain and relief;[75]
- a belief that analgesia makes diagnosis difficult;
- a belief that opioid dose should relate to disease severity rather than pain intensity;
- HCPs' fear of side effects and addiction, particularly when the analgesia is an opioid[47, 82] or the patient has a history of drug abuse;[75]
- a lack of knowledge amongst HCPs regarding the terms addiction, physical dependence, psychological dependence, and tolerance. This can result in the withholding of analgesia.[8]

Progression of acute to persistent pain

Acute pain may progress to persistent pain following surgery, trauma, infection (e.g. acute herpes zoster), or following an episode of musculoskeletal pain.[61] Although variable in its quality, evidence is beginning to demonstrate that psychological and social factors play important roles in the transition from acute to persistent pain[36, 83] and may have more of an impact on disability than biomechanical factors.[36] The psychological variables involved in the transition from acute to persistent pain are thought to be[36]

- cognitive factors (for example attitudes, cognitive style, fear-avoidance beliefs, interpretation of pain);
- passive coping;
- pain cognitions (for example catastrophizing);

- mood (notably depression and anxiety);
- self-perceived poor health status.

Psychosocial factors that are associated with the risk of developing long-term pain and disability following an episode of acute LBP are called "yellow flags"[84] (**Box 15.5**).

Although differences exist between LBP and pain in other areas, yellow flags are thought to be applicable to populations other than those with low back pain.[85] Guidelines have been developed[84] to help HCPs identify their patients' psychosocial yellow flags and provide interdisciplinary interventions that facilitate recovery and prevent or reduce long-term disability. Unfortunately, some HCPs misuse the identification of yellow flags to formulate the patient and their problems within an unhelpful framework that suggests functional or psychosomatic pain or even evidence of malingering, which is not their purpose.[84]

FEAR-AVOIDANCE AND CATASTROPHIZING

The relationship between fear-avoidance (**Box 15.2**), catastrophizing, and disability has been investigated, mainly in persistent pain.[40, 86, 87, 88] Research findings are beginning to suggest that some people hold fear-avoidance beliefs and have a tendency to catastrophize even if they have not experienced an episode of LBP or they are experiencing their first acute episode. Clinical studies have indicated that higher levels of catastrophizing in the very early stages of acute pain onset is associated with reports of greater pain intensity[86] and is predictive of self-reported disability at six months[89] and one year.[90] Studies that have investigated catastrophizing prior to an episode of acute pain have provided mixed evidence with regards to whether pain intensity reports are associated with catastrophizing before or during the experience of acute pain.[91]

HCPs BELIEFS

HCPs' beliefs influence their practice, and this may impact on the persistence of pain and level of disability of their patients.[92] Despite recommendations to avoid bed rest in the management of acute back pain,[18, 93, 94, 95, 96, 97] [I] some HCPs do not follow the guidelines.[98, 99, 100, 101] Beliefs that physical activity may be harmful and should be avoided in LBP continue to be prevalent amongst general practitioners.[102] A study involving physical therapists reported that despite recognizing predictors of chronic disability in patients with acute pain, 34.5 percent of physical therapists advised these patients not to work. The greater the physical therapists' perception of severe spinal pathology, the more likely they were to give this advice.[98] HCPs' beliefs may also influence their patients' beliefs. A study has shown that patients with LBP who have fear-avoidance beliefs have seen rheumatologists who also have extensive fear-avoidance beliefs about the relationship between work activities and back pain.[103]

PSYCHOLOGICAL INTERVENTIONS

Many people with acute pain do not require formal psychological interventions. High quality care aimed at the management of anxiety is sufficient for many. Should the level of threat become unmanageable for the patient, then more comprehensive psychological interventions may be required.

A meta-analysis[104][III] of 191 studies addressed the effects of three types of interventions in the context of surgery:

- **healthcare information** (information on preparation for surgery, timing of procedures and pain, functions and roles of HCPs and ways to self-manage);
- **skills teaching** (exercises, relaxation, hypnosis, cognitive reappraisal);
- **psychosocial support** (identifying/alleviating concerns, reassurance, problem-solving, encouraging questions).

Although significant small to moderate beneficial effects were found on recovery, postoperative pain, psychological distress, and length of hospital stay, there were methodological problems with the review: it did not assess

---

Box 15.5 Yellow flags

Yellow flags are the psychosocial factors that have been found to predict poor outcome following an episode of acute LBP and are associated with the development of long-term pain and disability. These include

- the belief that back pain is harmful and/or disabling;
- reduced activity levels due to fear of increased pain;
- tendency to low mood and withdrawal from social interaction;
- expectations that recovery will be facilitated purely by passive treatments rather than active participation;
- problems with claim and compensation;
- history of back pain, time off, other claims;
- problems at work, poor job satisfaction;
- heavy work, unsociable hours;
- overprotective family or lack of support;
- treatment that does not fit best practice.

whether these improvements were of clinical relevance; it included nonrandomized trials; and it was unable to state which specific interventions were effective because it analyzed many types of intervention together. This meta-analysis was published in 1992. There does not appear to be a more recent published meta-analysis or systematic review that addresses the efficacy of a range of non-medical interventions for postoperative pain. The more recent studies that are discussed below have tended to focus on one intervention.

The provision of information

Although some may not interpret providing information to patients as a psychological intervention, it is an essential foundation when addressing the needs of patients with acute pain. The majority of research that addresses the provision of information for acute pain focuses on the effects of procedural and sensory information on pain intensity following surgical and medical procedures. Procedural information describes what will happen during an intervention and sensory information describes the possible sensory experiences.[61] Procedural and sensory information can be provided separately or in combination. Reviews of their effectiveness have produced mixed findings. However, a summary of the evidence[105] based on a systematic review[106][I] states that

- providing a combination of sensory and procedural information preoperatively significantly reduces postoperative pain, distress, and negative affect;
- providing sensory information alone has similar, but not as strong, effects and is more effective than providing procedural information alone which does not provide any significant benefits over a control group.

A combination of sensory and procedural information may be more effective because procedural information provides "a map of specific events" and sensory information "facilitates their interpretation as nonthreatening."[106][I]

A more recent meta-analysis[107][I] has reported that

- procedural information reduces postoperative pain;
- sensory information does not reduce postoperative pain.

Because differences exist between patients in the amount of information they want and need to manage the perioperative situation, HCPs must be sensitive to, and assess the needs of, each individual rather than providing the same information by the same means to every patient. Some patients can be given too much information and when required to make decisions they feel more anxious and report more pain, especially if avoidance is their usual

means of coping. To help HCPs determine the type and detail of information to provide, their assessment of the patient should include[61]

- beliefs concerning the cause of the pain;
- knowledge, expectations, and preferences for pain management;
- expectations of outcomes of treatment;
- the level of pain reduction the patient requires to resume reasonable activities;
- views about the amount of procedural and sensory information they would like;
- coping responses for stress and pain.

HCPs must also consider the context in which they provide information. It is best given in the context of an ongoing relationship and in an environment where the patient is able to attend to what is being discussed, does not feel rushed, and feels able to ask questions and seek clarification.

HCPs education

The biopsychosocial model suggests that the patient's context influences their pain perception and beliefs. HCPs are an essential part of this context. Their beliefs and style and content of their communication play a pivotal role in how patients respond to their pain. HCPs need to receive education about, and support in, the following:

- The promotion of postoperative pain as preventable rather than inevitable,[11] Some HCPs consider pain to be an unavoidable postoperative problem and therefore its reduction is often not a priority for them.[108]
- Awareness that taking into account psychological factors when formulating a patient's pain experience is not an indication that the pain is "emotionally derived."[10] Psychological and physical processes are involved in all pain perception for all people.
- Awareness that a patient's meanings and beliefs about pain are subjective. They must not be dismissed if they differ from those of the HCP or do not appear to fit with an objective view of the patient's condition and situation. Even a minor hospital procedure can be accompanied by a high level of anxiety, anticipation of pain, worries about survival and recovery, concerns about the home situation, and memories of previous hospital experiences.[109]
- Awareness that words used benignly by HCPs can be interpreted by the patient as meaning serious pathology and/or future serious problems and can increase the patient's level of perceived threat.[110]
- Communication skills to help HCPs and patients work collaboratively and to enable patients to understand their options, communicate their

preferences, and share responsibility for their pain management.[77]

- Skills to listen and respond appropriately to a patient's anxiety about pain experiences.
- Skills to recognize patients who are at risk of their acute pain developing into chronic problems.
- The provision of appropriate information in line with current guidelines.
- The ability to explore patients' unhelpful beliefs and concerns as opposed to providing reassurance which may have the counterproductive and paradoxical effect of strengthening patients' fears.[110, 111]

Despite evidence to suggest that staff education programs can improve the management of pain,[112, 113, 114][III], [115][III], [116][III] these may not be effective in altering the practice of some HCPs. Postoperative pain assessment and documentation can still be inadequate in the clinical environment following HCPs' education.[117] One study concluded that despite a hospital policy of regular pain assessment using validated tools, a pain scale was used in only 12.6 percent of cases.[77] HCPs' fear-avoidance beliefs or the advice they give to patients concerning physical and occupational activities are not always modified with education sessions.[102, 103] It is essential that education programs are rigorously developed and continuously evaluated[108] and if they are proven not to change HCPs' beliefs and practice then alternative and possibly more complex interventions may be required.[103]

Attentional techniques

There is evidence to suggest that some attentional techniques (**Box 15.6**) reduce postoperative pain and the amount of analgesia used.[119][II], [120][III] However, this is not so for all techniques. For example, a systematic review concluded that focusing on music alone does not reduce pain levels in people undergoing surgery or invasive procedures.[121][I] A study comparing music with focusing on pain site during the changing of burns dressings concluded that focusing on the site was more effective in reducing pain during this procedure.[122][II] Focusing on the pain's sensory elements during a painful procedure may alter pain perception and reduce pain in people who wish to have a high level of control but perceive themselves as having low level of control.[123][II], [124][II]

Relaxation

Although relaxation has become popular as a pain-relieving intervention for acute pain, summaries of the available evidence state there is little to suggest that it is beneficial in the perioperative setting,[61] that "convincing evidence for the efficacy of relaxation [for acute pain] is lacking" and "more trials of better quality are needed."[125]

In 1996, a review of 21 trials (19 controlled trials of which 11 were randomized) evaluated the effects of several different methods of relaxation and/or types of music on postoperative pain.[120][III] It concluded that 10 out of 13 studies reported a significant reduction in affective pain and four out of four in observed pain. There was a less significant reduction in reported pain (6 out of 12 studies) and no significant reduction in opioid intake (5 out of 15 studies). Methodological problems cast doubt on the validity of the results.[125] Some treatment groups were small and some were not randomized. The majority did not report on pre-intervention between group differences in pain, some did not report controlling for any between group differences and there were a variety of pain measures used (sensory, affective, and unidimensional pain and self-reported and observed pain). Many studies did not supervise relaxation practice by the participants and their relaxation skills were not assessed.

A systematic review in 1998 assessed seven studies (six postoperative and one during a femoral angioplasty) addressing the effectiveness of relaxation techniques.[126] The authors could not conduct a meta-analysis due to a lack of primary data and a number of the trials being methodologically flawed. Three trials reported significantly less pain and/or pain distress in those who practiced relaxation. Four did not demonstrate a beneficial effect of relaxation.

A more recent systematic review of randomized trials studying the effect of relaxation on pain intensity reported similar findings to previous reviews: many studies had weaknesses in their methodology which limited the ability to draw conclusions about the effectiveness of relaxation.

Some studies have reported beneficial effects of relaxation. A meta-analysis of randomized controlled trials assessing a variety of methods of **psychological** preparation for surgery reported that relaxation was

---

Box 15.6 Attentional techniques

Attentional techniques aim to[61]

- alter attention in relation to the pain;
- modify the experience of the pain;
- achieve a change in emotional state.

There are two main categories of attentional techniques.

1. Switching attention to a stimulus other than pain, for example imagery, sensations, noise, and smells.
2. Retuning attention towards the pain "so that aspects are attended to which are less distressing and interruptive."[118]

associated with a reduction in pain intensity, negative affect, the use of analgesia, length of hospital stay and costs, and an improvement in clinical indices of recovery, physiological indices, and patient satisfaction.[107][I] A meta-analysis of studies evaluating relaxation for people with cancer undergoing acute medical interventions (chemotherapy, radiotherapy, and bone marrow transplant) suggested that relaxation strategies were associated with a reduction in treatment-related pain.[127][I]

Hypnosis

Comparing studies and drawing conclusions about the effectiveness of hypnosis (**Box 15.7**) in reducing acute pain is difficult given the variable nature of hypnotic procedures,[128] the small numbers of participants, and the absence of controls.[129] A meta-analysis of randomized controlled trials of different methods of psychological preparation for adults prior to surgery reported that hypnosis does not reduce pain intensity or medication use.[107][I] A more recent review of studies that evaluated the effectiveness of pre- and postoperative hypnosis in both randomized and nonrandomized studies reported mixed but more encouraging results.[129] Significantly less pain was reported by groups of patients following orthopedic hand surgery,[130][III] excisional breast biopsy,[131][II] plastic surgery,[132][III], [133][III] thyroid surgery,[134][III] and percutaneous vascular and renal procedures,[135][III] but not following various gynecological procedures,[136][II] breast surgery,[137][II] and radial keratotomy.[138][III] A significantly lower amount of analgesia was required intra- or postoperatively in breast[137][II] and thyroid,[134][III] but not head and neck[139][III] and maxillofacial surgery.[140][III] Other studies and reviews have concluded that hypnosis is superior to attention or standard care control conditions for acute pain associated with procedures such as burn wound care, bone marrow aspiration,[141] and child birth.[142][I]

It has been argued that the data in reviews of hypnosis must be treated with caution because not every patient can be hypnotized, many are small nonrandomized studies, and there is great variability in the techniques and definitions used.[129, 143]

Cognitive-behavioral therapy

Evidence is emerging to suggest that the psychological and social factors that play a significant role in the transition of acute pain to a chronic problem may be present before the first episode of pain or the first consultation with an HCP. These factors could be used to identify those at risk and guide cognitive-behavioral interventions (**Box 15.8**) to help prevent the development of permanent disability[144, 145][II], [146, 147, 148] Some have suggested that these interventions should focus on catastrophizing and fear in the same manner as interventions for persistent pain.[44][III], [63][III]

Box 15.7 Hypnosis

Although definitions of hypnosis vary according to the theoretical perspective taken, it can be considered to be a state of focused attention where one is absorbed in creative imagination and dissattends to outside stimuli. This state is often thought of as one that people naturally experience, for example when absorbed in a book or film. Once this state is achieved, the details of the procedure differ depending on the therapist's theoretical stance. In this state, people can respond more easily to suggestions that are given by someone externally or that people give to themselves using imaginal rehearsal (this involves visualization and mental rehearsal of steps to take and/or goals to achieve).

Box 15.8 Cognitive-behavioral therapy

Cognitive-behavioral therapy is a psychological intervention that addresses the relationship between people's cognitions (thoughts), emotions, behavior, and bodily sensations. The cognitive-behavioral model proposes that people create meanings and beliefs about themselves, their lives, the world, and other people. This includes physical symptoms experienced. Meanings, beliefs, emotions, behaviors, and bodily sensations all influence each other. More specifically to pain, the meaning people hold for their pain, and their subsequent cognitive, emotional, and behavioral responses to their pain can increase distress and, in the long term, disability.

Cognitive-behavioral interventions are appropriate when meanings and beliefs are having a detrimental impact on psychological and physical functioning. Cognitive-behavioral therapists work collaboratively with the patient to elicit the meanings they hold (for example, "Having to have this operation means I must have cancer and this means I will die" or "My pain means that something is badly damaged") and help them to become aware of their unhelpful beliefs, thoughts, thought processes, and behaviors that may be reinforcing the patient's difficulties. The therapist and patient work together to gather evidence that helps the patient generate alternative, more helpful beliefs and meanings and to change behaviors.

Despite growing evidence to support the provision of psychological interventions for acute pain, many patients continue to receive medical interventions (such as analgesics or physical therapy[149]) in isolation and with increasing intensity should initial attempts fail.[150] One study reported that people's physical function and sick leave did not improve over seven months despite receiving high levels of medical health care for spinal pain during this time.[151] A review of interventions for acute pain to prevent long-term back and neck pain problems revealed disappointing outcomes for lumbar supports, back and neck schools, use of ergonomics, and risk factor modification. Exercise was the only effective preventative intervention of those evaluated.[152][I] The lack of these interventions' effectiveness may be due to their focus being on pain and function rather than the psychological factors known to be associated with the risk of developing persistent pain (for example, fear-avoidance beliefs and catastrophizing).[151]

Some trials of psychosocial interventions for acute pain have not supported their use. A clinical trial[153] did not find significant beneficial effects of a minimal intervention strategy (MIS) provided by general medical practitioners for acute or subacute LBP when compared with care as usual. The MIS involved:

- the exploration of psychosocial prognostic factors (causal beliefs, fear-avoidance beliefs, catastrophizing, unhelpful behaviors such as avoidance, reactions from significant others, and physical and psychosocial factors at work);
- the provision of information about the cause, course, and treatment of LBP;
- the provision of information about the interaction between psychosocial factors, cognitions, emotions, behavior, and pain;
- collaborative goal setting by the patient and GP around resuming activities or work;
- discussion of time-contingent use of analgesia;
- a booklet based on the *Back Book*.[154]

The intervention for the "care as usual" group followed the Dutch College of General Practitioners' guidelines for LBP[155] advising analgesia and gradual uptake of activities, and recommendations on reactivation and home exercises. This group did not receive guidance on psychosocial factors. Unfortunately, this study had been cited as evidence that psychosocial interventions do not reduce the risk of persistent pain and disability in an acute pain population. However, there are significant methodological problems with this study:

- Patients who had elevated scores on the psychosocial measures were not identified. There may have been significance between group differences on these measures.

- The study did not assess whether, or to what extent, psychosocial factors were addressed in the usual care group.
- The practitioners had only five hours of training, which is an inadequate amount of time to learn what can be a complex intervention. Clinicians who have been formally trained in psychosocial interventions receive a significantly greater amount of training.
- The skills of the practitioners were not evaluated and the study did not assess whether the practitioners had carried out the interventions as required.
- Seventy percent of the patients in the MIS group had only one 20-minute consultation in which psychosocial issues were addressed. This may not have been sufficient to enable some patients to use and generalize the information.
- A significant part of the MIS intervention was examination and activity advice. Although essential, this may have been inadequate for people who required a cognitive-behavioral intervention, with a cognitive behaviorally trained clinician, to address catastrophizing, pain-related fear, and avoidance[86] with the aim of reducing their risk of long term disability.[156]

Cognitive-behavioral interventions for acute pain do not consist of one technique but are multimodal. Depending on the patient's needs they may include education about pain, goal setting, graded exercise, pacing of activities, relaxation, specific cognitive and behavioral techniques, and problem solving. Although some have specific aims such as return to work,[157] a more general aim of these interventions (whether in the perioperative setting or in the prevention of acute pain developing into chronic problems) would be to alter patients' beliefs and behavior in relation to their pain; reduce fear and avoidance (**Box 15.2**); enhance coping; reduce distress; and prevent long-term disability.[158][II] Randomized controls trials show that an early intervention cognitive-behavioral group approach for those with pain in the acute phase demonstrates significantly better results in preventing disability when compared with control groups.[157, 159][II], [160][III], [161][II], [162][II] These interventions also reduce sick leave and healthcare use[158][II] and produce long-term health and economic benefits.[163][II] Cognitive-behavioral interventions for people who have experienced episodes of acute back pain but who have not yet accessed the healthcare system reduce the risk of disability three-fold, sick leave three-fold, significantly reduce fear-avoidance beliefs, and increase the number of pain-free days.[164][II]

Although this work is promising, some essential work is still required:[22, 156]

- Those at risk need to be identified with reliable screening instruments.

- Further knowledge is required regarding which patients respond, at what time point, and with what interventions.[145][II], [165]
- The interventions need to be refined and controlled studies are needed to evaluate their effectiveness.[18]

USING ASSESSMENT PATIENT SATISFACTION TO EVALUATE PAIN INTENSITY

It is essential that the effectiveness of interventions for pain intensity is evaluated. Using a visual analog scale to assess pain intensity is extremely common although problems exist with this method.[166] It is acknowledged that the multidimensional nature of pain should be reflected in the outcome measures used. In an attempt to do this, a measure of patient satisfaction with postoperative care is often used as a means to assess the effectiveness of pain management. However, many patients report being satisfied with their postoperative care despite experiencing moderate or severe postoperative pain.[71, 167, 168, 169] For example, one study[170] reported that 76 percent of patients reported moderate to severe postoperative pain, yet 81 percent reported being satisfied with their pain management. Another reported that although more than half of patients stated that postoperative pain interfered with their sleep and daily activities, and more than one-third reported that it interfered with their normal sexual functioning, most were satisfied with the management of their pain.[4]

Although patient satisfaction is influenced by a reduction in pain intensity, it is influenced by many other factors including:[171]

- perception of high levels of support;[172]
- lower levels of depression;[172]
- higher levels of internal locus of control;[173]
- beliefs that the HCP appears caring[174] and is making efforts to provide pain relief;[175]
- perceptions of the quality of HCPs communication;[176]
- confidence and trust in the HCP;[177]
- a desire to please the HCP;[8]
- the drug side effects experienced.[8]

These factors and the paradoxical relationship between pain experienced and satisfaction suggests that satisfaction ratings do not fully reflect the patient's experience of their pain management and should not be use to report its effectiveness.[4, 178, 179] Although it is important to assess patient satisfaction, the assessment of pain management requires a multidimensional assessment.[178]

CONCLUSION

Medical interventions can be helpful in reducing acute pain. However, acute pain, notably postoperative pain and the progression of acute pain to persistent pain, continues to be a problem in the healthcare system. Given that psychological variables are involved in the processing of and responses to pain, psychological interventions may be useful in reducing acute pain. Research is enabling clinicians to consider such interventions. However, the amount of research is relatively small when compared with that for persistent pain, and the results are inconsistent. This inconsistency may be due to methodological problems in the studies and the heterogeneity (for example, etiology, pain site, type of surgery) of acute pain. An effective psychological intervention for acute pain of one cause may not be effective for another. Research to date suggests that psychological interventions may reduce postoperative pain and prevent the transition from acute pain to chronic problems. However, many studies conclude that further research is required. This research is needed to ascertain which psychologically based interventions are appropriate for which population (taking account of the pain's etiology, the patient's psychosocial characteristics, and the risk factors present) and at what time point.

Even with sound research available, it is important that HCPs are skilled in developing a comprehensive understanding of the patient and their pain that includes psychosocial variables. This will help them to offer appropriate individualized pain management that is sensitive to the patient's needs.[8, 180]

REFERENCES

* 1. The Royal College of Anaesthetists and The Pain Society. *Pain management service; Good practice.* London: The Royal College of Anaesthetists and The Pain Society, 2003.

2. Linton SJ, Hellsing AL, Andersson D. A controlled study of the effects of an early intervention on acute musculoskeletal problems. *Pain.* 1993; **54**: 353–9.

3. Dolin SJ, Cashman JN, Bland JM. Effectiveness of acute postoperative pain management: I. Evidence from published data. *British Journal of Anaesthesia.* 2002; **89**: 409–23.

4. Strassels SA, McNicol E, Wagner AK *et al.* Persistent postoperative pain, health-related quality of life, and functioning 1 month after hospital discharge. *Acute Pain.* 2004; **6**: 95–104.

5. Apfelbaum JL, Chen C, Mehta SS, Gan TJ. Postoperative pain experience: results from a national survey suggest postoperative pain continues to be undermanaged. *Anesthesia and Analgesia.* 2003; **97**: 534–40.

* 6. International Association for the Study of Pain, European Federation of IASP Chapters (fact sheet). 2004. Unrelieved pain is a major global healthcare problem. Accessed August 13, 2006. Available from: www.painreliefhumanright.com/pdf/04a_global_day_fact_sheet.pdf.

7. Brown AK, Christo PJ, Wu CL. Strategies for postoperative pain management. *Best Practice and Research Clinical Anaesthesiology.* 2004; **18**: 703–17.

8. Thomas T, Robinson C, Champion D *et al.* Prediction and assessment of the severity of post-operative pain and of satisfaction with management. *Pain.* 1998; **75**: 177–85.

9. Wu CL, Naqibuddin M, Rowlingson AJ *et al.* The effect of pain on health-related quality of life in the immediate postoperative period. *Anesthesia and Analgesia.* 2003; **97**: 1078–85.

10. Macrae WA. Chronic pain after surgery: Advances in pain. *British Journal of Anaesthesia.* 2001; **87**: 88–98.

11. Visser EJ. Chronic post-surgical pain: Epidemiology and clinical implications for acute pain management. *Acute Pain.* 2006; **8**: 73–81.

12. Crombie IK, Davies HT, Macrae WA. Cut and thrust: antecedent surgery and trauma among patients attending a chronic pain clinic. *Pain.* 1998; **76**: 167–71.

13. Davies HTO, Crombie IK, Macrae WA, Rogers KM. Pain clinic patients in Northern Britain. *Pain Clinic.* 1992; **5**: 129–35.

14. Tasmuth T, Estlander AM, Kalso E. Effect of present pain and mood on the memory of past postoperative pain in women treated surgically for breast cancer. *Pain.* 1996; **68**: 343–7.

15. Kehlet H, Hole K. Effect of postoperative analgesia on surgical outcome. *British Journal of Anaesthesia.* 2001; **87**: 62–72.

16. Carli F, Mayo N, Klubien K *et al.* Epidural analgesia enhances functional exercise capacity and health-related quality of life after colonic surgery. *Anesthesia.* 2002; **97**: 540–9.

17. Rawal N. Analgesia for day-case surgery. *British Journal of Anaesthesia.* 2001; **87**: 73–87.

18. Koes B W, van Tulder M W, Thomas S. Diagnosis and treatment of low back pain. *British Medical Journal.* 2006; **332**: 1430–4.

19. Nachemson AL. Newest knowledge of low back pain. *Clinical Orthopedics.* 1992; **279**: 8–20.

∗ 20. Waddell G. *The back pain revolution.* Edinburgh: Churchill Livingstone, 1998: 438.

21. Nachemson A, Jonsson E (eds). *Neck and back pain: The scientific evidence of causes, diagnosis, and treatment.* Philadelphia: Lippincott Williams and Wilkins, 2000: 495.

∗ 22. Grotle M, Brox JI, Veierød MB *et al.* Clinical course and prognostic factors in acute low back pain: Patients consulting primary care for the first time. *Spine.* 2005; **30**: 976–82.

23. Reid S, Haugh LD, Hazard RG, Tripathi M. Occupational low back pain: recovery curves and factors associated with disability. *Journal of Occupational Rehabilitation.* 1997; **7**: 1–14.

24. Commission on the Provision of Surgical Services. Report of the working party on pain after surgery. London: Royal College of Surgeons of England and College of Anaesthetists, 1990.

25. Department of Health. *The provision of services for acute post-operative pain in Scotland.* Edinburgh: HMSO, 1996.

26. A Report by the American Society of Anesthesiologists Task Force on Pain Management, Acute Pain Section. Practice guidelines for acute pain management in the perioperative setting. *Anesthesiology.* 1995; **82**: 1071–81.

27. Agency for Health Care Policy and Research. Acute pain management: Operative or medical procedures and trauma. *Clinical practice guidelines.* Rockville, MD: AHCPR, 1992.

28. Nagi H. Acute pain services in the United Kingdom. *Acute Pain.* 2004; **5**: 89–107.

∗ 29. Melzack R, Wall PD. Pain mechanisms: A new theory. *Science.* 1965; **150**: 171–9.

∗ 30. Melzack R. Evolution of the neuromatrix theory of pain. The Prithvi Raj Lecture: presented at the third world congress of world institute of pain, Barcelona 2004. *Pain Practice.* 2005; **5**: 85–94.

∗ 31. Price DD. Psychological and neural mechanisms of the affective dimension of pain. *Science.* 2000; **288**: 1769–72.

∗ 32. Coghill RC, McHaffie JG, Yen Y. Neural correlates of interindividual differences in the subjective experience of pain. *Proceedings of the National Academy of Sciences.* 2003; **100**: 8538–42.

∗ 33. Engel GL. The need for a new medical model: A challenge for biomedicine. *Science.* 1977; **196**: 129–36.

∗ 34. Waddell G. *The back pain revolution*, 2nd edn. Edinburgh: Churchill Livingstone, 2004.

∗ 35. Main C, Williams ACdeC. ABC of psychological medicine. *British Medical Journal.* 2002; **325**: 534–7.

∗ 36. Linton SJ. A review of psychological risk factors in back and neck pain. *Spine.* 2000; **25**: 1148–56.

∗ 37. Sullivan MJ, Thorn B, Haythornthwaite J *et al.* Theoretical perspectives on the relation between catastrophizing and pain. *Clinical Journal of Pain.* 2001; **17**: 52–64.

38. Granot M, Ferber SG. The roles of pain catastrophizing and anxiety in the prediction of postoperative pain intensity: A prospective study. *Clinical Journal of Pain.* 2005; **21**: 439–45.

∗ 39. Vlaeyen JWS, Kole-Snijders AMJ, Boeren RGB, van Eek H. Fear of movement/(re)injury in chronic low back pain and its relation to behavioral performance. *Pain.* 1995; **62**: 363–72.

40. Crombez G, Eccleston C, Baeyens F *et al.* Attention to chronic pain is dependent upon pain-related fear. *Journal of Psychosomatic Research.* 1999; **47**: 403–10.

41. Crombez G, Van Damme S, Eccleston C. Hypervigilance to pain: an experimental and clinical analysis. *Pain.* 2005; **116**: 4–7.

42. Waddell G, Newton M, Henderson I *et al.* A Fear-Avoidance Beliefs Questionnaire (FABQ) and the role of fear-avoidance beliefs in chronic low back pain and disability. *Pain.* 1993; **52**: 157–68.

43. Munafo MR, Stevenson J. Selective processing of threat-related cues in day surgery patients and prediction of post-operative pain. *British Journal of Health Psychology.* 2003; **8**: 439–49.

44. Pavlin DJ, Sullivan MJ, Freund PR, Roesen K. Catastrophizing: a risk factor for postsurgical pain. *Clinical Journal of Pain*. 2005; **21**: 83–90.

45. Katz J, Poleshuck EL, Andrus CH *et al*. Risk factors for acute pain and its persistence following breast cancer surgery. *Pain*. 2005; **119**: 16–25.

46. Keogh E, Hughes S, Ellery D *et al*. Psychosocial influences on women's experience of planned elective cesarean section. *Psychosomatic Medicine*. 2005; **68**: 167–74.

47. Kalkman CJ, Visser K, Moen J *et al*. Preoperative prediction of severe postoperative pain. *Pain*. 2003; **105**: 415–23.

48. Caumo W, Schmidt AP, Schneider CN *et al*. Preoperative predictors of moderate to intense acute postoperative pain in patients undergoing abdominal surgery. *Acta Anaesthesiologica Scandinavica*. 2002; **46**: 1265–71.

49. Boeke S, Duivenvoorden HJ, Verhage F, Zwaveling A. Prediction of postoperative pain and duration of hospitalization using two anxiety measures. *Pain*. 1991; **45**: 293–7.

50. Vaughn F, Wichowski H, Bosworth G. Does preoperative anxiety level predict postoperative pain? *AORN Journal*. 2007; **85**: 589–94.

51. Carr E, Brockbank K, Allen S, Strike P. Patterns and frequency of anxiety in women undergoing gynaecological surgery. *Journal of Clinical Nursing*. 2006; **15**: 341–52.

52. Kain ZN, Sevarino FB, Alexander GM *et al*. Preoperative anxiety and postoperative pain in women undergoing hysterectomy: A repeated-measures design. *Journal of Psychosomatic Research*. 2000; **49**: 417–22.

53. Caumo W, Schmidt AP, Schneider CN *et al*. Risk factors for postoperative anxiety in adults. *Anaesthesia*. 2001; **56**: 720–8.

54. Pan PH, Coghill R, Houle TT *et al*. Multifactorial preoperative predictors for postcesarean section pain and analgesic requirement. *Anesthesiology*. 2006; **104**: 417–25.

55. Wallace LM. Pre-operative state anxiety as a mediator of psychological adjustment to and recovery from surgery. *British Journal of Medical Psychology*. 1986; **59**: 253–61.

56. Speilberger CD, Gorsuch RL, Lushene R. *Manual for the state-trait anxiety inventory*, 1st edn. Palo Alto, CA: Consulting Psychiatry Press, 1983.

57. Kain ZN, Sevarino FB, Rinder C *et al*. Preoperative anxiolysis and postoperative recovery in women undergoing abdominal hysterectomy. *Anesthesiology*. 2001; **94**: 415–22.

58. Bauer K, Dom P, Ramirez A, O'Flaherty J. Preoperative intravenous midazolam: benefits beyond anxiolysis. *Journal of Clinical Anesthesia*. 2004; **16**: 177–83.

59. Caumo W, Hidalgo MP, Schmidt AP *et al*. Effect of pre-operative anxiolysis on postoperative pain response in patients undergoing total abdominal hysterectomy. *Anaesthesia*. 2002; **57**: 740–6.

60. Kain ZN, Sevarino FB, Pincus S *et al*. Attenuation of the preoperative stress response with midazolam: Effects on postoperative outcomes. *Anesthesiology*. 2000; **93**: 141–7.

∗ 61. Australian and New Zealand College of Anaesthetists and Faculty of Pain Medicine. *Acute pain management: scientific evidence*, 2nd edn. Melbourne: ANZCA, 2005.

62. Özalp G, Sarioglu R, Tuncel G *et al*. Preoperative emotional states in patients with breast cancer and postoperative pain. *Acta Anaesthesiologica Scandinavica*. 2003; **47**: 26–9.

63. Jacobsen PB, Butler RW. Relation of cognitive coping and catastrophizing to acute pain and analgesic use following breast cancer surgery. *Journal of Behavioral Medicine*. 1996; **19**: 17–29.

∗ 64. Crombez G, Vlaeyen JW, Heuts PH, Lysens R. Pain-related fear is more disabling than pain itself: evidence on the role of pain-related fear in chronic back pain disability. *Pain*. 1999; **80**: 329–39.

65. James JE, Hardardottir I. Influence of attention focus and trait anxiety on tolerance of acute pain. *British Journal of Health Psychology*. 2002; **7**: 149–62.

66. Van Damme S, Lorenz J, Eccleston C *et al*. Fear-conditioned cues of impending pain facilitate attentional engagement. *Neurophysiologie Clinique*. 2004; **34**: 33–9.

67. Pincus T, Morley S. Cognitive-processing bias in chronic pain: a review and integration. *Psychological Bulletin*. 2001; **127**: 599–617.

68. Van Damm S, Crombez G, Eccleston C. Disengagement from pain: the role of catastrophic thinking about pain. *Pain*. 2004; **107**: 70–6.

69. Boston A, Sharpe L. The role of threat-expectancy in acute pain: effects on attentional bias, coping strategy effectiveness and response to pain. *Pain*. 2005; **119**: 168–75.

70. Smith WB, Gracely RH, Safer MA. The meaning of pain: cancer patient's rating and recall of pain intensity and affect. *Pain*. 1998; **78**: 123–9.

71. Owen H, McMillan V, Rogowski D. Postoperative pain therapy: a survey of patients' expectations and their experiences. *Pain*. 1990; **41**: 303–7.

72. Brydon CW, Ashbury AJ. Attitudes to pain and pain relief in adult surgical patients. *Anaesthesiology*. 1996; **51**: 279–81.

73. Hallström I, Elander G, Rooke L. Pain and nutrition as experienced by patients with hip fracture. *Journal of Clinical Nursing*. 2000; **9**: 639–46.

74. Carr ECJ. Refusing analgesics: using continuous improvement to improve pain management in a surgical ward. *Journal of Clinical Nursing*. 2002; **11**: 743–52.

75. Bookbinder M, Coyle N, Kiss M *et al*. Implementing national standards for cancer pain management: program model and evaluation. *Journal of Pain and Symptom Management*. 1996; **12**: 334–47.

76. Chumbley GM, Hall GM, Salmon P. Patient-controlled analgesia: an assessment by 200 patients. *Anaesthesia*. 1998; **53**: 216–21.

77. Manias E, Botti M, Bucknall T. Patients' decision-making strategies for managing postoperative pain. *Journal of Pain*. 2006; **7**: 428–37.

78. Williams DC, Golding J, Phillips K, Towell A. Perceived control, locus of control and preparatory information: effects on the perception of an acute pain stimulus. *Personality and Individual Differences.* 2004; **36**: 1681–91.

79. Green CR, Tait AR. Attitudes of healthcare professionals regarding different modalities used to manage acute postoperative pain. *Acute Pain.* 2002; **4**: 15–21.

80. Rosenberger PH, Jokl P, Cameron A, Ickovics JR. Shared decision making, preoperative expectations, and postoperative reality: Differences in physician and patient predictions and ratings of knee surgery outcomes. *Arthroscopy: The Journal of Arthroscopic and Related Surgery.* 2005; **21**: 562–9.

81. Salmon P, Manyande A. Good patients cope with their pain: postoperative analgesia and nurses' perceptions of their patients' pain. *Pain.* 1996; **68**: 63–8.

82. Bennett D, Carr D. Opiophobia as a barrier to the treatment of pain. *Journal of Pain and Palliative Care Pharmacotherapy.* 2002; **16**: 105–9.

83. Pincus T, Burton AK, Vogel S, Field AP. A systematic review of psychological factors as predictors of chronicity/disability in prospective cohorts of low back pain. *Spine.* 2002; **27**: 109–20.

∗ 84. Kendall NAS, Linton SJ, Main CJ. *Guide to assessing psycho-social yellow flags in acute low back pain: Risk factors for long-term disability and work loss.* Wellington: Accident Compensation Corporation and the New Zealand Guidelines Group, 1997.

85. Bongers PM, de Winter CR, Kompier MA, Hildebrandt VH. Psychosocial factors at work and musculoskeletal disease. *Scandinavian Journal of Work, Environment and Health.* 1993; **19**: 297–312.

86. Buer N, Linton SJ. Fear-avoidance beliefs and catastrophizing: occurrence and risk factor in back pain and ADL in the general population. *Pain.* 2002; **99**: 485–91.

87. Sullivan MJ, Rodgers WM, Wilson PM *et al.* An experimental investigation of the relation between catastrophizing and activity intolerance. *Pain.* 2002; **100**: 47–53.

88. van den Hout JH, Vlaeyen JW, Houben RM *et al.* The effects of failure feedback and pain-related fear on pain report, pain tolerance, and pain avoidance in chronic low back pain patients. *Pain.* 2001; **92**: 247–57.

89. Picavet HS, Vlaeyen JW, Schouten JS. Pain catastrophizing and kinesiophobia: predictors of chronic low back pain. *American Journal of Epidemiology.* 2002; **156**: 1028–34.

90. Burton AK, Tillotson KM, Main CJ, Hollis S. Psychosocial predictors of outcome in acute and subchronic low back trouble. *Spine.* 1995; **20**: 722–8.

91. Edwards R, Fillingim RB, Maixner W *et al.* Catastrophizing predicts changes in thermal pain responses after resolution of acute dental pain. *Journal of Pain.* 2004; **5**: 164–70.

∗ 92. Linton SJ, Vlaeyen J, Ostelo R. The back pain beliefs of health care providers: are we fear-avoidant? *Journal of Occupational Rehabilitation.* 2002; **12**: 223–32.

93. Abenhaim L, Rossignol M, Valat JP *et al.* The role of activity in the therapeutic management of back pain. Report of the International Paris Task Force on Back Pain. *Spine.* 2000; **25**: 1–33.

94. ANAES. Diagnostic and therapeutic management of common lumbago and sciatica of less than 3 months duration. Recommendations of the ANAES. Agence Nationale d'Accreditation et d'Evaluation en Sante. *Journal de Radiologie.* 2000; **81**: 1665–6.

95. Ostelo RWJG, van Tulder MW, Vlaeyen JWS *et al.* Behavioural treatment for chronic low-back pain. *Cochrane Database of Systematic Reviews.* 2000; **CD002014**.

96. Clinical Standards Advisory Group. *Back Pain: Report of a CSAG Committee on Back Pain.* London: HMSO, 1994.

97. Waddell G, Feder G, Lewis M. Systematic reviews of bed rest and advice to stay active for acute low back pain. *British Journal of General Practice.* 1997; **47**: 647–52.

98. Bishop A, Foster NE. Do physical therapists in the United Kingdom recognize psychosocial factors in patients with acute low back pain? *Spine.* 2005; **30**: 1316–22.

99. Gonzalez-Urzelai V, Palacio-Elua L, Lopez-de-Munain J. Routine primary care management of acute low back pain: adherence to clinical guidelines. *European Spine Journal.* 2003; **12**: 589–94.

100. Dey P, Simpson CW, Collins SI *et al.* Implementation of RCGP guidelines for acute low back pain: a cluster randomised controlled trial. *British Journal of General Practice.* 2004; **54**: 33–7.

101. Rozenberg S, Allaert FA, Savarieau B *et al.* Compliance among general practitioners in France with not to prescribe bed rest for acute low back pain. *Joint Bone Spine.* 2004; **71**: 56–9.

102. Coudeyre E, Rannou F, Tubach F *et al.* General practitioners' fear-avoidance beliefs influence their management of patients with low back pain. *Pain.* 2006; **124**: 330–7.

103. Poiraudeau S, Rannou F, Baron G *et al.* Fear-avoidance beliefs about back pain in patients with subacute low back pain. *Pain.* 2006; **124**: 305–11.

104. Devine EC. Effects of psychoeducational care for adult surgical patients: a meta-analysis of 191 studies. *Patient Education and Counselling.* 1992; **19**: 129–42.

∗105. Bandolier. Preoperative information-giving interventions and pain. Available from: www.jr2.ox.ac.uk/bandolier/booth/painpag/Acutrev/Other/AP061.html (accessed 17th August 2006).

106. Suls J, Wan CK. Effects of sensory and procedural information on coping with stressful medical procedures and pain: a meta-analysis. *Journal of Consulting and Clinical Psychology.* 1989; **57**: 372–9.

107. Johnston M, Vogele C. Benefits of psychological preparation for surgery: a meta-analysis. *Annals of Behavioral Medicine.* 1993; **15**: 245–56.

108. Dalton JA, Blau W, Lindley C *et al.* Changing acute pain management to improve patient outcomes: An

educational approach. *Journal of Pain and Symptom Management.* 1999; **17**: 277–87.

109. Kiecolt-Glaser JK, Page GG, Marucha PT *et al.* Psychological influences on surgical recovery: perspectives from psychoneuroimmunology. *American Psychologist.* 1998; **53**: 1209–18.

*110. Vlaeyen JWS. Are we "fear-avoidant"? *Pain.* 2006; **124**: 240–1.

111. Modic MT, Obuchowski NA, Ross JS *et al.* Acute low back pain and radiculopathy: MR imaging findings and their prognostic role and effect on outcome. *Radiology.* 2005; **237**: 597–604.

112. Harmer M, Davies KA. The effect of education, assessment and a standard prescription on postoperative pain management. *Anaesthesia.* 1998; **53**: 424–30.

113. Rainville J, Carlson N, Polatin P *et al.* Exploration of physicians' recommendations for activities in chronic low back pain. *Spine.* 2000; **25**: 2210–20.

114. Buchbinder R, Jolley D, Wyatt M. Population based intervention to change back pain beliefs and disability: three part evaluation. *British Medical Journal.* 2001; **322**: 1516–20.

115. Buchbinder R, Jolley D. Population based intervention to change back pain beliefs and disability: three year follow up population survey. *British Medical Journal.* 2004; **328**: 321.

116. Li LC, Bombardier C. Physical therapy management of low back pain: an exploratory survey of therapist approaches. *Physical Therapy.* 2001; **81**: 1018–28.

117. Dalton JA, Carlson J, Blau W *et al.* Documentation of pain assessment and treatment: how are we doing? *Pain Management Nursing.* 2001; **2**: 54–64.

118. Morley S, Shapiro D, Biggs J. Developing manuals for the cognitive behavioural treatment of chronic pain. 1999. A prototype manual for one aspect of a complex treatment and an evaluation of the methodology. Accessed June 14, 2006. Available from: www.leeds.ac.uk/medicine/ psychiatry/staff/morley_docs/Attention%20Management %20Training%20in%20Chronic%20Pain.htm.

119. Voss JA, Good M, Yates B. Sedative music reduces anxiety and pain during chair rest after open-heart surgery. *Pain.* 2004; **112**: 197–203.

120. Good M. Effects of relaxation and music on postoperative pain: a review. *Journal of Advanced Nursing.* 1996; **24**: 905–14.

121. Evans D. The effectiveness of music as an intervention for hospital patients: a systematic review. *Journal of Advanced Nursing.* 2002; **37**: 8–18.

122. Haythornthwaite JA, Lawrence JW, Fauerbach JA. Brief cognitive intervention for burn pain. *Annals of Behavioral Medicine.* 2001; **23**: 42–9.

123. Logan HL, Baron RS, Kohout F. Sensory focus as therapeutic treatments for acute pain. *Psychosomatic Medicine.* 1995; **57**: 475–84.

124. Baron RS, Logan H, Hoppe S. Emotional and sensory focus as mediators of dental pain among patients differing in

desired and felt dental control. *Health Psychology.* 1993; **12**: 381–9.

*125. Bandolier. Relaxation techniques for acute pain management. Accessed August 17, 2006. Available from: http://www.jr2.ox.ac.uk/bandolier/booth/painpag/Acutrev/ Other/AP018.html.

126. Seers K, Carroll D. Relaxation techniques for acute pain management: a systematic review. *Journal of Advanced Nursing.* 1998; **27**: 466–75.

127. Luebbert K, Dahme B, Hasenbring M. The effectiveness of relaxation training in reducing treatment-related symptoms and improving emotional adjustment in acute non-surgical cancer treatment: a meta-analytical review. *Psycho-Oncology.* 2001; **10**: 490–502.

128. Ellis JA, Spanos NP. Cognitive behavioural interventions for children's distress during bone marrow aspirations and lumbar punctures: a critical review. *Journal of Pain and Symptom Management.* 1994; **9**: 96–108.

129. Wobst AHK. Hypnosis and surgery: Past, present, and future. *Anesthesia and Analgesia.* 2007; **104**: 1199–208.

130. Mauer MH, Burnett KF, Ouellette EA *et al.* Medical hypnosis and orthopedic hand surgery: pain perception, postoperative recovery, and therapeutic comfort. *International Journal of Clinical Experimental Hypnosis.* 1999; **47**: 144–61.

131. Montgomery GH, Weltz CR, Seltz M, Bovbjerg DH. Brief presurgery hypnosis reduces distress and pain in excisional breast biopsy patients. *International Journal of Clinical and Experimental Hypnosis.* 2002; **50**: 17–32.

132. Faymonville ME, Mambourg PH, Joris J *et al.* Psychological approaches during conscious sedation. Hypnosis versus stress reducing strategies: a prospective randomized study. *Pain.* 1997; **73**: 361–7.

133. Faymonville ME, Fissette J, Mambourg PH *et al.* Hypnosis as adjunct therapy in conscious sedation for plastic surgery. *Regional Anesthesia.* 1995; **20**: 145–51.

134. Defechereux T, Degauque C, Fumal I *et al.* Hypnosedation, a new method of anesthesia for cervical endocrine surgery. Prospective randomized study. *Annales de Chirurgie.* 2000; **125**: 539–46.

135. Lang EV, Benotsch EG, Fick LJ *et al.* Adjunctive nonpharmacological analgesia for invasive medical procedures: a randomised trial. *Lancet.* 2000; **355**: 1486–90.

136. van der Laan WH, van Leeuwen BL, Sebel PS *et al.* Therapeutic suggestion has no effect on postoperative morphine requirements. *Anesthesia and Analgesia.* 1996; **82**: 148–52.

137. Enqvist B, Bjorklund C, Englman M, Jakobsson J. Preoperative hypnosis reduces postoperative vomiting after surgery of the breasts. A prospective, randomized and blinded study. *Acta Anaesthesiologica Scandinavica.* 1997; **41**: 1028–32.

138. John Jr ME, Parrino JP. Practical hypnotic suggestion in ophthalmicsurgery. *American Journal of Opthalmology.* 1983; **96**: 540–2.

139. Rapkin DA, Straubing M, Holroyd JC. Guided imagery, hypnosis and recovery from head and neck cancer surgery: an exploratory study. *International Journal of Clinical and Experimental Hypnosis.* 1991; **39**: 215–26.

140. Enqvist B, von Konow L, Bystedt H. Pre- and perioperative suggestion in maxillofacial surgery: effects on blood loss and recovery. *International Journal of Clinical and Experimental Hypnosis.* 1995; **43**: 284–94.

141. Patterson DR, Jensen MP. Hypnosis and clinical pain. *Psychological Bulletin.* 2003; **129**: 495–521.

142. Cyna AM, McAuliffe GL, Andrew M. Hypnosis for pain relief in labour and childbirth: a systematic review. *British Journal of Anaesthesia.* 2004; **93**: 505–11.

143. Stewart JH. Hypnosis in contemporary medicine. *Mayo Clinic Proceedings.* 2005; **80**: 511–24.

144. Koes BW, van Tulder MW, Ostelo R *et al.* Clinical guidelines for the management of low back pain in primary care. *Spine.* 2001; **26**: 2504–14.

145. Linton SJ. Early identification and intervention in the prevention of musculoskeletal pain. *American Journal of Industrial Medicine.* 2002; **41**: 433–42.

*146. Boersma K, Linton SJ. Screening to identify patients at risk profiles of psychological risk factors for early intervention. *Clinical Journal of Pain.* 2005; **21**: 38–43.

147. Boersma K, Linton SJ. Early identification of patients at risk of developing persistent back problem: The predictive validity of The Örebro Musculoskeletal Pain Questionnaire. *Clinical Journal of Pain.* 2003; **19**: 80–6.

148. Pulliam CB, Gatchel RJ, Gardea MA. Psychosocial differences in high risk versus low risk acute low-back pain patients. *Journal of Occupational Rehabilitation.* 2001; **11**: 43–52.

149. Linton SJ. Do psychological factors increase the risk for back pain in the general population in both a cross-sectional and prospective analysis? *European Journal of Pain.* 2005; **9**: 355–61.

*150. Boersma K, Linton SJ. How does persistent pain develop? An analysis of the relationship between psychological variables, pain and function across stages of chronicity. *Behaviour Research and Therapy.* 2005; **43**: 1495–507.

151. Boersma K, Linton SJ. Psychological processes underlying the development of a chronic pain problem: A prospective study of the relationship between profiles of psychological variables in the fear–avoidance model and disability. *Clinical Journal of Pain.* 2006; **22**: 160–6.

*152. Linton SJ, van Tulder MW. Preventive interventions for back and neck pain problems: What is the evidence? *Spine.* 2001; **26**: 778–87.

153. Jellema P, van der Windt DAMW, van der Horst HE *et al.* Should treatment of (sub) acute low back pain be aimed at psychosocial prognostic factors? Results of a cluster-randomised clinical trial in general practice. *British Medical Journal.* 2005; **331**: 84–90.

154. Roland M, Waddell G, Klaber-Moffett J *et al. The back book*, 2nd edn. Norwich: Stationery Office, 2002.

155. Faas A, Chavannes AW, Koes BW *et al.* NGH-Standaard Lage-Rugpijn. *Huisarts en Wetenschap.* 1996; **39**: 18–31.

156. Linton SJ, Gross D, Schultz IZ *et al.* Prognosis and the identification of workers risking disability: Research issues and directions for future research. *Journal of Occupational Rehabilitation.* 2005; **15**: 459–74.

157. Marhold C, Linton SJ, Melin L. A cognitive-behavioral return-to-work program: effects on pain patients with a history of long-term versus short-term sick leave. *Pain.* 2001; **91**: 155–63.

158. Linton SJ, Andersson T. Can chronic disability be prevented? A randomized trial of a cognitive-behavioral intervention and two forms of information for spinal pain patients. *Spine.* 2000; **25**: 2825–31.

159. Von Korff M, Moore JE, Lorig K *et al.* A randomized trial of a lay-led self-management group intervention for back pain patients in primary care. *Spine.* 1998; **23**: 2608–15.

160. Elders LAM, van der Beek AJ, Burdork A. Return to work after sickness absence due to back disorders: A systematic review of intervention strategies. *International Archives of Occupational and Environmental Health.* 2000; **73**: 339–48.

161. Moore JE, Von Korff M, Cherkin D *et al.* A randomized trial of a cognitive-behavioral program for enhancing back pain self care in a primary care setting. *Pain.* 2000; **88**: 145–53.

162. Taimela S, Takala EP, Asklöf T *et al.* Active treatment of chronic neck pain: A prospective randomized intervention. *Spine.* 2000; **25**: 1021–7.

163. Linton SJ, Nordin E. A 5-year follow-up evaluation of the health and economic consequences of an early cognitive behavioral intervention for back pain: A randomized controlled trial. *Spine.* 2006; **31**: 853–8.

164. Linton SJ, Ryberg M. A cognitive-behavioral group intervention as prevention for persistent neck and back pain in a non-patient population: A randomized controlled trial. *Pain.* 2001; **90**: 83–90.

165. Turner JA, Jensen MP, Romano JM. Do beliefs, coping, and catastrophizing independently predict functioning in patients with chronic pain? *Pain.* 2000; **85**: 115–25.

166. Williams ACdeC, H Oakley Davies, Chadury Y. Simple pain rating scales hide complex idiosyncratic meanings. *Pain.* 2000; **85**: 457–63.

167. Cohen FL. Postsurgical pain relief: patients' status and nurses' medication choices. *Pain.* 1980; **9**: 265–74.

168. Donovan BD. Patients attitudes to postoperative pain relief. *Anaesthesia and Intensive Care.* 1983; **11**: 125–9.

169. Lavies N, Hart L, Rounsefell B, Runciman W. Identification of patient, medical and nursing staff attitudes to postoperative opioid analgesia: stage 1 of a longitudinal study of postoperative analgesia. *Pain.* 1992; **48**: 313–9.

170. Svensson I, Sjöström B, Haljamäe H. Influence of expectations and actual pain experiences on satisfaction with postoperative pain management. *European Journal of Pain.* 2001; **5**: 125–33.

171. Jensen MP, Mendoza T, Hanna DB *et al.* The analgesic effects that underlie patient satisfaction with treatment. *Pain.* 2004; **110**: 480–7.

172. Jamison RN, Taft K, O'Hara JP, Ferrante FM. Psychosocial and pharmacologic predictors of satisfaction with

intravenous patient-controlled analgesia. *Anesthesia and Analgesia.* 1993; **77**: 121–5.

173. Johnson LR, Magnami B, Chan V, Ferante FM. Modifiers of patient-controlled analgesia efficacy. Locus of control. *Pain.* 1999; **39**: 17–22.

174. Jamison RN, Ross MJ, Hoopman P *et al.* Assessment of postoperative pain management: patient satisfaction and perceived helpfulness. *Clinical Journal of Pain.* 1997; **13**: 229–36.

175. Dawson R, Spross JA, Jablonski ES *et al.* Probing the paradox of patients' satisfaction with inadequate pain management. *Journal of Pain and Symptom Management.* 2002; **23**: 211–20.

176. Riley JL, Meyers CD, Robinson ME *et al.* Factors predicting orofacial pain patient satisfaction with improvement. *Journal of Orofacial Pain.* 2001; **15**: 29–35.

177. McCracken LM, Klock PA, Mingay DJ *et al.* Assessment of satisfaction with treatment for chronic pain. *Journal of Pain and Symptom Management.* 1997; **14**: 292–9.

178. Miaskowski C, Nichols R, Brody R, Synold T. Assessment of patient satisfaction using the American Pain Society's Quality Assurance Standards on acute and cancer-related pain. *Journal of Pain and Symptom Management.* 1994; **9**: 5–11.

179. Cepeda MS, Africano JM, Polo R *et al.* What decline in pain intensity is meaningful to patients with acute pain? *Pain.* 2003; **105**: 51–7.

180. Daniel HC, Van Der Merwe J. Cognitive behavioural approaches and neuropathic pain. In: Cervero F, Jensen TS (eds). *Handbook of clinical neurology.* Edinburgh: Elsevier, 2006: 855–68.

16

Psychological interventions for acute pediatric pain

CHRISTINA LIOSSI AND LINDA S FRANCK

KEY LEARNING POINTS

- Psychological factors play an important role in shaping pain perception in children. These factors include personality (temperament), mood (anxiety, depression), and cognitions (attitudes, beliefs, meanings, expectancies, memories of previous painful experiences).
- Comprehensive assessment of the psychological factors that shape pain perception is imperative to maximize the success of pain management interventions.
- Psychological interventions are useful for the management of acute pediatric pain, although evidence for their efficacy varies depending on type of pain.

- For procedure-related pain, particularly needle procedures, distraction, hypnosis, and cognitive-behavior therapy are evidence-based interventions.
- For postoperative pain, preparation, guided imagery, and cognitive behavior therapy are promising.
- For acute pain due to illness or injury, cognitive behavior therapy is promising.
- How parents feel and what they think and do influences their child's pain perception and response. Parents need to be included in pain management interventions.

INTRODUCTION

The most common type of pain experienced by children is acute pain resulting from injury, illness, or, in many cases, necessary medical procedures. Healthy children undergo immunizations repeatedly throughout their childhood. Currently, the Advisory Committee on Immunization Practices (www.csc.gov/nip/acip), the American Academy of Family Physicians (www.aafp.org), and the Canadian Paediatric Society (www.cps.ca) recommend over 20 various immunizations before the age of 18 years. A variety of medical conditions can result in different levels of pain for

children from mild to extreme. These include, but are not limited to, burns, otitis media, pharyngitis, acute headaches, orthopedic injuries, some cancers, sickle cell crises, and procedures such as venepunctures, lumbar punctures, and bone marrow aspirations. This chapter will focus on:

- **Procedure-related pain.** Defined as pain caused by a diagnostic or treatment procedure in the conscious patient (e.g. venepuncture, lumbar puncture, dental). These procedures, although sometimes perceived as intensely painful by children, are not necessarily tissue damaging or invasive (e.g. physiotherapy).

- **Acute postoperative pain.** Defined as pain after a surgical procedure, sometimes associated with drains, chest or nasogastric tubes, or related to postoperative mobilization and resumption of daily activities.
- **Acute pain due to an illness or injury.** Defined as disease-related physiological processes that cause tissue damage and acute or recurrent pain (e.g. sickle cell crisis, fractures with osteogenesis imperfecta, cancer) of less than three months duration.

SIGNIFICANCE OF THE PROBLEM

There is now a substantial body of research affirming that children who have been repeatedly exposed to anxiety-provoking painful medical events are at increased risk for developing adult dysfunctional cognitions and avoidant attitudes toward health care.[1] In some cases, serious mental health problems, such as posttraumatic stress can occur. Posttraumatic stress is characterized by severe memories of the traumatic event; avoidance of people, places, and things that remind the child of the trauma; poor sleep and nightmares; and difficulty feeling calm and in control. In a study of over 300 cancer survivors and their parents,[2] distressing recollections of pain and painful procedures were prominent, in both mothers' and children's accounts, supporting the notion that poorly managed pain during procedures contributes to long-term psychological difficulties for children and their parents. Relatively sophisticated theories have been developed that explain these risk mechanisms and give direction to specific approaches for clinical intervention.[3]

In recent years, great progress has been made in the use of pharmacological analgesia to prevent and treat children's acute pain. However, as yet there are no perfect analgesics that provide complete pain relief without risk or side effects. Thus, the risks of analgesics may outweigh the benefit for some acute pain situations, they may provide incomplete analgesia, or have bothersome side effects such that children or parents refuse them.[4] Furthermore, pharmacological analgesia does not adequately address the emotional, cognitive, and behavioral components that are integral to pain perception. Consequently, effective pain management requires an interdisciplinary approach and must include behavioral, psychological, and physical techniques, which can be used alone or in combination with pharmacologic treatment.

This chapter summarizes current knowledge about the theoretical, empirical, and clinical characteristics of certain psychological interventions, and aims to encourage practitioners working with children to make informed choices in their treatment selection, and understand the potential risks, as well as benefits, of specific treatment choices for their young patients. The chapter begins by briefly discussing a model of acute pediatric pain and the general assessment strategy that is required when evaluating children experiencing pain. It continues by presenting relevant developmental and cultural considerations. Following this, psychological interventions that are widely used in clinical practice and have been empirically investigated in acute pain management with children (such as preparation, relaxation, distraction, hypnosis, and multicomponent cognitive-behavioral programs) are presented in detail. For each intervention the available evidence supporting its efficacy for postoperative, procedure-related, and illness-related acute pain is discussed. The chapter concludes by reviewing the state of the knowledge regarding the role of parents in pediatric pain perception and management.

PSYCHOLOGICAL INFLUENCES ON CHILDREN'S ACUTE PAIN

Most researchers agree that many factors can influence a child's response to pain including historical events (previous personal and family experience with pain), environmental, developmental, sociocultural, psychological (cognitive, emotional, behavioral), and contextual.[5, 6, 7] Identifying psychological factors associated with acute pain not only has theoretical value, but is vital for the development and refinement of effective treatments. **Figure 16.1** presents a model of acute pediatric pain based on the biobehavioral model of pain[5, 8] and recent research findings. The main child-related factors contributing to pain perception and response are briefly discussed below.

Anxiety

Preoperative anxiety in young children undergoing surgery is associated with a more painful postoperative recovery and a higher incidence of sleep and other behavioral problems.[9][IV]

Anxiety sensitivity

Anxiety sensitivity is the fear of arousal-related somatic sensations, arising from beliefs that these sensations have harmful consequences (e.g. fear of palpitations arising from beliefs that cardiac sensations lead to heart attacks).[10] Lipsitz and colleagues[11] found that youngsters with noncardiac chest pain had higher levels of anxiety symptoms and anxiety sensitivity compared to youngsters with benign heart murmurs.

Expectancies

Expectancies are beliefs about a future state of affairs and arise from knowledge about outcome contingencies. They are subjective probabilities and vary in certainty.[12] Palermo and Drotar[13] in their model of postoperative pain propose that a child's postoperative pain report is a product of background variables (age, surgery severity, medication

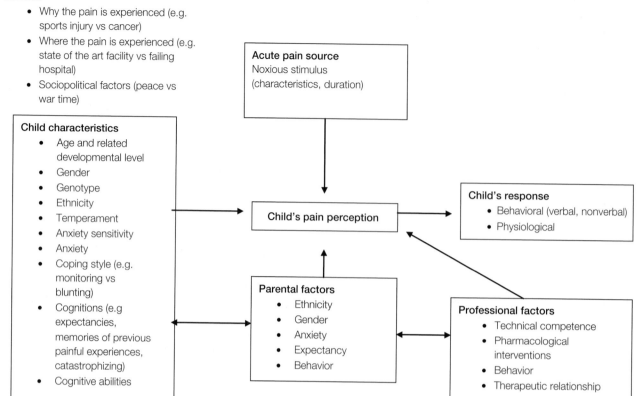

Figure 16.1 A model of acute pediatric pain.

received), anticipatory emotions (anxiety), and expectations about pain and analgesia. Logan and Rose[14] found that there is self-fulfilling prophesy in adolescents' postoperative pain experience, wherein teens who expect to have high levels of postoperative pain ultimately report more pain and use more opioid (via patient-controlled analgesia (PCA)) than those who expect lower levels of pain.

Temperament

Temperament is the behavior style or the "how" of behavior as contrasted with the abilities, or "what" of behavior, and the motivations, or "why" of behavior.[15] A more pain-sensitive temperament has been associated with increased reports of pain and anxiety during painful medical procedures. Chen and colleagues[16] found that pain sensitivity moderated the effectiveness of a psychological intervention in reducing observer-related distress during lumbar punctures. Children with higher pain sensitivity who received the intervention showed greater decreases in distress and systolic blood pressure than did children with lower pain sensitivity. In the control group, those with high pain sensitivity showed greater increases in these variables over time. In a postoperative setting, Helgadottir and Wilson[17] found that after tonsillectomy children who were more temperamentally active and had lower

temperamental thresholds, had more negative moods, were distractible, and reported higher pain intensity.

Catastrophizing

Catastrophizing is defined as "an exaggerated negative mental set brought to bear during actual or anticipated pain experience."[18] Bennett-Branson and Craig[19] found that coping strategy use, perceived self-efficacy, and frequency of catastrophizing thoughts were significantly predictive of children's postoperative pain, affective distress, and physical recovery. Parental anxiety was positively related to child anxiety, and inversely related to child self-efficacy and frequency of cognitive coping.

Coping style

In the cognitive–social model of health-information processing, developed by Miller,[20, 21] the style of information processing where individuals typically cope with threat by distracting themselves and avoiding threatening cues is called "blunting." Blunters should respond best to pain management strategies such as distraction, which require them to direct their attention away from the noxious event or stimulus. In contrast, individuals who typically search for and tune into threatening material and attend closely to physical sensations, termed "monitors" by Miller and colleagues,[21] should do best with pain management strategies such as sensation monitoring, which allow them to monitor or attend to the pain situation, while cognitively reconceptualizing the noxious stimulation in an objective, less affectively arousing manner.[21, 22]

Memory

Children's memories of painful experiences can have long-term consequences for their reaction to later painful events and their acceptance of later healthcare interventions.[23] Chen and colleagues[16] demonstrated that at any given age, children with greater exaggeration in negative memory of anxiety and pain, report higher distress during a future lumbar puncture.

DEVELOPMENTAL CONSIDERATIONS

Children and adolescents experience the same amount of pain as adults do for similar procedures and in many cases

even more. For example, in athletes scheduled for arthroscopic anterior cruciate ligament reconstructive surgery using the patella autograft procedure, adolescents reported greater pain intensity, higher state anxiety, and greater pain catastrophizing (particularly helplessness and ruminations) than did adults.[24]

Children's understanding of pain and its relief is thought to follow Piagetian developmental stages (see **Table 16.1**), therefore pain measurement and management needs to be developmentally appropriate.[27] For example, in one study, children who received age-appropriate information about their upcoming medical procedure displayed less overt distress than those receiving age-advanced information.[28][III]

ETHNIC AND CULTURAL CONSIDERATIONS

Cultural competence in treatment is critical to adapting psychological treatment paradigms to clients from diverse cultural, religious, and racial/ethnic groups. Different cultural groups are likely to have varying norms regarding many relevant issues, such as the role of the family, styles

Table 16.1 Developmental considerations in relation to psychological interventions for children's pain.

Developmental stage	Cognitive abilities	Understanding of pain	Psychological interventions
Preoperational (2–7 years)	Learns to use language and to represent objects by images and words Thinking is still egocentric: has difficulty taking the viewpoint of others Classifies objects by a single feature, e.g. groups together all the red blocks regardless of shape or all the square blocks regardless of color	Pain is understood as an aversive sensory experience Children chose action over thought strategies to deal with negative emotions[25]	Children benefit from interventions that are active, concrete, and outward focused, e.g. simple electronic toys that make animal noises, recite a sentence, or play a tune when the child touches them may be effective distractors[26]
Concrete operational (7–11 years)	Can think logically about objects and events Achieves conservation of number (age 6 years), mass (age 7 years), and weight (age 9 years) Classifies objects according to several features and can order them in series along a single dimension, such as size.	Incomplete understating of the psychosocial nature of pain Self-regulatory abilities are developing Limitations of domain-specific knowledge, memory, and motivation	Use of a narrative rather than a rationalistic paradigm is preferable In a story, abstract concepts can become concrete, and analogy and metaphor can be used to demonstrate reasoning
Formal operational (11 years and over)	Can think logically about abstract propositions and test hypotheses systematically Becomes concerned with the hypothetical, the future, and ideological problems	Pain is understood as a psychosocial experience Has the ability for self-reflection and perspective taking, and can understand causality	Children can benefit from verbally based, abstract, and introspective interventions, e.g. reframing beliefs by realistically appraising an aversive situation and their ability to cope with it

of coping with adverse life events, the cultural meaning of pain, the meaning of certain adverse life events such as illness, manners of trust and mistrust, stigma associated with disease, and reliance on informal sources of help and care.

Unfortunately, only a few studies have specifically addressed cultural and ethnic issues in children's pain. Pfefferbaum and colleagues[29] found a decrease in observed and reported distress with increasing age in children undergoing lumbar punctures or bone marrow aspirations, regardless of ethnic groups. Hispanic parents, however, reported significantly higher levels of anxiety than did Ango-American parents. Jones and colleagues[30] found few ethnic differences in parents' desire to be present during their child's painful medical procedures with most parents overall preferring to remain present even for highly invasive procedures. Interestingly, ethnic differences were established in the parents' desire to have the physician decide whether the parent should stay, with black parents less likely to want the physician to decide and English-speaking Hispanic parents more likely to want the physician to decide.

MANAGEMENT

A basic principle of all clinical practice is that assessment should precede the introduction of interventions. Pain can be measured using self-report, behavioral observation,[31] or physiologic measures, depending on the age of the child and his or her communication capabilities.[27, 32] Pain assessment is discussed in more detail elsewhere in this volume (see Chapter 38, Pain assessment in children in the *Practice and Procedures* volume of this series). Accurate acute pain assessment requires consideration of the plasticity and complexity of children's pain perception (see **Figure 16.1**), the influence of psychological and developmental factors discussed above (see above under Psychological influences on children's acute pain), and the appreciation of the potential severity and specific types of pain experienced.[7] There are at present no composite measures of these key factors, and assessment of anxiety, temperament, catastrophizing, and pain coping style are all measured with different instruments, all demonstrating good reliability and validity.

Psychological interventions for acute pain include a wide variety of physiological, behavioral, and cognitive techniques aimed at reducing pain and pain-related distress through the modulation of thoughts, behaviors, and sensory information.[33] Over the past two decades, the psychological management of children experiencing acute pain and their parents has received much attention by both the clinical and research communities. A large and rich clinical treatment literature has developed, describing interventions that are theoretically sound and have good clinical utility. Many of these treatments have been used by practitioners for some time, and are well accepted in the

field. Most important, there is now a growing research literature testing the efficacy of these interventions with pediatric populations. Pediatric procedures, particularly needle procedures, have typically been used as a paradigm through which acute pain interventions have been studied. Though much research remains to be done, the efficacy of at least some treatments is supported theoretically, clinically, and empirically.

The approach to the management of acute pain varies according to the origin of the pain and the estimated intensity and duration of the expected pain. As a general principle, a quiet environment, calm adults, and clear, confident instructions increase the likelihood that the specific psychological strategy selected will be effective.

PREPARATION

Preparation includes specific interventions to provide information and reduce anxiety. Leventhal and Johnson,[34] in their Self-Regulation Theory, propose that reactions to threatening situations are influenced by cognitive factors; therefore individuals should be able to consciously influence the experience associated with such situations. Providing three types of information is central to the Self-Regulation Theory: information is provided about the procedure itself (i.e. steps that children must perform and steps that healthcare professionals will perform); the sensations the patient can expect to feel (e.g. sharp scratch, numbness); and about how to cope with the procedure.

A meta-analysis of predominantly adult studies[35][I] involving different stressful medical procedures and various indicators of physical and psychological comfort showed that a combination of procedural and sensory preparation was significantly better than control on all measures (negative affect, self-rated pain, other-rated pain/distress). Effect sizes were larger for the combination than either sensory or procedural information alone, suggesting that this is the most powerful intervention. Suls and Wan[35] explain the effectiveness of such information with their dual-process preparation hypothesis. The procedural information specifies events on which sensory information can be mapped; the sensory information assures that the anticipation of the procedural events is not interpreted in threatening terms.

For pediatric patients, research suggests that psychological preparation for surgery generally improves psychological adjustment and the prepared patients require less pain medication during recovery. When preparatory information also includes instruction or training on coping with postoperative pain, prepared patients require significantly less analgesia than control patients.[36][II], [37] In a recent study, more specifically concerning venepuncture in children, Kolk and colleagues[38][II] found that distress before and during venepuncture was significantly reduced if parents themselves applied the anesthetic cream and read their child a simple story containing information about the venepuncture procedure and the sensations the child was likely to experience. However, a recent meta-analysis[39][I] of 28 trials with 1951 participants receiving various psychological interventions for procedure-related pain management commented that while there may be preliminary evidence to support the efficacy of information/preparation there is not enough evidence at this time to make strong conclusions.

A growing body of literature suggests that preparatory interventions for stressful medical procedures are most effective when they conform to the patient's preferred way of coping.[40, 41, 42, 43, 44, 45] The literature examining individual differences in information processing or coping styles in response to pain management interventions has been more limited. The few available studies have also found that participants report less pain[46] and less physiological arousal during a painful procedure[47] when the content of the information provided in the intervention is matched to their coping style. However, there is some evidence that individuals react better to a distraction strategy in the early stages of coping with pain, regardless of their individual coping style, whereas the effectiveness of sensation monitoring strategies may be more apparent in chronic pain situations, during which sustained distraction is less feasible.[48, 49]

Based on available evidence, psychological preparation can improve acute pain management and postoperative recovery. However, the type of preparation should be matched to the child's coping style and stage of the procedure.

DISTRACTION

Attentional or cognitive strategies used to process information presented by painful stimuli appear to modulate (diminish or magnify) the salience of these events.[50, 51] Attentional capacity during painful episodes may be diverted away from pain and occupied by focusing on information irrelevant to the noxious stimulus (see **Box 16.1** for examples of distraction techniques). Alternatively, attention can be focused away from noxious stimulation by suppressing awareness of it. Suppression of pain, like distraction, entails directing attention away from a stimulus but, unlike distraction, does not involve thinking about things other than pain. A number of studies have examined distraction during painful procedures with good results.[52, 53, 54, 55, 56, 57, 58, 59, 60]

Leventhal[61] and Cioffi[62] have argued that thinking differently about pain may have longer-term effects than not thinking about the pain at all, because thinking about noxious events in a way that elaborates their benign content may provide a template for evaluating the next unpleasant event. Distraction may avoid making salient the worst emotionally charged elements of pain, but it does not provide a method of changing the meaning of

---

Box 16.1 Distraction techniques

Mental exercises Count back from 1000 in 7s; think of an animal beginning with each letter of the alphabet in turn; remember your favorite baseball game in detail; try to come up with some of your own mental exercises.

Pleasant memories and fantasies Imagine vividly concrete memories of a past experience (e.g. an enjoyable holiday) and fantasies (what will you do with the new bicycle that you get for Christmas?)

Counting thoughts Note the occurrence of any thoughts that go through your mind (for example, by marking a mark on a piece of paper) and put them to one side rather than letting them influence the way you feel. *Note to the healthcare professional: Counting thoughts is designed to promote distance from negative thinking.*

Focus on an object Focus your attention on an object and describe it to yourself in as much detail as possible, e.g. Where exactly is it? How big is it? What is it made of? Exactly how many of them are there? What is it for? Alternatively, describe your wider surroundings (e.g. room you're in).

---

what is happening. This has been proposed to account for some failures of distraction to provide analgesia,[63] and may also translate into relatively greater protection against future painful events for those who focus on sensory information during pain.[61] Fanurik and colleagues[64] found that children who were blunters in a matched (distraction) condition showed an increase in pain tolerance relative to baseline, whereas monitors using sensation monitoring showed no change from baseline.

Based on available evidence, distraction is effective in procedure-, particularly needle-related pain management.[39][I]

RELAXATION

McCaffery and Beebe[65] define relaxation as "a state of relative freedom from both anxiety and skeletal muscle tension, a quieting or calming of the mind and muscles." This situation is characterized by decreased muscle tone, lower heart and respiratory rates, normal blood pressure, decreased skin resistance and intense, slow alpha-waves in the brain.[65, 66, 67] There are different types of relaxation including tension-release,[68] autogenic,[69] and meditation.[70] **Box 16.2** describes a simple relaxation exercise and how it could be presented to a young patient.

The choice of relaxation technique depends on the pain problem, the patient's preferences and abilities, availability of professional expertise, and available time.

Box 16.2 Relaxation techniques

1. Choose a quiet place where you won't be interrupted.
2. Before you start, do a few gentle stretching exercises to relieve muscular tension.
3. Make yourself comfortable, either sitting or lying down.
4. Start to breathe slowly and deeply, in a calm and effortless way.
5. Gently tense, then relax, each part of your body, starting with your feet and working your way up to your face and head.
6. As you focus on each area, think of warmth, heaviness, and relaxation.
7. Push any distracting thoughts to the back of your mind; imagine them floating away.
8. Stay like this for about 20 minutes, then take some deep breaths and open your eyes, but stay sitting or lying for a few moments before you get up.

Box 16.3 Diaphragmatic breathing techniques

Learning to breathe from your diaphragm is a skill you were born with and have most probably lost. Babies naturally breathe from their diaphragms, and so do you when you are asleep. Diaphragmatic breathing may take some practice to relearn and once you have the skill again you can reduce the tension in your body rapidly by breathing this way for 5 minutes. To perform this exercise while sitting in a chair:

1. Sit comfortably, with your knees bent and your shoulders, head, and neck relaxed.
2. Place one hand on your upper chest and the other just below your rib cage. This will allow you to feel your diaphragm move as you breathe.
3. Tighten your stomach muscles, letting them fall inward as you exhale through pursed lips. The hand on your upper chest must remain as still as possible.

You may notice an increased effort will be needed to use the diaphragm correctly. At first, you'll probably get tired while doing this exercise. Keep at it, because with continued practice, diaphragmatic breathing will become easy and automatic.

At first, practice this exercise 5–10 minutes about three or four times per day. Gradually increase the amount of time you spend doing this exercise, and perhaps even increase the effort of the exercise by placing a book on your abdomen.

Patterson[71] points out that progressive muscle relaxation generally requires lengthy and frequent training before the technique is sufficiently mastered. Certain patient populations, burned children for example, are often too exhausted and ill to invest the time or have the discipline required to learn these techniques. Taal[72] expresses further objections to this technique because the muscles must be tensed before they can be relaxed. Muscle tension in burned parts of the body can further increase pain during wound care. In other words, even a simple technique, such as progressive muscle relaxation, can be inappropriate for specific patient populations. More benefit for these patients can be expected from the use of alternative techniques, such as meditation or autogenic relaxation.[71, 72]

Although approximately 43–58 percent of pediatric hospitals in the USA use relaxation across a variety of acute pain situations,[73] uncertainty exists in the pediatric pain literature regarding the efficacy of relaxation as a sole analgesic in acute pain management. This is also reflected in the adult pain literature (see Chapter 15, Psychological therapies – adults). Based on available evidence, the efficacy of relaxation as a sole technique for acute pain management is limited. However, it may be useful in combination with other psychological and pharmacologic interventions.

BREATHING TECHNIQUES

Simple breathing relaxation techniques are particularly useful in pain management, are easy and quick to learn,

can be employed immediately by the patient, and involve no risk.[74] However, even though breathing techniques are widely used in practice and form part of many relaxation interventions and multicomponent cognitive behavioral treatment programs, the individual effect of breathing exercises on acute pain has not been investigated. A recent literature review of 11 studies[74][V] using breathing exercises in the management of acute pain in general, and procedural pain in adult burn patients in particular, found insufficient evidence to establish the efficacy of breathing exercises in adult patients.

Box 16.3 describes a simple breathing exercise and how it could be presented to a young patient. Generally, given the lack of empirical evidence, the choice of a breathing technique, the moment to teach it, and how to coach the patient depend on the experience, background, and clinical judgment of the health professional. There is a lack of evidence of the effectiveness of breathing techniques as a single intervention in acute pain management.

HYPNOSIS

Hypnosis is a psychological state of heightened awareness and focused attention, in which critical faculties are reduced and susceptibility and receptiveness to ideas is greatly enhanced. Hypnosis is usually introduced to the patient as a suggestion for an imaginative experience. Hypnotic induction procedures traditionally involve suggestions to relax, although relaxation is not necessary for hypnosis, particularly with children who respond better to more active inductions. During hypnosis, the healthcare professional makes suggestions for changes in subjective experience, alterations in perception, sensation, emotion, thought, or behavior (see **Box 16.4** for examples of hypnotic inductions and suggestions).[75, 76]

Children have blurred boundaries between fantasy and reality which makes them particularly good candidates for hypnotic interventions. They are open to new experiences and find hypnosis interesting. The therapist guides the individual to concentrate and observe the suggested images as they are forming, and this promotes a feeling of being active and creative in the therapeutic process. Such an approach results in a kind of "playful" engagement between the therapist and the child as she imagines and awaits the images and emotions that emerge during a given exercise.[77] Unlike adults, children usually move and talk during hypnosis without this meaning that they are resisting the intervention. Young patients can also easily be taught and learn self-hypnosis.[78]

Hypnotic suggestions for analgesia are usually targeted towards both the sensory and affective dimensions of pain. Rainville and colleagues[79] pointed to the critical role that the nature of the hypnotic suggestion plays in pain management. Specifically, in a functional magnetic resonance imaging (fMRI) study suggestions for sensory reductions of pain resulted in decreased activity in the somatosensory cortex, and suggestions for affective pain reduction led to decreased activity in the arterior cingulate cortex (ACC), a part of the brain that processes emotion and suffering-related information.

Theoretical conceptualizations of hypnosis have been fiercely debated in the past and range from the ones that maintain that hypnosis represents a cognitive process distinct from normal day-to-day cognitive processes (i.e. the neodissociative[80] or dissociated control views[81]) to the social–cognitive models that suggest that the operative variables in hypnosis include contextual cues in the social environment, patient and subject expectancies, demand characteristics of the setting or situation, and role enactment.[82] The neodissociative model regards hypnosis as a state in which one or more forms of consciousness is split off from the rest of mental processing. Bowers and colleagues maintained that subsystems of control in the brain can be activated directly rather than through higher level executive control. In other words, the strategies subjects used to reduce pain were evoked automatically without any type of conscious strategy.[83, 84] According to the social–cognitive models, on the other hand, neither hypnotic induction nor the existence of an altered state of consciousness are necessary for hypnotic responding, including responses to suggestions for pain relief.[85] Hypnotic analgesia is thought to reduce pain instead through cognitive–behavioral mechanisms, in which changes in cognitions are thought to alter the affective states associated with pain.[85] This conceptualization is consistent with the evidence that cognitive–behavioral interventions reduce both acute[86][V], [87][I] and chronic clinical pain.[88][I] More recent theorists have suggested that attempting to explain the effects of hypnosis solely in terms of one school of thought presents distinctions that are too arbitrary.[82, 89] See Chapter 15, Psychological therapies – adults, for further evaluation of hypnosis in adult patients.

The findings from acute studies demonstrate consistent clinical effects with hypnotic analgesia that are superior to attention or standard care control conditions.[87][I], [90] Hypnosis has achieved status as an empirically validated, possibly efficacious intervention in the management of pediatric procedure-related pain,[91] according to the criteria devised by the American Psychological Association to judge the efficacy of psychological interventions.[92] All studies conducted to date[93, 94, 95, 96, 97, 98, 99, 100, 101, 102, 103] [II] found hypnosis effective in reducing the pain and anxiety of young patients during painful medical procedures, such as lumbar punctures, bone marrow aspirations, and voiding cystourethrography.

Limited support is available in the pediatric literature that hypnosis significantly lowers postoperative pain and anxiety ratings and contributes to shorter hospital stays. Lambert[104][II] randomly assigned 52 children (matched for sex, age, and diagnosis) to an experimental or control group. Significantly lower postoperative pain ratings and shorter hospital stays occurred for children in the

---

Box 16.4 Hypnotic techniques

Simple induction technique Just think about how you feel when you are building a Lego house at home; just let yourself feel that way now.

Topical anesthesia Just imagine painting numbing medicine on to that part of your body.

Moving pain away from the self Imagine for a while that that arm (or other body part) doesn't belong to you, isn't part of you … see it just floating out there by itself.

Directing attention to pain itself Imagine that you have come from another planet far deep in the universe where there is no pain … you have never experienced pain before … notice the discomfort very carefully … what sensations you have … how does it make you feel …

experimental group. State anxiety was decreased for the hypnosis group and increased postoperatively for the control group. This is in contrast to the adult literature in which a meta-analysis of 38 randomized controlled trials of different methods of psychological preparation prior to surgery reported that hypnosis did not reduce pain intensity or medication use.[105] [I]

Individual responsiveness to hypnotic suggestions varies. Four out of five studies[93, 98, 100, 101, 102] that have examined the relationship between the child's hypnotizability and pain relief during painful medical procedures reported a significant positive relationship between hypnotizability and clinical benefit following hypnosis treatment.

Based on available evidence, there is strong support for the efficacy of hypnosis in procedure-related pain management and a recent meta-analysis concluded that hypnosis is the most promising psychological intervention.[39]

GUIDED IMAGERY

Guided imagery is a self-regulatory technique that capitalizes on young patients' active imagination. Activities such as role-playing, pretending, and daydreaming are natural elements of children's play. Guided imagery was developed and refined by Roberto Assagioli[106] and involves paying attention to cognitively generated mental images. The child uses his or her imagination to create mental images, using as many senses as possible, to alter the pain experience. Naparstek[107] describes guided imagery as "a gentle but powerful technique that focuses and directs the imagination." She maintains that it is more than visualization (and since only approximately 55 percent of people are able to visualize strongly, this is worth bearing in mind); rather it involves all the senses. Naparstek[107] further elaborates that the body recognizes all sensory images as real, whether fact or fantasy. Research using positron emission tomography (PET) and fMRI methodologies[108] suggests that the neuronal processes underlying perception are also used in imagery "and can engage mechanisms used in memory, emotion and motor control" (p. 635). Furthermore, these researchers maintain, "there is much evidence that imagery of emotional events activates the autonomic nervous system and the amygdala. That is, visualizing an object has much the same effects on the body as actually seeing the object" (p. 641).

During a guided imagery session, a state of deep relaxation is usually induced using a relaxation technique which allows the child to then be guided in actively creating images that facilitate resolution of symptoms, such as pain. Imagery themes that may enhance safety include soothing environments (beach scenes, warmth of the sun, familiar places where the individual has felt safe), the construction of a protective structure, or the inclusion of a trusted individual. Two types of imagery can be incorporated in imagery exercises: directive, in which the

---

Box 16.5 Guided imagery techniques

Direct

Imagine your pain has a certain size, shape, and color … What does it feel like? Is it rough or smooth? Does it stay in one place or move around?… Allow the pain to melt and turn to a liquid the same size, shape, and color as before… let the liquid flow down to your arm or leg and let it flow out of your fingertips or toes. Watch it as it flows out of the room, out of the hospital, down the street.

Indirect

Ask the child to close their eyes, take several deep breaths, and relax. Introduce the exercise by giving them some background on the situation they will be visualizing. Encourage them to make use of all their senses as they imagine – sight, sound, physical sensations, and emotions. Suggest an image to children one sentence at a time, and pause for several seconds after each sentence to allow them time to process what you are saying and to visualize the picture. As images occur spontaneously, direct the child's attention by asking questions, e.g. "How do you feel here?", "When you observe this image, what feelings come forward?"

---

image is specifically described ("imagine being on a school trip") and nondirective, in which less specific description allows for the formation of more personalized and spontaneous imagery ("imagine being outdoors"; "find some special place") (see **Box 16.5** for suggestions of guided imagery exercises). Some children experience difficulty with a nondirective suggestion and prefer the more direct approach. Images range from the concrete, such as objects or people, to the more abstract, such as a color or metaphor.

A number of factors may influence success with guided imagery, including imaging ability (the ability to create vivid mental images and to experience those images as if they were almost real) and outcome expectancy (an individual's expectation regarding the effects of a particular intervention on pain). Although related, guided imagery differs from hypnosis in that the child, through imagery, attempts to create his own solution to the problem rather than the therapist offering suggestions and alternatives for change.

The evidence for the efficacy of guided imagery in acute pain management is limited. A recent randomized controlled trial[109][II] investigated imagery administered pre- and postoperatively, as a supplement to routine analgesics, for reduction of pain and anxiety after tonsillectomy and adenoidectomy in the ambulatory setting and at home in 73 children aged 7–12 years. After controlling for trait anxiety (i.e. personality-related anxiety) and for opioid and nonopioid analgesic intake one to four hours before pain measurement, the investigators found significantly lower self-reported pain and situation-related anxiety one to four hours after surgery in the imagery group, but not 22–27 hours after surgery.

Based on available evidence, there is strong theoretical support on guided imagery and one clinical trial suggesting efficacy for acute pain management.

COMBINED COGNITIVE AND BEHAVIORAL INTERVENTIONS

The most widely practiced and researched interventions in acute pain management are cognitive and behavioral. Cognitive behavioral interventions are based on the premise that symptoms develop and are maintained, at least in part, by maladaptive cognitions, as well as conditioned and learned behavioral responses.[110] Emphasis is given to the interdependence of thoughts, behaviors, feelings, as well as physiological responses. For the purpose of this review, cognitive interventions are defined as interventions which involve identifying and altering negative thinking styles related to anxiety about the painful situation, and replacing them with more positive beliefs and attitudes, leading to more adaptive behavior and coping styles.[111] Behavioral interventions are defined as interventions based on principles of behavioral science, as well as learning principles by targeting specific behaviors.[111] For pain management, cognitive and behavioral techniques are aimed at assisting the child develop and apply coping skills in order to manage the pain and distress, and when developmentally appropriate, to help the child comprehend how thoughts and behaviors can alter their experience of pain.[112] The treatment also focuses on conditioned emotional associations to memories and reminders of traumatic medical experiences, distorted cognitions about the event(s), and negative attributions about self, others, and the world. Treatment plans are based on comprehensive assessments and are individually tailored to address the patients' specific needs. The rationale for the use of cognitive and behavioral techniques is fully explained to young patients and their parents so that they can be active participants in developing and applying interventions in session, at home, and at the clinic. Parents are included in the treatment process to enhance support for the child, reduce parental distress, and teach appropriate strategies to manage child reactions. Cognitive–behavioral interventions are popular because the emphasis is goal directed, short term, teaching coping skills, promoting self-control, and enhancing self-efficacy.[113] Box 16.6 describes some of the commonly used cognitive–behavioral interventions in the management of acute pain in children.

Box 16.6 Cognitive–behavioral therapy interventions

Reframing

Reframing involves helping the child to modify or restructure how they perceive their difficulties, and the context in which they take place, in a different way. Aims to modify or restructure a child's view or perception of pain.

Modeling and rehearsal

Live or videotaped demonstration by another child of coping strategies relevant to the situation that the young patient is in.

Thought stopping

When the child begins to think about the painful experience refuses to allow negative thoughts to continue and gain strength by some positive and defined action (e.g. visualize a STOP sign in your mind's eye; saying "stop" out loud).

Positive self-statements

"I've had this procedure before and I coped successfully."

Cognitive and behavioral interventions may modulate pain, altering pain transmission and pain perception, by distracting attention from the pain stimulus, producing relaxation, or influencing mood or emotional context.[114] The evaluation of the current literature regarding the efficacy of combined interventions is complicated by the range of techniques that are combined in different permutations and the lack of clear specifications of therapeutic activity and integrity checks. Distraction, relaxation training, imagery, breathing exercises, desensitization, preparation, modeling,[115] rehearsal, reinforcement, making positive coping statements, and coaching a child to engage in such strategies are all examples of some of the interventions that are frequently used to help decrease pain and distress in children and are included in multicomponent cognitive–behavioral programs.[16] A number of studies[37, 100, 116, 117, 118] have tested the efficacy of these programs for procedure-related pain with good results. A recent meta-analysis[39][I] for needle procedures concluded that taken together the evidence for these interventions shows that they are not effective in reducing self-reported pain, observer-reported pain, self-reported distress, or heart rate. However, combined cognitive and behavioral interventions are effective at reducing other reported distress and behavioral measures of distress. Similarly, in children undergoing a voiding cystourethrogram,[119][II] it was found that children who received a cognitive–behavioral intervention displayed fewer distress behaviors and greater coping behaviors, and were rated as more cooperative than children receiving standard care. However, children's fear and pain ratings did not differ significantly between groups. Research also supports the efficacy of memory modification via suggestive post-event interviews. An intervention that targeted children's memories of their most recent lumbar puncture reduced anticipatory physiological and self-report distress ratings relative to a control group at post-intervention.[120][II]

Cognitive and behavioral interventions, tested with younger children (2–12 years) undergoing minor surgery indicate that strategies such as relaxation,[121][V] role play,[122][IV], [123][II] film modeling,[124][II] and training in coping skills[125][II] are effective for reducing preoperative fear, anxiety, and distress. In older adolescents, LaMontagne and colleagues[126][II] conducted a randomized controlled trial with adolescents undergoing major orthopedic surgery, exploring the efficacy of a videotaped intervention (information only, coping only, information plus coping, or control). It was found that information plus coping was most effective for reducing postoperative anxiety in adolescents with high preoperative anxiety. Coping instruction led to less postoperative anxiety and pain for adolescents aged 13 years and younger. The control group reported the highest levels of pain. Recently, Kain and colleagues[127][II] found that the family-centered preoperative ADVANCE preparation program (family-centered behavioral preparation) is effective in the reduction of preoperative anxiety and improvement in postoperative outcomes (exhibited a lower incidence of emergence delirium after surgery, required significantly less analgesia in the recovery room, and were discharged from the recovery room earlier). In a review of psychosocial interventions for pain in sickle cell disease, cognitive–behavioral techniques were considered as "probably efficacious" for sickle cell pain.[128][I]

Based on the available evidence, combined cognitive and behavioral interventions in children undergoing needle procedures reduce other reported distress and behavioral measures of distress. Some combinations of cognitive and behavioral interventions, but not all, reduce self-reported pain and distress. There is also good evidence for the efficacy of combined interventions designed to prepare children and adolescents for surgery.

PARENTAL INVOLVEMENT IN ACUTE PAIN MANAGEMENT

Theoretical models emphasize the role of parenting in the development, maintenance, and amelioration of child anxiety.[129, 130, 131, 132, 133] Some models[129, 131, 132] hypothesize that when parents are highly controlling in contexts when it is developmentally appropriate for children to act independently (e.g. attending elementary school), children may experience decreased self-efficacy, and thus, increased anxiety,[134] for example, about their ability to

function on their own within their environments. Conversely, some models[129] have hypothesized that parental encouragement of children's autonomy and independence (e.g. in novel contexts) may augment children's perceptions of mastery over the environment, leading to anxiety reduction.

In the pediatric pain literature, a number of studies point to the role that parents play in shaping their child's pain perception and response. Frank and colleagues[135] found that during immunization, maternal behavior accounted for 53 percent of the variance in child distress behavior. Certain parental behaviors are associated with child coping and others with child distress when children undergo painful medical procedures. Parenting behaviors, such as agitation, provision of reassurance, empathic comments, giving control, excessive explanations and apologies to their children, have been shown to be associated with (and indeed precede) elevated distress and increased pain intensity during medical procedures[136, 137, 138] and experimentally induced pain.[139] Humor, commands to use coping strategies, and nonprocedural talk are associated with increases in a child's coping. There is experimental evidence that maternal modeling of pain behaviors can result in elevated pain perception in their children and particularly their daughters.[140] Dahlquist and colleagues[141] demonstrated the influence of speech function on pain distress. Their results showed that vague commands by caregivers were positively associated with child distress during painful procedures. Liossi and colleagues[142] showed that parental expectancies are highly predictive of experienced pain in children undergoing lumbar punctures. Taken together these results lend support to the theoretical models that emphasize the importance of parental control and behavior in the development, maintenance, and/or amelioration of pain reactions, but the results do not clarify the direction of effects or the specific process involved. These remain important questions for future research. It is possible that when parents fail to provide children with the opportunity to experience control in age-appropriate contexts, children may not develop a sense of self-efficacy, thereby increasing their sense of vulnerability to threat and heightened anxiety.

Children's pain while in hospital is one of the foremost concerns of parents and they can potentially contribute to more effective pain management for their children.[143] Parent involvement in pain management has resulted in parents acting as helpful agents in treating children's pain problems, while enhancing the parents' feelings of usefulness and competency in the process. At home, parents are expected to manage children's pain, but are often given inadequate instruction at discharge and no follow-up support.[144] Postoperative pain is a significant post-hospital behavior problem at four weeks and has been shown to adversely affect children's attitudes towards doctors and nurses.[144] Parents who have been educated regarding expected child posthospital behavior problems and who have been given instructions on how they can assist in the care of their children have reported less negative mood states, less depression, and fewer negative outcomes in their children.[145]

Parents are often anxious not only about their child's distress but also about their own ability to support and comfort their child through a painful experience. Thus, parents need to be included in interventions and helped to control their own anxiety which in turn will ensure less anxiety being communicated to the child. Simple educational leaflets can give useful information and more extensive training programs can teach parents what to do.[146]

CONCLUSIONS

Psychological factors play an important role in shaping pain perception in children and comprehensive assessment of the psychological factors that shape pain perception is imperative to maximize the success of pain management interventions. Psychological interventions are useful for the management of acute pediatric pain, although evidence for their efficacy varies depending on type of pain. For procedure-related pain, particularly needle procedures, distraction, hypnosis, and cognitive–behavior therapy are evidence-based interventions. For postoperative pain, preparation, guided imagery, and cognitive–behavior therapy are promising. For acute pain due to illness or injury, cognitive–behavior therapy is promising. How parents feel and what they think and do influences their child's pain perception and response. Parents need to be included in pain management interventions.

Children with acute pain require proactive psychological treatment approaches aiming to reduce current pain, prevent pain in the future, and reduce risk for subsequent physical or psychological morbidity. In recent years, a wide range of behavioral and cognitive techniques have been found to be efficacious for helping children to cope with acute pain. However, although a number of strategies are promising, there have been relatively few attempts to customize treatments on the basis of patient characteristics. Rather, patients tend to be treated with a one size fits all approach, which may actually undermine their natural coping style and artificially underestimate the apparent efficacy of a particular pain management strategy.[147]

REFERENCES

1. Pate JT, Blount RL, Cohen LL, Smith AJ. Childhood medical experiences and temperament as predictors of adult functioning in medical situations. *Children's Health Care*. 1996; **25**: 281–98.
2. Kazak AE, Barakat LP, Meeske K *et al.* Posttraumatic stress, family functioning, and social support in survivors of childhood leukemia and their mothers and fathers. *Journal of Consulting and Clinical Psychology*. 1997; **65**: 120–9.
3. Kazak AE, Kassam-Adams N, Schneider S *et al.* An integrative model of pediatric medical traumatic stress. *Journal of Pediatric Psychology*. 2006; **31**: 343–55.
4. Weisman SJ, Bernstein B, Schechter NL. Consequences of inadequate analgesia during painful procedures in children. *Archives of Pediatrics and Adolescent Medicine*. 1998; **152**: 147–9.
5. McGrath PA. *Pain in children: nature, assessment, and treatment*. New York: Guilford Press, 1990.
6. Liossi C. Acute procedural pain management. In: Schmidt RF, Willis WD (eds). *Encyclopedia of pain*. Berlin: Springer-Verlag, 2007.
* 7. McGrath PA, Brigham MC. The assessment of pain in children and adolescents. In: Turk DC (ed.). *Handbook of pain assessment*. New York: Guilford Press, 1992: 295–314.
8. Varni JW, Blount RL, Waldron SA, Smith AJ. Management of pain and distress. In: Roberts MC (ed.). *Handbook of pediatric psychology*, 2nd edn. New York: Guilford, 1995: 105–23.
9. Kain ZN, Mayes LC, Caldwell-Andrews AA *et al.* Preoperative anxiety, postoperative pain, and behavioral recovery in young children undergoing surgery. *Pediatrics*. 2006; **118**: 651–8.
10. Taylor S. *Anxiety sensitivity: theory, research, and treatment of the fear of anxiety*. London: Lawrence Erlbaum Associates, 1999: 370.
11. Lipsitz JD, Masia-Warner C, Apfel H *et al.* Anxiety and depressive symptoms and anxiety sensitivity in youngsters with noncardiac chest pain and benign heart murmurs. *Journal of Pediatric Psychology*. 2004; **29**: 607–12.
12. Kirsch I. Response expectancy as a determinant of experience and behavior. *American Psychologist*. 1985; **40**: 1189–202.
13. Palermo TM, Drotar D. Prediction of children's postoperative pain: the role of presurgical expectations and anticipatory emotions. *Journal of Pediatric Psychology*. 1996; **21**: 683–98.
14. Logan DE, Rose JB. Is postoperative pain a self-fulfilling prophecy? Expectancy effects on postoperative pain and patient-controlled analgesia use among adolescent surgical patients. *Journal of Pediatric Psychology*. 2005; **30**: 187–96.
15. Thomas A, Chess S. *Temperament and development*. New York: Bunner/Mazel, 1977.
16. Chen E, Joseph MH, Zeltzer LK. Behavioral and cognitive interventions in the treatment of pain in children. *Pediatric Clinics of North America*. 2000; **47**: 513–25.
17. Helgadottir HL, Wilson ME. Temperament and pain in 3 to 7-year-old children undergoing tonsillectomy. *Journal of Pediatric Nursing*. 2004; **19**: 204–13.
18. Sullivan MJ, Thorn B, Haythornthwaite JA *et al.* Theoretical perspectives on the relation between catastrophizing and pain. *Clinical Journal of Pain*. 2001; **17**: 52–64.
19. Bennett-Branson SM, Craig KD. Postoperative pain in children: Developmental and family influences on

spontaneous coping strategies. *Canadian Journal of Behavioural Science Revue Canadienne des Sciences du Comportement*. 1993; **25**: 355–83.

20. Miller SM. Monitoring and blunting: validation of a questionnaire to assess styles of information seeking under threat. *Journal of Personality and Social Psychology*. 1987; **52**: 345–53.

21. Miller SM, Shoda Y, Hurley K. Applying cognitive-social theory to health-protective behavior: breast self-examination in cancer screening. *Psychological Bulletin*. 1996; **119**: 70–94.

22. Leventhal H, Everhart D. Emotion, pain, and physical illness. In: Izard CE (ed.). *Emotions in personality and psychopathology*. New York: Plenum, 1979: 263–98.

* 23. von Baeyer CL, Marche TA, Rocha EM, Salmon K. Children's memory for pain: overview and implications for practice. *Journal of Pain*. 2004; **5**: 241–9.

24. Stanish WD, Tripp DA, Coady C, Biddulph M. Injury and pain in the adolescent athlete. In: Finley GA, McGrath PJ (eds). *Acute and procedure pain in infants and children*. Progress in Pain Research and Management, 20. Seattle: IASP Press, 2001.

25. Harter S. Developmental and dynamic changes in the nature of the self-concept: Implications for child psychotherapy. In: Shirk SR (ed.). *Cognitive development and child psychotherapy*. New York: Plenum Press, 1988.

26. Dahlquist LM. *Pediatric pain management*. New York: Kluwer Academic/Plenum Publishers, 1999.

* 27. Gaffney A, McGrath PJ, Dick BD. Measuring pain in children: Developmental and instrument issues. In: Schechter CB N, Yaster M (eds). *Pain in infants, children, and adolescents*, 2nd edn. Baltimore: Williams & Wilkins, 2003.

28. Rasnake LK, Linscheid TR. Anxiety reduction in children receiving medical care: developmental considerations. *Journal of Developmental and Behavioral Pediatrics*. 1989; **10**: 169–75.

29. Pfefferbaum B, Adams J, Aceves J. The influence of culture on pain in Anglo and Hispanic children with cancer. *Journal of the American Academy of Child and Adolescent Psychiatry*. 1990; **29**: 642–7.

30. Jones M, Qazi M, Young KD. Ethnic differences in parent preference to be present for painful medical procedures. *Pediatrics*. 2005; **116**: e191–7.

* 31. von Baeyer CL, Spagrud LJ. Systematic review of observational (behavioral) measures of pain for children and adolescents aged 3 to 18 years. *Pain*. 2007; **127**: 140–50.

32. Franck LS, Greenberg CS, Stevens B. Pain assessment in infants and children. *Pediatric Clinics of North America*. 2000; **47**: 487–512.

33. Anderson C, Zeltzer L, Fanuric D. Procedural pain. In: Schechter NL, Berde CB, Yaster M (eds). *Pain in infants, children and adolescents*. Baltimore, MD: Williams & Wilkins, 1993: 435–58.

34. Leventhal H, Johnson JE. In: Woolridge P (ed.). *Behavioral science and nursing theory*. St Louis: Mosby, 1983: 54–127.

35. Suls J, Wan CK. Effects of sensory and procedural information on coping with stressful medical procedures and pain: a meta-analysis. *Journal of Consulting and Clinical Psychology*. 1989; **57**: 372–9.

36. Langer EJ, Janis IL, Wolfer JA. Reduction of psychological stress in surgical patients. *Journal of Experimental Social Psychology*. 1975; **11**: 155–65.

* 37. Powers SW. Empirically supported treatments in pediatric psychology: procedure-related pain. *Journal of Pediatric Psychology*. 1999; **24**: 131–45.

* 38. Kolk AM, van Hoof R, Fiedeldij Dop MJ. Preparing children for venepuncture. The effect of an integrated intervention on distress before and during venepuncture. *Child: Care, Health and Development*. 2000; **26**: 251–60.

* 39. Uman LS, Chambers CT, McGrath PJ, Kisely S. Psychological interventions for needle-related procedural pain and distress in children and adolescents. *Cochrane Database of Systematic Reviews*. 2006; **CD005179**.

40. Davis TM, Maguire TO, Haraphongse M, Schaumberger MR. Preparing adult patients for cardiac catheterization: informational treatment and coping style interactions. *Heart and Lung*. 1994; **23**: 130–9.

41. Gattuso SM, Litt MD, Fitzgerald TE. Coping with gastrointestinal endoscopy: self-efficacy enhancement and coping style. *Journal of Consulting and Clinical Psychology*. 1992; **60**: 133–9.

42. Miller SM, Mangan CE. Interacting effects of information and coping style in adapting to gynecologic stress: should the doctor tell all? *Journal of Personality and Social Psychology*. 1983; **45**: 223–36.

43. Miller SM, Buzaglo JS, Simms SL *et al*. Monitoring styles in women at risk for cervical cancer: Implications for the framing of health-relevant messages. *Annals of Behavioral Medicine*. 1999; **21**: 27–34.

44. Watkins LO, Weaver L, Odegaard V. Preparation for cardiac catheterization: tailoring the content of instruction to coping style. *Heart and Lung*. 1986; **15**: 382–9.

45. Williams-Piehota P, Pizarro J, Schneider TR *et al*. Matching health messages to monitor-blunter coping styles to motivate screening mammography. *Health Psychology*. 2005; **24**: 58–67.

46. Martelli MF, Auerbach SM, Alexander J, Mercuri LG. Stress management in the health care setting: matching interventions with patient coping styles. *Journal of Consulting and Clinical Psychology*. 1987; **55**: 201–7.

47. Bonk VA, France CR, Taylor BK. Distraction reduces self-reported physiological reactions to blood donation in novice donors with a blunting coping style. *Psychosomatic Medicine*. 2001; **63**: 447–52.

48. Roth S, Cohen LJ. Approach, avoidance, and coping with stress. *American Psychologist*. 1986; **41**: 813–9.

49. Suls J, Fletcher B. The relative efficacy of avoidant and nonavoidant coping strategies: a meta-analysis. *Health Psychology*. 1985; **4**: 249–88.

50. Michael ES, Burns JW. Catastrophizing and pain sensitivity among chronic pain patients: moderating effects of sensory and affect focus. *Annals of Behavioral Medicine.* 2004; **27**: 185–94.

51. Valet M, Sprenger T, Boecker H *et al.* Distraction modulates connectivity of the cingulo-frontal cortex and the midbrain during pain – an fMRI analysis. *Pain.* 2004; **109**: 399–408.

52. Cassidy KL, Reid GJ, McGrath PJ *et al.* Watch needle, watch TV: Audiovisual distraction in preschool immunization. *Pain Medicine.* 2002; **3**: 108–18.

53. Fanurik D, Koh JL, Schmitz ML. Distraction techniques combined with EMLA: Effects on IV insertion pain and distress in children. *Childrens Health Care.* 2000; **29**: 87–101.

54. Fowler-Kerry S, Lander JR. Management of injection pain in children. *Pain.* 1987; **30**: 169–75.

55. Gonzalez JC, Routh DK, Armstrong FD. Effects of maternal distraction versus reassurance on children's reactions to injections. *Journal of Pediatric Psychology.* 1993; **18**: 593–604.

56. Kleiber C, Craft-Rosenberg M, Harper DC. Parents as distraction coaches during i.v. insertion: a randomized study. *Journal of Pain and Symptom Management.* 2001; **22**: 851–61.

57. Press J, Gidron Y, Maimon M *et al.* Effects of active distraction on pain of children undergoing venipuncture: Who benefits from it? *Pain Clinic.* 2003; **15**: 261–9.

58. Tak JH, van Bon WH. Pain- and distress-reducing interventions for venepuncture in children. *Child: Care, Health and Development.* 2006; **32**: 257–68.

59. Vessey JA, Carlson KL, McGill J. Use of distraction with children during an acute pain experience. *Nursing Research.* 1994; **43**: 369–72.

60. Zabin MA. 'Modification of children's behavior during bloodwork procedures'. Unpublished doctoral dissertation, West Virginia University, 1982.

61. Leventhal H. I know distraction works even though it doesn't! *Health Psychology.* 1992; **11**: 208–9.

62. Cioffi D. Beyond attentional strategies: cognitive-perceptual model of somatic interpretation. *Psychological Bulletin.* 1991; **109**: 25–41.

63. Eccleston C. The attentional control of pain: methodological and theoretical concerns. *Pain.* 1995; **63**: 3–10.

64. Fanurik D, Zeltzer LK, Roberts MC, Blount RL. The relationship between children's coping styles and psychological interventions for cold pressor pain. *Pain.* 1993; **53**: 213–22.

65. McCaffery M, Beebe A. *Pain, clinical manual for nursing practice.* London: Mosby, 1994.

66. Bulechek GM, McCloskey JC. *Nursing interventions, essential nursing treatments.* Philadelphia: WB Saunders Company, 1992.

67. Watt-Watson J, Donovan MI. *Pain management, nursing perspective.* St Louis: Mosby-Year Book Inc., 1992.

68. Jacobson E. *Progressive relaxation.* Chicago: Chicago University Press, 1938.

69. Schultz JH, Luthe W. *Autogenic methods.* Autogenic therapy, 1. New York: Grune & Stratton, 1969.

70. Perez-De-Albeniz A, Holmes J. Meditation: Concepts, effects and uses in therapy. *International Journal of Psychotherapy.* 2000; **5**: 49–59.

71. Patterson DR. Practical applications of psychological techniques in controlling burn pain. *Journal of Burn Care and Rehabilitation.* 1992; **13**: 13–8.

72. Taal LA. *The psychological aspects of burn injuries.* Maastricht: Shaker Publishing, 1998.

73. O'Byrne KK, Peterson L, Saldana L. Survey of pediatric hospitals' preparation programs: evidence of the impact of health psychology research. *Health Psychology.* 1997; **16**: 147–54.

74. de Jong AEE, Gamel C. Use of a simple relaxation technique in burn care: literature review. *Journal of Advanced Nursing.* 2006; **54**: 710–21.

75. Green JP, Barabasz AF, Barrett D, Montgomery GH. Forging ahead: the 2003 APA Division 30 definition of hypnosis. *International Journal of Clinical and Experimental Hypnosis.* 2005; **53**: 259–64.

∗ 76. Liossi C. *Procedure-related cancer pain in children.* Oxford: Radcliffe Medical Press, 2002.

77. Liossi C, Mystakidou K. Clinical hypnosis in palliative care. *European Journal of Palliative Care.* 1996; **3**: 56–8.

78. Gardner GG, Olness K. *Hypnosis and hypnotherapy with children.* New York: Grune & Stratton, 1981.

79. Rainville P, Carrier B, Hofbauer RK *et al.* Dissociation of sensory and affective dimensions of pain using hypnotic modulation. *Pain.* 1999; **82**: 159–71.

80. Hilgard ER, Hilgard JR. *Hypnosis in the relief of pain.* New York: Brunner/Mazel, 1994.

81. Bowers KS, LeBaron S. Hypnosis and hypnotizability: implications for clinical intervention. *Hospital and Community Psychiatry.* 1986; **37**: 457–67.

82. Kirsch I, Lynn SJ. The altered state of hypnosis – changes in the theoretical landscape. *American Psychologist.* 1995; **50**: 846–58.

83. Bowers KS. Unconscious influences and hypnosis. In: Singer JL (ed.). *Repression and dissociation: Implications for personality theory, psychopathology and health.* Chicago: University of Chicago Press, 1990: 143–78.

84. Bowers KS. Imagination and dissociation in hypnotic responding. *International Journal of Clinical and Experimental Hypnosis.* 1992; **40**: 253–75.

85. Chaves JF. Hypnosis in pain management. In: Rhue JW, Lynn SJ, Kirsch I (eds). *Handbook of clinical hypnosis.* Washington DC: American Psychiatric Association, 1993: 511–32.

86. Carr DB, Goudas LC. Acute pain. *Lancet.* 1999; **353**: 2051–8.

∗ 87. Montgomery GH, DuHamel KN, Redd WH. A meta-analysis of hypnotically induced analgesia: how effective is hypnosis? *International Journal of Clinical and Experimental Hypnosis.* 2000; **48**: 138–53.

88. Thorn BE, Cross TH, Walker BB. Meta-analyses and systematic reviews of psychological treatments for chronic pain: Relevance to an evidence-based practice. *Health Psychology*. 2007; **26**: 1–9.

89. Kihlstrom JF. Hypnosis: a sesquicentennial essay. *International Journal of Clinical and Experimental Hypnosis*. 1992; **40**: 301–14.

90. Patterson DR, Jensen MP. Hypnosis and clinical pain. *Psychological Bulletin*. 2003; **129**: 495–521.

91. Liossi C. Management of paediatric procedure-related cancer pain. *Pain Reviews*. 1999; **6**: 279–302.

92. Chambless DL, Hollon SD. Defining empirically supported therapies. *Journal of Consulting and Clinical Psychology*. 1998; **66**: 7–18.

93. Hilgard JR, LeBaron S. Relief of anxiety and pain in children and adolescents with cancer: quantitative measures and clinical observations. *International Journal of Clinical and Experimental Hypnosis*. 1982; **30**: 417–42.

94. Zeltzer L, LeBaron S. Hypnosis and nonhypnotic techniques for reduction of pain and anxiety during painful procedures in children and adolescents with cancer. *Journal of Pediatrics*. 1982; **101**: 1032–5.

95. Kellerman J, Zeltzer L, Ellenberg L, Dash J. Adolescents with cancer. Hypnosis for the reduction of the acute pain and anxiety associated with medical procedures. *Journal of Adolescent Health Care*. 1983; **4**: 85–90.

96. Katz ER, Kellerman J, Ellenberg L. Hypnosis in the reduction of acute pain and distress in children with cancer. *Journal of Pediatric Psychology*. 1987; **12**: 379–94.

97. Kuttner L, Bowman M, Teasdale M. Hypnotic versus active cognitive strategies for alleviation of procedural distress in pediatric oncology patients. *Journal of Developmental and Behavioral Pediatrics*. 1988; **9**: 374–82.

98. Wall VJ, Womack W. Hypnotic versus active cognitive strategies for alleviation of procedural distress in pediatric oncology patients. *American Journal of Clinical Hypnosis*. 1989; **31**: 181–91.

99. Hawkins P, Liossi C, Ewart B, Hatira P. Hypnosis in the alleviation of procedure related pain and distress in paediatric oncology patients. *Contemporary Hypnosis*. 1998; **15**: 199–207.

100. Liossi C, Hatira P. Clinical hypnosis versus cognitive behavioral training for pain management with pediatric cancer patients undergoing bone marrow aspirations. *International Journal of Clinical and Experimental Hypnosis*. 1999; **47**: 104–16.

101. Liossi C, Hatira P. Clinical hypnosis in the alleviation of procedure-related pain in pediatric oncology patients. *International Journal of Clinical and Experimental Hypnosis*. 2003; **51**: 4–28.

102. Liossi C, White P, Hatira P. Randomized clinical trial of local anesthetic versus a combination of local anesthetic with self-hypnosis in the management of pediatric procedure-related pain. *Health Psychology*. 2006; **25**: 307–15.

103. Butler LD, Symons BK, Henderson SL et al. Hypnosis reduces distress and duration of an invasive medical procedure for children. *Pediatrics*. 2005; **115**: e77–85.

104. Lambert SA. The effects of hypnosis/guided imagery on the postoperative course of children. *Journal of Developmental and Behavioral Pediatrics*. 1996; **17**: 307–10.

*105. Johnston M, Vogele C. Benefits of psychological preparation for surgery: A meta-analysis. *Annals of Behavioral Medicine*. 1993; **15**: 245–56.

106. Assagioli R. *Psychosynthesis: A manual of principles and techniques*. New York: Hobbs, Dorman and Company, 1965.

107. Naparstek B. *Staying well with guided imagery*. New York: Warner Books, 1994.

108. Kosslyn SM, Ganis G, Thompson WL. Mental imagery: against the nihilistic hypothesis. *Trends in Cognitive Sciences*. 2003; **7**: 109–11.

109. Huth MM, Broome ME, Good M. Imagery reduces children's post-operative pain. *Pain*. 2004; **110**: 439–48.

110. Brewin CR. Cognitive change processes in psychotherapy. *Psychological Review*. 1989; **96**: 379–94.

111. Barlow DH, Durand VM. *Abnormal psychology: an integrative approach*. California: Brooks/Cole Publishing Company, 1999.

112. Keefe FJ, Dunsmore J, Burnett R. Behavioral and cognitive-behavioral approaches to chronic pain: recent advances and future directions. *Journal of Consulting and Clinical Psychology*. 1992; **60**: 528–36.

113. Kendall PC, Panichelli-Mindel SM. Cognitive-behavioral treatments. *Journal of Abnormal Child Psychology*. 1995; **23**: 107–24.

114. Villemure C, Bushnell MC. Cognitive modulation of pain: how do attention and emotion influence pain processing? *Pain*. 2002; **95**: 195–9.

115. Greenbaum PE, Melamed BG. Pretreatment modeling. A technique for reducing children's fear in the dental operatory. *Dental Clinics of North America*. 1988; **32**: 693–704.

116. Cohen LL, Blount RL, Panopoulos G. Nurse coaching and cartoon distraction: an effective and practical intervention to reduce child, parent, and nurse distress during immunizations. *Journal of Pediatric Psychology*. 1997; **22**: 355–70.

117. Cohen LL, Bernard RS, Greco LA, McClellan CB. A child-focused intervention for coping with procedural pain: are parent and nurse coaches necessary? *Journal of Pediatric Psychology*. 2002; **27**: 749–57.

118. Tyc VL, Leigh L, Mulhern RK et al. Evaluation of a cognitive-behavioral intervention for reducing distress in pediatric cancer patients undergoing magnetic resonance imaging procedures. *International Journal of Rehabilitation and Health*. 1997; **3**: 267–79.

119. Zelikovsky N, Rodrigue JR, Gidycz CA, Davis MA. Cognitive behavioral and behavioral interventions help young children cope during a voiding cystourethrogram. *Journal of Pediatric Psychology*. 2000; **25**: 535–43.

120. Chen E, Zeltzer LK, Craske MG, Katz ER. Alteration of memory in the reduction of children's distress during repeated aversive medical procedures. *Journal of Consulting and Clinical Psychology*. 1999; **67**: 481–90.

121. Kain ZN, Caldwell-Andrews A, Wang SM. Psychological preparation of the parent and pediatric surgical patient. *Anesthesiology Clinics of North America*. 2002; **20**: 29–44.

122. Hatava P, Olsson GL, Lagerkranser M. Preoperative psychological preparation for children undergoing ENT operations: a comparison of two methods. *Paediatric Anaesthesia*. 2000; **10**: 477–86.

123. Kain ZN, Mayes LC, Caramico LA. Preoperative preparation in children: a cross-sectional study. *Journal of Clinical Anesthesia*. 1996; **8**: 508–14.

124. Pinto RP, Hollandsworth Jr JG. Using videotape modeling to prepare children psychologically for surgery: influence of parents and costs versus benefits of providing preparation services. *Health Psychology*. 1989; **8**: 79–95.

125. Kain ZN, Caramico LA, Mayes LC *et al.* Preoperative preparation programs in children: a comparative examination. *Anesthesia and Analgesia*. 1998; **87**: 1249–55.

126. LaMontagne LL, Hepworth JT, Cohen F, Salisbury MH. Cognitive-behavioral intervention effects on adolescents' anxiety and pain following spinal fusion surgery. *Nursing Research*. 2003; **52**: 183–90.

127. Kain ZN, Caldwell-Andrews AA, Mayes LC *et al.* Family-centered preparation for surgery improves perioperative outcomes in children: a randomized controlled trial. *Anesthesiology*. 2007; **106**: 65–74.

*128. Chen E, Cole SW, Kato PM. A review of empirically supported psychosocial interventions for pain and adherence outcomes in sickle cell disease. *Journal of Pediatric Psychology*. 2004; **29**: 197–209.

129. Chorpita BF, Barlow DH. The development of anxiety: the role of control in the early environment. *Psychological Bulletin*. 1998; **124**: 3–21.

130. Dadds MR, Roth JH. Family processes in the development of anxiety problems. In: Vasey MW, Dadds MR (eds). *The developmental psychopathology of anxiety*. New York: Oxford University Press, 2001: 278–303.

131. Krohne HW. Parental childrearing and anxiety development. In: Hurrelmann K, Losel F (eds). *Health hazards in adolescence*. New York: Walter de Gruyter, 1990: 115–30.

132. Rapee RM. The development of generalized anxiety. In: Vasey MW, Dadds MR (eds). *The developmental psychopathology of anxiety*. New York: Oxford University Press, 2001: 481–503.

133. Vasey MW, Dadds MR. An introduction to the developmental psychopathology of anxiety. In: Vasey MW, Dadds MR (eds). *The developmental psychopathology of anxiety*. New York: Oxford University Press, 2001: 3–26.

134. Wood JJ. Parental intrusiveness and children's separation anxiety in a clinical sample. *Child Psychiatry and Human Development*. 2006; **37**: 73–87.

135. Frank NC, Blount RL, Smith AJ *et al.* Parent and staff behavior, previous child medical experience, and maternal anxiety as they relate to child procedural distress and coping. *Journal of Pediatric Psychology*. 1995; **20**: 277–89.

136. Blount RL, Corbin SM, Sturges JW *et al.* The relationship between adults behavior and child coping and distress during Bma Lp procedures – a sequential analysis. *Behavior Therapy*. 1989; **20**: 585–601.

137. Blount RL, Bunke VL, Zaff JF. The integration of basic research, treatment research, and clinical practice in pediatric psychology. In: Drotar D (ed.). *Handbook of research in pediatric and clinical child psychology. Practical strategies and methods*. Dordrecht: Kluwer Academic Publishers, 2000: xiii, 557.

138. Dahlquist LM, Power TG, Carlson L. Physician and parent behavior during invasive pediatric cancer procedures: relationships to child behavioral distress. *Journal of Pediatric Psychology*. 1995; **20**: 477–90.

139. Chambers CT, Craig KD, Bennett SM. The impact of maternal behavior on children's pain experiences: an experimental analysis. *Journal of Pediatric Psychology*. 2002; **27**: 293–301.

140. Goodman JE, McGrath PJ. Mothers' modeling influences children's pain during a cold pressor task. *Pain*. 2003; **104**: 559–65.

141. Dahlquist LM, Pendley JS, Power TG *et al.* Adult command structure and children's distress during the anticipatory phase of invasive cancer procedures. *Childrens Health Care*. 2001; **30**: 151–67.

142. Liossi C, White P, Franck L, Hatira P. Parental pain expectancy as a mediator between child expected and experienced procedure-related pain intensity during painful medical procedures. *Clinical Journal of Pain*. 2007; **23**: 392–9.

143. Kristensson-Hallstrom I. Strategies for feeling secure influence parents' participation in care. *Journal of Clinical Nursing*. 1999; **8**: 586–92.

144. Kotiniemi LH, Ryhanen PT, Valanne J *et al.* Postoperative symptoms at home following day-case surgery in children: a multicentre survey of 551 children. *Anaesthesia*. 1997; **52**: 963–9.

145. Melnyk BM, Alpert-Gillis L, Feinstein NF *et al.* Creating opportunities for parent empowerment: program effects on the mental health/coping outcomes of critically ill young children and their mothers. *Pediatrics*. 2004; **113**: e597–607.

146. Power N, Liossi C, Franck L. Helping parents to help their child with procedural and everyday pain: practical, evidence-based advice. *Journal for Specialists in Pediatric Nursing*. 2007; **12**: 203–9.

147. Turk DC. Customizing treatment for chronic pain patients: who, what, and why. *Clinical Journal of Pain*. 1990; **6**: 255–70.

PART III

MANAGEMENT – CLINICAL SITUATIONS

17

Postoperative pain management following day surgery

GIRISH P JOSHI

KEY LEARNING POINTS

- Patient education is critical in improving postoperative pain management as it reduces anxiety, allows realistic expectation, and improves patient satisfaction.
- Preventative analgesia, particularly with nonopioids (e.g. nonsteroidal anti-inflammatory drugs (NSAIDs), paracetamol, and local anesthetics), reduces intraoperative and postoperative opioid requirements, and potentially lower opioid-related side effects as well as improves postoperative pain relief.
- Multimodal analgesia regimens improve pain relief, and reduce opioid requirements and opioid-related side effects.
- Opioids should be used sparingly as opioid-related side effects delay recovery and return to daily living.

- Regional analgesia techniques, particularly perineural infusion of local anesthetic, reduce intraoperative anesthetic and analgesic requirements, provide for a rapid and smooth recovery, and facilitate early mobilization and discharge.
- Nonsteroidal anti-inflammatory drugs (nonselective NSAIDs or COX-2 selective inhibitors) should be used if there are no contraindications.
- Incorporation of evidence-based procedure specific pain management guidelines into clinical pathways may improve postoperative pain management and surgical outcome.

INTRODUCTION

It is estimated that ambulatory surgery constitutes 60–65 percent of all surgical procedures performed in the United States. With increases in the surgical workload,[1] the practice of ambulatory surgery is expected to expand further. Our ability to provide adequate postoperative pain relief is one of the major determinants for performing a surgical procedure on an outpatient basis. Therefore, with more extensive and potentially more painful surgical procedures being performed on an outpatient basis, there is an increased need for prolonged dynamic postoperative pain relief,[2, 3] particularly after discharge home.[4]

The adverse pathophysiological and psychological consequences of unrelieved pain are well recognized:[5]

- increased postanesthesia care unit (PACU) stay;
- increased phase II unit stay;
- delayed discharge home;
- unanticipated hospital admission;
- increased contact with family practitioner;
- delayed return to daily living function;
- decreased patient satisfaction.

Uncontrolled pain may be associated with a prolonged PACU stay, delayed discharge from an ambulatory facility, and unanticipated hospital admission.[6, 7, 8] Inadequate postoperative pain control was also the most frequent reason for patients to contact their family practitioner after discharge from hospital.[9] In addition, unrelieved pain may also delay return to normal daily activities after outpatient surgery.[10, 11] Furthermore, recent data suggest that inadequately treated acute pain can become chronic, leading to persistent postoperative pain.[5, 12] Importantly, the presence of postoperative symptoms, including pain, contributes to patient dissatisfaction with their surgical experience.[13] Therefore, it is imperative that postoperative pain be managed appropriately and aggressively. In spite of emphasis on provision of adequate analgesia, treatment of postoperative pain continues to be a major challenge with numerous studies indicating that postoperative pain is not always adequately treated.[14, 15]

One of the important reasons for suboptimal pain management is inadequate or improper application of available analgesic therapies, which may partly be due to the significant amount of new and conflicting information that is being increasingly made available. Evidence-based guidelines may be used to guide clinical practice and improve patient care.[16, 17, 18] However, one of the major limitations of these pain management guidelines is that they are derived from multiple surgical procedures with different pain characteristics (e.g. location, intensity, type, and duration) and different consequences of inadequate pain relief.[19] In addition, the risks and benefits of different analgesic techniques differ between surgical procedures. Also, some analgesic techniques are applicable to specific surgical procedures (e.g. intra-articular and intraperitoneal techniques for joint surgery and abdominal surgery, respectively).

Some pain guidelines use the number needed to treat (NNT) values (i.e. number of patients that achieve at least a 50 percent pain relief as compared to placebo)[18] to determine the choice of analgesic. However, the NNT values are derived from a variety of surgical procedures and the efficacy of an analgesic may vary depending upon the type of surgical procedure. For example, paracetamol (acetaminophen) is less effective in relieving pain after orthopedic procedures than after dental procedures (i.e. NNT 1.87 versus 3.77, respectively).[20] Furthermore, efficacy of combinations of analgesics varies significantly between surgical procedures. For example, the combination of paracetamol and NSAIDs provided improved analgesic efficacy after mild-to-moderate surgical procedures, but its benefits were smaller for more extensive surgical procedures.[21] In addition, the clinical relevance of a 50 percent decrease in pain (i.e. definition of NNT) may be different with an initial pain score of 80 on a 100-point visual analog scale (VAS) as compared to an initial score of 30. Therefore, it is clear that NNT may not necessarily be valid in all types of surgery, as well as all intensities of pain.[20]

PROCEDURE-SPECIFIC PAIN MANAGEMENT

The limitations of conventional pain management guidelines suggest that pain guidelines should be specific for surgical procedures.[19, 22] To date, there are two initiatives that provide procedure-specific postoperative pain guidelines, one from the United States Veterans Administration (VA), the Department of Defence, and the University of Iowa (www.oqp.med.va.gov/cpg/cpg.htm)[23] and the other from the Procedure-specific Postoperative Pain Management (PROSPECT) group (www.postoppain.org).[22] The VA procedure-specific guidelines have been constructed based upon a systematic review of the literature in a variety of procedures and interpreted by a consensus group to provide the guidelines for overall recommendations for specific analgesic interventions.

The PROSPECT group is a collaboration of international anesthesiologists and surgeons that provides evidence-based recommendations derived from systematic reviews of the literature (using the Cochrane Collaboration of randomized controlled trials of analgesic, anesthetic, and surgical interventions affecting postoperative pain) for the specific type of surgery.[24] In addition, these procedure-specific systematic reviews are supplemented with evidence from other similar surgical procedures (i.e. transferable evidence) and clinical practice information (i.e. practical guidelines from the PROSPECT Working Group).[25] The recommendations available online (www.postoppain.org) are arranged into pre-, intra-, and postoperative sections, which are presented as folders in the "tree" structure. Within the folders, evidence and clinical practice are presented as arguments for and against an analgesic, anesthetic, or operative technique, together with links to abstracts. The detailed information allows the readers to make their own decisions based on their practice.[26, 27]

PREOPERATIVE CONSIDERATIONS

Planning for postoperative pain management should begin in the preoperative period.[28] Often patients complain that they did not receive any information on the degree of expected pain and the plan to control pain.[29, 30]

Patient education regarding the degree of pain that they might expect, the pain assessment tools, and the modalities of pain treatment that might be utilized, should reduce their anxiety and fear of unrelieved pain. Reduced patient anxiety may reduce the incidence of postoperative pain.[31][III] In addition, patients have to be made aware of the importance of communicating their analgesic needs. Furthermore, it is important that the general practitioners/family physicians/primary care physicians are adequately educated regarding the management of pain after discharge home.[32]

TIMING OF ANALGESIC ADMINISTRATION (PREEMPTIVE OR PREVENTATIVE ANALGESIA TECHNIQUES)

Tissue injury from surgical procedure produces alterations in the chemical profile and structure, as well as function, of neurons, which may increase the sensitivity to pain.[33, 34] Peripheral sensitization of nociceptors and subsequent barrage of nerve impulses entering the spinal cord results in hyperexcitability in dorsal horn neurons and central sensitization leading to reduced pain threshold and amplification of the pain response.[33, 34] Preemptive analgesia (i.e. analgesic intervention before noxious stimuli) attempts to reduce peripheral and central sensitization, and prevent the consequent amplification and prolongation of pain. Although preemptive analgesia has been overwhelmingly demonstrated in animal studies,[33, 34] clinical studies have provided conflicting results.[35, 36, 37, 38, 39] The lack of benefit of preemptive analgesia may be due to deficiencies in the study designs. Most clinical trials used single analgesic dose (preoperative versus postoperative administration) and/or had a short duration of analgesic treatment. In addition, most studies have evaluated unimodal analgesia techniques (e.g. local anesthesia alone or NSAIDs alone) rather than multimodal analgesia techniques.[40] An optimal preemptive analgesic technique would prevent the establishment of neural sensitization caused by incisional and inflammatory injuries; it would begin prior to the surgical injury and continue until the inflammation is resolved.

Until clinical studies confirm the benefits of preemptive analgesia, it is crucial to prevent pain on emergence from anesthesia (may be called "preventative analgesia"). Therefore, the timing of analgesic administration still remains critical. Analgesics should be administered such that the peak effects occur prior to emergence from anesthesia. Because ambulatory surgical procedures often tend to be of short duration, it is better to administer the analgesic as early as possible and preferably preoperatively.[40] Preventative analgesia, particularly with nonopioids (e.g. NSAIDs, paracetamol, and local anesthetics), should reduce intraoperative and postoperative opioid requirements, and potentially lower opioid-related side effects, as well as improve postoperative pain relief.

For more detail on preemptive and preventive analgesia, see Chapter 9, Preventive analgesia and beyond: current status, evidence, and future directions.

MULTIMODAL ANALGESIA TECHNIQUES

With advances in our understanding of the pathophysiology of postoperative pain, it is now clear that pain is a complex phenomenon and several mechanisms play a role in pain perception.[33, 34][I] Because pain is multifactorial, its management requires a multimodal therapy.[40, 41, 42] Therefore, it is recommended that a combination of several analgesics that have different mechanisms of action be utilized whenever possible.[40, 41, 42] Although it is generally accepted that multimodal analgesia regimens improve pain relief and reduce opioid requirements and opioid-related side effects, this has not resulted in improved postoperative outcome.[40] Furthermore, several studies reporting reduced opioid requirements have not been able to demonstrate a reduction in opioid-related side effects.[40, 41, 42] Although the reasons for the lack of benefits are not yet clear, it may be due to inappropriate (or irrational) combinations of analgesics or techniques. Also, benefits of multimodal analgesia techniques may only be realized if they are integrated with a multimodal postoperative rehabilitation program.[40]

An ideal analgesic technique after ambulatory surgery should be effective, intrinsically safe with minimal side effects, and be easily managed outside the hospital. The analgesic modalities commonly used for postoperative pain management include opioids, local analgesic techniques, paracetamol, and cyclooxygenase (COX) enzyme inhibitors such as NSAIDs or COX-2-selective inhibitors. Recently, there has been increased interest in using analgesic adjuncts such as N-methyl-D-aspartate (NMDA) receptor antagonists (e.g. ketamine and dextromethorphan), alpha-2 agonists (e.g. clonidine and dexmedetomidine), corticosteroids, and anticonvulsants (e.g. gabapentin and pregabalin) (Table 17.1).

Opioids

Opioids are highly efficacious analgesics particularly suited for moderate-to-severe pain and still remain the mainstay for perioperative analgesia. Chung et al.[6] found that patients receiving smaller intraoperative doses of fentanyl on a μg/kg basis, and those undergoing longer operations had a higher incidence of severe pain in the PACU. This suggests that adequate intraoperative opioid administration is necessary. However, the role of opioids in ambulatory surgery remains controversial.[43, 44] Recent data suggest that clinically relevant tolerance to opioids can occur within hours of their intraoperative use,[45, 46] which may reduce their postoperative analgesic efficacy. Furthermore, opioids cause a dose-dependent increase in

Table 17.1 Analgesic options for ambulatory surgery.

Analgesic options		
Paracetamol		
Nonsteroidal anti-inflammatory drugs or cyclooxygenase specific inhibitors		
Local/regional anesthetic techniques		
Opioids		
Tramadol		
Analgesic adjuncts	NMDA receptor antagonists	Ketamine
		Dextromethrophan
	Alpha-2 receptor agonists	Clonidine
		Dexmedetomidine
	Steroids	
	Anticonvulsants	Gabapentin
		Pregabalin

adverse effects including nausea, vomiting, sedation, dizziness, bladder dysfunction, and constipation, all of which may contribute to a delayed recovery.[47, 48, 49, 50, 51, 52][II] Interestingly, the increased use of perioperative opioids after the emphasis on adequate pain relief (i.e. "pain as the fifth vital sign") by the Joint Commission for Accreditation of Healthcare Organizations (JCAHO) in the United States[53] has been reported to increase postoperative opioid-related side effects.[54] However, others found that reduced opioid requirements did not reduce opioid-related side effects.[55, 56] The lack of reduction in opioid-related side effects may have resulted from the studies having inadequate study design and smaller sample sizes. Nevertheless, opioids should be used sparingly and non-opioid analgesic techniques should be used whenever possible.[44][II]

Local analgesic techniques

Local anesthetic techniques are simple and provide excellent dynamic pain relief, as well as reduce opioid requirements, which may reduce opioid-related side effects.[57, 58] In addition, if used intraoperatively, these techniques decrease the intraoperative anesthetic and analgesic requirements, provide for a rapid and smooth recovery, and facilitate early mobilization and discharge.[59, 60, 61, 62][I] A wide variety of local anesthetic techniques can be used to provide intra- and postoperative pain relief (**Table 17.2**). Although the potential benefits of local anesthetic techniques have been well recognized, these techniques have been underutilized.

Wound infiltration and topical application of local anesthetics

Infiltration of the surgical wound with local anesthetic can provide excellent analgesia that outlasts the duration

Table 17.2 Local anesthetic techniques.

Local anesthetic techniques	Specific blocks
Wound infiltration	
Field block	Ilioinguinal/iliohypogastric nerves
Upper extremity blocks	Intravenous regional block
	Brachial plexus block
	Wrist block
	Digital block
Lower extremity blocks	Lumbar plexus block
	Femoral nerve block
	Sciatic nerve block
	Popliteal nerve block
	Ankle block
Paravertebral block	
Intracavity local anesthetic administration	Intra-articular administration
	Intraperitoneal administration

of action of the local anesthetic.[26, 27, 63] Interestingly, a systematic review of published literature found that except for inguinal hernia repair surgery, there was a lack of evidence for analgesic efficacy of a single incisional local anesthetic injection.[64] Overall, wound infiltration with long-acting local anesthetics reduces wound pain and is therefore recommended for routine use.[26, 27][I] Although it has been suggested that infiltration of local anesthetic subfascially or injection at the level of the parietal peritoneum provides more effective pain relief compared with subcutaneous infiltration,[65] the evidence is limited and therefore cannot be recommended at this time. Similar to wound infiltration, instillation or aerosol application of local anesthetics in the surgical wound has also been found to provide analgesia and reduce postoperative opioid requirements;[66] however, the evidence is limited and therefore this use is not recommended. Despite its limitations, local anesthetic infiltration of the surgical wound is beneficial and should be performed whenever possible.[26, 27, 67][II]

Intra-articular analgesia

Intra-articular administration of long-acting local anesthetics in patients undergoing joint surgery has been shown to improve pain relief, reduce opioid requirements, and facilitate early recovery and mobilization.[68][I] A systematic review of intra-articular local anesthesia for pain relief after arthroscopic knee surgery found that although the pain relief was small-to-moderate and of short duration, it may be of clinical significance in the ambulatory setting.[68] One of the concerns with this technique is systemic absorption of local anesthetic leading to systemic adverse events.[69] However, the plasma bupivacaine concentrations after intra-articular instillation of 25–40 mL of bupivacaine 0.5 percent have been reported to be within a safe range.[70]

The demonstration of an increased number of opioid receptors on peripheral nerve terminals in the inflammatory models has led to the concept of peripheral opioid analgesia.[71] Peripheral administration of smaller doses of morphine (1–5 mg) has been reported to provide effective postoperative pain relief.[72, 73, 74] Quantitative systematic reviews of published studies found that a single injection of intra-articular morphine (morphine glucuronide) had mild analgesic effects for up to 24 hours, and the analgesic effect was best evident when the pain intensity was moderate to severe.[73, 74][I] With reports of benefits of local anesthetics as well as morphine, the combination of intra-articular bupivacaine and morphine is increasingly used, even in patients undergoing painful joint procedures (e.g. joint replacement surgery).[75, 76][II]

Many investigators have used an arthroscopic model to evaluate the peripheral analgesic properties of nonopioid analgesics (e.g. ketorolac, clonidine, steroids, neostigmine bromide). Because NSAIDs reduce prostaglandin levels at the peripheral nerve sites, they should provide analgesia when injected intra-articularly. Intra-articular administration of ketorolac 60 mg with bupivacaine 0.25 percent provided significant analgesia after knee arthroscopy.[77] However, one of the concerns with the use of intra-articular NSAIDs is the possibility of reduction in chondrocyte biosynthesis and cartilage destruction. Similarly, steroids have also been administered intra-articularly to reduce surgically induced inflammation and improve postoperative pain relief.[78] Intra-articular clonidine in combination with local anesthetics has also been reported to provide effective pain relief.[79] Recent experimental studies suggest that the cholinergic mediated neuropathways can modulate pain transmission.[80] Neostigmine, an anticholinergic drug, can cause hyperpolarization of neurons, reduction in the release of pronociceptive

neurotransmitters, and/or activation of the nitric oxide-cyclic guanosine monophosphate pathway and, thereby, might provide antinociception by elevating endogenous levels of acetylcholine.[80] Intra-articular administration of neostigmine 500 μg has been reported to reduce pain scores and time to rescue analgesics.[81] However, the overall benefits of adding ketorolac, steroids, clonidine, or neostigmine to intra-articular injection of local anesthetic and morphine remains controversial and is not recommended at this time.[82]

Intraperitoneal instillation of local anesthetics

Another simple and effective method of reducing the intensity of postlaparoscopic pain is intraperitoneal instillation of long-acting local anesthetic drugs.[26, 27, 67][I] However, high volumes of more dilute concentrations of local anesthetics may not provide significant pain relief.[27] This would suggest that both the timing and concentration of the local anesthetic are important in achieving effective pain relief with this technique. Significant pain relief after laparoscopic cholecystectomy was observed when 15–20 mL of bupivacaine 0.5 percent with or without epinephrine (adrenaline) was administered into the hepatodiaphragmatic space, near and above the hepatoduodenal ligament and above the gallbladder or gallbladder bed.[26, 27] A recent systematic review of published literature found that intraperitoneal local anesthetic administration provided effective postoperative pain relief.[67][I] Although adverse effects from bupivacaine 150–200 mg with or without epinephrine are rare, caution was recommended.[67]

Peripheral nerve blocks and field blocks

It is well accepted that field blocks or peripheral nerve blocks are highly effective in reducing anesthetic and analgesic requirements in day surgery.[57, 58, 59, 60, 61, 62][II] Because orthopedic surgical procedures have been shown to be associated with significant postoperative pain,[6] the utilization of peripheral nerve blocks for these procedures without general anesthesia may be highly beneficial in reducing the need for hospitalization, allowing early ambulation and return to daily activities.[59, 60, 61, 62][II]

However, one of the major limitations of single injections of local anesthetic is the short duration of analgesia.[83] Because it is difficult to anticipate the degree of pain at the time of discharge in patients who have received single-shot local anesthetic injection, there might be higher pain after discharge.[83] In addition, the abrupt termination of the analgesic effect may lead to an increased perception of pain after recovery from the neural blockade.[62] Therefore, the overall benefits of single-shot local anesthetic techniques may be similar to those after general anesthesia.[83]

Continuous local anesthetic infusion in wound and perineural space

The duration of analgesia can be increased by infusion of local anesthetics through a catheter placed in the layers of the skin or in the perineural space.[84, 85, 86, 87, 88, 89, 90, 91, 92, 93] Elastometric balloon pumps or portable mechanical infusion pumps allow self-administration of local anesthetic solution (i.e. patient-controlled regional analgesia) at home. Infusion in the surgical wound with long-acting local anesthetic is an easy and effective analgesic technique for superficial surgical procedures, breast surgery (e.g. breast augmentation or reduction), relatively minor shoulder surgery, and minor abdominal surgery.[57, 67][II]

The efficacy of continuous perineural (brachial plexus, lumbar plexus, femoral, sciatic, and popliteal nerve) infusion is well documented for ambulatory surgery.[84, 85, 86, 87, 88, 89, 90, 91, 92][II] Recent studies have evaluated their use in this setting.[84, 85, 86, 87, 88, 89, 90, 91, 92] This has enabled prompt discharge with excellent pain control and few side effects after painful and complex procedures. In addition, this technique diminishes breakthrough pain that patients can experience following resolution of a single-injection block. Other benefits of these techniques include reduced sleep disturbances and preserved cognitive function. Perineural local anesthetic infusion may allow more vigorous postoperative physical therapy. Furthermore, the use of continuous infusion techniques should allow more extensive and painful surgical procedures to be performed on an ambulatory surgical basis.[84, 85, 86, 87, 88, 89, 90, 91, 92]

Recently, Ilfeld et al.[90] reported that the use of continous interscalene nerve block decreases the time to discharge home after total shoulder arthroplasty, a procedure that is otherwise performed on an inpatient basis. Similarly, Capadevila et al.[91] reported that continuous perineural local anesthetic infusion with patient-controlled administration in patients undergoing ambulatory orthopedic procedures improved pain relief and optimized functional recovery. Because of the ease of performance and its safety, femoral nerve block remains one of the most commonly performed lower extremity peripheral nerve blocks. It can provide excellent pain relief after knee procedures, but preserves hip flexion. The sciatic nerve block can also be used for knee and hip procedures, however, the majority of studies have used the sciatic nerve as an adjunct to femoral or lumbar plexus blocks. Combined femoral and sciatic nerve blocks have been shown to reduce pain and opioid requirements after anterior cruciate liagament surgery performed on an ambulatory surgical basis.[92] Recently, paravertebral blocks have been utilized as they provide similar benefits as epidural analgesia but without its potential adverse effects (**Table 17.3**).[87] In contrast to epidural infusion, patients with a continuous local anesthetic infusion through a paravertebral catheter can be discharged home.

Table 17.3 Indications of paravertebral blocks.

Indications	
Breast surgery	
Mastectomy	
Breast augmentation/reduction	
Abdominal wall herniorrhaphy	
Minilaparotomy	
Laparoscopic Nissen's fundoplication	
Orthopedic surgery	Shoulder/elbow surgery
	Iliac crest bone grafting

Perineural local anesthetic infusion is generally well tolerated by day surgery patients.[93] Although there is a risk of catheter migration and potential local anesthetic toxicity, this risk is minimal.[89] Other concerns include patient injury related to the insensate extremity, particularly after discharge home, as well as masking of surgery-related nerve injury and compartment syndrome.[89] In addition, there is also a concern of increased potential for surgical wound infection due to the presence of a catheter; however, a large series of peripheral local anesthetic infusions has not reported an increased incidence of infection.[89] Most importantly, appropriate patient selection, education, and follow up are crucial with continuous catheter techniques in an unmonitored environment.

Nevertheless, there is clearly a need for refinement of peripheral nerve block techniques and development of more effective methods for continuous administration after discharge (i.e. less bulky infusion devices and improved technology to reduce failure). The use of ultrasound to guide catheter placement may reduce failure rate as well as some of the complications associated with these regional techniques.[94] Further studies are necessary to clarify the clinical significance of the timing of local anesthetic blockade, as well as the dose and volume of local anesthetics.

It is now recognized that the inflammatory responses to injury (e.g. increase in cytokines) are not modified by neural blockade. Peripheral sensitization induces COX-2 expression in the central nervous system (CNS) through neuronal activity arising from the sensory fibers innervating the inflamed tissue (this can be blocked using local anesthetic technique) and a humoral response through a signal molecule (probably pro-inflammatory cytokines IL-6) that enters the circulation, crosses the blood–brain barrier, and elevates IL-1β (this can be blocked by a COX-2 inhibitor).[34] Therefore, the combination of COX-2 inhibitors (i.e. NSAIDs and COX-2 selective inhibitors) with local/regional analgesia may be a more appropriate regimen to improve postoperative pain relief.[95][II]

Paracetamol

Paracetamol is generally recognized as a safe and effective drug with a favorable side effect profile,[96, 97, 98][I] and is a widely used over-the-counter analgesic and antipyretic drug. Although the mechanism of action of paracetamol is poorly understood, it is thought to act by inhibition of COX-3 isoenzyme and subsequent reduced prostanoid release in the CNS.[99, 100] Paracetamol is devoid of some of the side effects of nonselective (traditional) NSAIDs, such as gastrointestinal ulceration and hemorrhage, cardiorenal adverse effects, and impaired platelet aggregation.[96] Furthermore, unlike nonselective NSAIDs and COX-2 selective inhibitors, paracetamol does not appear to have clinically significant effects on bone and ligament healing.[2] Although it is generally considered safe, paracetamol is associated with liver toxicity,[101] particularly in patients with compromised hepatic function, severe alcoholism, cirrhosis, or hepatitis. In addition, recent data suggest that higher doses of paracetamol may also have gastrointestinal and cardiovascular adverse effects similar to nonselective NSAIDs.[102, 103] Importantly, patients should be warned that commonly used opioid combinations may contain paracetamol. Furthermore, paracetamol displays an analgesic ceiling effect similar to nonselective NSAIDs and COX-2 selective inhibitors.[104] Of note, paracetamol has weak anti-inflammatory activity and may not block the inflammatory pain response. Of note, paracetamol has a weak anti-inflammatory action and may not block the inflammatory pain response. It is a weak analgesic, and as the sole agent may not provide adequate pain relief. However, it may be combined with other analgesics to provide superior pain relief and reduce opioid requirements.[21, 105, 106]

The availability of an injectable form of paracetamol (and prodrug, propacetamol) has expanded the knowledge of the pharmacodynamics of paracetamol in terms of the relationship between plasma level, peak concentrations, and clinical efficacy. Compared with oral formulations, parenteral paracetamol has a predictable onset and duration of action.[107] Intravenous paracetamol 1 g possesses a similar analgesic efficacy to 2 g of the prodrug of paracetamol, propacetamol. The initial dose of injectable paracetamol can be given intraoperatively followed by oral administration after discharge home.

NSAIDs and COX-2-selective inhibitors

With improved understanding of pain mechanisms, and the realization that tissue injury and subsequent inflammation causes the induction of COX-2 expression both at the peripheral and the central nervous system sites, leading to peripheral and central sensitization,[34] as well as the widespread acceptance of the concept of multimodal analgesia,[40] anti-inflammatory drugs have been increasingly used in the management of perioperative pain.[100, 108, 109, 110] There is no evidence that a particular route of NSAID administration (e.g. intravenous versus oral) is superior for perioperative use,[109][I] because oral availability of most NSAIDs is high. However, bioavailability

after rectal administration is low.[109] Therefore, NSAIDs should preferably be administered orally if patients can swallow and the choice of NSAID would depend upon the duration of analgesia, the propensity for side effects, and cost. Of note, NSAIDs exhibit a "ceiling effect" with respect to their maximum analgesic effect,[111] and they have weaker analgesic properties than opioids or local anesthetic techniques.

Despite numerous benefits, nonselective NSAIDs are not routinely used perioperatively,[6, 7] probably because of concerns regarding their potential adverse effects such as impaired coagulation (and increased perioperative bleeding), gastric irritation, renal dysfunction, and cardiovascular complications (**Table 17.4**). Overall, NSAIDs appear to be safe and well tolerated in patients undergoing ambulatory surgery. Nevertheless, NSAIDs should be used with caution in patients with preexisting coagulation defects or those undergoing certain surgical procedures (e.g. tonsillectomy and plastic surgery).[112, 113] Similarly, these drugs are best avoided in patients with pre-existing renal dysfunction, hypovolemia, sepsis, or end-stage cirrhosis of the liver.[114, 115] Although the gastrointestinal adverse effects of short-term use of nonselective NSAIDs appears to be safe,[112, 116] they should be used with caution in patients at high risk of gastrointestinal complications. Finally, NSAIDs should be used with caution in the elderly and in patients at high cardiac risk.[117]

The COX-2-selective inhibitors were developed to target the COX-2 enzyme while sparing the COX-1 enzyme, avoiding the COX-1-related adverse effects of nonselective NSAIDs (e.g. gastrointestinal and platelet dysfunction). Of note, the COX-2-selective inhibitors have similar analgesic efficacy as nonselective NSAIDs, and exhibit a "ceiling effect" with respect to their maximum analgesic effect. It is suggested that the COX-2-selective inhibitors may have an advantage over nonselective NSAIDs because they do not affect platelet function and reduce the risk of gastrointestinal complications, and may be safely administered preoperatively.[118, 119, 120, 121] In addition, the COX-2-selective inhibitors do not appear to inhibit bone healing.[122]

Table 17.4 Adverse effects of nonselective nonsteroidal anti-inflammatory drugs.

Adverse effects	
Gastrointestinal	Dyspepsia
	Diarrhea
	Peptic ulcer and hemorrhage
Renal	Acute renal failure
	Decreased renal blood flow
	Decreased glomerular filtration
Hemostatic	Inhibition of platelet aggregation
	Increased bleeding time
Immunological	Anaphylaxis, aspirin-induced asthma

Parecoxib, a prodrug of valdecoxib, is the first injectable COX-2 selective inhibitor approved in Europe and Australia for short-term (less than ten days) treatment of moderate-to-severe postoperative pain. It is currently undergoing phase III clinical trials for approval by the United States Food and Drug Administration.[123, 124, 125] Numerous studies have reported on the analgesic and opioid-sparing efficacy of parecoxib.[118] In addition, some studies have reported opioid-related side effects and superior quality of postoperative recovery as well as a faster return to normal activity and greater patient satisfaction.[123, 124, 125][II]

Recently, there have been increasing concerns that anti-inflammatory drugs have cardiovascular adverse effects. Published meta-analysis of randomized trials and systematic reviews of observational trials of long-term use of anti-inflammatory drugs have reported that there is a significant risk of cardiovascular events with rofecoxib, but celecoxib in commonly used doses (< 200 mg/day) may not increase the risk.[126, 127, 128][I] In addition, there may be increased risks with nonselective NSAIDs.[126, 127] With respect to short-term use, a large study in patients undergoing major surgical procedures did not find an increased incidence of cardiovascular adverse events with short-term use of parecoxib and valdecoxib.[125] A post-hoc pooled analysis of cardiovascular safety data from all randomized, placebo-controlled parecoxib studies in major surgery ($n = 19$), which included two coronary artery bypass grafting studies and 17 noncardiac surgery studies, was performed to achieve the greatest statistical power.[129] The data indicated that the incidence of cardiovascular adverse events after short-term use of parecoxib 20–80 mg (0.44 percent) were similar to that with placebo (0.37 percent). However, none of the studies conducted so far were specifically designed to examine the cardiovascular outcomes and patients included in the noncardiac studies had a low cardiovascular risk. Therefore, further study is required to determine the safety cardiovascular profile in patients with high cardiovascular risk. In the meantime, anti-inflammatory drugs should be avoided in patients at high cardiac risk (e.g. previous myocardial infarction, unstable angina, congestive heart failure, and known or suspected atherosclerotic disease). The Food and Drug Administration of the United States has imposed a "boxed warning" of increased cardiovascular risks with both nonselective NSAIDs and COX-2 selective inhibitors.

Alpha–2 receptor agonists

Alpha-2 receptor agonists (e.g. clonidine and dexmedetomidine) have hypnotic, sedative, sympatholytic, and analgesic properties via central actions in the locus ceruleus and in the dorsal horn of the spinal cord.[130, 131] They improve analgesia and reduce opioid requirements; however, they are limited by their side effects including bradycardia, hypotension, and excessive sedation. Nevertheless, the addition of clonidine to the local anesthetic solution for peripheral nerve blocks has been reported to enhance and prolong analgesia.[57][II]

Dexmedetomidine is a more selective alpha-2 agonist with a shorter duration of action. Because it provides analgesia without respiratory depression, it may be beneficial in patients at risk of postoperative respiratory depression and airway obstruction (e.g. morbid obesity, obstructive sleep apnea, and airway abnormalities). One of the limitations of dexmedetomidine is that a short duration of action may lead to increased pain after discontinuation of the infusion unless other longer-acting analgesics are administered. The role of dexmedetomidine in the ambulatory setting is as yet unclear.

Glucocorticoids

Because perioperative pain is primarily an inflammatory phenomenon,[34] anti-inflammatory drugs such as steroids may play a role in pain management. Although the mechanisms of analgesic effects of steroids are as yet unclear, their anti-inflammatory properties and inhibition of prostaglandin and leukotriene production may play some role.[132] Several studies have reported analgesic effects of a single doses of steroid administered intraoperatively.[132, 133, 134, 135] Concerns of perioperative steroids include increased infection rate, gastrointestinal side effects, and delayed wound healing.[132] However, single doses of steroids have not been found to cause any significant adverse effects. Of note, the studies have been small and have not included patients at risk. In addition to analgesic properties, steroids also have antiemetic properties that could be highly beneficial in the ambulatory setting.[134][II]

NMDA receptor antagonists

Because NMDA receptors have been implicated in the development of central sensitization,[34, 136]), NMDA antagonists (i.e. ketamine and dextromethorphan) have been used to provide postoperative analgesia.[137, 138, 139, 140] Low doses of ketamine have been shown to reduce opioid requirements, prolong opioid analgesia, and improve pain relief.[136, 137, 138, 139, 140] However, routine use of ketamine, in the outpatient setting, remains controversial because of the potential adverse effects (e.g. hemodynamic and psychomimetic effects). Dextromethorphan, a popular antitussive ingredient, is an isomer of the codeine analog levorphanol.[141, 142] Because it is available in both intravenous and oral formulation, it can be used to maintain NMDA receptor blockade after discharge home.[141, 142] Although intravenous dextromethorphan has been shown to be beneficial,[141, 142][I] the efficacy of the oral formation remains controversial.

Further research is necessary to determine the appropriate dose, timing, and duration of administration of NMDA antagonists, as well as the benefits of their combination with other analgesics.

Anticonvulsants

Gabapentin and pregabalin are anticonvulsants with analgesic properties and have been widely used for the treatment of neuropathic pain. Their mechanism of analgesic action is through the modulation of the presynaptic alpha-2 delta subunits of the calcium channels in the spinal cord and brain.[143] Recent studies have evaluated the efficacy of these drugs in the management of postoperative pain.[144, 145, 146, 147] Gabapentin 1200 mg administered prior to radical mastectomy was found to reduce movement-related pain and opioid requirements.[145] Another study evaluating the analgesic effects of gabapentin 1200 mg and mexiletine 600 mg after breast surgery for cancer found that both gabapentin and mexiletine equally reduced analgesic requirements at rest; however, gabapentin was more effective in reducing pain after movement.[146] A recent systematic review evaluating the perioperative use of gabapentin and pregabalin concluded that these drugs might have beneficial analgesic properties in the perioperative period.[147] However, all the studies have had a small sample size and have a short duration of follow up. Therefore, larger studies of longer duration are required before routine use of gabapentin or pregabalin can be recommended for postoperative pain management.

PAIN CONTROL IN THE EARLY POSTOPERATIVE PERIOD

Pain relief in the immediate postoperative period is critical to facilitate discharge home. With increased emphasis on the sparing use of opioids in the intraoperative period,[44] patients may arrive in PACU in pain if nonopioids are not administered at appropriate times prior to emergence.[6] Patients complaining of pain in the recovery room may receive parenteral and/or oral analgesics, depending upon the severity of pain. The rapid recovery associated with the availability of short-acting anesthetic drugs and the use of prophylactic antiemetics makes it possible for patients to tolerate oral medications in the early postoperative period. Oral analgesics (opioid and/or nonopioid) may be used in the early recovery period if the patient is in mild-to-moderate pain and is not experiencing nausea or vomiting.

Patients not tolerating oral analgesics could receive intravenous NSAIDs, if there are no contraindications. However, it may be necessary to use opioids if the pain is severe or if NSAIDs are not adequate. The choice of parenteral opioid could be short acting (e.g. fentanyl) or longer acting (e.g. morphine). Fentanyl has a faster onset, and its use may provide more effective pain control in the early postoperative period. On the other hand, morphine provides a longer duration of analgesia, but its slower onset may result in the administration of extra doses and thereby increase side effects (e.g. sedation, nausea, and vomiting). It is generally believed that morphine should not be used in ambulatory surgery patients because of the concerns of increased postoperative nausea and vomiting. However, the use of fentanyl in the PACU might lead to recurrence of pain in the phase II unit, and delayed discharge home and increase the need for hospitalization, particularly if oral analgesics are not administered or are not tolerated.

Claxton et al.[148] compared the analgesic efficacy and the incidence of opioid-related side effects of equipotent doses of morphine (1–2 mg) and fentanyl (12.5–25 μg) repeated every five minutes. These authors found that morphine and fentanyl in equipotent doses were comparable in treating postoperative pain in the PACU. However, these regimens did not provide rapid analgesia, as it took over 20 minutes to achieve a significant decrease in baseline pain scores. Morphine provided more sustained analgesia than fentanyl, but it was associated with a higher incidence of nausea and vomiting after discharge home.[148] On the other hand, patients receiving fentanyl required additional oral analgesia during the second phase of recovery. Therefore, these authors suggested that if fentanyl is used to provide analgesia in the PACU, oral analgesics should be administered as supplements to provide more prolonged pain relief. If oral analgesics are not administered, morphine may be a better choice. Of note, local anesthetic techniques should be considered an option and utilized in the immediate postoperative period if oral or parenteral analgesics do not provide adequate pain relief.

PAIN CONTROL AFTER DISCHARGE HOME

Patients undergoing day-case procedures require an analgesic technique that is effective, devoid of side effects, intrinsically safe, and easily managed at home. With more extensive and painful surgical procedures being performed on an outpatient basis, pain management after discharge is increasingly becoming more challenging. After discharge home, oral paracetamol, NSAIDs or opioids (e.g. codeine, oxycodone, and hydrocodone), either alone or in combination, are frequently used to provide postoperative pain relief. Regular dosing with analgesic medications provides superior analgesia as this prevents the pain from becoming severe and decreases the incidence of breakthrough pain.

Moderate-to-severe pain not responding to nonopioid analgesics should be treated with a combination of paracetamol or NSAIDs and opioids, which may prove more effective than either drug alone. A quantitative systematic review of randomized controlled trials evaluating the analgesic efficacy of paracetamol administered either alone or in combination with codeine found that paracetamol is an effective analgesic, and that the addition of codeine 60 mg produces worthwhile additional pain relief, even in single doses.[149] Controlled-release preparations of oxycodone have been reported to provide superior analgesia, because they allow greater convenience, improve patient compliance, and provide uninterrupted nighttime sleep.[150, 151] However, controlled-release preparations should never be used on an "as needed" basis because it may take as long as four hours to attain peak analgesia. The slow onset of analgesia also makes it difficult to titrate to the degree of pain.

Tramadol, a synthetic, centrally acting analgesic, is a weak opioid agonist, with selectivity for the μ-receptor, and a weak inhibitor of the reuptake of norepinephrine and serotonin.[152] Unlike other opioids, tramadol does not have clinically significant respiratory effects. In many countries, tramadol is not a controlled substance because it has low abuse and addiction potential. The adult dose of tramadol is 50–100 mg every four to six hours with a maximum of 400 mg per day. The availability of controlled-release tramadol makes it an attractive alternative to controlled-release oxycodone. Although it is generally well tolerated, side effects include nausea, vomiting, dizziness, and drowsiness. Tramadol has a potential to cause seizures, and it should therefore be used with caution in patients with increased intracranial pressures and in patients receiving neuroleptic drugs. It is also contraindicated in patients receiving monoamine oxidase inhibitors.

Sometimes patients are reluctant to use analgesics, and consider them as a last resort. Therefore, it is necessary to educate patients that it is preferable not to allow pain to become severe, as it is easier to "control" pain if it is treated at an early stage. Patients should also be informed about nonpharmacologic ways of alleviating postoperative pain, such as the application of ice, elevation of the operated extremity, and wearing loose-fitting clothing.

SURGICAL CONSIDERATIONS

Several studies have found that the type of surgical procedure is a significant predictor of severity of postoperative pain.[6, 14] Certain procedures (e.g. orthopedic and urologic procedures) produce more pain than other surgical procedures.[6, 14] The surgical technique may also affect the degree of postoperative pain. Minimally invasive surgical techniques are associated with smaller incisions, which may reduce tissue trauma and decrease postoperative pain. Nevertheless, the pain after laparoscopic procedures can sometimes be severe and may last for several days.[26, 27] The type of pain after laparoscopic procedures is primarily visceral in origin (versus somatic

pain after open surgery). Higher insufflation pressures should be avoided, as they can significantly increase the severity of postoperative pain.[153] Subphrenic and shoulder pain after laparoscopic procedures appears to arise from diaphragmatic and phrenic nerve irritation due to insufflated carbon dioxide. This pain tends to be aggravated by ambulation and may persist for several days after surgery.

Pain after laparoscopic tubal ligation is usually more severe than that after diagnostic laparoscopy. The deep pelvic pain after tubal ligation might be due to tubal spasm following their occlusion or due to uterine contractions resulting from prostaglandin release secondary to tubal trauma and ischemia. Administration of an antispasmodic drugs (e.g. glycopyrronium bromide (glycopyrrolate) 0.3 mg, i.v.) at induction of anesthesia significantly reduced pain scores in the immediate postoperative period, decreased the requirements for analgesics, and improved the quality of recovery after daycase laparoscopic sterilization.[154] Also, sequential avulsion of the long saphenous vein reduces postoperative pain, as compared to stripping.[155] Similarly, tension-free hernia repair using a laparoscopic technique or a mesh-plug is less painful.[156, 157] It has been suggested that infection of hemorrhoidectomy wounds may influence postoperative pain and analgesic requirement through inflammatory swelling and edema.[158] Administration of metronidazole in ambulatory surgery patients undergoing hemorrhoidectomy has been shown to decrease the degree of pain, increase patient satisfaction, and allow for an earlier return to work.[159]

FUTURE DEVELOPMENTS

With a better understanding of pain mechanisms it may be possible to develop novel drugs with long-lasting, peripheral analgesic effects, and negligible adverse effects.[34] The availability of longer-acting, slow-release preparations, which incorporate local anesthetics or opioids into liposomes (or microspheres), can extend the duration of action and enhance the efficacy of local anesthetic techniques.[160, 161, 162] Novel delivery systems that are less invasive and provide continuous delivery preventing analgesic gaps (i.e. breakthrough pain) have been investigated. Intranasal analgesics (e.g. intranasal ketorolac and nicotine) are being evaluated.[163] Patient-controlled analgesia systems that deliver small doses of fentanyl (40 μg) every ten minutes by iontophoresis has been shown to provide pain relief similar to a standard intravenous morphine PCA regimen.[164, 165] Although this transdermal system is not currently approved for non-inpatient use, it may be used as an adjunct with non-opioids for the control of moderate-to-severe pain. Future analgesic techniques may also include use of bradykinin and substance-P antagonists and leukotriene synthesis blockers used as a part of balanced analgesia regimens.

SUMMARY

The management of pain after ambulatory surgery poses some unique challenges for the practitioner. The goal of pain management should be to minimize pain not only at rest, but also during mobilization and physical therapy. Local anesthetic techniques, preferably perineural infusion, should be utilized whenever possible because they allow a more rapid recovery and discharge. In addition, local anesthetic techniques provide pain relief until the onset of oral analgesics. Whenever possible, local anesthetic techniques may be combined with NSAIDs initiated prior to surgery and continued until tissue inflammation is resolved. Furthermore, it is imperative that these analgesics are administered on a regular "round-the-clock" basis with, opioids used as "rescue" analgesics or "as needed" basis. The role of alpha-2-adrenergic agonists (e.g. clonidine and dexmedetomidine), NMDA receptor antagonists (e.g. ketamine), and anticonvulsants (e.g. gabapentin and pregabalin) in the day surgery setting needs to be clarified by further investigation, which also focuses on patient outcome and cost-effective related issues.

An important reason for suboptimal pain management is inadequate or improper application of available information. The procedure-specific guidelines that are incorporated into clinical pathways for specific surgical procedures may improve postoperative pain management and surgical outcome. It is also necessary to improve the instructions given to the patients and their families regarding the treatment of pain after discharge. Finally, it is important to integrate the analgesic therapy into the surgical care as a continuum from the preoperative period through the convalescence period, which will require close cooperation between the anesthesiologists and surgeons.

REFERENCES

1. Liu JH, Etzioni DA, O'Connell JB et al. The increasing workload of surgery. *Archives of Surgery*. 2004; **139**: 423–8.

* 2. Joshi GP. Multimodal analgesia techniques for ambulatory surgery. *International Anesthesiology Clinics*. 2005; **43**: 215–18.

3. Joshi GP. Pain management after ambulatory surgery. *Ambulatory Surgery*. 1999; **7**: 3–12.

4. Wu CL, Berenholtz SM, Pronovost PJ, Fleisher LA. Systematic review and analysis of postdischarge symptoms after outpatient surgery. *Anesthesiology*. 2002; **96**: 994–1003.

* 5. Joshi GP, Ogunnaike B. Consequences of inadequate postoperative pain relief and chronic persistent postoperative pain. *Anesthesiology Clinics of North America*. 2005; **23**: 21–36.

6. Chung F, Ritchie E, Su J. Postoperative pain in ambulatory surgery. *Anesthesia and Analgesia*. 1997; **85**: 808–16.

7. Pavlin DJ, Chen C, Penaloza DA et al. Pain as a factor complicating recovery and discharge after ambulatory surgery. *Anesthesia and Analgesia*. 2002; **95**: 627–34.

8. Fortier J, Chung F, Su J. Unanticipated admission after ambulatory surgery – a prospective study. *Canadian Journal of Anaesthesia*. 1998; **45**: 612–19.

9. Ghosh S, Sallam S. Patient satisfaction and postoperative demands on hospital and community services after day surgery. *British Journal of Surgery*. 1994; **81**: 1635–8.

10. Wu CL, Naqibuddin M, Rowlingson AJ et al. The effect of pain on health-related quality of life in the immediate postoperative period. *Anesthesia and Analgesia*. 2003; **97**: 1078–85.

11. Mattila K, Toivonen J, Janhunen L et al. Postdischarge symptoms after ambulatory surgery: first-week incidence, intensity, and risk factors. *Anesthesia and Analgesia*. 2005; **101**: 1643–50.

* 12. Kehlet H, Jensen TS, Woolf C. Persistent postsurgical pain: risk factors and prevention. *Lancet*. 2006; **367**: 1618–25.

13. Tong D, Chung F, Wong D. Predictive factors in global and anesthesia satisfaction in ambulatory surgical patients. *Anesthesiology*. 1997; **87**: 856–64.

14. Rawal N, Hylander J, Nydahl PA et al. Survey of postoperative analgesia following ambulatory surgery. *Acta Anaesthesiologica Scandinavica*. 1997; **41**: 1017–22.

15. Apfelbaum JL, Chen C, Shilpa S, Gan TJ. Postoperative pain experience: results from a national survey suggest postoperative pain continues to be undermanaged. *Anesthesia and Analgesia*. 2003; **97**: 534–40.

* 16. American Society of Anesthesiologists Task Force on Acute Pain Management. Practice guidelines for acute pain management in the perioperative setting. *Anesthesiology*. 2004; **100**: 1573–81.

* 17. Australian and New Zealand College of Anaesthetists, Faculty of Pain Medicine. *Acute pain management: Scientific evidence*, 2nd edn. Melbourne: Australian and New Zealand College of Anaesthetists, 2005. Also available online at: www.anzca.edu.au/resources/books-and-publications.

* 18. Moore A, Edwards J, Barden J, McQuay H. *Bandolier's little book of pain*. Oxford: Oxford University Press, 2003.

19. Rowlingson JC, Rawal N. Postoperative pain guidelines targeted to the site of surgery. *Regional Anesthesia and Pain Medicine*. 2003; **284**: 265–7.

20. Gray A, Kehlet H, Bonnet F, Rawal N. Predicting postoperative analgesia outcomes: NNT league tables or procedure-specific evidence? *British Journal of Anaesthesia*. 2005; **94**: 710–14.

21. Hyllested M, Jones S, Pedersen JL, Kehlet H. Comparative effect of acetaminophen, NSAIDs or their combination in postoperative pain management: a qualitative review. *British Journal of Anaesthesia*. 2002; **88**: 199–214.

* 22. Kehlet H. Procedure specific postoperative pain management. *Anesthesiology Clinics of North America*. 2005; **23**: 209–10.

* 23. Rosenquist RW, Rosenberg J, and United States Veterans Administration. Postoperative pain guidelines. *Regional*

Anesthesia and Pain Medicine. 2003; **28**: 279–88 (www.oqp.med.va.gov/cpg/cpg.htm).

* 24. PROSPECT: Procedure-specific postoperative pain management. Last accessed February 20, 2008. Available from: www.postoppain.org.

25. Neugebauer E, Wilkinson R, Kehlet H, on behalf of the PROSPECT Group. Transferable evidence in support of reaching a consensus. *German Journal of Evidence and Quality in Healthcare.* 2007; **101**: 419–26.

* 26. Kehlet H, Gray AW, Bonnet F, on behalf of the PROSPECT Group. A procedure-specific systematic review and consensus recommendations for postoperative analgesia following laparoscopic cholecystectomy. *Surgical Endoscopy.* 2005; **19**: 1396–415.

* 27. Bisgaard T. Analgesic treatment after laparoscopic cholecystectomy. A critical assessment of the evidence. *Anesthesiology.* 2006; **104**: 835–46.

28. Doyle CE. Preoperative strategies for managing postoperative pain at home after day surgery. *Journal of Perianesthesia Nursing.* 1999; **14**: 373–9.

29. Scott NB, Hodson M. Public perceptions of postoperative pain and its relief. *Anaesthesia.* 1997; **52**: 438–42.

30. McGrath B, Elgendy H, Chung F et al. Thirty percent of patients have moderate to severe pain 24 hr after ambulatory surgery: a survey of 5,703 patients. *Canadian Journal of Anaesthesia.* 2004; **51**: 886–91.

31. Slappendel R, Weber E, Bugter M, Dirksen R. The intensity of preoperative pain is directly correlated with the amount of morphine needed for postoperative analgesia. *Anesthesia and Analgesia.* 1999; **88**: 146–8.

32. Robaux S, Bouaziz H, Cornet C et al. Acute postoperative pain management at home after ambulatory surgery: a French pilot survey of general practitioners' views. *Anesthesia and Analgesia.* 2002; **95**: 1258–62.

* 33. Brennan TJ, Zahn PK, Pogatzki-Zahn EM. Mechanisms of incisional pain. *Anesthesiology Clinics of North America.* 2005; **23**: 1–20.

* 34. Woolf CJ. Pain: moving from symptom control towards mechanism-specific pharmacologic management. *Annals of Internal Medicine.* 2004; **140**: 441–51.

35. Woolf CJ, Chong M. Preemptive analgesia – treating postoperative pain by preventing the establishment of central sensitization. *Anesthesia and Analgesia.* 1993; **77**: 362–79.

36. Dahl JB, Kehlet H. The value of pre-emptive analgesia in the treatment of postoperative pain. *British Journal of Anaesthesia.* 1993; **70**: 434–9.

37. Kissin I. Preemptive analgesia. *Anesthesiology.* 2000; **93**: 1138–43.

* 38. Moiniche S, Kehlet H, Dahl JB. A qualitative and quantitative systematic review of preemptive analgesia for postoperative pain relief. *Anesthesiology.* 2002; **96**: 725–41.

* 39. Ochroch EA, Mardini IA, Gottschalk A. What is the role of NSAIDs in pre-emptive analgesia? *Drug.* 2004; **63**: 2709–23.

* 40. Joshi GP. Multimodal analgesia techniques and postoperative rehabilitation. *Anesthesiology Clinics of North America.* 2005; **23**: 185–202.

41. Jin F, Chung F. Multimodal analgesia for postoperative pain control. *Journal of Clinical Anesthesia.* 2001; **13**: 524–39.

42. Kehlet H, Werner M, Perkins F. Balanced analgesia. What is it and what are its advantages in postoperative period? *Drugs.* 1999; **58**: 793–7.

43. Kehlet H, Rung GW, Callesen T. Postoperative opioid analgesia: time for a reconsideration? *Journal of Clinical Anesthesia.* 1996; **8**: 441–5.

44. Kehlet H. Postoperative opioid sparing to hasten recovery: what are the issues? *Anesthesiology.* 2005; **102**: 1083–5.

45. Chia YY, Liu K, Wang JJ et al. Intraoperative high dose fentanyl induces postoperative fentanyl tolerance. *Canadian Journal of Anaesthesia.* 1999; **46**: 872–7.

46. Guignard B, Bossard AE, Coste C et al. Acute opioid tolerance: intraoperative remifentanil increases postoperative pain and morphine requirement. *Anesthesiology.* 2000; **93**: 409–17.

47. Wheeler M, Oderda GM, Ashburn MA, Lipman AG. Adverse events associated with postoperative opioid analgesia: a systemic review. *Journal of Pain.* 2002; **3**: 159–80.

48. Zhao SZ, Chung F, Hanna DB et al. Dose-response relationship between opioid use and adverse effects after ambulatory surgery. *Journal of Pain and Symptom Management.* 2004; **28**: 35–46.

49. Dolin SJ, Cashman JN. Tolerability of acute postoperative pain management: nausea, vomiting, sedation, pruritis, and urinary retention. Evidence from published data. *British Journal of Anaesthesia.* 2005; **95**: 584–91.

50. Remy C, Marret E, Bonnet F. Effects of acetaminophen on morphine side-effects and consumption after major surgery: meta-analysis of randomized controlled trials. *British Journal of Anaesthesia.* 2005; **94**: 505–13.

51. Marret E, Kurdi O, Zufferey P, Bonnet F. Effects of nonsteroidal antiinflammatory drugs on patient-controlled analgesia morphine side effects: meta-analysis of randomized controlled trials. *Anesthesiology.* 2005; **102**: 1249–60.

52. Roberts GW, Becker TB, Carlsen HH et al. Postoperative nausea and vomiting are strongly influenced by postoperative opioid use in a dose-related manner. *Anesthesia and Analgesia.* 2005; **101**: 1343–8.

53. Frasco PE, Sprung J, Trentman TL. The impact of the joint commission for accreditation of healthcare organizations pain initiative on perioperative opiate consumption and recovery room length of stay. *Anesthesia and Analgesia.* 2005; **100**: 162–8.

54. Smetzer JL, Cohen MR. Pain scales don't weigh every risk. *Journal of Pain and Palliative Care Pharmacotherapy.* 2003; **17**: 67–70.

55. Romsing J, Moiniche S, Mathiesen O, Dahl JB. Reduction of opioid-related adverse events using opioid-sparing analgesia with COX-2 inhibitors lacks documentation: a

systematic review. *Acta Anaesthesiologica Scandinavica.* 2005; **49**: 133–42.

56. van den Bosch JE, Kalkman CJ, Vergouwe Y *et al.* Assessing the applicability of scoring systems for predicting postoperative nausea and vomiting. *Anaesthesia.* 2005; **60**: 323–31.

57. Joshi GP. Recent developments in regional anesthesia for ambulatory surgery. *Current Opinion in Anaesthesiology.* 1999; **12**: 643–7.

58. Nielsen KC, Steele SM. Outcome after regional anesthesia in the ambulatory setting – is it really worth it? *Best Practice and Research. Clinical Anaesthesiology.* 2002; **16**: 145–57.

59. Williams BA, Kentor ML, Vogt MT *et al.* Economics of nerve block pain management after anterior cruciate ligament reconstruction: potential hospital cost savings via associated postanesthesia care unit bypass and same-day discharge. *Anesthesiology.* 2004; **100**: 697–706.

60. Hadzic A, Arliss J, Kerimoglu B *et al.* A comparison of infraclavicular nerve block versus general anesthesia for hand and wrist day-case surgeries. *Anesthesiology.* 2004; **101**: 127–32.

61. Hadzic A, Williams BA, Karaca PE *et al.* For outpatient rotator cuff surgery, nerve block anesthesia provides superior same-day recovery over general anesthesia. *Anesthesiology.* 2005; **102**: 1001–07.

62. Wilson AT, Nicholson E, Burton L, Wild C. Analgesia for day-case shoulder surgery. *British Journal of Anaesthesia.* 2004; **92**: 414–15.

63. Dahl JB, Moiniche S, Kehlet H. Wound infiltration with local anesthetics for postoperative pain relief. *Acta Anaesthesiologica Scandinavica.* 1994; **38**: 7–14.

64. Moiniche S, Mikkelsen S, Wetterslev J, Dahl JB. A qualitative systematic review of incisional local anesthesia for postoperative pain relief after abdominal operations. *British Journal of Anaesthesia.* 1998; **81**: 377–83.

65. Yndgaard S, Holst P, Bjerre-Jepsen K *et al.* Subcutaneously versus subfascially administered lidocaine in pain treatment after inguinal herniotomy. *Anesthesia and Analgesia.* 1994; **79**: 324–7.

66. Spittal MJ, Hunter SJ. A comparison of bupivacaine instillation and inguinal field block for pain control after herniorrhaphy. *Annals of the Royal College of Surgeons of England.* 1992; **74**: 85–8.

67. Striujs P, Kerkhoffs G. *Ankle sprain.* BMJ Clinical Evidence. London: BMJ, last updated September 1, 2007; cited February 2008. Available from: http:// clinicalevidence.bmj.com/ceweb/conditions/msd/1115/ 1115_background.jsp.

68. Moiniche S, Mikkelsen S, Wetterslev J, Dahl JB. A systematic review of intra-articular local anesthesia for postoperative pain relief after arthroscopic knee surgery. *Regional Anesthesia and Pain Medicine.* 1999; **24**: 430–7.

69. Hoeft MA, Rathmell JP, Dayton MR *et al.* Continuous, intra-articular infusion of bupivacaine after total-knee arthroplasty may lead to potentially toxic serum levels of

local anesthetic. *Regional Anesthesia and Pain Medicine.* 2005; **30**: 414–15.

70. Kaeding CC, Hill JA, Katz J, Benson L. Bupivacaine use after knee arthroscopy: pharmacokinetics and pain control study. *Arthroscopy.* 1990; **6**: 33–9.

71. Joshi GP, McCarroll SM, Cooney CM *et al.* Intra-articular morphine for pain relief after knee arthroscopy. *Journal of Bone and Joint Surgery.* 1992; **74-B**: 749–51.

72. Joshi GP, McCarroll SM, O'Brien TM, Lenane P. Intraarticular analgesia following knee arthroscopy. *Anesthesia and Analgesia.* 1993; **76**: 333–6.

73. Kalso E, Tramer MR, Carroll D *et al.* Pain relief from intra-articular morphine after knee surgery: a qualitative systemic review. *Pain.* 1997; **71**: 127–34.

∗ 74. Gupta A, Bodin L, Holmstrom B, Berggren L. A systematic review of peripheral analgesic effects of intraarticular morphine. *Anesthesia and Analgesia.* 2001; **93**: 761–70.

75. Lombardi AV, Berend KR, Mallory TH *et al.* Soft tissue and intra-articular injection of bupivacaine, epinephrine, and morphine has a beneficial effect after total knee arthroplasty. *Clinical Orthopaedics and Related Research.* 2004; **428**: 125–30.

76. Crawford F. *Plantar heel pain and fasciitis.* BMJ Clinical Evidence. London: BMJ, last updated May 1, 2006; cited February 2008. Available from: http:// clinicalevidence.bmj.com/ceweb/conditions/msd/1111/ 1111.jsp

77. Reuben SS, Connelly NR. Postoperative analgesia for outpatient arthroscopic knee surgery with intraarticular bupivacaine and ketorolac. *Anesthesia and Analgesia.* 1995; **80**: 1154–7.

78. Wang JJ, Ho ST, Lee SC *et al.* Intraarticular triamcinolone acetonide for pain control after arthroscopic knee surgery. *Anesthesia and Analgesia.* 1998; **87**: 1113–16.

79. Joshi W, Reuben SS, Kilaru PR *et al.* Postoperative analgesia for outpatient arthroscopic knee surgery with intraarticular clonidine and/or morphine. *Anesthesia and Analgesia.* 2000; **90**: 1102–06.

80. Xu Z, Tong C, Eisenach JC. Acetylcholine stimulates the release of nitrix oxide from rat spinal cord. *Anesthesiology.* 1996; **85**: 107–11.

81. Yang LC, Chen L-M, Wang C-J, Beurkle H. Postoperative analgesia by intraarticular neostigmine in patients undergoing knee arthroscopy. *Anesthesiology.* 1998; **88**: 334–9.

82. Habib AS, Gan TJ. Role of analgesic adjuncts in postoperative pain management. *Anesthesiology Clinics of North America.* 2005; **23**: 85–107.

83. McCartney CJ, Brull R, Chan VW *et al.* Early but no long-term benefit of regional compared general anesthesia for ambulatory hand surgery. *Anesthesiology.* 2004; **101**: 461–7.

84. Rawal N, Allvin R, Axelsson K *et al.* Patient-controlled regional anesthesia (PCRA) at home. *Anesthesiology.* 2002; **96**: 1290–6.

∗ 85. Enneking FK, Ilfeld BM. Major surgery in the ambulatory environment: continuous catheters and home infusions.

Best Practice and Research. Clinical Anaesthesiology. 2002; **16**: 285–94.

86. Liu SS, Salinas FV. Continuous plexus and peripheral nerve blocks for postoperative analgesia. *Anesthesia and Analgesia.* 2003; **96**: 263–72.

∗ 87. Evans H, Steele SM, Nielsen KC *et al.* Peripheral nerve blocks and continuous catheter techniques. *Anesthesiology Clinics of North America.* 2005; **23**: 141–62.

∗ 88. Ilfeld BM, Enneking FK. Continuous peripheral nerve blocks at home: a review. *Anesthesia and Analgesia.* 2005; **100**: 1822–33.

∗ 89. Boezaart AP. Perineural infusion of local anesthetics. *Anesthesiology.* 2006; **104**: 872–80.

90. Ilfeld BM, Vandenborne K, Duncan PW *et al.* Ambulatory continous interscalene nerve blocks decrease the time to discharge readiness after total shoulder arthroplasty. *Anesthesiology.* 2006; **105**: 999–1007.

91. Capdevila X, Dadure C, Bringuier S *et al.* Effect of patient-controlled perinerual analgesia on rehabilitation and pain after ambulatory orthopedic surgery. A multicenter randomized trial. *Anesthesiology.* 2006; **105**: 566–73.

92. Williams BA, Kentor ML, Vogt MT *et al.* Femoral-sciatic nerve blocks for complex outpatient knee surgery are associated with less postoperative pain before same-day discharge: a review of 1,200 consecutive cases from the period 1996–1999. *Anesthesiology.* 2003; **98**: 1206–13.

93. Ilfeld BM, Esener DE, Morey TE, Enneking FK. Ambulatory perineural infusion: the patients' perspective. *Regional Anesthesia and Pain Medicine.* 2003; **28**: 418–23.

∗ 94. Marhofer P, Gerher M, Kapral S. Ultrasound guidance in regional anaesthesia. *British Journal of Anaesthesia.* 2005; **94**: 7–17.

95. Buvanendran A, Kroin JS, Tuman KJ *et al.* Effects of perioperative administration of a selective cyclooxygenase 2 inhibitor on pain management and recovery of function after knee replacement: a randomized controlled trial. *Journal of the American Medical Association.* 2003; **290**: 2411–18.

96. Kehlet H, Werner MU. Role of paracetamol in the acute pain management. *Drugs.* 2003; **63**: 15–22.

∗ 97. Barden J, Edwards J, Moore A, McQuay H. Single dose oral paracetamol (acetaminophen) for postoperative pain. *Cochrane Database of Systematic Reviews.* 2004; **CD004602**.

98. Moore A, Collins S, Carroll D. *et al.* Single dose paracetamol (acetaminophen), with and without codeine, for postoperative pain. *Cochrane Database of Systematic Reviews.* 1999; **CD001547**.

99. Botting RM. Mechanism of action of acetaminophen: is there a cyclooxygenase 3? *Clinical Infectious Diseases.* 2000; **5** (Suppl. 31): S202–10.

100. Chandrasekharan NV, Dai H, Roos KL *et al.* COX-3, a cyclooxygenase-1 variant inhibited by acetaminophen and other analgesic/antipyretic drugs: Cloning, structure, and expression. *Proceedings of the National Academy of Sciences of the United States of America.* 2002; **99**: 13926–31.

101. Larson AM, Polson J, Fontana RJ *et al.* Acetaminophen-induced acute liver failure: results of a United States multicenter, prospective study. *Hepatology.* 2005; **42**: 1364–72.

102. Garcia Rodriguez LA, Hernandez-Diaz S. Relative risk of upper gastrointestinal complications among users of acetaminophen and nonsteroidal anti-inflammatory drugs. *Epidemiology.* 2001; **12**: 570–6.

103. Chan AT, Manson JE, Albert CM *et al.* Nonsteroidal anti-inflammatory drugs, acetaminophen, and risk of cardiovascular events. *Circulation.* 2006; **113**: 1578–87.

104. Hahn TW, Mogensen T, Lund C *et al.* Analgesic effect of i.v. paracetamol: possible ceiling effect of paracetamol in postoperative pain. *Acta Anaesthesiologica Scandinavica.* 2003; **47**: 138–45.

105. Miranda HF, Puig MM, Prieto JC, Pinardi G. Synergism between paracetamol and nonsteroidal anti-inflammatory drugs in experimental acute pain. *Pain.* 2006; **121**: 22–8.

106. Romsing M, Moiniche S, Dahl JB. Rectal and parenteral paracetamol, and paracetamol in combination with NSAIDs for postoperative analgesia. *British Journal of Anaesthesia.* 2002; **88**: 215–26.

107. Holmer Pettersson P, Owall A, Jakobsson J. Early bioavailability of paracetamol after oral or intravenous administration. *Acta Anaesthesiologica Scandinavica.* 2004; **48**: 867–70.

108. Kehlet H, Mather LE. The value of non-steroidal antiinflammatory drugs in postoperative pain. *Drugs.* 1992; **44**: 1–63.

109. Tramer MR, Williams JE, Carroll D *et al.* Comparing analgesic efficacy of non-steroidal anti-inflammatory drugs given by different routes in acute and chronic pain: a quantitative systematic review. *Acta Anaesthesiologica Scandinavica.* 1998; **42**: 71–9.

110. Forrest JB, Camu F, Greer IA *et al.* Ketorolac, diclofenac, and ketoprofen are equally safe for pain relief after major surgery. *British Journal of Anaesthesia.* 2002; **88**: 227–33.

111. O'Hara DA, Fragen RJ, Kinzer M, Pemberton D. Ketorolac tromethamine as compared with morphine sulphate for the treatment of postoperative pain. *Clinical Pharmacology and Therapeutics.* 1987; **41**: 556–61.

112. Strom BL, Berlin JA, Kinman JL *et al.* Parenteral ketorolac and risk of gastrointestinal and operative site bleeding. *Journal of the American Medical Association.* 1996; **275**: 376–82.

113. Moiniche S, Romsing J, Dahl JB, Tramer MK. Non-steroidal anti-inflammatory drugs and the risk of operative bleeding after tonsillectomy – a quantitative systematic review. *Anesthesia and Analgesia.* 2003; **96**: 68–77.

114. Kenny GNC. Potential renal, haematological and allergic adverse effects associated with nonsteroidal anti-inflammatory drugs. *Drugs.* 1992; **44**: 31–7.

115. Feldman HI, Kinman JL, Berlin JA *et al.* Parenteral ketorolac: the risk for acute renal failure. *Annals of Internal Medicine.* 1997; **126**: 193–9.

116. Kehlet H, Dahl JB. Are perioperative nonsteroidal anti-inflammatory drugs ulcerogenic in the short term? *Drugs*. 1992; **44**: 38–41.

∗117. Graham DJ. COX-2 inhibitors, other NSAIDs, and cardiovascular risk. The seduction of common sense. *Journal of the American Medical Association*. 2006; **296**: 1653–6.

∗118. Gajraj NM, Joshi GP. Role of cyclooxygenase-2 inhibitors in postoperative pain management. *Anesthesiology Clinics of North America*. 2005; **23**: 49–72.

∗119. Romsing J, Moiniche S. A systemic review of COX-2 inhibitors compared with traditional NSAIDs, or different COX-2 inhibitors for post-operative pain. *Acta Anaesthesiologica Scandinavica*. 2004; **48**: 525–46.

120. Gilron I, Milne B, Hong M. Cyclooxygenase-2 inhibitors in postoperative pain management. *Anesthesiology*. 2003; **99**: 1198–208.

121. Joshi GP. Valdecoxib for the management of chronic and acute pain. *Expert Review of Neurotherapeutics*. 2005; **5**: 11–24.

∗122. Gajraj NM. The effect of cyclooxygenase-2 inhibitors on bone healing. *Regional Anesthesia and Pain Medicine*. 2003; **28**: 456–65.

123. Joshi GP, Viscusi E, Gan TJ et al. Effective treatment of laparoscopic cholecystectomy pain with intravenous followed by oral COX-2 specific inhibitor. *Anesthesia and Analgesia*. 2004; **98**: 336–42.

124. Gan TJ, Joshi GP, Viscusi E et al. Presurgical parenteral and oral COX-2 specific inhibitors improve quality of recovery following laparoscopic cholecystectomy. *Anesthesia and Analgesia*. 2004; **98**: 1665–73.

∗125. Nussmeier NA, Whelton AA, Brown MT et al. Safety and efficacy of the cyclooxygenase-2 inhibitors parecoxib and valdecoxib after noncardiac surgery. *Anesthesiology*. 2006; **104**: 518–26.

∗126. Kearney PM, Baigent C, Godwin J et al. Do selective cyclo-oxgenase 2 inhibitors and traditional non-steroidal anti-inflammatory drugs increase the risk of atherothrombosis? Meta-analysis of randomized trials. *British Medical Journal*. 2006; **332**: 1302–08.

∗127. McGettigan P, Henry D. Cardiovascular risk and inhibition of cyclooxygenase. A systematic review of the observational studies of selective and nonselective inhibitors of cyclooxygenase 2. *JAMA*. 2006; **296**: 1633–44.

∗128. Zhang J, Ding EI, Song Y. Adverse effects of cyclooxygenase 2 inhibitors on renal and arrhythmia events. Meta-analysis of randomized trials. *Journal of the American Medical Association*. 2006; **296**: 1619–32.

∗129. Schug SA, Camu F, Joshi GP et al. Cardiovascular safety of cyclo-oxygenase selective inhibitor parecoxib sodium: review of pooled data from surgical studies. *European Journal of Anaesthesiology*. 2006; **23** (Suppl. 37): A-849.

130. Maze M, Tranquilli W. Alpha-2 adrenoceptor agonists: defining the role in clinical anesthesia. *Anesthesiology*. 1991; **74**: 581–605.

131. Wilhelm S, Maze M. Controversial issues in adult and pediatric ambulatory anesthesia: is there a role for the alpha-2 agonists in conscious sedation with adults and pediatric ambulatory surgical practice? *Current Opinion in Anaesthesiology*. 2000; **13**: 619–24.

132. Gilron I. Corticosteroids in postoperative pain management: future research directions for a multifaceted therapy. *Acta Anaesthesiologica Scandinavica*. 2004; **48**: 1221–2.

133. Aasboe V, Raeder JC, Groegaard B. Betamethasone reduces postoperative pain and nausea after ambulatory surgery. *Anesthesia and Analgesia*. 1998; **87**: 319–23.

134. Holte K, Kehlet H. Perioperative single-dose glucocorticoid administration – pathophysiological effects in clinical implications. *Journal of the American College of Surgeons*. 2002; **195**: 694–711.

135. Romundstad L, Breivik H, Roald H et al. Methylprednisolone reduces pain, emesis, and fatigue after breast augmentation surgery: a single-dose, randomized, parallel-group study with methylprednisolone 125 mg, parecoxib 40 mg, and placebo. *Anesthesia and Analgesia*. 2006; **102**: 418–25.

136. Stubhaug A, Breivik H, Eide PK et al. Mapping of punctuate hyperalgesia surrounding a surgical incision demonstrates that ketamine is a powerful suppressor of central sensitization to pain following surgery. *Acta Anaesthesiologica Scandinavica*. 1997; **41**: 1124–32.

137. Petrenko AB, Yamakura T, Baba H, Shimoji K. The role of N-methyl-D-aspartate (NMDA) receptors in pain: a review. *Anesthesia and Analgesia*. 2003; **97**: 1108–16.

138. McCartney CJ, Sinha A, Katz J. A qualitative systematic review of the role of N-methyl-D-aspartate receptor antagonists in preventative analgesia. *Anesthesia and Analgesia*. 2004; **98**: 1385–400.

139. Subramaniam K, Subramaniam B, Steinbrook RA. Ketamine as adjuvant analgesic to opioids: a qualitative and quantitative systematic review. *Anesthesia and Analgesia*. 2004; **99**: 482–95.

∗140. Himmelseher S, Durieux ME. Ketamine for perioperative pain management. *Anesthesiology*. 2005; **102**: 211–20.

∗141. Duedahl TH, Romsing J, Moiniche S, Dahl JB. A qualitative systematic review of peri-operative dextromethorphan in post-operative pain. *Acta Anaesthesiologica Scandinavica*. 2006; **50**: 1–13.

142. Weinbroum AA, Rudick V, Paret G, Ben-Abraham R. The role of dextromethorphan in pain control. *Canadian Journal of Anaesthesia*. 2000; **47**: 585–96.

143. Gee NS, Brown JP, Dissanayake VU et al. The novel anticonvulsant drug, gabapentin (Neurontin), binds to the alpha2delta subunit of a calcium channel. *Journal of Biological Chemistry*. 1996; **271**: 5768–76.

144. Gilron I. Is gabapentin a broad-spectrum analgesic? *Anesthesiology*. 2002; **97**: 537–9.

145. Dirks J, Fredensborg BB, Christensen D et al. A randomized study of the effects of single dose of gapapentin versus placebo on postoperative pain and morphine consumption after mastectomy. *Anesthesiology*. 2002; **97**: 560–4.

146. Fassoulaki A, Patris K, Sarantopoulos C, Hogan Q. The analgesic effect of gabapentin and mexiletine after breast surgery for cancer. *Anesthesia and Analgesia*. 2002; **95**: 985–91.

*147. Dahl JB, Maithiesen O, Moiniche S. Protective premedication: an option with gabapentin and related drugs? A review of gabapentin and pregabalin in the treatment of postoperative pain. *Acta Anaesthesiologica Scandinavica*. 2004; **48**: 1130–6.

148. Claxton AR, McGuire G, Chung F, Cruise C. Evaluation of morphine versus fentanyl for postoperative analgesia after ambulatory surgical procedures. *Anesthesia and Analgesia*. 1997; **84**: 509–14.

149. Moore A, Collins S, Carroll D, McQuay H. Paracetamol with or without codeine in acute pain: a qualitative systematic review. *Pain*. 1997; **70**: 193–201.

150. Sunshine A, Olson NZ, Rivera J *et al*. Analgesic efficacy of controlled-release oxycodone in postoperative pain. *Journal of Clinical Pharmacology*. 1996; **36**: 595–603.

151. Reuben SS, Connelly NR, Maciolek H. Postoperative analgesic with controlled-release oxycodone for outpatient anterior cruciate ligament surgery. *Anesthesia and Analgesia*. 1999; **88**: 1286–91.

152. Broome IJ, Robb HM, Raj N *et al*. The use of tramadol following day-case oral surgery. *Anaesthesia*. 1999; **54**: 289–92.

153. Wallace DH, Serpell MG, Baxter JN, O'Dwyer PJ. Randomized trial of different insufflation pressures for laparoscopic cholecystectomy. *British Journal of Surgery*. 1997; **84**: 455–8.

154. Guard BC, Wiltshire SJ. The effect of glycopyrrolate on postoperative pain and analgesic requirements following laparoscopic sterilisation. *Anaesthesia*. 1996; **51**: 1173–5.

155. Khan B, Khan S, Greany MG, Blair SD. Prospective randomized trial comparing sequential avulsion with stripping of the long saphenous vein. *British Journal of Surgery*. 1996; **83**: 1559–62.

156. Bringman S, Ramel S, Heikkinen T-J *et al*. Tension-free inguinal hernia repair: TEP versus mesh-plug versus Lichtenstein. *Annals of Surgery*. 2003; **237**: 142–7.

157. Callesen T, Bech K, Nielsen R *et al*. Pain after groin hernia repair. *British Journal of Surgery*. 1998; **85**: 1412–14.

158. Limb RI, Rudkin GE, Luck AJ *et al*. The pain of haemorrhoidectomy: a prospective study. *Ambulatory Surgery*. 2000; **8**: 129–34.

159. Carapeti EA, Kamm MA, McDonald PJ, Phillips RK. Double-blind randomised controlled trial of effect of metronidazole on pain after day-case haemorrhoidectomy. *Lancet*. 1998; **351**: 169–72.

160. White JL, Durieux ME. Clinical pharmacology of local anesthetics. *Anesthesiology Clinics of North America*. 2005; **23**: 73–84.

161. Curley J, Castillo J, Hotz J *et al*. Prolonged regional nerve blockade. Injectable biodegradable bupivacaine/polyester microspheres. *Anesthesiology*. 1996; **84**: 1401–10.

162. Grant GJ, Vermeulen K, Zakowski MI *et al*. Prolonged analgesia and decreased toxicity with liposomal morphine in a mouse model. *Anesthesia and Analgesia*. 1994; **79**: 706–09.

163. Flood P, Daniel D. Intranasal nicotine for postoperative pain treatment. *Anesthesiology*. 2004; **101**: 1417–21.

164. Chelly JE, Grass J, Houseman TW *et al*. The safety and efficacy of a fentanyl patient-controlled transdermal system for acute postoperative analgesia: a multicenter, placebo-controlled trial. *Anesthesia and Analgesia*. 2004; **98**: 4427–33.

165. Viscusi ER, Reynolds L, Chung F *et al*. Patient-controlled transdermal fentanyl hydrochloride vs intravenous morphine pump for postoperative pain. *A randomized controlled trial. Journal of the American Medical Association*. 2004; **291**: 1333–41.

18

Acute pain management in the intensive care unit

R SCOTT SIMPSON

KEY LEARNING POINTS

- There are many barriers to adequate pain assessment in the intensive care unit (ICU).
- The implementation of formalized pain assessment and management can significantly improve patient outcomes.
- Sedatives and analgesics are complementary, but not interchangable.
- Current evidence suggests that sedatives are easily over-dosed, and analgesics are frequently under-dosed.

- Dose adjustments of analgesics and sedatives are necessary in moderate to severe organ failure.
- Continuous renal replacement therapy may not clear drugs or metabolites that are normally cleared by intermittent hemodialysis.
- ICU practitioners should talk reassuringly to their patients whenever possible during emergency procedures, as lack of awareness is not guaranteed.

The greatest improvement to our clinical care is likely to be found by applying and refining existing knowledge of current treatments before searching for new frontiers or discoveries.

Dr J Bonica[1]

INTRODUCTION

Intensive care units (ICUs) are constantly evolving. Technological advances in equipment have completely changed the manner in which business is done, making possible that which was previously unthinkable. Only ten years ago, pain management in the ICU consisted of little more than a syringe of a benzodiazepine and opioid mixture, infused rapidly enough to keep the patient tolerant of the ventilator. In the modern ICU, not all patients are ventilated, not everyone who is ventilated is intubated, and those who are intubated are connected to ventilators that can almost read their thoughts. The relative needs for sedation and analgesia have changed dramatically. Daily interruption of sedation and analgesia has been shown to reduce the duration of mechanical ventilation and the incidence of nosocomial respiratory infections, shortening ICU admission, and improving overall survival.[2][II], [3][II], [4][III] On the other hand, it has been consistently demonstrated that approximately 60 percent of ICU survivors recall experiences of moderate to severe pain during their admission,[5][III], [6][III], [7][III], [8,9][III], [10] prompting a call to make pain the "fifth vital sign."[11] The message – patients generally need less sedation and more analgesia.

The complete abolition of all pain in ICU is basically unrealistic, but this is not an excuse to be complacent about pain that can be avoided.[5, 7, 8, 9, 12, 13] Patient comfort is ranked second only to prognosis in the concerns of family members visiting the ICU, yet formal training of clinicians in the use of sedation and analgesia is generally given lower priority than most other aspects of ICU care.[14, 15][V], [16, 17, 18] Analgesia prescription is often relegated to unit "routine," in the same manner as gastric protection, thromboembolism prophylaxis, and nutrition, in a "one-style-suits-all" fashion. Although simple protocols for analgesics are one way of ensuring that the needs of the majority are promptly attended, it may be necessary to deviate from the algorithm on occasions. With new therapeutic alternatives becoming available, the development and use of more comprehensive protocols has merit, but any protocol needs to be applied and used appropriately.[19, 20, 21][II] ICU therapies require a team to function cohesively for effective delivery, including discretionary adjustments according to individual patient needs, but failure to comply at any level of the hierarchy of care may jeopardize the end result. It can be difficult to keep the whole team focused on placing pain management as a high priority, especially when other more exciting or attractive therapies and innovations are beckoning for attention. Each ICU needs a "pain management champion" to keep the team on track.[22] Health administrators also have vested interests in establishing good pain management in ICU. Per patient, per episode, ventilator-associated pneumonia (VAP) adds an estimated additional $US40,000 and 6.1 days to the ICU length of stay (LOS), at an overall mortality of 60 percent; approximately double the baseline risk.[23][II], [24][I] Changes in the approach to sedation and analgesia have reduced the incidence of VAP and LOS by as much as 50 percent in controlled trials, with a significant saving of money, resources, and lives.[2][II], [21][II], [25] With both the costs of ICU care and the demand for ICU beds constantly increasing, there are new imperatives to "fast-track" patients. Systematic review has identified a wide range of factors which impact on the ability to implement fast-track strategies safely, and excellent pain management is a key element.[26]

There are very few data examining the impact of good or bad acute pain management in the longer-term rehabilitation of ICU survivors. The more painful and traumatic the experience, the more likely it will lead to the development of a longstanding and debilitating chronic pain syndrome.[5, 27][IV], [28][III] Survival is the yardstick of current ICU outcome measures, but survival to a life of chronic pain and misery is arguably the worst possible outcome, and does not alter the statistics.

Another major role of the ICU is end-of-life care. In the developed world, nearly 40 percent of all deaths occur in hospital, with more than half of these in ICU.[29][II] Death in ICU is now more commonly the result of a decision to withhold or withdraw life-sustaining therapy, than an unexpected event. There is usually ample opportunity to ensure that patients are at least comfortable as they die.[30, 31]

SOURCES OF PAIN IN ICU

Pain is, by definition, an individual, subjective experience with nociceptive, emotional, and possibly neuropathic elements.[32] Pain may be related to the disease, trauma, or surgery that brings the patient to ICU in the first instance, it can be a consequence of treatments administered, or it may arise from complications which develop. Potentially painful procedures include endotracheal intubation and extubation, dressing and suturing of wounds, and insertion and removal of tubes and lines including vascular access, chest drains, surgical drains, and intracranial pressure monitors.[9][III], [12, 13][II], [33, 34, 35][IV], [36][III], [37][IV], [38][IV] Procedural pain is usually intense but short-lived, and logically calls for the use of short-acting intravenous analgesics or local anesthesia. Time constraints can put pressure on clinicians to omit this step in care, as borne out by one large study which indicated that less than 40 percent of patients having procedures were appropriately medicated.[12]

Routine nursing care involves essential but potentially uncomfortable interventions, including endotracheal suctioning, washes, and turns.[9, 39, 40] Joint and muscle pains may be associated with immobility, awkward posture, pressure points, and pressure sores. The occiput, heels, and sacrum are vulnerable sites that need careful surveillance.

Pain is not necessarily proportional to the nociceptive stimulus. Anxiety, fear, and feelings of helplessness are known to intensify pain, and are commonly exhibited in ICU patients.[41] The ICU environment is not often tranquil, and therefore not usually conducive to providing patients with adequate rest. Analgesia and anxiolysis have a role for all patients in ICU, regardless of the cause of admission and how "painless" the procedures that are performed. ICU staff must strive to maintain a caring and compassionate approach in order to reduce anxiety and make suffering more bearable. Patients' experiences can actually be turned from negative to positive if they feel cared for.[36][III], [42][IV], [43][IV], [44][IV], [45] The patient who suddenly awakens with pain as they are turned in the bed may panic and lose coordination with their ventilator, and suffer hypoxia or unscheduled extubation.[40, 45] Providing advanced notice to patients about proposed interventions, combined with pre-emptive use of appropriate sedative and analgesic medication if there is any sign of distress, is an easy strategy to adopt with little extra effort.

PAIN ASSESSMENT IN ICU PATIENTS

The Achilles' heel of pain assessment in ICU is the communication gap between patients and caregivers.

There are many reasons for this, broadly categorized as physical barriers, patient factors, staff factors, and system factors. The most obvious physical barrier is the endotracheal tube, which prevents talking. Nevertheless, many patients can communicate well with nods, facial expressions, and hand signals. Severe motor weakness inhibits the ability to write or use sign language, and is a specific consequence of critical illness polyneuropathy-myopathy, other neuromuscular disease, central neural trauma, or the use of muscle relaxants.[46, 47, 48] Excessive sedation will also impair communications.

Patient factors include delirium, cultural mores, and language deficits. Common causes of delirium are electrolyte imbalances, hypo- and hyperthermia, sepsis, concussion, alcohol and drug withdrawal, hypoxia, and sleep deprivation.[49][III] In pediatrics, there are additional issues associated with young age, stage of development, and maturity, making reliable pain assessment more of an art than a science (see Chapter 38, Pain assessment in children in the *Practice and Procedures* volume of this series). A child lying still and silent in the bed is not behaving normally, and clinicians need to actively seek a reason for pain.

Staff factors in communication may be related to diversion of their attention, poor time management, lack of knowledge or understanding, or indifference to pain and suffering.

System factors include inadequate staffing levels for nursing workloads, absence of appropriate pain assessment tools in routine ICU activity, and lack of staff education programs.[5][III]

When assessing pain, ICU clinicians rely heavily on indirect autonomic and behavioral indicators.[50] Tachycardia, diaphoresis, tachypnea, grimacing, abnormal posturing, and increased muscle tension may all be caused by pain, but are not pain-specific. Conversely, the presence of a normal heart rate and blood pressure does not exclude the presence of pain, especially if cardiovascular responses are blunted by medications or disease. Nor are pupillary changes and responses entirely reliable. Mydriasis may be a result of pain, atropine or catecholamine administration, direct trauma, seizures, or raised intracranial pressure, while miosis can be due to pontine dysfunction, metabolic syndromes or organophosphate intoxication, but can also occur in response to opioids, although the presence of miosis does not guarantee an in the absence of an analgesic effect.[51][V] Association between autonomic responses and noxious stimuli increases the likelihood of pain as the cause, but it can be difficult to discriminate pain from agitation, anxiety, or delirium.

Following the hypothesis that pain assessment accuracy would be optimal if performed by a family member who knew the patient, the SUPPORT study showed a 75 percent agreement between observer assessments and patient reports for the presence or absence of pain. However, there was less agreement in terms of severity of pain, with an equal tendency for observers to both overestimate and underestimate pain at least 50 percent of the time.[52][III]

ICU pain scores

More formalized pain assessment in critically ill patients is possible, using a variety of scoring systems, most of which have been developed and validated for specific patient populations.[5][III], [34, 53][II], [54][IV], [55, 56, 57, 58, 59, 60][III], [61, 62] An example is provided in **Table 18.1**. There are also many versions of "sedation scales" in use, which inherently assess analgesia.[14, 19, 59, 65, 66][V], [67][IV], [68, 69][IV], [70][V], [71][III], [72, 73, 74][IV], [75][III], [76, 77, 78][III], [79][I], [80][III]. An example is shown in **Table 18.2**. A common feature of these scales is to derive an aggregate total score by accumulating points in several categories of behavioral and/or autonomic physiological observations, as there is no single clinical discriminator with appropriate sensitivity and sufficient specificity for pain alone. Pain and sedation assessment scales encourage regular assessment of the patient. Used in conjunction with response algorithms they reduce the chance of significant treatment differences from one staff shift to the next, and increase the likelihood that a patient will receive timely intervention.[53][III] Prospective, randomized data indicate that the implementation of formalized pain assessment and management can significantly improve ICU outcomes.[21][II], [25, 81][III] An assessment scale and action protocol which works well in one ICU may not necessarily apply in another with a different case-mix, so incorporation of these scales into widespread routine practice is bound to be a gradual process as individual unit evaluation continues.[82] Regular, formalized pain assessment is rapidly becoming a "standard of care."[83]

Pain monitors?

Computer-processed bispectral analysis (BIS), a modified form of electroencephalogram (EEG), has a proven role in evaluating the state of arousal or awareness in patients receiving general anesthesia.[78][III], [84, 85][III], [86][III], [87][V], [88][IV] BIS is influenced by the choice of sedative agents, the underlying illness, and other environmental factors, leading to considerable variation in responses and practical problems excluding background noise. At this point BIS in ICU is still experimental, and although it provides additional information, BIS must be interpreted in context with other clinical signs.[74][IV], [78][III], [84, 85][III], [87][V], [88][IV], [89][IV] Whether BIS can be used to differentiate pain from agitation or delirium is currently unresolved.[90]

SEDATION AND ANALGESIA

Sedation and analgesia are usually paired together in ICU for practical reasons, and are therefore often confused

Table 18.1   Behavioral Pain Assessment Scale.

For patients unable to provide a self report of pain: Scored 0–10 clinical observations			
Face	0 Face muscles relaxed	1 Face muscle tension, frown, grimace	2 Frequent to constant frown, clenched jaw	Face score:
Restlessness	0 Quiet relaxed appearance, normal movement	1 Occasional restless movement, shifting position	2 Frequent restless movement, may include extremities or head	Restlessness score:
Muscle tone[a]	0 Normal muscle tone, relaxed	1 Increased tone, flexion of fingers and toes	2 Rigid tone	Muscle tone score:
Vocalization[b]	0 No abnormal sounds	1 Occasional moans, cries, whimpers or grunts	2 Frequent or continuous moans, cries, whimpers or grunts	Vocalization score:
Consolability	0 Content, relaxed	1 Reassured by touch or talk. Distractible	2 Difficult to comfort by touch or talk	Consolability score:
Behavioral Pain Assessment Scale total (0–10)			/10

[a]Assess muscle tone in patients with spinal cord lesions or injury at a level above the lesion or injury. Assess patients with hemiplegia on the unaffected side.
[b]This item cannot be measured in patients with artificial airways. How to use the pain assessment behavioral scale: Observe behaviours and mark appropriate numbers for each category. Total the numbers in the pain assessment behavioral score column. Zero = no evidence of pain. Mild pain = 1–3. Moderate pain = 4–5. Severe uncontrolled pain is ≥ 6. This adult scale is very similar in style and content to the "FLACC" scale used in pediatrics, and the "COMFORT" scale, which includes physiological parameters of respiration, heart rate variability, and blood pressure.[63, 64] Note that this scale, and others like it, cannot be used for patients receiving neuromuscular blocking drugs. Adapted with permission from Ref. 53.

Table 18.2   The Richmond Agitation-Sedation Assessment Scale (RASS).

Score	Term	Description
+4	Combative	Overtly combative, violent, immediate danger to staff
+3	Very agitated	Pulls or removes tube(s) or catheter(s); aggressive
+2	Agitated	Frequent nonpurposeful movement, fights ventilator
+1	Restless	Anxious but movements not aggressive or vigorous
0	Alert and calm	
−1	Drowsy	Not fully alert but has sustained awakening (eye opening/eye contact) to voice (> 10 seconds)
−2	Light sedation	Briefly awakens with eye contact to voice (< 10 seconds)
−3	Moderate sedation	Movement or eye opening to voice (but no eye contact)
−4	Deep sedation	No response to voice, but movement or eye opening to physical stimulation
−5	Unarousable	No response to voice or physical stimulation

This scale is not applicable to patients receiving neuromuscular blockers. © American Thoracic Society. Adapted with permission from Ref. 80.

with one another. An ideal ICU sedative regimen maintains good analgesia and allows patients to retain sufficient mental clarity to be calm and cooperative without being psychologically traumatized.[91] For the majority of patients the actual drugs used are less important than the manner in which they are administered.[25] The management of sedation in ICU has been extensively reviewed.[92]

There is evidence that daily interruption of sedation decreases length of stay in ICU, reduces morbidity associated with ventilation, and improves long-term psychological outcomes.[2][II], [3][II], [4][III] Implementation of

another assessment-focused protocol has been similarly successful.[21][II] Collectively, these studies indicate that regular clinical assessment of sedation and analgesia facilitates dose titration to an appropriate therapeutic level. Modern ventilators are infinitely more responsive to patients' voluntary efforts than older machines, greatly reducing the discomfort associated with being artificially ventilated, especially using pressure support modes (CPAP, BiPAP) or airway pressure release settings (APRV).[40]

There are some conditions for which deep sedation is part of essential therapy, and interruption for patient assessment should only be considered under strictly controlled circumstances, if at all. These conditions are diverse and include critically raised intracranial pressure, refractory seizures, tetanus, hyperpyrexia, extensive burns with skin grafting, patients on extracorporeal membrane oxygenation (ECMO), and patients with problematic ventilator dysynchrony, such as those with severe acute respiratory distress syndrome (ARDS) or asthma ventilated to permissive hypercapnia.[40] Any patient who is administered neuromuscular blockade should also receive concurrent sedative and analgesic medications, empirically.

Sedative versus analgesic drugs

Sedatives are primarily hypnotic (sleep inducing) and anxiolytic agents. Analgesics are primarily designed to relieve pain. Strong analgesics often have some hypnotic effect, but most sedatives have no analgesic properties. Failure to appreciate this can lead to inappropriate prescription or omission. In 2001 an extensive survey of Italian ICUs found that 35 percent of postsurgical ICU patients received no analgesia at all in the first 48 hours of their admission, only 51 percent received an opioid and, of these, 42 percent had only one bolus dose of short-acting agent.[93][III] Another study reached the extraordinary conclusion that analgesic use was associated with an increased length of stay in a medical ICU.[94] The study groups were clearly biased, with strong indicators of more severe illness in the analgesic recipients, but the most concerning feature of this study was that only 36 percent of the patients had any analgesia prescribed.[82, 94]

Modulation of nociception is believed to be vital for the prevention of peripheral and central pathophysiological changes that lead to augmented acute pain responses and chronic pain states. The presence of coma does not exclude the need for antinociceptive medication in the presence of a recognizable noxious stimulus.[93][III] Amnesia is far more reliably achieved with a benzodiazepine–opioid combination than with a benzodiazepine alone, and tolerance to analgesics develops less rapidly than with isolated infusions.[95, 96] Amnesia may not always be desirable, however, as posttraumatic stress disorders appear to be more common in patients with large memory deficits following ICU admission.[97, 98][V], [99][III] Delirium is a recognized consequence of nonanalgesic sedative administration in the presence of pain.[100][III]

ANALGESICS

Details of the pharmacology of opioid and nonopioid analgesic agents are to be found in Chapter 3, Clinical pharmacology: opioids; Chapter 4, Clinical pharmacology: traditional NSAIDs and selective COX-2 inhibitors; Chapter 5, Clinical pharmacology: paracetamol and compound analgesics; and Chapter 6, Clinical pharmacology: other adjuvants.

Most analgesics given in ICU are delivered by i.v. infusion, with additional bolus administration as needed. An understanding of infusion kinetics and the influences of age, end-organ disease, and polypharmacy is essential,[101, 102, 103, 104, 105][III], [106, 107, 108, 109][V], [110][V], [111] but is unfortunately outside the scope of this chapter. All ICU staff should understand why increasing a morphine (or fentanyl) infusion from 2 to 4 mL/h, 15 minutes before an intervention is a gesture that comforts the provider more than the receiver.

Broadening category of "analgesic"

Research in the use of newer agents with primary analgesic and secondary sedative properties, particularly dexmedetomidine, has raised the profile of all analgesic prescription in ICU. Adjunctive analgesics such as anticonvulsants, antidepressants, and antiarrhythmic agents are rarely used purely for pain in ICU, although they may have a role in neuropathic pain states.[112, 113, 114, 115]

Opioids

Opioids are the principal strong analgesics used in ICU. The choice of agent is usually determined by unit protocols, prescriber familiarity, or the specific indications.[107] Morphine, fentanyl, and alfentanil are widely employed, with remifentanil and sufentanil holding niche applications. With chronic high-dose exposure, hyperalgesia and agitation may be a consequence of opioid intoxication, rather than under-dosing.[116, 117] Slow-release enteral preparations may have roles at later stages of ICU admission.

Nonopioid analgesics

PARACETAMOL (ACETAMINOPHEN)

Paracetamol is a centrally acting analgesic used to treat mild to moderate pain and pyrexia.[118] Severe hepatotoxicity can occur when standard doses are given to patients with liver dysfunction.[119] The Rumack–Matthew nomogram is not applicable to patients with chronic overdosage.[120, 121]

NONSTEROIDAL ANTI-INFLAMMATORY DRUGS

The role of nonsteroid anti-inflammatory drugs (NSAIDs) in ICU is limited by their potential side effects (see Chapter 4, Clinical pharmacology: traditional NSAIDs and selective COX-2 inhibitors). Cyclooxygenase (COX) may have an important role in the resolution of acute lung injury, so its inhibition by NSAIDs is theoretically detrimental.[122] Carefully supervised use of NSAIDs may provide excellent analgesia in the setting of uncomplicated adult and pediatric cardiothoracic surgery, improving the tolerance of chest drains and tubes, and permitting rapid weaning from ventilation.[123][III], [124][II]

ALPHA–2 ADRENOCEPTOR AGONISTS

Clonidine and dexmedetomidine have analgesic, sedative, and anxiolytic properties. Both can be used to ameliorate drug withdrawal symptoms, facilitate the weaning of opioids in dependent patients, and to augment opioid analgesic effects in tolerant patients.[125, 126][I] These effects are possibly mediated by the cellular expression of μ-α_2 receptor heterodimers, which diminish the effects of either agonist alone but enhance synergy when they are given together.[127] Dexmedetomidine improves patient–ventilator synchrony following cardiac and thoracic surgery, providing analgesia and "cooperative sedation" without causing respiratory depression.[126, 128][V], [129, 130][II], [131] There are case reports of prolonged infusions, without detriment, including 65 pediatric burns patients with a mean duration of use of 11 days.[132, 133][IV] The principal side effects are bradycardia and hypotension, more common after a loading dose administration.[134] At steady state these effects are of the order of 10–15 percent below baseline.[135][IV] There is no rebound hypertension observed after abrupt cessation of the infusion, even after prolonged administration.[136][III] The analgesic properties of dexmedetomidine are modest. In a postsurgical case series, comparison of propofol and dexmedetomidine, the latter group had a 60–70 percent reduction in their fentanyl requirements.[137][II] In adult thoracic surgery, the addition of i.v. dexmedetomidine to epidural analgesia led to a significant reduction in the requirements for rescue opioids.[138][II] Pediatric experience is accumulating.[110][V], [139, 140, 141][III], [142] There is an incentive to find a suitable alternative to propofol because of the "propofol infusion syndrome".[110, 143, 144] Dexmedetomidine has also been used to facilitate abrupt termination of opioids in chronically exposed children, following cardiac transplantation.[145]

KETAMINE

Ketamine is a potent analgesic in subanesthetic doses, and has been shown to reduce morphine requirements and decrease nausea and vomiting rates in perioperative studies.[146][I], [147][I] Ketamine may prevent opioid tolerance and dependence, hyperalgesia, and withdrawal symptoms.[148] Overall, the collection of small studies of ketamine use in ICU is insufficient evidence to draw firm conclusions or make recommendations about its role.[110, 148, 149, 150, 151]

Drug withdrawal symptoms

Sedatives and analgesics are commonly stopped in order to awaken and extubate patients. For patients not previously exposed to these drugs, infusions of less than five days duration can usually be ceased without consequence. After longer infusions, or for patients chronically habituated to sedatives and analgesics, abrupt cessation may precipitate a withdrawal syndrome, manifest as a variable constellation of hyper-alertness, tachycardia, hypertension, tachypnea, pupillary dilation, diaphoresis, increased intestinal peristalsis with cramping pain, and a spectrum of insomnia, confusion, agitation, or delirium.[152, 153, 154, 155, 156][I], [157] Slower weaning of the agents is necessary. Withdrawal symptoms may be attenuated by coadministration of α_2-adrenoceptor agonists, or substitution therapy with long-acting agents such as methadone.[125, 145, 157, 158, 159, 160]

Physiology and pharmacology in critical illness

The main issue relevant to pain management is the redistribution of organ blood flow in shock states. Vital organ perfusion is preserved at the expense of other circulations, increasing the percentage of intravenously delivered drug reaching the brain, heart, and lungs. Dose alterations may be necessary.

Significant alteration in circulating cytokines is common in critical illness, causing increased capillary permeability and interstitial extravasation of plasma. Fluid resuscitation often causes massive expansion of the extracellular fluid space. This changes the volume of distribution of many water-soluble drugs, such as neuromuscular blockers and morphine. Dose increases may be needed to maintain a therapeutic effect.

ORGAN FAILURE

Organ failure is common in ICU. Its impact on acute pain management has been comprehensively reviewed.[161]

Kidney

Renal dysfunction causes reduced clearance and prolongation of the effects of many drugs, including some analgesics and their metabolites. Alfentanil, fentanyl, remifentanil, sufentanil, buprenorphine, and ketamine are least affected.[161] Morphine, hydromorphone, methadone, oxycodone, tramadol, clonidine, amitriptyline, and bupivacaine have all been used safely at reduced doses. Morphine glucuronides may accumulate in oliguric renal failure, increasing the risk of prolonged sedation, respiratory depression, profound intestinal stasis, and myoclonus. Norpethidine, a pethidine (meperidine) metabolite with neuro-excitatory serotonergic effects, is exclusively renally cleared, and this drug is rarely used in ICU.[161]

Paracetamol is safe provided it is not part of a compound analgesic that contains salicylates or NSAIDs.[161]

RENAL REPLACEMENT THERAPY

Extracorporeal renal replacement therapy (dialysis and ultrafiltration) is less efficient than functioning kidneys at clearing plasma of drugs and their metabolites. Data on drug removal by dialysis refer only to standard intermittent hemodialysis and filtration (IHD), which may cause hypotension or even circulatory collapse in some ICU patients. Continuous renal replacement therapy (CRRT), using equipment designed for ICU use, induces less hypotension but needs to run for up to 24 hours to achieve a similar effect as four hours of IHD. Slow low efficiency dialysis (SLED) is a hybrid method that is more efficient than CRRT and less hemodynamically destabilizing than IHD. Evidence for the clearance of certain drugs by IHD has been empirically extrapolated to CRRT or SLED, but there are few supporting data.[162]

Because of the multiple techniques employed in CRRT, the variability in individual patient circumstances, and the lack of *in vivo* data, the information displayed in **Table 18.3** can only be used as a guide.[162]

Liver

In mild forms of hepatic dysfunction there is rarely a need to adjust analgesic or sedative drug doses. In liver failure, these drugs must be prescribed with extreme caution. Analgesics and adjuvants which should be specifically avoided are paracetamol, valproic acid, carbamazepine, amitriptyline, and methadone.[119, 161] In critical illness the liver reduces its synthesis of albumin in favor of production of higher levels of alpha-1-glycoprotein, globulins, and other acute phase reactants. The pharmacokinetics of highly protein bound drugs may be altered.

Other organs

Microvascular "failure" causes many patients to develop generalized edema, excess total body water, and compartmental fluid shifts that may alter drug distribution, either lessening, or potentiating their actions. This creates an inconstant relationship between plasma levels and tissue concentrations. Plasma level surveillance is common ICU practice with drugs such as antibiotics, anticoagulants, and anticonvulsants, either to monitor therapeutic benefits, or to avoid potentially toxic effects related to high plasma levels. Currently, there are no cheap commercial assays for analgesics or sedative agents.

REGIONAL BLOCKS IN ICU

The aim of any regional technique is to provide excellent analgesia while preserving or enhancing respiratory function, cardiovascular stability, and cognition through the avoidance of systemic medication.

Epidural and intrathecal blocks

Epidural analgesia is commonly used in the management of major thoracic, abdominal, and lower limb surgery and trauma. For details of the technique and a review of studies looking at patient outcomes with epidural analgesia compared with opioid analgesia, please see Chapter 13, Epidural and spinal analgesia. Very few large trials have included ICU patients.

HEMOSTASIS

Critical illness is regularly associated with dysfunction of the liver, spleen, kidneys, and bone marrow, and the use of anticoagulants and platelet inhibitors. Throughout the duration of epidural use, and particularly at the time of insertion or removal of the epidural catheter, attention

Table 18.3 The effect of dialysis on plasma clearance of analgesic and adjunctive medications.

Cleared >30%	Not cleared by dialysis		No data available
Paracetamol	Alfentanil	Ketamine	Hydromorphone
Gabapentin	Baclofen	Pethidine	Ketoralac
Norpethidine[a]	Buprenorphine	Methadone	Naloxone
Mexilitene	Carbamazepine	Morphine glucuronides	Oxymorphone
Morphine[a]	Chlorpromazine	Naltrexone	Piroxicam
Oxycodone[a]	Clonidine	Sufentanil	
Pentazocine	Codeine	Local anesthetics	
Tramadol[a]	Dexmedetomidine	NSAIDs	
Valproic acid[a]	Fentanyl	Tricyclic antidepressants	

[a]Denotes clearance only with nonstandard high sieving coefficient dialysis filters ($K_f > 8$ mL/mmHg/min).
Due to the variability of circuits, filters, and modes of CRRT, the list may not be applicable.
Adapted with permission from Ref. 162.

must be paid to the coagulation status and platelet function. Timing of administration of drugs affecting hemostasis must be taken into account, and consensus guidelines are available.[163]

HYPOTENSION

An effective epidural will cause some peripheral vasodilation, reducing systemic vascular resistance. Intravenous fluid supplementation prevents and corrects hypotension in the majority of cases. Liberal fluid use has been shown to negatively influence pulmonary outcomes in ICU, although this is a general finding that does not specifically pertain to epidural use.[164][II] Vasopressors may be a preferred method of maintaining blood pressure. Epidurals are contraindicated in shocked and unresuscitated patients.

SEPSIS

Sepsis is common in ICU. Opinions vary on how epidurals should be managed in sepsis. In a survey of British anesthesiologists and intensivists, the majority of respondents favored removal of epidural catheters in culture-positive sepsis, but not in the presence of so-called culture negative sepsis, or systemic inflammatory response syndrome (SIRS).[165] The pathophysiological consequences of sepsis or SIRS are identical, affecting organ function, coagulation, and platelet adhesion. Drotrecogin alfa (activated protein C (a-PC), has been shown in phase III trials to significantly reduce mortality in adults with severe sepsis.[166] The rate of hemorrhagic complications in septic patients rises from a baseline of 2 to 3.5 percent when a-PC is used.[166][III], [167][III] The need to simultaneously prescribe this agent and perform neuraxial blockade is unlikely; should a patient become septic with an epidural catheter in place, the safe interval for its removal before or after a-PC administration is unknown.

Thoracic paravertebral block (TPVB)

Thoracic paravertebral block (TPBV) is a useful unilateral technique for analgesia after thoracic trauma or surgery.[168, 169, 170] Repeated percutaneous injection may be performed, or an indwelling catheter placed for bolus drug administration or continuous infusion. TPVB has less hemodynamic effect than an epidural or intrathecal blockade.[168, 171][III] Pneumothorax occurs in approximately 0.5 percent.[171] The overall failure rate is about 10 percent, consistent with most forms of regional blockade, although higher success rates are seen with catheters placed by the surgeon at the time of operation.[172] TPVB has been compared with epidural, intercostal, and interpleural analgesia in adult thoracic surgery in a series of

papers at one center, showing TPVB to be the superior modality.[173][II], [174, 175][III], [176] In pediatric studies, TPVB has been shown to be safe and effective, with prolonged analgesic benefit.[170, 171][III], [177, 178] TPVB will ablate somatosensory-evoked potentials and prevent hormonal stress responses to thoracic surgery, unlike epidural blockade which does neither.[172, 178] There is hope that TPVB may prevent chronic post-thoracotomy pain, which remains debilitating in up to 50 percent of patients five years after thoracic surgery.[178, 179]

Intercostal blocks

Perioperative intercostal blockade, using surgically placed catheters and continuous infusion, has been shown to be as effective as continuous epidural block following unilateral thoracotomy, with less time taken to place the catheter, less need for urinary catheterization, and less hypotension.[180][III] Intercostal blocks may also facilitate the insertion and removal of chest drains. Care needs to be taken to avoid inadvertent local anesthetic toxicity with multiple level injections.

Interpleural blocks

This can be performed as a percutaneous procedure, or by instillation of local anesthetic through an existing intrapleural drain. The results are generally disappointing in adult practice, with lasting benefit in less than 30 percent of cases, and minimal effect on pulmonary dynamics.[181] There is more success in children.[182][IV] The pleura will rapidly absorb local anesthetic, and toxicity is a significant risk.

Other peripheral nerve blocks

Other peripheral nerve blocks may be used in ICU. For details, see Chapter 12, Continuous peripheral neural blockade for acute pain.

ACUTE ANALGESIA AND THE DYING PATIENT

Definitions

A significant percentage of patients admitted to ICU will die before leaving hospital, depending on individual unit acuity, age range, and case-mix.[29][II] "Withdrawal of care," and its corollary term "withholding treatment," describes an active decision not to indulge in life-prolonging therapies, but care of the patient continues in all other aspects. "Palliation" refers to the alleviation of unpleasant symptoms in a patient who is terminally ill, although death may not be immediately imminent. This is subtly different, and some seemingly aggressive treatments may still be provided in an ICU setting. A palliative approach requires a change of mind-set for members of the ICU team.[31] The emphasis shifts from one of using all available therapies to preserve life, which is the common foundation of ICU care, to one of optimizing the enjoyment of remaining life, and possibly extending it a little at the same time.[183]

Practicalities of analgesia in end-of life care

There are excellent reviews and guideline documents written by expert committees and representative authorities detailing the practical and ethical issues of end-of-life care.[31, 184, 185, 186, 187, 188, 189, 190] The sequence of events often moves considerably faster in the ICU than in hospice or ward settings. Proactive, collaborative decision making and open communication is essential, and physicians often need to take the lead to initiate discourse with families.[191] Patients and families may also benefit from contact by a palliative care team with broader expertise in psychosocial and spiritual matters.[185, 192, 193, 194][IV], [195]

New directions in organ donation, particularly donation after cardiac death (DCD), are raising some ethical challenges regarding the appropriateness of analgesic and sedative use at the end-of-life.[196, 197] Analgesic and sedative drugs must also be adequately cleared before any clinical determination of brain death can be made for more conventional organ donation.[198]

Palliative analgesia

The patient should receive analgesia doses titrated to their individual need, rather than applying any particular formula, and dose requirements can be surprisingly high. A "double effect principle" is widely accepted for palliative analgesia. This provides legal justification for the moral and medical indications of continuing to administer strong analgesia for patient comfort, acknowledging that some potential side effects, such as respiratory depression, may be detrimental, or even hasten death.[187, 199, 200] Anxiolytics may also be used to relieve suffering, following the same principle, even if they sedate the patient.[201] The intentional prescription of sedative and analgesic overdoses to accelerate death is not sanctioned by this principle, and is illegal in most countries.

SPECIFIC PAIN MANAGEMENT IN ICU

Pain management in emergency resuscitation

Shocked patients do not tolerate the vasodilatory effects of most anesthetic agents, nor the physiological consequences of intubation and ventilation. These are partly offset by aggressive resuscitation using i.v. fluids, inotropes, and vasopressors. The choice of drugs, their dosage, and timing often needs to be modified. Unfortunately, not all "unstable" patients are unaware. There is, however, a world of difference between awareness and painful, frightening awareness. Opioids like fentanyl may be gradually titrated in concert with fluid resuscitation and invasive monitoring, and small doses of benzodiazepines used for additional amnesia and anxiolysis. Ketamine is another agent with analgesic and anesthetic properties that has been advocated in emergency situations because of its sympathomimetic effects, although care with dosing is also necessary. ICU practitioners should talk reassuringly to their patients whenever possible during emergency procedures, as sedative drugs are imperfect and lack of awareness is not guaranteed.[202]

Thoracic surgery

Thoracotomy has a significant and prolonged adverse effect on pulmonary mechanics, and although the reasons for this are multifactorial, pain is believed to be the most relevant factor.[181] Analgesia is aimed at preserving the functional residual capacity of the lung, maintaining the ability to cough, and facilitating early mobilization, thus preventing atelectasis, infection, and thromboembolism. Thoracic paravertebral block is reported to provide the best analgesic effect and pulmonary mechanical advantage.[181, 203][I]

Cardiac surgery

Adult cardiac surgery is changing with the proliferation of percutaneous catheter treatments, keeping many "healthier" cardiac bypass patients away from the ICU environment. The majority of research on cardiac bypass surgery has been carried out prior to this era. The average patient presenting for cardiac surgery now has multiple comorbidities, and existing data may not apply. Combination therapy with diclofenac and paracetamol improved pain scores, and significantly reduced fentanyl requirements and side effects in patients undergoing cardiac bypass grafting.[124][II] Epidural block in cardiac surgery remains controversial, with the main debate centered on the risk of neuraxial hematoma in association with perioperative anticoagulation.[204, 205] The technique mandates specific strategies to rapidly detect and treat neuraxial complications in order to maintain safety.

Neuropathic pain

Neuropathic pain is particularly predictable in the setting of major nerve injury, such as traumatic amputation, spinal cord injury, and limb plexus avulsion, but is also a feature of Guillain–Barré syndrome (GBS) and critical illness polyneuropathy.[113, 114, 206] The hallmark features are those of ongoing pain in the absence of a recognizable stimulus, dysesthesia, allodynia, and hyperpathia, and pain that is resistant to opioid therapy.[32] Pathophysiological neural changes gradually become established, often leading to disabling chronic pain. Theoretically, early intervention may be preventative.[113] "Antineuropathic" analgesics include ketamine, tricyclic antidepressants, anticonvulsants, and α-2 agonists[113, 148] (see Chapter 6, Clinical pharmacology: other adjuvants). Early referral to a multidisciplinary chronic pain unit is recommended for all patients identified as having neuropathic pain in ICU as treatment is specialized, and likely to need to be prolonged.

Guillain–Barré syndrome

Severe cases are admitted to ICU for airway protection and ventilation because of loss of laryngeal, bulbar, thoracic, and diaphragmatic muscle function. Consciousness is not affected. Common complications are deep vein thrombosis, pulmonary embolism, cardiac arrhythmias, and gut dysfunction.[207] Pain is experienced in the acute phase of GBS by about 70 percent of cases as a result of sensory nerve involvement, pressure necrosis, myopathy, constipation, and procedural interventions.[208, 209] Backache, headache, joint, and muscle pain, and paresthesiae are common. Early plasmapheresis or immunoglobulin administration will shorten the duration of this illness and the associated pain.[210] There is no benefit of combining these treatments. Recovery often takes three to six months, or longer.[207, 211, 212, 213] Enquire about pain early in the presentation, before communication is impaired by motor weakness.[214] In small randomized controlled trials, gabapentin and carbamazepine were effective for neuropathic pain in GBS, with gabapentin performing marginally better.[215][III], [216][III] The management of pain in these patients is discussed in Chapter 23, Acute pain and medical disorders.

CONCLUSION

Pain management in ICU uses the same principles and the same drugs as pain management in other hospital settings. Organ failure and critical illness physiology will influence choice and dose of analgesic drugs. Morphine is still the most commonly used agent. Barriers to communication, including sedatives, make assessment of pain difficult. The appropriate application of specific pain assessment tools and response algorithms has been shown to improve patient outcomes in ICU. Regular patient assessment permits careful titration of existing drugs to a level that provides a very satisfactory outcome in the majority of patients. Optimal pain management requires a complete working knowledge of the pharmacokinetics and toxicity profiles of all opioid and nonopioid analgesics. Regional block techniques may be useful and warrant further study in the ICU setting. Simple strategies that can be instituted immediately, at no cost, include the use of procedural local anesthesia, talking to sedated patients as if they are awake, and minimizing "doom and gloom" discussions at the bedside. New ventilators have revolutionized the way in which sedation and analgesia is managed in ICU. The emphasis should probably favor more analgesia, and less sedation.

ACKNOWLEDGMENTS AND DISCLOSURES

My sincere thanks to Ms Shanti Nadaraja and Mrs Jenny Jolley, Librarians at the Australian and New Zealand College of Anaesthetists, for their excellent assistance in collecting many of the articles in the reference list.

No financial or other professional disclosures, or conflicts.

REFERENCES

1. Frenette L. The acute pain service. *Critical Care Clinics.* 1999; **15**: 143–50.

* 2. Kress JP, Pohlman AS, O'Connor MF et al. Daily interruption of sedative infusions in critically ill patients undergoing mechanical ventilation. *New England Journal of Medicine.* 2000; **342**: 1471–7.

* 3. Schweickert WD, Gehlbach BK, Pohlman AS et al. Daily interruption of sedative infusions and complications of critical illness in mechanically ventilated patients. *Critical Care Medicine.* 2004; **32**: 1272–6.

4. Kress JP, Gehlbach B, Lacy M et al. The long-term psychological effects of daily sedative interruption on critically ill patients. *American Journal of Respiratory and Critical Care Medicine.* 2003; **168**: 1457–61.

5. Carroll KC, Atkins PJ, Herold GR et al. Pain assessment and management in critically ill postoperative and trauma patients: a multisite study. *American Journal of Critical Care.* 1999; **8**: 105–17.

6. Desbiens NA, Wu AW. Pain and suffering in seriously ill hospitalized patients. *Journal of the American Geriatrics Society.* 2000; **48**: S183–6.

7. Desbiens NA, Wu AW, Broste SK et al. Pain and satisfaction with pain control in seriously ill hospitalized adults: findings from the SUPPORT research investigations. For the SUPPORT investigators. Study to Understand Prognoses and Preferences for Outcomes and Risks of Treatmentm. *Critical Care Medicine.* 1996; **24**: 1953–61.

8. Dasta JF. Drug prescribing issues in the intensive care unit: finding answers to common questions. *Critical Care Medicine.* 1994; **22**: 909–12.

9. Puntillo KA. Dimensions of procedural pain and its analgesic management in critically ill surgical patients. *American Journal of Critical Care*. 1994; **3**: 116–22.

10. Stannard D, Puntillo K, Miaskowski C *et al.* Clinical judgment and management of postoperative pain in critical care patients. *American Journal of Critical Care*. 1996; **5**: 433–41.

11. Lanser P, Gesell S. Pain management: the fifth vital sign. *Healthcare Benchmarks*. 2001; **8**: 68–70, 62.

12. Puntillo KA, Wild LR, Morris AB *et al.* Practices and predictors of analgesic interventions for adults undergoing painful procedures. *American Journal of Critical Care*. 2002; **11**: 415–29.

13. Puntillo KA, White C, Morris AB *et al.* Patients' perceptions and responses to procedural pain: results from Thunder Project II. *American Journal of Critical Care*. 2001; **10**: 238–51.

* 14. Sessler CN. Sedation scales in the ICU. *Chest*. 2004; **126**: 1727–30.

15. Twite MD, Rashid A, Zuk J *et al.* Sedation, analgesia, and neuromuscular blockade in the pediatric intensive care unit: survey of fellowship training programs. *Pediatric Critical Care Medicine*. 2004; **5**: 521–32.

16. Mularski RA. Pain management in the intensive care unit. *Critical Care Clinics*. 2004; **20**: 381–401, viii.

17. Devlin J. Pain assessment in the seriously ill patient: can family members play a role? *Critical Care Medicine*. 2000; **28**: 1660–1.

18. Devlin JW, Tanios MA, Epstein SK. Intensive care unit sedation: waking up clinicians to the gap between research and practice. *Critical Care Medicine*. 2006; **34**: 556–7.

19. Hynes-Gay P, Leo M, Molino-Carmona S *et al.* Optimizing sedation and analgesia in mechanically ventilated patients – an evidence-based approach. *Dynamics*. 2003; **14**: 10–13.

* 20. Park G, Coursin D, Ely EW *et al.* Commentary. Balancing sedation and analgesia in the critically ill. *Critical Care Clinics*. 2001; **17**: 1015–27.

* 21. Chanques G, Jaber S, Barbotte E *et al.* Impact of systematic evaluation of pain and agitation in an intensive care unit. *Critical Care Medicine*. 2006; **34**: 1691–9.

22. Stenger K, Schooley K, Moss L. Moving to evidence-based practice for pain management in the critical care setting. *Critical Care Nursing Clinics of North America*. 2001; **13**: 319–27.

* 23. Cocanour CS, Peninger M, Domonoske BD *et al.* Decreasing ventilator-associated pneumonia in a trauma ICU. *Journal of Trauma*. 2006; **61**: 122–9.

* 24. Safdar N, Dezfulian C, Collard HR *et al.* Clinical and economic consequences of ventilator-associated pneumonia: a systematic review. *Critical Care Medicine*. 2005; **33**: 2184–93.

* 25. Hamill-Ruth RJ. Managing pain and agitation in the critically ill – are we there yet? *Critical Care Medicine*. 2006; **34**: 1838–9.

26. Cheng DC, Barash PG. Is fast-track intensive care unit management still on the express track? *Critical Care Medicine*. 2006; **34**: 1826–8.

27. Boyle M, Murgo M, Adamson H *et al.* The effect of chronic pain on health related quality of life amongst intensive care survivors. *Australian Critical Care*. 2004; **17**: 104–13.

28. Desbiens NA, Wu AW, Alzola C *et al.* Pain during hospitalization is associated with continued pain six months later in survivors of serious illness. The SUPPORT Investigators. Study to understand prognoses and preferences for outcomes and risks of treatments. *American Journal of Medicine*. 1997; **102**: 269–76.

29. Angus DC, Barnato AE, Linde-Zwirble WT *et al.* Use of intensive care at the end of life in the United States: an epidemiologic study. *Critical Care Medicine*. 2004; **32**: 638–43.

30. Prendergast TJ, Luce JM. Increasing incidence of withholding and withdrawal of life support from the critically ill. *American Journal of Respiratory and Critical Care Medicine*. 1997; **155**: 15–20.

* 31. Truog RD, Cist AF, Brackett SE *et al.* Recommendations for end-of-life care in the intensive care unit: The Ethics Committee of the Society of Critical Care Medicine. *Critical Care Medicine*. 2001; **29**: 2332–48.

32. Pain terms: a list with definitions and notes on usage. Recommended by the IASP Subcommittee on Taxonomy. *Pain*. 1979; **6**: 249.

33. Graf C, Puntillo K. Pain in the older adult in the intensive care unit. *Critical Care Clinics*. 2003; **19**: 749–70.

34. Shannon K, Bucknall T. Pain assessment in critical care: what have we learnt from research. *Intensive and Critical Care Nursing*. 2003; **19**: 154–62.

35. Stanik-Hutt JA, Soeken KL, Belcher AE *et al.* Pain experiences of traumatically injured patients in a critical care setting. *American Journal of Critical Care*. 2001; **10**: 252–9.

36. Stein-Parbury J, McKinley S. Patients' experiences of being in an intensive care unit: a select literature review. *American Journal of Critical Care*. 2000; **9**: 20–7.

37. Gardner G, Elliott D, Gill J *et al.* Patient experiences following cardiothoracic surgery: an interview study. *European Journal of Cardiovascular Nursing*. 2005; **4**: 242–50.

38. Paiement B, Boulanger M, Jones CW *et al.* Intubation and other experiences in cardiac surgery: the consumer's views. *Canadian Anaesthetists' Society Journal*. 1979; **26**: 173–80.

39. Turner P, Glass C, Grap MJ. Care of the patient requiring mechanical ventilation. *Medical-Surgical Nursing*. 1997; **6**: 68–73, 76, 94.

* 40. Burchardi H. Aims of sedation/analgesia. *Minerva Anestesiologica*. 2004; **70**: 137–43.

41. Szokol JW, Vender JS. Anxiety, delirium, and pain in the intensive care unit. *Critical Care Clinics*. 2001; **17**: 821–42.

42. Ballard N, Robley L, Barrett D et al. Patients' recollections of therapeutic paralysis in the intensive care unit. *American Journal of Critical Care.* 2006; **15**: 86–94.

43. Berger I, Waldhorn RE. Analgesia, sedation and paralysis in the intensive care unit. *American Family Physician.* 1995; **51**: 166–72.

44. Cheng EY. Recall in the sedated ICU patient. *Journal of Clinical Anesthesia.* 1996; **8**: 675–8.

45. Mohta M, Sethi AK, Tyagi A et al. Psychological care in trauma patients. *Injury.* 2003; **34**: 17–25.

46. Bolton CF. Neuromuscular manifestations of critical illness. *Muscle and Nerve.* 2005; **32**: 140–63.

47. Hund E. Neurological complications of sepsis: critical illness polyneuropathy and myopathy. *Journal of Neurology.* 2001; **248**: 929–34.

48. Latronico N, Peli E, Botteri M. Critical illness myopathy and neuropathy. *Current Opinion in Critical Care.* 2005; **11**: 126–32.

49. Ely EW, Inouye SK, Bernard GR et al. Delirium in mechanically ventilated patients: validity and reliability of the confusion assessment method for the intensive care unit (CAM-ICU). *Journal of the American Medical Association.* 2001; **286**: 2703–10.

50. Slaughter A, Pasero C, Manworren R. Unacceptable pain levels. *American Journal of Nursing.* 2002; **102**: 75, 77.

51. Sanders KD, McArdle P, Lang Jr JD. Pain in the intensive care unit: recognition, measurement, management. *Seminars in Respiratory and Critical Care Medicine.* 2001; **22**: 127–36.

52. Desbiens NA, Mueller-Rizner N. How well do surrogates assess the pain of seriously ill patients? *Critical Care Medicine.* 2000; **28**: 1347–52.

53. Erdek MA, Pronovost PJ. Improving assessment and treatment of pain in the critically ill. *International Journal for Quality in Health Care.* 2004; **16**: 59–64.

54. Blenkharn A, Faughnan S, Morgan A. Developing a pain assessment tool for use by nurses in an adult intensive care unit. *Intensive and Critical Care Nursing.* 2002; **18**: 332–41.

55. Brinker D. Sedation and comfort issues in the ventilated infant and child. *Critical Care Nursing Clinics of North America.* 2004; **16**: 365–77, viii–ix.

56. Coleman MM, Solarin K, Smith C. Assessment and management of pain and distress in the neonate. *Advances in Neonatal Care.* 2002; **2**: 123–36.

57. Hall SJ. Paediatric pain assessment in intensive care units. *Intensive and Critical Care Nursing.* 1995; **11**: 20–5.

58. Kwekkeboom KL, Herr K. Assessment of pain in the critically ill. *Critical Care Nursing Clinics of North America.* 2001; **13**: 181–94.

59. Li D, Puntillo K. What is the current evidence on pain and sedation assessment in nonresponsive patients in the intensive care unit? *Critical Care Nurse.* 2004; **24**: 68, 70, 72–3.

60. McNair C, Ballantyne M, Dionne K et al. Postoperative pain assessment in the neonatal intensive care unit. *Archives of Disease in Childhood. Fetal and Neonatal.* 2004; **89**: F537–41.

61. Morton NS. Pain assessment in children. *Paediatric Anaesthesia.* 1997; **7**: 267–72.

62. Oakes LL. Assessment and management of pain in the critically ill pediatric patient. *Critical Care Nursing Clinics of North America.* 2001; **13**: 281–95.

63. Ambuel B, Hamlett KW, Marx CM et al. Assessing distress in pediatric intensive care environments: the COMFORT scale. *Journal of Pediatric Psychology.* 1992; **17**: 95–109.

64. Merkel SI, Voepel-Lewis T, Shayevitz JR et al. The FLACC: a behavioral scale for scoring postoperative pain in young children. *Pediatric Nursing.* 1997; **23**: 293–7.

65. Chamorro C, Borrallo JM, Silva JA. Rational guidelines on the provision of analgesia, sedation, and neuromuscular blockade in critical care. *Critical Care Medicine.* 2001; **29**: 1096–8.

66. Crippen DW. The role of sedation in the ICU patient with pain and agitation. *Critical Care Clinics.* 1990; **6**: 369–92.

67. Devlin JW, Boleski G, Mlynarek M et al. Motor Activity Assessment Scale: a valid and reliable sedation scale for use with mechanically ventilated patients in an adult surgical intensive care unit. *Critical Care Medicine.* 1999; **27**: 1271–5.

* 68. Devlin JW, Fraser GL, Kanji S et al. Sedation assessment in critically ill adults. *Annals of Pharmacotherapy.* 2001; **35**: 1624–32.

69. Ely EW, Truman B, Shintani A et al. Monitoring sedation status over time in ICU patients: reliability and validity of the Richmond Agitation-Sedation Scale (RASS). *Journal of the American Medical Association.* 2003; **289**: 2983–91.

70. Fraser GL, Riker RR. Monitoring sedation, agitation, analgesia, and delirium in critically ill adult patients. *Critical Care Clinics.* 2001; **17**: 967–87.

71. Ista E, van DM, Tibboel D et al. Assessment of sedation levels in pediatric intensive care patients can be improved by using the COMFORT "behavior" scale. *Pediatric Critical Care Medicine.* 2005; **6**: 58–63.

72. Jacobi J, Fraser GL, Coursin DB et al. Clinical practice guidelines for the sustained use of sedatives and analgesics in the critically ill adult. *Critical Care Medicine.* 2002; **30**: 119–41.

73. Riker RR, Fraser GL. Monitoring sedation, agitation, analgesia, neuromuscular blockade, and delirium in adult ICU patients. *Seminars in Respiratory and Critical Care Medicine.* 2001; **22**: 189–98.

74. Riker RR, Fraser GL, Simmons LE et al. Validating the Sedation-Agitation Scale with the Bispectral Index and Visual Analog Scale in adult ICU patients after cardiac surgery. *Intensive Care Medicine.* 2001; **27**: 853–8.

75. Riker RR, Picard JT, Fraser GL. Prospective evaluation of the Sedation-Agitation Scale for adult critically ill patients. *Critical Care Medicine.* 1999; **27**: 1325–9.

76. Riker RR, Fraser GL. Sedation in the intensive care unit: refining the models and defining the questions. *Critical Care Medicine.* 2002; **30**: 1661–3.

77. Shapiro BA, Warren J, Egol AB *et al.* Practice parameters for intravenous analgesia and sedation for adult patients in the intensive care unit: an executive summary. Society of Critical Care Medicine. *Critical Care Medicine.* 1995; **23**: 1596–600.

78. Simmons LE, Riker RR, Prato BS *et al.* Assessing sedation during intensive care unit mechanical ventilation with the Bispectral Index and the Sedation-Agitation Scale. *Critical Care Medicine.* 1999; **27**: 1499–504.

∗ 79. Vender JS, Szokol JW, Murphy GS *et al.* Sedation, analgesia, and neuromuscular blockade in sepsis: an evidence-based review. *Critical Care Medicine.* 2004; **32**: S554–61.

∗ 80. Sessler CN, Gosnell MS, Grap MJ *et al.* The Richmond Agitation-Sedation Scale: validity and reliability in adult intensive care unit patients. *American Journal of Respiratory and Critical Care Medicine.* 2002; **166**: 1338–44.

∗ 81. Jaber S, Chanques G, Altairac C *et al.* A prospective study of agitation in a medical-surgical ICU: incidence, risk factors, and outcomes. *Chest.* 2005; **128**: 2749–57.

82. Hamill-Ruth RJ. Use of analgesics in the intensive care unit: who says it hurts? *Critical Care Medicine.* 2002; **30**: 2597–8.

83. New JCAHO standards for pain management. *Texas Nursing.* 2001; **75**: 7.

84. Dasta JF, Kane SL, Gerlach AT *et al.* Bispectral Index in the intensive care setting. *Critical Care Medicine.* 2003; **31**: 998–9.

85. Ely EW, Truman B, Manzi DJ *et al.* Consciousness monitoring in ventilated patients: bispectral EEG monitors arousal not delirium. *Intensive Care Medicine.* 2004; **30**: 1537–43.

86. Forestier F, Hirschi M, Rouget P *et al.* Propofol and sufentanil titration with the bispectral index to provide anesthesia for coronary artery surgery. *Anesthesiology.* 2003; **99**: 334–46.

87. Fraser GL, Riker RR. Bispectral index monitoring in the intensive care unit provides more signal than noise. *Pharmacotherapy.* 2005; **25**: 19S–27S.

88. Tobias JD, Berkenbosch JW. Tolerance during sedation in a pediatric ICU patient: effects on the BIS monitor. *Journal of Clinical Anesthesia.* 2001; **13**: 122–4.

89. Twite MD, Zuk J, Gralla J *et al.* Correlation of the Bispectral Index Monitor with the COMFORT scale in the pediatric intensive care unit. *Pediatric Critical Care Medicine.* 2005; **6**: 648–53.

90. Hamill-Ruth RJ, Marohn ML. Evaluation of pain in the critically ill patient. *Critical Care Clinics.* 1999; **15**: 35–vi.

91. Lavery GG. Optimum sedation and analgesia in critical illness: we need to keep trying. *Critical Care.* 2004; **8**: 433–4.

92. Kress JP, Hall JB. Sedation in the mechanically ventilated patient. *Critical Care Medicine.* 2006; **34**: 2541–6.

93. Bertolini G, Minelli C, Latronico N *et al.* The use of analgesic drugs in postoperative patients: the neglected problem of pain control in intensive care units. An observational, prospective, multicenter study in 128 Italian intensive care units. *European Journal of Clinical Pharmacology.* 2002; **58**: 73–77.

94. Freire AX, Afessa B, Cawley P *et al.* Characteristics associated with analgesia ordering in the intensive care unit and relationships with outcome. *Critical Care Medicine.* 2002; **30**: 2468–72.

95. Puntillo K, Casella V, Reid M. Opioid and benzodiazepine tolerance and dependence: application of theory to critical care practice. *Heart and Lung.* 1997; **26**: 317–24.

96. Shafer A, White PF, Schuttler J *et al.* Use of a fentanyl infusion in the intensive care unit: tolerance to its anesthetic effects? *Anesthesiology.* 1983; **59**: 245–8.

97. Kress JP, Hall JB. Delirium and sedation. *Critical Care Clinics.* 2004; **20**: 419–33, ix.

98. Jones C, Griffiths RD, Humphris G. Disturbed memory and amnesia related to intensive care. *Memory.* 2000; **8**: 79–94.

99. Jones C, Griffiths RD, Humphris G *et al.* Memory, delusions, and the development of acute posttraumatic stress disorder-related symptoms after intensive care. *Critical Care Medicine.* 2001; **29**: 573–80.

100. Pandharipande P, Shintani A, Peterson J *et al.* Lorazepam is an independent risk factor for transitioning to delirium in intensive care unit patients. *Anesthesiology.* 2006; **104**: 21–6.

101. Bailey JM. Context-sensitive half-times: what are they and how valuable are they in anaesthesiology? *Clinical Pharmacokinetics.* 2002; **41**: 793–9.

102. Bodenham A, Park GR. Alfentanil infusions in patients requiring intensive care. *Clinical Pharmacokinetics.* 1988; **15**: 216–26.

103. Hughes MA, Glass PS, Jacobs JR. Context-sensitive half-time in multicompartment pharmacokinetic models for intravenous anesthetic drugs. *Anesthesiology.* 1992; **76**: 334–41.

104. Jacqz-Aigrain E, Burtin P. Clinical pharmacokinetics of sedatives in neonates. *Clinical Pharmacokinetics.* 1996; **31**: 423–43.

105. Katz R, Kelly HW. Pharmacokinetics of continuous infusions of fentanyl in critically ill children. *Critical Care Medicine.* 1993; **21**: 995–1000.

106. Lotsch J. Pharmacokinetic–pharmacodynamic modeling of opioids. *Journal of Pain and Symptom Management.* 2005; **29**: S90–103.

107. Mastronardi P, Cafiero T. Rational use of opioids. *Minerva Anestesiologica.* 2001; **67**: 332–7.

108. Nickel EJ, Smith T. Analgesia in the intensive care unit. Pharmacologic and pharmacokinetic considerations. *Critical Care Nursing Clinics of North America.* 2001; **13**: 207–19.

109. Scholz J, Steinfath M, Schulz M. Clinical pharmacokinetics of alfentanil, fentanyl and sufentanil. *An update. Clinical Pharmacokinetics.* 1996; **31**: 275–92.

110. Tobias JD. Sedation and analgesia in the pediatric intensive care unit. *Pediatric Annals.* 2005; **34**: 636–45.

111. Volles DF, McGory R. Pharmacokinetic considerations. *Critical Care Clinics.* 1999; **15**: 55–75.

112. Beydoun A. Neuropathic pain: from mechanisms to treatment strategies. *Journal of Pain and Symptom Management.* 2003; **25**: S1–3.

113. Chong MS, Bajwa ZH. Diagnosis and treatment of neuropathic pain. *Journal of Pain and Symptom Management.* 2003; **25**: S4–11.

114. Harden N, Cohen M. Unmet needs in the management of neuropathic pain. *Journal of Pain and Symptom Management.* 2003; **25**: S12–17.

115. Kalso E. Sodium channel blockers in neuropathic pain. *Current Pharmaceutical Design.* 2005; **11**: 3005–11.

116. Mercadante S, Ferrera P, Villari P et al. Hyperalgesia: an emerging iatrogenic syndrome. *Journal of Pain and Symptom Management.* 2003; **26**: 769–75.

∗117. Crain SM, Shen KF. Antagonists of excitatory opioid receptor functions enhance morphine's analgesic potency and attenuate opioid tolerance/dependence liability. *Pain.* 2000; **84**: 121–31.

118. Graham GG, Scott KF. Mechanism of action of paracetamol. *American Journal of Therapeutics.* 2005; **12**: 46–55.

119. Gould TH, Cockings JG, Buist M. Postoperative acute liver failure after therapeutic paracetamol administration. *Anaesthesia and Intensive Care.* 1997; **25**: 153–5.

120. James LP, Wilson JT, Simar R et al. Evaluation of occult acetaminophen hepatotoxicity in hospitalized children receiving acetaminophen. Pediatric Pharmacology Research Unit Network. *Clinical Pediatrics.* 2001; **40**: 243–8.

121. Sivilotti ML, Good AM, Yarema MC et al. A new predictor of toxicity following acetaminophen overdose based on pretreatment exposure. *Clinical Toxicology.* 2005; **43**: 229–34.

122. Fukunaga K, Kohli P, Bonnans C et al. Cyclooxygenase 2 plays a pivotal role in the resolution of acute lung injury. *Journal of Immunology.* 2005; **174**: 5033–9.

123. Gupta A, Daggett C, Drant S et al. Prospective randomized trial of ketorolac after congenital heart surgery. *Journal of Cardiothoracic and Vascular Anesthesia.* 2004; **18**: 454–7.

124. Fayaz MK, Abel RJ, Pugh SC et al. Opioid-sparing effects of diclofenac and paracetamol lead to improved outcomes after cardiac surgery. *Journal of Cardiothoracic and Vascular Anesthesia.* 2004; **18**: 742–7.

125. Jasinski DR, Johnson RE, Kocher TR. Clonidine in morphine withdrawal. Differential effects on signs and symptoms. *Archives of General Psychiatry.* 1985; **42**: 1063–6.

∗126. Aantaa R, Jalonen J. Perioperative use of alpha 2-adrenoceptor agonists and the cardiac patient. *European Journal of Anaesthesiology.* 2006; **23**: 361–72.

∗127. Gupta A, Decaillot FM, Devi LA. Targeting opioid receptor heterodimers: strategies for screening and drug development. *AAPS Journal.* 2006; **8**: E153–9.

128. Chrysostomou C, Di FS, Manrique AM et al. Use of dexmedetomidine in children after cardiac and thoracic surgery. *Pediatric Critical Care Medicine.* 2006; **7**: 126–31.

129. Hall JE, Uhrich TD, Barney JA et al. Sedative, amnestic, and analgesic properties of small-dose dexmedetomidine infusions. *Anesthesia and Analgesia.* 2000; **90**: 699–705.

130. Martin E, Ramsay G, Mantz J et al. The role of the alpha2-adrenoceptor agonist dexmedetomidine in postsurgical sedation in the intensive care unit. *Journal of Intensive Care Medicine.* 2003; **18**: 29–41.

131. Maze M, Scarfini C, Cavaliere F. New agents for sedation in the intensive care unit. *Critical Care Clinics.* 2001; **17**: 881–97.

∗132. Riker RR, Fraser GL. Adverse events associated with sedatives, analgesics, and other drugs that provide patient comfort in the intensive care unit. *Pharmacotherapy.* 2005; **25**: 8S–18S.

133. Walker J, MacCallum M, Fischer C et al. Sedation using dexmedetomidine in pediatric burn patients. *Journal of Burn Care and Research.* 2006; **27**: 206–10.

134. Coursin DB, Coursin DB, Maccioli GA. Dexmedetomidine. *Current Opinion in Critical Care.* 2001; **7**: 221–6.

135. Ickeringill M, Shehabi Y, Adamson H et al. Dexmedetomidine infusion without loading dose in surgical patients requiring mechanical ventilation: haemodynamic effects and efficacy. *Anaesthesia and Intensive Care.* 2004; **32**: 741–5.

136. Shehabi Y, Ruettimann U, Adamson H et al. Dexmedetomidine infusion for more than 24 hours in critically ill patients: sedative and cardiovascular effects. *Intensive Care Medicine.* 2004; **30**: 2188–96.

137. Elbaradie S, El Mahalawy FH, Solyman AH. Dexmedetomidine vs. propofol for short-term sedation of postoperative mechanically ventilated patients. *Journal of the Egyptian National Cancer Institute.* 2004; **16**: 153–8.

138. Wahlander S, Frumento RJ, Wagener G et al. A prospective, double-blind, randomized, placebo-controlled study of dexmedetomidine as an adjunct to epidural analgesia after thoracic surgery. *Journal of Cardiothoracic and Vascular Anesthesia.* 2005; **19**: 630–5.

139. Munoz R, Berry D. Dexmedetomidine: promising drug for pediatric sedation? *Pediatric Critical Care Medicine.* 2005; **6**: 493–4.

140. Tobias JD, Berkenbosch JW. Initial experience with dexmedetomidine in paediatric-aged patients. *Paediatric Anaesthesia.* 2002; **12**: 171–5.

141. Tobias JD, Berkenbosch JW. Sedation during mechanical ventilation in infants and children: dexmedetomidine versus midazolam. *Southern Medical Journal.* 2004; **97**: 451–5.

142. Tobias JD, Berkenbosch JW, Russo P. Additional experience with dexmedetomidine in pediatric patients. *Southern Medical Journal.* 2003; **96**: 871–5.

143. Miller LJ, Wiles-Pfeifler R. Propofol for the long-term sedation of a critically ill patient. *American Journal of Critical Care.* 1998; **7**: 73–6.

∗144. Mistraletti G, Donatelli F, Carli F. Metabolic and endocrine effects of sedative agents. *Current Opinion in Critical Care.* 2005; **11**: 312–17.

145. Finkel JC, Johnson YJ, Quezado ZM. The use of dexmedetomidine to facilitate acute discontinuation of opioids after cardiac transplantation in children. *Critical Care Medicine*. 2005; **33**: 2110–12.

*146. Bell RF, Dahl JB, Moore RA *et al.* Perioperative ketamine for acute postoperative pain. *Cochrane Database of Systematic Reviews*. 2006; **CD004603**.

*147. Bell RF, Dahl JB, Moore RA *et al.* Peri-operative ketamine for acute post-operative pain: a quantitative and qualitative systematic review (Cochrane review). *Acta Anaesthesiologica Scandinavica*. 2005; **49**: 1405–28.

148. Visser E, Schug SA. The role of ketamine in pain management. *Biomedicine and Pharmacotherapy*. 2006; **60**: 341–8.

149. Annetta MG, Iemma D, Garisto C *et al.* Ketamine: new indications for an old drug. *Current Drug Targets*. 2005; **6**: 789–94.

150. Ivani G, Vercellino C, Tonetti F. Ketamine: a new look to an old drug. *Minerva Anestesiologica*. 2003; **69**: 468–71.

151. Tobias JD, Martin LD, Wetzel RC. Ketamine by continuous infusion for sedation in the pediatric intensive care unit. *Critical Care Medicine*. 1990; **18**: 819–21.

152. Clinical practice guidelines for the sustained use of sedatives and analgesics in the critically ill adult. *American Journal of Health-system Pharmacy*. 2002; **59**: 150–78.

*153. Anand KJ, Ingraham J. Pediatric. Tolerance, dependence, and strategies for compassionate withdrawal of analgesics and anxiolytics in the pediatric ICU. *Critical Care Nurse*. 1996; **16**: 87–93.

154. Carr DB, Todres ID. Fentanyl infusion and weaning in the pediatric intensive care unit: toward science-based practice. *Critical Care Medicine*. 1994; **22**: 725–7.

155. Chamorro C, Romera MA, Martinez JL. Withdrawal syndrome and tolerance to sedatives and analgesics in intensive care unit patients. *Critical Care Medicine*. 1999; **27**: 2602–4.

*156. Tobias JD. Tolerance, withdrawal, and physical dependency after long-term sedation and analgesia of children in the pediatric intensive care unit. *Critical Care Medicine*. 2000; **28**: 2122–32.

157. Zapantis A, Leung S. Tolerance and withdrawal issues with sedation. *Critical Care Nursing Clinics of North America*. 2005; **17**: 211–23.

158. Tobias JD. Subcutaneous administration of fentanyl and midazolam to prevent withdrawal after prolonged sedation in children. *Critical Care Medicine*. 1999; **27**: 2262–5.

159. Tobias JD, Schleien CL, Haun SE. Methadone as treatment for iatrogenic narcotic dependency in pediatric intensive care unit patients. *Critical Care Medicine*. 1990; **18**: 1292–3.

160. Baddigam K, Russo P, Russo J *et al.* Dexmedetomidine in the treatment of withdrawal syndromes in cardiothoracic surgery patients. *Journal of Intensive Care Medicine*. 2005; **20**: 118–23.

*161. Murphy EJ. Acute pain management pharmacology for the patient with concurrent renal or hepatic disease. *Anaesthesia and Intensive Care*. 2005; **33**: 311–22.

162. Johnson C, Simmons W. *Dialysis of drugs 2006*. Amgen: Nephrology Pharmacy Associates Inc., 2006.

*163. Horlocker TT, Wedel DJ, Benzon H *et al.* Regional anesthesia in the anticoagulated patient: defining the risks (the second ASRA Consensus Conference on Neuraxial Anesthesia and Anticoagulation). *Regional Anesthesia and Pain Medicine*. 2003; **28**: 172–97.

164. Wiedemann HP, Wheeler AP, Bernard GR *et al.* Comparison of two fluid-management strategies in acute lung injury. *New England Journal of Medicine*. 2006; **354**: 2564–75.

165. Low JH. Survey of epidural analgesia management in general intensive care units in England. *Acta Anaesthesiologica Scandinavica*. 2002; **46**: 799–805.

166. Kanji S, Devlin JW, Piekos KA *et al.* Recombinant human activated protein C, drotrecogin alfa (activated): a novel therapy for severe sepsis. *Pharmacotherapy*. 2001; **21**: 1389–402.

167. Dhainaut JF, Laterre PF, LaRosa SP *et al.* The clinical evaluation committee in a large multicenter phase 3 trial of drotrecogin alfa (activated) in patients with severe sepsis (PROWESS): role, methodology, and results. *Critical Care Medicine*. 2003; **31**: 2291–301.

168. Karmakar MK. Thoracic paravertebral block. *Anesthesiology*. 2001; **95**: 771–80.

169. Richardson J, Lonnqvist PA. Thoracic paravertebral block. *British Journal of Anaesthesia*. 1998; **81**: 230–8.

170. Lonnqvist PA. Continuous paravertebral block in children. Initial experience. *Anaesthesia*. 1992; **47**: 607–9.

171. Lonnqvist PA, MacKenzie J, Soni AK *et al.* Paravertebral blockade. Failure rate and complications. *Anaesthesia*. 1995; **50**: 813–15.

172. Lonnqvist PA. Entering the paravertebral space age again? *Acta Anaesthesiologica Scandinavica*. 2001; **45**: 1–3.

173. Richardson J, Sabanathan S, Mearns AJ *et al.* A prospective, randomized comparison of interpleural and paravertebral analgesia in thoracic surgery. *British Journal of Anaesthesia*. 1995; **75**: 405–8.

174. Sabanathan S, Richardson J, Mearns AJ. Management of pain in thoracic surgery. *British Journal of Hospital Medicine*. 1993; **50**: 114–20.

175. Richardson J, Sabanathan S, Jones J *et al.* A prospective, randomized comparison of preoperative and continuous balanced epidural or paravertebral bupivacaine on post-thoracotomy pain, pulmonary function and stress responses. *British Journal of Anaesthesia*. 1999; **83**: 387–92.

176. Richardson J, Sabanathan S, Shah RD *et al.* Pleural bupivacaine placement for optimal postthoracotomy pulmonary function: a prospective, randomized study. *Journal of Cardiothoracic and Vascular Anesthesia*. 1998; **12**: 166–9.

177. Shah R, Sabanathan S, Richardson J *et al.* Continuous paravertebral block for post thoracotomy analgesia in

children. *Journal of Cardiovascular Surgery.* 1997; **38**: 543–6.

178. Lonnqvist PA. Pre-emptive analgesia with thoracic paravertebral blockade? *British Journal of Anaesthesia.* 2005; **95**: 727–8.

179. Karmakar MK, Ho AM. Postthoracotomy pain syndrome. *Thoracic Surgery Clinics.* 2004; **14**: 345–52.

180. Luketich JD, Land SR, Sullivan EA *et al.* Thoracic epidural versus intercostal nerve catheter plus patient-controlled analgesia: a randomized study. *Annals of Thoracic Surgery.* 2005; **79**: 1845–9.

181. Richardson J, Sabanathan S, Shah R. Post-thoracotomy spirometric lung function: the effect of analgesia. A review. *Journal of Cardiovascular Surgery.* 1999; **40**: 445–56.

182. Tobias JD, Martin LD, Oakes L *et al.* Postoperative analgesia following thoracotomy in children: interpleural catheters. *Journal of Pediatric Surgery.* 1993; **28**: 1466–70.

*183. Fisher MM. God, medicine and ethics. *Critical Care and Resuscitation.* 2001; **3**: 277–9. 2006.

184. Baggs JG, Norton SA, Schmitt MH *et al.* The dying patient in the ICU: role of the interdisciplinary team. *Critical Care Clinics.* 2004; **20**: 525–40, xi.

185. Burns JP, Rushton CH. End-of-life care in the pediatric intensive care unit: research review and recommendations. *Critical Care Clinics.* 2004; **20**: 467–85, x.

*186. Cist AF, Truog RD, Brackett SE *et al.* Practical guidelines on the withdrawal of life-sustaining therapies. *International Anesthesiology Clinics.* 2001; **39**: 87–102.

*187. Hawryluck LA, Harvey WR, Lemieux-Charles L *et al.* Consensus guidelines on analgesia and sedation in dying intensive care unit patients. *BMC Medical Ethics.* 2002; **3**: E3.

188. Masri C, Farrell CA, Lacroix J *et al.* Decision making and end-of-life care in critically ill children. *Journal of Palliative Care.* 2000; **16** (Suppl.): S45–52.

189. Rubenfeld GD. Principles and practice of withdrawing life-sustaining treatments. *Critical Care Clinics.* 2004; **20**: 435–51, ix.

190. Thompson BT, Cox PN, Antonelli M *et al.* Challenges in end-of-life care in the ICU: statement of the 5th International Consensus Conference in Critical Care: Brussels, Belgium, April 2003: executive summary. *Critical Care Medicine.* 2004; **32**: 1781–4.

*191. Cassell J. The elephant in the living room. Ethics as a screen for covering one's butt. *Critical Care and Resuscitation.* 2005; **7**: 244–5. 2006.

192. Baker R, Wu AW, Teno JM *et al.* Family satisfaction with end-of-life care in seriously ill hospitalized adults. *Journal of the American Geriatrics Society.* 2000; **48**: S61–9.

193. Carlet J, Thijs LG, Antonelli M *et al.* Challenges in end-of-life care in the ICU. Statement of the 5th International Consensus Conference in Critical Care: Brussels, Belgium, April 2003. *Intensive Care Medicine.* 2004; **30**: 770–84.

194. Hofmann JC, Wenger NS, Davis RB *et al.* Patient preferences for communication with physicians about end-of-life decisions. SUPPORT Investigators. Study to Understand Prognoses and Preference for Outcomes and Risks of Treatment. *Annals of Internal Medicine.* 1997; **127**: 1–12.

195. Rubenfeld GD, Curtis JR. Beyond ethical dilemmas: improving the quality of end-of-life care in the intensive care unit. *Critical Care.* 2003; **7**: 11–12.

196. Bernat JL, D'Alessandro AM, Port FK *et al.* Report of a national conference on donation after cardiac death. *American Journal of Transplantation.* 2006; **6**: 281–91.

197. Baron L, Shemie SD, Teitelbaum J *et al.* Brief review: history, concept and controversies in the neurological determination of death. *Canadian Journal of Anaesthesia.* 2006; **53**: 602–8.

198. Pearson IY. Australia and New Zealand Intensive Care Society Statement and Guidelines on Brain Death and Model Policy on Organ Donation. *Anaesthesia and Intensive Care.* 1995; **23**: 104–8.

199. Hawryluck LA, Harvey WR. Analgesia, virtue, and the principle of double effect. *Journal of Palliative Care.* 2000; **16** (Suppl.): S24–30.

200. Truog RD, Arnold JH, Rockoff MA. Sedation before ventilator withdrawal: medical and ethical considerations. *Journal of Clinical Ethics.* 1991; **2**: 127–9.

201. Krakauer EL, Penson RT, Truog RD *et al.* Sedation for intractable distress of a dying patient: acute palliative care and the principle of double effect. *Oncologist.* 2000; **5**: 53–62.

202. Dewland P, Dewland J. At the coalface, but on the receiving end. *Journal of Medical Ethics.* 1999; **25**: 541–6.

*203. Davies RG, Myles PS, Graham JM. A comparison of the analgesic efficacy and side-effects of paravertebral vs epidural blockade for thoracotomy – a systematic review and meta-analysis of randomized trials. *British Journal of Anaesthesia.* 2006; **96**: 418–26.

204. Chaney MA. Intrathecal and epidural anesthesia and analgesia for cardiac surgery. *Anesthesia and Analgesia.* 2006; **102**: 45–64.

205. Djaiani G, Fedorko L, Beattie WS. Regional anesthesia in cardiac surgery: a friend or a foe? *Seminars in Cardiothoracic and Vascular Anesthesia.* 2005; **9**: 87–104.

206. Werhagen L, Budh CN, Hultling C *et al.* Neuropathic pain after traumatic spinal cord injury – relations to gender, spinal level, completeness, and age at the time of injury. *Spinal Cord.* 2004; **42**: 665–73.

207. Hund EF, Borel CO, Cornblath DR *et al.* Intensive management and treatment of severe Guillain–Barré syndrome. *Critical Care Medicine.* 1993; **21**: 433–46.

208. Khatri A, Pearlstein L. Pain in Guillain–Barré syndrome. *Neurology.* 1997; **49**: 1474.

209. Pentland B, Donald SM. Pain in the Guillain–Barré syndrome: a clinical review. *Pain.* 1994; **59**: 159–64.

210. van der Meche FG, Schmitz PI. A randomized trial comparing intravenous immune globulin and plasma exchange in Guillain–Barré syndrome. Dutch

Guillain–Barré Study Group. *New England Journal of Medicine*. 1992; **326**: 1123–9.

211. Bernsen RA, de Jager AE, van der Meche FG *et al*. How Guillain–Barré patients experience their functioning after 1 year. *Acta Neurologica Scandinavica*. 2005; **112**: 51–6.

212. Bernsen RA, Jager AE, Schmitz PI *et al*. Long-term sensory deficit after Guillain–Barré syndrome. *Journal of Neurology*. 2001; **248**: 483–6.

213. Khan F. Rehabilitation in Guillain–Barré syndrome. *Australian Family Physician*. 2004; **33**: 1013–17.

214. Gregory MA, Gregory RJ, Podd JV. Understanding Guillain–Barré syndrome and central nervous system involvement. *Rehabilitation Nursing*. 2005; **30**: 207–12.

215. Pandey CK, Raza M, Tripathi M, *et al*. The comparative evaluation of gabapentin and carbamazepine for pain management in Guillain–Barré syndrome patients in the intensive care unit. *Anesthesia and Analgesia*. 2005; **101**: 220–5, table.

216. Tripathi M, Kaushik S. Carbamazepine for pain management in Guillain–Barré syndrome patients in the intensove care unit. *Critical Care Medicine*. 2000; **28**: 655–8.

19

Acute pain management in the emergency department

ANNE-MAREE KELLY AND BARRY D GUNN

KEY LEARNING POINTS

PRINCIPLES

- Pain management in emergency departments (ED) requires a system for quantification of pain, initiation of therapy, and reassessment.
- As a general rule, the approach to analgesia in EDs should be simple before complex, specific before nonspecific, and local before general.
- When opioids are required for severe pain, parenteral administration is usually indicated in the initial phases of ED care and the intravenous (i.v.) route is preferred when practical.
- Opioid-tolerant patients are likely to require higher doses of opioid in order to achieve analgesia. Opioids should not be withheld from any patient where there is an apparently genuine cause for pain.
- Ketamine may be a useful adjunct to i.v. opioids in patients who are requiring high doses of opioids in very painful conditions, such as severe burns.

ANALGESIA FOR SPECIFIC CONDITIONS

- There is no evidence to support the withholding of opioid analgesia in patients suffering abdominal pain.
- Nonsteroidal anti-inflammatory drugs (NSAID) are effective for treating the pain of renal and biliary colic, but require about 30 minutes to be effective.

- Oral NSAIDs, including aspirin, are useful for treating mild to moderate traumatic and musculoskeletal pain and mild migraine.
- For severe migraine, the evidence suggests that the most effective agents are the phenothiazines (chlorpromazine and prochlorperazine) and the triptans (sumatriptan and related agents).
- For fractures of the femoral neck, titrated i.v. opioids are appropriate for initial pain control. Femoral nerve or "three-in-one" local anesthetic blocks (either as a single injection or by a catheter) may be a useful opioid-sparing adjunct. Skin traction does not provide superior analgesia to positioning.
- Regarding local anesthetic infiltration for wound analgesia/anesthesia, infiltration via the wound rather than the surrounding skin has been shown to reduce the pain of infiltration as has warming of the injected solution.
- Topical anesthetic preparations have been shown to be effective alternatives to infiltration of local anesthesia for selected simple lacerations.
- There is no clearly superior method of analgesia for fracture/dislocation reduction.

INTRODUCTION

Pain is the single most common reason for presentation to emergency departments (ED). Causes are both medical and surgical and severity ranges from mild to very severe. Despite its prevalence, there is strong evidence that patients in ED around the world receive suboptimal pain management.[1]

Before discussing the evidence, it is important to clarify how it was chosen. Two approaches were considered: including all the data for a particular condition (i.e. data derived from both ED and non-ED settings) or restricting the analysis to data obtained from studies of ED patients. The latter approach is appealing because ED patients are suffering from undifferentiated illness, so a disease-based approach does not always mimic the clinical context. In addition, there is some evidence that ED patients may be different from other patients, for example in that they may have already tried self-medication before coming to the ED.[2, 3][II] Unfortunately, high quality trials in the ED setting alone are uncommon for most conditions. We have decided to use data derived from ED-based studies if it is of sufficient quality and/or there is reasonable evidence that the ED population with a given painful condition is different from the general outpatient population. Where there is no ED-specific data of sufficient quality, data from other settings have been incorporated.

Some of the available evidence and best practice regarding pain management in the ED has recently been summarized in guidelines[4] and publications.[5] These are useful sources for reference.

PRINCIPLES

Choice of analgesia

As a general rule, the choice of analgesia should be the simplest, most condition-specific, and most local that is effective. For example, for a patient suffering myocardial ischemia, an appropriate initial analgesic is nitroglycerin, although it has no intrinsic analgesic properties. For a patient with a crushed digit, although nitrous oxide or systemic opioid may be needed in the short term, a digital nerve block is highly effective ongoing analgesia and may additionally facilitate wound repair. For a patient suffering pain due to an envenomation, treatment of the envenomation rather than, or concurrent with, systemic analgesia is indicated. There is not sufficient space to provide a condition by condition list, however the principles of simple before complex, specific before nonspecific, and local before general, coupled with regular reassessment of the adequacy of analgesia usually prove effective.

Systems for analgesia delivery

There is evidence that analgesia in ED is often neither timely nor adequate.[1] Children, the elderly, the cognitively impaired, and some ethnic groups appear to be at increased risk of poor pain management.[1, 6]

A system to deliver timely and effective analgesia requires the following elements: a process to quantify and document pain at regular intervals (e.g. using pain scores), a process to initiate appropriate therapy, and a process to monitor response to initial therapy and provide additional analgesia as required. The design of such a system will depend on factors such as overall staffing levels and its match to workload, patient characteristics such as age, ethnicity mix, and urgency distribution, mix of medical, nursing and assistant staff, level of training of staff, local legislative restrictions, and safety concerns.

Examples of system design to achieve this include assessment of pain intensity at the time of triage and integrating it as part of the assignment of triage (treatment priority) categories and development of pain management guidelines to direct choice of agent and route of administration for selected conditions. Where legislative and hospital policies allow, analgesia can be initiated at the time of triage for patients who are expected to have to wait before medical treatment. This may take the form of topical anesthesia for a wound[7][II] or oral medication.[8][V] For patients suffering severe pain, a titrated intravenous (i.v.) opioid protocol can be effective,[9][IV], [10][V] as can nurse-initiated titrated i.v. opioids for selected conditions.[11][III]

Analgesia at the extremes of age

Data suggest that children and the elderly receive poorer pain management in ED than adults.[1, 6] Reasons for this are unclear and probably multifactorial. In some centers, there appears to be reluctance to treat children with parenteral analgesics and/or to delay i.v. insertion for analgesia until topical anesthetic has been employed. Neither of these is justified. Children suffering severe pain should receive appropriate analgesia without delay. Details of pediatric analgesia are discussed in Chapter 27, Acute pain management in children. Regarding the elderly, some concerns appear to be centered on the risks of sedation and hypotension. Although physiological changes make responses to analgesia different in the elderly, this is insufficient justification for under-analgesia. This group is ideally served by titrated doses of opioids as described under Systemic analgesia.

SYSTEMIC ANALGESIA

Opioids

Opioid analgesics are frequently required in ED for the treatment of severe pain. They are discussed in detail in

Chapter 3, Clinical pharmacology: opioids, so only issues specifically related to their use in ED will be covered here.

There are a range of opioids commonly used in ED for analgesia, including short-acting agents, such as fentanyl, as well as the more traditional agents, morphine and pethidine (meperidine). Generally, morphine is preferred to pethidine because of the lack of euphoric effect and slightly higher potency. The long-taught adages that morphine should not be used to treat renal or biliary colic for fear of exacerbating pain are not borne out by evidence and should be disregarded.[12][II]

In most cases, parenteral administration is indicated in the initial phases of ED care. In selected cases, oral agents can be substituted for ongoing analgesia once initial control has been obtained. Examples include management of cancer pain crises and preoperative management of fracture pain. Given the risks of addiction, care should be taken in prescribing opioids for outpatient use unless there is a definite diagnosis, alternatives are not available/appropriate and there is a longer-term pain management plan.

Given the individual variability in dose requirement and the delay to onset of action of intramuscular (i.m.) opioids, the i.v. route is generally preferred with dose titrated to effect. It is recognized that titrated i.v. dosing requires appropriate training and sufficient staff to appropriately monitor patients. This is not always possible in ED and when this is the case, i.m. dosing may be safer but is likely to be less effective. A dose of 0.1–0.15 mg/kg of morphine would be an appropriate initial dose in this circumstance.

For i.v. opioids, doses should be adjusted for age (lower doses are advised in patients aged over 65 years) and weight and titrated to effect (see Chapter 28, Acute pain management in the elderly patient). For an adult male aged 40 years and weighing about 80 kg, an indicative initial dose of morphine would be 0.05 mg/kg (i.e. 4 mg) with incremental doses of 0.025 mg/kg (i.e. 2 mg) at five- to ten-minute intervals until pain is controlled. For an elderly female aged 80 years and weighing 60 kg, an indicative initial dose would be 0.025 mg/kg (i.e. 1.5 mg) with increments of 1 mg (approximately 0.0125 mg/kg) at the intervals defined above. Fentanyl has also be shown to be effective when administered i.v. by titration.[13][II] Patients require close observation for sedation and hypotension. Hypotension has been reported to occur in 4.9 percent of patients when titrated regimens are used.[14] [IV] Respiratory depression, although a possibility, is extremely rare when titrated regimens with monitoring of vital signs, sedation, and pain score are used.[14][IV] It is important to remember that patients with hemodynamic compromise may be more prone to the hypotensive effects of opioids and both initial and incremental doses should be reduced.

Opioid-tolerant patients, such as those taking illicit opioids, patients on opioid management programs such as methadone programs, and patients taking opioids to manage chronic pain, are likely to require higher doses of opioid in order to achieve analgesia; however, the rapid titration approach is still recommended as long as it allows for an appropriately higher total dose. Opioids should not be withheld from any patient where there is an apparently genuine cause for pain. The misconception that therapeutic opioids "feed a habit" is ill founded (see also Chapter 30, The opioid-tolerant patient, including those with a substance abuse disorder).

Intranasal (i.n.) opioids including fentanyl and diacetylmorphine (diamorphine) have been trialled in the ED and prehospital settings and have been shown to be effective.[15][IV], [16][II] Median dose requirements of fentanyl in children are 1.5 μg/kg.[15]

Although patient-controlled analgesia (PCA) has been shown to be safe when used in the ED for patients with defined pathology,[17][II], [18][IV] its overall place in ED is still being defined. PCA has the advantage of being responsive to patient's pain, but as pain is a significant factor in diagnosis, knowing that a higher than expected dose of analgesia is being required might influence investigation, diagnosis, and disposition. PCA may mask this. Based on current evidence, PCA in ED should probably be reserved for patients who have a defined diagnosis and ongoing analgesia needs.

Tramadol

Tramadol, a synthetic opioid, has been suggested as an option for treatment of severe pain of any cause, renal colic, dental problems, migraine, and musculoskeletal conditions. Evidence of its effectiveness in acute, non-postoperative pain is not convincing.

In the ED setting, for patients with severe pain from trauma, i.v. tramadol was shown to have similar effectiveness to i.v. morphine.[19][II] For patients with right lower quadrant pain, tramadol provided statistically better analgesia than placebo, but the effect size was small (7 mm difference on a 100 mm visual analog scale (VAS)) and probably not of clinical significance.[20][II] For renal colic, it has been shown to be less effective than pethidine[21][II] and similarly effective to ketorolac 30 mg, although ketorolac had a more rapid onset of action.[22][II] For dental pain, a meta-analysis suggests tramadol to have similar effectiveness to codeine 60 mg, but to be less effective than full dose nonsteroidal anti-inflammatory drugs (NSAID) or codeine/aspirin (acetylsalicylic acid) or acetaminophen (paracetamol) preparations.[23][II] For musculoskeletal pain, oral tramadol has been shown to be less effective than hydrocodone/acetaminophen[24][II] and parenteral tramadol has been shown to have similar effectiveness to parenteral diclofenac.[25][II] Oral acetaminophen/tramadol combinations have been shown to have similar efficacy to oral ibuprofen 400 mg.[26][II] For treatment of migraine, tramadol has a reported clinical success rate of 59 percent,[27, 28][II] significantly inferior to other available treatments.

Based on available evidence, tramadol is not more effective than morphine/pethidine for severe pain or than NSAIDs or codeine/aspirin or acetaminophen combinations for moderate pain. It is not highly effective for any specific condition. Thus its place in the ED pain armamentarium remains in doubt. It may be a useful alternative in patients for whom NSAIDs are contraindicated or who are codeine intolerant.

Nonsteroidal anti-inflammatory agents

Oral NSAIDs, including aspirin, are useful for treating mild to moderate traumatic and musculoskeletal pain (see Chapter 24, Acute musculoskeletal pain). NSAIDs are also effective for treating the pain of renal and biliary colic, as the mechanisms of pain production include prostaglandin release, but require about 30 minutes to be effective, even when given parenterally. This is discussed further under Renal colic and Biliary colic.

Nitrous oxide

Nitrous oxide, in a variety of mixtures with oxygen, is used widely in both pediatric and adult ED (see Chapter 6, Clinical pharmacology: other adjuvants). For adults, self-administration via a demand valve is usual while for children continuous flow systems are more appropriate. Nitrous oxide has been shown to be effective analgesia and anxiolysis for minor procedures in both adults and children.[29, 30, 31, 32][II], [33][IV] It may also be useful as a temporizing measure while more definitive analgesia is instituted, e.g. insertion of a digital nerve block for finger injury.

Ketamine

The pharamacology of ketamine is discussed in Chapter 6, Clinical pharmacology: other adjuvants. It has been shown to reduce opioid requirements in the treatment of acute pain. Although there is no specific evidence from the ED setting, ketamine may be a useful adjunct to i.v. opioids in patients who are requiring high doses of opioids in very painful conditions, such as severe burns.

ANALGESIA FOR SPECIFIC CONDITIONS

Abdominal pain

Abdominal pain is common in ED and causes range from benign to life-threatening. Traditionally, there had been reluctance to provide strong analgesics to patients with abdominal pain for the fear of masking the signs of intra-abdominal pathology. This notion, stemming from

Cope's 1921 publication *Diagnosis of the acute abdomen*,[34] predates the availability of accurately titratable opioid solutions and opioid reversal agents. It is now recognized that early appropriate analgesia is important for both patient comfort and physician assessment. Choice of agent and route of administration will depend on the level of pain being reported, the clinical state, and the possible cause of pain.

There is now convincing evidence to support the early use of analgesia in the assessment and management of patients with abdominal pain. In adult patients, it has been shown that opioid analgesia does not reduce the ability to make an accurate surgical diagnosis.[35, 36, 37][II] In some studies, it has been suggested that early analgesia actually improves the accuracy of surgical diagnosis.[35, 36] [II] Clinical signs of peritonism are not masked by appropriate opioid analgesia.[36][II] A meta-analysis of prospective trials of ED patients with abdominal pain receiving opioid analgesia found that there were no adverse outcomes or diagnostic delays in patients who received analgesia.[38][I]

Evidence in pediatric patients similarly supports provision of analgesia for patients with abdominal pain.[39, 40] [II] The provision of analgesia did not impair the ability to make a diagnosis by pediatric emergency physicians or surgeons.

Despite this evidence, attitudes are changing slowly. There is still reluctance among some clinicians to prescribe analgesia for both adult and pediatric ED patients with abdominal pain.[41, 42, 43][III] Attitudes reported by surgeons suggest that they believe that analgesia should be delayed until surgical review has occurred.[44][III]

If abdominal pain is severe, opioids are often required. Although it has previously been recommended that pethidine be used in preference to morphine, particularly for renal and biliary colic due to the theoretical risk of spasm, there is no evidence to support this position.[12]

Renal colic

Patients with acute renal colic usually present to ED with severe pain.[45] Patients are often distressed and require rapidly administered analgesia.

The pathological basis of the pain of renal colic is increasing wall tension from the obstructing calculus that causes localized release of prostaglandins, that in turn induce vasodilation and diuresis that further increase pain.[46, 47]

Most of the evidence regarding the ED management of renal colic examines the use of opioid analgesics, NSAIDs, or both. Unfortunately, studies use differing doses of drugs and routes of administration making it difficult to compare them. In particular, in some studies, the drugs that are being compared are not in equipotent dosages.

Titrated i.v. opioids have traditionally been the mainstay of treatment and provide rapid analgesia.[48][II]

Incremental doses should be given as described above under Opioids. It was thought that pethidine caused less smooth muscle spasm, but this has not been found to be clinically relevant.[12][II] Morphine is the analgesic of preference for reasons described above under Opioids.

NSAIDs provide effective analgesia for renal colic and act by inhibiting prostaglandin synthesis – the basis of the pain. In comparing NSAIDs and opioids, the evidence shows that patients treated with opioids have a lower pain score than a NSAID-treated group at ten minutes, but there was no difference between groups at 30 minutes.[48] [II] Given that renal colic often causes severe pain, this earlier onset of analgesia with opioids is likely to be clinically relevant to patients. A significant problem with NSAID–opioid comparisons is that they often compare the response to a single dose of an NSAID with a single bolus of an i.v. opioid. However, considerable variability in opioid requirement has been documented,[49][V] so comparisons of single doses may not be reflective of everyday clinical practice.[46]

With respect to the effectiveness of injectable NSAIDs, ketorolac 30 mg i.m. was reported to be as effective as pethidine 100 mg i.m., with no difference in the proportion of patients improving at one hour between groups.[50] [II] Fifty-six percent of patients treated with ketorolac required supplementary opioid analgesia. Intravenous ketorolac 60 mg was compared with i.v. pethidine 50 mg i.v. and a combination of both and it was reported that ketorolac was more effective at reducing pain at 30 minutes than pethidine.[51][II] This comparison is, however, biased as the doses of agents being compared were not equipotent. Approximately 75 percent of all patients studied required supplementary opioid analgesia. Based on this evidence, ketorolac as a single agent in either a 30- or 60-mg dose could not be recommended for treatment of moderate–severe renal colic. Some evidence suggests that rectal NSAIDs are as effective as i.v. NSAIDs.[52]

Some evidence questions whether NSAIDs have any role in the acute ED management of renal colic. Neither NSAIDs (indomethacin and diclofenac) nor the cyclo-oxygenase-2 inhibitor rofecoxib have been shown to reduce narcotic requirements in patients with renal colic.[45][III], [53][II]

NSAIDs (both oral and rectal) are effective in managing pain after ED discharge, decreasing the frequency and severity of recurrent episodes of pain.[54, 55][II]

No high quality trials evaluating the effectiveness of anti-muscarinic medications such as hyoscine-N-butyl-bromide (scopolamine) as single agents in renal colic could be identified. When studied in combination with other agents (opioids or NSAIDs), the evidence does not show a difference in additional analgesic requirements when patients are or are not treated with adjuvant anti-muscarinic medications.[56, 57, 58][II] Anti-muscarinic agents are not recommended for the treatment of acute renal colic in the ED.

Biliary colic

So-called "biliary colic" is caused by impaction of a gallstone in Hartmann's pouch of the gall bladder or in the cystic duct.[59, 60] This leads to a series of events causing cellular injury which result in release of lysosomal enzymes, phospholipase, lecithin, and prostaglandins causing pain and inflammation.

Patients with biliary colic often report severe pain. The choices for analgesia are opioids, NSAIDs, anticholinergic medications, or a combination of these.

Patients with severe pain or who are vomiting should be treated with parenteral opioids.[61] For reasons discussed above under Opioids, titrated i.v. dosing is recommended. Historically, pethidine has been the analgesic of choice for biliary colic. This is based on the belief that morphine may increase pain by causing contraction/spasm of the sphincter of Oddi, whereas pethidine does not have this effect. Unfortunately, this is based on intraoperative manometry studies[62, 63] and did not examine clinical outcomes. To date, there are no data directly comparing the effectiveness and side effects of these agents, so neither can be recommended above the other.

NSAIDs are also effective in treating the pain of biliary colic, having their action by inhibition of prostaglandin synthesis. Intramuscular diclofenac has been shown to be more effective than placebo.[60][III], [64][II] Ketorolac 60 mg i.m. has been found to be as effective as i.m. pethidine (1.5 mg/kg up to 100 mg).[65][II] Intravenous ketorolac 30 mg was found to provide similar analgesia at 30 minutes, one and two hours to pethidine 50 mg i.v.[61][II] with a lower incidence of nausea. Most of these studies have compared effectiveness at 30 minutes or longer. It is known that NSAIDs require at least 15–30 minutes for onset of analgesia even if given parenterally.[66][II] So for severe pain, it is appropriate to use titrated i.v. opioids initially followed by NSAIDs.

For those with mild pain, analgesia should be tailored accordingly with NSAIDs being the treatment of choice, unless contraindicated.

A short course of NSAIDs may decrease the risk of progression to cholecystitis as prostaglandin synthesis is reduced.[60][III]

Anticholinergic drugs are of little benefit in the ED management of biliary colic.[67, 68, 69][II] Glycopyrrolate showed no benefit over placebo.[69][II] Hyoscine-N-butyl-bromide, long a favored treatment for biliary colic, gave less pain relief when compared with NSAIDs.[67, 68][II] The onset of action of hyoscine-N-butylbromide was also slower and there were more recurrent episodes of pain in patients given hyoscine-N-butylbromide.

Ischemic cardiac chest pain

There is a little high-quality evidence comparing treatments for acute ischemic cardiac pain. Recommendations in this section are based on evidence where available, published evidence-based consensus guidelines[70, 71] and the principle as described previously of using specific agents before nonspecific ones.

Initial treatment for suspected ischemic cardiac chest pain should be with aspirin (as an anti-platelet agent, rather than an analgesic) and nitroglycerin, usually administered sublingually. Should pain persist or hypotension, potential interactions (e.g. with sildenafil), or other adverse effects limit nitroglycerin use, i.v. morphine titrated to effect is recommended.[70][II] Concern has been raised about the safety of i.v. morphine in this condition. One registry study has suggested that patients who receive morphine within the first 24 hours of presentation with an acute coronary syndrome have higher in-hospital mortality.[72][IV] This result must, however, be regarded with caution as it was based on retrospective registry data. It does, however, highlight that current analgesia pathways in cardiac pain are not based on robust evidence.

Urgent efforts should be made to determine whether the patient has clinical and electrocardiogram (ECG) criteria for emergent reperfusion as reperfusion treats the pain but, more importantly, reduces mortality and morbidity.[71]

Although in theory, supplemental oxygen might be considered indicated on the basis that it might limit damage by increasing myocardial oxygen supply, it has not been shown to impact the hard outcomes of myocardial ischemia, morbidity, and mortality.[70][II], [73][I] That said, there is general agreement that supplemental oxygen should be applied to patients who are hypoxic or in respiratory distress, with the aim of achieving oxygen saturations of greater than 90 percent.[70][II]

Nitroglycerin or diltiazem administered as i.v. infusions are options if pain is difficult to control. Intravenous nitroglycerin, at infusion rates of 5–50 µg/minute, has been reported to reduce episodes of chest pain in patients with clinical unstable angina when compared to placebo.[74][II] There is some evidence that, in patients who have suffered myocardial infarction, i.v. nitroglycerin may reduce infarct size.[75][IV] These data, however, predate the use of reperfusion therapies. Intravenous diltiazem, at a dose titrated to effect of between 1 and 5 µg/kg per minute, has been reported to be effective in 94 percent of patients with few side effects.[76][III] When compared to intravenous nitroglycerin in small studies, intravenous diltiazem is reported to result in less refractory angina than intravenous nitroglycerin.[77, 78, 79][III] Bradycardia may occur, but is usually resolved by reducing the infusion rate.[76] There is no convincing evidence that either drug by infusion reduces mortality.

Beta-blockers may have a place in selected patients who do not achieve control of chest pain with the above agents. The rationale for their use is that they reduce myocardial oxygen demand by reducing heart rate and contractility. The reduction in heart rate also results in a greater proportion of diastole in the cardiac cycle, thus theoretically allowing more coronary perfusion time. Cohort studies of

esmolol and metoprolol infusions have reported reduction in pain intensity and frequency.[80][II], [81][III], [82][IV] When compared to titrated i.v. morphine, both treatments resulted in significant reductions in pain, but morphine was effective faster.[80][II] Indicative doses of esmolol are 2–24 mg/minute titrated to reduce the heart rate and systolic blood pressure product by 20–25 percent. Indicative doses of metoprolol are 2.5–5 mg every five to ten minutes as intermittent boluses or 3 mg/minute as an infusion titrated to heart rate, blood pressure, and effect. Beta-blockage is contraindicated in patients with bradycardia, advanced atrioventricular block, hypotension, significant pulmonary congestion, or severe chronic obstructive airways disease.

Migraine

Only a small proportion of migraine sufferers present to ED for treatment. Evidence suggests that as much as 80 percent of them have tried their usual medications before attending ED,[2, 3, 83] making them different from the general migraine population. Choice of treatment in the ED will depend on whether the sufferer has tried their usual medication, the presence of nausea, and/or vomiting, and previous allergies or reactions. For many ED patients, parenteral treatment is the most appropriate choice.

Interpreting the evidence regarding ED treatment of migraine is challenging as the majority of the studies have small sample sizes, compare different agents, or combinations of agents, are set in different treatment settings (e.g. home, GP, clinic, ED), and test a variety of outcomes. Because the ED migraine population appears to be different from the general outpatient population, the data presented here are based on studies in ED unless otherwise stated. Non-ED migraine treatment options and treatment of mild migraine are discussed in Chapter 34, Headache in the *Chronic Pain* volume of this series.

For mild to moderate migraine without nausea and vomiting in patients who have not tried an anti-migraine agent for this episode, aspirin in a dose of 1000 mg or the combination of aspirin 600 mg and metoclopramide 10 mg orally may be effective.[84, 85][II] Acetaminophen has not been shown to be superior to placebo.[86][II]

For severe migraine, the evidence suggests that the most effective agents are the triptans (sumatriptan and related agents) and phenothiazines (chlorpromazine and prochlorperazine) (see **Table 19.1**). Metoclopramide and ketorolac are also commonly used. The pooled clinical success rates and number needed to treat from published ED studies are shown in **Table 19.1**. Only agents with an aggregate of 50 patients or more have been included. Pediatric studies have been excluded.

Opioids are not indicated for the treatment of migraine, despite being commonly used in some countries.[87][IV] There are no placebo-controlled studies demonstrating their effectiveness in this context. Only one small clinical trial[2][II] has investigated the effectiveness of

Table 19.1 Pooled effectiveness data from emergency department studies of the treatment of migraine.

Agent	No. of studies	Total patients	Clinical success rate (%)	NNT: Clinical success[a]
Chlorpromazine	6	171	85	1.7
Prochlorperazine	4	113	79	1.9
Sumatriptan	5	659	69	2.3
Metoclopramide	5	169	67	2.4
Ketorolac	6	155	66	2.4
Tramadol	2	174	59	2.9

[a]Calculated as 1/% success of active agent – % success placebo (assumes placebo success of 25%).

pethidine without adjuvant anti-emetic or phenothiazine, reporting a clinical success rate of 56 percent. This is considerably lower than other available treatments. Any benefit must also be balanced against the potential for the development of dependence.

In the ED setting, non-oral preparations of triptans are usually required. Clinical trials of sumitriptan in the ED setting have reported clinical success rates of approximately 71 percent.[88, 89][II] There are also a significant number of non-responders (up to 25 percent).[88][II] It is important to note that triptans are contraindicated in patients with a history of ischemic heart disease, uncontrolled hypertension, or the concomitant use of ergot preparations.

The mechanism by which chlorpromazine and other phenothiazines act in migraine remains uncertain, but is most likely the result of a combination of actions. Dosing regimens of chlorpromazine include 25 mg in 1-L normal saline over 30–60 minutes, repeated if necessary, or bolus doses of 12.5 mg intravenously, repeated every 20 minutes as needed to a maximum dose of 37.5 mg accompanied by intravenous saline to avert postural hypotension. Prochlorperazine is administered at a dose of 12.5 mg intravenously. Haloperidol administered as 5 mg in 500 mL normal saline has been reported to given siginificant pain relief in more than 80 percent of patients in two small randomized controlled trials.[90, 91][II] All agents may cause sedation, akathesia, or uncommonly, dystonia.

Other agents that have been tried in the ED management of migraine are ergot alkaloids (e.g. dihydroergotamine), lidocaine (lignocaine), magnesium, dexamethasone, octreotide, and valproic acid. Interpretation of the evidence is difficult because of the small sample sizes in most of these studies. Intravenous lidocaine[92] and subcutaneous octreotide[93] have not been shown to be superior to placebo. [II] Intravenous valproic acid (valproate sodium) has not been shown to elicit significant improvement and was inferior in effectiveness to prochlorperazine.[94][II] The effectiveness of dihydroergotamine is difficult to interpret because it is often used in combination with other agents (e.g. metoclopramide). However, it has also been shown to be less effective than chlorpromazine[95][II] and sumatriptan[96][II] in acute treatment, and to have a high rate (<55 percent) of unpleasant side effects.[95][II] The efficacy of intravenous magnesium sulfate (1 or 2 mg) remains unclear with

conflicting results.[97, 98, 99][II] Intramuscular droperidol has been shown to be moderately effective, but a 13 percent rate of akathisia[100][II] and a "black box" warning regarding side effects limit its utility.

Fractured neck of the femur

Fractured neck of the femur occurs most commonly in the elderly and available evidence suggests that provision of analgesia is poor.[1] One Australian study reported that only 49 percent of patients with fractured neck of femur received analgesia in the ED and that the median delay was 2.75 hours.[101][IV] A US study found that patients with fractured neck of the femur were less likely than other lower extremity fractures to receive analgesia in the prehospital setting (11 versus 32 percent).[102][IV] Reasons for this are not clear, but may include patient factors such as cognitive impairment, advanced age, and comorbidities and ED factors, such as assignment of low priority to this patient group.

In the early ED phase, titrated i.v. morphine is appropriate to gain initial pain control. Titration increments are usually smaller because of the sensitivity to opioids common in the elderly, but should occur at frequent intervals until pain is controlled.

Available evidence suggests that femoral nerve or "three-in-one" local anesthetic blocks can provide good analgesia for patients who have had surgery for fractures of the femoral neck. This approach may also be useful in the ED, either as single injections or via a catheter. Fletcher et al.[103][II] compared "three-in-one" femoral nerve block using bupivacaine plus i.v. morphine with i.v. morphine alone and found that the combination had a faster time to analgesia and lower morphine requirements in the first 24 hours.

Preoperative traction (skin or skeletal) has not been shown to provide an analgesia benefit when compared to support with pillows or similar.[104, 105, 106][II] In fact, the trend is towards increased pain if traction is used.[104, 105][II]

Wounds

Local anesthesia is often required for the treatment of wounds. Two routes of administration are in common use in the ED: local infiltration and topical application. Regional nerve blocks may also be appropriate in selected cases (see Chapter 12, Continuous peripheral neural blockade for acute pain).

For local anesthesia by infiltration, the choice between short-acting agents, such as lidocaine, or long-acting agents, such as bupivacaine, will depend on the duration of anesthesia required and whether analgesia post-procedure is desirable. Infiltration via the wound rather than the surrounding skin has been shown to reduce the pain of infiltration,[107, 108][II] as has warming of injected solution.[109, 110][II] There are conflicting data about whether buffering of lidocaine reduces the pain of infiltration.[111][II] Speed of injection does not appear to alter pain of infiltration.[111][II]

Topical anesthetic preparations such as ALA (epinephrine (adrenaline), lidocaine, amethocaine) have been shown to be effective alternatives to infiltration of local anesthesia for selected simple lacerations,[112, 113][II], [114] [III] It has also been shown to reduce the pain of infiltration when supplemental infiltration of anesthesia was required.[112]

In patients with sensitivity to local anesthetic agents, infiltration of diphenhydramine may provide adequate analgesia.[115][V]

Analgesia for fracture and dislocation reduction

Analgesia for the management of limb fractures and dislocations in the ED requires both pharmacological and nonpharmacological treatments. Nonpharmacological methods include splinting, traction devices, elevation, and mobility assistance devices, such as crutches for lower limb injuries.[116][II]

Reductions of displaced limb fractures and dislocations that are performed in the ED are either for definitive management of those that can be treated and discharged or interim management of the subset who will require fixation for definitive treatment, but require urgent reduction due to concerns regarding nerve injury, vascular compromise, skin integrity, blood loss, or pain control.

Initial pain management for patients with fractures or dislocations causing significant pain should be with titrated i.v. opioids at the doses previously described. Reasons for this are rapidity of pain control and maintenance of fasting status in patients who are likely to need sedation or anesthesia. This should not be delayed while awaiting x-ray confirmation of the injury.

Pharmacological treatment for reduction of fractures and dislocations in the ED usually requires sedation or anesthesia (local or regional), in addition to analgesia. Separation of these is difficult. A full discussion of procedural sedation in the ED is not within the remit of this chapter and local and regional blocks are discussed elsewhere. That said, this section addresses the principles involved and the evidence where it is available. As in other areas, there is very little high quality evidence comparing the different techniques of analgesia for fracture and dislocation reduction in the ED and the numbers in these studies are small.

The choice of method of analgesia will depend on the site of the injury (and its amenability to local regional anesthesia), patient age, the compliance of the patient, comorbidities, the urgency of the reduction, and the desired outcome (definitive reduction versus interim reduction).

Morphine, fentanyl, and pethidine are the opioids most commonly used in conscious sedation for fracture reduction in the ED. There is limited evidence evaluating the benefits of one over another when combined with a sedating agent. In a small study, Soysal et al.[117][II] have reported equal effectiveness of pethidine and fentanyl when combined with midazolam in adult fracture reduction.

Ketorolac, when added to a midazolam/fentanyl combination, did not result in significant additional analgesia nor did it provide significant opioid sparing.[118][II]

The dissociative anesthetic, ketamine, has been used as an alternative to opioid analgesia in fracture reduction in children. It has the advantage of being able to be administered i.v. or i.m. with usual initial doses 4 mg/kg for i.m. administration and 0.5–1 mg/kg for i.v. administration. One study has suggested that the combination of ketamine and midazolam is safer than fentanyl and midazolam in pediatric fracture and dislocation reduction in the ED, resulting in fewer respiratory complications, such as hypoxia.[119][II] That study also reported lower distress scores (scored by independent observers who reviewed videotapes of the procedures) and parental ratings of pain in the ketamine group. The only disadvantages to ketamine were an increased incidence of vomiting and a longer recovery time. Ketamine/midazolam has also been compared to nitrous oxide inhalation combined with hematoma block for the reduction for forearm fractures in children.[120][II] Both combinations resulted in minimal distress during the reduction procedure, but the nitrous oxide/hematoma block combination had less adverse effects and shorter recovery time.

Propofol has also been used in combination with opioids, in particular fentanyl, as analgesia/sedation for fracture reduction in both children and adults. A recent systematic review comparing propofol/fentanyl with ketamine/midazolam and fentanyl/midazolam concluded that ketamine/midazolam seemed to be more effective and have fewer adverse events than the other combinations.[121][I]

Forearm fractures

Hematoma block can be used for the ED reduction of both wrist and ankle fractures.[116, 122, 123][III] This involves injection of local anesthetic into the hematoma associated with the fracture. In comparison with conscious sedation without anesthesia, it has been reported that patients who underwent a hematoma block for fracture reduction had greater pain score reductions.[122, 123][III] The numbers in these studies are small, but in neither study were there any adverse effects from the local anesthetic agent nor were there any cases of osteomyelitis. Similar effectiveness to a ketamine/midazolam combination was reported when hematoma block was combined with nitrous oxide in children.[120][II]

Intravenous regional anesthesia (IVRA, also known as Bier's block) is an alternative method of anesthesia for forearm fracture reduction. It is relatively simple to perform, is low risk, has a rapid onset of action, rapid recovery, and does not depress conscious level and hence risk airway compromise.[124][IV] It does, however, require training and special equipment, but an anesthetist is not necessarily required. It also requires patient cooperation, so is not suitable for the very young or those with cognitive impairment. It has been used successfully in children as young as three years.[125][III] IVRA has been reported to be very effective as analgesia for reduction of wrist fractures[126] [II] and forearm fractures.[125][II] A recent Cochrane review reported that, when compared with hematoma block, IVRA provided better analgesia during fracture manipulation and enabled better and easier reduction of the fracture with a trend towards reduced risk of later redislocation or need for rereduction[127][I] (see Chapter 7, Clinical pharmacology: local anesthetics).

There is only one study comparing IVRA with nitrous oxide inhalational analgesia for fracture reduction. That small study (28 children) found that there was no difference in pain scores between the two groups, but was probably underpowered to detect a difference.[128][III]

Nerve blocks have been reported as being effective for the ED treatment of forearm fractures in both children and adults. These include axillary blocks[129][III] and combined median, ulnar, and radial nerve blocks at the elbow.[130][II] These also require training and experience in order to achieve acceptable success rates.

Shoulder dislocation

While conscious sedation is the most common analgesia used for the reduction of shoulder dislocations, there are two randomized trials reporting on the effectiveness of intra-articular lidocaine in this context. Typically, 20 mL of 1 percent lidocaine is used. Both studies report no difference in pain scores or procedural success when comparing intra-articular anesthesia to i.v. conscious sedation.[131, 132][II]

REFERENCES

1. Rupp T, Delaney KA. Inadequate analgesia in emergency medicine. *Annals of Emergency Medicine*. 2004; **43**: 494–503.

2. Larkin GL, Prescott JE. A randomized, double-blind, comparative study of the efficacy of ketorolac tromethamine versus pethidine in the treatment of severe migraine. *Annals of Emergency Medicine*. 1992; **21**: 919–24.

3. Shrestha M, Singh R, Moreden J, Hayes JE. Ketorolac vs chlorpromazine in the treatment of acute migraine without aura: A prospective, randomised, double-blind trial. *Archives of Internal Medicine*. 1996; **156**: 1725–8.

* 4. National Health and Medical Council. *Acute pain management: scientific evidence*, 2nd edn. Australia: National Health and Medical Council, 2005, Available from: www.anzca.edu.au/publications/acutepain.pdf.

* 5. Mace S, Ducharme J, Murphy M (eds). *Pain management and procedural sedation in the emergency department*. New York: McGraw-Hill, 2005.

6. Cone DC, Richardson LD, Todd KH *et al.* Health care disparities in emergency medicine. *Academic Emergency Medicine*. 2003; **10**: 1176–83.

7. Priestley S, Kelly AM, Chow L *et al.* Application of topical local anaesthetic at triage reduces treatment time for children with lacerations. *Annals of Emergency Medicine*. 2003: **42**: 34–40.

8. Tully M, Priestley S, Green D, Kelly AM. *Nurse-initiated oral analgesia administration standing order*. Australia: Emergency Departments of Western Health, 2003-2006.

9. Kelly AM. A process approach to improving pain management in the emergency department: Development and evaluation. *Journal of Accident and Emergency Medicine*. 2000; **17**: 185–7.

10. Green D, Kelly AM, Priestley S, Tully M. *Pain management package WH*. Australia: Emergency Departments of Western Health, Australia, 2003–2006.

11. Kelly AM, Brumby C, Barnes C. Nurse-initiated, titrated intravenous opioid analgesia reduces time to analgesia for selected painful conditions. *Canadian Journal of Emergency Medicine*. 2005; **7**: 149–54.

12. O'Connor A, Schug SA, Cardwell H. A comparison of the efficacy and safety of morphine and pethidine as analgesia for suspected renal colic in the emergency setting. *Journal of Accident and Emergency Medicine*. 2000; **17**: 261–4.

13. Galinski M, Dolveck F, Borron SW *et al.* A randomized, double-blind study comparing morphine with fentanyl in prehospital analgesia. *American Journal of Emergency Medicine*. 2005; **23**: 114–9.

14. Coman M, Kelly AM. Safety of a nurse-managed, titrated intravenous analgesia policy on the management of severe pain in the emergency department. *Emergency Medicine*. 1999; **11**: 128–32.

15. Borland ML, Jacobs I, Geelhoed G. Intranasal fentanyl reduces acute pain in children in the emergency department: a safety and efficacy study. *Emergency Medicine*. 2002; **14**: 275–80.

16. Kendall JM, Reeves BC, Latter VS. Nasal Diacetylmorphine Trial Group. Multicentre randomised controlled trial of nasal diacetylmorphine for analgesia in children and teenagers with clinical fractures. *BMJ*. 2001; **322**: 261–5.

17. Evans E, Turley N, Robinson N, Clancy M. Randomised controlled trial of patient controlled analgesia compared with nurse delivered analgesia in an emergency department. *Emergency Medicine Journal*. 2005; **22**: 25–9.

18. Brana A, Getti R, Mezaib K *et al*. Self-administered morphine algorithm in an emergency department observation unit. *Academic Emergency Medicine*. 2004; **11**: 495.

19. Vergnion M, Degesves S, Gareet L, Magotteaux V. Tramadol, an alternative to morphine for treating posttraumatic pain in the prehospital situation. *Anesthesia and Analgesia*. 2001; **92**: 1543–6.

20. Mahadevan L, Graff L. Prospective randomized study of analgesic use for ED patients with right lower quadrant abdominal pain. *American Journal of Emergency Medicine*. 2000; **18**: 753–6.

21. Eray O, Cete Y, Oktay C *et al*. Intravenous single-dose tramadol versus pethidine for pain relief in renal colic. *European Journal of Anaesthesiology*. 2002; **19**: 368–70.

22. Nicolas-Torralba JA, Rigabert Monteil M, Banon Perez V *et al*. Intramuscular ketorolac compared to subcutaneous tramadol in the initial emergency treatment of renal colic. *Archivos Españoles de Urología*. 1999; **52**: 435–7.

23. Moore PA, Crout RJ, Jackson DL *et al*. Tramadol hydrochloride: analgesic efficacy compared with codeine, aspirin with codeine, and placebo after dental extraction. *Journal of Clinical Pharmacology*. 1998; **38**: 554–60.

24. Turturro MA, Paris PM, Larkin GL. Tramadol versus hydrocodone-acetaminophen in acute musculo-skeletal pain: a randomised, double-blind clinical trial. *Annals of Emergency Medicine*. 1998; **32**: 139–43.

25. Hoogewijs J, Diltoer MW, Hubloue I *et al*. A prospective, open, single-blind, randomised study comparing four analgesics in the treatment of peripheral injury in the emergency department. *European Journal of Emergency Medicine*. 2000; **7**: 119–23.

26. McQuay H, Edwards J. Meta-analysis of single dose oral tramadol plus acetaminophen in acute postoperative pain. *European Journal of Anaesthesiology*. 2003; **28** (Suppl.): 19–22.

27. Silberstein SD, Freitag FG, Rozen TD *et al*. Tramadol/acetaminophen for the treatment of acute migraine pain: findings of a randomised, placebo-controlled trial. *Headache*. 2005; **45**: 1317–27.

28. Engindeniz Z, Demircan C, Karli N *et al*. Intramuscular tramadol versus diclofenac sodium for the treatment of acute migraine attacks in emergency department: a prospective, randomised, double-blind study. *Journal of Headache and Pain*. 2005; **6**: 143–8.

29. Gregory PR, Sullivan JA. Nitrous oxide compared with intravenous regional anesthesia in pediatric forearm fracture manipulation. *Journal of Pediatric Orthopedics*. 1996; **16**: 187–91.

30. Gamis AS, Knapp JF, Genski JA. Nitrous oxide analgesia in a pediatric emergency department. *Annals of Emergency Medicine*. 1989; **18**: 177–81.

31. Gerhardt RT, King KM, Wiegert RS. Inhaled nitrous oxide versus placebo as an analgesic and anxiolytic adjunct to peripheral IV cannulation. *American Journal of Emergency Medicine*. 2001; **19**: 492–4.

32. Burton JH, Auble TE, Fuchs SM. Effectiveness of 50% nitrous oxide/50% oxygen during laceration repair in children. *Academic Emergency Medicine*. 1998; **5**: 112–7.

33. Burnweit C, Diana-Zerpa JA, Nahmad MH *et al*. Nitrous oxide analgesia for minor pediatric surgical procedures: an effective alternative to conscious sedation. *Journal of Pediatric Surgery*. 2004; **39**: 495–9.

34. Cope Z. *The early diagnosis of the acute abdomen*. New York: Oxford University Press, 1921.

35. Attard AR, Corlett MJ, Kidner NJ *et al*. Safety of early pain relief for acute abdominal pain. *BMJ*. 1992; **305**: 554–6.

36. Pace S, Burke TF. Intravenous morphine for early pain relief in patients with acute abdominal pain. *Academic Emergency Medicine*. 1996; **3**: 1086–92.

37. Thomas SH, Silen W, Cheema F *et al*. Effects of morphine analgesia on diagnostic accuracy in Emergency Department patients with abdominal pain: a prospective, randomized trial. *Journal of the American College of Surgeons*. 2003; **196**: 18–31.

∗ 38. McHale PM, LoVecchio F. Narcotic analgesia in the acute abdomen – a review of prospective trials. *European Journal of Emergency Medicine*. 2001; **8**: 131–6.

39. Green R, Bulloch B, Kabani A *et al*. Early analgesia for children with acute abdominal pain. *Pediatrics*. 2005; **116**: 978–83.

40. Kim MK, Strait RT, Sato TT, Hennes HM. A randomized clinical trial of analgesia in children with acute abdominal pain. *Academic Emergency Medicine*. 2002; **9**: 281–7.

41. Wolfe JM, Lein DY, Lenkoski K, Smithline HA. Analgesic administration to patients with an acute abdomen: a survey of emergency medicine physicians. *American Journal of Emergency Medicine*. 2000; **18**: 250–3.

42. Kim MK, Galustyan S, Sato TT *et al*. Analgesia for children with acute abdominal pain: a survey of pediatric emergency physicians and pediatric surgeons. *Pediatrics*. 2003; **112**: 1122–6.

43. Green RS, Kabani A, Dostmohamed H, Tenenbein M. Analgesic use in children with acute abdominal pain. *Pediatric Emergency Care*. 2004; **20**: 725–9.

44. Nissman SA, Kaplan LJ, Mann BD. Critically reappraising the literature-driven practice of analgesia administration for acute abdominal pain in the emergency room prior to surgical evaluation. *American Journal of Surgery*. 2003; **185**: 291–6.

45. Ginifer C, Kelly AM. Administration of rectal indomethacin does not reduce the requirement for intravenous narcotic analgesia in acute renal colic. *European Journal of Emergency Medicine*. 1996; **3**: 92–4.

46. Labrecque M, Dostaler LP, Rouselle *et al*. Efficacy of nonsteroidal anti-inflammatory drugs in the treatment of acute renal colic. A meta-analysis. *Archives of Internal Medicine*. 1994; **27**: 1381–7.

47. Holdgate A, Pollock T. Systematic review of the relative efficacy of non-steroidal anti-inflammatory drugs and opioids in the treatment of acute renal colic. *BMJ*. 2004; **12**: 328:1401.

48. Cordell WH, Larson TA, Lingeman JE *et al*. Indomethacin suppositories versus intravenously titrated morphine for the treatment of ureteral colic. *Annals of Emergency Medicine*. 1994; **23**: 262–9.

49. Kelly AM. Nurse-managed analgesia for renal colic pain in the emergency department. *Australian Health Review*. 2000; **23**: 185–9.

50. Sandhu DP, Iacovou JW, Fletcher MS *et al*. A comparison of intramuscular ketorolac and pethidine in the alleviation of renal colic. *British Journal of Urology*. 1994; **74**: 690–3.

51. Cordell WH, Wright SW, Wolfson AB *et al*. Comparison of intravenous ketorolac, pethidine, and both (balanced analgesia) for renal colic. *Annals of Emergency Medicine*. 1996; **28**: 151–8.

52. Lee C, Gnanasegaram D, Maloba M. Best evidence topic report. Rectal or intravenous non-steroidal anti-inflammatory drugs in acute renal colic. *Emergency Medicine Journal*. 2005; **22**: 653–4.

53. Engeler DS, Ackermann DK, Osterwalder JJ *et al*. A double-blind, placebo controlled comparison of the morphine sparing effect of oral rofecoxib and diclofenac for acute renal colic. *Journal of Urology*. 2005; **174**: 933–6.

54. Laerum E, Ommundsen OE, Grenseth JE *et al*. Oral diclofenac in the prophylactic treatment of recurrent renal colic. A double-blind comparison with placebo. *European Journal of Urology*. 1995; **28**: 108–11.

55. Kapoor DA, Weitzel S, Mowad JJ *et al*. Use of indomethacin suppositories in the prophylaxis of recurrent ureteral colic. *Journal of Urology*. 1989; **142**: 1428–30.

56. Holdgate A, Oh CM. Is there a role for antimuscarinics in renal colic? A randomized controlled trial. *Journal of Urology*. 2005; **174**: 572–5.

57. Jones JB, Giles BK, Brizendine EJ, Cordell WH. Sublingual hyoscyamine sulfate in combination with ketorolac tromethamine for ureteral colic: a randomized, double-blind, controlled trial. *Annals of Emergency Medicine*. 2001; **37**: 141–6.

58. Al-Waili NS, Saloom KY. Intravenous tenoxicam to treat acute renal colic: comparison with buscopan compositum. *Journal of the Pakistan Medical Association*. 1998; **48**: 370–2.

59. Moscati RM. Cholelithiasis, cholecystitis, and pancreatitis. *Emergency Medicine Clinics of North America*. 1996; **14**: 719–37.

60. Goldman G, Kahn PJ, Alon R, Wiznitzer T. Biliary colic treatment and acute cholecystitis prevention by prostaglandin inhibitor. *Digestive Diseases and Sciences*. 1989; **34**: 809–11.

61. Henderson SO, Swadron S, Newton E. Comparison of intravenous ketorolac and pethidine in the treatment of biliary colic. *Journal of Emergency Medicine*. 2002; **23**: 237–41.

62. Thune A, Baker RA, Saccone GT *et al*. Differing effects of pethidine and morphine on human sphincter of Oddi motility. *British Journal of Surgery*. 1990; **77**: 992–5.

63. Wu SD, Zhang ZH, Jin JZ *et al*. Effects of narcotic analgesic drugs on human Oddi's sphincter motility. *World Journal of Gastroenterology*. 2004; **10**: 2901–4.

64. Akriviadis EA, Hatzigavriel M, Kapnias D *et al*. Treatment of biliary colic with diclofenac: a randomized, double-blind, placebo-controlled study. *Gastroenterology*. 1997; **113**: 225–31.

65. Dula DJ, Anderson R, Wood GC. A prospective study comparing IM ketorolac with IM pethidine in the treatment of acute biliary colic. *Journal of Emergency Medicine*. 2001; **20**: 121–4.

66. Curry C, Kelly AM. Intravenous tenoxicam for the treatment of renal colic. *New Zealand Journal of Medicine*. 1995; **108**: 229–30.

67. Kumar A, Deed JS, Bhasin B *et al*. Comparison of the effect of diclofenac with hyoscine-N-butylbromide in the symptomatic treatment of acute biliary colic. *Australia and New Zealand Journal of Surgery*. 2004; **74**: 573–6.

68. Al-Waili N, Saloom KY. The analgesic effect of intravenous tenoxicam in symptomatic treatment of biliary colic: a comparison with hyoscine N-butylbromide. *European Journal of Medical Research*. 1998; **3**: 475–9.

69. Antevil JL, Buckley RG, Johnson AS *et al*. Treatment of suspected symptomatic cholelithiasis with glycopyrrolate: a prospective, randomized clinical trial. *Annals of Emergency Medicine*. 2005; **45**: 172–6.

∗ 70. Braunwald E, Antman EM, Beasley JW *et al*. ACC/AHA 2002 guideline update for the management of patients with unstable angina non-ST segment elevation myocardial infarction: a report of the American College of Cardiology/American Heart Association taskforce on practice guidelines (Committee on the Management of Patients with Unstable Angina). *Journal of the American College of Cardiology*. 2002; **40**: 1366–74.

∗ 71. Aroney C, Aylward P, Kelly AM *et al*. on behalf of Acute Coronary Syndrome Guidelines Working Group. Guidelines for the management of acute coronary syndromes 2006. *Medical Journal of Australia*. 2006; **184**: S1–30.

72. Meine TJ, Roe MT, Chen AY *et al*. Association of intravenous morphine use and outcomes in acute coronary syndromes: results from the CRUSADE Quality Improvement Initiative. *American Heart Journal*. 2005; **149**: 1043–9.

73. Nicholson C. A systematic review of the effectiveness of oxygen in reducing acute myocardial ischaemia. *Journal of Clinical Nursing*. 2004; **15**: 121–2.

74. Karlberg KE, Saldeen T, Wallin R *et al*. Intravenous nitroglycerin reduces ischaemia in unstable angina pectoris: a double-blind placebo-controlled study. *Journal of Internal Medicine*. 1998; **243**: 25–31.

75. Raos V, Jeren-Strujic B, Ljutic D *et al*. The effect of intravenous nitroglycerin therapy on infarct size in patients with acute myocardial infarction. *Acta Medica Croatica*. 1995; **49**: 5–14.

76. Bai R. Diltiazem Clinical Trial Task Group of Wuhan. Assessment of the efficacy, optimal dosage, and safety of diltiazem in early treatment of unstable angina pectoris. *Clinical Cardiology.* 2005; **28**: 343–8.

77. Gobel EJ, Hautvast RW, van Gilst WH *et al.* Randomised, double-blind trial of intravenous diltiazem versus nitrogycerin for unstable angina pectoris. *Lancet.* 1995; **346**: 1653–7.

78. Castro P, Corbalan R, Vergara I, Kunstmann S. (Diltiazem versus intravenous nitroglycerin in the treatment of unstable angina pectoris. *A randomized study*). *Revista Médica de Chile.* 1995; **123**: 823–9 (in Spanish).

79. Fiol M, Costa A, Suarez-Pinilla MA *et al.* (A comparative study of intravenous diltiazem and nitroglycerin in the treatment of unstable angina). *Revista Española de Cardiología.* 1992; **45**: 98–102 (in Spanish).

80. Everts B, Karlson BW, Abdon NJ *et al.* A comparison of metoprolol and morphine in the treatment of chest pain in patients with suspected acute myocardial infarction – the MEMO study. *Journal of Internal Medicine.* 1999; **245**: 133–41.

81. Everts B, Karlson BW, Herlitz J *et al.* Effects and pharmacokinetics of high dose metoprolol on chest pain in patients with suspected or definite acute myocardial infarction. *European Journal of Clinical Pharmacology.* 1997; **53**: 23–31.

82. Barth C, Ojile M, Pearson AC, Labovitz AJ. Ultra short-acting intravenous beta-adrenergic blockade as add-on therapy in acute unstable angina. *American Heart Journal.* 1991; **121**: 782–8.

83. Friedman BW, Corbo J, Lipton RB *et al.* A trial of metoclopramide vs sumatriptan for the emergency department treatment of migraines. *Neurology.* 2005; **64**: 463–8.

84. Lipton RB, Goldstein J, Baggish JS *et al.* Aspirin is efficacious for the treatment of acute migraine. *Headache.* 2005; **45**: 283–92.

85. Tfelt-Hansen P, Oleson J. Effervescent metoclopramide and aspirin (Migravess) versus effervescent aspirin or placebo for migraine attacks: a double-blind study. *Cephalalgia.* 1984; **4**: 107–11.

86. Leinisch E, Evers S, Kaempfe N *et al.* Evaluation of the efficacy of intravenous acetaminophen in the treatment of acute migraien attack: a double-blind, placebo controlled parallel group multicentre study. *Pain.* 2005; **117**: 396–400.

87. Vinson DR. Treatment patterns of isolated benign headaches in US emergency departments. *Annals of Emergency Medicine.* 2002; **39**: 215–22.

88. Akpunonu BE, Mutgi AB, Federman DJ *et al.* Subcutaneous sumatriptan for the treatment of acute migraine in patients admitted to the emergency department. *Annals of Emergency Medicine.* 1995; **25**: 464–9.

89. Wendt J, Cady R, Singer R *et al.* A randomized, double-blind, placebo-controlled trial of the efficacy and tolerability of a 4 mg dose of subcutaneous sumatriptan

for the treatment of acute migraine headaches in adults. *Clinical Therapeutics.* 2006; **28**: 517–26.

90. Monzillo PH, Nemoto PH, Costa AR, Sanvito WL. (Acute treatment of migraine in emergency room: comparative study between dexamethasone and haloperidol. Preliminary results. *Arquivos de Neuro-psiquiatria.* 2004; **62**: 513–8 (in Portugese).

91. Honkaniemi J, Liimatainen S, Rainesalo S, Sulavuori S. Haloperidol in the acute treatment of migraine: a randomised, double-blind, placebo-controlled study. *Headache.* 2006; **46**: 781–7.

92. Reutens DC, Fatovich DM, Stewart-Wynne EG, Prentice DA. Is intravenous lidocaine clinically effective in acute migraine? *Cephalalgia.* 1991; **11**: 245–7.

93. Levy MJ, Matharu MS, Bhola R *et al.* Octreotide is not effective in the acute treatment of migraine. *Cephalgia.* 2005; **25**: 48–55.

94. Tanen DA, Miller S, French T, Riffenburgh RH. Intravenous valproate versus prochloperazine for the emergency department treatment of acute migraine headache; A prospective, randomised, double-blind trial. *Annals of Emergency Medicine.* 2003; **41**: 847–53.

95. Bell R, Montoya D, Shuaib A, Lee MA. A comparative trial of three agents in the treatment of migraine headache. *Annals of Emergency Medicine.* 1990; **19**: 1079–82.

96. Winner P, Ricalde O, Le Force B *et al.* A double-blind study of subcutaneous dihydroergotamine vs subcutaneous sumatriptan in the treatment of acute migraine. *Archives of Neurology.* 1996; **53**: 180–4.

97. Demirkaya S, Vural O, Dora B, Topcuoglu MA. Efficacy of intravenous magnesium sulphate in the treatment of acute migraine attacks. *Headache.* 2001; **41**: 171–7.

98. Corbo J, Esses D, Bijur PE *et al.* Randomised clinical trial of intravenous magnesium sulphate as an adjunctive medication in the emergency department treatment of migraine. *Annals of Emergency Medicine.* 2001; **38**: 621–7.

99. Cete Y, Dora B, Ertan C *et al.* A randomized, prospective, placebo-controlled study of intravenous magnesium sulphate vs. metoclopramide in the management of acute migraine attacks in the emergency department. *Cephalagia.* 2005; **25**: 199–204.

100. Richman PB, Allegra J, Eskin B *et al.* A randomised clinical trial to assess the efficacy of intramuscular droperidol for the treatment of acute migraine headache. *American Journal of Emergency Medicine.* 2002; **20**: 39–42.

101. Vassiliadis J, Hitos K, Hill CT. Factors influencing prehospital and emergency department analgesia administration to patients with femoral neck fractures. *Emergency Medicine.* 2002; **14**: 261–6.

102. McEachin CC, McDermott JT, Swor R. Few emergency medical services patients with lower-extremity fractures receive prehospital analgesia. *Prehospital Emergency Care.* 2002; **6**: 406–10.

103. Fletcher AK, Rigby AS, Heyes FL. Three-in-one femoral nerve block as analgesia for fractured neck of femur in the

emergency department: a randomized, controlled trial. *Annals of Emergency Medicine.* 2003; **41**: 227–33.

104. Rosen JE, Chen FS, Hiebert R, Koval KJ. Efficacy of preoperative skin traction in hip fracture patients: a prospective, randomized study. *Journal of Orthopaedic Trauma.* 2001; **15**: 81–5.

105. Yip DK, Chan CF, Chiu PK et al. Why are we still using pre-operative skin traction for hip fractures? *International Orthopaedics.* 2002; **26**: 361–4.

106. Resch S, Bjarnetoft B, Thorngren KG. Preoperative skin traction or pillow nursing in hip fractures: a prospective, randomized study in 123 patients. *Disability and Rehabilitation.* 2005; **27**: 1191–5.

107. Kelly AM, Cohen M, Richards D. Minimizing the pain of local infiltration anesthesia for wounds by injection into the wound edges. *Journal of Emergency Medicine.* 1994; **12**: 593–5.

108. Bartfield JM, Sokaris SJ, Raccio-Robak N. Local anesthesia for lacerations: pain of infiltration inside vs outside the wound. *Academic Emergency Medicine.* 1998; **5**: 100–4.

109. Jones JS, Plzak C, Wynn BN, Martin S. Effect of temperature and pH adjustment of bupivacaine for intradermal anesthesia. *American Journal of Emergency Medicine.* 1998; **16**: 117–20.

110. Brogan Jr GX, Giarrusso E, Hollander JE et al. Comparison of plain, warmed, and buffered lidocaine for anesthesia of traumatic wounds. *Annals of Emergency Medicine.* 1995; **26**: 121–5.

111. Boyd R. Plain or buffered lidocaine for local anaesthetic. 2001; cited 1 August 2006. Available from: http://www.bestbets.org/cgi-bin/ bets.pl?record=00102.

112. Singer AJ, Stark MJ. Pretreatment of lacerations with lidocaine, epinephrine and tetracaine at triage: a randomised double blind trial. *Academic Emergency Medicine.* 2000; **7**: 751–6.

113. Smith GA, Strausbaugh SD, Harbeck-Weber C et al. Comparison of topical anesthetics with lidocaine infiltration during laceration repair in children. *Clinical Pediatrics.* 1998; **36**: 17–23.

114. Charters A. Topical anaesthesia before suturing children's minor lacerations: a critical review. *Accident and Emergency Nursing.* 1998; **6**: 180–3.

115. Pollack Jr CV, Swindle GM. Use of diphenhydramine for local anesthesia in '-caine' sensitive patients. *Journal of Emergency Medicine.* 1989; **7**: 611–4.

116. Kennedy RM, Luhmann JD, Luhmann SJ. Emergency department management of pain and anxiety related to orthopedic fracture care: a guide to analgesic techniques and procedural sedation in children. *Paediatric Drugs.* 2004; **6**: 11–31.

117. Soysal S, Karcioglu O, Demircan A et al. Comparison of pethidine plus midazolam and fentanyl plus midazolam in procedural sedation: a double-blind, randomized controlled trial. *Advances in Therapy.* 2004; **21**: 312–21.

118. Pierce MC, Fuchs S. Evaluation of ketorolac in children with forearm fractures. *Academic Emergency Medicine.* 1997; **4**: 22–6.

119. Kennedy RM, Porter FL, Miller JP, Jaffe DM. Comparison of fentanyl/midazolam with ketamine/midazolam for pediatric orthopedic emergencies. *Pediatrics.* 1998; **102**: 956–63.

120. Luhmann JD, Schootman M, Luhmann SJ, Kennedy RM. A randomized comparison of nitrous oxide plus hematoma block versus ketamine plus midazolam for emergency department forearm fracture reduction in children. *Paediatrics.* 2006; **118**: e1078–1086.

121. Migita RT, Klein EJ, Garrison MM. Sedation and analgesia for pediatric fracture reduction in the emergency department: a systematic review. *Archives of Pediatrics and Adolescent Medicine.* 2006; **160**: 46–51.

122. Furia JP, Alioto RJ, Marquardt JD. The efficacy and safety of the hematoma block for fracture reduction in closed, isolated fractures. *Orthopedics.* 1997; **20**: 423–6.

123. Alioto RJ, Furia JP, Marquardt JD. Hematoma block for ankle fractures: a safe and efficacious technique for manipulations. *Journal of Orthopaedic Trauma.* 1995; **9**: 113–6.

124. Thamizhavell RC, Shankar S. How safe is Biers Block in the accident and emergency department? *European Journal of Emergency Medicine.* 1996; **3**: 56–8.

125. Davidson AJ, Eyres RL, Cole WG. A comparison of prilocaine and lidocaine for intravenous regional anaesthesia for forearm fracture reduction in children. *Paediatric Anaesthesia.* 2002; **12**: 146–50.

126. Kendall JM, Allen P, Younge P et al. Haematoma block or Bier's block for Colles' fracture reduction in the accident and emergency department – which is best? *Journal of Accident and Emergency Medicine.* 1997; **14**: 352–6.

127. Handoll HHG, Madhok R, Dodds C. Anaesthesia for treating distal radial fracture in adults. *Cochrane Database of Systematic Reviews.* 2006; **CD003320**.

128. Gregory PR, Sullivan JA. Nitrous oxide compared with intravenous regional anesthesia in pediatric forearm fracture manipulation. *Journal of Pediatric Orthopedics.* 1996; **16**: 187–91.

129. Cramer KE, Glasson S, Mencio G, Green NE. Reduction of forearm fractures in children using axillary block anesthesia. *Journal of Orthopaedic Trauma.* 1995; **9**: 407–10.

130. Haasio J. Cubital nerve block vs haematoma block for the manipulation of Colles' fracture. *Annales Chirurgiae et Gynaecologiae.* 1990; **79**: 168–71.

131. Miller S, Cleeman E, Auerbach J, Flatow E. Comparison of intra-articular lidocaine and intravenous sedation for reduction of shoulder dislocations. *Journal of Bone and Joint Surgery.* 2002; **84**: 2135–9.

132. Matthews DE, Roberts T. Intraarticular lidocaine versus intravenous analgesic for reduction of acute anterior shoulder dislocations. A prospective randomized study. *American Journal of Sports Medicine.* 1995; **23**: 54–58.

FURTHER READING

Bigal ME, Bordini CA, Speciali JG. Intravenous chlorpromazine in the emergency department treatment of migraines: A randomised controlled trial. *Journal of Emergency Medicine.* 2002; **23**: 141–8.

Cameron JD, Lane PL, Speechley M. Intravenous chlorpromazine vs intravenous metoclopramide in acute migraine headache. *Academic Emergency Medicine.* 1995; **2**: 597–602.

Cete Y, Dora B, Ertan C *et al.* A randomized prospective placebo-controlled study of intravenous magnesium sulphate vs. metoclopramide in the management of acute migraine attacks in the Emergency Department. *Cephalalgia.* 2005; **25**: 199–204.

Coppola M, Yealy DM, Leibold RA. Randomized, placebo-controlled evaluation of prochlorperazine versus metoclopramide for emergency department treatment of migraine headache. *Annals of Emergency Medicine.* 1995; **26**: 541–6.

Davis CP, Torre PR, Schafer NC *et al.* Ketorolac as a rapid and effective treatment of migraine headache: evaluations by patients. *American Journal of Emergency Medicine.* 1993; **11**: 573–5.

Davis CP, Williams C, Barrett K, Peake D. Ketoroloc versus meperidine plus promethazine treatment of migraine headache: evaluation by patients. *American Journal of Emergency Medicine.* 1995; **13**: 146–50.

Duarte C, Dunaway F, Turner L *et al.* Ketoroloc versus meperidine and hydroxyzine in the treatment of acute migraine headache: A randomized, prospective, double-blind trial. *Annals of Emergency Medicine.* 1992; **21**: 1116–21.

Friedman BW, Corbo J, Lipton RB *et al.* A trial of metoclopramide vs sumatriptan for the emergency department treatment of migraines. *Neurology.* 2005; **64**: 643–8.

Friedman BW, Hochberg M, Esses D *et al.* A clinical trial of trimethobenzamide/diphenhydramine versus sumatriptan for acute migraines. *Headache.* 2006; **46**: 934–41.

Jones J, Sklar D, Dougherty J, White W. Randomized double-blind trial of intravenous prochlorperazine for the treatment of acute headache. *Journal of the American Medical Association.* 1989; **261**: 1174–6.

Kelly AM, Ardagh M, Curry C *et al.* Intravenous chlorpromazine versus intramuscular sumatriptan for acute migraine. *Journal of Accident and Emergency Medicine.* 1997; **14**: 209–11.

Lane PL, McLellan BA, Baggoley CJ. Comparative efficacy of chlorpromazine and meperidine with dimenhydrinate in migraine headache. *Annals of Emergency Medicine.* 1989; **18**: 360–5.

Miner JR, Smith SW, Moore J, Biros M. Sumatriptan for the treatment of undifferentiated primary headaches in the ED. *American Journal of Emergency Medicine.* 2007; **25**: 60–4.

Seim MB, March JA, Dunn KA. Intravenous ketorolac vs intravenous prochlorperazine for the treatment of migraine headaches. *Academic Emergency Medicine.* 1998; **5**: 573–6.

Tek DS, McClellan DS, Olshaker JS *et al.* A prospective, double-blind study of metoclopramide hydrochloride for the control of migraine in the emergency department. *Annals of Emergency Medicine.* 1990; **19**: 1083–7.

20

Acute pain management in field and disaster situations

CHESTER C BUCKENMAIER III

KEY LEARNING POINTS

- Historically, pain management in the field has been considered an unrealistic luxury.
- All anesthesiologists should be prepared to provide pain management in austere conditions since recent disasters and terror events underscore how fragile modern medical infrastructure can be.
- The challenges of austere environment pain management include weather, terrain, equipment, logistics, and personnel safety.
- The key resource for any effective acute pain response in war or disaster centers is the trained personnel that make up the acute pain service (APS) team.

- Successful pain management in the field requires multimodal analgesic therapy to reduce the unwanted side effects of each individual medication.
- Regional anesthesia can be utilized successfully in the field.
- Novel pain control technologies (e.g. iontophoresis, intranasal ketamine) have the potential to greatly enhance pain management.
- Effective acute pain management can significantly enhance the effectiveness of the healthcare response during war or disaster.

AN UNREALISTIC LUXURY?

During the battle of Chancellorsville in 1862, Confederate General Thomas J "Stonewall" Jackson was performing a late evening reconnaissance when he was shot in the left arm and right hand by musketry coming from his own soldiers. Suffering much from the pain of the wounds, he was brought to the field hospital of Dr Hunter McGuire by a horse-drawn field ambulance. During his transport, the general's pain was eased by drinking whiskey. Jackson was then transported on to the Confederate II Corps hospital during which more whiskey and some morphine were administered. Early the following morning, Dr McGuire amputated Jackson's left arm two inches below the shoulder. He was assisted in the operation by Dr JT Coleman who administered chloroform to the general for the amputation. As the general succumbed to the effects of the chloroform, he is reported to have murmured, "What an infinite blessing."[1]

This description of General Jackson's mortal wounding in 1863 illustrates many of the complex issues involved in managing pain in austere environments. The general received a traumatic wound in the field, during the chaos of war, while far from a field hospital. He required rapid transport to appropriate medical services over rough terrain which exacerbated the pain of the wound, further complicating the injury. Pain management strategies and technologies were inadequate during the general's transport and at the field hospital. Finally, physician understanding of pain mechanisms, treatment, and consequences were limited. While the treatment of traumatic wounds sustained during war or disaster has advanced significantly since the nineteenth century, improvement in acute pain therapy for traumatic injury has been far less dramatic.[2] Even now in the twenty-first century, the "infinite blessing" of effective acute pain management in field and disaster situations remains an elusive goal.

Friedrick Serturner, a German pharmacist, first isolated morphine from opium in 1805.[3] Morphine and other opioid drugs have played a major role in austere environment pain management ever since, particularly in the military. The preeminence and success of opioid medications in pain management is without question. However, their use is not without significant side effects[4, 5, 6] that are undesirable in the most advanced medical setting; they are potentially devastating in the field environment. Opioid use in austere environments is further complicated by international regulations governing transportation and use of these medications. Despite these drawbacks, morphine has essentially been the only answer for pain in austere conditions for over 200 years.

The reasons for the unhurried development of acute pain management technology for field applications are numerous. The science of understanding pain mechanisms and associated morbidity is relatively new. Multimodal pain treatment beyond morphine (e.g. new drugs, drug delivery technologies, adjunct therapies) remains controversial.[7] Before the advent of modern anesthesia practice, patients wholly depended upon speedy surgeons to limit suffering. Even after the discovery of ether, many surgeons considered anesthetic agents unnecessary, or even detrimental to a patient's recovery.[8] Historically, pain has been thought an unfortunate and unavoidable consequence of trauma and surgery. For many physicians practicing under harsh conditions, the treatment of pain must have seemed an unrealistic luxury. In the past few decades, attitudes concerning pain have changed radically from this antiquated view. Perhaps the most significant change in physician attitudes concerning pain science has been the realization that pain should be considered a disease state of the nervous system, rather then just a symptom of disease or trauma.[9] Emphasis on effective pain management within the United States medical community has been embodied by the Joint Commission on Accreditation of Healthcare Organizations labeling pain as "the fifth vital sign."[10]

In this chapter, the challenges and advantages of effective pain management in field and disaster situations will be explored. Additionally, recent advances, new technologies, and future possibilities in austere environment analgesia, beyond morphine, will be examined.

DEFINING AUSTERE ENVIRONMENTS – THE BATTLEFIELD IN YOUR BACKYARD

In the developed world, healthcare providers need only take the briefest moment to recognize the insulating cocoon of technology that surrounds them and facilitates their healthcare activities. From the moment of injury, the infrastructure of modern society imparts tremendous advantages to the trauma victim and to the healthcare providers caring for them. Patients in the developed world are rapidly transported by trained personnel to medical centers in motor vehicles or aircraft packed with lifesaving technology. Current urban transportation infrastructure (e.g. maintained roadways, communications towers, air traffic control) facilitates this fast response and travel. Upon arrival at the medical center, physicians and nurses have a cornucopia of devices, medications, and machines to diagnose, support, and maintain bodily functions. Modern infrastructure, providing clean tap water, artificial light on demand, climate control, and power for every electronic device, is at the ready for patient care. In short, the resources and infrastructure of the developed world impart significant advantages in the quality and availability of healthcare services following injury. The ability to manage pain with advanced technologies and techniques under these conditions is a realistic expectation of the physician and patient.

Recent events, such as the World Trade Center attack, Indian Ocean tsunami, London train bombing, Hurricane Katrina and South Asian earthquake, underscore how modern infrastructure is discouragingly fragile and easily disrupted. While the developed world's mastery of environment, upon which modern medicine depends, is truly awesome in its potential, the sudden loss of that infrastructure is a constant and unpredictable threat. Healthcare providers, complacent in the constancy of their modern technologic medical environment, in an instant may find themselves thrust into the austere environment realities faced daily by providers in the developing world. The healthcare crisis affecting thousands in the United States following Hurricane Katrina underscores the need for improved disaster medical planning.[11, 12] Battlefield or disaster medicine can literally arrive in the provider's own backyard without warning. For the unprepared, pain management issues that are difficult in the most modern settings can quickly become overwhelming. Conversely, effective medical planning and forethought for austere environment medicine, particularly in the management of casualty pain, can significantly lessen the impact man-made and natural disasters have on patients and healthcare providers alike.

CHALLENGES

The challenges of planning for and managing acute pain in an austere environment are myriad but can broadly be categorized into issues relating to:

- extremes in weather;
- extremes in terrain;
- facility and equipment;
- logistics;
- personnel safety.

Weather extremes are often the inciting condition that triggers the need for acute pain medicine services in an austere medical environment. The devastation of the major population center in New Orleans, Louisiana from Hurricane Katrina has continued to plague the city's medical infrastructure months after the disaster.[13] Any pain management plan must factor in the prolonged loss of basic services and facilities that might render the use of many common analgesic medications or procedures impractical or dangerous. Exposure to temperature extremes following a disaster in which climate control is lost can affect patient health, damage equipment, degrade medications, and adversely impact on healthcare provider performance.

Local geography and terrain are vital considerations in planning for pain management following a disaster. The

remoteness and mountainous topography of the South Asian earthquake or the sheer size of the devastation wrought by the Indian Ocean tsunami underscore the added complexity terrain can bring to healthcare efforts.[14, 15] Terrain extremes can impede or prevent health professionals from reaching patients, limit communication to areas outside the effected area, and curtail resupply of consumable medical supplies.

Many of the difficulties of providing healthcare in austere environments can be mitigated by transporting modern medical infrastructure into the disaster area, thus freeing the provider from local resource limitations. An example of this approach is the deployment by the United States military of a combat support hospital (CSH) (**Figure 20.1**), which provides services comparable to a modern civilian community hospital on the battlefield.[16] A civilian version of this type of facility called a deployable rapid assembly shelter and surgical hospital (DRASH) sponsored by the Federal Emergency Management Agency was deployed in December 2003 to Bam, Iran following a major earthquake.[17] While the CSH and DRASH represent a successful approach to austere environment medicine, the logistics required to place and support these facilities are likely beyond the capabilities of most disaster planners. Nevertheless, facilities of this type provide an excellent proving ground for new pain technologies and protocols designed for austere environment medicine. The success and failures in managing pain by these modern austere environment medicine facilities will serve as a guide for medical planners working to improve pain management in future times of war or disaster. The ability to provide effective pain management must be integral to deployable facility design and equipment selection for any austere environment medical mission. For reasons outlined later (see Advantages of effective pain management in field and disaster situations), acute

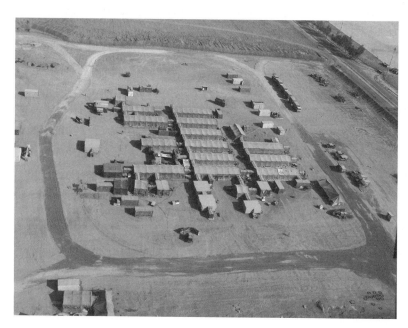

Figure 20.1 Twenty-first Combat Support Hospital, Balad, Iraq in 2003.

pain management should become a primary goal of disaster medical planning rather than an afterthought.

A popular adage in the United States military is "armchair generals think of strategy, whereas professionals study logistics." The success of any medical effort in time of war or disaster depends upon the ability to efficiently get medical personnel and material into the region of the austere environment medical mission. Having a trained acute pain physician on the scene without medications or equipment to employ in pain management essentially negates the advantages of having that medical asset. Medication and equipment selection for a particular mission is also of prime importance. Variables to consider when selecting pain management supplies and equipment include:

- medication storage and shelf-life requirements;
- size and weight of desired medications;
- medication side-effect profile;
- equipment environmental operating parameters, size, and weight;
- equipment power requirements (voltage, plug configuration, battery life);
- medication or equipment consumable requirements;
- available pain management protocols;
- special requirements for pain medication or equipment use based on mission constraints or interservice differences.

The last point has been particularly important in introducing new pain technologies to the modern battlefield for the United States military. For example, initial efforts to introduce continuous peripheral nerve block (CPNB) pumps and patient-controlled analgesia (PCA) pumps were thwarted due to interservice pump technology requirement differences between the army, air force, and navy. Pumps used in the army CSH for pain control could not follow the patient on air force medical evacuation flights because they had not undergone airworthiness certification for use on military aircraft.[18] The advantages of these advanced pain management techniques were lost if the soldier could not enjoy the benefits of the technology during long evacuation flights. In response to this issue, the triservice Military Advanced Regional Anesthesia and Analgesia (MARAA, www.arapmi.org) organization was formed as a committee of the Uniformed Services Society of Anesthesiologists (USAA – a component society of the American Society of Anesthesiologists).[19] This organization has improved interservice communication and decision-making for battlefield pain control and has been instrumental in coordinating the efforts of the three services in improving pain management for wounded soldiers. The MARAA committee is directly responsible for the establishment of battlefield CPNB pump and PCA pump technology for the United States military, particularly on medical evacuation flights. The triservice cooperation and communication demonstrated by MARAA in the current conflicts should serve as a model for other war or disaster logistics planners tasked with developing pain medicine responses that depend upon multiple and diverse agencies working together for success.

Finally, any plan for austere environment pain management must include healthcare provider safety as a key component. Healthcare providers participating in missions outside their home country should incorporate into their planning as much information about the mission country as possible to ensure appropriate clothing and personal safety. Medical planners can use *The world factbook*, updated annually by the Central Intelligence Agency (www.cia.gov/cia/publications/factbook), as a resource tool for finding detailed information on all countries. Unconventional nuclear, biological, or chemical (NBC) warfare is a potential threat in any community, as recent experience has demonstrated (Halabja, Iraq, gas attack 1988; Tokyo subway, sarin gas attack 1995; and anthrax mail attacks of 2001). Medical providers should educate themselves on available NBC personal protective equipment and seek opportunities to train with protective gear. Excellent resources for learning more about potential NBC threats can be found on the Internet from sources such as eMedicine (www.emedicinehealth.com/collections/CO1542) or the National Library of Medicine (www.nlm.nih.gov). Pain management missions can occur in areas experiencing extreme violence or war. Providers in these scenarios should integrate modern body armor and helmet use into their medical practice. Recent experience has demonstrated the effectiveness of modern body armor at reducing the lethality of war wounds.[20, 21, 22] In any austere medical environment, medical providers must maintain a high level of situational awareness so that potential threats to health and safety can be quickly identified and managed. Including additional personnel tasked solely with medical mission security is a sound approach to ensuring the medical response team's safety.

PAIN MANAGEMENT RESOURCES

Personnel

The absolute key resource for any plan to manage pain in an austere environment starts with selecting personnel trained and motivated to treat acute pain aggressively. Since 1985, efforts to improve perioperative pain management have centered on the development of acute pain service teams of healthcare professionals, usually directed by an anesthesiologist, who are organized and committed to the management of acute postsurgical pain.[23] The advantages of a dedicated acute pain service (APS) in improving patient analgesia following surgery and reducing gaps in patient pain care has caused numerous healthcare organizations, from many countries, to recommend guidelines for the creation of APS teams as an integral function of quality hospital care.[24, 25] However, application of APS guidelines are highly variable between hospitals.[26] The lack of consistency in APS procedures has made the impact of APS teams on surgical outcomes difficult to define. Nevertheless, the adoption of the APS model to austere environment pain management is a logical approach. Without medical personnel being tasked specifically with the APS function, pain treatment will revert to the low priority status it has traditionally been given by surgeons and anesthesiologists.[27] This is particularly true in the chaotic, high stress, mass casualty medical environment of the battlefield or disaster scene.

Protocols and guidelines

Pain medication pharmacology and clinical use guidelines have been described elsewhere within this text. Medication issues relating to the application of these same drugs in the field warrants additional comment. The dominance of morphine and other opioid medications in austere environment pain management has been noted earlier. Morphine remains the "gold standard" analgesic to which all other medications tend to be compared.[28, 29] The ease of morphine administration following the invention of hollow hypodermic needles and syringes in the 1850s enhanced use and acceptance of the drug as an effective treatment for traumatic pain. The use of morphine for pain was widespread during the American Civil War (1861–65) and French–German War (1870–71), but a lack of understanding concerning opioid use and side effects led to morphine addiction in many soldiers which was known as "soldier's disease."[30] Despite the potential for life-threatening side effects with the use of morphine in extreme environments, the success of opioids in treating pain in field medicine is beyond dispute. However, the challenge is developing acute pain protocols and pain technologies that emphasize the beneficial pain relief properties of opioids, while minimizing their side effects. Abraham Maslow (1908–70), an American psychologist stated, "If the only tool you have is a hammer, you tend to see every problem as a nail." This quote could be applied to the use of morphine by the United States military for much of its history until recently. Morphine has been the "hammer" historically applied to every battlefield pain situation since the Civil War. This reliance on morphine and other opioid medications is understandable since options for pain management in previous conflicts were limited, comprehension of pain mechanisms nascent, and casualties, when they survived, tended to remain static near the battlefield while they recovered.

Casualty care advances in patients coming from the conflicts in Iraq and Afghanistan have changed pain management attitudes and practices in the field environment. While the lethality of weapons and severity of wounds continues to increase, paradoxically, casualty survival has never been higher. United States military casualties from Iraq and Afghanistan currently have a 90 percent survival rate compared with only 76 percent during the Vietnam War (1961–73), 67 percent during the Civil War (1861–65), or 58 percent during the Revolutionary War (1775–83).[31] Many factors have contributed to increased casualty survival. These factors include emphasis on early advanced surgical care far forward, improved surgical and critical care techniques, availability of blood products; advances in body armor; and rapid ground and air evacuation to major medical facilities within and outside the war zone, among others.[32] The rapid movement of casualties in the current conflicts, in particular, has rendered pain management protocols that emphasize opioids less appealing. Modern combat casualty care now emphasizes rapid evacuation to progressively higher levels (**Table 20.1**) of medical care while providing critical care support at all times (including transport). Casualties that would typically remain within a war zone for days to weeks until they were stable for transport now are transported by plane to Germany from Iraq within 8 to 72 hours of injury.[33] The crowded, low light, deafening, jolting, and difficult monitoring environment of evacuation aircraft only magnify the difficulties in using opioid-only pain control therapy. Healthcare providers placed in this situation are less apt to use adequate doses of morphine over valid patient safety concerns. The high numbers of healthcare providers in the evacuation chain and long evacuation distances further complicate opioid use in these patients. Indeed, it

Table 20.1 Levels of medical care in the United States military.

Level[a]	Capabilities	Facility
Level I	Self aid, combat medic, battalion surgeon – advanced trauma life support	Battalion aid station
Level II	Resuscitation/stabilization surgery	Forward surgical teams
Level III	Full operating rooms and specialty care	Combat support hospital
Level IV	Full service hospital	Regional medical center
Level V	Reconstructive and restorative care	Tertiary medical center

[a]Levels I to III are located within a war or disaster operational zone. Levels IV and V are typically located outside the war or disaster operational zone.

was these very conditions and the significant pain that casualties were experiencing on evacuation flights that resulted in the author's deployment to Iraq to explore other pain management solutions.[34] The key to pain management in this, or any other austere medical environment following war or disaster is multimodal pain therapy, tailored to the austere medicine scenario, in which opioids are only part of the overall pain medication plan.

Analgesic medications (multimodal analgesia)

Multimodal analgesia refers to the concept of using multiple analgesics with different mechanisms of action that act synergistically to result in improved overall pain control, while attempting to minimize the unwanted side effects of each individual medication.[35] A significant advantage of multimodal analgesia in austere environments is the lower total dose of each drug needed. Though multimodal analgesic approaches do provide superior pain control and are opioid-sparing following surgery, evidence indicating that this approach reduces drug side effects or improves postoperative outcome is lacking.[36, 37] This controversy aside, multimodal analgesic practices continue to play an ever more important role in perioperative pain management.[38] The importance of multimodal analgesic approaches in field medicine is amplified since it offers a departure from opioid-only options.

Nonsteroidal anti-inflammatory drugs (NSAID) are an important class of medications for austere environment analgesia. Paracetamol (acetaminophen) is a medication from this class that lacks some of the side effects associated with other NSAIDs, such as impaired platelet function,[38] renal function,[39] or bone growth.[40] Though a weak analgesic when used alone, paracetamol enhances the analgesic effects of other NSAIDs[41] and morphine[42] when used concurrently. Oral NSAIDs block prostaglandin synthesis by inhibiting the cyclooxygenase enzyme, thus reducing the inflammatory response along with the nociceptive response following injury.[43] [I] The COX-2-selective drugs lack the antiplatelet effects of the nonspecific COX-inhibiting NSAIDs, but have similar analgesic effects.[44] [I] Prolonged use of the COX-2-specific drugs is currently controversial due to concerns over increased cardiovascular events. However, for short-term use in a field setting, the advantages of these medications as adjunct analgesics for reducing opioid requirements, far outweigh their disadvantages by decreasing the possibility of respiratory depression or over sedation. The long shelf-life, ease of transport, and small abuse potential of NSAIDs are additional benefits of these analgesics in an austere environment. Some United States military units have developed "wound packs" containing paracetamol, a COX-2-specific analgesic, and a fluroquinolone that the soldier is instructed to consume following a penetrating extremity wound.[45] While this approach is too new for comment on effectiveness, the concept of prepackaged pain medications for use under defined conditions during war or disaster warrants further research and development. Parenteral preparations of NSAIDs are also available that further the potential utility of these medications in field medicine.

Of the N-methyl-D-aspartate (NMDA) antagonists, ketamine is the most commonly used and well-known example for use in austere conditions. It has been used extensively and exclusively for anesthesia in war casualties in a variety of conflicts and conditions.[46, 47, 48] Ketamine's cardiovascular stimulating and bronchodilatory activity coupled with its profound amnestic and analgesic properties make it particularly useful. For perioperative pain management, ketamine has been shown to provide an additive analgesic effect with other medications when used preemptively,[49] in epidural catheters,[50, 51] and as an intravenous infusion following major surgery.[52] Small dose ketamine has been found to be a safe adjuvant to opioids when reduced narcotic use is desirable.[53] [I] A common concern among providers using ketamine is its association with "bad dreams," hallucinations, dizziness, dysphoria, disorientation, and confusion. In a recent review, no significant increase in these central nervous system symptoms was seen in patients receiving ketamine (via patient-controlled analgesia, intravenous infusion, continuous intravenous infusion, or epidural) compared with patients receiving opioids alone.[53] Nevertheless, in the high stress environment of war and disaster medicine, the use of ketamine should be judicious, low dose, and reserved for patients whose pain is not adequately controlled with other medications. Subanesthetic concentrations of ketamine at 0.5 mg/kg slow bolus injection before incision for painful procedures, followed by ketamine 0.25 mg/kg boluses at 30-minute intervals or a ketamine infusion of 500 µg/kg/hour has been proposed to reduce postoperative opioid requirements and diminish nervous system sensitization.[54] For operations lasting more than two hours, it is recommended that the ketamine dosing be stopped at least 60 minutes before the end of surgery to prevent prolonged emergence. Dextromethorphan is another weak NMDA receptor antagonist that has been shown to reduce opioid consumption when used orally and intramuscularly.[55] Additional clinical experience is needed before routine use of dextromethorphan can be recommended for the field.

Clonidine and dexmedetomidine are α_2-adrenergic agonists that can produce a significant analgesic effect when used alone or in combination with other analgesics, without the respiratory depression associated with opioids. Clonidine's analgesic properties have been demonstrated whether administered by the intravenous,[56] intrathecal,[57] epidural,[58] intra-articular[59] route, or as an adjunct to local anesthetics in peripheral nerve block.[60] [II] The versatility of clonidine in providing anesthesia in a variety of clinical scenarios suggests it would be a useful addition to any field medicine medication list. Infusion bolus doses of clonidine at 2–5 µg/kg which can be followed by a continuous infusion of 0.3 µg/kg/hour has been described for perioperative pain management.[61] Dose-related side effects of clonidine include hypotension, bradycardia, and sedation. Seven times more selective for α$_2$-adrenergic receptors though of shorter duration, dexmedetomidine has also been used for perioperative pain management though profound sedation can complicate its use.[62, 63] One important consideration when using these medications in austere conditions is their propensity to suppress thermoregulatory responses thus promoting the development of hypothermia.[64]

Anticonvulsant medications, such as gabapentin and pregabalin (along with the NMDA receptor antagonists already mentioned), are used in acute pain management as antihyperalgesic drugs to prevent the induction and maintenance of pain sensitization of the spinal cord dorsal horn and peripheral nerves following trauma.[65] In theory, preemptive analgesia, using a multimodal approach, can prevent or at least attenuate the unwanted neurophysiological and biochemical consequences of untreated pain.[66] Gabapentin at a total dose of 3000 mg in the first 24 hours following abdominal hysterectomy has been shown to significantly reduce morphine consumption with minimal side effects.[67] It has been suggested that gabapentin use with other analgesic medications may protect the patient from central sensitization to pain following surgery, though definitive evidence for this effect is currently lacking.[68] [II] Nevertheless, gabapentin and pregabalin are currently used routinely in the pain management of United States military casualties. Available evidence supports the inclusion of these medications in a field pain medicine plan.

Other nonopioid medications, such as adenosine, droperidol, magnesium, neostigmine, and opioid antagonists, among others, have been used successfully in the management of postsurgical pain. The clinical advantages and disadvantages of these unconventional therapies will require further clarification before recommendations for use in an austere medical environment can be made.

Regional anesthesia

Regional anesthesia has characteristics that make it particularly "field friendly" for both anesthesia and analgesia.[69] Regional anesthesia, beyond spinals and epidurals, has undergone a renaissance in the last 15 years with advances in peripheral nerve stimulation techniques, stimulating needles, peripheral nerve catheters, and more recently, ultrasound technology.[70, 71, 72, 73] Advantages of regional anesthesia include:[74, 75, 76, 77, 78]

- excellent operating conditions;
- profound perioperative analgesia;
- stable hemodynamics;
- limb-specific anesthesia;
- reduced need for other analgesics (opioids);
- improved postoperative alertness;
- reduced postoperative nausea and vomiting;
- rapid recovery from anesthesia;
- improved sleep and rehabilitation;
- preservation of protective airway reflexes;
- minimal side effects;
- reduced complications;
- simple, easily transported equipment.

When general anesthesia is used as the primary anesthetic in modern hospitals, the increased incidence of postoperative pain, nausea, vomiting, and drowsiness are the most frequently cited causes for prolonged postoperative stays following ambulatory surgery.[79, 80] Delayed recovery has economic significance in the developed world. In the resource- and personnel-constrained field environment, delayed patient recovery can have a profoundly negative impact on mission success and possibly increase patient morbidity. Regional anesthesia facilitates evacuation of alert patients, free of pain and nausea, who can be active proponents in their own recovery. This is a tremendous advantage in austere environment medicine since personnel and supply resources are freed for service on more acutely ill patients.

Single injection peripheral nerve block (PNB) can provide superior analgesia with fewer side effects when compared with other pain control methods.[81] [I] The site-specific mechanism of action for local anesthetics also complements the use of other pain medications in a multimodal pain treatment plan. Unfortunately, the benefits of PNB are lost with block regression in 10–18 hours when long-acting local anesthetics are used. This length of time is often inadequate to effectively manage pain following severe trauma or major surgery. This limitation can be overcome with the use of CPNB technology that allows placement of an infusion catheter next to targeted nerves for sustained infusions of local anesthetic. First described by Ansboro[82] in 1946, CPNB catheters have been demonstrated to provide effective surgical anesthesia,[83, 84] prolonged postoperative analgesia,[70, 85] reduced opioid requirements,[86] improved rehabilitation,[87, 88, 89] and safe application outside the hospital.[90] [II] The utility of CPNB in the combat casualty environment was first described in a soldier who sustained a left calf injury from a rocket propelled grenade in 2003.[91] He arrived at the combat support hospital within one hour of injury complaining of severe pain despite titration of morphine 18 mg intravenously prior to his arrival. A left lumbar plexus CPNB and a left sciatic nerve CPNB was placed before surgery which relieved his discomfort. The patient underwent surgery using the nerve blocks and light sedation. Postoperatively he was alert, pain free, and communicating with soldiers from his unit. The lumbar plexus and sciatic catheters were subsequently infused with 0.2 percent ropivacaine at 6 mL/hour and 10 mL/hour, respectively. He also had a patient-controlled bolus function for an additional 2 mL of local anesthetic every 20 minutes to the sciatic catheter as needed. These catheters controlled his pain during a 40-minute helicopter and five-hour flight during which he did not require any morphine. The pain was managed with catheters for an additional 16 days as he traveled back to the United States. During this time, the catheters were used to establish surgical blocks for five operative procedures and provide continuous perioperative analgesia. This case illustrates the advantages of CPNB technology for austere environment pain management: prolonged, titratable analgesia; access to reestablish dense nerve block if needed for surgery; and minimal requirements for opioids, which reduced sedation risk and monitoring requirements. Since this first report, hundreds of soldiers have had CPNB catheters placed for surgical anesthesia and perioperative pain management of their wounds. Many of these catheters have been placed in the austere medical conditions. In the author's experience as an anesthesiologist, it was not uncommon to receive multiple casualties. After unstable patients had been successfully managed in the operating room, stable patients waiting for operating room availability were given various CPNB blocks if their wounds were amenable. This provided preoperative pain management, facilitated operating room patient flow, and preserved anesthetic resources since general anesthesia was often avoided.

Stojadinovic et al.[92] recently outlined the advantages and safety of regional anesthesia in a series of 287 war casualties treated at Walter Reed Army Medical Center. In this trauma patient population, catheter-related complications were rare (11.9 percent), and mostly technical or minor in nature, for 1718 total catheter days. Patients with CPNB catheters used them for surgical anesthesia and perioperative analgesia for a mean of (S.D., range) of 9 (5, 1–34) days.

The advantages of advanced regional anesthetic techniques for managing pain in austere environments are clear, but the application of this technology does have some limitations. Presently, advanced regional anesthesia techniques are underutilized in the United States despite its notable advantages in perioperative pain control.[81] Anesthesiology resident training in regional anesthesia varies widely among training programs resulting in trainees having reduced confidence in their abilities to use advanced regional anesthesia.[93] Identification and availability of trained personnel to apply regional anesthesia during war or disaster can diminish its usefulness. This potential limitation can be mitigated with appropriate predisaster planning that ensures experienced providers are part of the military or disaster pain management response. The use of regional anesthesia also requires some specialized equipment (**Figure 20.2**). A discussion of the PNB and CPNB techniques for various clinical situations is available through many excellent textbooks on the subject.[94, 95] **Table 20.2** provides information on standard adult ropivacaine dosages for single injection and CPNB blocks used by the author in field situations.

Novel pain control methods and equipment

Considerable effort has been made to find alternative pain control methods, other than intravenous morphine, for

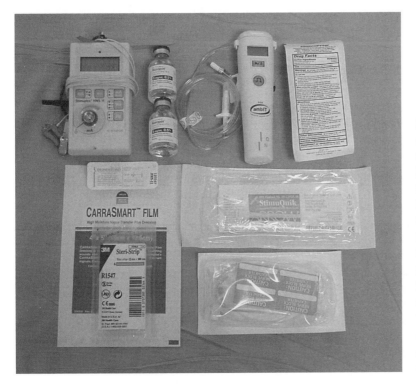

Figure 20.2 Advanced regional anesthesia equipment. Equipment for single injection or continuous peripheral nerve block displayed on top. Items include Stimuplex™ HNS-11 nerve stimulator (B Braun Medical Inc., Bethlehem, PA, USA), Naropin™ 0.5% (ropivacaine HCL, AstraZeneca, Wilmington, DE, USA), Ambit™ infusion pump (Sorenson Medical), Chloraprep™ (Medi-Flex Hospital Products, Inc., Overland Park, KS, USA), Dermabond™ (Ethicon Inc., Cornelia, GA, USA), Steri-Strip™ (3M Health Care, St Paul, MN, USA), CarraSmart™ (Carrington Laboratories, Inc., Irving, TX, USA), StimuQuick™ insulated peripheral block needle (Arrow International Inc., Reading, PA, USA), and Contiplex™ Tuohy continuous nerve block set (B Braun Medical Inc.).

Table 20.2 Standard adult ropivacaine dosages for single injection and continuous regional anesthesia at Walter Reed Army Medical Center.

Regional anesthesia technique	Adult single injection dose of ropivacaine[a]	Continuous infusion of 0.2% ropivacaine	Patient-controlled bolus rate of 0.2% ropivacaine[b]	Notes
Interscalene	35–40 mL of 0.5% ropivacaine	8–10 mL	2 mL bolus/20-min lockout	Often supplemented with an intercostal brachial nerve block
Supraclavicular	35–40 mL of 0.5% ropivacaine	8–10 mL	2 mL bolus/20-min lockout	Shortest latency block of the brachial plexus
Infraclavicular	35–40 mL of 0.5% ropivacaine	10–12 mL	2 mL bolus/20-min lockout	Catheter techniques less effective compared with supraclavicular catheters
Axillary	40 mL of 0.5% ropivacaine	10–12 mL	2 mL bolus/20-min lockout	Catheter techniques less common
Paravertebral	3–5 mL of 0.5% ropivacaine per level blocked	8–10 mL	2 mL bolus/20-min lockout	Catheters effective in thoracic region only
Lumbar plexus (posterior approach)	35–40 mL of 0.5% ropivacaine	8–10 mL	2 mL bolus/20-min lockout	Epidural spread is a concern
Femoral	20–30 mL of 0.5% ropivacaine	8–10 mL	2 mL bolus/20-min lockout	Catheter techniques less effective compared with lumbar plexus catheters
Sciatic (anterior or posterior approach)	20–30 mL of 0.5% ropivacaine	8–10 mL	2 mL bolus/20-min lockout	Proximal approaches to the sciatic nerve preferable for catheters
Sciatic (lateral or popliteal approach)	35–40 mL of 0.5% ropivacaine	10–12 mL	2 mL bolus/20-min lockout	Catheter techniques less common
Lumbar plexus or femoral + sciatic	50–60 mL of 0.5% ropivacaine between both sites	5–10 mL for both catheters	2 mL bolus/20-min lockout on one catheter	Infusion rates divided between catheters based on distribution of patient's pain
Epidural	20–25 mL of 0.5% ropivacaine	6–10 mL	2 mL bolus/20-min lockout	Opioids often added to infusions
Spinal	5–15 mg of 1.0% ropivacaine	NA	NA	Opioids often added to injections

Information is based on the author's experience with ropivacaine in a successful and busy regional anesthesia practice.
[a]Mepivacaine 1.5% can be used in place of ropivacaine at the volumes noted when a shorter duration block is desirable.
[b]Occasionally, 5 mL bolus per 30-minute lockout is used in selected patients. Generally, total infusion (continuous plus bolus) >20 mL/h are avoided.
NA, not applicable.
Reprinted with permission from Buckenmaier III CC, Bleckner LL. Anaesthetic agents for advanced regional anesthesia: A North American perspective. *Drugs.* 2005: **65**; 745–59.

pain management in battlefield scenarios. Though the effectiveness of intravenous morphine is without question, the equipment and expertise to establish intravenous access may be lacking in battlefield or natural disaster situations. A possible alternative is transdermal delivery of fentanyl. One delivery device that has promise in acute pain management is the patient-controlled transdermal delivery system (PCTS) for fentanyl hydrochloride.[96] [III] The credit card-sized device is placed on the patient's skin with adhesive and activated by the patient pushing a button. The device then delivers a 40-μg fentanyl dose over a ten-minute period through a process of iontophoresis (introduction of medication into tissue through means of an electric current). Unlike transdermal fentanyl

patches that continuously deliver medication passively and are inappropriate for opioid-naive patients, the PCTS is similar to a PCA machine and the two devices have been shown to be equivalent for perioperative pain control following major surgery.[97]

Oral transmucosal fentanyl is another possible delivery method that has potential for use in austere environment pain control. In 2003, 22 soldiers were treated following mild injury with oral fentanyl lozenges (1600 μg) in a field setting.[98] [V] Oral fentanyl was effective in this setting, though three soldiers complained of nausea and one required naloxone for hypoventilation, emphasizing that novel delivery systems for opioids do not eliminate the potential dangerous side effects of these drugs.

Intranasal ketamine has received substantial attention for pain control following injury in the field. Opioid use for pain can significantly degrade a soldier's ability to continue the mission due to its sedative effects. Theoretically, low-dose ketamine delivered intranasally reduces pain without substantially degrading performance. While intranasal ketamine has been used successfully in chronic pain patients for breakthrough pain with minimal side effects, its abuse potential and possible cognitive effects in a high stress environment, such as a battlefield, warrants further study before recommendations on use in austere environments can be made.[99, 100] [V]

Efforts continue to develop longer-acting local anesthetics by combining them with polymers or liposomes.[101] The advantage in the field of a local anesthetic effect that lasts for several days, without the need for CPNB or an infusion pump, is clear. Unfortunately, no agent of this type is currently available for human use.

Basic vital sign monitoring equipment is essential for any healthcare provider managing pain in austere conditions. Many automated, portable, rugged, battery-operated patient monitors are available for this purpose, but this equipment should be supplemented with manual monitoring equipment to cover inevitable malfunctions. One extremely useful patient monitor for field applications is the compact Nonin Onyx 9500[TM] pulse oximeter (Nonin Medical Inc., Plymouth, MN, USA). This pocket-sized device supports rapid checking of numerous patient pulses and oxygen saturations under the most difficult field conditions.

Recent advances in electronic infusion pump technology have facilitated the introduction of CPNB and PCA to the modern battlefield. Presently, the Stryker PainPump 2[TM] (Stryker Corporation, Kalamazoo, MI, USA) used for CPNB infusions and Sorenson ambiT[TM] (Sorenson Medical, West Jordan, UT, USA) used for PCA are the only pain pumps currently approved for pain management during aeromedical evacuation in the United States military. The ability of electronic pumps to function with consistent infusion rates at extremes of temperature and pressure favors electronic pump devices in harsh environments. Electronic pumps have the added advantage of programmability for infusion adjustment that other pneumatic pump devices lack.

ADVANTAGES OF EFFECTIVE PAIN MANAGEMENT IN FIELD AND DISASTER SITUATIONS

Maladaptive pain and the patient stress response

Woolf[102] has suggested that pain can be divided into two broad categories: adaptive and maladaptive. Adaptive pain enhances survival by warning the patient of impending injury and promoting healing following injury. An example would be a stubbed toe that results in minor but persistent pain for a few days, causing the patient to protect the toe from further injury while it heals. Maladaptive pain occurs when the nervous system expression of this protective mechanism becomes pathologic, due to overwhelming noxious stimuli or other factors, and pain becomes a disease state. Traumatic amputation of a foot from an explosive device, with severe phantom pain that persists for years following the injury is an example. Understanding that pain is not just a symptom of disease, but at times a disease process in itself, is a fundamental change occurring in medicine that explains the new emphasis on effective pain control whether in the modern hospital or in the field. Regardless of the conditions in which health care is being provided, inadequate acute pain control is associated with a myriad of physiologic changes that can significantly increase patient morbidity and possibly mortality (**Table 20.3**). Evidence suggests that untreated or poorly treated acute pain, and the proinflammatory and immunosuppressive responses associated with it, may result in deleterious health effects for months or even years after the initial pain insult.[103] Pain is a disease state of the nervous system and deserves the same attention to management that is given any other disease state known to medicine.

Improved patient condition for evacuation

Modern healthcare systems in the developed world are well equipped to minimize the impact of the physiologic stress pain places on a patient and can deal with consequences of this stress. This is not the case in austere environments where seemingly minor problems arising from untreated pain, like nausea, vomiting, urinary retention, or impaired immune function, among many others, can balloon into devastating complications in the resource-constrained and chaotic medical environments typical of war or disaster. Effective pain management is critical for maximizing the success of the medical response to disaster.

Anger, increased anxiety, sensitivity to external stimuli, withdrawal from interpersonal contact, and self-absorption eventually leading to depression and despair, are among the negative psychological responses associated with uncontrolled pain.[7, 104, 105] Paolini,[106] in his fictional work *Eldest*, provides an insightful description of the emotional impact intractable pain can have on a patient:

> I have a new name for pain. What's that? The Obliterator. Because when you're in pain, nothing else can exist. Not thought. Not emotion. Only the drive to escape the pain. When it's strong enough, the Obliterator strips us of everything that makes us who we are, until we're reduced to creatures less than animals, creatures with a single desire and goal: escape.

Table 20.3 Consequences of unrelieved pain.

Organ systems	Physiologic responses
Cardiovascular	Increased heart rate, peripheral vascular resistance, arterial blood pressure, and myocardial contractility resulting in increased cardiac work, myocardial ischemia, and infarction
Pulmonary	Respiratory and abdominal muscle spasm (splinting), diaphragmatic dysfunction, decreased vital capacity, impaired ventilation and ability to cough, atelectasis, increased ventilation/perfusion mismatch, hypoventilation, hypoxemia, hypercarbia, increased postoperative pulmonary infection
Gastrointestinal	Increased gastrointestinal secretions and smooth muscle sphincter tone, reduced intestinal motility, ileus, nausea, and vomiting
Renal	Oliguria, increased urinary sphincter tone, urinary retention
Coagulation	Increased platelet aggregation, venostasis, increased deep vein thrombosis, thromboembolism
Immunologic	Impaired immune function, increased infection, tumor spread or recurrence
Muscular	Muscle weakness, limitation of movement, muscle atrophy, fatigue
Psychological	Anxiety, fear, anger, depression, reduced patient satisfaction
Overall recovery	Delayed recovery, increased need for hospitalization, delayed return to normal daily living, increased healthcare resource

Reprinted with permission from Joshi GP, Ogunnaike BO. Consequences of inadequate postoperative pain relief and chronic persistent postoperative pain. *Anesthesiology Clinics of North America.* 2005; **23**: 21–36.

In the author's experience, many soldiers have echoed similar sentiments when describing the impact of pain during their evacuation and recovery. In the turmoil of war or disaster medicine, a self-absorbed patient whose attention is confined to their pain, cannot assist in their own health care. The burden of these patients, in all aspects of care and evacuation is greatly magnified. Through effective pain control, the healthcare provider is creating an improved patient condition for stabilizing care and evacuation following disaster. An alert, interactive, pain-free patient will ease the burden of providing an effective medical response in austere conditions. Personnel training and resource allocation toward achieving this goal is an investment in medical resources that will return multiple dividends. Effective pain management is an austere medical mission force multiplier.

ROLE OF THE ACUTE PAIN SERVICE TEAMS IN AUSTERE ENVIRONMENT MEDICINE

Effective pain management for austere medical missions assumes the deployment of trained medical personnel and equipment needed to run an acute pain service within the disaster medical response infrastructure. While anesthesiologists are a natural choice for leading the APS team due to their focus on perioperative pain relief, the responsibility for managing pain should not fall to the anesthesiologist by default as an "extra" or "assumed" duty.[107] The austere medicine APS should be seen as an additional requirement that necessitates supplementary staffing specifically for the pain mission. Despite the recent advances in pain management by the United States military, the lack of APS teams has significantly hampered continued improvement of pain management in austere

medical environments. The forethought by military or civilian medical planners in including APS teams in the disaster medicine plan will impart significant advantages to the medical response team. For example, the anesthesiologist leading the APS team will be available to assist with triage in mass casualty scenarios. As mentioned previously, anesthesiologists serving in this capacity can manage the pain of many patients waiting for operating room availability, often using regional anesthetic techniques that can also be used to provide surgical anesthesia for the operative procedure, thus facilitating patient flow. The APS team also provides a reserve of providers (anesthesia, nursing, etc.) that can assist with critical care medicine during mass casualty situations. The advantages of the APS team in relieving suffering and preparing patients to be active participants in their own recovery and evacuation is clear.

Training the austere environment APS team

A simple but effective approach for developing a pain management response in times of disaster is the establishment of pain treatment protocols that all responding healthcare providers can use regardless of their level of pain training. This may be the only option if APS teams are not part of the medical disaster response plan. Hocking and de Mello[108, 109] have provided basic and more advanced pain management guidelines for battlefield analgesia and these protocols can serve as a template for medical planners if APS teams are not an option. For these pain protocols to be effective, response teams must train with the protocols and incorporate them into standard operating procedures.

The expertise needed to establish austere environment APS teams begins with existing hospital-based teams.

New pain technologies and medications must first demonstrate efficacy and safety on the hospital wards before being considered for austere environment missions. The type of austere environment (military or civilian) that the APS team will be responding to will dictate planning, preparation, and training. Undoubtedly one of the best ways to train APS teams, short of an actual disaster, is through healthcare missions to medically underserved areas of the world. These missions have proven extremely valuable for training military anesthesiology residents in austere environment anesthesia and in exercising new pain management techniques and in equipment for use in austere conditions.[74]

CONCLUSIONS

This chapter has outlined current trends and future possibilities for managing acute pain during war or disaster. Our understanding of pain and its consequences has advanced greatly since General "Stonewall" Jackson quaffed whiskey to ease his suffering. Unfortunately, despite these advances, the necessity for and responsibility of pain management in austere medical environments remains inadequately defined. If events during this first decade of the twenty-first century are any guide, the need for effective pain management in austere conditions is great and concepts of effective pain control following war or disaster are the concern of all physicians, civilian and military. As stated by John J Bonica in *The management of pain*, "The proper management of pain remains, after all, the most important obligation, the main objective, and the crowning achievement of every physician."[107]

REFERENCES

1. Farwell B. *Stonewall: A biography of General Thomas J. Jackson.* New York: WW Norton, 1992: 492–526.
2. Van AH, Buerkle H. Acute pain services: transition from the Middle Ages to the 21st century. *European Journal of Anaesthesiology.* 1998; **15**: 253–4.
3. Hamilton GR, Baskett TF. In the arms of Morpheus the development of morphine for postoperative pain relief. *Canadian Journal of Anaesthesia.* 2000; **47**: 367–74.
4. Taylor S, Voytovich AE, Kozol RA. Has the pendulum swung too far in postoperative pain control? *American Journal of Surgery.* 2003; **186**: 472–5.
* 5. Wheeler M, Oderda GM, Ashburn MA, Lipman AG. Adverse events associated with postoperative opioid analgesia: a systematic review. *Journal of Pain.* 2002; **3**: 159–80.
6. Kehlet H, Rung GW, Callesen T. Postoperative opioid analgesia: time for a reconsideration? *Journal of Clinical Anesthesia.* 1996; **8**: 441–5.
* 7. Joshi GP, Ogunnaike BO. Consequences of inadequate postoperative pain relief and chronic persistent

postoperative pain. *Anesthesiology Clinics of North America.* 2005; **23**: 21–36.
8. Condon-Rall ME. A brief history of military anesthesia. In: Zajtchuk R, Grande CM (eds). *Anesthesia and perioperative care of the combat casualty.* Zajtchuk R, Bellamy RF (eds). *Textbook of Military Medicine.* Washington DC: Office of the Surgeon General, 1995: 855–96.
9. Basbaum AI. Spinal mechanisms of acute and persistent pain. *Regional Anesthesia and Pain Medicine.* 1999; **24**: 59–67.
10. Lanser P, Gesell S. Pain management: the fifth vital sign. *Healthcare Benchmarks.* 2001; **8**: 68–70.
11. Rosenbaum S. US health policy in the aftermath of Hurricane Katrina. *Journal of the American Medocal Association.* 2006; **295**: 437–40.
12. deBoisblanc BP. Black Hawk, please come down: reflections on a hospital's struggle to survive in the wake of Hurricane Katrina. *American Journal of Respiratory and Critical Care Medicine.* 2005; **172**: 1239–40.
13. Berggren RE, Curiel TJ. After the storm – health care infrastructure in post-Katrina New Orleans. *New England Journal of Medicine.* 2006; **354**: 1549–52.
14. Brennan RJ, Waldman RJ. The south Asian earthquake six months later – an ongoing crisis. *New England Journal of Medicine.* 2006; **354**: 1769–71.
15. Carballo M, Daita S, Hernandez M. Impact of the tsunami on healthcare systems. *Journal of the Royal Society of Medicine.* 2005; **98**: 390–5.
16. Beitler AL, Wortmann GW, Hofmann LJ, Goff Jr JM. Operation Enduring Freedom: the 48th Combat Support Hospital in Afghanistan. *Military Medicine.* 2006; **171**: 189–93.
17. Owens PJ, Forgione Jr A, Briggs S. Challenges of international disaster relief: use of a deployable rapid assembly shelter and surgical hospital. *Disaster Management and Response.* 2005; **3**: 11–16.
18. McCullum K. A new kind of pain management. *Military Medicine/NBC Technology.* 2006; **10**: 38–41.
19. Croll SM, Shockey SM. Advances in battlefield pain control. *ASA Newsletter.* 2006; **70**: 26–8.
20. Mabry RL, Holcomb JB, Baker AM *et al.* United States army rangers in Somalia: an analysis of combat casualties on an urban battlefield. *Journal of Trauma.* 2000; **49**: 515–28.
21. Gondusky JS, Reiter MP. Protecting military convoys in Iraq: an examination of battle injuries sustained by a mechanized battalion during Operation Iraqi Freedom II. *Military Medicine.* 2005; **170**: 546–9.
22. Peleg K, Rivkind A, Haronson-Daniel L. Does body armor protect from firearm injuries?. *Journal of the American College of Surgeons.* 2006; **202**: 643–8.
23. Werner MU, Soholm L, Rotboll-Nielsen P, Kehlet H. Does an acute pain service improve postoperative outcome? *Anesthesia and Analgesia.* 2002; **95**: 1361–72.
* 24. American Society of Anesthesiologists Task Force on Acute Pain Management. Practice guidelines for acute pain management in the perioperative setting: an updated report by the American Society of Anesthesiologists Task

Force on Acute Pain Management. *Anesthesiology.* 2004; **100**: 1573–81.

∗ 25. Rawal N. Organization, function, and implementation of acute pain service. *Anesthesiology Clinics of North America.* 2005; **23**: 211–25.

26. Stamer UM, Mpasios N, Stuber F, Maier C. A survey of acute pain services in Germany and a discussion of international survey data. *Regional Anesthesia and Pain Medicine.* 2002; **27**: 125–31.

27. Rawal N. Acute pain services revisited – good from far, far from good? *Regional Anesthesia and Pain Medicine.* 2002; **27**: 117–21.

28. McCartney CJ, Ahtsham N. Use of opioid analgesics in the perioperative period. In: Shorten G, Carr DB, Harmon D et al. (eds). *Postoperative pain management – an evidence-based guide to practice.* Philadelphia, PA: Saunders Elsevier, 2006: 137–47.

29. Goodsell DS. The molecular perspective: morphine. *Stem Cells.* 2005; **23**: 144–5.

30. Sabatowski R, Schafer D, Kasper SM et al. Pain treatment: a historical overview. *Current Pharmaceutical Design.* 2004; **10**: 701–16.

31. Gawande A. Casualties of war – military care for the wounded from Iraq and Afghanistan. *New England Journal of Medicine.* 2004; **351**: 2471–5.

32. Montgomery SP, Swiecki CW, Shriver CD. The evaluation of casualties from Operation Iraqi Freedom on return to the continental United States from March to June 2003. *Journal of the American College of Surgeons.* 2005; **201**: 7–12.

33. Peake JB. Beyond the purple heart – continuity of care for the wounded in Iraq. *New England Journal of Medicine.* 2005; **352**: 219–22.

34. Silberman S. The painful truth. Anonymous. *Wired.* 2005; **13**: 112–23.

35. Jin F, Chung F. Multimodal analgesia for postoperative pain control. *Journal of Clinical Anesthesia.* 2001; **13**: 524–39.

∗ 36. Joshi GP. Multimodal analgesia techniques and postoperative rehabilitation. *Anesthesiology Clinics of North America.* 2005; **23**: 185–202.

37. Romsing J, Moiniche S, Mathiesen O, Dahl JB. Reduction of opioid-related adverse events using opioid-sparing analgesia with COX-2 inhibitors lacks documentation: a systematic review. *Acta Anaesthesiologica Scandinavica.* 2005; **49**: 133–42.

38. Joshi GP. Multimodal analgesia techniques for ambulatory surgery. *International Anesthesiology Clinics.* 2005; **43**: 197–204.

39. Giovanni G, Giovanni P. Do non-steroidal anti-inflammatory drugs and COX-2 selective inhibitors have different renal effects? *Journal of Nephrology.* 2002; **15**: 480–8.

40. Glassman SD, Rose SM, Dimar JR et al. The effect of postoperative nonsteroidal anti-inflammatory drug administration on spinal fusion. *Spine.* 1998; **23**: 834–8.

41. Issioui T, Klein KW, White PF et al. Cost-efficacy of rofecoxib versus acetaminophen for preventing pain after ambulatory surgery. *Anesthesiology.* 2002; **97**: 931–7.

42. Schug SA, Sidebotham DA, McGuinnety M et al. Acetaminophen as an adjunct to morphine by patient-controlled analgesia in the management of acute postoperative pain. *Anesthesia and Analgesia.* 1998; **87**: 368–72.

∗ 43. White PF. The changing role of non-opioid analgesic techniques in the management of postoperative pain. *Anesthesia and Analgesia.* 2005; **101**: S5–22.

44. Gajraj NM, Joshi GP. Role of cyclooxygenase-2 inhibitors in postoperative pain management. *Anesthesiology Clinics of North America.* 2005; **23**: 49–72.

45. Wedmore IS, Johnson T, Czarnik J, Hendrix S. Pain management in the wilderness and operational setting. *Emergency Medicine Clinics of North America.* 2005; **23**: 585–601, xi–xii.

∗ 46. Bonanno FG. Ketamine in war/tropical surgery (a final tribute to the racemic mixture). *Injury.* 2002; **33**: 323–7.

47. Read D, Ashford B. Surgical aspects of Operation Bali Assist: initial wound surgery on the tarmac and in flight. *ANZ Journal of Surgery.* 2004; **74**: 986–91.

48. Shah RK, Singh RP, Prasad N. Sedation with ketamine: a safe and effective anaesthetic agent for children in the developing world. *Nepal Medical College Journal.* 2003; **5**: 9–13.

49. Launo C, Bassi C, Spagnolo L et al. Preemptive ketamine during general anesthesia for postoperative analgesia in patients undergoing laparoscopic cholecystectomy. *Minerva Anestesiologica.* 2004; **70**: 727–34.

50. Chia YY, Liu K, Liu YC et al. Adding ketamine in a multimodal patient-controlled epidural regimen reduces postoperative pain and analgesic consumption. *Anesthesia and Analgesia.* 1998; **86**: 1245–9.

51. Wu CT, Yeh CC, Yu JC et al. Pre-incisional epidural ketamine, morphine and bupivacaine combined with epidural and general anaesthesia provides pre-emptive analgesia for upper abdominal surgery. *Acta Anaesthesiologica Scandinavica.* 2000; **44**: 63–8.

52. Weinbroum AA. A single small dose of postoperative ketamine provides rapid and sustained improvement in morphine analgesia in the presence of morphine-resistant pain. *Anesthesia and Analgesia.* 2003; **96**: 789–95.

∗ 53. Subramaniam K, Subramaniam B, Steinbrook RA. Ketamine as adjuvant analgesic to opioids: a quantitative and qualitative systematic review. *Anesthesia and Analgesia.* 2004; **99**: 482–95.

54. Himmelseher S, Durieux ME. Ketamine for perioperative pain management. *Anesthesiology.* 2005; **102**: 211–20.

55. Habib AS, Gan TJ. Role of analgesic adjuncts in postoperative pain management. *Anesthesiology Clinics of North America.* 2005; **23**: 85–107.

56. Bernard JM, Hommeril JL, Passuti N, Pinaud M. Postoperative analgesia by intravenous clonidine. *Anesthesiology.* 1991; **75**: 577–82.

57. De KM, Lavand'homme P, Waterloos H. The short-lasting analgesia and long-term antihyperalgesic effect of intrathecal clonidine in patients undergoing colonic surgery. *Anesthesia and Analgesia*. 2005; **101**: 566–72.

58. Forster JG, Rosenberg PH. Small dose of clonidine mixed with low-dose ropivacaine and fentanyl for epidural analgesia after total knee arthroplasty. *British Journal of Anaesthesia*. 2004; **93**: 670–7.

59. Brill S, Plaza M. Non-narcotic adjuvants may improve the duration and quality of analgesia after knee arthroscopy: a brief review. *Canadian Journal of Anaesthesia*. 2004; **51**: 975–8.

60. Hutschala D, Mascher H, Schmetterer L *et al*. Clonidine added to bupivacaine enhances and prolongs analgesia after brachial plexus block via a local mechanism in healthy volunteers. *European Journal of Anaesthesiology*. 2004; **21**: 198–204.

61. Marinangeli F, Ciccozzi A, Donatelli F *et al*. Clonidine for treatment of postoperative pain: a dose-finding study. *European Journal of Pain*. 2002; **6**: 35–42.

62. Arain SR, Ruehlow RM, Uhrich TD, Ebert TJ. The efficacy of dexmedetomidine versus morphine for postoperative analgesia after major inpatient surgery. *Anesthesia and Analgesia*. 2004; **98**: 153–8.

63. Hofer RE, Sprung J, Sarr MG, Wedel DJ. Anesthesia for a patient with morbid obesity using dexmedetomidine without narcotics. *Canadian Journal of Anaesthesia*. 2005; **52**: 176–80.

64. Talke P, Tayefeh F, Sessler DI *et al*. Dexmedetomidine does not alter the sweating threshold, but comparably and linearly decreases the vasoconstriction and shivering thresholds. *Anesthesiology*. 1997; **87**: 835–41.

* 65. Dahl JB, Moiniche S. Pre-emptive analgesia. *British Medical Bulletin*. 2004; **71**: 13–27.

* 66. Kehlet H, Jensen TS, Woolf CJ. Persistent postsurgical pain: risk factors and prevention. *Lancet*. 2006; **367**: 1618–25.

67. Dierking G, Duedahl TH, Rasmussen ML *et al*. Effects of gabapentin on postoperative morphine consumption and pain after abdominal hysterectomy: a randomized, double-blind trial. *Acta Anaesthesiologica Scandinavica*. 2004; **48**: 322–7.

* 68. Dahl JB, Mathiesen O, Moiniche S. 'Protective premedication': an option with gabapentin and related drugs? A review of gabapentin and pregabalin in in the treatment of post-operative pain. *Acta Anaesthesiologica Scandinavica*. 2004; **48**: 1130–6.

69. *Emergency war surgery*, 3rd United States revision. Washington DC: Borden Institute, 2004: 9.1–9.12.

70. Buckenmaier III CC, Xenos JS, Nilsen SM. Lumbar plexus block with perineural catheter and sciatic nerve block for total hip arthroplasty. *Journal of Arthroplasty*. 2002; **17**: 499–502.

71. Buckenmaier III CC. Anaesthesia for outpatient knee surgery. Best practice and research. *Clinical Anaesthesiology*. 2002; **16**: 255–70.

72. Klein SM, Buckenmaier III CC. Ambulatory surgery with long acting regional anesthesia. *Minerva Anestesiologica*. 2002; **68**: 833–41.

73. Plunkett AR, Brown DS, Rogers JM, Buckenmaier III CC. Supraclavicular continuous peripheral nerve block in a wounded soldier: when ultrasound is the only option. *British Journal of Anaesthesia*. 2006; **97**: 715–7.

* 74. Buckenmaier III CC, Lee EH, Shields CH *et al*. Regional anesthesia in austere environments. *Regional Anesthesia and Pain Medicine*. 2003; **28**: 321–7.

75. Chelly JE, Greger J, Gebhard R *et al*. Continuous femoral blocks improve recovery and outcome of patients undergoing total knee arthroplasty. *Journal of Arthroplasty*. 2001; **16**: 436–45.

76. Ilfeld BM, Morey TE, Enneking FK. Continuous infraclavicular brachial plexus block for postoperative pain control at home: a randomized, double-blinded, placebo-controlled study. *Anesthesiology*. 2002; **96**: 1297–304.

77. Hadzic A, Williams BA, Karaca PE *et al*. For outpatient rotator cuff surgery, nerve block anesthesia provides superior same-day recovery over general anesthesia. *Anesthesiology*. 2005; **102**: 1001–07.

78. Yazigi A, Madi-Gebara S, Haddad F *et al*. Intraoperative myocardial ischemia in peripheral vascular surgery: general anesthesia vs combined sciatic and femoral nerve blocks. *Journal of Clinical Anesthesia*. 2005; **17**: 499–503.

79. Chung F, Mezei G. Factors contributing to a prolonged stay after ambulatory surgery. *Anesthesia and Analgesia*. 1999; **89**: 1352–9.

80. Pavlin DJ, Rapp SE, Polissar NL *et al*. Factors affecting discharge time in adult outpatients. *Anesthesia and Analgesia*. 1998; **87**: 816–26.

* 81. Evans H, Steele SM, Nielsen KC *et al*. Peripheral nerve blocks and continuous catheter techniques. *Anesthesiology Clinics of North America*. 2005; **23**: 141–62.

82. Ansboro F. Method of continuous brachial plexus block. *American Journal of Surgery*. 1946; **71**: 716–22.

83. Grant SA, Nielsen KC, Greengrass RA *et al*. Continuous peripheral nerve block for ambulatory surgery. *Regional Anesthesia and Pain Medicine*. 2001; **26**: 209–14.

84. Klein SM, Grant SA, Greengrass RA *et al*. Interscalene brachial plexus block with a continuous catheter insertion system and a disposable infusion pump. *Anesthesia and Analgesia*. 2000; **91**: 1473–8.

85. Capdevila X, Pirat P, Bringuier S *et al*. Continuous peripheral nerve blocks in hospital wards after orthopedic surgery: a multicenter prospective analysis of the quality of postoperative analgesia and complications in 1,416 patients. *Anesthesiology*. 2005; **103**: 1035–45.

86. Richman JM, Liu SS, Courpas G *et al*. Does continuous peripheral nerve block provide superior pain control to opioids? A meta-analysis. *Anesthesia and Analgesia*. 2006; **102**: 248–57.

87. Capdevila X, Barthelet Y, Biboulet P *et al*. Effects of perioperative analgesic technique on the surgical outcome

and duration of rehabilitation after major knee surgery. *Anesthesiology.* 1999; **91**: 8–15.

88. Singelyn FJ, Deyaert M, Joris D *et al.* Effects of intravenous patient-controlled analgesia with morphine, continuous epidural analgesia, and continuous three-in-one block on postoperative pain and knee rehabilitation after unilateral total knee arthroplasty. *Anesthesia and Analgesia.* 1998; **87**: 88–92.

89. Capdevila X, Dadure C, Bringuier S *et al.* Effect of patient-controlled perineural analgesia on rehabilitation and pain after ambulatory orthopedic surgery: a multicenter randomized trial. *Anesthesiology.* 2006; **105**: 566–73.

90. Greengrass RA, Nielsen KC. Management of peripheral nerve block catheters at home. *International Anesthesiology Clinics.* 2005; **43**: 79–87.

∗ 91. Buckenmaier CC, McKnight GM, Winkley JV *et al.* Continuous peripheral nerve block for battlefield anesthesia and evacuation. *Regional Anesthesia and Pain Medicine.* 2005; **30**: 202–05.

∗ 92. Stojadinovic A, Auton A, Peoples GE *et al.* Responding to challenges in modern combat casualty care: innovative use of advanced regional anesthesia. *Pain Medicine.* 2006; **7**: 330–8.

93. Smith MP, Sprung J, Zura A *et al.* A survey of exposure to regional anesthesia techniques in American anesthesia residency training programs. *Regional Anesthesia and Pain Medicine.* 1999; **24**: 11–16.

94. Brown DL. *Atlas of regional anesthesia*, 3rd edn. Philadelphia: Elsevier, 2006: 1–438.

95. Hadzic A, Vloka JD. *Peripheral nerve blocks: principles and practice*, 1st edn. New York: McGraw-Hill, 2004: 1–365.

96. Koo PJ. Postoperative pain management with a patient-controlled transdermal delivery system for fentanyl. *American Journal of Health-System Pharmacy.* 2005; **62**: 1171–6.

97. Viscusi ER, Reynolds L, Chung F *et al.* Patient-controlled transdermal fentanyl hydrochloride vs intravenous morphine pump for postoperative pain: a randomized controlled trial. *Journal of American Medical Association.* 2004; **291**: 1333–41.

98. Kotwal RS, O'Connor KC, Johnson TR *et al.* A novel pain management strategy for combat casualty care. *Annals of Emergency Medicine.* 2004; **44**: 121–7.

99. Bell RF, Kalso E. Is intranasal ketamine an appropriate treatment for chronic non-cancer breakthrough pain? *Pain.* 2004; **108**: 1–2.

100. Carr DB, Goudas LC, Denman WT *et al.* Safety and efficacy of intranasal ketamine for the treatment of breakthrough pain in patients with chronic pain: a randomized, double-blind, placebo-controlled, crossover study. *Pain.* 2004; **108**: 17–27.

101. Kuzma PJ, Kline MD, Calkins MD, Staats PS. Progress in the development of ultra-long-acting local anesthetics. *Regional Anesthesia.* 1997; **22**: 543–51.

∗102. Woolf CJ. Pain: moving from symptom control toward mechanism-specific pharmacologic management. *Annals of Internal Medicine.* 2004; **140**: 441–51.

∗103. Meiler SE. Long-term outcome after anesthesia and surgery: remarks on the biology of a newly emerging principle in perioperative care. *Anesthesiology Clinics.* 2006; **24**: 255–78.

104. Feeney SL. The relationship between pain and negative affect in older adults: anxiety as a predictor of pain. *Journal of Anxiety Disorders.* 2004; **18**: 733–44.

∗105. Janssen SA, Spinhoven P, Arntz A. The effects of failing to control pain: an experimental investigation. *Pain.* 2004; **107**: 227–33.

106. Paolini C. *Eldest.* Inheritance, book 2, 1st edn. New York: Alfred A Knopf, 2006: 400–01.

107. Bridenbaugh LD. The 1990 John J. Bonica lecture. Acute pain therapy – whose responsibility? *Regional Anesthesia.* 1990; **15**: 219–22.

∗108. Hocking G, de Mello WF. Battlefield analgesia – a basic approach. *Journal of the Royal Army Medical Corps.* 1996; **142**: 101–02.

∗109. Hocking G, de Mello WF. Battlefield analgesia: an advanced approach. *Journal of the Royal Army Medical Corps.* 1999; **145**: 116–8.

21

Acute pain management in the developing world

MATTHEW HJ SIZE AND IAIN H WILSON

KEY LEARNING POINTS

- Untreated acute pain in the developing world is a major problem, causing immeasurable misery and morbidity.
- The reasons for poor management of acute pain are many and vary from country to country.
- Simple, cheap, and effective measures can make a big difference to patients.

INTRODUCTION

Pain is a feature of many of the most common conditions presenting to doctors in the developing world, yet many patients do not have access to the basic human right of analgesia. Patients present with pain secondary to trauma, especially following road traffic accidents (RTA) and acts of violence (including land mine injuries and gunshot wounds), but also pain from labor, and medical and surgical disease.

The lack of infrastructure and resources that characterize the developing world makes estimating the magnitude of the problem almost impossible. There are few data on the incidence or prevalence of pain, or its treatment. It is troubling to note how few studies focus on the diseases that are most prevalent in the developing world, and the treatments available for them. Therefore, much of this chapter is based on inference from the data that are available and the personal experience of the authors.

INCIDENCE AND PREVALENCE OF PAIN

The World Health Organization (WHO) collects data on the burden of disease globally and, although it does not list pain as a separate entity, many of the leading causes of disease have pain as a major feature.

Trauma

In 2001, the WHO described injuries as the hidden epidemic. Road traffic accidents are the tenth most common cause of death in low- to middle-income countries.[1] More importantly, RTAs, violence, and self-inflicted injury are among the top ten leading causes of ongoing morbidity, as measured by disability adjusted life years. In some developing countries, they account for a third of the disease burden in male adults between 15 and 44 years.[1] The problem of RTA-related trauma is increasing in Sub-Saharan Africa and South East Asia. The vast majority of these victims will suffer severe pain as a result of their injuries.

Obstetrics

Labor is universally associated with pain. Birth rates are higher in the developing world and the lack of obstetric services means that obstructed labor and uterine rupture are much more common than in the developed world. Ninety-nine percent of all maternal deaths occur in the developing world and there is a 500-fold difference in maternal mortality between the worst of the developing countries (one in six) and best of the more developed world (1 in 29,800).[2] The lack of obstetric services demonstrated by these figures means that analgesia is often unavailable for normal or abnormal labor. However, despite the general lack of medical facilities in many developing countries, cesarean section is still the most common surgical procedure performed in the developing world.[3]

Surgery

Accurately quantifying the number of surgical procedures is very difficult in resource-poor regions. However, it is known that rates of major surgical operations in Sub-Saharan Africa are 70–500 per 100,000 population per year. Corresponding figures in high-income industrialized countries are 5000–9000.[4] The majority of nonobstetric surgical procedures in Sub-Saharan Africa are operative management of injuries, abdominal emergencies, hernia repair, and hydrocele repair. The lack of surgical and anesthetic services results in large quantities of surgical pathology being untreated; those patients who are treated have often travelled long distances and present with advanced pathology. As a result, a high proportion of emergency surgery ensues. Thus, it must be assumed that levels of preoperative pain from the underlying condition and postoperative pain are high.

AVAILABILITY AND EFFECTIVENESS OF ANALGESIA

In the majority of cases, pain relief for patients in the developing world is poor or nonexistent. The consequences of this untreated pain are not just humanitarian. Poor pain management leads to prolonged recovery, immobility, and an increase in cardiac, respiratory, and gastrointestinal complications. These in turn increase the burden on an already overstretched healthcare system and increase morbidity and mortality. In addition, chronic pain conditions may be increased leading to a further decrease in the quality of life and further humanitarian and economic suffering.

This acute deprivation is certainly widespread in Sub-Saharan Africa. Even when doctors and resources can

be accessed, pain relief still seems to be poor. Preoperative pain relief was evaluated in 100 patients in the accident and emergency department of the University Hospital in Ibadan, Nigeria; many were victims of trauma. Analgesia was not prescribed in around half of the patients, two-thirds of whom were in severe pain. Even when analgesia was prescribed, it was often inadequate; for example, 81 percent of those patients who were given preoperative analgesia had moderate to severe residual pain.[5] When assessing 149 postoperative patients in the same hospital, moderate to unbearable pain was reported in over two-thirds of patients at 24 hours and half at 48 hours.[6] Likewise, in obstetrics, a study in Benin City, Nigeria, found that only 39 percent of women received any form of labor analgesia in a large teaching hospital, despite the fact that 85 percent of the women requested it when asked.[7] In many smaller hospitals, analgesia is simply not an option. As all three of these studies are reported from large teaching hospitals, they may represent the better resourced centers. Conditions in more rural settings are largely unrecorded, but can be expected to be considerably worse.

When war and political instability are also present in a region, access to any health care – let alone analgesia – can be difficult, or even impossible. Dr Phil Lacoux of Médicins Sans Frontières (MSF) has recently highlighted the problems of providing analgesia in emergency situations.[8] His work in Sierra Leone and Sri Lanka has shown that analgesia is understandably often neglected, but also that even simple measures can have surprisingly good results.

BARRIERS TO ACUTE PAIN RELIEF

The "developing world" is an umbrella term that encompasses a wide range of countries united only by their lack of capital resources, poor infrastructure, and often political instability. In each country, differences in population, geography, resources, politics, and culture result in diverse problems in providing analgesia and variable attempts at solutions.

Population and geography

Despite rapidly increasing urbanization, the populations of developing countries are still generally predominately rural-based. Health services in these areas are often inadequate and cover vast areas. Poor roads and lack of transport hinder the distribution of medicine and equipment. Extremes of weather and high frequency of natural disasters further stretch these services. In contrast, the urban population often live in overcrowded conditions with poor sanitation and often scarcely better access to medical care.

Resources

To date, anesthesia and analgesia have received minimal funding and investment in countries where generalized lack of resources and trained staff mean that providing any health care is difficult. The magnitude of this problem has at least been recognized within the more developed world, and the International Society for the Prevention of Pain (ISAP) has been working in conjunction with the WHO to increase awareness of the problem and to improve access to pain relief to people in the developing world.[9] Many of these countries are already overburdened by diseases such as HIV/AIDS, tuberculosis, and malaria; analgesia is often still seen as a very low priority. **Table 21.1** shows the vast differences in spending on health care, numbers of doctors, and basic health indices between the developing and more developed world.

Resources usually taken for granted in more developed countries may be a luxury in the developing world. A recent survey of anesthetic facilities in 80 hospitals in Uganda found that 44 percent did not have running water all the time and 80 percent did not have a reliable source of electricity.[10] Only 45 percent always had access to morphine or pethidine (meperidine). The fact that access to running water was virtually the same as access to opioid drugs illustrates the complexity of the situation. Limited funding often means that money is spent on short-term urgent priorities, rather than on long-term planning. Budgeting is often hampered by fluctuating exchange rates causing escalation of the price of even basic items. These problems, coupled with charitable donations, can result in imbalances, such as patients having access to computed tomography (CT) scanning, but no access to simple drugs, such as paracetamol.

In many areas, the problems associated with the general lack of resources are further compounded by poor management, corruption, and lack of training. This leads to available resources being poorly utilized. These phenomena are by no means confined to the developing world; however, in these resource-poor settings, the affects are more acutely felt by staff and patients.

Evidence of the importance of good management can be seen in the success of mission hospitals in many parts of the world. These hospitals often survive on similar budgets to the government hospitals that they support. However, because of their smaller size, careful management, and accountability, they often produce a much better service for patients.

Storage and transport of drugs

Most commonly used analgesic drugs do not require refrigeration, but can be ruined by the heat and humidity present in many developing countries. More importantly, transport, fuel, a driver, and passable roads are required to transport drugs from the cities into rural hospitals. Tragically, this basic lack can lead to drugs sitting unused in warehouses. Poor hospital/healthcare management also has a role to play; it is not uncommon to find that drugs are going out of date in a warehouse because no one knows that they are there or where they should be sent.

Opioid availability

Opioids are essential in the management of moderate and severe pain. However, opioid availability and use is not uniform across the globe. Morphine is a low-cost, effective analgesic; in 1999, 87 percent of the world's morphine was consumed by ten major industrial countries (Australia, Canada, Denmark, France, Germany, Japan, Spain, Sweden, United Kingdom, and United States). The remaining 85 percent of the world population consumed 13 percent.[11]

Globally, the average consumption of morphine is 5.9 mg per capita. The figure is approximately 20–75 mg per capita in industrial nations. In comparison, mean consumption is 0.7[12] in Africa, 5.66 in Latin America,[13]

Table 21.1 Health economic data for a number of developed and developing nations.

Country	GDP per capita Int$	Life expectancy at birth M/F	Child mortality M/F per 1000	Total health expenditure Int$	Total health expenditure as % of GDP	Physicians per 1000 population
USA	39,901	75/80	8/7	5711	15.2	2.56
UK	31,308	76/81	6/5	2389	8	2.30
Bangladesh	2098	62/63	81/73	68	3.4	0.26
Belize	7151	65/72	44/33	309	4.5	1.05
Bolivia	2762	63/66	70/68	176	6.7	1.22
Vietnam	3298	69/74	24/22	164	5.4	0.53
Laos	1878	58/60	88/78	56	3.2	0.59
Uganda	1088	48/52	144/132	75	7.3	0.08
Malawi	519	41/41	179/172	46	9.3	0.02

Source: WHO website, www.who.int.

and 1.05 mg per capita in Asia[11] (**Figure 21.1**). However, these data represent only a crude estimate of global usage obtained from data of opioids purchased by these countries; they provide no information on how the morphine was used, i.e. whether it was given for palliative care or acute pain, or whether it was given in sufficient dosage. Nevertheless, whilst there is no particular level that can be declared adequate or inadequate, the figures highlight the lack of opioid analgesics available in the developing world.

The WHO and the International Narcotics Control Board (INCB), who collate these data, are mainly interested in the use of opioids in palliative care. The introduction of the WHO analgesic ladder in 1986 and various other publications and initiatives[14, 15, 16] has led to an increase in opioid usage overall. However, the majority of these increases have been in the more developed world with minimal increases in the developing world.[11, 12, 13]

Globally, morphine is the most available opioid,[13] although pethidine is also extensively used, especially for acute pain. Thus, pethidine data may better represent usage of opioids for acute pain. **Table 21.2** shows the regional data for pethidine.

There are many barriers to opioid use in the developing world. There is a general fear of opioid medication with exaggerated concern over risks of side effects, addiction, misuse, and abuse. There is very little evidence to confirm these fears. In India, a palliative care nongovernmental organization, which dispensed 13.6 kg of morphine to 1723 patients on an outpatient basis, found no episodes of loss and theft and only minor errors in stock position representing 0.007 percent of the total opioids dispensed.[17]

At a governmental level, import restrictions may be overly restrictive and the laws regarding prescribing and dispensing opioids may make it virtually impossible to get opioids to patients. Forty-three percent of governments that responded to the INCB survey said that they require physicians to report to the government those patients who are prescribed opioid analgesics.[11] Opioid

Table 21.2 Regional consumption of pethidine in milligrams per capita for 1999.

Region	Per capita consumption of pethidine (mg/capita)
Global mean	3.90
African regional mean	1.60
Latin America mean	6.56
Asian regional mean	0.75

Source: Refs 11, 12, 13.

legislation can therefore have a massive effect on opioid consumption. In India, the introduction of the Narcotic Drugs and Psychotropic Substances Act, a piece of legislation that resulted in a massive increase in the bureaucracy associated with purchasing opioids, led to a fall in consumption of morphine of 97 percent, from 716 kg in 1985 to 18 kg in 1997.[17]

In summary, the principal barriers to opioid availability are:

- fear of addiction;
- fear of misuse;
- fear of side effects;
- restrictive national opioid legislation;
- lack of infrastructure;
- lack of finance;
- lack of prescribers.

Drug administration

Even when a drug is available in a clinic or hospital, actually getting it to the patient may still prove challenging. Even in the more developed world, analgesics are under-prescribed by doctors, under-administered by nurses, and under-requested by patients. These factors are also present in the developing world, but to a much greater extent.

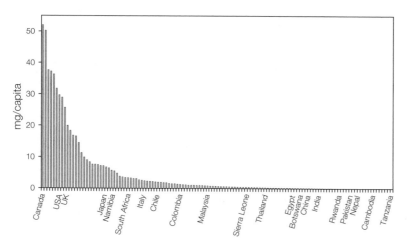

Figure 21.1 Morphine consumption in milligrams per capita. Source: Pain and Policy Studies Group. Availability of opioid analgesics in Asia: Consumption trends, Resources, Recommendations. University of Wisconsin Pain and Policy Studies Group/WHO Collaborating Center for Policy and Communications in Cancer Care, Madison, WI, USA. Prepared for 17th Study Programme for Overseas Experts on Drug Abuse and Narcotics Control, Tokyo, Japan, 26 June 2002 (monograph).

PRESCRIBING PROBLEMS

Doctors, nurses, or clinical officers may have received minimal or no training in the importance of analgesia and may have little practical idea of appropriate medications or techniques; drugs may thus never even be prescribed. There are severe shortages of medical staff in the developing world, partly due to lack of training and also due to doctors emigrating in search of better pay and living conditions.[18] The vast burden of clinical work is often performed by nonmedically trained healthcare workers who, at best, will only have received a basic training in analgesia yet perform valuable work with minimal resources. Desperate for more information and training, they are often unable to access the additional support required to improve their knowledge and clinical skills.

ADMINISTRATION PROBLEMS

Whilst nurses remain primarily responsible for dispensing drugs as they do in more developed countries, their wider function in developing countries is often very different. Wards are normally massively understaffed to the extent that one nurse may care for 50–80 patients, even more at night. Patient advocates, often the family of the patient, who stay with the patient on the ward, provide the majority of basic care, such as washing and feeding. It is normally left up to the patient or the patient's advocate to collect and then administer the prescribed drugs at the appropriate times from the nurse. Huge queues form at these times and those patients with no advocate may not receive any treatment.

The all-to-familiar lack of training is also a problem for nurses and it is a sad reality that those who are well trained or well motivated are lured into working in more developed countries, leaving undertrained and demotivated colleagues behind. This may result in patients in pain being ignored by nurses who are either not present due to staff shortages, or too overstretched or demotivated to help even when the drugs are present. Since this has been the way of practice for long periods of time, changing expectations, attitudes, and treatments can prove difficult.

This situation is sharply illustrated by an audit of postoperative analgesia in the Queen Elizabeth Central Hospital, Malawi, a government-funded university teaching hospital with 1000 beds. Despite the majority of patients having pethidine prescribed every four to six hours, it was found that the senior nurse (the only nurse with keys to the controlled drug cupboard) was only available during two ward rounds per day (midday and midnight). At other times, no opioid analgesia was available; the hospital had no paracetamol or nonsteroidal anti-inflammatory drugs (NSAID) in the pharmacy (Goddia, 2004, unpublished data).

Poor training also leads to fear of side effects in both medical and nursing staff which in turn leads to a culture of nonintervention: if you do nothing, no one can blame you. Arguably, a fatalistic attitude pervades: the common perception is that pain is to be expected and if death occurs secondary to an untreated condition, nature has taken its course. Poor outcomes then perpetuate this attitude and erode further the expectation of staff of their ability to treat pain.

PATIENT FACTORS

Given the poor quality of medical care and low quantities of analgesia available in the majority of the developing world, it is unsurprising to find that patients have low knowledge, expectations, and a distrust of western medicine. Many patients will have no knowledge of western medical care; 37 percent of patients in labor in a Nigerian teaching hospital had no knowledge of the possibility of labor analgesia on admission.[7] Many may have preferred to rely on traditional medicine, or use it in combination with whatever western medicine was offered. Little is known about interactions between the two, although the WHO is currently undertaking research into the use of traditional medicine globally.[19]

Because of the severely limited resources, hospitals gain a reputation as a place to die rather than a place to be cured. As a result, patients often wait until traditional medicine has failed and then present with advanced pathology. This results in a higher death rate and perpetuates the poor reputation of the hospital. Lack of adequate analgesia leads patients to believe that severe pain is to be expected after injury or surgery; as a result, they do not seek or expect analgesia and are also less likely to submit freely to necessary surgery or treatment, unless the pain or disability related to the underlying condition is severe. Should a visiting doctor from a developing country try to assess pain and intervene, he or she may not speak local languages, and may have little experience of local health beliefs. This hampers pain assessment and can be compounded by the translator having similar health beliefs to the patient.

In many African cultures, any form of illness is seen as a curse or spell placed upon the patient by either an individual or malevolent spirit. Traditional healers in this situation focus on identifying the culprit and reversing the spell. In these cultures, it may be difficult to impose modern medicine on the patient.

PRACTICAL TECHNIQUES AND SOLUTIONS

This section focuses on practical techniques for the delivery and administration of analgesia that can be used in the developing world. All of the techniques used in the more developed world and found to be effective may be used. However, given the lack of resources in the developing world, some techniques may be more appropriate than others. Improvements are most likely to result from application of simple techniques introduced with effective training and supplies.

Pain assessment

Despite the shortage of nursing staff on the wards, assessment of pain should become a basic observation along with pulse and blood pressure. Assessment tools need to be simple to use and understand. All techniques require the ability to explain the concept in the local language. Verbal rating scales require directly translatable words, something that may be difficult to acquire. Numerical scales require the patient to have a degree of numeracy. Visual analog scales do not require a degree of numeracy or literacy, but may be a difficult concept to explain. Scales that require observation of patient characteristics or behavior may be useful where communication is difficult.

Therapeutic interventions

These can take the form of psychological, pharmacological, or local anesthetic-based techniques.

PSYCHOLOGICAL INTERVENTION

Patient information and reassurance is an important component of pain management. Many patients in pain receive no explanation as to the underlying cause, treatment options, and prognosis of their condition. This approach results in a helpless, dependent patient who may assume that the pain indicates that their underlying problem is much more serious.

PHARMACOLOGICAL THERAPY

The WHO has outlined a standard approach to cancer pain in the developing world with the analgesic ladder coupled to some basic principles (**Figure 21.2**).[20][V] It has shown that good quality pain relief is achievable with minimal resources and minimal cost. Unlike chronic cancer pain, acute pain tends to be most severe at the time of the insult and then diminishes. As a result, the World Federation of Societies of Anaesthesiologists (WFSA) has produced a modified analgesic ladder for acute pain (**Figure 21.3**).[21][V] This is similar to the WHO ladder, but in reverse. Starting with strong parenteral opioids and or local anesthetic, there is then a step down to oral opioids and finally to NSAIDs and paracetamol alone.

This ladder should be coupled with some basic principles of acute pain management:

- Assessment:
  - cause of the pain;
  - severity of the pain;
  - patient factors, allergies, contraindications;
  - routes available: oral, intravenous, rectal.
- Treatment:
  - Local anesthetic techniques should be used when possible.
  - Adequate analgesic drugs should be prescribed regularly with extra drugs available for breakthrough pain.
  - Use the oral route where possible.
  - Use nonopioid drugs for their opioid-sparing effects.

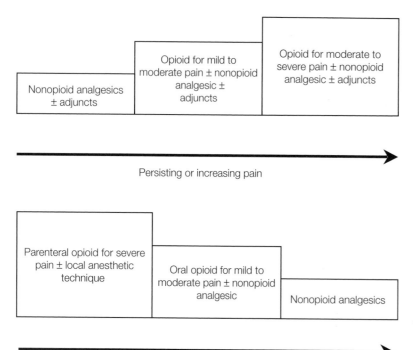

Figure 21.2   World Health Organization analgesic ladder. Redrawn from *Cancer pain relief: with a guide to opioid availability*, 2nd edn. Geneva: World Health Organization, 1996: 13–36, with permission.

Figure 21.3   World Federation of Societies of Anaesthesiologists (WFSA) analgesic ladder. Redrawn from Charlton E. The management of post-operative pain. *Update in Anaesthesia.* 1997; **7**: 1-7, with permission.

The WHO also produces a list of drugs that it believes are essential for the treatment of priority diseases which includes a section on analgesics and local anesthetics as shown in **Table 21.3**.[22] Increasingly, the WHO is trying to base its choices on evidence and there are few surprises: all of the drugs have been used for many years and most are backed by a considerable number of trials.[23]

Ketamine is the main anesthetic drug used in areas of the developing world where access to trained anesthetic staff is limited. It provides profound analgesia and dissociative anesthesia. In lower doses (for example, 0.1–0.5 mg/kg i.v.), it can be used as an analgesic. Classically, it has been used for short periods of intense pain, such as during dressing changes for burns. Its use is limited mainly by unpleasant emergence phenomenon. However, it may have a role when other forms of potent analgesic, such as opioids are unavailable. There are sporadic case reports of the use of mixtures of dilute ketamine, tramadol, and diclofenac added to liter bags of Hartmann's solution and administered over eight hours to provide analgesia for postoperative pain relief after laparotomy.[24] Whilst not a technique that can be recommended in all situations, it provided good analgesia to patients in an extremely resource-poor area.

Modes of delivery

In most cases, the oral route is the most convenient; it requires no training and no equipment. Unfortunately, it is common in acute pain secondary to surgery or trauma for the enteral route to be unavailable. Per rectum medication can be used when the oral route is not available, but cultural perceptions may hinder acceptance of this route. Few medications are absorbed sublingually.

When the enteral route is unavailable, intramuscular injection is most commonly used, requiring minimal training and with minimal complications. Intravenous administration of drugs, especially opioids, is possible, but careful training and monitoring is required to avoid complications. Loading with intravenous morphine during sugery, when postoperative pain is anticipated is practical.

The benefits of patient-controlled analgesia (PCA) have been demonstrated in the more developed world, but a lack of equipment and the need for careful ward monitoring of these devices mean that in many developing countries they cannot be used.

LOCAL ANESTHESIA

Local anesthetic techniques can provide excellent postoperative pain relief and generally their use should be encouraged. However, there are important limitations in the developing world due to the side effects of some of the treatments.

Spinal anesthesia is often a mainstay in the developing world. When appropriate preservative-free opioids are available, the intrathecal administration of these drugs can prolong analgesia long after the anesthetic effect has passed. However, there are risks of excessive sedation and respiratory depression that may be difficult to detect and manage safely in resource-poor wards. Where

Table 21.3 WHO essential drugs that can be used in acute pain.

Drug	Dose
Anesthetic medications	
Ketamine	Injection 50 mg (as hydrochloride)/ml in 10-ml vial.
Local anesthetics	
Bupivacaine	Injection 0.25%, 0.5% (hydrochloride) in vial.
	Injection for spinal anesthesia, 0.5% (hydrochloride) in 4-ml ampoule to be mixed with 7.5% glucose solution
Lidocaine	Injection 1%, 2% (hydrochloride) in vial.
	Injection for spinal anesthesia, 5% (hydrochloride) in 2-ml ampoule to be mixed with 7.5% glucose solution.
	Topical forms, 2–4% (hydrochloride)
Lidocaine + epinephrine (adrenaline) injection	1%, 2% (hydrochloride) + epinephrine 1:200,000 in vial; dental cartridge 2% (hydrochloride) + epinephrine 1:80,000
Analgesics, antipyretics, nonsteroidal anti-inflammatory drugs (NSAIDs)	
Acetylsalicylic acid	Tablet 100–500 mg; suppository 50–150 mg
Ibuprofen	Tablet 200 mg, 400 mg
Paracetamol	Tablet 100–500 mg; suppository 100 mg; syrup 125 mg/5 mL
Codeine	Tablet 30 mg (phosphate)
Morphine	Injection 10 mg in 1-mL ampoule (sulfate or hydrochloride); oral solution 10 mg (hydrochloride or sulfate)/5 mL; tablet 10 mg (sulfate)

Source: World Health Organization. *Essential medicines. WHO model list*, 14th edn. Geneva: World Health Organization, 2005.

high-dependency unit (HDU) facilities can be provided, these techniques are effective and easy to implement.

Epidural anesthesia is used in a number of developing countries, although continuous infusions of drugs via epidural catheters to prolong analgesia is often impossible due to lack of equipment, expertise, and staff to monitor the effects. Where HDU facilities are available, combinations of preservative opioids and local anesthetics provide very effective pain relief.

Single shot caudal analgesia for lower limb and perineal surgery in children is very practical, and where preservative-free ketamine is available, a prolonged effect may be produced by a combination of bupivacaine and ketamine (0.5 mg/kg). Clonidine (1 µg/kg) has also been used in combination with local anesthetic and is equally effective, but produces some sedation and should not be used for patients under three months of age.[25][II]

Plexus blockade can provide very useful anesthesia and analgesia where the expertise and equipment exists to provide them. These blocks can provide excellent analgesia in the immediate postoperative period and may produce analgesia lasting up to 24 hours. Many blocks are simply learned or taught, but their reliability is considerably improved by the use of a nerve stimulator. It is often difficult to prolong analgesia unless continuous infusions through sterile catheters via infusion pumps can be provided. Additionally, the techniques require training for ward staff and careful postoperative monitoring.

Local infiltration of wounds with a long-acting local anesthetic, such as bupivicaine, provides a degree of postoperative analgesia and should be encouraged.

Long-acting local anesthetics, such as bupivacaine, are essential to prolong analgesia after a procedure. However, lidocaine is generally cheaper and more commonly available. The use of opioids, ketamine, and ephedrine, in addition to local anesthetic in central neuroaxial or plexus blocks may prolong useful analgesia. However, care must be taken to ensure sterility of the drugs used, especially as many drugs are presented in multiple-use ampoules, and to avoid drug formulations containing preservative.

Drug cost and availability

Most of the commonly used analgesic medications are well established and manufactured "off licence," allowing inexpensive production. If therapies are limited to these simple established medications (for example, paracetamol, NSAIDs, morphine), expense should be minimal. Costs will obviously be affected by the ability to produce a drug locally, import taxes, and the costs of distribution. The WHO estimates that if barriers to access morphine in the developing world could be removed, then a reasonable estimate of the cost of morphine would be 1 US cent per milligram.[26] Recent research has shown that the current situation in those developing countries that do have access to morphine is very different. A survey

of opioid cost in 2003 showed that opioid drugs were considerably more expensive in the developing world when compared with the more developed world (median cost of a 30-day supply of an opioid was US$ 112 compared with US$ 53). This is equivalent to 36 percent of gross national product per capita per month for the developing world compared with only 3 percent for the developed world – a ten-fold difference.[27]

There are no cost-effectiveness analyses of analgesic interventions in acute pain in the developing world. If similar trends are seen in the developing world as in the more developed world, then it may be expected that, in a postoperative setting, good analgesia may result in reduced hospital stay, decreased postoperative complications, and a more rapid return to activity. These must lead to cost savings in an already over-stretched healthcare system and are likely to offset the costs of simple analgesic drugs.

In many countries, drugs that are available commercially in pharmacies may not be available in hospitals. In these cases, patients with sufficient funds can be asked to purchase their own analgesic drugs. Alternatively, charitable funds can be used to purchase drugs to use within the hospital. In private hospital systems, most drugs are available. Unfortunately, few patients have access to these. Where supplies of drugs are inadequate, donations from the developed world can be very important. However, these drugs should be appropriate and not out of date.

AN APPROACH TO ANALGESIA IN A DEVELOPING COUNTRY AS A VISITING EXPERT

It is not uncommon for overseas visitors to be asked their opinion on how to resolve difficulties with a range of clinical situations. Whenever this occurs, a knowledge of the local situation and the barriers to change should be taken into account so that effective local solutions are suggested rather than impractical concepts. The following approach is suggested:

- Consult with local staff at different levels.
- Find out what happens currently.
- Find out why other techniques are not used:
  - equipment?
  - drugs?
  - knowledge?
- Start with a simple strategy.
- Implement basic first steps.
- Teach staff.
- Assess whether implementation has been effective.
- Audit your results.
- Do not expect to make major changes in the short term, e.g. government policy on opioids, staff levels on wards.
- Solutions adopted by local staff will last after you have left. Techniques dependent on the expert visitor will stop after they have left!

Box 21.1 Case study: Malawi

Country statistics

- Population: 12.8 million
- Rural:urban: 85%:15%
- GDP per capita: US$519
- Life expectancy: 41 years
- Spending on medical care:
  - Per capita per year: US$46
  - % of GDP: 9.3
- No. physicians per 1000 population: 0.02

Healthcare system

Government healthcare system free to all, supplemented by mission hospitals

Queen Elizabeth Central Hospital (QECH) Blantyre

- Main teaching hospital in commercial capital
- Tertiary referral hospital for southern Malawi
- 1000 beds, over 100% bed occupancy
- Departments: Medicine, Surgery, Orthopaedics, Paediatrics, Opthalmology, Obstetrics and Gynaecology.

Case 1

- Fit 30-year-old man
- RTA minibus versus bicycle
- Open fractured tibia and fibula for open reduction, debridement, and fixation
- Preoperative analgesia:
  - Nil despite long journey from crash site in back of police truck to local hospital then transfer from local hospital.
  - Intramuscular pethidine on ward at QECH.
- Anesthesia:
  - Spinal with bupivicaine if available (5% lidocaine readily available, but very short acting) or general anesthesia with 50 mg meperidine as analgesia.

- Postoperative analgesia:
  - Pethidine 50 mg i.m. as needed
- Short-term ways to improve analgesia:
  - Patient's family to buy paracetamol or NSAIDs (costs may be prohibitive).
  - Department to use charitable funds to buy bupivicaine to allow use of long-acting regional techniques.
- Long-term ways to improve analgesia:
  - Improve training of clinical officers in the district hospital and QECH.
  - Improve drug supplies to hospital.
  - Improve staffing on wards.

Case 2

- 19-year-old female in labor for 36 hours
- Diagnosis: cephalopelvic disproportion
- Plan: cesarean section
  - Labor analgesia: Nil
  - Anesthetic: spinal 5% lidocaine heavy
  - Postoperative analgesia: i.m. pethidine 50 mg
- Short-term ways to improve analgesia:
  - supplies to get heavy bupivacaine and local infiltration;
  - patient's family to buy paracetamol or NSAIDs (costs often prohibitive).
- Long-term ways to improve analgesia:
  - improve training of clinical officers and midwives in the district hospital and QECH;
  - improve drug supplies to hospital;
  - improve staffing on wards.

Box 21.1 uses two case studies from Malawi to illustrate some of the problems that may be faced in a developing country and suggests some possible solutions.

CONCLUSIONS

The more developed world clearly has a responsibility to improve the care of people in the developing world. Improved funding is an important part of the solution, but only alongside the adoption of simple, cost-effective, and appropriate techniques. Basic drugs need to be kept in production and healthcare managers must ensure

regular supplies are always available in clinical areas. Staff at all levels need to be trained in the use of specific techniques and challenged to change beliefs that pain is a necessary evil. Patients also need to be encouraged to become more aware that pain is treatable, while politicians should carry the banner that unrelieved pain is unacceptable.

REFERENCES

1. Mathers CD, Lopez AD, Murray CJL. The burden of disease and mortality by condition: data, methods, and results for

2001. In: Lopez AD, Mathers CD, Ezzati M *et al.* (eds). *Global burden of disease and risk factors*. New York: The World Bank and Oxford University Press, 2006: 45–180.

2. Graham WJ, Cairns J, Bhattacharya S *et al.* Maternal and perinatal conditions. In: Jamison DT, Breman JG, Measham AR *et al.* (eds). *Disease control priorities in developing countries*, 2nd edn. New York: The World Bank and Oxford University Press, 2006: 499–529.

3. Fenton PM. The epidemiology of district surgery in Malawi. *East Central Africa Journal of Surgery*. 1997; **3**: 33–41.

4. Nordberg E. Surgical operations in eastern Africa: a review with conclusions regarding the need for further research. *East African Medical Journal*. 1990; **67** (Suppl. 3): 1–28.

5. Aisuodionoe-Shadrach OI, Olapade-Olaopa EO, Soyannwo OA. Preoperative analgesia in emergency surgical care in Ibadan. *Central African Journal of Medicine*. 2001; **47**: 70–4.

6. Faponle AF, Soyannwo OA, Ajayi IO. Postoperative pain therapy: a survey of prescribing patterns and adequacy of analgesia in Ibadan, Nigeria. *West African Journal of Medicine*. 1999; **18**: 207–10.

7. Imarengiaye CO, Ande AB. Demand and utilisation of labour analgesia service by Nigerian women. *Journal of Obstetrics and Gynaecology*. 2006; **26**: 130–2.

8. Moszynski P. Pain control often neglected in war areas. *BMJ*. 2004; **328**: 1398.

9. Bond M, Breivik H. Why pain control matters in a world full of killer diseases. *Pain: Clinical Updates*. 2004; **12**: 1–4.

✱ 10. Hodges SC, Okello M, Mijumbi C *et al.* Anaesthesia services in developing countries: defining the problems. *Anaesthesia*. 2007; **62**: 4–11.

11. Pain and Policy Studies Group. Availability of opioid analgesics in Asia: consumption trends, resources, recommendations. University of Wisconsin Pain and Policy Studies Group/WHO Collaborating Center for Policy and Communications in Cancer Care, Madison, WI. Prepared for 17th Study Programme for Overseas Experts on Drug Abuse and Narcotics Control, Tokyo, Japan, 26 June 2002 (monograph).

12. Pain and Policy Studies Group. Availability of opioid analgesics in Africa and the world. University of Wisconsin Pain and Policy Studies Group/WHO Collaborating Center for Policy and Communications in Cancer Care, Madison, WI. Prepared for A Community Health Approach to Palliative Care for HIV/AIDS and Cancer Patients in Africa Gaborone, Botswana, 9–12 July 2002 (monograph).

13. Pain and Policy Studies Group. Availability of opioid analgesics in Latin America and the world. University of

Wisconsin Pain and Policy Studies Group/WHO Collaborating Center for Policy and Communications in Cancer Care, Madison, WI. Prepared for 1st Congress of the Latin American Association of Palliative Care, 7th Latin American Course on Medicine and Palliative Care, Guadalajara, Mexico, 20–22 March 2002 (monograph).

14. World Health Organization. *Cancer pain relief: with a guide to opioid availability*, 2nd edn. Geneva: World Health Organization, 1996.

15. World Health Organization. *Achieving balance in national opioid control policy: guidelines for assessment*. Geneva: World Health Organization, 2000.

16. International Narcotics Control Board. Availability of opiates for medical needs. In: Anon. Report of the International Narcotics Control Board for 1995. New York: United Nations, 1996.

17. Rajagopal MR, Joranson DE, Gilson AM. Medical use, misuse, and diversion of opioids in India. *Lancet*. 2001; **358**: 139–43.

18. Eastwood J, Conroy RE, Naicker S *et al.* Loss of health professionals from sub-Saharan Africa: The pivotal role of the UK. *Lancet*. 2005; **365**: 1893–900.

19. World Health Organization. *WHO traditional medicine strategy, 2002–2005*. Geneva: World Health Organization, 2002.

✱ 20. World Health Organization. *Cancer pain relief: with a guide to opioid availability*, 2nd edn. Geneva: World Health Organization, 1996: 13–36.

✱ 21. Charlton E. The management of post operative pain. *Update in Anaesthesia*. 1997; **7**: 1–7.

22. World Health Organization. *Essential medicines. WHO model list*, 14th edn. Geneva: World Health Organization, 2005.

23. Wifen F. An evidence base for WHO 'essential analgesics'. *World Anaesthesia News*. 2000; **5**: 3–5.

24. King C. Postoperative analgesia in rebel territory in Cote d'Ivoire. *Anaesthesia*. 2005; **60**: 419.

25. Berg S. Paediatric and neonatal anaesthesia. In: Allman K, Wilson I (eds). *Oxford handbook of anaesthesia*, 2nd edn. Oxford: Oxford University Press, 2006: 784–7.

26. Foley KM, Wagner JL, Joranson DE, Gelband H. Pain control for people with cancer and AIDS. In: Jamison DT, Breman JG, Measham AR *et al.* (eds). *Disease control priorities in developing countries*, 2nd edn. New York: The World Bank and Oxford University Press, 2006: 981–93.

27. De Lima L, Sweeney C, Palmer JL, Bruera E. Potent analgesics are more expensive for patients in developing countries: a comparative study. *Journal of Pain and Palliative Care Pharmacotherapy*. 2004; **18**: 59–70.

22

Acute pain management in burns

JOHN KINSELLA AND COLIN P RAE

KEY LEARNING POINTS

- Burn pain can be divided into three categories: background, breakthrough, and procedural, which require separate treatment strategies.
- The intensity of burn pain is unpredictable, often severe and inadequately treated.
- Intravenous opioids, titrated to effect, are the mainstay of acute management.
- Peripheral and central mechanisms contribute to burn pain and the development of chronic pain.

- Multimodal analgesia should be utilized, including the use of antineuropathic agents such as tricyclic antidepressants and anticonvulsants.
- There is interest in the use of agents to reduce central sensitization or "wind up."
- A biopsychsocial model should be used when managing chronic burn pain.

INTRODUCTION

Pain is an almost inevitable consequence of burns and is often undertreated.[1] The intensity of pain that will be experienced after a burn injury by an individual is unpredictable.[2] Burn pain has three major components: background pain (pain at rest), breakthrough pain (e.g. pain following activities such as turning in bed or walking), and procedural pain (e.g. pain during wound care procedures). It is characterized by primary and secondary hyperalgesia.[3] Pain may still be present long after the burn has healed, causing continued impairment of function. The likelihood of developing chronic pain and associated psychological morbidity can be reduced with appropriate and aggressive acute pain control.[4] In this chapter, the mechanisms and time-course of burn pain are described and the various strategies available to treat burn pain are discussed.

MECHANISMS OF BURN PAIN

- Severity of burn pain cannot be predicted from depth or area of burn.
- Burn pain is divided into background, breakthrough, and procedural pain.
- Severity of pain is linked to psychological morbidity.

Burn injury

Cutaneous burns remain a common cause of accidental injury. In the UK, there were 532 fire deaths and 14,400 nonfatal injuries in 2004.[5] The number of fires in the UK and worldwide is falling. For example, fire and burn deaths in the United States declined approximately 60 percent from 1971 to 1998.[6] The mortality of burn injuries has declined significantly due to advances in treatment. In 1984, the total body surface area burn lethal to 50 percent of patients was 65 percent. This had improved to 81 percent by the early 1990s.[7]

Burn injury causes local cell death. This is followed by variable amounts of healing, regeneration, scarring, and contraction. Modern surgical management is directed at accurate assessment of depth of burn, early surgery, and excision of necrotic tissue to reduce infection, and early wound closure to promote maximal functional and esthetic recovery.[8] Much attention is directed to factors that influence survival, such as resuscitation, smoke inhalation, and intensive care. Pain management is also of considerable importance.

Burn wound depth is important because of the potential damage to nerve endings and the subsequent pain sensation. The depth of burn wound may be classified[8] as:

- superficial, in which the epidermal damage heals within a week;
- superficial partial thickness, in which the epidermis is completely destroyed along with more superficial dermis. As most adnexal structures survive, this injury heals within two weeks without scarring;
- deep partial thickness, in which epidermis and substantial parts of dermis including nerve endings are destroyed, leading to incomplete healing over several weeks;
- full thickness, in which all skin elements including nerve endings are destroyed with variable involvement of underlying structures.

In theory, depth may be used to predict the amount of pain that is likely to be experienced. In practice, there is no reliable way of predicting pain intensity from the characteristics of the burn injury.[2] Pain from superficial partial thickness burns may be severe, as nerve endings are damaged but continue to function. The pain is variable and exacerbated by contact with different surfaces and when the affected areas are cleaned and dressed. In deep partial thickness burns, not all nerve endings are destroyed, so the ability to detect pain remains. Pain should, in theory, be absent in full-thickness burns as the nerve endings are destroyed. Surprisingly, patients with full-thickness burns tend to have the most pain.[9] This can be explained by the increased frequency and intensity of therapeutic procedures that the burn patient has to undergo and the presence of complex chronic pain with a neuropathic or sympathetically maintained component due to nerve endings growing back into the granulating area. The remote unburned skin sites that are used for donor skin may be as painful, or more painful, than burned areas.[10]

Characteristics of pain after burn injury

Initially, at the time of burn injury, there is an immediate and massive stimulation of nociceptors in the damaged skin, which may be experienced as pain, irrespective of the depth of the burn.

INFLUENCE OF LEVEL OF CONSCIOUSNESS

As the patient's consciousness may be impaired at the time of injury – owing to factors commonly associated with burns injuries, including alcohol, smoke inhalation, epilepsy, and head injury – appreciation of this pain will vary. Interestingly, a significant proportion of patients who remain conscious after major burns, experience no pain in the early stages. It is thought that psychological factors play a major part in this response.

PERIPHERAL MECHANISMS

A number of polymodal cutaneous nociceptors sensitive to heat have been identified. C-fibers responsive to mechanical and heat stimulation predominate, but two A-fiber nociceptors are also sensitive to heat and mechanical stimuli. Once the skin is damaged by the burn, the response to further stimuli is altered by the development of increased sensitivity to pain both in the burned skin and in the surrounding, apparently normal, skin.[11] This is the result of the development of primary and secondary hyperalgesia.[3] Primary hyperalgesia is due to sensitization and continued stimulation of peripheral nociceptors by a number of inflammatory mediators, such as substance P, bradykinin, histamine, and calcitonin gene related peptide.[12] In the area of primary hyperalgesia, there is increased sensitivity to both mechanical and thermal stimuli. Even normally nonpainful stimuli such as light pressure may be painful (allodynia).[13] Some patients have spontaneous pain.

CENTRAL MECHANISMS

Secondary hyperalgesia is thought to be due to changes within the dorsal horn of the spinal cord leading to sensitization and lowering of the thresholds of neurons involved in pain transmission within the dorsal horn. It has been demonstrated that these wide dynamic range neurons increase their receptive field in response to peripheral stimulation following tissue damage.[14] Thus, the apparently normal skin surrounding a burn may demonstrate abnormal sensitivity to painful (hyperalgesia) and normally nonpainful (allodynia) stimuli. The initial injury and repeated painful insults lead to central sensitization or spinal cord "wind up" and further amplification of the pain. The development of spinal cord wind up and secondary hyperalgesia has been extensively investigated in the search for more effective analgesia.[15, 16] The use in the experimental situation of preinjury local analgesics with lidocaine (lignocaine) only has a mild effect on the development of hyperalgesia.[17][III] Prolonged application of local anesthetic cream to the injured area does not affect subsequent hyperalgesia.[18][III] Much of the hypersensitivity and dysesthesia decreases as the burn wound heals.[2] Although bradykinin is thought to have a role in this process, these findings can be reproduced in the presence of kininogen deficiency, which indicates that other mechanisms are also involved.[19] Following thermal injury, a peripheral antinociceptive effect of morphine can be demonstrated. The practical relevance for this in managing burn pain is unclear.[20] Gabapentin reduces hyperalgesia induced by burn injury.[21][III] This may open up new avenues for pain relief following burns. The efficacy of N-methyl-D-aspartate (NMDA) antagonists such as ketamine, memantine, and dextromorphan in preventing secondary hyperalgesia confirms that central sensitization plays an important role in pain management.[22][II], [23][II], [24][II] In addition to local and spinal cord changes, a number of other factors also affect the patient's experience and response to burn pain and form the basis for psychological and distraction therapies.

NOCICEPTIVE AND NEUROPATHIC PAIN

Patients with a burn injury often have pain symptoms and signs consistent with a diagnosis of neuropathic pain. It is important to recognize neuropathic pain as it may be more effectively treated with adjunctive analgesics, such as tricyclic antidepressants and anticonvulsants.

Background, breakthrough, and procedural pain

Practically, the pain experienced by burns patients can be divided into three categories: background, breakthrough, and procedural pain. Background pain is experienced continually. It correlates poorly with the severity of the burn. It remains fairly constant in the absence of major interventions, may be significant and requires treatment.[2] If it is not treated adequately it predisposes to the development of chronic pain and anxiety about the severity of procedural pain. It can usually be managed by relatively simple analgesic regimens. Background pain tends to be worse in the first week after injury and usually decreases with time.[25] Minor routine activity may lead to further pain. Some patients also describe spontaneous pain more consistent with a diagnosis of neuropathic pain.

Procedures including physiotherapy, dressing changes, and surgery are associated with short lasting, acute pain which requires much more intense analgesia. The pain of some procedures may be so severe that general anesthesia is needed.[9]

Evolution of burn pain

Effective pain management following burn injury is made more difficult by the unpredictable severity and nature of pain over time.[2, 9] Background pain will usually gradually reduce as the burn wounds heal and skin cover is achieved. In some patients though, pain appears to increase with time.[10] This may be due to complications such as infection or the development of neuropathic or complex regional pain syndromes. In one study, more than 80 percent of patients still had tingling, stiffness, cold sensations, or numbness and 35 percent complained of pain in the scarred tissue one year after the injury.[2] In one study, more than half of the patients with symptoms over a year after the burn have impairment of daily living as a result. Approximately half still had significant pain after an average of 12 years from time of injury.[26] Long-term sequelae include sensory loss, abnormal pain sensation, and chronic pain syndromes, especially in those areas that have been grafted or where the burn was deep.[27]

Effect of psychological factors on burn pain

Psychological factors may greatly influence the patient's appreciation of, and response to, pain. The psychological consequences of the burn, combined with the premorbid psychological state of the patient, may lead to severe psychological problems that may be long lasting.[28] Depression may increase the patient's report of pain.[2] Patients who exhibit the greatest posttraumatic stress experience greater levels of pain at rest and during procedures.[29, 30] Patients who experience severe pain during procedures have an increased risk of psychological morbidity.[31] Careful attention to pain management is especially important following burn injury in children.[32]

ASSESSMENT OF BURN PAIN

Pain has been managed for years without formal assessment of severity or recording of response to treatment. Pain measurement tools have commonly been used in research, but it is only relatively recently that routine assessment of pain in clinical practice has become widespread.

For detailed assessment, the most widely used technique is the McGill Pain Questionnaire.[2, 33] This is accepted as a good test for pain that is relatively stable. Owing to the length of time it takes to complete, its role in measuring acute or rapidly changing pain is limited.

The use of observations made by medical or nursing staff caring for the burned patient is limited by the lack of good correlation between staff and patient assessments of pain.[34, 35] The effects of analgesics may be overestimated by nurses.[36] Similarly, retrospective patient reports of pain do not accurately measure the severity of present pain. Ideally, it is best to have the patient report their pain at the time. The measurement tools used should be as simple as possible, as measurements will need to be repeated on a regular basis. In some centers, the multicultural mix of patients with different languages and cultural backgrounds makes pain reporting difficult.

Pain scoring systems commonly used are:

- verbal rating;
- verbal numerical;
- visual analog.

Simple verbal rating scores of pain (e.g. none, mild, moderate, severe) are commonly used as changes are easy to interpret. However, they are more difficult to analyze and to use for interpatient comparisons. In our experience, scores with more than five categories can lead to confusion. To overcome these problems, visual analog or verbal numerical rating scales can be used. These are easier to deal with statistically but have practical difficulties. A visual analog scale ruler/thermometer can be used for children or if there are language problems.[37, 38] Other quantitative scores such as the Children's Hospital of Eastern Ontario Pain Score (CHEOPS) may be used by nurses for pediatric patients.[39] Pain measurement is essential if analgesic protocols are to be adapted to the needs of individual patients. The scoring system used is less important than the consistent application of a score that is recorded at frequent intervals for background pain and during procedures.

Simple, widely applied, and regularly used measurements of pain are recommended.

TREATMENT OF BURN PAIN

Following the burn injury, patients are subjected to a number of maneuvers that may be painful. These include removal from the fire, resuscitation, transportation to a hospital, assessment, and urgent procedures, such as intravenous access, control of the airway, urethral catheter insertion, radiographs, escharotomies, and transport to the burns unit or intensive care unit. Pain management is an important issue during all these maneuvers. Initially, the patient's pain may be severe or surprisingly mild, but the severity is rarely recorded. The perception of pain by the patient may also be affected by alcohol, a post-ictal state, prescribed or recreational drugs, or other causes of altered levels of consciousness, such as smoke inhalation, hypoxia, or hypotension.

The management of burn pain, before formal assessment and stabilization, is very difficult to study. Recommendations are therefore based on observations and clinical experience. Simple measures, such as cooling[40][III] and covering the burn and immobilizing the patient, may suffice. Local cooling, however, does not prevent the development of hyperalgesia in humans.[41] Once appropriately trained personnel are available, on site or on arrival in the hospital, then parenteral opioid administration becomes the most widely used form of analgesia for patients with all but the most trivial burns. At this

stage, opioids should be administered intravenously as the intramuscular or subcutaneous routes are unreliable, particularly where hypovolemia and vasoconstriction are present. Irrespective of the opioid chosen, titration of small intravenous bolus doses is the most effective way to obtain pain relief. Once control is obtained, infusions or patient-controlled analgesia (PCA)[42, 43, 44][II] systems may be used. Analgesia can be provided by inhalation of a mixture of oxygen and nitrous oxide, in varying concentrations. Entonox, a 50:50 mixture of oxygen and nitrous oxide, is available in some countries,[45][III] but if smoke inhalation or another reason for hypoxia is present 100 percent oxygen will be needed. In addition to drug therapy, other essential approaches include reassurance and compassion, cooling of the burn wound,[46][III] positioning, and suitable support or beds that minimize pressure on the wound. Dressing the wound with a transparent cover such as clear plastic film allows repeated inspection in the early stages without removing the dressing. Fear, anxiety, awareness of their injury and injury to others, loss of property, and feelings of guilt or despair may exacerbate distress at this stage, especially if the injury was a result of attempted suicide.

Following initial resuscitation, an attempt should be made to distinguish between background pain and pain associated with procedures. A plan should be developed to treat each type of pain. Background pain may initially be treated with intravenous opioids by continuous infusion or PCA. Later, once adequate analgesia has been obtained and oral intake resumed, oral opioids and other oral analgesic agents may be used.[46][III] Multimodal analgesia using drugs with different mechanisms of action, such as paracetamol (acetamoniphen), nonsteroidals, local anesthetics opioids, and adjunctive analgesics improves analgesia and reduces side effects.

A separate plan is required for more severe procedural pain. This can vary from a slight increase in therapy for background pain to the use of short-acting potent opioids such as alfentanil[47][III] or remifentanil, local anesthetic blocks, or general anesthesia. In addition, a variety of psychological and supportive techniques in conjunction with drug-based management have been tried.[48][II], [49][II]

Opioids

Intravenous opioids remain the most popular method of reducing burn pain.[50, 51] Morphine has been widely used and investigated in this setting. The pharmacokinetics of morphine, and that of its principle active metabolites, do not differ significantly between patients with and patients without burns; as a result, similar doses can be used.[52][III], [53][III] In common with other opioids, morphine has sedative and antitussive properties and, depending on the route of administration, it has a relatively long duration of action. The metabolites of morphine, especially morphine-6-glucuronide, may play an active role in analgesia, especially when morphine is used for prolonged periods.[54] Morphine is commonly used as PCA for burn pain.[42, 43, 44][II] PCA is a useful method of adjusting dose to requirements as the pain levels may change quite rapidly due to movement and procedures, but there may also be a gradual increase in opioid requirements with time. As PCA is reliant on a patient's ability to use the equipment, fixed rate infusions have been used post-operatively in burns patients but seem to provide an initially inferior level of analgesia when the pain is most intense.[55][III]

Other opioids which are more commonly used during anesthesia have been to treat procedural pain. The more rapid onset, increased lipid solubility, and ease of titration of these drugs are potential advantages, although the potential respiratory depression from these potent analgesics is a concern. PCA fentanyl has been used to treat postoperative burn pain and it has also been successfully used by the intranasal route in pediatric patients.[56][III], [57][II] A randomized crossover study of patient-controlled intranasal fentanyl and oral morphine for burns dressing changes in adult patients found them to have similar efficacy and safety.[58] Two case series have described the successful use of alfentanil during dressing changes with no significant respiratory depression.[47][III], [59][III] Remifentanil, which is very rapid acting, has been used during burn surgery[60] and it may be feasible to use this outside the operating theater, although the safety of this drug in that setting would need to be established.

Pethidine (meperidine) may be administered by PCA, but problems with norpethidine (normeperidine) toxicity can occur, especially with high doses, prolonged use, or renal impairment.[61] Methadone administration has been described for burn pain, but its long and unpredictable half-life makes rapid titration difficult. It may be useful if there is a neuropathic component to the pain as there is evidence that it has activity at the NMDA receptor.[62][IV]

The use of agonist–antagonist drugs and partial agonists in order to reduce pure agonist-related side effects has also been described. Nalbuphine has been shown to be as effective as morphine for the relief of burn debridement pain, and has also been used successfully for prehospital analgesia.[63][IV], [64][IV] These drugs may be more expensive than pure agonists, but the ceiling on the respiratory depressant effect has potential advantages.

Other drugs, such as benzodiazepines, may be used in combination with opioids to provide greater degrees of anxiolysis; however, the risk of respiratory depression is greater.[65][III] Lorazepam, when combined with morphine, has been shown to improve analgesia in patients who have more severe pain.[66][IV]

Despite the widespread use of opioids to treat burn pain, psychological opioid addiction is unlikely to develop as a consequence of treating burn pain, although a physical dependence may occur.[67] Opioids are also theoretically associated with depression of immune function and in one retrospective study opioid usage was associated with an increased risk of infection in patients with small burns.[68] It has also been noted that the increasing dosage of opioids used to treat burn pain has been associated with an increase in fluid requirements, however a causal link between the two observations is lacking.[69] It could be that improved resuscitation has been matched by an improved understanding of the analgesic requirements in burns patients.

Nonopioid analgesia

A variety of nonopioid drugs has been investigated for the treatment of burn pain.[70, 71] In one study of burns centers where opioids were not used it was observed that the pain relief obtained with nonopioids was similar to that obtained with opioids.[72][II] In addition, there may be a reluctance to administer opioids to elderly patients with burns because of the increased risk of side effects.[73]

Nonsteroidal anti-inflammatory drugs (NSAIDs) have been used successfully to treat pain or reduce opioid requirements in a variety of acute pain conditions. The use of parenteral nonsteroidal anti-inflammatory agents, such as ketorolac, has been described to treat burn pain.[74][IV] It was also postulated that the use of ketorolac was associated with other benefits due to the anti-inflammatory effects in the burn patient.[75][IV] Caution is required in the presence of hypovolemia or renal injury as the use of NSAIDs in burns patients has been associated with deteriorating renal function.[76] The fear of causing or exacerbating gastrointestinal ulceration following burn injury should also limit the use of NSAIDs. Despite the potential of a lesser gastrointestinal risk with cyclooxygenase-2-selective inhibitors drugs, these drugs have significant cardiovascular and renal risks.[77] As a result, there are no prospective trials of these drugs as analgesics in burns patients that allow conclusions to be made regarding their potential clinical role.

Experimental burn pain can be relieved using NMDA antagonists such as ketamine.[78] Unfortunately, high-dose ketamine is associated with unpleasant side effects, such as hallucinations and dysphoria. Low-dose ketamine may be an effective analgesic and may reduce opioid requirements.[79][I] It is an attractive option as the action of ketamine on the NMDA receptor has been shown to reduce central sensitization and the development of secondary hyperalgesia in animal models of neuropathic pain. Experience in small trials and larger case series provides reasonable evidence that ketamine is effective and safe for the management of burn pain.[80][IV] As ketamine is stereoselective, S ketamine may prove to be a superior analgesic and its successful use has been described in one pediatric case series.[81][III]

Other pharmacological interventions commonly used for the treatment of neuropathic pain – such as tricyclic antidepressants, anticonvulsants, including gabapentin, and membrane stabilizers – are increasingly used, but evidence for their efficacy in burn injury is lacking. Clonidine, an alpha-2 agonist, produces analgesia when given systemically.[82][III] Analgesia is prolonged when it is added to epidural mixtures of local anesthetic and opioids.[83][II] A case report has suggested that it can be used to successfully treat burn pain that is responding poorly to opioids.[84][V] In a small, prospective, randomized placebo-controlled study, clonidine reduced the requirements for fentanyl in burn pain.[85][II]

The use of intravenous lidocaine (lignocaine) to provide analgesia may be extremely effective in burn patients, especially if there is a neuropathic component; however, concerns regarding side effects may be the reason why this effective technique has not gained more widespread acceptance.[86][V]

Local anesthesia

There may be a number of reasons why a local or regional anesthetic technique may be inappropriate in a significant number of burns patients. Both the donor and burn areas may extend beyond the area covered by a single technique, and there may be a reluctance to perform these procedures in patients at risk of sepsis. Both topical and subcutaneous applications of local anesthetic have been used for the treatment of burn pain.[17][II], [87][IV]

Inhalation anesthetic agents

The use of these agents at subanesthetic concentrations has possible advantages such as ease of delivery, predictable elimination, and freedom from the need for prolonged fasting. Methoxyflurane and trichloroethylene have both been shown to provide useful analgesia for burn dressings.[88][V] Methoxyflurane use is limited by the risk of serious nephrotoxicity[89] and trichloroethylene was withdrawn as agents undergoing less biotransformation were introduced. Halothane, enflurane, and nitrous oxide were subsequently used as inhalational agents for burn dressings.[90, 91] Concerns regarding halothane hepatotoxicity and enflurane use in patients at risk of convulsions have tended to reduce the utilization of these agents. With repeated exposure, nitrous oxide-induced bone marrow suppression may occur, mediated by inhibition of methionine synthetase. It has been suggested that patients receiving repeated exposures to nitrous oxide should receive vitamin B_{12} and folinic acid supplements.[92] Neuropathy may also occur in the absence of hematological evidence of bone marrow suppression, especially if there is vitamin B_{12} deficiency.[93, 94, 95][V] Concerns over repeated exposure of patients and staff to nitrous oxide should limit its clinical utility. Currently, the use of low-dose isoflurane and desflurane for short procedures is being investigated because of their minimal metabolism and the rapid recovery of patients after using these agents.[96][II]

General anesthesia

Although opioids alone or in combination with other drugs and techniques may provide worthwhile relief for rest pain and pain during some procedures, there are procedures for which the provision of adequate pain relief in the conscious patient is impossible. Many of the procedures required are unsuitable for the awake patient. Therefore, general anesthesia will be required.

No single technique has gained widespread acceptance as the gold standard. Altered pharmacokinetics and pharmacodynamics, difficult airway, problems of monitoring, and maintenance of body temperature in the face of long procedures with large blood loss present obvious difficulties. Also, reluctance to use muscle relaxants, because of the sensitivity to suxamethonium (succinyl choline) and resistance to nondepolarizing drugs, affects the type of anesthetic given.[97, 98]

If possible, repeated general anesthesia should be avoided to prevent recurrent exposure to volatile agents and to minimize the interruption of feeding due to repeated fasting. However, a large series of patients having wound debridement or dressing changes under anesthesia suggest that these can be carried out safely with minimal disruption to nutrition.[99, 100] In an attempt to keep the postoperative sequelae of anesthesia to a minimum, the use of short-acting, rapidly metabolized agents such as alfentanil and propofol has been investigated.[101] As in other types of surgery, this technique is associated with a quick recovery, which may have advantages in burns patients. In children, the use of ketamine is popular owing to the cardiovascular stability and airway safety. In adults, it is associated with unpleasant dreams. The drug is well tolerated in children and is used for operative procedures and dressing changes.[102, 103] Ketamine has profound analgesic effects and can be given by the intramuscular, rectal, or intravenous routes.[104]

Nonpharmacological approaches

Hypnosis has been used for the treatment of burn pain, and it has been shown to reduce procedural pain in a small study using historical controls.[105][IV] However, lack of prospective randomized trials makes it difficult to compare this therapy with conventional drug treatment.[106] When used in combination with opioids, no benefit could be demonstrated for the use of hypnosis, lorazepam, or both compared with opioid alone.[107][II] This may suggest that these techniques are suitable for mild pain as an alternative to drug therapy. Other studies suggest that it is patients with severe pain that show some benefit from hypnosis.[108] An additional problem is that only a proportion of patients are susceptible to hypnosis.[109]

The use of auricular electrical stimulation, which is similar to acupuncture, can reduce procedural pain.[110]

[IV] Therapeutic touch techniques can be shown to reduce pain scores, but not analgesic requirements, in burn patients.[111][V] Massage therapy is associated with decreased pain and less depression.[112][V] Music therapy has a positive effect on pediatric patients' pain and anxiety during donor site dressing changes.[113, 114][V]

Mild pain can be reduced using a number of cognitive and behavioral techniques. Techniques include watching television or videos,[115][V] talking about pain, and the use of virtual reality distraction therapy using gaming consoles.[116, 117] These techniques were not effective for severe pain.[118] These psychological coping strategies may be employed by experienced burn unit staff.[119] In children, parental involvement may reduce the pain and anxiety associated with procedures.[120][V] The relative failure of nonpharmacological therapies in severe pain has also been demonstrated in children.[121] Fear avoidance behavior is common in recovered burn patients and the incidence correlates with severity of pain symptoms and psychological distress.[122] As a result of the high incidence of psychiatric morbidity in burn patients and the association of psychological morbidity with severe pain, psychological support is important. Psychologists and psychiatrists are therefore essential members of the burn care team.[123]

Burn wound dressings

The goals of burn therapy are to achieve skin cover over the uninfected burn wound, healing with good cosmetic and functional result, and a reduction of and finally relief from pain and discomfort. Unfortunately, this goal may take some time to achieve, and in the meantime the wound must be covered. Recent discussions of new burn dressings have included consideration of their effect on the patient's pain. The use of honey as a burns dressing has been reported to lead to improved results and less pain. The low cost and easy availability may make such simple biological dressings acceptable where resources are very limited, but such therapy is unlikely to be acceptable where other topical creams are available.[124][V] A variety of dressings such as Biobrane or hydrocolloidal dressings have been described as being associated with increased patient comfort.[125][III], [126]

Pain relief in practice

The quality of evidence for the efficacy of treatments of burn pain is poor, with a large number of small studies, pilot studies, and case reports, but relatively few large randomized controlled trials. This is a reflection of the difficulties in studying this group of patients. The systematic undertreatment of pain in burns units should be avoided. Different strategies are required to treat background, breakthrough, and procedural pain. Owing to the unpredictable severity of the pain, its regular measurement is required with frequent adjustment of doses and drugs used.

REFERENCES

* 1. Gallagher G, Rae CP, Kinsella J. Treatment of pain in severe burns. *American Journal of Clinical Dermatology.* 2000; **1**: 329–35.

* 2. Choiniere M, Melzack R, Rondeau J *et al.* The pain of burns: characteristics and correlates. *Journal of Trauma.* 1989; **29**: 1531–9.

3. Gustorff B, Anzenhofer S, Sycha T *et al.* The sunburn pain model: The stability of primary and secondary hyperalgesia over 10 hours in a crossover setting. *Anesthesia and Analgesia.* 2004; **98**: 173–7.

4. Saxe G, Stoddard F, Courtney D *et al.* Relationship between acute morphine and the course of PTSD in children with burns. *Journal of American Acadamy Child Adolescent Psychiatry.* 2001; **40**: 915–21.

5. Gamble J, Avery L. Fire Statistics Monitor last updated 28 February 2006. 2005: 2. Available from: www.communities.gov.uk/publications/fire/firestatisticsmonitor2.

6. American Burn Association. National Burn Repository 2005 Report, Version 2. Last updated 2006, cited February 2008. Available from: www.ameriburn.org/NBR2005.pdf.

7. Saffle JR, Davis B, Williams P. Recent outcomes in the treatment of burn injury in the United States: A report from the American Burn Association Patient Registry. *Journal of Burn Care and Rehabilitation.* 1995; **16** (3 pt 1): 219–32.

* 8. Scott JR, Watson SB. *Clinical anaesthesiology: Burns.* London: Ballière Tindall, 1997: 473–4.

9. Atchison N, Osgood P, Carr D, Szyfelbein S. Pain during burn dressing change in children: relationship to burn area, depth and analgesic regimens. *Pain.* 1991; **47**: 41–5.

10. Osgood PF, Szyfelbein SK. Management of burn pain in children. *Pediatric Clinics North America.* 1989; **36**: 1001–13.

11. Pedersen JL, Andersen OK, Arendt-Nielsen L, Kehlet H. Hyperalgesia and temporal summation of pain after heat injury in man. *Pain.* 1998; **74**: 189–97.

12. Imokawa H, Ando K, Kubota T *et al.* Study on the kinetics of bradykinin level in the wound produced by thermal injury in the ear burn model in mice. *Nippon-Yakurigaku-Zasshi.* 1992; **99**: 445–50.

13. Coderre TJ, Melzack R. Cutaneous hyperalgesia: contribution of peripheral and central mechanisms to the increase in pain sensitivity after injury. *Brain Research.* 1987; **404**: 95–106.

14. Kawamata M, Watanabe H, Nishikawa K *et al.* Different mechanisms of development and maintenance of experimental incision-induced hyperalgesia in human skin. *Anesthesiology.* 2002; **97**: 550–9.

15. Nozaki-Taguchi N, Yaksh T. Spinal and peripheral [mu] opioids and the development of secondary tactile allodynia after thermal injury. *Anesthesia and Analgesia*. 2002; **94**: 968–74.

16. Oatway M, Reid A, Sawynok J. Peripheral antihyperalgesic and analgesic actions of ketamine and amitriptyline in a model of mild thermal injury in the rat. *Anesthesia and Analgesia*. 2003; **97**: 168–73.

17. Dahl JB, Brennum J, Arendt-Nielsen L et al. The effect of pre- versus postinjury infiltration with lidocaine on thermal and mechanical hyperalgesia after heat injury to the skin. *Pain*. 1993; **53**: 43–51.

18. Pedersen JL, Callesen T, Moiniche S, Kehlet H. Analgesic and anti-inflammatory effects of lignocaine-prilocaine (EMLA) cream in human burn injury. *British Journal of Anaesthesia*. 1996; **76**: 806–10.

19. Raja SN, Campbell JN, Meyer RA, Colman RW. Role of kinins in pain and hyperalgesia: psychophysical studies in a patient with kininogen deficiency. *Clinical Science*. 1992; **83**: 337–41.

20. Koppert W, Likar R, Geisslinger G et al. Peripheral antihyperalgesic effect of morphine to heat, but not mechanical, stimulation in healthy volunteers after ultraviolet-b irradiation. *Anesthesia and Analgesia*. 1999; **88**: 117–22.

21. Gustorff B, Hoechtl K, Sycha T et al. The effects of remifentanil and gabapentin on hyperalgesia in a new extended inflammatory skin pain model in healthy volunteers. *Anesthesia and Analgesia*. 2004; **98**: 401–7.

22. Schulte H, Sollevi A, Segerdahl M. The synergistic effect of combined treatment with systemic ketamine and morphine on experimentally induced windup-like pain in humans. *Anesthesia and Analgesia*. 2004; **98**: 1574–80.

23. Wiech K, Kiefer R, Topfner S et al. A placebo-controlled randomized crossover trial of the N-methyl-D-aspartic acid receptor antagonist, memantine, in patients with chronic phantom limb pain. *Anesthesia and Analgesia*. 2004; **98**: 408–13.

24. Ilkjaer S, Dirks J, Brennum J et al. Effect of systemic N-methyl-D-aspartate receptor antagonist (dextromethorphan) on primary and secondary hyperalgesia in humans. *Britsh Journal of Anaesthesia*. 1997; **79**: 600–5.

25. Jonsson CE, Holmsten A, Dahlstrom L, Jonsson K. Background pain in burn patients: routine measurement and recording of pain intensity in a burn unit. *Burns*. 1998; **24**: 448–54.

* 26. Dauber A, Osgood P, Breslau AJ et al. Chronic persistent pain after severe burns: A survey of 358 burn survivors. *Pain Medicine*. 2002; **3**: 6–17.

27. Malenfant A, Forget R, Amsel R et al. Tactile, thermal and pain sensibility in burned patients with and without chronic pain and paresthesia problems. *Pain*. 1998; **77**: 241–51.

28. Wiechman SA, Ptacek JT, Patterson DR et al. Rates, trends, and severity of depression after burn sijuries. *Journal of Burn Care and Rehabilitation*. 2001; **22**: 417–24.

29. Taal LA, Faber AW. Post-traumatic stress, pain and anxiety in adult burn victims. *Burns*. 1997; **23**: 545–9.

* 30. Byers JF, Bridges S, Kijek J, LaBorde P. Burn patients' pain and anxiety experiences. *Journal of Burn Care and Rehabilitation*. 2001; **22**: 144–9.

31. Willebrand M, Andersson G, Ekselius L. Prediction of psychological health after an accidental burn. *Journal of Trauma-Injury Infection and Critical Care*. 2004; **57**: 367–74.

* 32. Stoddard FJ, Sheridan RL, Saxe GN et al. Treatment of pain in acutely burned children. *Journal of Burn Care and Rehabilitation*. 2002; **23**: 135–56.

33. Melzack R. The McGill Pain Questionnaire: major properties and scoring methods. *Pain*. 1975; **1**: 277–99.

34. Rae CP, Gallagher G, Watson S, Kinsella J. An audit of patient perception compared with medical and nursing staff estimation of pain during burn dressing changes. *European Journal of Anaesthesiology*. 2000; **17**: 43–45.

35. Choiniere M, Melzack R, Girard N et al. Comparisons between patients' and nurses' assessment of pain and medication efficacy in severe burn injuries. *Pain*. 1990; **40**: 143–52.

36. Geisser ME, Bingham HG, Robinson ME. Pain and anxiety during burn dressing changes: concordance between patients' and nurses' ratings and relation to medication administration and patient variables. *Journal of Burn Care and Rehabilitation*. 1995; **16**: 165–71.

37. McGrath PJ, Unruh AM. The measurement and assessment of pain. In: McGrath PJ, Unruh AM (eds). *Pain in children and adolescents*. New York, NY: Elsevier, 1987.

38. Choiniere M, Auger F, Letarjet J. Visual analogue thermometer: a valid and useful instrument for measuring pain in burned patients. *Burns*. 1994; **20**: 229–36.

39. Fields DR, Cervero F (eds). *Advances in pain research and therapy*. New York: Raven Press, 1985: 375–402.

40. Davies JW. Prompt cooling of burned areas: a review of benefits and the effector mechanisms. *Burns Including Thermal Injury*. 1982; **9**: 1–6.

41. Werner MU, Lassen B, Pedersen JL, Kehlet H. Local cooling does not prevent hyperalgesia following burn injury in humans. *Pain*. 2002; **98**: 297–303.

42. Kinsella J, Glavin R, Reid WH. Patient controlled analgesia in burn patients. *Burns*. 1988; **14**: 500–3.

43. Choiniere M, Grenier R, Paquette C. Patient-controlled analgesia: a double-blind study in burn patients. *Anaesthesia*. 1992; **47**: 467–72.

44. Gaukroger PB, Chapman MJ, Davey RB. Pain control in paediatric burns: the use of patient controlled analgesia. *Burns*. 1991; **17**: 396–9.

45. Donen N, Tweed WA, White D et al. Pre-hospital analgesia with Entonox. *Canadian Anaesthesia Society Journal*. 1982; **29**: 275–9.

* 46. Alexander L, Wolman R, Blache C et al. Use of morphine sulfate (MS Contin) in patients with burns: a pilot study. *Journal of Burn Care and Rehabilitation*. 1992; **13**: 581–3.

47. Gallagher G, Rae CP, Kenny GN, Kinsella J. The use of a target-controlled infusion of alfentanil to provide

analgesia for burn dressing changes: a dose finding study. *Anaesthesia.* 2000; **55**: 1159–63.

48. Hoffman HG, Doctor JN, Patterson DR *et al.* Virtual reality as an adjunctive pain control during burn wound care in adolescent patients. *Pain.* 2000; **85**: 305–9.

* 49. Haythronthwaite JA, Lawrence JW, Fauerbach JA. Brief cognitive interventions for burn pain. *Annals of Behavioural Medicine.* 2001; **23**: 42–9.

50. Braam MJ, Bath AP, Spauwen PH, Bailie FB. Survey of analgesia regimens in burns centres in the UK. *Burns.* 1994; **20**: 360–2.

51. Martin-Herz SP, Patterson DR, Honari S *et al.* Pediatric pain control practices of North American Burn Centers. *Journal of Burn Care and Rehabilitation.* 2003; **24**: 26–36.

52. Herman RA, Veng-Pedersen P, Miotto J *et al.* Pharmacokinetics of morphine sulfate in patients with burns. *Journal of Burn Care and Rehabilitation.* 1994; **15**: 95–103.

53. Perreault S, Choiniere M, du Souich PB *et al.* Pharmacokinetics of morphine and its glucuronidated metabolites in burn injuries. *Annals of Pharmacotherapy.* 2001; **35**: 1588–92.

54. Langlade A, Carr DB, Serrie A *et al.* Enhanced potency of intravenous, but not intrathecal, morphine and morphine-6-glucuronide after burn trauma. *Life Science.* 1994; **54**: 1699–709.

55. Garcia Barreiro J, Rodriguez A, Cal M *et al.* Treatment of postoperative pain for burn patients with intravenous analgesia in continuous perfusion using elastomeric infusors. *Burns.* 2005; **31**: 67–71.

56. Prakash S, Fatima T, Pawar M. Patient-controlled analgesia with fentanyl for burn dressing changes. *Anesthesia and Analgesia.* 2004; **99**: 552–5.

57. Borland ML, Bergesio R, Pascoe EM *et al.* Intranasal fentanyl is an equivalent analgesic to oral morphine in paediatric burns patients for dressing changes: a randomised double blind crossover study. *Burns.* 2005; **31**: 831–7.

58. Finn J, Wright J, Fong J *et al.* A randomised crossover trial of patient controlled intranasal fentanyl and oral morphine for procedural wound care in adult patients with burns. *Burns.* 2004; **30**: 262–8.

59. Sim KM, Hwang NC, Chan YW, Seah CS. Use of patient-controlled analgesia with alfentanil for burns dressing procedures: a preliminary report of five patients. *Burns.* 1996; **22**: 238–41.

60. Lopez Navarro AM, Peiro C, Matoses S *et al.* General anesthesia by infusion of remifentanil for debridement and grafting of large burns in 3 pediatric patients. *Revista Espanola de Anestesiologia y Reanimacion.* 2004; **51**: 47–50.

61. McHugh GJ. Norpethidine accumulation and generalized seizure during pethidine patient-controlled analgesia. *Anaesthesia and Intensive Care.* 1999; **27**: 289–91.

62. Altier N, Dion D, Boulanger A, Choiniere M. Successful use of methadone in the treatment of chronic neuropathic

pain arising from burn injuries: a case-study. *Burns.* 2001; **27**: 771–5.

63. Chambers JA, Guly HR. Prehospital intravenous nalbuphine administered by paramedics. *Resuscitation.* 1994; **27**: 153–8.

64. Lee JJ, Marvin JA, Heimbach DM. Effectiveness of nalbuphine for relief of burn debridement pain. *Journal of Burn Care and Rehabilitation.* 1989; **10**: 241–6.

65. Sheridan RL, McEttrick M, Bacha G *et al.* Midazolam infusion in pediatric patients with burns who are undergoing mechanical ventilation. *Journal of Burn Care and Rehabilitation.* 1994; **15**: 515–8.

66. Patterson DR, Ptacek JT, Carrougher GJ, Sharar SR. Lorazepam as an adjunct to opioid analgesics in the treatment of burn pain. *Pain.* 1997; **72**: 367–74.

67. Perry S, Heidrich G. Management of pain during debridement: a survey of U.S. burn units. *Pain.* 1982; **13**: 267–80.

68. Schwacha MG, McGwin Jr G, Hutchinson CB *et al.* The contribution of opiate analgesics to the development of infectious complications in burn patients. *American Journal of Surgery.* 2006; **192**: 82–6.

69. Sullivan SR, Friedrich JB, Engrav LH *et al.* "Opioid creep" is real and may be the cause of "fluid creep". *Burns.* 2004; **30**: 583–90.

* 70. Patterson DR. Non-opioid-based approaches to burn pain. *Journal of Burn Care and Rehabilitation.* 1995; **16**: 372–6.

* 71. Esselman PC, Thombs BD, Magyar-Russell G, Fauerbach JA. Burn rehabilitation: State of the science. *American Journal of Physical Medicine and Rehabilitation.* 2006; **85**: 383–413.

72. Foertsch CE, O'Hara MW, Kealey GP *et al.* A quasi-experimental, dual-center study of morphine efficacy in patients with burns. *Journal of Burn Care and Rehabilitation.* 1995; **16**: 118–26.

73. Honari S, Patterson DR, Gibbons J *et al.* Comparison of pain control medication in three age groups of elderly patients. *Journal of Burn Care and Rehabilitation.* 1997; **18**: 500–4.

74. Tran HT, Ackerman BH, Wardius PA *et al.* Intravenous ketorolac for pain management in a ventilator-dependent patient with thermal injury. *Pharmacotherapy.* 1996; **16**: 75–8.

75. Enkhbaatar P, Murakami K, Shimoda K *et al.* Ketorolac attenuates cardiopulmonary derangements in sheep with combined burn and smoke inhalation injury. *Clinical Science.* 2003; **105**: 621–8.

76. Jonsson CE, Ericsson F. Impairment of renal function after treatment of a burn patient with diclofenac, a non-steroidal antiinflammatory drug. *Burns.* 1995; **21**: 471–3.

* 77. Moore RA, Derry S, Phillips CJ, McQuay HJ. Nonsteroidal anti-inflammatory drugs (NSAIDs), cyxlooxygenase-2 selective inhibitors (coxibs) and gastrointestinal harm: review of clinical trials and clinical practice. *BMC Musculoskeletal Disorders.* 2006; **7**: 79.

78. Schulte H, Sollevi A, Segerdahl M. The synergistic effect of combined treatment with systemic ketamine and

morphine on experimentally induced windup-like pain in humans. *Anesthesia & Analgesia*. 2004; **98**: 1574–80.

79. Bell RF, Dahl JB, Moore RA, Kalso E. Peri-operative ketamine for acute post-operative pain: a quantitative and qualitative systematic review (Cochrane review). *Acta Anaesthesiologica Scandinavica*. 2005; **49**: 1405–28.

80. Owens VF, Palmieri T, Comroe C et al. Ketamine: A safe and effective agent for painful procedures in the pediatric burn patient. *Journal of Burn Care and Research*. 2006; **27**: 211–6.

81. Heinrich M, Wetzstein V, Muensterer OJ, Till H. Conscious sedation: Off-label use of rectal S(+)-ketamine and midazolam for wound dressing changes in paediatric heat injuries. *European Journal of Pediatric Surgery*. 2004; **14**: 235–9.

82. Nader ND, Ignatowski TA, Kurek CJ et al. Clonidine suppresses plasma and cerebrospinal fluid concentrations of TNF-alpha during the perioperative period. *Anesthesia and Analgesia*. 2001; **93**: 363–9.

83. De Negri P, Ivani G, Visconti C et al. The dose–response relationship for clonidine added to a postoperative continuous epidural infusion of ropivacaine in children. *Anesthesia and Analgesia*. 2001; **93**: 71–6.

84. Lyons B, Casey W, Doherty P et al. Pain relief with low-dose intravenous clonidine in a child with severe burns. *Intensive Care Medicine*. 1996; **22**: 249–51.

85. Viggiano M, Badetti C, Roux F et al. Controlled analgesia in a burn patient: fentanyl sparing effect of clonidine. *Annales Françaises d'Anesthésie et de Réanimation*. 1998; **17**: 19–26.

86. Jonsson A, Cassuto J, Hanson B. Inhibition of burn pain by intravenous lignocaine infusion. *Lancet*. 1991; **20**: 151–2.

87. Brofeldt BT, Cornwell P, Doherty D et al. Topical lidocaine in the treatment of partial-thickness burns. *Journal of Burn Care and Rehabilitation*. 1989; **10**: 63–8.

88. Laird SM, Gray BM. Intermittent inhalation of methoxyflurane and trichloroethylene as analgesics for burn dressing procedures. *British Journal of Anaesthesia*. 1971; **43**: 149–59.

89. Lawson NW, Eggers Jr GW. Methoxyflurane and renal failure. *Southern Medical Journal*. 1971; **64**: 924–8.

90. Filkins SA, Cosgrave P, Marvin JA. Self administered anaesthetic: a method of pain control. *Journal of Burn Care and Research*. 1981; **2**: 33–4.

91. Firn S. Enflurane analgesia. *Journal of the Royal Society of Medicine*. 1982; **75** (Suppl. 1): 36–8.

92. Weimann J. Toxicity of nitrous oxide. *Best Practice and Research. Clinical Anaesthesiology*. 2003; **17**: 47–61.

93. Schilling RF. Is nitrous oxide a dangerous anaesthetic for vitamin B12 deficient subjects? *Journal of the American Medical Association*. 1986; **255**: 1605–06.

94. Berger JJ, Modell JH, Sypert GW. Megaloblastic anaemia and brief exposure to nitrous oxide – a causal relationship. *Anesthesia and Analgesia*. 1988; **75**: 577–82.

95. Holloway K, Alberico A. Postoperative myeloneuropathy: a preventable complication in patients with Vit B12 deficiency. *Journal of Neurosurgery*. 1990; **72**: 732–6.

96. Thompson N, Murray S, MacLennan F et al. A randomised controlled trial of intravenous versus inhalational analgesia during outpatient oocyte recovery. *Anaesthesia*. 2000; **55**: 770–3.

97. Martyn J. Clinical pharmacology and drug therapy in the burned patient. *Anesthesiology*. 1986; **65**: 67–75.

* 98. Black RG, Kinsella J. Anaesthetic management for burns patients. *British Journal of Anaesthesia*. 2001; **1**: 1–4.

99. Dimick P, Helvig E, Heimbach D et al. Anesthesia-assisted procedures in a burn intensive care unit procedure room: benefits and complications. *Journal of Burn Care and Rehabilitation*. 1993; **14**: 446–9.

100. Powers PS, Cruse CW, Daniels S, Stevens BA. Safety and efficacy of debridement under anesthesia in patients with burns. *Journal of Burn Care and Rehabilitation*. 1993; **14**: 176–80.

101. Reyneke CJ, James MF, Johnson R. Alfentanil and propofol infusions for surgery in the burned patient. *British Journal of Anaesthesia*. 1989; **63**: 418–22.

102. Groeneveld A, Inkson T. Ketamine: a solution to procedural pain in burned children. *Canadian Nurse*. 1992; **88**: 28–31.

103. Demling RH, Ellerby S, Jarrett F. Ketamine analgesia for tangential excision of burn eschar: a burn unit procedure. *Journal of Trauma*. 1978; **18**: 269–70.

*104. White PF, Way WL, Trevor AJ. Ketamine, its pharmacology and therapeutic uses. *Anaesthesiology*. 1982; **56**: 119–36.

105. Patterson DR, Questad KA, de-Lateur BJ. Hypnotherapy as an adjunct to narcotic analgesia for the treatment of pain for burn debridement. *American Journal of Clinical Hypnosis*. 1989; **31**: 156–63.

*106. Van-der-Does AJ, Van-Dyck R. Does hypnosis contribute to the care of burn patients? Review of the evidence. *General Hospital Psychiatry*. 1989; **11**: 119–24.

107. Everett JJ, Patterson DR, Burns GL et al. Adjunctive interventions for burn pain control: comparison of hypnosis and ativan: the 1993 Clinical Research Award. *Journal of Burn Care and Rehabilitation*. 1993; **14**: 676–83.

108. Patterson DR, Adcock RJ, Bombardier CH. Factors predicting hypnotic analgesia in clinical burn pain. *International Journal of Clinical and Experimental Hypnosis*. 1997; **45**: 377–95.

109. Gilboa D, Borenstein A, Seidman DS, Tsur H. Burn patients' use of autohypnosis: making a painful experience bearable. *Burns*. 1990; **16**: 441–4.

110. Lewis SM, Clelland JA, Knowles CJ et al. Effects of auricular acupuncture-like transcutaneous electric nerve stimulation on pain levels following wound care in patients with burns: a pilot study. *Journal of Burn Care and Rehabilitation*. 1990; **11**: 322–9.

111. Turner JG, Clark AJ, Gauthier DK, Williams M. The effect of therapeutic touch on pain and anxiety in burn patients. *Journal of Advanced Nursing*. 1998; **28**: 10–20.

112. Field T, Peck M, Krugman S et al. Burn injuries benefit from massage therapy. *Journal of Burn Care and Rehabilitation*. 1998; **19**: 241–4.

113. Whitehead-Pleaux AM, Baryza MJ, Sheridan RL. The effects of music therapy on pediatric patients' pain and

anxiety during donor site dressing change. *Journal of Musical Therapy.* 2006; **43**: 136–53.

114. Ferguson SL, Voll KV. Burn pain and anxiety: the use of music relaxation during rehabilitation. *Journal of Burn Care and Rehabilitation.* 2004; **25**: 8–14.

115. Miller AC, Hickman LC, Lemasters GK. A distraction technique for control of burn pain. *Journal of Burn Care and Rehabilitation.* 1992; **13**: 576–80.

116. Haik J, Tessone A, Nota A *et al.* The use of video capture virtual reality in burn rehabilitation: the possibilities. *Journal of Burn Care and Research.* 2006; **27**: 195–7.

117. Hoffman HG, Patterson DR, Magula J *et al.* Water-friendly virtual reality pain control during wound care. *Journal of Clinical Psychology.* 2004; **60**: 189–95.

118. Blew AF, Patterson DR, Quested KA. Frequency of use and rated effectiveness of cognitive and behavioural coping responses to burn pain. *Burns.* 1989; **15**: 20–2.

119. Patterson DR. Practical applications of psychological techniques in controlling burn pain. *Journal of Burn Care and Rehabilitation.* 1992; **13**: 13–18.

120. George A, Hancock J. Reducing pediatric burn pain with parent participation. *Journal of Burn Care and Rehabilitation.* 1993; **14**: 104–7.

121. Foertsch CE, O'Hara MW, Stoddard FJ, Kealey GP. Treatment-resistant pain and distress during pediatric burn-dressing changes. *Journal of Burn Care and Rehabilitation.* 1998; **19**: 219–24.

122. Sgroi MI, Willebrand M, Ekselius L *et al.* Fear-avoidance in recovered burn patients: association with psychological and somatic symptoms. *Journal of Health Psychology.* 2005; **10**: 491–502.

∗123. Watkins PN, Cook EL, May SR, Still JM. The role of the psychiatrist in the team treatment of the adult patient with burns. *Journal of Burn Care and Rehabilitation.* 1992; **13**: 19–27.

124. Subrahmanyam M. Topical application of honey in treatment of burns. *British Journal of Surgery.* 1991; **78**: 497–8.

125. Gerding RL, Emerman CL, Effron D *et al.* Outpatient management of partial-thickness burns: Biobrane versus 1% silver sulfadiazine. *Annals of Emergency Medicine.* 1990; **19**: 121–4.

∗126. Smith Jr DJ, Thomson PD, Garner WL, Rodriguez JL. Burn wounds: infection and healing. *American Journal of Surgery.* 1994; **167**: 46S–8S.

23

Acute pain and medical disorders

ERIC J VISSER AND C ROGER GOUCKE

KEY LEARNING POINTS

- Acute neuropathic pain associated with neurological disorders may be treated with antidepressants, anticonvulsants, opioids, or tramadol. In cases of severe pain, intravenous administration of opioids, tramadol, low-dose ketamine, or lidocaine may be useful for "rescue analgesia."
- Gabapentin, opioids, plasma exchange, immunoglobulin therapy, and possibly steroids are effective in the treatment of acute pain in Guillain–Barré syndrome. Supplemental analgesia includes tramadol, paracetamol, nonsteroidal anti-inflammatory drugs (NSAIDs), intravenous low-dose ketamine or lidocaine (lignocaine), physical therapies, and comfort measures.
- In patients with acute abdominal pain, parenteral opioids provide rapid and effective analgesia and do not interfere with the diagnostic process.
- Pethidine should be avoided in the treatment of acute pain associated with abdominal disorders, sickle cell anemia, and the porphyrias. The accumulation of nor-pethidine, (particularly with high-dose pethidine administration and in renal impairment) may produce adverse neurological sequelae, such as an altered mental state, myoclonus, and seizures. There is no advantage to using pethidine (meperidine) in terms of reducing abdominal pain (due to smooth muscle spasm or colic) or nausea and vomiting and the risk of opioid addiction is higher.
- Intravenous low-dose ketamine may improve analgesia in patients with acute abdominal pain that is poorly responsive to opioids (including tolerance) or where

there is visceral hyperalgesia (e.g. chronic abdominal pain disorders).
- In renal and biliary colic, intravenous NSAIDs, and to a lesser extent opioids, provide effective "first line" analgesia; anticholinergic smooth muscle relaxants such as hyoscine N-butylbromide and atropine are ineffective. In renal colic, ondansetron, transcutaneous electrical nerve stimulation (TENS), intranasal desmopressin, or medical expulsive therapies may also improve pain relief.
- Antispasmodic agents and peppermint oil are effective analgesics in irritable bowel syndrome (IBS).
- NSAIDs are the most effective analgesics for primary dysmenorrhea, although aspirin, paracetamol (acetaminophen), TENS, and abdominal compression are also beneficial; vitamin B1 and vitamin E provide effective prophylaxis against pain and blood loss.
- Most forms of acute orofacial pain are treated effectively by NSAIDs, cyclooxygenase (COX)-2 selective inhibitors, aspirin, paracetamol, opioids, or tramadol, either alone or in combination. Steroids reduce pain in acute pharyngitis and antibiotics reduce pain marginally in pharyngitis, acute otitis media, and sinusitis.
- Intravenous opioids, nitroglycerine, and inhaled nitrous oxide in oxygen are effective analgesics for acute ischemic chest pain.
- During a sickle cell crisis, parenteral or oral opioids, NSAIDs, paracetamol, and nitrous oxide provide effective analgesia; steroids, nitric oxide, and disease-modifying agents may also improve pain relief.

- In acute porphyria, pain management is based on ceasing triggers, early administration of hematin, high-dose dextrose, and possibly cimetidine and the use of intravenous and (later) oral opioid analgesia. Paracetamol, hyoscine N-butylbromide, gabapentin, nitrous oxide, and TENS may also be

- beneficial as part of a multimodal analgesia approach.
- This chapter aims to provide scientific evidence for the treatment of acute pain associated with medical disorders and is not intended to detail their primary management.

ACUTE PAIN ASSOCIATED WITH NEUROLOGICAL DISORDERS

Acute pain associated with neurological disorders is usually neuropathic in etiology, although nociceptive pain may also occur, such as painful muscular spasms in multiple sclerosis or shoulder subluxation pain after a stroke. There is minimal specific evidence to guide the management of acute pain associated with many neurological disorders; treatments are largely based on evidence from studies of chronic neuropathic pain. Associated psychosocial problems and physical disabilities should be managed within a multidisciplinary framework. The management of acute pain associated with headache and herpes zoster will be discussed in Chapter 34, Headache and Chapter 32, Herpes zoster pain including shingles and postherpetic neuralgia both in the *Chronic Pain* volume of this series.

Central post-stroke pain

Central post-stroke pain develops in 8.4 percent of stroke patients, usually within a few months.[1] There are no specific data for treatment of acute pain in this condition; however, persistent pain may be treated with tricyclic antidepressants such as amitriptyline[2][I], [3][I] or anticonvulsants such as lamotrigine.[4][II] Gabapentin may also be effective, based on evidence of benefit in the treatment of spinal cord injury pain.[5] Post-stroke patients may also develop acute musculoskeletal pain, particularly a shoulder pain syndrome associated with subluxation, requiring treatment based on physical therapies, such as shoulder stabilization or TENS, and analgesia, such as paracetamol, NSAIDs, or COX-2 selective inhibitors, opioids, tramadol, and suprascapular nerve or shoulder joint injections with local anesthetic and steroid. An acute flare-up of peripheral limb pain may herald the development of a superimposed complex regional pain syndrome (CRPS).

Multiple sclerosis

Multiple sclerosis (MS) is associated with persistent central pain in 28 percent of patients with 20 percent

reporting musculoskeletal pain such as back pain or muscle spasms.[1] Acute paroxysmal "tic-like" pains in various parts of the body have been described as an initial presenting symptom or may develop during the course of the disease.[6] Carbamazepine is effective in treating trigeminal neuralgia and has been suggested as the drug of choice for this and other paroxysmal pains in MS.[3][I], [7][I] Other anticonvulsants may be of benefit but specific data are lacking. The cannabinoid dronabinol was effective in treating MS-related neuropathic pain in a single small randomized controlled trial (RCT).[3][I] A Cochrane review concluded there was no clear data to direct the use of anti-spasticity drugs such as baclofen for acute pain in MS.[8][I] Readers are directed to Chapter 33, Management of painful spasticity in the *Chronic Pain* volume of this series.

Guillain–Barré syndrome

Guillain–Barré syndrome (GBS) is an acute inflammatory sensorimotor polyneuropathy affecting both adults and children. Ninety percent of patients report pain at some stage during their illness, usually within the first eight weeks, with half describing their pain as "horrible," "distressing," or "excruciating." The most common reports are of deep, aching, back and leg pains, and limb dysesthesiae, however, painful paresthesiae, meningism, headache (autonomic dysreflexia), muscle and joint pains, and visceral pain are also described.[9, 10] The distal-to-proximal spread of limb pain that commonly characterizes peripheral neuropathies is not usually seen.[11] The back and legs pains usually resolve within ten weeks; however, 5–10 percent of patients are left with persisting limb dysesthesiae despite recovery of motor function.[10] Patients with GBS are often nursed in an intensive care setting and may require sedation or tracheal cannulation, making pain assessment difficult.

Gabapentin is the treatment of choice for acute pain in GBS, significantly improving pain scores and reducing fentanyl requirements[12][II] and being more effective than carbamazepine.[13][II] However, early treatment with carbamazepine also improves analgesia and reduces requirements for pethidine and sedation.[14][II] Intravenous low-dose ketamine[15, 16][II], [17][II], [18][II] or lidocaine infusions[16][II], [17][II], [19][I], [20][II], [21][II] and possibly opioids[3][I], [22][II] tramadol,[3][I] or lamotrigine[23][II] may also be useful in the treatment of acute neuropathic pain in GBS, based on evidence of benefit in other neuropathic pain disorders, including spinal cord injury pain.

Musculoskeletal pain may be treated with analgesics including paracetamol, NSAIDs, COX-2-selective inhibitors, and physical therapies. A multimodal analgesia approach may be useful. Opioids may worsen respiratory failure and muscular weakness or paralysis may negate the use of patient-controlled analgesia (PCA) devices.

Disease-modifying approaches such as plasma exchange[24][I] or immunoglobulin therapy[25][I] are both equally effective in the treatment of acute GBS, resulting in shortened disease duration and improved outcomes, including pain. Intravenous methylprednisolone hastens recovery when added to immunoglobulin therapy; however, steroids alone do not clearly affect GBS outcomes and oral prednisolone may even slow the rate of recovery.[26][I] Case reports show that steroids may provide rapid resolution of severe backache during the acute phase of GBS.[27]

Acute headache in GBS may be due to primary disorders such as tension-type headache or migraine or secondary to autonomic dysreflexia with acute hypertension, immunoglobulin or steroid therapy,[28] meningism, post-dural puncture headache, temporal arteritis,[29] or hydrocephalus.[30] A case report describes cerebrospinal fluid drainage via a lumbar intrathecal catheter as an effective treatment for intractable headache associated with GBS.[31]

Comfort measures such as air mattresses, cushioning and turns, padding of exposed peripheral nerves, physical therapies, bladder, bowel, pressure-area, eye and mouth care are all of vital importance in the management of acute pain in GBS. The psychosocial impacts of GBS, including prolonged hospitalization, must be considered and treated within a multidisciplinary framework.

Acute pain associated with peripheral neuropathies

Painful peripheral neuropathy has a variety of etiologies, including diabetes mellitus, nutritional disorders, toxins (e.g. alcohol), medications (e.g. chemotherapy), trauma, and surgery. A nutritional deficiency, metabolic disorder, or "toxic effect" should always be considered where the diagnosis is unclear. Acute, severe neuropathic limb pain associated with autonomic features may herald the onset of a CRPS. Intravenous low-dose ketamine or lidocaine infusions,[16][II], [19][I], [32][II] opioids, or tramadol[3][I] may be useful rescue treatments for severe, acute peripheral neuropathic pain.

Chronic alcohol intake may result in a toxic polyneuropathy involving the sensory, motor, and autonomic components of the nervous system, most likely due to thiamine deficiency and/or a direct neurotoxic effect of ethanol. Classically, alcoholic neuropathy presents as a slowly progressive, symmetrical, painful peripheral neuropathy, principally affecting the lower limbs in a "stocking (and glove) distribution." A "burning feet syndrome" associated with allodynia, lancinating pains, and sensorimotor disturbance is common. Alcoholic neuropathy may also present in a rapidly progressive acute form, sometimes mimicking GBS.[33] Acute pain management is based on alcohol abstinence (and the treatment of withdrawal), administration of parenteral thiamine, and provision of analgesia, including the use of antineuropathic agents such as mexiletine.[34] There is a trend toward improvement in pain with thiamine supplementation[35] and lumbar sympathectomy has also been used successfully for pain management.[36]

Acute pain in patients with human immunodeficiency virus Infection

Infection with the human immunodeficiency virus (HIV) and the subsequent development of acquired immune deficiency syndrome (AIDS) is an ever-growing global epidemic, particularly in sub-Saharan Africa and Asia. In 2004, nearly 40 million people worldwide were HIV positive. In patients with HIV/AIDS, pain is a common and progressive symptom, affecting approximately 25 percent with early stage disease, 50–75 percent with AIDS, and almost all patients in the terminal phase.[37, 38, 39] The $CD4^+$ T-cell count does not predict the number of symptoms including pain or the severity of distress.[40]

Pain may be due to the effects of the virus (which is neurotropic) or infective or neoplastic processes associated with immunodeficiency such as tuberculosis or Kaposi's sarcoma. Pain may also be due to treatment-related adverse effects such as antiretroviral neuropathy, physical debilitation (in patients with end-stage AIDS) or unrelated co-morbidities.[41, 42]

HIV-related pain may occur at multiple sites, increasing in number throughout the course of the disease. Common presentations include abdominal pain (26 percent), throat pain (20 percent), multifactorial headaches (17–63 percent), chest pain, anorectal pain, arthralgias and myalgias (5 percent), back pain (5 percent), and pain related to acute herpes zoster (5 percent) or GBS. Twenty-five percent of HIV patients develop (often painful) peripheral neuropathies, most commonly a distal symmetrical polyneuropathy (DSP) usually affecting the lower limbs, associated with paresthesiae, abnormal sensory testing, and absent ankle jerks.[43] HIV-associated neuropathy may present at the time of primary infection, at seroconversion, or during advanced stages of the disease.[44, 45] Increased age, immunosuppression, poor nutritional status, and the presence of chronic disease are associated with a higher incidence of peripheral nerve dysfunction in patients with HIV.[46]

TREATMENT OF HIV/AIDS-RELATED ACUTE PAIN

Initially, management of acute pain in HIV/AIDS should be directed at diagnosis and treatment of the underlying cause. Disease-specific therapy, psychosocial interventions, and physical modalities should accompany standard analgesic treatments.[42, 47] Unfortunately, HIV/AIDS-related pain is often undertreated, due to patient and clinician-related barriers,[48, 49, 50, 51, 52] particularly in patients who are female, non-caucasians, substance abusers, poorly educated, or those with higher levels of psychosocial distress.[53] There is a higher incidence of substance abuse, including opioids, in patients with HIV/AIDS. These patients report more pain and psychological distress and may be difficult to treat because of problems such as opioid tolerance or addiction.

The treatment of acute pain in HIV/AIDS should parallel the treatment of acute cancer pain, following the World Health Organization's analgesic ladder.[54] Breakthrough pain is defined as pain that breaks through an existing, effective analgesic regimen.[55] Urgent and rapid titration with an opioid analgesic is usually required; intravenous[56][II] or transmucosal fentanyl[57][II] are both highly effective for the treatment of breakthrough pain.

Oral controlled-release opioids provide effective analgesia with minimal side effects in the treatment of severe HIV-related pain;[58] however, transdermal fentanyl may be superior with lower pain scores and improved daily function.[59] Fifteen to twenty percent of AIDS patients require parenteral opioids for maintenance and breakthrough analgesia during the terminal phase of their disease.[60, 61, 62]

Potentially complex drug interactions should be considered whenever prescribing opioids (particularly methadone or pethidine), benzodiazepines, antidepressants, or anticonvulsants in HIV/AIDS patients on antiretroviral, antibiotic, or antifungal therapies. Ritonavir decreases the metabolism of fentanyl[63][II] leading to accumulation and increases the concentration of pethidine's clinically active metabolite, norpethidine, leading to possible neurotoxicity including seizures.[64][III] Ritonavir also increases the metabolism of methadone and buprenorphine, but without clinical relevant effects. Lopinavir, rifampicin, and rifabutin all increase opioid metabolism (particularly methadone), possibly inducing withdrawal symptoms in patients on opioid maintenance therapy.[65][III] Fluconazole potentiates the effects of methadone and, conversely, methadone inhibits the metabolism of zidovudine, thereby increasing the bioavailability and toxicity of this antiviral agent.

Bupropion,[3][I] lamotrigine,[3][I], [66][II] gabapentin,[67][II], [68] or acetyl L-carnitine[69] may be effective in treating HIV-related painful peripheral neuropathy. In contrast, amitriptyline,[3][I], [70][II], [71][II] topical 5 percent lidocaine,[72][II] mexiletine,[3][I], [70][II], [73][II] topical capsaicin,[74] Peptide-T,[75][II] vibratory counterstimulation,[76][III] and acupuncture[71][II] were ineffective. Although not studied specifically in HIV/AIDS, intravenous ketamine or lidocaine infusions, tramadol, or opioids may be useful in the treatment of severe, acute neuropathic pain. Although there is good evidence that cannabinoids are ineffective in the treatment of acute pain, approximately 30 percent of patients attending an HIV treatment clinic used cannabis for symptom relief, reporting a 90 percent improvement in muscle pain and painful peripheral neuropathy.[77] There is limited evidence that cannabinoids may be effective in the treatment of some forms of peripheral neuropathic pain, although not specifically HIV-related neuropathy.[3][I]

ACUTE ABDOMINAL PAIN

The purpose of this section is not to provide an exhaustive list of all the surgical and nonsurgical causes of abdominal pain and their management, but rather to provide evidence for acute pain management approaches. Acute abdominal pain may originate from visceral or somatic structures or may be referred. Recurrent acute abdominal pain may be a manifestation of a chronic visceral pain syndrome, such as chronic pancreatitis, recurrent renal calculosis, or irritable bowel syndrome. Neuropathic pain, abdominal wall disorders, such as rectus sheath nerve entrapment, or medical conditions such as diabetic ketoacidosis, hypercalcemia, herpes zoster, porphyria, or abdominal migraine should be considered. Patients with recurrent acute or chronic abdominal pain, particularly pelvic pain in women, may have significant psychosocial issues and would benefit from comprehensive multidisciplinary pain assessment. Abdominal pain is a common presenting complaint in opioid-seeking patients, particularly in primary care settings such as the emergency room (ER) and substance abuse issues should be considered.

Early accurate diagnosis is obviously important if surgical intervention is to be curative, e.g. appendicitis, perforated, or infarcted bowel. When considering such conditions as acute back pain, the concept of "red and yellow flags" has been accepted. We believe these terms might also be useful when reviewing patients with abdominal pain. The identification of red flags alerts the team to acute surgical pathology.

Red flags for surgical acute abdominal pain include:

- weight loss;
- history of malignancy;
- history of previous abdominal surgery or pathology;
- rebound tenderness or guarding;
- biochemical/hematological abnormalities.

Patients with acute abdominal pain are often admitted to hospital for observation, assessment, and further investigation including laparoscopy. Easter et al.,[78] reporting on 131 laparoscopies performed for investigation of acute or chronic pain and cancer staging, found that 4 out of 7 (57 percent) patients with acute pain and 37 out of 70 (53 percent) with chronic pain had positive findings. These findings affected treatment options in 71 and 39 percent of the patients, respectively.

Of equal importance is the identification of psychosocial yellow flags. Psychosocial issues have long been recognized as important contributors to abdominal pain and have been extensively studied.

Psychosocial yellow flags in recurrent acute and chronic abdominal pain include:

- depression;
- sexual or physical abuse.

Abdominal migraine

Abdominal migraine (AM) is a functional neurogastrointestinal disorder most commonly presenting in male children between the ages of 2 and 11. It is characterized by recurrent attacks of acute abdominal pain and/or vomiting and sometimes headache and may be precipitated by migraine triggers such as stress (parental separation, school), fasting, or sleep deprivation. There may be a prodromal or aura phase associated with listlessness, drowsiness, mood disturbance, or headache. The abdominal pain is typically located diffusely in the periumbilical region and is described as burning or aching in nature, associated with nausea, vomiting, pallor, flushing, and occasionally fever. A typical episode lasts at least four hours and children are completely asymptomatic between attacks.[79, 80] Organic causes for the symptoms, such as appendicitis, need to be excluded before treatment is commenced.

Prophylaxis includes avoiding trigger factors and the use of dietary measures. Although there are no specific data, an episode of AM should be treated using comfort measures, rest, and simple analgesia including paracetamol, NSAIDs, or an antihistamine if the oral route is reliable. Pizotifen is effective for the prophylaxis and treatment of AM[81][II] and there are case reports of benefit with propranolol, cyproheptadine, tritpans, clonidine, or sodium valproate.[82]

Analgesia in acute abdominal pain

Abdominal pain is the most frequent presenting complaint in patients attending the ER in the United States. Until recently, it was believed that analgesia masked the signs and symptoms of abdominal pathology and should be withheld until a diagnosis was established. However, a recent RCT demonstrated that intravenous morphine provides rapid and effective analgesia for acute abdominal pain and was no different to placebo in terms of diagnostic accuracy.[83][II]

A summary of eight randomized, placebo-controlled trials confirmed that opioid analgesia does not affect diagnostic accuracy in adults or children presenting with acute abdominal pain in primary care situations.[83][II], [84][II]

Based on these data, it has become increasingly accepted practice that analgesia should not be withheld for acute abdominal pain in order to facilitate a diagnosis. However, there are still some concerns with this approach, particularly in young children or nonverbal adults, or where there are difficulties in accessing timely surgical review or appropriate diagnostic imaging. Patients who have little or no abdominal pain after receiving analgesia also present a management dilemma.[85]

Patients with acute abdominal pain but no surgically treatable pathology are often managed conservatively by restricting oral intake (including oral analgesics), nasogastric drainage, intravenous fluid replacement, and provision of analgesia. In this situation, intravenous opioids should be administered, preferably using a PCA device. In patients on long-term opioid therapy prior to admission, a background infusion may be necessary to prevent withdrawal, together with a higher bolus dose because of tolerance. Once the acute pain has settled, parenteral opioids should be weaned and the oral route used as soon as gut function is restored. Co-analgesics, such as paracetamol or NSAIDs, may be useful as part of a multimodal approach, although the adverse effects of these drugs on liver, gut, and renal function should be considered.

Pethidine should be avoided because of the adverse neurological effects of its renally excreted metabolite norpethidine, including confusion, myoclonus, or seizures, and because of a higher abuse potential.[86] Tramadol has an advantage in causing less gastrointestinal stasis,[87][II], [88][II] but there may be dose limitations in patients with severe pain.

Intravenous low-dose ketamine, given either by bolus doses or infusion, may be useful in severe, acute abdominal pain that is poorly responsive to opioids,[89][II] particularly in tolerant patients[90, 91][II] or in visceral pain states such as acute-on-chronic pancreatitis.[92][II], [93][II]

Renal colic

Renal colic is common, particularly in older males and during warmer months, with an overall incidence of 1/1000, accounting for 1 percent of all ER visits.[94] Most patients are discharged from the ER within a few hours of treatment, with approximately 5 percent requiring admission and 15 percent re-attending within a few days because of continuing symptoms.[95] Renal colic is a common presenting complaint in patients seeking opioids (particularly pethidine) for an addiction, so an index of suspicion must be held. In some cases, renal colic is a recurrent acute condition or it may be associated with a chronic renal (visceral) pain disorder, such as loin pain hematuria.

Parenteral analgesia is very effective in renal colic with 74 percent of patients becoming pain free soon after initial treatment, usually in the ER.[95] Although NSAIDs and opioids both provide effective analgesia, NSAIDs are superior with less vomiting, decreased requirements for rescue analgesia,[96][I] and a lower incidence of recurrent symptoms in ER patients.[97][II], [98][II] The onset of analgesia is fastest when NSAIDs are given intravenously,[99][I] although suppositories may also be effective.[100][II] The oral route is less reliable and effective; oral rofecoxib or diclofenac administered regularly over 24 hours did not reduce morphine requirements in acute renal colic.[101][II] When administering NSAIDs or COX-2-selective inhibitors in renal colic, the patient's renal function must be considered, particularly if there is ureteric obstruction.

Although pethidine is commonly administered for renal colic in the belief that it causes less smooth muscle spasm and nausea, there is no difference between intravenous pethidine or morphine[102][II] in the quality of analgesia and the incidence of nausea is higher with pethidine.[96][I]

Anticholinergic smooth muscle relaxants, such as atropine or hyoscine-N-butylbromide, fail to provide effective analgesia in renal colic, when administered alone or in combination with NSAIDs,[103][II] opioids,[104][II] or metamizole.[105][I]

Metamizole is an effective analgesic in renal colic, particularly via the intravenous route. Limited data indicates that a single dose metamizole is of similar efficacy to other analgesics used in renal colic, although intramuscular metamizole was less effective than 75 mg of diclofenac.[105][I]

Intravenous ondansetron (8 mg) produced analgesia in 42 percent of patients with renal colic but was less effective than 75 mg of intramuscular diclofenac.[106][II] Intranasal desmopressin is also an effective analgesic, either alone or in combination with intramuscular diclofenac.[107][II]

TENS applied over the painful flank reduces pain scores, anxiety, and nausea in patients with renal colic[108][II] and acupuncture may also be beneficial based on limited data.[109]

Although it is common clinical practice to promote diuresis in patients with renal colic, a single RCT demonstrated that intravenous fluid therapy (3 L over six hours) had no effect on pain outcomes or stone transition at six hours.[110][I]

The distal ureter contains specific adrenoceptor subtypes that produce smooth muscle relaxation. Medical (renal calculus) expulsive therapy, using the specific alpha blocker tamsulosin for up to two weeks, significantly reduced calculus expulsion time, hospitalizations for recurrent colic, and possibly analgesia requirements, although further research is ongoing.[111] Tamsulosin was superior to comparative smooth muscle relaxants such as phloroglucinol or nifedipine in terms of increased stone expulsion and a reduction in analgesia requirements, surgical interventions, duration of hospital stay, and days off work.[112][II] There are no clear data on the effects of urgent lithotripsy or surgical interventions on acute renal colic.

In summary, acute renal colic should be treated using a multimodal analgesia approach based on first-line administration of intravenous (or rectal) NSAIDs and/or titrated intravenous opioids, supplemented by paracetamol, metamizole (dipyrone), ondansetron, TENS, and possibly acupuncture. Inhalation of nitrous oxide in oxygen or methoxyflurane may provide short-term analgesia, particularly in the ER, without specific evidence in renal colic. For persisting or severe acute pain, opioid PCA and/or intravenous low-dose ketamine may be beneficial, the latter based on evidence of efficacy in patients with opioid tolerance or visceral pain. Intranasal desmopressin or medical expulsive therapy with tamsulosin may also be beneficial. There is no clear indication for the use of pethidine, anticholinergic smooth muscle relaxants or fluid diuresis in the treatment of renal colic.

Biliary colic and acute pancreatitis

All opioids increase sphincter of Oddi tone and bile duct pressures based on animal and human experimental data,[113] although morphine increased sphincter contractions more than pethidine during cholecystectomy.[114][II] There are no clinical studies comparing opioids in the treatment of biliary colic or acute pancreatitis-related pain; however, the use of morphine, fentanyl, or hydromorphone is appropriate. Pethidine offers no clear clinical advantage and may be associated with serious adverse effects (see below under Opioids).[113]

Parenteral NSAIDs (ketorolac, tenoxicam, or diclofenac) are at least as effective as parenteral opioids and more effective than anticholinergic smooth muscle relaxants (hyoscine-N-butylbromide) in providing analgesia for biliary colic[115][II], [116][II], [117][II], [118][II], [119][II] and may also prevent progression to cholecystitis.[115][II], [116][II], [119][II] Metamizole is more effective than tramadol or smooth muscle relaxants (butylscopolamine).[120][II] Glycopyrronium bromide (glycopyrrolate)[121][II] and atropine[122][II]) were no more effective than placebo in relieving acute biliary tract pain. Perhaps not surprisingly, these are similar findings to the efficacy of these drugs in the treatment of renal colic. A single RCT demonstrated faster resolution of acute biliary colic and right upper quadrant tenderness in patients who were administered glucagon.[123][II]

Expedient cholecystectomy is advocated for crescendo biliary colic. TENS and comfort measures, such as heat packs, may be helpful, but there are no data to support their effectiveness.

Acute pancreatitis can be a severe life-threatening illness, although 85 percent of cases are benign and self limiting, usually resolving within a week. The most common causes are cholelithiasis or ethanol abuse and elevated serum amylase levels are usually diagnostic. Apart from abdominal symptoms, systemic manifestations may also occur, including sepsis. The treatment of acute pancreatitis is largely supportive with therapy aimed at reducing pancreatic secretions (by restricting oral intake and using nasogastric drainage), replacing fluid and electrolyte losses, blood sugar control and occasionally the use of antibiotics, or endoscopic, surgical, or critical care management. Treatment of alcohol withdrawal may be required in patients with alcohol-induced pancreatitis, which may complicate pain management. Acute pancreatitis-related pain may be a "one-off" event or an acute exacerbation of a chronic visceral pain syndrome such as chronic pancreatitis.

Patients with recurrent acute or chronic pancreatitis-related pain may be treated with long-term opioids, associated with complications such as tolerance and addiction and in some cases alcohol abuse. Abdominal pain due to "pancreatitis" is a common presenting complaint in patients seeking opioids for addiction, so an index of suspicion must be maintained.

Although there are no specific data for pain management in acute pancreatitis, the use of parenteral opioids, preferably via a PCA device (during fasting) and multimodal analgesia including regular paracetamol (if liver function is normal), and possibly a COX-2-selective inhibitor, may be appropriate. Although traditionally used as the first-line opioid in pancreatitis, pethidine should be avoided as there is no clear clinical or pharmacological advantage in terms of reduced biliary spasm or colic.[113] In addition, the administration of higher doses of pethidine (greater than 10 mg/kg per day) over several days, as is common in acute pancreatitis, is associated with accumulation of norpethidine and the possible development of adverse psychocognitive effects, myoclonus, or seizures, particularly in patients at risk of alcohol withdrawal. Fentanyl PCA has been used extensively with good effect in the treatment of acute pain in pancreatitis and may be the opioid of choice (Visser EJ, personal communication). Tramadol may also be effective with less gastrointestinal stasis and possibly less biliary spasm; however, its usefulness may be limited by dose restrictions or the risk of seizures associated with alcohol withdrawal.

Parenteral NSAIDs may improve analgesia in acute pancreatitis, particularly if there is biliary colic. However, caution should be exercised if the patient is systemically unwell or at risk of gastrointestinal or pancreatic hemorrhage or renal impairment. Apart from renal considerations, a parenteral COX-2-selective inhibitor may be preferable as there is no bleeding risk and the rate of acute peptic ulceration is similar to placebo if used for less than five days.[124][II]

In patients with severe acute pain that is poorly responsive to opioids or where there is visceral hyperalgesia (chronic pancreatitis), intravenous low-dose ketamine may be effective although there are no specific data to support this approach in acute pancreatitis.

Chronic pancreatitis develops in up to 10 percent of acute cases and may be difficult to diagnose. In a review of the diagnostic criteria, Clain and Pearson comment that "chronic pancreatitis is not a single well-defined entity but rather it is a condition with multiple causes, a complex, not well defined pathogenesis and a variety of clinical presentations". Normal serum amylase levels do not exclude the diagnosis.[125] Patients with chronic pancreatitis may have diabetes and therefore related pain disorders such as painful peripheral neuropathy or, rarely, acute abdominal pain due to diabetic ketoacidosis. Psychosocial and substance abuse issues (including alcohol) are common in this group of patients and may impact on acute pain management.

Irritable bowel syndrome and inflammatory bowel disorders

Irritable bowel syndrome (IBS) is a common, functional gastrointestinal or visceral hypersensitivity disorder affecting 2.6 percent of the population, particularly females,[126] and is frequently associated with other complex pain syndromes such as functional dyspepsia, fibromyalgia, headaches, or dysmenorrhea. IBS is characterized by recurrent, episodic gastrointestinal symptoms, principally defecation-related abdominal pain and intestinal dysfunction (constipation, diarrhea, or both) and is diagnosed clinically using Rome III criteria.[127] Although 70 percent of patients with IBS do not seek medical attention, they frequently use over-the-counter medications[128] and symptoms may significantly affect a patient's health-related quality of life.[129] Psychosocial factors such as anxiety and depression are common in IBS and may impact on acute pain management.

Smooth muscle relaxants[130][I] or peppermint oil[131][I] provide effective acute pain relief in IBS. However, there are no specific data for opioids, tramadol, NSAIDs, or paracetamol, including over-the-counter medications, in the treatment of IBS pain. Preventive treatments such as antidepressants or anti-bulking agents are not supported by high level evidence,[132][I] although citalopram[133][II] or fluoxetine[134][II] may reduce pain and constipation. The partial 5HT4 receptor agonist tegaserod reduces IBS-related constipation and possibly pain (in females),[135][I] whereas the 5HT3 antagonist alosetron is effective where diarrhea predominates.[136][I] Cognitive-behavioral therapy was no better than standard care in the treatment of IBS, including pain.[137][II]

Crohn's disease and ulcerative colitis are chronic inflammatory bowel disorders with systemic manifestations. They may present with acute abdominal pain due to flare up of chronic visceral pain or acute surgical pathology including enterocolitis, intestinal obstruction, intraabdominal infection, or postsurgical pain following laparotomy. Other causes of acute pain include stomal ulceration or perianal pathology, such as fistulae or fissures. Some patients require acute pain relief for seronegative polyarthropathy which is commonly associated with inflammatory bowel disease.

Although there are no specific data, the treatment of acute abdominal pain in inflammatory bowel disease is based on multimodal analgesia including opioids, tramadol, paracetamol, intravenous low-dose ketamine, NSAIDs, or COX-2-selective inhibitors (only with due consideration of the potential gastrointestinal or renal adverse effects) and comfort measures, including TENS and heat packs. Steroids may be prescribed for an exacerbation of inflammatory bowel disease, although there is no clear evidence that they reduce acute abdominal pain. Because of the chronic and recurrent nature of these conditions, chronic abdominal pain may develop which is often associated with significant psychosocial problems and long-term opioid use, thus complicating acute pain management.

Acute dyspepsia and esophageal spasm

The most common cause of upper gastrointestinal symptoms is non-ulcer dyspepsia (NUD) and yet the pathophysiology of this condition is poorly characterized and the optimum treatment is uncertain. NUD is frequently classified as a functional gastrointestinal disorder; however, dyspepsia may be related to gastroesophageal reflux or gastritis. Patients with functional dyspepsia have higher levels of anxiety, depression, and neuroticism, although there are insufficient data to determine if they respond to psychological therapies.[138][I] Esophageal spasm is a related upper gastrointestinal acute pain disorder where increased lower esophageal smooth muscle spasm is associated with dysphagia and epigastric or retrosternal pain, occasionally mimicking acute coronary ischemia.

Viscous benzocaine or lidocaine were equally effective in the treatment of acute dyspepsia.[139][II] The so-called GI cocktail, a combination of antacid, compounded hyoscyamine (atropine and hyoscine), and viscous lidocaine was no more effective than antacid alone in the treatment of severe dyspepsia in the emergency department.[140][II] Other therapies such as *Helicobacter pylori* eradication, H2 blockers, and "pro-kinetics" may be beneficial in treating NUD, but further trials are required; antacids or sucralfate were only of marginal benefit.[141][I], [142][I]

For the treatment of acute pain in esophageal spasm, nifedipine, glyceryl trinitrate, or the application of TENS over the anterior chest wall may be useful; there were no specific data for antispasmodics, antacids, or topical local anesthetics. Diazepam or tricyclic antidepressants may improve symptoms during recurrent, acute episodes. Botulinum toxin injection or dilatation of the lower esophagus are effective long-term treatments.[143]

Primary dysmenorrhea and Mittelschmerz

Primary dysmenorrhea (PD) is one of the most common acute pain disorders, affecting up to 60 percent of premenopausal women, with the same percentage reporting pain as moderate or severe and a large proportion reporting interference with daily activities, including missing school or work. Younger age, smoking, non-use of the oral contraceptive pill, and nulliparity are risk factors for PD.[144] Although most women do not seek medical attention for the disorder, many resort to use of over-the-counter medications or complementary therapies to treat the symptoms. NSAIDs, including naproxen, ibuprofen, and mefenamic acid are highly effective in the treatment of dysmenorrhea with ibuprofen having the least adverse effects.[145][I] The COX-2-selective inhibitors lumiracoxib and rofecoxib are effective once-daily treatments.[146][II] Aspirin and paracetamol were less effective than NSAIDs.[147][I]

High frequency TENS and possibly acupuncture may be effective in PD based on the results of a small number of RCTs[148][I] and a lower abdominal wall pressure garment is also effective in reducing menstrual pain and analgesia use.[149][II] As preventive therapies, vitamin B1[150][I] and vitamin E[151][II] significantly reduce pain and blood loss in PD.

Mittelschmerz is mid-cycle lower abdominal pain linked to ovulation, which affects 1–3 percent of premenopausal women, most commonly in their late teens or twenties. It presents with mild to moderate unilateral or bilateral iliac fossa pain, lasting hours to days. The pain is usually mild, but it may be severe when there is peritoneal irritation and there may be associated nausea, vomiting, or shoulder tip pain. A severe episode may herald gynecological pathology, such as an intraperitoneal hemorrhage or torsion of an ovarian cyst. Moderate pain is treated with rest and comfort measures, such as heat and simple analgesia.

ACUTE CARDIAC PAIN

Acute coronary syndrome refers to a range of acute myocardial ischemic states including unstable angina and myocardial infarction. Typically, myocardial ischemia causes central chest pain, which may radiate into the arm, neck, or jaw; nontypical presentations may occur, particularly in the elderly patient. Analgesia begins with restoration of coronary perfusion and myocardial oxygenation, including the use of supplemental oxygen.

Intravenous morphine is the mainstay of effective and rapid analgesia for acute coronary syndromes, often requiring surprisingly low doses. Independent predictors of increased morphine requirements include suspicion or confirmation of infarction, ST changes on the admission electrocardiogram, male sex, and a history of angina or cardiac failure.[152] Intravenous morphine or alfentanil are equally effective in relieving acute ischemic chest pain, however, the onset of analgesia is faster with alfentanil.[153] [II] Morphine is similar to buprenorphine[154][II] and pethidine[155][II] and superior to metoprolol[156][II] in terms of analgesia and adverse effects. Intravenous tramadol provides adequate analgesia with minimal changes in clinical cardiorespiratory parameters in acute myocardial infarction,[157][III] although it may reduce the left ventricular stroke work index.[158][III]

Nitroglycerine is effective in relieving acute ischemic chest pain; however, the analgesic response does not predict a diagnosis of active coronary artery disease.[159] In patients with chest pain due to cocaine-induced acute coronary syndrome, the addition of intravenous diazepam or lorazepam to treatment with sublingual nitroglycerine provides superior analgesia.[160][II], [161][II]

Nitrous oxide in oxygen is effective in relieving acute ischemic chest pain with a significant reduction in beta-endorphin levels.[162][II] NSAIDs are effective in the treatment of acute pain due to pericarditis.[163]

ACUTE OROFACIAL PAIN

Acute orofacial pain is most commonly due to pharyngitis, dental, sinus, glandular, or otic disease; however, it may also be associated with chronic facial pain syndromes (e.g. trigeminal neuralgia) or be referred from adjacent regions such as the cervical spine or the thorax. A thorough history (including dental) and examination (particularly of the oral cavity and cranial nerves) is essential in the assessment of acute orofacial pain. Recurrent or persistent orofacial pain may be neuropathic in etiology and is frequently associated with significant psychosocial problems, requiring multidisciplinary pain assessment and management.

Acute dental pain

Based on third molar extraction models, paracetamol, aspirin, opioids, or tramadol (either alone or in combination), NSAIDs or COX-2-selective inhibitors all provide effective analgesia for acute dental pain,[164][I], [165][I] However, NSAIDs or COX-2-selective inhibitors provide superior pain relief with less adverse effects than opioids or tramadol and are the treatment of choice.[166][I] NSAIDs and emergency pulpectomy, but not antibiotics, provide effective pain relief in acute apical periodontitis.[167][I]

Acute pharyngitis and mucositis

Acute sore throat due to pharyngitis is usually the result of viral (including infectious mononucleosis) or streptococcal infection and is effectively treated with NSAIDs or COX-2-selective inhibitors, aspirin, paracetamol, tramadol, or opioids, either alone or in combination, based on studies of post-tonsillectomy pain[168][II] and data from a topical review.[169] A single dose of ibuprofen (200–400 mg) reduced sore throat intensity by 32–80 percent at four hours compared with placebo. Paracetamol (approximately 15 mg per kg) reduced pain by 31–50 percent at three hours.[168][II] Aspirin was also effective in the treatment of sore throat and other symptoms associated with an upper respiratory tract infection[170][II] and the addition of caffeine further improved analgesia for sore throat.[171][II] Topical agents such as local anesthetic gargles may be helpful. Benzydamine HCl 0.15 percent anti-inflammatory spray reduced the mean pain score for sore throat by 42 percent compared with placebo[169][I] and flurbiprofen lozenges provided effective pain relief without any adverse effects.[172][II]

Steroid therapy with oral dexamethasone,[173][II] either as a single dose or three daily doses,[174][II] or intramuscular betamethasone[175][II] significantly reduced pain on swallowing and the duration of symptoms in patients (including children) with moderate to severe pharyngitis, particularly those with proven streptococcal infection on bacterial culture. However, another RCT using oral dexamethasone in children failed to support this finding[176] [II] and the effectiveness and safety of steroids for symptom control in infectious mononucleosis is not yet clear.[177][I] A single dose of intravenous steroid improved throat pain, trismus, and fever in patients treated with antibiotics and needle aspiration for peri-tonsillar abscess.[178][II]

Antibiotics for sore throat reduced pain, headache, and fever by 50 percent on day three and shortened the duration of symptoms by 16–24 hours. The number needed to treat (NNT) to prevent one sore throat with antibiotics on day three was 5.0 (4.5–5.8) and 14.2 (11.5–20.6) at one week.[179][I]

Acute oral ulceration due to trauma (physical, chemical, thermal), infection (e.g. herpes simplex), drugs, radiation, or chemotherapy may be extremely painful and debilitating. Mucosal analgesia may be achieved by topical application of eutectic mixture of local anesthetics (EMLA®) cream or 5 percent lidocaine gel.[180][II]

In treating acute oropharangeal pain associated with cancer-related mucositis, opioid PCA is effective[181][I] and morphine provides better analgesia with less dose escalation then hydromorphone or sufentanil.[182][II] Topical doxepin[183][II]) or ketamine solutions[184] also provide effective analgesia and intravenous ketamine "burst therapy" is effective in mucositis pain that is refractory to opioid analgesia.[185][V] Allopurinol mouthwash, vitamin E, immunoglobulin, and human placental extract may improve outcomes in acute mucositis, but the evidence is inconclusive.[181][I] Topical lidocaine, chlorhexidine, or sulcrafate solutions were no more effective than simple salt and soda water mixtures.

Sinusitis and otitis media

There are only limited data to direct the choice of analgesia in patients with acute sinusitis or otitis media. It is appropriate to use NSAIDs, COX-2-selective inhibitors, paracetamol, weak opioids, or tramadol, based on evidence for the treatment of acute dental pain. Administration of penicillin V decreased pain scores over three days in patients with severe sinusitis.[186][II] In children with otitis media, antibiotics provided a small improvement in pain after two days[187][I] and there was a trend to reduced pain using topical naturopathic or local anesthetic ear drops.[188][I]

ACUTE PAIN ASSOCIATED WITH HEMATOLOGICAL OR METABOLIC DISORDERS

Sickle cell disease, hemophilia, and the acute porphyrias may present with recurrent episodes of severe, acute pain. Opioids are the mainstay of analgesia in these conditions. Because of their relapsing nature, patients with these conditions may develop chronic pain, requiring long-term opioid therapy with all the attendant complications. Rational use of opioid analgesia, disease-modifying therapies, and patient-specific pain management with multidisciplinary support, as appropriate, offers the best chance of effective pain relief.

Hemophilia

Hemophilia A and B are inherited disorders of coagulation. In hemophilia A, there is a deficiency of factor VIII; in hemophilia B, there is a deficiency of factor IX. In both disorders, spontaneous and post-traumatic hemorrhages occur, the frequency and extent of which are proportional to the level of clotting factor deficiency.

Bleeding into restricted spaces, such as muscles, joints, and internal organs is a frequent cause of acute pain. In hemophilic arthropathy, the most common sites of pain are the ankles (45 percent), knees (39 percent), spine (14 percent), and elbows (7 percent);[189] septic arthritis is a frequent complication.[190] Hemophilia patients may also suffer acute pain due to procedures such as intravenous cannulation, joint aspiration, and surgery or the effects of co-morbid disease, such as HIV/AIDS.

Many hemophilia patients use Factor VIII to decrease pain associated with a bleeding episode;[189] higher-dose Factor VIII replacement reduces the number of patients

with restricted joint movement after an acute hemarthrosis.[191][II] Joint aspiration may reduce acute pain and improve function.[192] Early physiotherapy is recommended if there is any delay in restoring joint function, in order to minimize the risk of chronic hemophilic arthropathy.[193]

Although there is no specific evidence, analgesics, steroids, cold therapy, and bandaging are used to treat acute pain in hemophilic arthropathy. Intravenous access for analgesia may be difficult in these patients because of "poor veins" and intramuscular analgesics should be avoided due to the risk of intramuscular hematomas. However, the use of immediate-release oral opioids and promising new methods of sublingual, intranasal, and intrapulmonary delivery may decrease the need for intravenous opioid administration.

NSAIDs are used for pain relief in hemophilic arthropathy but there are no data in acute hemarthrosis. Ibuprofen has been used successfully to control joint pain and stiffness in hemophiliacs without significant changes in platelet function, bleeding time, frequency of joint hemorrhages, or frequency of factor infusions.[194][II], [195, 196] COX-2-specific inhibitors may be of advantage due to a lack of platelet inhibitory effects.

Sickle cell disease

Sickle cell disease is an inherited disorder (autosomal dominant) of abnormal hemoglobin production which most commonly affects patients of African, Middle-Eastern, or Mediterranean ancestry and is particularly prevalent in the United States. Hemoglobin S polymerizes when deoxygenated, causing rigidity of erythrocytes, blood hyperviscosity, and occlusion of the microcirculation, with resultant tissue ischemia and infarction. Sickle cell disease usually presents with painful vaso-occlusive crises, occurring either spontaneously or due to low oxygen tension, dehydration, infection, temperature change, menstruation, stress, or fatigue.

A sickle cell crisis most commonly affects multiple bony sites or joints (due to avascular necrosis of bone marrow) resulting in severe pain lasting for hours to weeks, usually in the low back, legs, knees, arms, or chest.[197] Crises involving abdominal organs, such as the spleen, gut, liver, or gallbladder may present as an acute surgical abdomen. Priapism is not uncommon and renal colic may develop due to renal papillary necrosis and hematuria. An "acute chest syndrome" presents with chest pain, cough, dyspnea, and fever with hypoxemia, leukocytosis, and pulmonary infiltrates on a chest radiograph. Other causes of acute pain include ischemic leg ulcers or central pain associated with stroke or spinal cord infarction.

Most patients with sickle cell disease attend the ER during a crisis with a mean of 7.4 visits per year and an admission rate of 30 percent;[198] however, the frequency and severity of crises varies greatly between patients and over time. In the United States, the development of dedicated sickle cell anemia day wards for the treatment of acute crises has significantly reduced the rate of inpatient admissions. Because patients attend a wide variety of healthcare providers at different times, an individualized pain management plan in the form of a letter, card, or portfolio carried by the patient at all times is recommended.[199]

Patients suffering frequent painful sickle cell crises may develop chronic pain, opioid dependency, and psychosocial problems, such as mood disorders or interruption of schooling or work life, requiring a multidisciplinary pain management approach.[200, 201] Pain is frequently under-treated due to "distraction" by more urgent medical problems, a lack of objective clinical signs at the time of pain onset, or issues surrounding opioid analgesia including concerns about addiction.[202]

The management of an acute sickle cell crisis consists of resuscitation, oxygen therapy, hydration, organ failure support, treatment of infection, occasionally surgery (e.g. amputation), and multimodal analgesia based on intravenous or oral opioid therapy.[203]

According to a Cochrane review, there is not enough evidence to allow clarification of the most effective analgesia approach during an acute sickle cell crisis and further research is required.[204][I]

OXYGEN

Although commonly prescribed during a sickle cell crisis, supplemental oxygen has no effect on the duration or intensity of pain or opioid consumption[205][II], [206][II], although the frequency of painful crises was higher in children suffering nocturnal oxygen desaturations.[207]

OPIOIDS

The titration of intravenous opioids for acute pain management during a sickle cell crisis is similar in concept to treating breakthrough cancer pain. Intravenous opioid loading improves the efficacy of subsequent PCA and oral therapies[199] in sickle cell crisis pain and a continuous morphine infusion is more effective than intermittent bolus doses.[205][II] The absorption of intramuscular or subcutaneous opioids during a sickle cell crisis may be reduced due to impaired microcirculation in the dermis or muscles.[208]

Although intravenous opioid PCA is the mainstay of acute pain management in sickle cell disease, oral opioids are also effective. Oral sustained-release morphine is just as effective as parenteral morphine[204][I] and the use oral opioids at home reduced the number of ER visits and hospital admissions for sickle cell pain.[209, 210] The use of inpatient morphine PCA, rapidly converted to an oral sustained-release form for home use, reduced the length of

hospital stay by 23 percent and subsequent ER visits and readmissions by approximately 50 percent, compared with inpatients treated with intramuscular pethidine.[211][III]

Intravenous morphine and pethidine are the most commonly administered analgesics for sickle cell pain in the ER.[203] However, pethidine should be avoided because of the potential accumulation of norpethidine and the subsequent risk of seizures in patients who often require high doses for several days and may have renal impairment. The incidence of pethidine-induced seizures in patients with sickle cell disease is estimated at 0.4–2.6 percent.[208, 212, 213]

In patients with severe opioid-resistant or visceral pain, intravenous low-dose ketamine may improve analgesia, although there are no specific data for this approach in the treatment of sickle cell pain.[214]

Patients with frequent acute or chronic sickle cell-related pain may require long-term opioid therapy with all the associated difficulties in pain management. Children with sickle cell anemia who underwent laparoscopic cholecystectomy, reported higher pain scores, used twice as much morphine PCA and remained in hospital nearly twice as long as children without the disease having the same procedure, possibly due to a complex interaction of pain sensitization, opioid tolerance, and psychosocial factors.[215]

NSAIDS

NSAIDs (oral and intravenous) are effective analgesics during sickle cell crises and reduce opioid requirements.[216, 217] However, not all studies support their efficacy and further research is required.[218][II], [219][II] Extreme care should be taken in administering NSAIDs where there is renal impairment due to renal vaso-occlusive disease, dehydration, or severe systemic illness.

INHALED NITROUS OXIDE

Inhaled nitrous oxide in 50 percent oxygen, used for limited periods, may provide effective and rapid analgesia for acute sickle cell pain, particularly in primary care settings.[199]

INHALED NITRIC OXIDE

Defective nitric oxide (NO) mechanisms in the vascular endothelium may contribute to sickle cell vaso-occlusion. Inhaled NO may be beneficial in the treatment of acute painful crises in children; however, further studies are required.[220][II]

CORTICOSTEROIDS

Parenteral corticosteroids reduced analgesia requirements and hospital stay without major side effects during sickle cell crises[204][I] and a short course of high-dose intravenous methylprednisolone reduced the duration of severe pain in children. However, patients receiving corticosteroids suffered more rebound attacks after therapy was discontinued[221][II] and other potential risks such as the acceleration of avascular necrosis or infection may limit their usefulness.

EPIDURAL ANALGESIA

Epidural analgesia has used been effectively in sickle cell patients with severe acute pain that was unresponsive to high-dose opioids, NSAIDs, and adjunctive measures.[222]

OTHER APPROACHES

Other analgesic treatments include physical therapies such as heat and TENS.[223] Education improves knowledge and engenders a more positive attitude in patients with sickle cell disease; however, the benefits of psychological therapies such as relaxation in managing an acute crisis requires further research.[224][I]

THE PREVENTION OF PAINFUL SICKLE CELL CRISES

The incidence of painful sickle cell crises is reduced by Niprisan (a phyto-medicinal anti-sickling agent), zinc, piracetam (which prevents red blood cell dehydration),[225][II], [226][II] and hydroxyurea (induces fetal hemoglobin production); the latter also reduces the frequency of blood transfusions and life-threatening complications (including acute chest syndrome).[227][I]

Acute pain associated with the porphyrias

The acute porphyrias are a group inherited disorders of heme biosynthesis (acute intermittent porphyria, variegate porphyria, and hereditary coproporphyria being the most common, autosomal dominant forms), leading to the accumulation of neurotoxic aminolaevulinic acid (ALA) and porphyrin metabolites. These metabolic neurotoxins produce widespread peripheral (motor weakness), visceral (abdominal pain), and autonomic neuropathy (tachycardia) and central nervous system (CNS) toxicity (neuropsychiatric symptoms, seizures, brain stem, and pituitary dysfunction) and in some cases cutaneous photosensitivity.[228]

The acute porphyrias are rare with a combined prevalence of 1/20,000, although the variegate form affects 3/1000 South African Caucasians of Dutch descent. Attacks usually commence around the time of puberty and are most common in women of child-bearing age, with most patients averaging four to six episodes per lifetime.

The acute porphyrias are notoriously difficult to diagnose, on average requiring four visits to a primary care facility before a diagnosis is confirmed.[229] They are also great mimics of other medical disorders such as acute abdominal pathology, sepsis, polyneuropathy, or GBS; lead poisoning may induce a rare porphyria-variant.[230] The most common symptoms are recurrent diffuse abdominal pain (85–95 percent), vomiting (43–88 percent), constipation (48–84 percent), pain in the extremities, back, neck, chest, or head (50–70 percent), paresis (42–68 percent), altered mental state (40–58 percent) and convulsions (10–20 percent) along with tachycardia (64–85 percent), and hypertension (36–55 percent).

Abdominal pain is usually the result of visceral neuropathy and secondary bladder or bowel dysfunction (such as colic or urinary retention), although patients may also have acute postsurgical pain if an exploratory laparotomy was performed. Hypoesthesia, pain, and motor weakness due to peripheral neuropathy classically affects the "bathing trunk" area over the back, buttocks, and thighs. Dark urine is usually present and the diagnosis is confirmed by the presence and raised urinary, plasma, or fecal porphobilinogen and ALA levels. Hyponatremia is a common biochemical abnormality due to pituitary dysfunction and inappropriate secretion of antidiuretic hormone.

An episode of acute porphyria is usually precipitated by factors that induce hepatic heme or cytochrome P450 synthesis, most commonly drugs (alcohol, barbiturates, anticonvulsants, rifampicin, or steroid hormones) but also smoking, physical exertion, stress, fasting, menstruation, and pregnancy.[228]

The management of acute porphyria is the same for the three common variants and is based on confirming the diagnosis, stopping triggers, supportive medical therapy including resuscitation (seizures, bulbar or respiratory paralysis), disease modification, and analgesia. The psychosocial sequelae of an acute attack, particularly psychiatric symptoms and prolonged hospitalization, requires input from appropriate disciplines.

Disease modification, including the administration of intravenous heme arginate (Hematin) (3 mg/kg/daily, for four days),[231][II], high-dose dextrose (usually via an intravenous infusion: 0.1–0.2 g/kg/h)[228] or cimetidine[232] early in an attack, may decrease the duration and severity of symptoms, including pain, by reducing ALA synthetase activity and the subsequent production of "neurotoxic" ALA and porphyrins. A central venous catheter is indicated when administering intravenous hematin or dextrose as both produce phlebitis. Large volumes of dextrose may exacerbate hyponatremia. Hematin may cause a coagulopathy and rarely fever, aches, malaise, renal impairment, or circulatory collapse. Administration of hematin in albumin reduces phlebitis and coagulopathy and may enhance the drug's efficacy.[228]

The potential for analgesic drugs to precipitate an acute attack is a practical concern and an up-to-date reference of safe drugs should be consulted.[228] The mainstay of analgesia in acute porphyria is intravenous opioid therapy, preferably using a PCA device with either morphine, fentanyl, or hydromorphone.[228] Pethidine[233] and tramadol should be avoided because of seizure risk. Opioid analgesia may be complicated in patients with altered consciousness or mental state or when there is respiratory failure due to neuromuscular paralysis. Constipation is common and aperients may be required. An episode of acute porphyria may last for weeks; if gastro-intestinal function is reliable and the pain has stabilized, conversion to an oral opioid is appropriate.

Paracetamol may be used, however, the safety of NSAIDs or COX-2-specific inhibitors has not been established and are listed as unsafe in some reviews.[228] Hyoscine N-butylbromide is safe to use; however, it may not be effective in the treatment of colic. Droperidol is the antiemetic of choice in acute porphyria as metoclopramide is contraindicated and the safety of 5HT3 antagonists is as yet unclear. Nitrous oxide in oxygen may be useful for short-term analgesia[228, 234] and a case report describes using TENS to treat abdominal pain during acute porphyria.[235] Epidural analgesia was effective in the treatment of abdominal pain in a patient with acute intermittent porphyria (Visser EJ, personal communication) although the use of regional techniques in these patients (who may develop polyneuropathy, paralysis, or autonomic instability) is a concern.

Although the acute porphyrias produce acute and (if untreated) chronic neuropathic pain, standard anti-neuropathic pain medications such as the tricyclic antidepressants and some anticonvulsants (carbamazepine, valproate, and phenytoin) are contraindicated, although gabapentin is safe and possibly effective.[228] The use of intravenous lidocaine or low-dose ketamine for analgesia is controversial and essentially untested in acute porphyria. Intravenous low-dose ketamine was used effectively on two occasions in a patient with acute intermittent porphyria without obvious adverse effects (Visser EJ, personal communication). Ketamine does not induce ALA synthetase in rats[236] and has been used to induce anesthesia in porphyria patients without apparent problems. However, a case report noted raised porphyrin levels in a patient after induction with ketamine, thus highlighting some concerns.[237]

In summary, pain management in acute porphyria is based on ceasing triggers, early administration of hematin, high-dose dextrose, and possibly cimetidine (disease-modifying agents), and the use of intravenous and (later) oral opioid analgesia. Paracetamol, hyoscine N-butyl bromide, gabapentin, nitrous oxide, or TENS are safe and possibly effective. There may be a place for intravenous low-dose ketamine or regional analgesia, although the safety of these approaches has not been established in acute porphyria. Psychosocial support is vital in these patients who often have psychiatric symptoms or require recurrent or prolonged hospitalization.

ACKNOWLEDGMENT

This chapter is adapted and expanded from Roche SI and Goucke CR. Management of acutely painful medical conditions. In: Rowbotham DJ and Macintyre PE (eds). *Clinical Pain Management: Acute Pain*, 1st edn. London: Hodder Arnold, 2003: 369–92.

REFERENCES

1. Wall PD, Melzack R (eds). *Textbook of pain*, 4th edn. Edinburgh: Churchill Livingstone, 1999: 905.
2. McQuay HJ, Tramer M, Nye BA et al. A systematic review of antidepressants in neuropathic pain. *Pain*. 1996; **68**: 217–27.
* 3. Finnerup NB, Otto M, McQuay HJ et al. Algorithm for neuropathic pain treatment: An evidence based proposal. *Pain*. 2005; **118**: 289–305.
4. Vestergaard K, Andersen G, Gottrup H et al. Lamotrigine for central poststroke pain: a randomized controlled trial. *Neurology*. 2001; **56**: 184–90.
* 5. Nicholson BD. Evaluation and treatment of central post stroke pain syndromes. *Neurology*. 2004; **63**: S30–6.
6. Moulin DE, Foley KM, Ebers GC. Pain syndromes in multiple sclerosis. *Neurology*. 1988; **38**: 1840–4.
* 7. Wiffen PJ, McQuay HJ, Moore RA. Carbamazepine for acute and chronic pain. *Cochrane Database of Systematic Reviews*. 2005; **CD005451**.
8. Shakespeare DT, Boggild M, Young C. Anti-spasticity agents for multiple sclerosis. *Cochrane Database of Systematic Reviews*. 2003; **CD001332**.
9. Moulin DE. Pain in central and peripheral demyelinating disorders. *Neurologic Clinics*. 1998; **16**: 889–98.
* 10. Moulin DE, Hagen N, Feasby TE et al. Pain in Guillain–Barré syndrome. *Neurology*. 1997; **48**: 328–31.
11. Khatri A, Pearlstein L. Pain in Guillain–Barré syndrome. *Neurology*. 1997; **49**: 1474.
12. Pandey CK, Bose N, Garg G et al. Gabapentin for the treatment of pain in Guillain–Barré syndrome: a double-blinded, placebo-controlled, crossover study. *Anesthesia and Analgesia*. 2002; **95**: 1719–23.
13. Pandey CK, Raza M, Tripathi M et al. The comparative evaluation of gabapentin and carbamazepine for pain management in Guillain–Barré syndrome patients in the intensive care unit. *Anesthesia and Analgesia*. 2005; **101**: 220–5.
14. Tripathi M, Kaushik S. Carbamazapine for pain management in Guillain–Barré syndrome patients in the intensive care unit. *Critical Care Medicine*. 2000; **28**: 655–8.
15. Parisod E. Management of pain in a patient with Guillain–Barré syndrome. *ANZCA Bulletin*. 2002; **11**: 53–61.
16. Kvarnstrom A, Karlsten R, Quiding H et al. The effectiveness of intravenous ketamine and lidocaine on

peripheral neuropathic pain. *Acta Anaesthesiologica Scandinavica*. 2003; **47**: 868–77.

17. Kvarnstrom A, Karlsten R, Quiding H, Gordh T. The analgesic effect of intravenous ketamine and lidocaine on pain after spinal cord injury. *Acta Anaesthesiologica Scandinavica*. 2004; **48**: 498–506.

18. Eide PK, Stubhaug A, Stenehjem AE. Central dysesthesia pain after traumatic spinal cord injury is dependent on N-methyl-D-aspartate receptor activation. *Neurosurgery*. 1995; **37**: 1080–7.

* 19. Kalso E, Tramer MR, McQuay HJ, Moore RA. Systemic local-anaesthetic-type drugs in chronic pain: a systematic review. *European Journal of Pain*. 1998; **2**: 3–14.

20. Finnerup NB, Biering-Sorensen F, Johannesen IL *et al.* Intravenous lidocaine relieves spinal cord injury pain: a randomized controlled trial. *Anesthesiology*. 2005; **102**: 1023–30.

21. Attal N, Gaude V, Brasseur L *et al.* Intravenous lidocaine in central pain: a double-blind, placebo-controlled, psychophysical study. *Neurology*. 2000; **54**: 564–74.

22. Attal N, Guirimand F, Brasseur L *et al.* Effects of IV morphine in central pain: a randomized placebo-controlled study. *Neurology*. 2002; **58**: 554–63.

23. Finnerup NB, Sindrup SH, Bach FW *et al.* Lamotrigine in spinal cord injury pain: a randomized controlled trial. *Pain*. 2002; **96**: 375–83.

24. Raphael JC, Chevret S, Hughes RA, Annane D. Plasma exchange for Guillain–Barré syndrome. *Cochrane Database of Systematic Reviews*. 2002; **CD001798**.

25. Hughes RA, Raphael JC, Swan AV, van Doorn PA. Intravenous immunoglobulin for Guillain–Barré syndrome. *Cochrane Database of Systematic Reviews*. 2006; **CD002063**.

26. Hughes RA, Swan AV, van Koningsveld R, van Doorn PA. Corticosteroids for Guillain–Barré syndrome. *Cochrane Database of Systematic Reviews*. 2006; **CD001446**.

27. Kabore R, Magy L, Boukhris S *et al.* Contribution of corticosteroid to the treatment of pain in the acute phase of Guillain–Barré syndrome. *Revue Neurologique*. 2004; **160**: 821–3.

28. Odaka M, Tatsumoto M, Hoshiyama E *et al.* Side effects of combined therapy of methylprednisolone and intravenous immunoglobulin in Guillain–Barré syndrome. *European Neurology*. 2005; **53**: 194–6.

29. Roca B, Ferrer D, Calvo B. Temporal arteritis and Guillain–Barré syndrome. *Southern Medical Journal*. 2002; **95**: 1081–2.

30. Ersahin Y, Mutluer S, Yurtseven T. Hydrocephalus in Guillain–Barré syndrome. *Clinical Neurology and Neurosurgery*. 1995; **97**: 253–5.

31. Pyati S, Razis PA, Desai P. Headache in Guillain–Barré syndrome. *Journal of Neurosurgical Anesthesiology*. 2004; **16**: 294–5.

32. Gottrup H, Bach FW, Juhl G, Jensen TS. Differential effect of ketamine and lidocaine on spontaneous and mechanical

evoked pain in patients with nerve injury pain. *Anesthesiology*. 2006; **104**: 527–36.

33. Vandenbulcke M, Janssens J. Acute axonal polyneuropathy in chronic alcoholism and malnutrition. *Acta Neurologica Belgica*. 1999; **99**: 198–201.

34. Nishiyama K, Sakuta M. Mexiletine for painful alcoholic neuropathy. *Internal Medicine*. 1995; **34**: 577–9.

35. Woelk H, Lehrl S, Bitsch R, Kopcke W. Benfotiamine in treatment of alcoholic polyneuropathy: an 8-week randomised controlled study (BAP I study). *Alcohol and Alcoholism*. 1998; **33**: 631–8.

36. Galer BS, Lipton RB, Kaplan R *et al.* Bilateral burning foot pain: monitoring of pain, sensation and autonomic function during successful treatment with sympathetic blockade. *Journal of Pain and Symptom Management*. 1991; **6**: 92–7.

* 37. Singer EJ, Zorilla C, Fahy-Chandon B *et al.* Painful symptoms reported by ambulatory HIV infected men in a longitudinal study. *Pain*. 1993; **54**: 15–9.

38. Breitbart W, McDonald MV, Rosenfeld B *et al.* Pain in ambulatory AIDS patients. I. Pain characteristics and medical correlates. *Pain*. 1996; **68**: 315–21.

39. Kimball LR, McCormick WC. The pharmacologic management of pain and discomfort in persons with AIDS near the end of life: use of opioid analgesia in the hospice setting. *Journal of Pain and Symptom Management*. 1996; **11**: 88–94.

40. Vogl D, Rosenfeld B, Breitbart W *et al.* Symptom prevalence, characteristics and distress in AIDS outpatients. *Journal of Pain and Symptom Management*. 1999; **18**: 253–62.

41. O'Neill WM, Sherrard JS. Pain in human immunodeficiency virus disease: a review. *Pain*. 1993; **54**: 3–14.

42. Glare P. Pain in patients with HIV infection: issues for the new millennium. *European Journal of Pain*, **5** (suppl A): 2001: 43–8.

* 43. Hewitt DJ, McDonald M, Portenoy RK *et al.* Pain syndromes and etiologies in ambulatory AIDS patients. *Pain*. 1997; **70**: 117–23.

44. Wulff EA, Wang AK, Simpson DM. HIV-associated peripheral neuropathy: epidemiology, pathophysiology and treatment. *Drugs*. 2000; **59**: 1251–60.

45. Dalakas MC, Cupler EJ. Neuropathies in HIV infection. *Ballières Clinical Neurology*. 1996; **5**: 199–218.

46. Tagliati M, Grinnell J, Godbold J *et al.* Peripheral nerve function in HIV infection: clinical, electrophysiologic, and laboratory findings. *Archives of Neurology*. 1999; **56**: 84–9.

47. Jacox A, Carr DB, Payne R. New clinical-practice guidelines for the management of pain in patients with cancer. *New England Journal of Medicine*. 1994; **330**: 651–5.

48. Breitbart W, Rosenfeld BD, Passik SD *et al.* The undertreatment of pain in ambulatory AIDS patients. *Pain*. 1996; **65**: 243–9.

49. Larue F, Fonatine A, Colleau SM. Underestimation and undertreatment of pain in HIV disease: a multicenter study. *British Medical Journal*. 1997; **314**: 23–8.

50. Breitbart W, Passik S, McDonald MV *et al.* Pain-related barriers to pain management in ambulatory AIDS patients. *Pain.* 1998; **76**: 9–16.

51. Breitbart W, Kaim M, Rosenfeld B. Clinicians' perceptions of barriers to pain management in AIDS. *Journal of Pain and Symptom Management.* 1999; **18**: 203–12.

52. Frich LM, Borgbjerg FM. Pain and pain treatment in AIDS: a longitudinal study. *Journal of Pain and Symptom Management.* 2000; **19**: 339–47.

53. Breitbart W, Passik S, McDonald MV *et al.* Patient-related barriers to pain management in ambulatory AIDS patients. *Pain.* 1998; **76**: 9–16.

✱ 54. Breitbart W. Pain in AIDS. In: Jensen TS, Turner JA, Wiesenfeld-Hallin Z (eds). *Proceedings of the 8th World Congress on Pain. Progress in Pain Research and Management*, Vol. 8. Seattle: IASP Press, 1997.

55. McQuay HJ, Jadad AR. Incident pain. *Cancer Surveys.* 1994; **21**: 17–24.

56. Soares LG, Martins M, Uchoa R. Intravenous fentanyl for cancer pain: a "fast titration" protocol for the emergency room. *Journal of Pain and Symptom Management.* 2003; **26**: 876–81.

57. Farrar J, Cleary J, Rauck R *et al.* Oral transmucosal fentanyl citrate: randomised, double-blinded, placebo-controlled trial for treatment of breakthrough pain in cancer patients. *Journal of the National Cancer Institute.* 1998; **90**: 611–6.

58. Kaplan R, Conant M, Cundiff D *et al.* Sustained-release morphine sulfate in the management of pain associated with acquired immunodeficiency syndrome. *Journal of Pain and Symptom Management.* 1996; **12**: 150–60.

59. Newshan G, Lefkowitz M. Transdermal fentanyl for chronic pain in AIDS: a pilot study. *Journal of Pain and Symptom Management.* 2001; **21**: 69–77.

60. Dixon P, Higginson I. AIDS and cancer pain treated with slow release morphine. *Postgraduate Medical Journal.* 1991; **67**: S92–4.

61. Kimball LR, McCormick WC. The pharmacologic management of pain and discomfort in persons with AIDS near the end of life: use of opioid analgesia in the hospice setting. *Journal of Pain and Symptom Management.* 1996; **11**: 88–94.

62. Frich LM, Borgbjerg FM. Pain and pain treatment in AIDS: a longitudinal study. *Journal of Pain and Symptom Management.* 2000; **19**: 339–47.

63. Olkkola KT, Palkama VJ, Neuvonen PJ. Ritonavir's role in reducing fentanyl clearance and prolonging its half-life. *Anesthesiology.* 1999; **91**: 681–5.

64. Piscitelli SC, Kress DR, Bertz RJ *et al.* The effect of ritonavir on the pharmacokinetics of meperidine and normeperidine. *Pharmacotherapy.* 2000; **20**: 549–53.

65. McCance-Katz EF, Rainey PM, Friedland G, Jatlow P. The protease inhibitor lopinavir-ritonavir may produce opiate withdrawal in methadone-maintained patients. *Clinical Infectious Diseases.* 2003; **37**: 476–82.

66. Simpson DM, Olney R, McArthur JC *et al.* A placebo controlled trial of lamotrigine for painful HIV-associated neuropathy. *Neurology.* 2000; **54**: 2115–9.

67. Hahn K, Arendt G, Braun JS *et al.* A placebo-controlled trial of gabapentin for painful HIV-associated sensory neuropathies. *Journal of Neurology.* 2004; **251**: 1260–6.

68. La Spina I, Porazzi D, Maggiolo F *et al.* Gabapentin in painful HIV-related neuropathy: a report of 19 patients, preliminary observations. *European Journal of Neurology.* 2001; **8**: 71–5.

69. Scarpini E, Sacilotto G, Baron P *et al.* Effect of acetyl-l-carnitine in the treatment of painful peripheral neuropathies in HIV+ patients. *Journal of the Peripheral Nervous System.* 1997; **2**: 250–2.

70. Kieburtz K, Simpson D, Yiannoutsos C *et al.* A randomised trial of amitriptyline and mexiletine for painful neuropathy in HIV infection. AIDS clinical trial group 242 protocol team. *Neurology.* 1998; **51**: 1682–8.

71. Shlay JC, Chaloner K, Max MB *et al.* Acupuncture and amitriptyline for pain due to HIV-related peripheral neuropathy: a randomized controlled trial. Terry Beirn Community Programs for Clinical Research on AIDS. *Journal of the American Medical Association.* 1998; **280**: 1590–5.

72. Estanislao L, Carter K, McArthur J *et al.* A randomized controlled trial of 5% lidocaine gel for HIV-associated distal symmetric polyneuropathy. *Journal of Acquired Immune Deficiency Syndromes.* 2004; **37**: 1584–6.

73. Kemper CA, Kent G, Burton S, Deresinski SC. Mexiletine for HIV-infected patients with painful peripheral neuropathy: a double-blind, placebo-controlled, crossover treatment trial. *Journal of Acquired Immune Deficiency Syndromes and Human Retrovirology.* 1998; **19**: 367–72.

74. Paice JA, Ferrans CE, Lashley FR *et al.* Topical capsaicin in the management of HIV associated peripheral neuropathy. *Journal of Pain and Symptom Management.* 2000; **1**: 45–52.

75. Simpson DM, Dorfman D, Olney RK *et al.* Peptide T in the treatment of painful distal neuropathy associated with AIDS: results of a placebo-controlled trial. The Peptide T Neuropathy Study Group. *Neurology.* 1996; **47**: 1254–9.

76. Paice JA, Shott S, Oldenburg FP *et al.* Efficacy of a vibratory stimulus for the relief of HIV associated neuropathic pain. *Pain.* 2000; **84**: 291–6.

77. Woolridge E, Barton S, Samuel J *et al.* Cannabis use in HIV for pain and other medical symptoms. *Journal of Pain and Symptom Management.* 2005; **29**: 358–67.

78. Easter DW, Cuschieri A, Nathanson LK *et al.* The utility of diagnostic laparoscopy for abdominal disorders. *Archives of Surgery.* 1992; **127**: 379–83.

79. Merskey H, Bogduk N (eds). *Classification of chronic pain*, 2nd edn. Seattle: IASP Press, 1994: 160.

80. International Classification of Headache Disorders, 2nd edn. *Cephalalgia* 2004; **24** (Suppl. 1): 30–31.

81. Symon DN, Russell G. Double blind placebo controlled trial of pizotifen syrup in the treatment of abdominal migraine. *Archives of Disease in Childhood.* 1995; **72**: 48–50.

✷ 82. Russell G, Abu-Arafeh I, Symon DN. Abdominal migraine: evidence for existence and treatment options. *Paediatric Drugs.* 2002; **4**: 1–8.

✷ 83. Gallagher EJ, Esses D, Lee C *et al.* Randomized clinical trial of morphine in acute abdominal pain. *Annals of Emergency Medicine.* 2006; **48**: 150–60.

84. Thomas SH, Silen W, Cheema F *et al.* Effects of morphine analgesia on diagnostic accuracy in Emergency Department patients with abdominal pain: a prospective, randomized trial. *Journal of the American College of Surgeons.* 2003; **196**: 18–31.

✷ 85. Knopp RK, Dries D. Analgesia in acute abdominal pain: what's next? *Annals of Emergency Medicine.* 2006; **48**: 161–3.

86. Zacny JP, Galinkin JL. Psychotropic drugs used in anesthesia practice: abuse liability and epidemiology of abuse. *Anesthesiology.* 1999; **90**: 269–88.

87. Wilder-Smith CH, Hill L, Wilkins J *et al.* Effects of morphine and tramadol on pain and gastrointestinal motility after abdominal surgery. *Anesthesiology.* 1999; **91**: 639–47.

88. Lim AW, Schug SA. Tramadol versus morphine as oral step down analgesia after post operative epidural analgesia. *Regional Anesthesia and Pain Medicine.* 2001; **26**: S133.

89. Weinbroum AA. A single small dose of postoperative ketamine provides rapid and sustained improvement in morphine analgesia in the presence of morphine-resistant pain. *Anesthesia and Analgesia.* 2003; **96**: 789–95.

90. Bell RF. Low-dose subcutaneous ketamine infusion and morphine tolerance. *Pain.* 1999; **83**: 101–3.

91. Eilers H, Philip LA, Bickler PE *et al.* The reversal of fentanyl-induced tolerance by administration of "small-dose" ketamine. *Anesthesia and Analgesia.* 2001; **93**: 213–4.

92. Strigo IA, Duncan GH, Bushnell MC *et al.* The effects of racemic ketamine on painful stimulation of skin and viscera in human subjects. *Pain.* 2005; **113**: 255–64.

93. Willert RP, Woolf CJ, Hobson AR *et al.* The development and maintenance of human visceral pain hypersensitivity is dependent on the N-methyl-D-aspartate receptor. *Gastroenterology.* 2004; **126**: 683–92.

94. Chauhan V, Eskin B, Allegra JR, Cochrane DG. Effect of season, age, and gender on renal colic incidence. *American Journal of Emergency Medicine.* 2004; **22**: 560–3.

95. Lindqvist K, Hellstrom M, Holmberg G *et al.* Immediate versus deferred radiological investigation after acute renal colic: a prospective randomized study. *Scandinavian Journal of Urology and Nephrology.* 2006; **40**: 119–24.

96. Holdgate A, Pollock T. Nonsteroidal anti-inflammatory drugs (NSAIDs) versus opioids for acute renal colic. *Cochrane Database of Systematic Reviews.* 2005; **CD004137**.

97. Kapoor DA, Weitzel S, Mowad JJ *et al.* Use of indomethacin suppositories in the prophylaxis of recurrent ureteric colic. *Journal of Urology.* 1989; **142**: 1428–30.

98. Laerum E, Ommundsen OE, Gronseth JE *et al.* Oral diclofenac in the prophylactic treatment of recurrent renal

colic. A double-blind comparison with placebo. *European Urology.* 1995; **28**: 108–11.

99. Tramer MR, Williams JE, Carroll D *et al.* Comparing analgesic efficacy of non-steroidal anti-inflammatory drugs given by different routes in acute and chronic pain: a qualitative systematic review. *Acta Anaesthesiologica Scandinavica.* 1998; **42**: 71–9.

100. Lee C, Gnanasegaram D, Maloba M. Best evidence topic report. Rectal or intravenous non-steroidal anti-inflammatory drugs in acute renal colic. *Emergency Medicine Journal.* 2005; **22**: 653–4.

101. Engeler DS, Ackermann DK, Osterwalder JJ *et al.* A double-blind, placebo controlled comparison of the morphine sparing effect of oral rofecoxib and diclofenac for acute renal colic. *Journal of Urology.* 2005; **174**: 933–6.

102. O'Connor A, Schug SA, Cardwell H. A comparison of the efficacy and safety of morphine and pethidine for suspected renal colic in the emergency setting. *Journal of Accident and Emergency Medicine.* 2000; **17**: 261–4.

103. Jones JB, Giles BK, Brizendine EJ *et al.* Sublingual hyoscyamine sulfate in combination with ketorolac tromethamine for ureteral colic: a randomised double-blind, controlled trial. *Annals of Emergency Medicine.* 2001; **37**: 141–6.

104. Holdgate A, Oh CM. Is there a role for antimuscarinics in renal colic? A randomized controlled trial. *Journal of Urology.* 2005; **174**: 572–5.

105. Edwards JE, Meseguer F, Faura C *et al.* Single dose dipyrone for acute renal colic pain. *Cochrane Database of Systematic Reviews.* 2002; **CD003867**.

106. Ergene U, Pekdemir M, Canda E *et al.* Ondansetron versus diclofenac sodium in the treatment of acute ureteral colic: a double blind controlled trial. *International Urology and Nephrology.* 2001; **33**: 315–9.

107. Lopes T, Dias JS, Marcelino J *et al.* An assessment of the clinical efficacy of intranasal desmopressin spray in the treatment of renal colic. *BJU International.* 2001; **87**: 322–5.

108. Mora B, Giorni E, Dobrovits M *et al.* Transcutaneous electrical nerve stimulation: an effective treatment for pain caused by renal colic in emergency care. *Journal of Urology.* 2006; **175**: 1737–41.

109. Lee YH, Lee WC, Chen MT *et al.* Acupuncture in the treatment of renal colic. *Journal of Urology.* 1992; **147**: 16–18.

110. Worster A, Richards C. Fluids and diuretics for acute ureteric colic. *Cochrane Database of Systematic Reviews.* 2005; **CD004926**.

111. De Sio M, Autorino R, Di Lorenzo G *et al.* Medical expulsive treatment of distal-ureteral stones using tamsulosin: a single-center experience. *Journal Endourology.* 2006; **20**: 12–16.

112. Dellabella M, Milanese G, Muzzonigro G. Randomised trial of the efficacy of tamsulosin, nifedipine and phoroglucinol in medical expulsive therapy of distal ureteral calculi. *Journal of Urology.* 2005; **174**: 167–72.

113. Thompson DR. Narcotic analgesia effects on the sphincter of Oddi: a review of data and the therapeutic implications in treating pancreatitis. *American Journal of Gastroenterology*. 2001; **96**: 1266–72.

114. Thune A, Baker RA, Saccone GT *et al.* Differing effects of pethidine and morphine on sphincter of Oddi motility. *British Journal of Surgery*. 1990; **77**: 992–5.

115. Goldman G, Kahn PJ, Alon R *et al.* Biliary colic treatment and acute cholecystitis prevention by prostaglandin inhibitor. *Digestive Diseases and Sciences*. 1989; **34**: 809–11.

116. Al-Waili N, Saloom KY. The analgesic effect of intravenous tenoxicam in symptomatic treatment of biliary colic: a comparison with hyoscine-N-butylbromide. *European Journal of Medical Research*. 1998; **14**: 475–9.

117. Dula DJ, Anderson R, Wood GC. A prospective study comparing i.m. ketorolac with i.m. meperidine in the treatment of acute biliary colic. *Journal of Emergency Medicine*. 2001; **20**: 121–4.

118. Henderson SO, Swadron S, Newton E. Comparison of intravenous ketorolac and meperidine in the treatment of biliary colic. *Journal of Emergency Medicine*. 2002; **23**: 237–41.

119. Kumar A, Deed JS, Bhasin B *et al.* Comparison of the effect of diclofenac with hyoscine-N-butylbromide in the symptomatic treatment of acute biliary colic. *ANZ Journal of Surgery*. 2004; **74**: 573–6.

120. Schmieder G, Stankov G, Zerle G *et al.* Observer-blind study with metamizole versus tramadol and butylscopolamine in acute biliary colic pain. *Arzneimittelforschung*. 1993; **43**: 1216–21.

121. Antevil JL, Buckley RG, Johnson AS *et al.* Treatment of suspected symptomatic cholelithiasis with glycopyrrolate: a prospective, randomized clinical trial. *Annals of Emergency Medicine*. 2005; **45**: 172–6.

122. Rothrock SG, Green SM, Gorton E. Atropine for the treatment of biliary tract pain: a double-blind, placebo-controlled trial. *Annals of Emergency Medicine*. 1993; **22**: 1324–7.

123. Stower MJ, Foster GE, Hardcastle JD. A trial of glucagon in the treatment of painful biliary tract disease. *British Journal of Surgery*. 1982; **69**: 591–2.

124. Harris SI, Kuss M, Hubbard RC *et al.* Upper gastrointestinal safety evaluation of parecoxib sodium, a new parenteral cyclooxygenase-2-specific inhibitor, compared with ketorolac, naproxen and placebo. *Clinical Therapeutics*. 2001; **23**: 1422–8.

125. Clain JE, Pearson RK. Diagnosis of chronic pancreatitis. Is a gold standard necessary? *Surgical Clinics of North America*. 1999; **79**: 829–45.

126. Bommelaer G, Poynard T, Le Pen C *et al.* Prevalence of irritable bowel syndrome (IBS) and variability of diagnostic criteria. *Gastroenterologie Clinique et Biologique*. 2004; **28**: 554–61.

127. Drossman DA. Functional versus organic: an inappropriate dichotomy for clinical care. *American Journal of Gastroenterology*. 2006; **101**: 1172–5.

128. Drossman DA, Whitehead WE, Toner BB *et al.* What determines severity among patients with painful functional bowel disorders? *American Journal of Gastroenterology*. 2000; **95**: 974–80.

129. Amouretti M, Le Pen C, Gaudin AF *et al.* Impact of irritable bowel syndrome (IBS) on health-related quality of life (HRQOL). *Gastroenterologie Clinique et Biologique*. 2006; **30**: 241–6.

130. Poynard T, Regimbeau C, Benhamou Y. Meta-analysis of smooth muscle relaxants in the treatment of irritable bowel syndrome. *Alimentary Pharmacology and Therapeutics*. 2001; **15**: 355–61.

131. Pittler MH, Ernst E. Peppermint oil for irritable bowel syndrome: a critical review and meta analysis. *American Journal of Gastroenterology*. 1998; **93**: 1131–5.

132. Quartero AO, Meineche-Schmidt V, Muris J *et al.* Bulking agents, antispasmodic and antidepressant medication for the treatment of irritable bowel syndrome. *Cochrane Database of Systematic Reviews*. 2005; **CD003460**.

133. Tack J, Broekaert D, Fischler B *et al.* A controlled cross-over study of the selective serotonin reuptake inhibitor citalopram in irritable bowel syndrome. *Gut*. 2006; **55**: 1095–103.

134. Vahedi H, Merat S, Rashidioon A *et al.* The effect of fluoxetine in patients with pain and constipation-predominant irritable bowel syndrome: a double-blind randomized-controlled study. *Alimentary Pharmacology and Therapeutics*. 2005; **22**: 381–5.

135. Evans BW, Clark WK, Moore DJ, Whorwell PJ. Tegaserod for the treatment of irritable bowel syndrome. *Cochrane Database of Systematic Reviews*. 2004; **CD003960**.

136. Lesbros-Pantoflickova D, Michetti P, Fried M *et al.* Meta-analysis: The treatment of irritable bowel syndrome. *Alimentary Pharmacology and Therapeutics*. 2004; **20**: 1253–69.

137. Boyce PM, Talley NJ, Balaam B *et al.* A randomized controlled trial of cognitive behavior therapy, relaxation training, and routine clinical care for the irritable bowel syndrome. *American Journal of Gastroenterology*. 2003; **98**: 2209–18.

138. Soo S, Moayyedi P, Deeks J *et al.* Psychological interventions for non-ulcer dyspepsia. *Cochrane Database of Systematic Reviews*. 2005; **CD002301**.

139. Vilke GM, Jin A, Davis DP, Chan TC. Prospective randomized study of viscous lidocaine versus benzocaine in a GI cocktail for dyspepsia. *Journal of Emergency Medicine*. 2004; **27**: 7–9.

140. Berman DA, Porter RS, Graber M. The GI cocktail is no more effective than plain liquid antacid: a randomized, double blind clinical trial. *Journal of Emergency Medicine*. 2003; **25**: 239–44.

141. Moayyedi P, Soo S, Deeks J *et al.* Pharmacological interventions for non-ulcer dyspepsia. *Cochrane Database of Systematic Reviews*. 2004; **CD001960**.

142. Moayyedi P, Soo S, Deeks J *et al.* Eradication of *Helicobacter pylori* for non-ulcer dyspepsia. *Cochrane Database of Systematic Reviews*. 2006; **CD002096**.

*143. Storr M, Allescher H-D, Classen M. Current concepts on pathophysiology, diagnosis and treatment of diffuse oesophageal spasm. *Drugs*. 2001; **61**: 579–91.

144. Burnett MA, Antao V, Black A et al. Prevalence of primary dysmenorrhea in Canada. *Journal of Obstetrics and Gynaecology Canada*. 2005; **27**: 765–70.

145. Marjoribanks J, Proctor ML, Farquhar C. Nonsteroidal anti-inflammatory drugs for primary dysmenorrhoea. *Cochrane Database of Systematic Reviews*. 2003; **CD001751**.

146. Bitner M, Kattenhorn J, Hatfield C et al. Efficacy and tolerability of lumiracoxib in the treatment of primary dysmenorrhoea. *International Journal of Clinical Practice*. 2004; **58**: 340–5.

147. Zhang WY, Li Wan Po A. Efficacy of minor analgesics in primary dysmenorrhoea: a systematic review. *British Journal of Obstetrics and Gynaecology*. 1998; **105**: 780–9.

148. Proctor ML, Smith CA, Farquhar CM, Stones RW. Transcutaneous electrical nerve stimulation and acupuncture for primary dysmenorrhoea. *Cochrane Database of Systematic Reviews*. 2002; **CD002123**.

149. Taylor D, Miaskowski C, Kohn J. A randomized clinical trial of the effectiveness of an acupressure device (relief brief) for managing symptoms of dysmenorrhea. *Journal of Alternative and Complementary Medicine*. 2002; **8**: 357–70.

150. Wilson ML, Murphy PA. Herbal and dietary therapies for primary and secondary dysmenorrhoea. *Cochrane Database of Systematic Reviews*. 2001; **CD002124**.

151. Ziaei S, Zakeri M, Kazemnejad A. A randomised controlled trial of vitamin E in the treatment of primary dysmenorrhoea. *BJOG*. 2005; **112**: 466–9.

152. Everts B, Karlson BW, Herlitz J, Hedner T. Morphine use and pharmacokinetics in patients with chest pain due to suspected or definite acute myocardial infarction. *European Journal of Pain*. 1998; **2**: 115–25.

153. Silfvast T, Saarnivaara L. Comparison of alfentanil and morphine in the pre-hospital treatment of patients with acute ischaemic-type chest pain. *European Journal of Emergency Medicine*. 2001; **8**: 275–8.

154. Weiss P, Ritz R. Analgesic effect and side effects of buprenorphine in acute coronary heart disease. A randomised double blind comparison with morphine. *Anasthesie Intensivtherapie, Notfallmedizin*. 1988; **23**: 309–12.

155. Nielsen JR, Pedersen KE, Dahlstrom CG et al. Analgetic treatment in acute myocardial infarction. A controlled clinical comparison of morphine, nicomorphine and pethidine. *Acta Medica Scandinavica*. 1984; **215**: 349–54.

156. Everts B, Karlson B, Abdon NJ et al. A comparison of metoprolol and morphine in the treatment of chest pain in patients with suspected acute myocardial infarction – the MEMO study. *Journal of Internal Medicine*. 1999; **245**: 133–41.

157. Rettig G, Kropp J. Analgesic effect of tramadol in acute myocardial infarct. *Therapie der Gegenwart*. 1980; **119**: 705–7.

158. Stankov S. Haemodynamic effects of tramadol and morphine in patients with acute myocardial infarction (abstract). In: 7th World Congress on Pain, August 22–27 1993, Paris. Seattle: IASP, 1995: 293.

159. Henrikson CA, Howell EE, Bush DE et al. Chest pain relief by nitroglycerin does not predict active coronary artery disease. *Annals of Internal Medicine*. 2003; **139**: 979–86.

160. Baumann BM, Perrone J, Hornig SE et al. Randomized, double blind, placebo controlled trial of diazepam, nitroglycerin or both for the treatment of patients with potential cocaine associated acute coronary syndromes. *Academic Emergency Medicine*. 2000; **7**: 878–5.

161. Honderick T, Williams D, Seaberg D et al. A prospective randomised, controlled trial of benzodiazepine and nitroglyerine or nitroglycerine alone in the treatment of cocaine associated acute coronary syndromes. *American Journal of Emergency Medicine*. 2003; **21**: 39–42.

162. O'Leary U, Puglia C, Friehling TD et al. Nitrous oxide anaesthesia in patients with ischaemic chest discomfort: effect on beta endorphin levels. *Journal of Clinical Pharmacology*. 1987; **27**: 957–61.

163. Schifferdecker B, Spodick DH. Nonsteroidal anti-inflammatory drugs in the treatment of pericarditis. *Cardiology in Review*. 2003; **11**: 211–7.

164. Barden J, Edwards JE, McQuay HJ, Andrew Moore R. Pain and analgesic response after third molar extraction and other postsurgical pain. *Pain*. 2004; **107**: 86–90.

165. Edwards JE, Mc Quay HJ, Moore RA. Combination analgesic efficacy; individual patient data meta-analysis of single dose oral tramadol plus acetaminophen in acute post operative pain. *Journal of Pain and Symptom Management*. 2002; **23**: 121–30.

166. Ahmad N, Grad HA, Haas DA et al. The efficacy of non opioid analgesics for post operative dental pain: a meta-analysis. *Anesthesia Progress*. 1997; **44**: 119–26.

167. Sutherland S, Matthews DC. Emergency management of acute apical periodontitis in the permanent dentition: a systematic review of the literature. *Journal of the Canadian Dental Association*. 2003; **69**: 160.

168. Romsing J, Ostergaard D, Drozdziewicz D et al. Diclofenac or acetaminophen for analgesia in paediatric tonsillectomy outpatients. *Acta Anaesthesiologica Scandinavica*. 2000; **44**: 291–5.

*169. Thomas M, Del Mar C, Glasziou P. How effective are treatments other than antibiotics for acute sore throat? *British Journal of General Practice*. 2000; **50**: 817–20.

170. Eccles R, Loose I, Jawad M, Nyman L. Effects of acetylsalicylic acid on sore throat pain and other pain symptoms associated with acute upper respiratory tract infection. *Pain Medicine*. 2003; **4**: 118–24.

171. Schachtel BP, Fillingim JM, Lane AC et al. Caffeine as an analgesic adjuvant. A double-blind study comparing aspirin with caffeine to aspirin and placebo in patients with sore throat. *Archives of Internal Medicine*. 1991; **151**: 733–7.

172. Miller K. Relief of sore throat with the anti-inflammatory throat lozenge flurbiprofen 8.75 mg: a randomised,

double-blind, placebo-controlled study of efficacy and safety. *International Journal of Clinical Practice.* 2000; **54**: 490–6.

173. Olympia RP, Khine H, Avner JR. Effectiveness of oral dexamethasone in the treatment of moderate to severe pharyngitis in children. *Archives of Pediatrics and Adolescent Medicine.* 2005; **159**: 278–82.

174. Niland ML, Bonsu BK, Nuss KE, Goodman DG. A pilot study of 1 versus 3 days of dexamethasone as add on therapy in children with streptococcal pharyngitis. *Pediatric Infectious Disease Journal.* 2006; **25**: 477–81.

175. Marvez-Valls EG, Ernst AA, Gray J, Johnson WD. The role of betamethasone in the treatment of acute exudative pharyngitis. *Academic Emergency Medicine.* 1998; **5**: 567–72.

176. Bulloch B, Kabani A, Tenenbein M. Oral dexamethasone for the treatment of pain in children with acute pharyngitis: a randomized, double-blind, placebo-controlled trial. *Annals of Emergency Medicine.* 2003; **41**: 601–8.

177. Candy B, Hotopf M. Steroids for symptom control in infectious mononucleosis. *Cochrane Database of Systematic Reviews.* 2006; **CD004402**.

178. Ozbek C, Aygenc E, Tuna EU *et al.* Use of steroids in the treatment of peritonsillar abscess. *Journal of Laryngology and Otology.* 2004; **118**: 439–42.

179. Del Mar CB, Glasziou PP, Spinks AB. Antibiotics for sore throat. *Cochrane Database of Systematic Reviews.* 2004; **CD000023**.

180. Vickers ER, Punnia-Moorthy A. A clinical evaluation of three topical anaesthetic agents. *Australian Dental Journal.* 1992; **37**: 266–70.

181. Worthington HV, Clarkson JE, Eden OB. Interventions for treating oral mucositis for patients with cancer receiving treatment. *Cochrane Database of Systematic Reviews.* 2004; **CD001973**.

182. Coda BA, O'Sullivan B, Donaldson G *et al.* Comparative efficacy of patient-controlled administration of morphine, hydromorphone, or sufentanil for the treatment of oral mucositis pain following bone marrow transplantation. *Pain.* 1997; **72**: 333–46.

183. Epstein JB, Epstein JD, Epstein MS *et al.* Oral doxepin rinse: the analgesic effect and duration of pain reduction in patients with oral mucositis due to cancer therapy. *Anesthesia and Analgesia.* 2006; **103**: 465–70.

184. Slatkin NE, Rhiner M. Topical ketamine in the treatment of mucositis pain. *Pain Medicine.* 2003; **4**: 298–303.

185. Jackson K, Ashby M, Goodchild C. Subanesthetic ketamine for cancer pain: by insisting on level I/II evidence, do we risk throwing the baby out with the bath water? *Journal of Pain and Symptom Management.* 2005; **29**: 328–30.

186. Hansen JG, Schmidt H, Grinsted P. Randomised double blind placebo controlled trial of penicillin V in the treatment of acute maxillary sinusitis in adults in general practice. *Scandinavian Journal of Primary Health Care.* 2000; **18**: 44–7.

187. Glasziou PP, Del Mar CB, Sanders SL, Hayem M. Antibiotics for acute otitis media in children. *Cochrane Database of Systematic Reviews.* 2004; **CD000219**.

188. Foxlee R, Johansson A, Wejfalk J *et al.* Topical analgesia for acute otitis media. *Cochrane Database of Systematic Reviews.* 2006; **CD005657**.

189. Wallny T, Hess L, Seuser A *et al.* Pain status of patients with severe haemophilic arthropathy. *Haemophilia.* 2001; **7**: 453–8.

190. Gilbert S. Hemophilia: the changing role of the orthopedic surgeon in the era of HIV infection. *Southeast Asian Journal of Tropical Medicine and Public Health.* 1993; **24**: 30–3.

191. Aronstam A, Wassef M, Hamad Z *et al.* A double-blind controlled trial of two dose levels of factor VIII in the treatment of high risk haemarthroses in haemophilia A. *Clinical Laboratory and Haematology.* 1983; **5**: 157–63.

192. Baker CL. Acute haemarthrosis of the knee. *Journal of the Medical Association of Georgia.* 1992; **81**: 301–05.

193. Aronstam A. Prevention of haemophilic arthropathy. *Folia Haematologica.* 1990; **117**: 499–504.

194. Steven MM, Small M, Pinkerton L *et al.* Non-steroidal anti-inflammatory drugs in haemophilic arthritis: a clinical and laboratory study. *Haemostasis.* 1985; **15**: 204–09.

195. Hasiba U, Scranton PE, Lewis JH, Spero JA. Efficacy and safety of ibuprofen for hemophilic arthropathy. *Archives of Internal Medicine.* 1980; **140**: 1583–5.

196. Thomas P, Hepburn B, Kim HC, Saidi P. Non-steroidal anti-inflammatory drugs in the treatment of hemophilic arthropathy. *American Journal of Hematology.* 1982; **12**: 131–7.

197. Ballas SK, Delengowski A. Pain measurement in hospitalized adults with sickle cell painful episodes. *Annals of Clinical and Laboratory Science.* 1993; **23**: 358–61.

198. Epstein K, Yuen E, Riggio JM. Utilization of the office, hospital and emergency department for adult sickle cell patients: a five-year study. *Journal of the National Medical Association.* 2006; **98**: 1109–13.

*199. Rees DC, Olujohungbe AD, Parker NE *et al.* Guidelines for the management of the acute painful crisis in sickle cell disease. *British Journal of Haematology.* 2003; **120**: 744–52.

200. Yale SH, Nagib N, Guthrie T. Approach to the vaso-occlusive crisis in adults with sickle cell disease. *American Family Physician.* 2000; **61**: 1349–56.

201. Cooper GS, Armitage KB, Ashar B *et al.* Design and implementation of an inpatient disease management program. *American Journal of Managed Care.* 2000; **6**: 793–801.

202. Labbe E, Herbert D, Haynes J. Physicians' attitude and practices in sickle cell disease pain management. *Journal of Palliative Care.* 2005; **21**: 246–51.

203. Silbergleit R, Jancis MO, McNamara RM. Management of sickle cell pain crisis in the emergency department at teaching hospitals. *Journal of Emergency Medicine.* 1999; **17**: 625–30.

204. Dunlop RJ, Bennett KC. Pain management for sickle cell disease. *Cochrane Database of Systematic Reviews*. 2006; **CD003350**.

205. Robieux IC, Kellner JD, Coppes MJ et al. Analgesia in children with sickle cell crisis: comparison of intermittent opioids vs. continuous intravenous infusion of morphine and placebo-controlled study of oxygen inhalation. *Pediatric Hematology and Oncology*. 1992; **9**: 317–26.

206. Zipursky A, Robieux IC, Brown EJ et al. Oxygen therapy in sickle cell disease. *American Journal of Pediatric Hematology/Oncology*. 1992; **14**: 222–8.

207. Hargrave DR, Wade A, Evans JPM et al. Nocturnal oxygen saturation and painful sickle cell crises in children. *Blood*. 2003; **101**: 846–8.

208. Murphy JG, Gibson G. Serum concentrations of meperidine in patients with sickle crisis. *Annals of Emergency Medicine*. 1986; **15**: 433–8.

209. Conti C, Tso E, Browne B. Oral morphine protocol for sickle cell crisis pain. *Maryland Medical Journal*. 1996; **45**: 33–5.

210. Friedman EW, Webber AB, Osborn HH, Schwartz S. Oral analgesia for the treatment of painful crisis in sickle cell anemia. *Annals of Emergency Medicine*. 1986; **15**: 787–91.

211. Brookoff D, Polomano R. Treating sickle cell pain like cancer pain. *Annals of Internal Medicine*. 1992; **116**: 364.

212. Nadvi SZ, Sarnaik S, Ravindranath Y. Low frequency of meperidine-associated seizures in sickle cell disease. *Clinical Pediatrics*. 1999; **38**: 459–62.

213. Liu JE, Gzesh DJ, Ballas SK. The spectrum of epilepsy in sickle cell anemia. *Journal of the Neurology Sciences*. 1994; **123**: 6–10.

214. Visser E, Schug SA. The role of ketamine in pain management. *Biomedicine and Pharmacotherapy*. 2006; **60**: 341–8.

215. Crawford MW, Galton S, Naser B. Postoperative morphine consumption in children with sickle-cell disease. *Paediatric Anaesthesia*. 2006; **16**: 152–7.

216. Perlin E, Finke H, Castro O et al. Enhancement of pain control with ketorolac tromethamine in patients with sickle cell vaso-occlusive crisis. *American Journal of Hematology*. 1994; **46**: 43–7.

217. Eke FU, Obamyonyi A, Eke NN, Oyewo EA. An open comparative study of dispersible piroxicam versus acetylsalicylic acid for the treatment of osteoarticular painful attack during sickle cell crisis. *Tropical Medicine and International Health*. 2000; **5**: 81–4.

218. Hardwick WE, Givens TG, Monroe KW et al. Effect of ketorolac in pediatric sickle cell vaso-occlusive pain. *Pediatric Emergency Care*. 1999; **15**: 179–82.

219. Wright SW, Norris RL, Mitchell TR. Ketorolac for sickle cell vaso-occlusive crisis pain in the emergency department: lack of narcotic sparing effect. *Annals of Emergency Medicine*. 1992; **21**: 925–8.

220. Weiner DL, Hibberd PL, Betit P et al. Preliminary assessment of inhaled nitric oxide for acute vaso-occlusive crisis in pediatric patients with sickle cell disease. *Journal of the American Medical Association*. 2003; **289**: 1136–42.

221. Griffin TC, McIntire D, Buchanan GR. High dose intravenous methylprednisolone therapy for pain in children and adolescents with sickle cell disease. *New England Journal of Medicine*. 1994; **330**: 733–7.

222. Yaster M, Tobin JR, Billett C et al. Epidural analgesia in the management of severe vaso-occlusive sickle cell crisis. *Pediatrics*. 1994; **93**: 310–5.

223. Yaster M, Kost-Byerly S, Maxwell LG. The management of pain in sickle cell disease. *Pediatric Clinics of North America*. 2000; **47**: 699–709.

224. Anie KA, Green J. Psychological therapies for sickle cell disease and pain. *Cochrane Database of Systematic Reviews*. 2002; **CD001916**.

225. Wambebe C, Khamofu H, Momoh JA et al. Double-blind, placebo-controlled, randomised cross-over clinical trial of NIPRISAN in patients with Sickle Cell Disorder. *Phytomedicine*. 2001; **8**: 252–61.

226. Riddington C, De Franceschi L. Drugs for preventing red blood cell dehydration in people with sickle cell disease. *Cochrane Database of Systematic Reviews*. 2002; **CD003426**.

227. Davies S, Olujohungbe A. Hydroxyurea for sickle cell disease. *Cochrane Database of Systematic Reviews*. 2001; **CD002202**.

*228. Anderson KE, Bloomer JR, Bonkovsky HL et al. Recommendations for the diagnosis and treatment of the acute porphyrias. *Annals of Internal Medicine*. 2005; **142**: 439–50.

229. Liu YP, Lien WC, Fang CC et al. ED presentation of acute porphyria. *American Journal of Emergency Medicine*. 2005; **23**: 164–7.

230. Bonkovsky HL. Neurovisceral porphyrias; what a hematologist needs to know. *Hematology/the Education Program of the American Society of Hematology*. 2005: 24–30.

231. Herrick AL, McColl KE, Moore MR et al. A Controlled trial of haem arginate in acute hepatic porphyria Lancet. 1989; **1**: 1295–7.

232. Rogers PD. Cimetidine in the treatment of acute intermittent porphyria. *Annals of Pharmacotherapy*. 1997; **31**: 365–7.

233. Deeg MA, Rajamani K. Normeperidine-induced seizures in hereditary coproporphyria. *Southern Medical Journal*. 1990; **83**: 1307–8.

234. Stoelting RK, Dierdorf SF (eds). *Anaesthesia and co-existing disease*, 3rd edn. New York: Churchill Livingstone, 1993: 375–7.

235. Kaada B, Romslo I. Use of transcutaneous nerve stimulation in the attacks of acute intermittent porphyria. *International Journal of Biochemistry*. 1985; **17**: 235–50.

236. Harrison GG, Moore MR, Meissner PN. Porphyrinogenicity of etomidate and ketamine as continuous infusions. Screening in the DCC-primed rat model. *British Journal of Anaesthesia*. 1985; **57**: 420–3.

237. Kanbak M. Ketamine in porphyria. *Anesthesia and Analgesia*. 1997; **84**: 1395.

Acute musculoskeletal pain

MILTON L COHEN

KEY LEARNING POINTS

- A functional taxonomy based on mechanism of production of clinical features and anatomical origin of pain is presented.
- The most useful diagnostic test for acute articular problems is aspiration and laboratory analysis of synovial fluid.
- Not only can imaging not demonstrate the presence of pain, but also the presence itself of anatomical abnormality establishes neither the anatomical origin nor the mechanism of musculoskeletal pain.
- Infiltration of local anesthetic into soft tissues as a diagnostico-therapeutic maneuver in musculoskeletal pain conveys no insight into the mechanism of production of pain but highlights the importance of

contextual (placebo) effect in assessment and treatment.
- The mainstay of management of acute inflammatory articular pain is anti-inflammatory medication
- The mainstay of management of acute noninflammatory joint pain is attention to biomechanical factors and the use of analgesic medication
- The evidence base for the management of acute nonarticular noninflammatory pain is disappointing: the approach includes consideration of rest, modification of activities, use of external supports, exercises, analgesic medications, "anti-inflammatory" medications (topical and oral), and injections.

INTRODUCTION

Despite the ubiquity in the community of musculoskeletal problems, acute and chronic, the discipline of musculoskeletal medicine suffers from a knowledge base that is yet to become coherent as it stems from a variety of different conceptual bases. Thus, the "turf" will be claimed by medical practitioners trained in fields as diverse as family medicine, orthopedic surgery, rheumatology, rehabilitation medicine, and manual medicine, by those trained in schools of osteopathy or chiropractic, and by other health professionals trained in physiotherapy or acupuncture or a variety of complementary therapies.

This has had several consequences which confound a rational, evidence-based approach to the practice of musculoskeletal medicine. Paramount among these is the problem of nomenclature. As the diagnostic labeling of a clinical problem entails a working hypothesis of its biological nature and implies the therapeutic pathway to be followed, the profusion of labels used by the different practitioner groups has thrown up a challenge to the standardization of names, to sharing of the knowledge base, and to the execution of therapeutic studies. For example, what is to be understood by the label "frozen shoulder" or "tennis elbow"?; is "adhesive capsulitis" or "lateral epicondylitis," respectively, the preferred term?;

what is the evidence that those entities ending in "-itis" are truly inflammatory in pathogenesis?; how is one to deal with the label "arthritis" being applied to any and all joint problems?

Irrespective of conventional or traditional labeling, the challenge remains of determining the mechanism of production of symptoms and signs in clinical musculoskeletal presentations. A label that implies inflammation denotes that the problem is nociceptive, that is, there is a local process in the tissue of complaint that excites nociceptive afferent nerves. However, it is now recognized that tissues can be the sites of pain and indeed of tenderness (hyperalgesia/allodynia) even when there is no discernible peripheral pathological process. This is the phenomenon of neuropathic pain, or pain due to disease, damage, or dysfunction of the nociceptive afferent pathways themselves.[1] Yet, overwhelmingly, the treatment of musculoskeletal problems is predicated on addressing peripheral pathology. This is by no means inappropriate in acute situations of, for example, trauma or infection, but as there is no distinct boundary between acute and chronic pain, and as the evidence has accumulated that sustained nociception over time can induce changes in central nervous system processing, the focus on peripheral mechanisms only was bound to prove inadequate. Indeed, it can be argued that the profusion of remedies available for musculoskeletal pain reflects the paradoxical "everything works and nothing works" state of the art. This is apparent in the lack of consensus regarding biological mechanisms in musculoskeletal pain.

Arising from these two related areas of controversy are the difficulties in reliability and validity of clinical assessment, including clinical investigation, of musculoskeletal problems. Diagnostic uncertainty compromises the internal validity of clinical trials. It is small wonder then that high-quality therapeutic studies on homogeneous clinical populations are hard to find. It follows that therapeutics as well as diagnosis may be based more on tradition than on scientifically driven insight.

This chapter on acute musculoskeletal pain will attempt to present an integrated view of the field via a functional taxonomy which provides a rational basis for therapy. The evidence base for therapy is overwhelming in some areas (such as the knee) and essentially absent in others (such as the ankle). While some generalizations can be made from this literature, major deficiencies in the knowledge base remain.

MECHANISM-BASED TAXONOMY

The conditions under consideration clinically fall into two mechanisms, inflammation and other, the latter taken to include mechanical and neuropathic.

Inflammation is a well-defined clinicopathological phenomenon. As a definitive mechanism, it can be characterized further by etiology: in the absence of trauma, the considerations include infection, crystal (monosodium urate, calcium pyrophosphate dihydrate), or acute exacerbation of chronic inflammatory disease such as rheumatoid arthritis.

The concept of "mechanical" joint pain is less secure, implying simultaneously that pain is not directly attributable to joint pathoanatomy, but rather that it is associated with abnormal joint movement, usually hypomobility. The neurophysiological basis for the observed phenomena – the transduction of abnormal mechanoception into nociception – is not well understood. The clinical observation is that restoration of normal joint movement may be associated with reduction in pain. "Normal" joint movement refers to the combination of the physiological movements able to be performed actively and accessory movements which can be demonstrated only passively. An example is the so-called "drawer" sign, said to reflect laxity of the anterior cruciate ligament in the knee. The physiological movements of the knee joint are of course flexion and extension in the sagittal plane about a transverse axis running through the joint. However, this axis is not stable in position. The "drawer" test in fact elicits passive femorotibial glide: this movement cannot be elicited actively but is a component of physiological movement as, in addition to rotating around the femoral condyles in flexion, the tibial condyles also glide posteriorly over them. The same principles apply to any concavo–convex synovial joint and form part of the conceptual basis for the schools of manual medicine and manipulative physiotherapy. Although a large pool of empirical observation supports the concept of joint pain of "mechanical" pathogenesis, placing movement-based interventions on an evidence base remains a challenge.

Neuropathic pain is that due to altered function of nociceptive pathways themselves, whether attributable to structural disease or to pathophysiological change. A neuropathic mechanism should be considered where there are no signs of nociceptive pathology, specifically inflammation, in the region of pain complaint, but where there is allodynia (pain in response to an innocuous stimulus) or hyperalgesia (increased pain in response to a noxious stimulus) to mechanical stimuli (touch, pressure, movement).

The above dichotomy of mechanism of pain can be combined with a dichotomy of anatomical origin of pain to construct a functional taxonomy (**Table 24.1**).

CLINICAL DIAGNOSIS

Clinical presentation

The presentation of acute musculoskeletal problems in limbs is characterized by acute pain and difficulty moving the affected part, resulting in compromised function.

Table 24.1 Functional taxonomy for musculoskeletal pain.

Site	Articular	Nonarticular
Mechanism		
Inflammatory	Infection	Infection (bursitis, cellulitis)
	Crystal	
	"Immunological"	
Noninflammatory	Symptomatic osteoarthrosis	Enthesopathy
	Osteonecrosis	Tendinopathy
	Hemarthrosis	"Mechanical"
	"Mechanical"	Neuropathic:
		Nerve entrapment/compression neuropathy
		Somatic referred pain
		"Regional" pain, local, or diffuse

Generally, the traditional signs of acute inflammation – heat, swelling, redness, allodynia – are valid in musculoskeletal tissues, especially when due to infection. Noninfective inflammation, such as in exacerbations of chronic inflammatory disease, may lack the erythema component and the calor component may not be impressive. The nature of tumor – fluid, soft tissue, or bone – leads to nuances in interpretation. In particular, tenderness (allodynia or hyperalgesia) alone, in the absence of other signs, does not lead to an inference of inflammation, as tenderness of clinically normal tissues (secondary allodynia/hyperalgesia) is characteristic of neuropathic pain. In most areas of musculoskeletal medicine, correlation among clinical history, clinical examination, investigations, and morphological findings is relatively imprecise. This is not necessarily a problem, especially in the acute situation.

The principles of clinical evaluation are to address these questions:

- What is the anatomical origin of the pain? (Articular versus nonarticular).
- What is the mechanism of the pain? (Inflammation versus noninflammation).
- What are the functional consequences of the pain? (Disability).
- What are the cognitive and affective components of the presentation? (Beliefs regarding diagnosis and prognosis; mood).

Clinical examination

Traditional teaching includes the following steps:

- inspection ("look");
- palpation ("feel") for temperature, tenderness (allodynia/hyperalgesia), and swelling;
- assessment of movement ("move"): passive/active/specific stressing of muscle groups.

To these can be added:

- signs of peripheral nerve dysfunction and/or signs of neuropathic pain such as evoked hyperesthetic phenomena;
- assessment of specific function of the affected part.

DIAGNOSTIC TESTS

Articular pain

SYNOVIAL FLUID ASPIRATION

The most useful and relevant diagnostic test for acute articular problems is aspiration of synovial fluid and laboratory investigation for:

- white cell count: the definitive test for inflammation;
- examination for crystals under polarized light microscopy: to identify monosodium urate or calcium pyrophosphate dihydrate crystals for gout and pseudogout, respectively;
- culture for and microbial sensitivity of bacteria.

BLOOD TESTS

The peripheral blood white cell count is a poor reflector of joint inflammation. A normal count does not exclude acute inflammation, especially infection. Exacerbations of chronic inflammatory arthritides, such as rheumatoid arthritis, may be associated with a modest neutrophil leukocytosis, but most commonly the white cell count is within the reference range.

- Mild normochromic normocytic anemia (secondary anemia) reflects activity in chronic disease.
- Mild thrombocytosis may also reflect inflammation.

- The erythrocyte sedimentation rate (ESR) is a time-honored but very nonspecific indirect indicator of inflammation. The main determinants of this *in vitro* phenomenon are the hematocrit of the sample of anticoagulated blood and the presence of proteins, the so-called acute-phase reactants, which promote red blood cells to form rouleaux. Foremost among the acute-phase reactants is fibrinogen, levels of which increase with age, which may account for the higher reference range for ESR in the elderly. Reliance on this test to determine inflammation, especially in the presence of anemia, is discouraged.
- C-reactive protein (CRP) is an α_2-globulin, elaborated as an acute-phase reactant. Its measurement and interpretation are not influenced by the hematocrit of the blood sample.

IMAGING STUDIES

There are two impediments to the utility of imaging studies in this context. First, imaging cannot demonstrate the presence of pain; second, the presence itself of anatomical abnormality (such as established osteoarthrosis) establishes neither the anatomical origin of pain nor its mechanism. Not only may damaged joints (osteoarthrosis) be asymptomatic but also anatomically normal joints can be painful. Generally speaking, plain radiography is of limited use in this situation. Radionuclide skeletal scans may identify regions of increased osteoblastic activity or increased vascularity, but these features do not identify the origin or mechanism of pain.

Techniques such as ultrasound, magnetic resonance imaging (MRI), and arthrography may be useful, depending upon

- the pretest probability of pathology (a clinical judgment);
- the sensitivity of the test (the ability of the test to detect the pathology if it is present);
- the specificity of the test (the ability of the test to exclude the pathology when it is absent).

These last indices of the test are usefully combined as the likelihood ratio, or the ratio between the true-positive rate and the false-positive rate, by which the pretest odds can then be multiplied. The literature here is complex; however, if the aim of the exercise is to distinguish inflammation from noninflammation, then imaging is of little use.

Nonarticular pain

BLOOD TESTS

In the absence of clinical features of inflammation, including infection, blood tests are rarely if ever of benefit. Noninflammatory mechanisms (mechanical and neuropathic) are not reflected in laboratory indices based on peripheral blood.

IMAGING

As mentioned above under Imaging studies, imaging is of limited utility in distinguishing inflammation from noninflammation, as the presence of swelling of soft tissue itself does not allow that inference. If the aim is to detect a periarticular structural derangement, then MRI is usually the modality of choice. The comments above regarding the use of the likelihood ratio are relevant here.

LOCAL DIAGNOSTIC TESTS

Infiltration of local anesthetic into soft tissues ("focal local") is popular as a diagnostico-therapeutic maneuver, the argument being that the anatomical origin of the pain is determined instantly and relief follows. Although this may work in some instances, it gives no insight into the mechanism of production of the pain and quite overlooks the contextual (placebo) component of an invasive procedure.[2] Such tests have not been subjected to systematic review.

MANAGEMENT OF ACUTE INFLAMMATORY JOINT PAIN

As a general principle, an inflamed joint should be aspirated for confirmation of inflammation and to search for possible bacterial or crystal etiology.

Septic arthritis, including bursitis and infection of prosthetic joints

Bacterial infection of these structures presents as typical acute inflammation. Systemic features may be present, especially in infants and young children. Infection of a prosthetic joint may present as an acute event or, more insidiously, with persistent pain, soft tissue swelling, or discharging sinus. Bacterial arthritis is a rheumatological emergency, as the chance of developing irreversible loss of joint function is 25–50 percent. Septic arthritis usually occurs following hematogenous seeding during bacteremia. Staphylococcal bacteria are the most common causes in adults, followed by group A beta-hemolytic streptococcal bacteria; *Hemophilus influenzae* and Gram-negative bacilli are the most common pathogens in neonates and children younger than five years. Disseminated gonococcal infection, often a cause of septic arthritis in young adults, tends to present with polyarthralgia, tenosynovitis, dermatitis, and fever rather than with joint effusion.[3]

The definitive diagnostic test is aspiration and culture of synovial fluid, which should be inoculated directly into blood culture bottles. The synovial fluid white cell count is usually very high with a polymorphonuclear predominance. Blood cultures themselves may be positive, especially in the presence of systemic features. Other tests performed on the peripheral blood, including ESR, CRP, and white cell count tend to be abnormal but nonspecific. Computed tomography (CT), MRI, and scintigraphy are more sensitive than plain radiography in early septic arthritis.

Acute septic bursitis occurs most commonly at the elbow and knee and may be accompanied by systemic features. Differentiation from inflammation of the underlying joint is clinical. Definitive diagnosis depends on aspiration and culture of bursal fluid.

Management of acute sepsis should be early and aggressive to prevent joint destruction, particularly in childhood, and mortality, particularly in the elderly and in patients with inflammatory joint disease or diabetes. The choice of antibiotic will of course depend upon the bacteriological findings. Antibiotic therapy is administered parenterally for up to four weeks, then orally for up to four weeks, depending upon the clinical situation.[3][V], [4][V] Aspiration of infected joints and bursae is recommended, by needle if possible, although arthroscopy for larger joints (shoulder, knee) may be required. Open surgical drainage is recommended for hip infections, especially in children. Treatment of infected joint prostheses usually requires removal of all foreign material.

Crystal arthritis

GOUT

The definitive diagnosis of acute gouty arthritis depends on the demonstration in synovial fluid of a neutrophil leukocytosis and intracellular crystals of uric acid. As synovial fluid is not always readily obtainable, the diagnosis may depend on inference in the appropriate clinical context. The possibility of sepsis must always be considered. Between attacks of acute gouty arthritis, urate crystals may be seen extracellularly in synovial fluid.

Treatment of acute gouty arthritis has two phases: relief of the acute inflammatory episode and prevention of recurrent episodes through control of hyperuricemia.

- For relief of the acute episode, any nonsteroidal anti-inflammatory drug (NSAID), except aspirin, orally in high dosage reducing over several days, is appropriate. Where there is a contraindication to NSAID therapy, oral prednisolone 20–50 mg reducing to 0 mg over several days or intra-articular corticosteroid can be considered.[5][V] Traditionally, colchicine in high doses has been used in this situation but it is poorly tolerated, being associated with severe diarrhea, nausea, and vomiting.[6][III] Colchicine in low dose (0.5 mg twice a day) may be useful as an adjunct to other treatments. Colchicine should be used with great care, especially in the elderly or patients with renal impairment, as diarrhea can be severe. No more than 6 mg of colchicine should be taken in 24 hours. There are no systematic comparisons of NSAIDs, corticosteroids, or colchicine in this situation.[7][I]. Drugs which alter plasma urate (aspirin, uricosuric agents, allopurinol) should not be used in the acute stage.

- Interval therapy, used to prevent recurrent episodes of gout, is not indicated in all patients. Attention should be given to risk factors, including obesity, alcohol excess, and drugs which impair urate excretion. In the absence of a history of tophi, impaired renal function, or urolithiasis, hypouricemic therapy may not be necessary. When indicated, either a xanthine oxidase inhibitor (allopurinol) or a uricosuric agent (probenecid, sulfinpyrazone) is introduced after acute inflammation has subsided. Colchicine 0.5 mg twice a day should be administered concurrently until plasma urate levels have stabilized to minimize the risk of inducing an acute episode.[8][II], [9][V] With this exception, there are no systematic studies on the effectiveness of strategies to prevent recurrent acute episodes of gout.[7][I]

CALCIUM CRYSTAL ARTHROPATHIES (CALCIUM PYROPHOSPHATE DIHYDRATE DEPOSITION DISEASE AND CALCIUM HYDROXYAPATITE DEPOSITION DISEASE)

Calcium pyrophosphate crystals may be associated with acute synovitis ("pseudogout"), which is a common cause of acute monoarthritis in the elderly, either as an acute event or as an "exacerbation" of osteoarthrosis. Basic calcium phosphate crystals may be associated with acute synovitis or, more commonly, as periarticular inflammation.[10]

As with gout, the definitive diagnosis of acute pseudogout arthritis depends on the demonstration of a neutrophil leukocytosis and crystals of calcium pyrophosphate dihydrate in synovial fluid.

Treatment of acute pseudogout follows the same principles as for acute gouty arthritis, with more emphasis on local joint treatment, specifically joint aspiration and intra-articular corticosteroid. Oral NSAIDs in high dosage reducing over several days may be appropriate in some patients but these must be used cautiously in the elderly or in patients with concurrent disease. Oral colchicine tends to be less effective than in gout.[11]

Exacerbations of chronic inflammatory diseases

In acute exacerbations of joint pain and/or swelling in a patient known to suffer from a chronic inflammatory arthropathy such as rheumatoid arthritis or one of the seronegative spondyloarthropathies, the possibility of sepsis must always be considered, as long-term anti-inflammatory therapy may modify some of the signs of acute inflammation. Such situations are best resolved by aspiration and culture of synovial fluid. Such aspiration will help the patient symptomatically and assist in determining whether the exacerbation is indeed inflammatory or due to joint damage, the synovial fluid white cell count being the discriminator. In a patient who is known to suffer from crystal arthropathy, joint aspiration is recommended where possible to help exclude sepsis and to perform local injection of depot corticosteroid.

Polyarticular exacerbations of chronic inflammatory disease may be best managed by revision of anti-inflammatory therapy, including the introduction of oral corticosteroids for short-term use. Mono- or oligo-articular exacerbations may respond to local joint injection with depot corticosteroid. In these situations, assessment and therapy are the province of the specialist.

MANAGEMENT OF ACUTE NONINFLAMMATORY JOINT PAIN

General considerations in the management of noninflammatory pain

A general approach to the management of noninflammatory musculoskeletal pain includes consideration of rest, modification of activities, use of external supports, exercises, analgesic medications, "anti-inflammatory" medications (topical and oral), and injections.

- Rest has intuitive appeal in the acute situation and may comprise immobilization or support of the painful part, avoidance of certain activities or postures or, in some circumstances, lying in bed. There is an inherent conflict between minimization of activity-related pain and the role of activity in facilitating normal function of musculoskeletal tissues. There is no consensus regarding this issue and little evidence on which to base generally applicable recommendations.
- Modification of activities to reduce biomechanical stresses addresses established or predictable risk factors, including those specifically applicable to the individual patient's predicament. The intuitive principle here tends not to be matched by evidence.
- The use of slings, supports, braces, or bandages may modify biomechanical stresses in conjunction with other measures. Their prescription is individual and not attributable to evidence-based rules. When associated with benefit, whether such devices work through biomechanical mechanisms or through placebo effect has not been determined.

- Exercises, active and passive, and a variety of physical modalities including heat and cold are usually prescribed. Two review articles have found it difficult to draw conclusions.[12][I], [13][I]
- The aim of drug therapy in acute noninflammatory musculoskeletal pain is symptom control.
  - Analgesic drugs include paracetamol (acetaminophen) alone at doses up to 4 g per day, or in combination with a weak opioid agonist such as codeine, or with stronger opioid drugs such as immediate-release morphine or oxycodone. In acute pain, single doses of paracetamol 600–650 mg are effective and the addition of codeine 60 mg enhances pain relief.[14][I] In the management of symptomatic osteoarthrosis of the knee (see below under Symptomatic osteoarthrosis), paracetamol alone has been shown to be superior to placebo[15][I], [16][I] and similar in efficacy to NSAIDs.[17][I]
  - Opioids: Apart from some single-dose efficacy studies, there are no controlled trials of opioid analgesics in acute musculoskeletal pain. This does not detract from their potential effectiveness. There is no *a priori* reason for not considering their use in situations where simple analgesics have failed.
  - NSAIDs: Despite the lack of evidence that inflammation is the relevant mechanism in what has been classified here as noninflammatory disorders, nonsteroidal anti-inflammatory drugs are used topically and systemically. In acute (mechanical) musculoskeletal conditions, topical ketoprofen, ibuprofen, or piroxicam have been shown to be significantly better than placebo for up to two weeks only and unassociated with an excess of adverse events.[18][I], [19][I] NSAIDs reduce pain intensity in symptomatic osteoarthritis of the knee compared with placebo but the size of the treatment effect is contentious.[20][I] Overall, the difference in effectiveness between paracetamol and NSAIDs in symptomatic osteoarthrosis is small, the latter appearing to be more effective in moderate-to-severe pain compared with milder pain.[15][I], [16][I], [17][I]
- Injections: The rationale for the use of local injections is that there is an anatomically localizable nociceptive process. When local anesthetic agent is used, the aims are to help with diagnosis and, if positive, with treatment. When depot corticosteroid agents are used, the presumption is that inflammation is the relevant mechanism. Although injection therapy is widely practiced, there is little support for its rationale or efficacy. Three problems confront the rational use of this approach. First is that of anatomical precision, which is of course linked with diagnostic uncertainty. Accuracy rates of 30 and 10–40 percent for intra-articular injections of

the knee and glenohumeral joint, respectively, and of 30 percent for the injections of the subacromial space, performed without radiological guidance, have been reported.[21][III], [22][III] The second problem is whether any observed outcome of the injected substance is due to its pharmaceutical property or due to physical effects. Third is the issue of the high potential contextual (placebo) effect of an invasive procedure itself.[2] Despite these major challenges to rationale, it is clinical experience that injections into potential spaces (joints, bursae) appear to help some patients. Unresolved issues include volume, dose, and technique of injection.

The issue of injecting a focally tender muscle with analgesic intent is based on the presumption that a site of nociception is being targeted, despite the fact that there is no evidence for such pathology. A similar argument applies to the injection of so-called "trigger points," the cornerstone of myofascial pain theory. Despite comprehensive refutation,[23] the practice continues in the absence of rationale or evidence.

Complications of injection include allergic reactions, local hemorrhage, and infection, and, in the case of corticosteroid injections, local tissue atrophy.

Symptomatic osteoarthrosis

Osteoarthrosis (osteoarthritis or OA) refers to a process of degradation and repair of articular cartilage ultimately leading to joint damage. Although most commonly idiopathic, it can also be the end result of other insults to synovial joints, including trauma and inflammatory arthritis. The process of cartilage damage is insidious and, when symptomatic, tends to be associated with persistent rather than acute pain.

However, a distinction has to be made between the presence of the pathological process of cartilage degradation (as usually reflected in the radiological signs of loss of "joint space" with reactive bone sclerosis) and clinical presentation. The prevalence of radiological OA increases with age: 70 percent of hands in the over 65 years age group and 60 percent of knees in the over 60 years age group. However, only 25–30 percent of affected joints become symptomatic. That is to say, the presence of OA neither predicts symptoms nor identifies the origin or mechanism of symptoms when they are present.[24]

This has particular implications in the context of acute joint pain. Acute pain in a known osteoarthrotic joint is unlikely due to the cartilage degradation process itself, but more likely to be due to biomechanical factors (altered movement or usage patterns), changes in subchondral bone, true inflammation (including sepsis or pyrophosphate crystal arthritis), loose body, or stress fracture. The approach is the same as that for a non-osteoarthrotic joint, namely aspiration if possible plus the approach

described above under General considerations in the management of noninflammatory pain.

"Mechanical" pain

Not only can osteoarthrotic joints be asymptomatic, but also anatomically normal joints may be painful. In the latter case the changes in joint biomechanics themselves may be responsible for pain, allodynia, and even swelling. Such pain, attributable to changes in movement, might be termed "mechanical" and attached to acutely symptomatic joints which do not have other signs suggestive of inflammation. Such an inference is further justified if the synovial fluid aspirate is typically acellular or mildly cellular ($< 1/\text{nL}$) with predominantly mononuclear count.

Hemarthrosis

Bleeding into a joint typically occurs in trauma and in patients with bleeding disorders, especially hemophilia. In the former case, the diagnosis is made on joint aspiration, which may also be therapeutic.

Osteonecrosis

Osteonecrosis[25] should be suspected when joint pain develops insidiously, especially on weight bearing, typically in the groin when a hip is involved, often with referral to the knee. When associated with painful limited passive joint movement and, in the case of the knee or shoulder, joint effusion, the conditions for an arthrosis are fulfilled. Diagnostic attention must exclude infection, which can be achieved only by joint aspiration. MRI is the most sensitive technique for detecting osteonecrosis.[26] However, the degree of bone or joint affection so demonstrated may be discordant with the clinical features. Bilateral changes may be seen when only one side has been affected clinically. Once there is plain radiological evidence of osteonecrosis, any chance of secondary prevention (i.e. of joint damage) has been lost. However, collapse of subchondral bone following osteonecrosis is not inevitable.

Osteonecrosis may be a cause of acute joint pain but usually has a spectrum of clinical presentation similar to that of osteoarthrosis. Specific management of early osteonecrosis (clinical findings and MRI positive; plain radiography or CT negative) remains undefined.

REGIONAL APPROACH TO ACUTE MUSCULOSKELETAL PAIN SYNDROMES

Acute shoulder pain

The shoulder region includes the synovial glenohumeral, acromioclavicular, and sternoclavicular joints and the extra-articular subacromial structures, especially the "rotator cuff" tendons and associated bursae. Shoulder region pain may also be referred from spinal or visceral structures.

ENTITIES

- Articular: taxonomy as in **Table 24.1** plus frozen shoulder, also known as "adhesive capsulitis" of the glenohumeral articulation.
- Nonarticular: impingement syndromes (subacromial bursitis, supraspinatus tendonitis/tears, rotator cuff tendonitis/tears).

CLINICAL FEATURES

The reliability and validity of elicited tenderness around the shoulder girdle is unknown. Range of shoulder movement on examination has been shown to be unreliable.[27][III] There is no firm evidence that any physical finding or group of signs is pathognomonic for a specific shoulder entity.[28][I] This has major implications for taxonomy, as described in **Table 24.1**.

INVESTIGATIONS

The utility of plain radiographs is limited by their inability to detect nonosseous lesions. Ultrasonography has better validity for full thickness than for partial thickness rotator cuff tears, but the demonstration of that pathology does not necessarily account for the pain. MRI has the greatest capacity to demonstrate structural abnormalities but again the demonstration of pathology does not reveal the cause or mechanism of the patient's pain. In particular, the prevalence of rotator cuff tears rises with age and does not correlate with symptoms.[29][III]

MANAGEMENT

- Articular entities. See above under Management of acute inflammatory joint pain and General considerations in the management of noninflammatory pain.
- Nonarticular entities:
  - Natural history: on the basis of a small number of prospective studies of nonhomogeneous patients with acute shoulder girdle pain, it seems that there is a 25–50 percent probability of recovery by six months, a 50 percent probability of recovery by 18 months, but a 50 percent chance of ongoing pain and functional compromise. Studies of relatively homogeneous patients with frozen shoulder suggest that major pain and disability resolve over a two to three year period.[28][I]
  - Exercise: active rather than passive exercises have been shown to be beneficial.[28][I], [30][I], [31][I]

- Physical modalities: whilst short-term therapeutic ultrasound may be of benefit, there is conflicting evidence regarding acupuncture and insufficient evidence regarding transcutaneous electrical nerve stimulation (TENS) or extracorporeal shock wave treatment (ESWT).[28][I]
- Pharmacotherapy: in a systematic review, NSAIDs were shown to have short-term (less than four weeks) superior efficacy in acute shoulder pain compared with placebo.[32][I] There is insufficient evidence concerning the efficacy of paracetamol or of oral corticosteroids.[28][I]
- Injection: subacromial corticosteroid injection is effective in delivering short-term relief.[28][I] Comparisons of corticosteroid injections with oral NSAIDs or physical therapies have yielded variable results.[32][I], [33][I], [34][I]
- Surgery: there are no published randomized controlled trials (RCTs) of the effectiveness of surgery for acute nontraumatic shoulder pain.[28][I]

These findings are sumarized in **Table 24.2**.

Acute elbow pain

The elbow region includes the humeroulnar and radiohumeral joints, the entheses (origins) of the extensor and flexor muscles of the forearm, and the cubital tunnel.

ENTITIES

- Articular. Taxonomy as in **Table 24.1**.
- Nonarticular:
  - lateral elbow pain (synonyms: lateral epicondylitis, tennis elbow, radial epicondylalgia, humeral epicondylalgia);
  - medial elbow pain (synonyms: medial epicondylitis, golfer's elbow, medial tennis elbow, medial epicondylalgia);
  - compression neuropathy of the ulnar nerve in the cubital tunnel;
  - acute olecranon bursitis.

CLINICAL FEATURES

No data concerning the reliability and validity of clinical features of diagnostic maneuvers for nonarticular entities have been published.[35][I]

INVESTIGATIONS

Imaging of articular entities is guided by the clinical picture; usually plain radiography will demonstrate articular or intraosseous pathology. There are no

Table 24.2 Evidence for interventions in acute shoulder pain.

Intervention	Detail	Beneficial?	Evidence level
Activity	Exercises	Benefit	[I]
	Passive therapy	Insufficient	[I]
Physical	Acupuncture	Conflicting	[I]
	Ultrasound (short-term)	Benefit	[I]
	Extracorporeal shock-wave therapy	Insufficient	No [I] or [II]
	Transcutaneous nerve stimulation	Insufficient	[I]
	Suprascapular nerve blocks	Insufficient	No [I] or [II]
Pharmacotherapy	Analgesics	Insufficient	No [I] or [II]
	Nonsteroidal anti-inflammatory drugs	Benefit	[I]
	Oral corticosteroids	Insufficient	No [I] or [II]
Injections	Subacromial corticosteroid injection	Benefit	[I]
Surgery	Surgery	Insufficient	No [I] or [II]

Adapted from: Australian Acute Musculoskeletal Pain Guidelines. Evidence-based Management of Acute Musculoskeletal Pain Online. Available at www.nhmrc.gov.au. Brisbane: Australian Academic Press, 2003.

controlled data out of which imaging of nonarticular entities can be recommended.

MANAGEMENT

- Articular entities. See above under Management of acute inflammatory joint pain and General considerations in the management of noninflammatory pain.
- Nonarticular entities:
  - Natural history: Lateral elbow pain is considered to be self-limiting, although symptoms can persist for more than 18 months. In one expectant trial in general practice, 80 percent of those with more than four weeks of elbow pain had recovered by 12 months.[36][I]
  - Rest or exercise: Two older systematic reviews of all treatments for lateral epicondylitis[37][I], [38][I] found rest to be a control intervention alone and not compared with other modalities. There is no consensus regarding rest or type, frequency, or duration of exercise.[35][I] There is insufficient evidence concerning the effects of braces compared with placebo or physiotherapy.[39][I]
  - Physical modalities: The older reviews failed to find evidence that ultrasound or laser treatment was better than placebo for lateral epicondylitis.[37][I], [38][I] A systematic review of the effects of needle acupuncture, laser acupuncture, or electroacupuncture generated insufficient evidence.[40][I] Three RCTs of ESWT found no difference from sham treatment at three months.[41][I], [42][II]
  - Pharmacological: Topical NSAIDs provide short-term (up to four weeks) improvement in pain compared with placebo.[43][I] There is limited evidence for the short-term effectiveness of oral

NSAIDs in reducing pain and improving function.[43][I] There are no published data with respect to medial epicondylitis.
  - Injection: There is limited evidence from one systematic review and two subsequent RCTs of short-term effectiveness of corticosteroid injections compared with placebo, local anesthetic, passive physiotherapy, or braces.[44][I], [45][II] In one study of medial epicondylitis, injection was superior to NSAIDs and physical therapy at six weeks.[46][III] However, there is no consensus as to the technique of injection, in terms of site or agents.[35][I]
  - Surgery: Operation for lateral epicondylitis is restricted to refractory cases which would be labeled chronic. There are no controlled data for any of the diverse surgical procedures which include "denervation" of the epicondyle, excision of "abnormal" tissue, and dissection of the common extensor origin off the lateral epicondyle.[47][I] Similar comments apply to medial epicondylitis.[35][I]

Acute wrist pain

The wrist region includes the radiocarpal, distal radioulnar, intercarpal and carpometacarpal joints, flexor and extensor tendons of the thumb and fingers, and the carpal tunnel.

ENTITIES

- Articular. Taxonomy as in **Table 24.1** plus:
  - Kienbock's disease (osteonecrosis of the lunate).
- Nonarticular:
  - carpal instability ("mechanical");
  - ulnar impaction syndrome;
  - tendon impairment: de Quervain's stenosing tenosynovitis.

CLINICAL FEATURES

The criterion standard for carpal instability is radiographic. No criterion standards are available for the labels of tendon impairment or ulnar impaction syndrome.

INVESTIGATIONS

Static plain radiographs may show diagnostic features of carpal instability but with low sensitivity.[48][IV]

MANAGEMENT

- Articular entities. See above under Management of acute inflammatory joint pain and General considerations in the management of noninflammatory pain.
- Nonarticular entities:
  - Natural history: Possibly 75 percent of patients with wrist pain defying specific diagnosis continue to experience pain.[49][I]
  - Rest or exercise; physical modalities: The general principles discussed above under General considerations in the management of noninflammatory pain may be followed in the absence of specific evidence.
  - Pharmacological: Data on the efficacy of anti-inflammatory drugs are not available.
  - Injection: Approximately 50 percent of a cohort of patients with de Quervain's tenosynovitis treated with corticosteroid injection achieved sustained benefit.[50][III]
  - Surgery: An option for chronic de Quervain's tenosynovitis resistant to therapy.[49][I]

Acute hip pain

The "hip" region, in colloquial parlance, usually refers to the buttock and lateral upper thigh. True hip joint pain, however, is usually felt in the groin and may also be felt in the anterior thigh to the knee. In broadening the "hip" region to include the "proximal hindquarter," the main considerations are the hip joint itself and referred pain from the lumbar spine. The sacroiliac joint, being properly part of the axial skeleton, will not be discussed here.

ENTITIES

- Articular. Taxonomy as in **Table 24.1** plus:
  - osteonecrosis of the femoral head;
  - undisplaced fracture of femoral neck.
- Nonarticular:
  - referred pain, greater trochanteric bursalgia.

CLINICAL FEATURES

Clinical localization of pain to the hip joint itself, based on painful limited joint movement is relatively uncontroversial. There are no data addressing validity, reliability, or criterion standards.

INVESTIGATIONS

Plain radiograph of the hip joint (anteroposterior pelvic view) may show articular pathology when suggested by clinical findings. MRI is superior to CT and plain radiography when osteonecrosis is suspected.

MANAGEMENT

Treatment follows the general principles outlined above under General considerations in the management of noninflammatory pain.

Acute knee pain

The knee region comprises the femorotibial and patellofemoral articulations, the patella and patellar ligament, the superior tibofibular joints, and the popliteal fossa including the hamstring tendons. Acute knee pain is most commonly caused by intrinsic knee disorders. The literature regarding knee disorders is enormous and features creative taxonomy. The difficulty of making an accurate, precise diagnosis may have contributed to the profusion of traditional labels. Most studies in the evidence-based literature have focused on acute anterior knee (or patellofemoral) pain.

ENTITIES

- Articular. Taxonomy as in **Table 24.1** plus:
  - a number of intra-articular mechanical derangements, including cruciate ligament and meniscal disruption, osteochondritis dissecans, and loose body formation;
  - problems relating to the patella and the patellofemoral articulation.
- Nonarticular:
  - prepatellar and infrapatellar bursitis;
  - Osgood–Schlatter disease (tibial tuberosity apophysitis);
  - traction apophysitis of the lower pole of the patella;
  - collateral ligament injury;
  - Pellegrini–Stieda disease, biceps tendinitis, pes anserine tenditis and bursitis, popliteus tendinitis, and popliteal cyst.

CLINICAL FEATURES

Studies have failed to show a link between individual symptoms and any specific pathology.[51][I] Reliability of most examination techniques is poor or unknown, with the exception of the assessment of cruciate ligament tears in the acutely injured and anesthetized knee.

INVESTIGATIONS

The Ottowa Knee Rule[52][III] for the use of conventional radiography in acute post-traumatic knee pain has been found to be reliable and valid. This rule states that a conventional radiograph is required for patients with acute knee injury who have any of the following findings: age 55 years or over; isolated tenderness of patella; tenderness at head of fibula; inability to flex to 90°; inability to bear weight. This rule is not applicable in patients younger than 18 years or in nontraumatic situations. There is no evidence for the use of plain radiography in situations of acute nontraumatic knee pain.

Although MRI has been studied extensively, it is difficult to conclude a relationship between clinical assessment, MRI, and arthroscopy in relation to efficacy and cost-effectiveness.[51][I] Both MRI and clinical examination are valid for anterior cruciate ligament tears.

Bone scan is sensitive but not specific for the detection of osteoarthritis, sepsis, inflammation, osteonecrosis, or Paget's disease.[53]

The knee is the easiest joint in the body to aspirate: the clinical suspicion of effusion is an indication for diagnostic aspiration.

MANAGEMENT

- Articular entities: The literature on the treatment of acute intra-articular mechanical derangements of the knee is extensive, as found in surgical sources, and is not reviewed here. The management of nontraumatic acute articular knee pain follows the principles outlined above under Management of acute noninflammatory joint pain.

The evidence base for the management of acute anterior knee pain (assumed to be noninflammatory) is summarized here and in **Table 24.3**.

- Natural history: Improvement, with a degree of persistence in most people.[51]
- Rest versus exercise: Maintenance of normal activity and performance of quadriceps strengthening techniques, especially eccentric, have been shown to be beneficial.[51][I], [54][I]
- Physical modalities: Whilst there is evidence of benefit in women from corrective foot orthoses, evidence of benefit from patellofemoral orthoses is conflicting.[51][I], [54][I] There is insufficient evidence for the effectiveness of patellar taping, therapeutic ultrasound or electrical stimulation, whilst laser therapy has been unassociated with benefit.[51][I]
- Pharmacotherapy: There is insufficient evidence for the effectiveness of analgesics or NSAIDs.
- Injections: Injection with corticosteroid or saline is associated with short-term benefit.

This evidence base provides a typical example of the adage that absence of evidence is not evidence of absence. Empirically in the clinic, treatment of acute noninflammatory anterior knee pain follows the principles outlined above under Management of acute

Table 24.3 Evidence for interventions in acute (anterior) knee pain.

Intervention	Detail	Beneficial?	Evidence level
Activity	Advice to stay active	Benefit	[II]
	Exercises (quadriceps, esp. eccentric)	Benefit	[I], [II]
Physical	Acupuncture	Insufficient	No [I] or [II]
	Electrical stimulation	Insufficient	No [I] or [II]
	Therapeutic ultrasound	Insufficient	[1]
	Laser therapy	No benefit	[I]
	Progressive resistance braces	Insufficient	[I]
	Patellar taping	Insufficient	[I], [II]
	Patellofemoral orthoses	Conflicting	[I]
	Corrective foot orthoses (in women)	Benefit	[I]
Pharmacotherapy	Analgesics (simple and opioid)	Insufficient	No [I] or [II]
	Nonsteroidal anti-inflammatory drugs	Insufficient	No [I] or [II]
Injection	Injection (treatment or saline)	Benefit	[II]

Adapted from: Australian Acute Musculoskeletal Pain Guidelines. Evidence-based Management of Acute Musculoskeletal Pain Online. Available at www.nhmrc.gov.au. Brisbane: Australian Academic Press, 2003.

noninflammatory joint pain, assisted by the evidence base. The emphasis in this bodily region is on distinguishing between the acutely painful knee and the acutely painful and swollen knee, the latter usually requiring aspiration to determine hemarthrosis, inflammation, or neither.

- Nonarticular (extra-articular) entities: Treatment follows the general principles outlined above under General considerations in the management of noninflammatory pain.

Acute ankle and foot pain

The ankle region includes the synovial tibiotalar (talocrural) and subtalar (talocalcaneal) joints and the extra-articular structures, especially the anterior tibial, peroneal, and posterior tibial tendons, the last passing through the "tarsal tunnel," which also contains the posterior tibial nerve. The foot comprises the tarsus, metatarsus, and phalanges, with associated flexor and extensor tendons and the plantar fascia (deep plantar ligament).

ENTITIES

- Articular: Taxonomy as in **Table 24.1**.
- Nonarticular:
  - tendinopathies (of the synovial tendon sheaths and tendo Achilles);
  - enthesopathy, especially of the plantar fascia ("plantar fasciitis");
  - stress fractures of the calcaneus and metatarsals in particular;
  - ankle "sprain" (injury to the lateral ligament complex)
  - symptomatic pes planovalgus (flat foot), manifest as metatarsalgia or hallux valgus with bursitis.

Other sources of acute foot pain include:

- peripheral vascular disease;
- peripheral neuropathy, including entrapment neuropathy of digital nerves (Morton's neuroma);
- referred pain from structures in the lumbar spine.

CLINICAL FEATURES

There are no data concerning reliability or validity or criterion standards for these extra-articular entities.

INVESTIGATIONS

Imaging of articular entities is guided by the clinical picture; usually plain radiography will demonstrate articular or intraosseous pathology. There are no controlled data from which imaging of nonarticular entities can be recommended.

MANAGEMENT

Management of articular entities follows the principles as above under Management of acute noninflammatory joint pain.

Management of nonarticular entities follows the general principles articulated above under General considerations in the management of noninflammatory pain. With respect to the treatment of ankle sprain, early mobilization with use of an external support is beneficial, whilst immobilization may be beneficial. Cold treatment and therapeutic ultrasound are unlikely to be beneficial, whilst the effectiveness of diathermy is unknown.[55][I] For plantar heel pain (including plantar fasciitis), corticosteroid injection alone or with local anesthetic is likely to be ineffective or harmful in the medium- to long-term, whilst injection of corticosteroid or local anesthetic in the short term, ultrasound, laser therapy, stretching exercises, custom-made insoles, and surgery are of unknown effectiveness.[56][I]

REFERENCES

1. Merskey H, Bogduk N (eds). *Classification of chronic pain,* 2nd edn. Seattle: IASP Press, 1994: 212.
2. Cohen ML. Placebo theory. In: Hutson M, Ellis R (eds). *Textbook of musculoskeletal medicine.* Oxford: Oxford University Press, 2006: 109–14.
* 3. Goldenberg DL. Septic arthritis. *Lancet.* 1998; **351**: 197–202.
4. Lidgren L. Septic arthritis and osteomyelitis. In: Hochberg MC, Silman AJ, Smolen J *et al.* (eds). *Rheumatology,* 3rd edn. Edinburgh: Mosby, 2003: 1055–65.
5. Emmerson BT. The management of gout. In: Hochberg MC, Silman AJ, Smolen J *et al.* (eds). *Rheumatology,* 3rd edn. Edinburgh: Mosby, 2003: 1929–36.
6. Ahern MJ, Reid C, Gordon TP *et al.* Does colchicine work? The results of the first controlled study in acute gout. *Australian and New Zealand Journal of Medicine.* 1987; **17**: 301–4.
7. Underwood M. Gout. *Clinical Evidence.* 2006; **15**: 1561–9.
8. Borstad GC, Bryant LR, Abel MP *et al.* Colchicine for prophylaxis of acute flares when initiating allopurinol for chronic gouty arthritis. *Journal of Rheumatology.* 2004; **31**: 2429–32.
9. Terkeltaub RA. Clinical practice. Gout. *New England Journal of Medicine.* 2003; **349**: 1647–55.
10. McCarthy GM. Basic calcium phosphate crystal deposition disease. In: Hochberg MC, Silman AJ, Smolen J *et al.* (eds). *Rheumatology,* 3rd edn. Edinburgh: Mosby, 2003: 1951–9.
11. Doherty M. Calcium pyrophosphate dihydrate crystal associated arthropathy. In: Hochberg MC, Silman AJ,

Smolen J (eds). *Rheumatology*, 3rd edn. Edinburgh: Mosby, 2003: 1937–50.

12. Feine JS, Lund JP. An assessment of the efficacy of physical therapy and physical modalities for the control of chronic musculoskeletal pain. *Pain*. 1997; **71**: 5–23.

13. Beckerman H, Bouter LM, van der Heijden BRA *et al.* Efficacy of physiotherapy for musculoskeletal disorders: what can we learn from research? *British Journal of General Practice*. 1993; **43**: 73–7.

* 14. Moore A, Collins S, Carroll D, McQuay H. Paracetamol with and without codeine in acute pain: a quantitative systematic review. *Pain*. 1997; **70**: 193–201.

15. Towheed T, Maxwell L, Judd M *et al.* Acetaminophen for osteoarthritis. *Cochrane Database of Systematic Reviews*. 2006; **1**: CD004257.

16. Zhang W, Jones A, Doherty M. Does paracetamol (acetaminophen) reduce the pain of osteoarthritis?: A meta-analysis of randomised controlled trials. *Annals of the Rheumatic Diseases*. 2004; **63**: 901–7.

17. Lee C, Straus WL, Balshaw R *et al.* A comparison of the efficacy and safety of nonsteroidal antiinflammatory agents versus acetaminophen in the treatment of osteoarthritis: A meta-analysis. *Arthritis and Rheumatism*. 2004; **51**: 746–54.

18. Mason L, Moore RA, Edwards JE *et al.* Topical NSAIDs for chronic musculoskeletal pain: systematic review and meta-analysis. *BMC Musculoskeletal Disorders*. 2004; **5**: 28.

19. Lin J, Zhang W, Jones A *et al.* Efficacy of topical non-steroidal anti-inflammatory drugs in the treatment of osteoarthritis: meta-analysis of randomised controlled trials. *British Medical Journal*. 2004; **329**: 324.

20. Bjordal JM, Ljunggren AE, Klovning A *et al.* Non-steroidal anti-inflammatory drugs, including cyclo-oxygenase-2 inhibitors, in osteoarthritic knee pain: meta-analysis of randomised placebo controlled trials. *British Medical Journal*. 2004; **329**: 1317.

21. Jones A, Regan M, Ledingham J *et al.* Importance of placement of intra-articular steroid injections. *British Medical Journal*. 1993; **307**: 1329–30.

22. Eustace JA, Brophy DP, Gibney RP *et al.* Comparison of the accuracy of steroid placement with clinical outcome in patients with shoulder symptoms. *Annals of the Rheumatic Diseases*. 1997; **56**: 59–63.

* 23. Quintner JL, Cohen ML. Referred pain of peripheral neural origin: an alternative to the "myofascial pain" construct. *Clinical Journal of Pain*. 1994; **10**: 243–51.

24. Dieppe PA, Lohmander LS. Pathogenesis and managment of pain in osteoarthritis. *Lancet*. 2005; **365**: 965–73.

25. Mazières B. Osteonecrosis. In: Hochberg MC, Silman AJ, Smolen J *et al.* (eds). *Rheumatology*, 3rd edn. Edinburgh: Mosby, 2003: 1877–90.

26. Mitchell MD, Kundel HL, Steinberg ME *et al.* Avascular necrosis of the hip: comparison of MR, CT and scintigraphy. *American Journal of Roentgenology*. 1986; **147**: 67–71.

27. Croft P, Pope D, Boswell R *et al.* Observer variability in measuring elevation and external rotation of the shoulder. *British Journal of Rheumatology*. 1994; **33**: 942–6.

* 28. Australian Acute Musculoskeletal Pain Guidelines Group. *Evidence-based management of acute musculoskeletal pain*. Brisbane: Australian Academic Press, 2003: 119–54. Available from: www.nhmrc.gov.au.

* 29. Chandnani V, Ho C, Gerharter J *et al.* MR findings in asymptomatic shoulders: a blind analysis using symptomatic shoulders as controls. *Clinical Imaging*. 1992; **16**: 25–30.

30. van der Heijden GJMG, van der Windt DAWM, de Winter AF. Physiotherapy for patients with soft tissue shoulder disorders. *British Medical Journal*. 1997; **315**: 25–9.

31. Green S, Buchbinder R, Hetrick S. Physiotherapy interventions for shoulder pain. *Cochrane Database of Systematic Reviews*. 2003; **CD004258**.

* 32. Green S, Buchbinder R, Glazier R, Forbes A. Systematic review of randomised controlled trials of interventions for painful shoulder; selection criteria, outcome assessment and efficacy. *British Medical Journal*. 1998; **316**: 354–60.

33. van der Heijden GJMG, van der Windt DAWM *et al.* Steroid injections for shoulder disorders: a systematic review of randomized clinical trials. *British Journal of General Practice*. 1996; **46**: 309–16.

34. Buchbinder R, Green S, Youd JM. Corticosteroid injections for shoulder pain. *Cochrane Database of Systematic Reviews*. 2003; **CD004016**.

35. Barnsley L, Bogduk N. *Australasian Faculty of Musculo-skeletal Medicine: Evidence-based guidelines for the management of acute elbow pain*. Newcastle, NSW: Newcastle Bone and Joint Institute, 1998.

36. Hudak PL, Cole DC, Haines AT. Understanding prognosis to improve rehabilitation: the example of lateral elbow pain. *Archives of Physical Medicine and Rehabilitation*. 1996; **77**: 568–93.

37. Labelle H, Guibert R, Joncas J *et al.* Lack of scientific evidence for the treatment of lateral epicondylitis of the elbow. An attempted meta-analysis. *Journal of Bone and Joint Surgery*. 1992; **74B**: 646–51.

38. Chandani A, Waldron D, Teng SS, Glasziou P. A systematic review of treatments for "tennis elbow". *Australian Association of Musculoskeletal Medicine*. 1997; **2**: 21–6.

39. Struijs PAA, Smidt N, Arola H *et al.* Orthotic devices for the treatment of tennis elbow. *Cochrane Database of Systematic Reviews*. 2002; **CD001821**.

40. Green S, Buchbinder R, Barnsley L *et al.* Acupuncture for lateral elbow pain. *Cochrane Database of Systematic Reviews*. 2002; **CD003527**.

41. Buchbinder R, Green S, White M *et al.* Shock wave therapy for lateral elbow pain. *Cochrane Database Systematic Reviews*. 2005; **CD003524**.

42. Speed C, Nichols D, Richards C *et al.* Extracorporeal shock wave therapy for lateral epicondylitis – a double blind randomized cotrolled trial. *Journal of Orthopaedic Research*. 2002; **20**: 895–8.

43. Green S, Buchbinder R, Barnsley L *et al.* Non-steroidal anti-inflammatory drugs (NSAIDs) for treating lateral elbow pain in adults. In: *Cochrane Database of Systematic Reviews.* 2002; **CD003686**.

44. Smidt N, Assendelft WJJ, van der Windt DAWM *et al.* Corticosteroid injections for lateral epicondylitis: a systematic review. *Pain.* 2002; **96**: 23–40.

45. Newcomer K, Laskowski E, Idank D *et al.* Corticosteroid injection in early treatment of lateral epicondylitis. *Clinical Journal of Sport Medicine.* 2001; **11**: 214–22.

46. Stahl S, Kaufman T. The efficacy of an injection of steroids for medial epicondylitis. *Journal of Bone and Joint Surgery.* 1997; **79A**: 1648–52.

47. Buchbinder R, Green S, Bell S *et al.* Surgery for lateral elbow pain in adults. *Cochrane Database of Systematic Reviews.* 2002; **CD003525**.

48. Truong NP, Mann FA, Gilula LA, Kang SW. Wrist instability series: increased yield with characteristic screening criteria. *Radiology.* 1994; **192**: 481–4.

49. Gray D, Bogduk N. *Australasian faculty of musculo-skeletal medicine: Evidence-based guidelines for the management of acute wrist pain.* Newcastle, NSW: Newcastle Bone and Joint Institute, 1998.

50. Anderson BC, Manthey R, Brouns MC. Treatment of De Quervain's tenosynovitis with corticosteroids. A prospective study of the response to local injection. *Arthritis and Rheumatism.* 1991; **34**: 793–8.

∗ 51. Australian Acute Musculoskeletal Pain Guidelines Group. *Evidence-based management of acute musculoskeletal pain.* Brisbane: Australian Academic Press, 2003: 155–81. Available from: www.nhmrc.gov.au.

52. Stiell IG, Greenberg GH, Wells GA *et al.* Prospective validation of a decision rule for the use of radiography in acute knee injuries. *Journal of the American Medical Association.* 1996; **275**: 611–15.

53. Lee YU, Sartoris DJ. Imaging of the knee. *Current Opinion in Orthopaedics.* 1995; **6**: 56–65.

54. Crossley K, Bennell K, Green S, McConnell J. A systematic review of physical interventions for patellofemoral pain syndrome. *Clinical Journal of Sport Medicine.* 2001; **11**: 103–10.

55. Striujs P, Kerkhoffs G. Ankle sprain. *BMJ Clinical Evidence.* 2005; **13**: 1366–76.

56. Crawford F. Plantar heel pain and fasciitis. *BMJ Clinical Evidence.* 2005; **13**: 1533–45.

25

Acute low back pain

MILTON L COHEN

KEY LEARNING POINTS

- Episodes of acute low back pain (LBP) are common and usually self-limiting, although 10 percent fail to resolve over six weeks to two months and the recurrence rate within one year is more than 50 percent.
- Approximately 95 percent of acute LBP is "nonspecific," in the sense that a specific etiological or pathological process will not be found.
- The clinical approach triad for acute LBP addresses:
  - Is the problem "mechanical" or not?
  - Is any associated pelvic girdle or lower limb pain radicular or somatic referred?
  - What other contributions to distress are there?
- Unless there is a suspicion of red flag conditions, laboratory investigations and radiographs can be deferred for four weeks.

- Psychological factors are more predictive of chronicity after acute LBP than clinical factors.
- Current anatomically based diagnostic terminology is inadequate to describe acute LBP.
- The evidence base for common interventions in LBP is constrained by most studies looking at populations with mixed duration of pain and not distinguishing between somatic referred and radicular pain when LBP is associated with radiating pain into the lower limbs.
- A pragmatic, evidence-assisted approach to management of acute LBP consists of the triad of assurance, activation, and analgesia.

INTRODUCTION

Low back pain (LBP) is common, confusing, and costly. The main source of the confusion (which feeds the mythology surrounding back pain) is the problem of clinical diagnostic terminology which stems from the biomedical imperative to identify an underlying structural lesion. However, not only is there poor concordance between symptoms and radiologically demonstrated pathology, but also approximately 85 percent of episodes are labeled as "nonspecific." That is, in the majority of cases a specific etiological or pathological diagnosis is not possible. Whilst it has been tempting to attribute acute low back pain to "disc degeneration" or to "facet joint arthritis," to name but two common labels, the mechanisms converting an age-related, usually asymptomatic, structural phenomenon into a clinical episode remain obscure. Although the prevalence of disc degeneration increases with age, the occurrence and associated disability of acute LBP peaks between the ages of 35 and 55 years, the middle working years of life.[1, 2]

This chapter will concern primarily so-called "nonspecific" acute LBP, being defined as an episode of pain felt in the lumbar spine and/or pelvic girdle of less than three months in duration. A clinical approach will be offered to identify "specific" biomedical conditions and psychosocial factors in presentation and outcome. Important in the physical assessment will be the distinction between radicular and somatic referred pain in the pelvic girdle and lower limb,[3] the former constituting a "red flag" condition. Management of such "red flag" conditions will not be discussed here. Integral to the assessment of psychosocial factors is the concept of "yellow flags," which identify risk factors for poor recovery.[4]

Despite the problem in terminology which attends LBP and the incomplete understanding underlying it, there is a place for diagnostic discipline. Given that "pain" is the presenting symptom, to recursively elevate that to a "diagnosis" is to avoid the clinical responsibility of identifying those factors in the biopsychosocial framework[5] that might contribute to that episode and thus may serve as a guide for instituting management. It will be suggested that, rather than "nonspecific LBP," a descriptive functional diagnostic label for the "biomedical" component be used, such as "mechanical lumbar spine impairment." This implies that the lumbar spine is the origin of pain and that the mechanism is neither inflammatory, infective, neoplastic, metabolic, nor neuropathic, but may be related to abnormal movement of the segment (although the transduction of that remains obscure).

Guidelines for the management of acute LBP were developed in a number of countries in the last decade;[6, 7, 8, 9, 10, 11, 12] this chapter seeks to update the evidence base underlying those. The limitations of extrapolating the results of randomized controlled trials (RCTs) to the patient who visits the primary care practitioner or specialist will be discussed.

EPIDEMIOLOGY

The natural histories of acute and recurrent low back pain are essentially benign in an impairment-based sense, although not so in a disability- or capacity-based context. In developed countries, around 60–80 percent of the population will experience LBP during their lifetime, with about 2–5 percent of the population at risk seeking medical attention or taking time off work.[2, 13, 14] The annual incidence of low back pain varies from 15 to 45 percent of adults, with 5 percent presenting with a new episode. The prevalence of low back pain (not necessarily distinguishing between acute and persistent) ranges from 10 to 45 percent.[15]

A survey in New Zealand found that 57 percent of men and 54 percent of women have had back pain during their lives, with 10 percent having LBP on any one day. Almost one-quarter felt that LBP had restricted their daily activities.[16] A UK survey[17] showed similar results, with a 67 percent lifetime prevalence, 43 percent annual prevalence, and 21 percent point prevalence among an adult population. Of these, 52 percent had not consulted a health professional, increasing to 71 percent of those with pain of less than two weeks duration. Those who did consult their doctor for acute pain were more likely to be unemployed or retired, to be given a diagnosis for their back pain and to have greater than the median worst pain. For those with pain of 2–12 weeks duration, a disability score greater than the median and externalized locus of control for pain management were the associated factors. A cross-sectional study[18] in a Danish population of people aged 12–41 years found that, by the age of 18 years in girls and 20 years in boys, more than 50 percent had experienced at least one back pain episode. A systematic review of the literature on LBP in the elderly[19] concluded that the prevalence of back pain in this population was not known with certainty and was not comparable with the younger population. There was wide variability in the reported prevalence, demonstrating the need for improved reporting of age information in studies.

Within the workforce, 50 percent or more will have back pain each year.[20] Almost one-quarter of patients with LBP will consult a health care practitioner, and, of these, 85 percent will have "nonspecific" LBP, the majority of the remainder having a diagnosis of a prolapsed intervertebral disk, for which the receipt of disability compensation does not necessarily reduce the rate of return to work.[21]

Episodes of acute low back pain are usually self-limiting, with 10 percent failing to resolve over six weeks to two months, but a recurrence rate of 50–80 percent within one year has been suggested. The risk of persistence of an acute episode to chronic low back pain is estimated at 2–7 percent.[22, 23] Risk factors for the development of acute LBP include heavy physical work, frequent bending, twisting, lifting, and prolonged static postures.[2]

There is evidence for an effect of psychosocial factors at work on the occurrence of back pain, particularly for low social support and low job satisfaction, but not for psychosocial factors in private life.[24] The possibility was raised of a positive association between low job satisfaction and the physical factors which have been reported as factors in LBP, including lifting, bending, twisting, and whole body vibration. In a study of 46 individuals with a high rate (73 percent) of asymptomatic disk abnormalities followed for five years, the physical job characteristics and psychological aspects of work were more powerful than magnetic resonance imaging (MRI) in predicting both medical consultations related to LBP and resultant work incapacity.[25]

Smoking has been associated with back pain in adolescents[26] and adults,[27, 28] although there were too few studies to relate smoking to structural factors such as disk degeneration or herniation. A review concluded that obesity should be considered as a possible weak indicator.[29] Studies are required to determine whether changing these lifestyle factors improves the outcome of acute LBP.

PRINCIPLES UNDERLYING CLINICAL EVALUATION

Neuroanatomy of the lumbar spine

There are several candidate structures for the origin of lumbar spinal pain. Nociceptive afferents supply the skin and subcutaneous tissues, adipose tissue, fasciae and ligaments, periosteum, dura mater, the adventitia of blood tissues, and the fibrous capsules of the apophyseal and sacroiliac joints.[30, 31, 32] These structures are innervated in a multisegmental, overlapping manner such that, for example, the L4/5 apophyseal joint receives innervation from the L4 and L5 segments and the L5 nerve supplies the L4/L5 and L5/S1 apophyseal joints.[31] This provides an anatomical substrate for the phenomenon of somatic referred pain. In routine clinical practice, precise diagnosis of the anatomical origin of LBP is not feasible and, indeed, in the absence of tools to influence nociception associated with altered spinal movement, may not matter. However, the clinician can make a reasonable inference as to the neuroanatomical segmental origin of pain and to the mechanism of pain production by assessment of spinal movement and mechanical allodynia over the spine (see below under Clinical approach to acute LBP).

Disease of the lumbar spine

Based on data from two prospective studies of patients with acute LBP from primary care for radiological study, the most common finding was normal in approximately 40 percent, with minor degenerative changes found in about 50 percent. Fracture (vertebral compression) ranged from 3 to 5 percent, whilst the prevalence of infection, tumor, and inflammatory disorders together was about 1 percent;[33, 34] 2199 patients). That is, approximately 95 percent of acute LBP is "nonspecific," in the sense that a specific etiological or pathological process will not be found.

Conversely, the correlation between pain and "degenerative" spinal conditions is low (relative risk <2.5;[35, 36] The prevalence in asymptomatic lumbar spines of anatomical abnormality, as shown by computed tomography (CT) or MRI, is about 30 percent.[37] It has been postulated that the degenerative changes in the intervertebral disks

which occur progressively with age result in forward tilting of the vertebrae and abnormal stresses on the apophyseal joints[23, 38] with subsequent osteoarthrosis and potential activation of nociception. An earlier study found that pain was associated with disk degeneration in just over 50 percent of cases, with no pain being reported in approximately 40 percent of individuals with similar degenerative changes.[13] Despite increasing disk degeneration with age, LBP and disability peaks around the age of 40 or during the middle working years of life.[1] Furthermore, there is wide variation between LBP and disability following physical impairment in individual patients.[1]

Psychosocial factors

There is increasing evidence that psychosocial factors are of more importance than medical factors and physical job factors in predicting the disability and chronicity associated with back pain.[39] A systematic review of psychological risk factors in back and neck pain has shown a link between psychosocial variables and the transition from acute to chronic pain disability, the presence of cognitive factors as risk factors for pain and disability, and the relationship between depression, anxiety, distress, and related emotions.[40]

The New Zealand *Guide to assessing psychosocial yellow flags in acute low back pain*[4] includes a systematic assessment of psychosocial risk factors, incorporating a screening questionnaire as well as suggested strategies for better management by primary care treatment providers for those with acute LBP who are at risk. These so-called "yellow flags," which may identify the risk of long-term disability, distress, and work have been classified into: attitudes and beliefs about back pain; behaviors; compensation issues; diagnosis and treatment issues; emotions; family; and work (**Box 25.1**). By reassessing patients for "yellow flag" factors where resolution of an acute episode of work-related LBP is slow, it may be possible to avoid the development of excess pain behavior, a sick role, inactivity syndromes, reinjuring, recurrences, complications, psychosocial sequelae, long-term disability, and work loss. However, stratification of

---

Box 25.1 Some psychosocial predictors of poor outcome

- Belief that back pain is harmful or severely disabling.
- Fear-avoidance behavior and reduced activity levels.
- Tendency to low mood and social withdrawal.
- Expectation that passive treatments rather than active participation will help.

back-injured workers, according to disability risk and treatment with practice guidelines, has not yet shown a significant impact on return to work, self-assessed pain, or satisfaction with health care,[41] although trials[40, 42, 43] do point to the relevance of the identification and management of psychosocial factors to reduce the long-term disability and hardship associated with acute back pain when that does not resolve with usual activity and confident reassurance by the health provider.

On the other hand, the "nonorganic" signs and symptoms originally described as screening tools to determine a poor outcome in patients with chronic pain have shown poor predictive value for determining which patients with acute work-related LBP would return to full work duty within four weeks with physical therapy.[44]

Prognosis

The natural history of LBP is dependent on the cohort being studied, with early (American) studies showing that approximately 40 percent of patients are well within one week, 60–85 percent within two weeks, and 90 percent within two months.[45] More recent (British) studies have suggested 90 percent resolution in two weeks[46] in a cohort of patients with pain of less than 72 hours duration. Another (British) study in primary care[47] found that although 90 percent of patients with LBP will have stopped consulting with symptoms within three months, only one-quarter will have completely recovered in terms of pain and disability in one year, although follow-up was incomplete. From the usual-care arm of a (Australian) study of patients in primary care with a median duration of acute LBP of 2.1 weeks, 49 percent had recovered completely at three months, 64 percent at six months, and 56 percent at 12 months.[48] A review of studies in primary care[49] concluded that although back pain usually improves considerably within a week of a primary care visit, it is common for less severe back pain to continue for one to three months, with long-term follow-up typically revealing a recurrent course and that chronic back pain is far from rare. Of relevance to this discussion is the observation that up to 70 percent of patients with acute LBP in the community do not consult their general practitioner.[17] If such patients were to be recruited into a study, the high spontaneous resolution rate would require a large cohort in order to show a statistically significant benefit from a therapeutic intervention.

Because of the difficulty in interpretation, the Cochrane Collaboration Back Review Group for spinal resources has developed method guidelines.[8] These guidelines include patient selection criteria, eligibility being specified to allow a match between the patient in the trial and the patient with back pain in the clinic. Such rigor in the methodology of the RCT increases the strength of the conclusions drawn from it, but it has the potential to be less applicable to the average patient

if the criteria are too exclusive. Proposed instruments for assessing outcome include measures of patient symptoms, function, general well-being, work disability, and satisfaction with care.[50, 51]

Reliable means of preventing the occurrence of back pain, particularly in industry, would be of particular social and economic benefit; however, studies have shown that interventions such as education[52] and lumbar corset did not lead to a reduction in LBP incidents or sick-leave,[53, 54] nor did a back school program lead to a reduction in recurrent episodes.[55] A review of preventive interventions for back and neck pain problems has confirmed these results, and has also shown that ergonomics and risk factor modification are either unhelpful or unproven. The only effective prevention appears to be exercises, although the methodology of the studies is weak and the effect is not strong.[24, 56, 57]

The influence of psychosocial factors on presentation, course, and prognosis has already been mentioned. Baseline job satisfaction significantly predicted variations in outcome scores at six months beyond the variations explained by control factors.[58] The outcome was poorer in those who always felt unwell and in those who were less well educated.[59] Older age and gender have also been found to be related to chronicity,[60] with a poor outcome being twice as common in women as in men. This study also found that premorbid factors associated with adverse outcome included psychological distress (as measured by the General Health Questionnaire), poor self-rated health, low levels of physical activity, smoking, and dissatisfaction with employment. Clinical factors associated with the episode of LBP, such as duration of symptoms, pain radiating to the leg, widespread pain, and restriction of spinal mobility, were also related to adverse outcome. Around 30 percent of episodes resulted in persistent disabling symptoms. In another study, higher levels of smoking were correlated with higher levels of back pain disability, lower physical functioning, and more severe low back pain.[61]

Those who are off work for a prolonged period have a reduced chance of ever returning to work, with up to 50 percent of patients with back pain out of work for six months never returning to work.[1] The return-to-work statistics are also dependent on the local employment rate[62] and workers' compensation infrastructure.[63] Despite this, advice to keep active and to remain at work if possible has been shown to improve the long-term outcome of back pain, including employment, although recurrences of pain (but not necessarily disability) commonly occur, regardless of initial treatment and maintenance regimens.

A summary of intervention studies found that employers who promptly offer appropriately modified duties can reduce time lost per episode of back pain by at least 30 percent, with newer studies of guideline-based approaches suggesting that a combination of all these approaches in a coordinated workplace-based care system can achieve a reduction of 50 percent in time lost due to back pain at no extra cost and, in some settings, with significant savings.[64]

CLINICAL APPROACH TO ACUTE LBP

The experience of pain reflects a complex interaction of somatic and psychosocial contributions. Those factors which convert a person with LBP into a patient with LBP are not well understood. Pain is "diagnosed" clinically, predominantly by history, with a contribution from physical examination. There is no test that measures the presence or extent of pain. Acute LBP may be present without structural disease and structural disease may be present without pain. With the exception of serious ("red flag") conditions, to which the main clinical alert is the history, identification of a specific cause of acute LBP is not necessary for effective management. Hence it may be more useful to determine, in broad terms, the mechanism of production of pain rather than trying to determine its anatomical origin.

Is the problem mechanical or not?

By introducing a mechanical/nonmechanical dichotomy in substitution for the "nonspecific"/"specific" dichotomy, it is intended to suggest firstly that abnormal spinal movement itself in the absence of an active disease process might be responsible for the pain and secondly that "nonmechanical" encompasses those medical diseases identified as "red flag" conditions, namely infection, inflammation, neoplastic disease, metabolic bone disease, and neural involvement. The presence of these latter "nonmechanical" conditions takes the patient out of the "nonspecific" algorithm into a process more resembling the biomedical model of disease assessment. In these conditions there will be other clues that the person is unwell and does not have a regional neuromusculoskeletal problem (**Table 25.1**).

The essential feature of LBP of presumed mechanical pathogenesis is painful limited spinal movements in the absence of systemic disease. This comprises the majority of presentations, including pain in anatomically normal spines and in spondylotic spines. Spondylosis – the combination of loss of intervertebral disk integrity and zygapophyseal osteoarthrosis[65] – is not an intrinsically symptomatic condition. Although the neurophysiological transduction of mechanical nociception is still being elucidated, the phenomena of altered intervertebral movement and mechanical allodynia may be useful "signs" leading to an inference of mechanical pain.

Physical examination consists of observation of spinal movement, gait and posture, palpation for allodynia, passive movement of lower limb joints, and screening of lower limb neurological function. Elicitation of allodynia by firm (nonnoxious) digital palpation over spinous processes and paraspinal structures may reproduce not only the pain of which the patient complaints, but also remote pelvic girdle or lower limb pain from which the anatomical level of origin may be inferred. The problems attending this fundamental clinical approach include absence of consensus on technique, variable interobserver reliability in elicitation of signs, poor construct validity regarding diagnosis, and poor predictive validity regarding treatment.[54] Nonetheless, if the purposes of examination are to facilitate reasonable inference of mechanism and to identify serious conditions, such an approach can be justified (**Table 25.2**).

Is any associated pelvic girdle or lower limb pain radicular or somatic referred?

This clinical distinction is important and has implications for investigation and for management, as the diagnosis of radicular pain takes the patient out of the mechanical or "nonspecific" LBP category and may require invasive treatment, in marked contrast to a diagnosis of somatic referred pain. Radicular pain is well-localized anatomically in a dermatomal distribution, is of dysesthetic

Table 25.1   "Red flags" suggesting potentially serious pathology underlying spinal pain.

From history	On examination
Significant trauma	Signs of lumbar radiculopathy
Weight loss	Features of cauda equina compression
History of cancer	Findings of visceral pathology
Fever	
Intravenous drug use, or exposure to human immunodeficiency virus (HIV)	
Steroid use	
Patients aged over 50 or under 20 years	
Severe unremitting pain	
Pain that is worse when the patient is lying down	

Table 25.2 Diagnostic framework for low back pain.

	Mechanical	Nonmechanical
Pain	Less localized Worse later in day Usually worst when sitting, least when lying, worse with movement	Usually localized No diurnal variation[a] Uninfluenced by posture or movement
Other features	Essentially well person	Weight loss Fever Peripheral arthritis Symptoms in other systems
Spinal movement	Painful limited movement usually of several segments	Normal, or reduced mobility of one or two segments
Allodynia/ hyperalgesia	Diffuse	Localized
Neurological signs in lower limbs	May be present	May be present
"Disease-based" entities	Anatomically normal spine Symptomatic disc failure: spondylosis, prolapse, spondylolisthesis, canal stenosis With limb pain: radicular, somatic referred	Infection: discitis, epidural abscess, meningitis Inflammatory: spondyloarthropathies (ankylosing spondylitis, psoriatic and reactive arthritis) Neoplastic: secondary carcinoma (breast, prostate, lung, melanoma) Metabolic: Paget's disease, osteoporotic vertebral fracture

[a]Except inflammatory disease: worse in mornings, eased by movement.

quality ("shooting," "burning," or "electrical") and is necessarily accompanied by features of disturbed axonal function such as myotomal weakness, dermatomal hypoesthesia, and reduction in deep tendon reflexes.[66] A particular example of such radiculopathy is so-called "cauda equina syndrome" when encroachment on the second, third, or fourth sacral nerve roots may produce perineal hypoesthesia and loss of sphincter function, in addition to pain. By contrast, somatic referred pain is poorly localized anatomically, is of dull or aching quality, and is unaccompanied by signs of axonal dysfunction (although there may be allodynia of deep tissues[67, 68]). Pain radiating to below the knee may be referred.[69, 70, 71, 72] Patterns of referral vary between individuals although commonly the spinal segmental origin can be ascertained.[67, 72] Low back pain, somatic referred pain, and radicular pain may occur together but their origins and mechanisms differ.

What other contributions to distress are there?

The experience of pain may be conceptualized as the outcome of interaction between somatic contributions as signaled by nociceptive pathways and affective, behavioral, and cognitive factors which reflect the individual's reaction to this unpleasant altered signaling, its perceived meaning, and the influence of society. A powerful example of the last of these is the apparent distinction made between instances of LBP which occur in the context of employment and those which do not.[5]

Frequently, distress appears to be in excess of any discernable somatic contribution. Of the many factors that potentially amplify the experience of pain, a common theme is beliefs concerning pathology and prognosis, especially those which might lead to fear-avoidance behavior, predicated on the assumption that pain incurred on movement heralds a disaster.[73] Affective consequences of a painful event, such as anxiety, depression, and anger, can also amplify pain.

These factors can be addressed through the use of simple open questions such as:

- "How is this pain interfering with your life?"
- "Has there been any change in your mood?"
- "What do you understand – or have been told – is (or might be) causing this pain?"

The responses to these or similar questions may help the clinician to allay unrealistic fears and expectations, to identify a mood disorder, and to tailor a treatment program to the individual patient.

Investigations

The AHCPR guidelines[6] suggest that a full blood count and erythrocyte sedimentation rate (ESR) should be performed only if there are features of red flag conditions. Other tests, such as calcium, alkaline phosphatase, prostate specific antigen, and serum protein electrophoresis, can be ordered depending on the circumstances such as a previous history of malignancy. Likewise, plain radiographs are useful only if the history and the examination suggest a red flag condition. Where there is a history of previous cancer or a suspicion of infection or of metabolic bone disease, nuclear medicine imaging is a useful screening test to guide additional imaging and biopsy.

In the absence of factors suggesting a red flag condition, laboratory tests and imaging can be deferred for four weeks because of the favorable natural history during this time and the need to avoid unnecessary radiation and expense. In addition, radiological interobserver error in some conditions, such as degenerative spondylolisthesis, facet joint arthrosis, and sacroiliac joint arthrosis, needs to be considered.[74]

The decision to image back pain patients should be informed by knowledge of the natural history, management options, and sensitivity and specificity of the imaging modality. Such an investigation should assist in the diagnosis of the patient and must also influence management.[75] For example, as 30 percent of people without low back symptoms will have significant abnormalities on MRI or CT,[37] these investigations should be reserved for people in whom cancer or infection is suspected, where there is persistent neurological deficit or symptomatic lumbar canal stenosis (although the last of these does not present with acute back pain), or where there is diagnostic uncertainty.

Diagnostic labeling

The current status of diagnostic labeling is based on anatomical concepts, according to the IASP taxonomy.[76] It has been suggested that, where there is no identifiable pathology, the terms "lumbar spinal pain of unknown origin" or "somatic lumbar spinal pain" be used.[54, 76] However, this elevates the symptom – pain – to the status of a diagnosis. Pain is, by definition, a highly complex phenomenon but clinical method invites identification of contributions – somatic and psychosocial if not also societal. Furthermore, in mechanical (or "nonspecific") spinal pain, the lack of concordance between anatomically defined disease and clinical presentation challenges that convention. An alternative proposition for the somatic component of "nonspecific" spinal pain is for it to be attributed to "(acute) mechanical lumbar spine impairment" with, if appropriate, "somatic referred pain in the lower limb." This labeling hypothesizes that abnormal function of the lumbar spine is relevant to nociception generated therein and the pain with which the patient presents. The addendum identifies the important distinction between somatic referred and radicular pain, the latter, being a "red flag" condition, taking the associated back pain out of the "nonspecific" category, even though the mechanisms are distinct. (It could be argued further that another

axis of diagnostic labeling could be added, to recognize the psychosocial or "nonsomatic" contributions to the presentation.)

Attempts have been made to classify nonspecific back pain to provide more homogeneous groups for further study, including natural history and response to treatment. The Quebec Task Force[7] developed a classification based on symptoms, their duration, and the working status of the patient at the time of the evaluation. Symptoms included pain without radiation, pain plus radiation to the proximal extremity, and pain plus radiation to the distal extremity, with the duration being less than seven days, between seven days and seven weeks, and longer than seven weeks. This concept was extended by Krause and Ragland,[77] who developed an eight-phase model of occupational disability. The initial four acute phases comprise: phase 1, nondisabling LBP episodes that are not reported; phase 2, a work-related injury or illness that is formally reported and that ends when the person takes time off work; phase 3, short-term disability of less than one week's duration; and phase 4, which is defined by work disability of one to seven weeks. It was claimed that this model overcomes the disadvantages of biomedical models of LBP and takes into account the social and dynamic nature of disability.

EVIDENCE-BASED EVALUATION OF MANAGEMENT

Studies have tended to look at populations with mixed duration of pain (acute and chronic) and with and without radiating pain to the lower limbs (not distinguishing between somatic referred and radicular pain) (**Table 25.3**).

Active physical therapy

ACTIVATION

Clinical evidence[78] found two systematic reviews:[79][I] search date 1996, six RCTs, 1957 people;[80][I]: search date 2003, 11 RCTs, 1963 people (excluding those with neurological signs) and one later RCT.[81][II], [82][II] The consensus from here and from the Australian Acute Musculoskeletal Pain Guidelines Group (AAMPGG)[54] is that advice to stay active is associated with a small beneficial effect on pain, rate of recovery, and function, compared with bed rest or with specific exercise regimens. This advice is also associated with reduced sick leave and persistent disability compared with no advice or with advice to rest and take analgesics. There is no evidence that performing normal activities of daily living within the limits of pain is harmful.

Table 25.3 Evidence for interventions in acute low back pain.

Intervention	Conclusion	Level of evidence
Activity		
Advice to stay active	Beneficial	[I], [II]
Bed rest	Conflicting evidence: Likely to be ineffective	[I], [II]
Back exercises	Insufficient evidence: Unlikely to be beneficial	[I], [II]
Back school	Insufficient evidence	[I], [II]
Physical		
Spinal manipulation	Conflicting evidence Likely short-term benefit	[I]
Acupuncture	Insufficient evidence	[I]
Massage	Insufficient evidence	No [I] or [II]
Lumbar supports	Insufficient evidence	No [I] or [II]
Traction	Insufficient evidence	No [I] or [II]
Transcutaneous electrical nerve stimulation	Insufficient evidence	No [I] or [II]
Pharmacotherapy		
Analgesics (simple)	Insufficient evidence	No [I] or [II]
Analgesics (compound and opioid)	Insufficient evidence	No [I] or [II]
Nonsteroidal anti-inflammatory drugs	Conflicting evidence Likely short-term benefit	[I]
Muscle relaxants	Conflicting Trade-off between benefit and harm	[I]
Injection		
Injection (facet joint, epidural, or soft tissue)	Insufficient evidence	No [I] or [II]
Cognitive behavioural		
Printed information	Beneficial	[II]
CBT	Insufficient evidence	No [I] or [II]
Multidisciplinary treatment in the workplace	Insufficient evidence	No [I] or [II]

Adapted from references 54 and 78.

BED REST

Clinical evidence[78] found a systematic review of 11 RCTs (search date 2003, 1963 people, distinction made between those with neurological deficit and thus with a "specific" diagnosis).[80][I] This review found that advice to rest in bed was associated with increased pain and poorer functional outcomes after three to four weeks and twelve weeks compared with advice to stay active. There was limited evidence of no significant difference in outcomes between advice to rest or to exercise, or in outcomes after three to seven days of bed rest. Adverse effects of bed rest include joint stiffness, muscle wasting, loss of bone mineral density, pressure sores, and venous thrombo-embolism.[79][I] Clinical evidence concludes that bed rest is likely to be ineffective or harmful.

The AAMPGG[54] concluded that, in mixed populations with low back pain, there was insufficient evidence that

bed rest was more effective than any other intervention (including no intervention) and there was conflicting evidence that bed rest was associated with increased disability and slower rate of recovery compared with staying active.[54]

BACK EXERCISES

Exercises prescribed for people with low back pain are diverse and may include stretching, flexion, extension, endurance, strengthening, alone or in combination. Exercise programs differ in their philosophy, content, and delivery. Taken together with the diversity in populations studied, outcome measures, and duration, it is difficult to draw conclusions on their effectiveness.

A systematic review (search date 2004, 11 RCTs) found no significant differences in pain or function between exercise and no treatment or between exercise and other conservative treatment.[55][I] However, in subacute LBP (6–12 weeks) occurring in an occupational setting, a graded exercise program may reduce time off work compared with usual care. Clinical evidence concludes that back exercises are unlikely to be beneficial.[78] The AAMPGG found conflicting evidence for the effectiveness of back exercises in reducing pain and disability compared with other active and passive modalities in mixed populations with low back pain. There is no evidence that back exercises cause harm.[54]

BACK SCHOOLS

Although a back school may be defined as a program of education and skills acquisition including exercises, supervised by a health professional, the format and content of such programs varies extensively. A systematic review,[55][I] search date 2003, four RCTs,[83] found the diversity prohibited analysis. There is insufficient evidence that back school is more effective than active, passive, or placebo therapies in people with acute low back pain.

Passive physical modalities

SPINAL MANIPULATION

Evaluation of the effectiveness of spinal manipulation is made difficult by the different techniques employed and methodological limitations of published studies. A systematic review,[84][I] search date 2000, 29 RCTs, found that spinal manipulative therapy reduced pain in the short term (less than six weeks) by 10 mm on a 100 mm pain visual analog scale (VAS) (95 percent CI 2–17 mm), but had no significant effect on functional outcomes or on longer term pain reduction. A later RCT[85][II], which compared manipulation, muscle relaxants, and placebo, found significantly reduced pain from chiropractic adjustment compared with sham at two and four weeks. The review found no differences in terms of pain or functional outcome between spinal manipulation, usual care, physical therapy, exercises, or back school. An earlier review concerning harm[86][I] found a low risk of potentially serious complications in skilled hands (cauda equina syndrome <1:1,000,000). Clinical evidence[78] concludes that spinal manipulation in the short term is likely to be beneficial; AAMPGG[54] considers that this evidence is conflicting, whilst there is insufficient evidence on which to compare spinal manipulation with other conservative treatments.

ACUPUNCTURE

A systematic review,[87][I] search date 2003, three RCTs, found insufficient evidence from which to draw conclusions, rendering the effectiveness of this treatment for acute LBP unknown. An earlier review found adverse effects to be rare although potentially serious, including infections, pneumothorax, and visceral trauma.[88][I]

MASSAGE

There are no controlled studies of the effectiveness of massage therapy in acute LBP. A systematic review,[89][I] search date 2001, nine RCTs, found moderate evidence that massage reduces pain intensity in the subacute period (4–12 weeks) comparable with the effects of exercise and manipulation.

LUMBAR SUPPORTS

Similarly, there are no controlled studies on the effect of lumbar supports in acute LBP. From studies of mixed populations with acute LBP, there is insufficient evidence for the effectiveness of lumbar supports compared with spinal manipulation, exercises, massage, transcutaneous electrical nerve stimulation (TENS), or simple analgesia.[53][I], [54]

TRACTION

Older reviews[8][I], [90][I] found no controlled studies on the effect of traction and conclude that there is insufficient evidence for its effectiveness compared with placebo and other treatments in mixed populations with acute LBP.

TENS

In mixed populations of acute LBP, there are no controlled studies on the effect of TENS in acute LBP and insufficient evidence for its effectiveness compared with other modalities.[91][I]

Pharmacotherapy

ANALGESICS: SIMPLE, COMPOUND, AND OPIOID

Paracetamol (acetaminophen) is readily available without prescription as an all-purpose analgesic agent. Clinical evidence[78] reports two systematic reviews[8][I], [92][I] that identified no RCTs of paracetamol compared with placebo. No significant differences have been found in clinical outcome comparing paracetamol, opioids, and nonsteroidal anti-inflammatory drugs (NSAIDs). At therapeutic doses (<4 g per day), adverse effects of paracetamol are rare, even in fasting patients and alcoholics.[93] Overdose of paracetamol may be associated with liver damage and secondary renal failure.[94] The most important clinical interaction involves paracetamol and warfarin; in patients who need anticoagulant and analgesic therapy, paracetamol is preferred to aspirin and nonselective and selective NSAIDs.[95]

There are no RCTs investigating the efficacy of opioid analgesics alone or with acetaminophen in acute LBP. In general, opioids have an increased risk of adverse effects compared with paracetamol alone.[96][I]

NSAIDS

Clinical evidence[78] cites one systematic review,[92][I] search date 1998, 45 RCTs, that pooled only for NSAIDs versus placebo. This review found significantly increased global improvement after one week in a mixed population. There was no difference among NSAIDs in outcomes. The same review found no difference between NSAIDs or muscle relaxants or opioids in terms of pain relief or overall improvement. Clinical evidence[78] concludes that NSAIDs are beneficial, whilst the AAMPGG[54] considers the evidence to be conflicting.

Adverse effects of NSAIDs include gastrointestinal bleeding and perforation, impaired renal function, interference with antihypertensive control, and worsening of cardiac failure.[6, 97][I], [98][III]

MUSCLE RELAXANTS

Muscle relaxants comprise a diverse group of agents acting on skeletal muscle directly or on the neuromuscular junction. The rationale is that muscle spasm contributes to acute LBP. A systematic review[99][I] found one poor quality RCT of (oral and parenteral) diazepam versus placebo. Meta-analysis of RCTs of oral non-benzodiazepine drugs (baclofen, cyclobenzaprine, orphenadrine, tizanidine) found reduced pain and global improvement at two to four days. No difference between muscle relaxants and placebo was found at four weeks.[85][II] Adverse effects of muscle relaxants are common, including dizziness, drowsiness, and nausea.[82]

Clinical evidence[78] considers that there is a trade-off between benefits and harms of muscle relaxants; the AAMPGG[54] considers the evidence to be conflicting.

Injections

SOFT TISSUE OR FACET JOINT

Injection therapy is predicated on the assumption that the anatomical origin of LBP can be readily identified and locally treated. Targets include "trigger points," ligaments, and apophyseal joints, but evidence for effectiveness in acute LBP is lacking.[6, 100][I]

EPIDURAL INJECTIONS

The literature on epidural steroids is complicated by mixed duration of pain and by mixed populations of patients with nonspecific LBP and radicular pain. Clinical evidence[78] found one review,[101][I] search date 1998, which found no RCTs on the use of epidural injections in people with acute LBP without leg pain.

Adverse effects of injection therapy are infrequent but include infection and hemorrhage (especially in the epidural space), intradural penetration, and headache.[6, 100][I], [101][I]

Cognitive modalities

PRINTED INFORMATION

Documents may provide evidence-based information on the nature and natural history of acute LBP, plus advice to stay active. The AAMPGG[54] cites level [II] evidence that "activity-focused" printed information reinforcing similar verbal advice was more effective than traditional brochures or no printed information. However, information received through the mail is less likely to have an effect than information provided in person.[41][II], [42][II], [102][II], [103][III], [104]

COGNITIVE-BEHAVIORAL THERAPY

Studies have not distinguished between acute and chronic populations, between specific and nonspecific conditions, and between varieties of behavioral therapies. A systematic review,[8][I] search date 1995, one RCT, found limited evidence that cognitive-behavioral therapy (CBT) reduced pain and disability at 9–12 months compared with traditional care. The AAMPGG[54] concludes that CBT reduces general disability in the long term compared with traditional care in mixed populations with back pain. However, there are no studies on CBT as a single intervention.

MULTIDISCIPLINARY PROGRAMS

A systematic review of inpatient and outpatient programs that included physician consultation and psychological, social work, or vocational input (excluding back schools) revealed two RCTs in subacute LBP,[105][I] search date 2002. Multidisciplinary treatment significantly reduced sick leave compared with usual care.

A PRAGMATIC APPROACH TO MANAGEMENT OF ACUTE LOW BACK PAIN

Guidelines and evidence-based medicine

Clinical guidelines are described as "systematically developed statements that assist practitioner and patient decisions about appropriate health care for specific clinical circumstances."[106] The Institute of Medicine stated that guidelines should be valid, reliable, clinically applicable, flexible, clear, developed with a multi-disciplinary process, scheduled for periodic review, and well documented. The first systematic large-scale review was that of the Quebec Task Force on Spinal Disorders,[7] which identified the size of the problem and the significant cost to the patient and to society which a delay in returning to work imposed. In addition to these factors, increasing evidence of inappropriate treatments and a growing body of clinical trial data resulted in the development of the Agency for Health Care Policy and Research guidelines.[6] The developers of these guidelines are reported as reviewing the abstracts of 10,317 studies and selecting 3918 articles for further evaluation. These comprehensive guidelines include the initial evaluation of patients who had acute low back problems, management of symptoms, including use of medications, spinal manipulations, and activity modifications, use of imaging studies, evaluations for surgery, surgery for herniated disks, and surgery for spinal stenosis. The scientific basis for the recommendations in the guidelines is made explicit and the strengths and weaknesses of the evidence are highlighted. In addition, the guidelines incorporated a preference-based approach,[9] which fulfilled the criteria for the outcome-based methodology but also explicitly assessed patient preferences for the relevant health outcomes.

The Clinical Standards Advisory Group (CSAG)[10] in the UK produced their own guidelines based on the US literature review, with a recommendation for a comprehensive biopsychosocial assessment at six weeks. More attention was placed on the dissemination of feedback from these guidelines to develop ownership, and in 1997 the Accident Rehabilitation and Compensation Insurance Corporation (ACC) and National Health Committee published the *New Zealand acute low back pain guide*[11] and the *Guide to assessing psychosocial yellow flags*,[4] with yellow flag conditions being those psychosocial risk factors for the development of chronicity and ongoing disability if not identified and addressed. Further clinical guidelines associated with a review of the evidence were produced in the UK in 1996.[12]

Clinical guidelines have been shown to demonstrate improvements in clinical practice and patient outcome in a variety of conditions, provided that attention is paid to appropriate implementation methodology.[107] Although there are barriers to the implementation of guidelines, because of patients' past experiences and preferences influencing general practitioners' practice,[108] benefit from their use has now been shown to occur in the area of back pain. A reduction in the rate of imaging and referrals for specialty advice was achieved by primary care physician education, without a fall in patient satisfaction. For those patients whose pain became chronic or complex, the implementation of a spine clinic resulted in visits to spine surgeons and the spine surgery rates falling by 50 and 35 percent, respectively.[109]

The results of this case study were replicated in a controlled study of 110 workers compensated for LBP for four to eight weeks, which showed an improvement in coordinated primary health care in a large community compared with a control group, with a trend toward an earlier return to work and statistically significant improvement in pain and function at six months, with three times less use of imagery at three months, and twice as much use of exercise at six months.[110]

These results were replicated in an interstate comparison in Australia, where a state-wide education program based on acute back pain evidence-based guidelines, including a mass media campaign, resulted in similar outcomes to a neighboring state at a reduced cost. This population-based primary prevention intervention improved beliefs about back pain in the general population and knowledge and attitudes among general practitioners, with a decrease in the number and rate of workers' compensation claims for back pain and a reduction in medical payments.[111]

Management of acute mechanical low back pain

Taking into account this state of the art regarding acute LBP, a rational approach to management can be proposed. In symptomatic mechanical lumbar spine impairment, the therapeutic targets are the pain itself ("distress") and the limitation of function ("disability"). Both medical and cognitive-behavioral approaches are involved. For nonmechanical ("specific") conditions associated with acute LBP, therapy directed towards the underlying disease process is added to this regimen.

The key elements of management are assurance, activation, and analgesia, and include:

- explain natural history, prognosis and principles of management;
- recommend minimal bed rest;
- prescribe adequate analgesia;
- correct ergonomics of spinal movement;
- pay attention to psychosocial factors;
- investigate where there are features of "red flag" conditions;
- reiterate regularly.

This has been presented as an algorithm in the *New Zealand acute low back pain guide* (**Figure 25.1**) These emphasize full reassessment at four weeks and at six weeks. If reasons for nonrecovery have not been identified, specialist referral is indicated. The use of a multidisciplinary team for an integrated management plan may be appropriate at this stage.

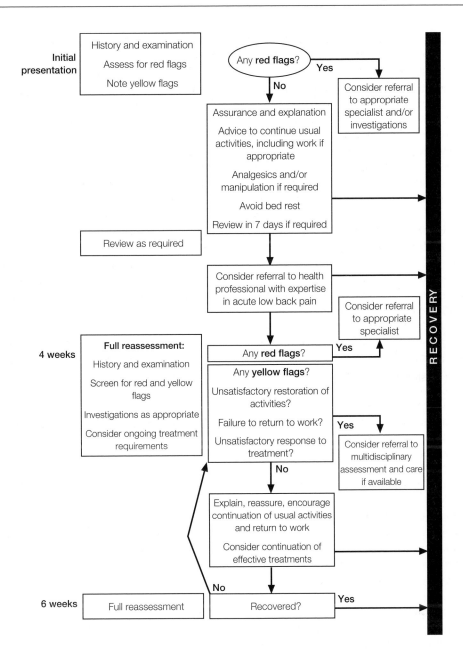

Figure 25.1 Management of acute low back pain – New Zealand guidelines. Reproduced with permission from ACC and the National Health Committee. *New Zealand acute low back pain guide*. Wellington: National Health Committee/ACC, 2004.

ACKNOWLEDGMENTS

This chapter is adapted and expanded from Gow P. Acute low back pain. In: Rowbotham DJ and Macintyre PE (eds). *Clinical pain management: acute pain*, 1st edn. London: Hodder Arnold, 405–22.

REFERENCES

∗ 1. Waddell G. A new clinical model for the treatment of low-back pain. *Spine*. 1987; **12**: 632–44.

2. Andersson GBJ. The epidemiology of spinal disorders. In: Frymoyer JW (ed.). *The adult spine: principles and practice*, 2nd edn. New York: Raven Press, 1997: 93–141.

3. Cohen ML. Cervical and lumbar pain. *Medical Journal of Australia*. 1996; **165**: 504–8.

∗ 4. Kendall NA, Linton SJ, Main CJ. *Guide to assessing psychosocial yellow flags in acute low back pain: Risk factors for long-term disability and work loss*. Wellington: National Health Committee/ACC, 1997.

5. Loeser JD. What is chronic pain? *Theoretical Medicine*. 1991; **12**: 213–35.

∗ 6. Bigos S, Bowyer O, Braen G. *et al*. Acute low back problems in adults. *Clinical Practice Guideline 14*. AHCPR

Publication No. 95-0642. Rockville, MD: Agency for Health Care Policy and Research, Public Health Service, US Department of Health and Human Services, 1994.

* 7. Spitzer WO. Scientific approach to the assessment and management of activity-related spinal disorders: a monograph for clinicians. Report of the Quebec Task Force on Spinal Disorders. *Spine*. 1987; **12**: S1-59.

* 8. van Tulder MW, Koes BW, Bouter LM. Conservative treatment of acute and chronic nonspecific low back pain: a systematic review of randomised controlled trials of the most common interventions. *Spine*. 1997; **22**: 2128-56.

   9. Owens DK. Spine update: patient preferences and the development of practice guidelines. *Spine*. 1998; **23**: 1073-9.

* 10. Rosen M, Breen A, Hamann W *et al. Report of a clinical standards advisory group committee on back pain.* London: HMSO, 1994.

  11. ACC and the National Health Committee. *New Zealand acute low back pain guide.* Wellington: National Health Committee/ACC, 2004.

* 12. Waddell G, McIntosh A, Lewis M *et al. Low back pain evidence review.* London: Royal College of General Practitioners, 1996.

* 13. Wood PH, Badley EM. Epidemiology of back pain. In: Jayson MI (ed.). *The lumbar spine and back pain*, 2nd edn. Tunbridge Wells: Pitman Medical, 1980: 29-55.

  14. Frymoyer JW, Cats-Baril WL. An overview of the incidence and costs of low back pain. *Orthopedic Clinics of North America*. 1991; **22**: 263-71.

  15. Waddell G. *The back pain revolution.* Edinburgh: Churchill Livingstone, 1998.

  16. Mann JI, Nye ER, Wilson B *et al.* Low back pain. In: *Life in New Zealand Commission Report.* Vol. V. *Health.* Dunedin: University of Otago, 1991: 33-8.

  17. Waxman R, Tennant A, Helliwell P. Community survey of factors associated with consultation for low back pain. *British Medical Journal*. 1998; **317**: 1564-7.

  18. Leboeuf-Yde C, Kyvik KO. At what age does low back pain become a common problem? A study of 29,424 individuals aged 12-41 years. *Spine*. 1998; **23**: 228-34.

* 19. Bressler HB, Keyes WJ, Rochon PA *et al.* The prevalence of low back pain in the elderly: a systematic review of the literature. *Spine*. 1999; **24**: 1813-19.

  20. Bigos SJ, Battie MC, Spengler DM *et al.* A prospective study of work perceptions and psychosocial factors affecting the report of back injury. *Spine*. 1991; **16**: 1-6.

  21. Atlas SJ, Chang Y, Kammann E *et al.* Long term disability and return to work among patients who have a herniated lumbar disc: the effect of disability compensation. *Journal of Bone and Joint Surgery*. 2000; **82A**: 4-15.

  22. Von Korff M, Deyo RA, Cherkin D *et al.* Back pain in primary care. *Spine*. 1993; **18**: 8545-62.

  23. Frymoyer JW. Back pain and sciatica. *New England Journal of Medicine*. 1988; **318**: 291-300.

* 24. Hoogendoorn WE, van Poppel MN, Bongers P *et al.* Systematic review of psychosocial factors at work and private life as risk factors for back pain. *Spine*. 2000; **25**: 2114-25.

* 25. Boos N, Semmer N, Elfering A *et al.* Natural history of individuals with asymptomatic disc abnormalities in magnetic resonance imaging: predictors of low back pain-related medical consultation and work incapacity. *Spine*. 2000; **25**: 1484-92.

  26. Feldman DE, Rossignol M, Shrier I *et al.* Smoking: a risk factor for development of low back pain in adolescents. *Spine*. 1999; **24**: 2492-6.

* 27. Goldberg MS, Scott SC, Mayo NE. A review of the association between cigarette smoking and the development of nonspecific back pain and related outcomes. *Spine*. 2000; **25**: 995-1014.

* 28. Scott SC, Goldberg MS, Mayo NE *et al.* The association between back pain and smoking in adults. *Spine*. 1999; **24**: 1090-8.

* 29. Leboeuf-Yde C. Body weight and low back pain: a systematic literature review of 56 journal articles reporting on 65 epidemiologic studies. *Spine*. 2000; **25**: 2114-15.

  30. Wyke B. Neurological aspects of low back pain. In: Jayson MI (ed.). *The lumbar spine and back pain*, 3rd edn. Edinburgh: Churchill Livingstone, 1987: 189-256.

  31. Bogduk N, Twomey LT. *Clinical anatomy of the lumbar spine.* Melbourne: Churchill Livingstone, 1987.

  32. Schwarzer AC, Aprill CN, Derby R *et al.* The relative contribution of the disc and zygapophyseal joint in chronic low back pain. *Spine*. 1994; **19**: 801-6.

  33. Suarez-Almazor ME, Belseck E, Russell AS, Mackel JV. Use of lumbar radiographs for the early diagnosis of low back pain: proposed guidelines would increase utilization. *Journal of the American Medical Association*. 1997; **277**: 1782-6.

  34. Hollingworth W, Todd CJ, King H *et al.* Primary care referrals for lumbar spine radiography: diagnostic yield and clinical guidelines. *British Journal of General Practice*. 2002; **52**: 475-80.

  35. Torgerson WR, Dotter WE. Comparative roentgenographic study of the asymptomatic and symptomatic lumbar spine. *Journal of Bone and Joint Surgery*. 1976; **56A**: 850-3.

  36. Van Tulder MW, Assendelft WJJ, Koes BW, Bouter LM. Spinal radiogaphic findngs and non-specific low back pain. A systematic review of observational studies. *Spine*. 1997; **22**: 427-34.

  37. Jensen MC, Brant-Zawadzki MN, Obucjowski N *et al.* Magnetic resonance imaging of the lumbar spine in people without back pain. *New England Journal of Medicine*. 1994; **331**: 69-73.

  38. Vernon Roberts B. Pathology of degenerative spondylosis. In: Jayson MI (ed.). *The lumbar spine and back pain*, 3rd edn. Edinburgh: Churchill Livingstone, 1987: 55-75.

  39. Cats-Baril WL, Frymoyer JW. Identifying patients at risk of becoming disabled because of low-back pain: the Vermont

Rehabilitation Engineering Center predictive model. *Spine*. 1991; **16**: 605–7.

∗ 40. Linton SJ. A review of psychological risk factors in back and neck pain. *Spine*. 2000; **25**: 1148–56.

41. Hazard RG, Haugh LD, Reid S *et al*. Early physician notification of patient disability risk and clinical guidelines after low back injury: a randomised clinical trial. *Spine*. 2000; **25**: 1925–31.

42. Burton AK, Waddell G, Tillotson KM *et al*. Information and advice to patients with back pain can have a positive effect: a randomized controlled trial of a novel educational booklet in primary care. *Spine*. 1999; **24**: 2484–91.

∗ 43. Linton SJ, Andersson T. Can chronic disability be prevented? A randomised trial of a cognitive-behaviour intervention and two forms of information for patients with spinal pain. *Spine*. 2000; **25**: 2825–31.

44. Fritz JM, Wainner RS, Hicks GE. The use of nonorganic signs and symptoms as a screening tool for return-to-work in patients with acute low back pain. *Spine*. 2000; **25**: 1925–31.

∗ 45. Quinet RJ, Hadler NM. Diagnosis and treatment of backache. *Seminars in Arthritis and Rheumatism*. 1979; **8**: 261–86.

46. Coste J, Delecoeuillerie G, Cohen de Lara A *et al*. Clinical course and prognostic factors in acute low back pain: an inception cohort study in primary care practice. *British Medical Journal*. 1994; **308**: 577–80.

47. Croft PR, Macfarlane GJ, Papageorgiou AC *et al*. Outcome of low back pain in general practice: a prospective study. *British Medical Journal*. 1998; **316**: 1356–9.

48. McGuirk B, King W, Govind J *et al*. The safety, efficacy, and cost-effectiveness of evidence-based guidelines for the management of acute low back pain in primary care. *Spine*. 2001; **26**: 2615–22.

∗ 49. von Korff M, Saunders K. The course of back pain in primary care. *Spine*. 1996; **21**: 2833–9.

50. Deyo RA, Battie M, Beurskens AJ *et al*. Outcome measures for low back pain research: a proposal for standardized use. *Spine*. 1998; **23**: 2003–13.

51. Bombardier C. Outcome assessments in the evaluation of treatment of spinal disorders: summary and recommendations. *Spine*. 2000; **25**: 3100–13.

∗ 52. Turner JA. Educational and behavioural interventions for back pain in primary care. *Spine*. 1996; **21**: 2851–9.

∗ 53. Jellema P, van Tulder MW, van Poppel MN. Lumbar supports for prevention and treatment of low back pain: a systematic review within the framework of the Cochrane Back Review Group. *Spine*. 2001; **26**: 377–86.

54. Australian Acute Musculoskeletal Guidelines Group. *Evidence-based management of acute musculoskeletal pain*. Brisbane: Australian Academic Press, 2003. http://www.nhmrc.gov.au

55. Hayden JA, van Tulder MW, Malmivaara A, Koes BW. Exercise therapy for treatment of non-specific low back pain. *Cochrane Database of Systematic Reviews*. 2005; CD000335.

∗ 56. Koes BW, Bouter LM, Beckerman H *et al*. Physiotherapy exercises and back pain: a blinded review. *British Medical Journal*. 1991; **302**: 1572–6.

∗ 57. Linton SJ, van Tulder MW. Preventive interventions for back and neck pain problems: what is the evidence? *Spine*. 2001; **26**: 778–87.

58. Williams RA, Pruitt SD, Doctor JN *et al*. The contribution of job satisfaction to the transition from acute to chronic low back pain. *Archives of Physical Medicine and Rehabilitation*. 1998; **79**: 366–74.

59. Deyo RA, Diehl AK. Psychosocial predictors of disability in patients with low back pain. *Journal of Rheumatology*. 1988; **15**: 1557–64.

60. Thomas E, Silman AJ, Croft PR *et al*. Predicting who develops chronic low back pain in primary care: a prospective study. *British Medical Journal*. 1999; **318**: 1662–7.

61. Oleske DM, Andersson GB, Lavender SA *et al*. Association between recovery outcomes for work-related low back disorders and personal, family, and work factors. *Spine*. 2000; **25**: 1259–6.

62. Brooker AS, Frank JW, Tarasuk VS. Back pain claim rates and the business cycle. *Social Science and Medicine*. 1997; **45**: 429–39.

63. McNaughton HK, Sims A, Taylor WJ. Prognosis for people with back pain under a no-fault 24-hour-cover compensation scheme. *Spine*. 2000; **25**: 1254–8.

64. Frank J, Sinclair S, Hogg-Johnson S *et al*. Preventing disability from work-related low-back pain. *Canadian Medical Association Journal*. 1998; **158**: 1625–31.

65. Vernon-Roberts B. Pathology of the intervertebral discs and apophyseal joints. In: Jayson MIV (ed.). *The lumbar spine and back pain*, 3rd edn. Edinburgh: Churchill Livingstone, 1997: 37–55.

66. Smyth MJ, Wright V. Sciatica and the intervertebral disc. An experimental study. *Journal of Bone and Joint Surgery*. 1959; **40A**: 1401–18.

67. Kellgren JH. On the distribution of pain arising from deep somatic structures with charts of segmental pain areas. *Clinical Science*. 1938; **4**: 35–46.

68. Feinstein B, Langton JNK, Jameson RM, Schiller F. Experiments on pain referred from deep somatic tissues. *Journal of Bone and Joint Surgery*. 1954; **36A**: 981–97.

69. Mooney V, Robertson J. The facet syndrome. *Clinical Orthopaedics and Related Research*. 1976; **115**: 149–56.

70. Fairbank JCT, Park WM, McCall IW, O'Brien JP. Apophyseal injections of local anaesthetic as a diagnostic aid in primary low back pain syndromes. *Spine*. 1981; **6**: 598–605.

71. Fukui S, Oheto K, Shiotani M *et al*. Distribution of referred pain from the lumbar zygapophyseal joints and dorsal rami. *Clinical Journal of Pain*. 1997; **13**: 303–7.

72. O'Neill CW, Kurgansky ME, Derby R, Ryan DP. Disc stimulation and patterns of referred pain. *Spine*. 2002; **27**: 2776–81.

73. Waddell G, Newton M, Henderson I *et al*. A Fear-Avoidance Beliefs Questionnaire and the role of fear-avoidance beliefs in chronic low back pain and disability. *Pain*. 1993; **52**: 157–68.

74. Espeland A, Korsbrekke K, Albrektsen G *et al*. Observer variation in plain radiography of the lumbosacral spine. *British Journal of Radiology*. 1998; **71**: 366–75.

75. Modic MT, Herzog RJ. Spinal imaging modalities: what's available and who should order them? *Spine*. 1994; **19**: 1764–5.

76. Merskey H, Bogduk N (eds). *Classification of chronic pain. Description of chronic pain syndromes and definitions of pain terms*, 2nd edn. Seattle: IASP Press, 1984.

77. Krause N, Ragland DR. Occupational disability due to low back pain: a new interdisciplinary classification based on a phase model of disability. *Spine*. 1994; **19**: 1011–20.

78. Koes BW, van Tulder MW. Low back pain (acute). *BMJ Clinical Evidence*. 2006; Web publication date April 1, 2006 (based on November 2004 search). Available from: www.clinicalevidence.bmj.com/ceweb/conditions/msd/1102/1102_contribdetails.jsp.

∗ 79. Waddell G, Feder G, Lewis M. Systematic reviews of bed rest and advice to stay active for acute low back pain. *British Journal of General Practice*. 1997; **47**: 647–52.

∗ 80. Hagen KB, Hilde G, Jamtvedt G *et al*. Bed rest for acute low back pain and sciatica. *Cochrane Database of Systematic Reviews*. 2004; **CD001254**.

81. Damush TM, Weinberger M, Perkins SM *et al*. Randomized trial of a self-management program for primary care patients with acute low back pain: short-term effects. *Arthritis and Rheumatism*. 2003; **49**: 179–86.

82. Damush TM, Weinberger M, Perkins SM *et al*. The long-term effects of a self-management program for inner-city primary care patients with acute low back pain. *Archives of Internal Medicine*. 2003; **163**: 2632–8.

83. Heymans MW, van Tulder MW, Esmail R *et al*. Back schools for non-specific low back pain. *Cochrane Database of Systematic Reviews*. 2004; **CD000261**.

84. Assendelft WJ, Morton SC, Yu EI *et al*. Spinal manipulative therapy for low back pain: a meta-analysis of effectiveness relative to other therapies. *Annals of Internal Medicine*. 2003; **138**: 871–81.

85. Hoiriis KT, Pfleger B, McDuffie FC *et al*. A randomized clinical trial comparing chiropractic adjustments to muscle relaxants for subacute low back pain. *Journal of Manipulative and Physiological Therapeutics*. 2004; **27**: 388–98.

86. Assendelft WJ, Bouter LM, Knipschild PG. Complications of spinal manipulation: a comprehensive review of the literature. *Journal of Family Practice*. 1996; **42**: 475–80.

87. Furlan AD, van Tulder MW, Cherkin DC *et al*. Acupuncture and dry-needling for low back pain. *Cochrane Database of Systematic Reviews*. 2005; **CD001351**.

88. Ernst E, White A. Life-threatening adverse reactions after acupuncture? A systematic review. *Pain*. 1997; **71**: 123–6.

89. Furlan AD, Brosseau L, Imamura M *et al*. Massage for low back pain. *Cochrane Database of Systematic Reviews*. 2002; **CD001929**.

90. Van der Heiden GJ, Beurskens AJ, Koes BW *et al*. The efficacy of traction for back and neck pain: a systematic, blinded review of randomized clinical trial methods. *Physical Therapy*. 1995; **75**: 93–104.

91. Pengel HM, Maher CG, Refshauge KM. Systematic review of conservative interventions for subacute low back pain. *Clinical Rehabilitation*. 2002; **16**: 811–20.

92. Van Tulder MW, Scholten RJ, Koes BW *et al*. Non-steroidal anti-inflammatory drugs (NSAIDs) for low back pain. *Cochrane Database of Systematic Reviews*. 2006; **CD000396**.

93. Strom BL. Adverse reactions to over-the-counter analgesics taken for therapeutic purposes. *Journal of the American Medical Association*. 1994; **272**: 1866–7.

94. Schnitzer TJ. Non-NSAID pharmacologial options for the management of chronic pain. *American Journal of Medicine*. 1998; **105** (Suppl 1B): S45–52.

95. Stockley IH (ed.). *Stockley's drug interactions*, 6th edn. London: Pharmaceutical Press, 2002.

96. De Craen AJ, Di Giulio G, Lampe-Schoenmaeckers AJEM *et al*. Analgesic efficacy and safety of paracetamol-codeine combinations versus paracetamol alone: a systematic review. *British Medical Journal*. 1996; **313**: 321–5.

∗ 97. Henry D, Lim LL-Y, Rodriguez LA *et al*. Variability in risk of gastrointestinal complications with individual non-steroidal anti-inflammatory drug: results of a collaborative meta-analysis. *British Medical Journal*. 1996; **312**: 1563–6.

98. Frishman WH. Effects of non-steroidal anti-inflammatory drug therapy on blood pressure and peripheral edema. *American Journal of Cardiology*. 2002; **89**: 18D–25D.

99. Van Tulder MW, Touray T, Furlan AD *et al*. Muscle relaxants for non-specific low back pain: a systematic review within the framework of the Cochrane collaboration. *Spine*. 2003; **28**: 1978–92.

∗100. Nelemans PJ, de Bie RA, de Vet HC *et al*. Injection therapy for subacute and chronic benign low back pain. *Spine*. 2001; **26**: 501–15.

101. Koes BW, Scholten RJPM, Mens JMA *et al*. Epidural steroid injections for low back pain and sciatica: an updated systematic review of randomized clinical trials. *Pain Digest*. 1999; **9**: 241–7.

∗102. Cherkin DC, Deyo RA, Battie M *et al*. A comparison of physical therapy, chiropractic manipulation, and provision of an educational booklet for the treatment of patients with low back pain. *New England Journal of Medicine*. 1998; **339**: 1021–9.

103. Cherkin DC, Deyo RA, Street JH *et al*. Pitfalls of patient education: limited success of a program for back pain in primary care. *Spine*. 1996; **21**: 345–55.

104. Hazard RG, Reid S, Haugh LED, McFarlane G. A controlled trial of an educational pamphlet to prevent disability after occupational low back injury. *Spine*. 2000; **25**: 1419–23.

105. Karjalainen K, Malmivaara A, van Tulder M *et al.* Multidisciplinary biopsychosocial rehabilitation for subacute low back pain among working adults. *Cochrane Database of Systematic Reviews.* 2003; **CD002193.**

106. Field MJ, Lohr KN (eds). *Clinical practice guidelines: Directions for a new program.* Washington, DC: National Academy Press, 1990.

∗107. Grimshaw J, Russell I. Effect of clinical guidelines on medical practice: a systematic review of rigorous evaluations. *Lancet.* 1993; **342:** 1317–21.

108. Schers H, Wensing M, Huijsmans Z *et al.* Implementation barriers for general practice guidelines on low back pain: a qualitative study. *Spine.* 2001; **26:** E348–53.

109. Klein B, Radecki RT, Foris MP *et al.* Bridging the gap between science and practice in managing low back pain: a comprehensive spine care system in a health maintenance organization setting. *Spine.* 2000; **25:** 738–40.

∗110. Rossignol M, Abenhaim L, Seguin P *et al.* Coordination of primary health care for back pain: a randomized controlled trial. *Spine.* 2000; **25:** 251–9.

111. Buchbinder R, Jolley D, Wyatt M. Population based intervention to change back pain beliefs and disability: three part evaluation. *BMJ.* 2001; **322:** 1516–20.

26

Pain in pregnancy, childbirth, and the puerperium

PHILIP HESS AND PEDRAM ALESHI

KEY LEARNING POINTS

- Childbirth represents one of the most intense pains that a woman may experience in her life.
- The pain of parturition is dynamic, with wide variation among parturients and during the course of labor.
- The pain of parturition generally parallels the course of labor, with early pain being primarily visceral and late pain being primarily somatic.
- Dysfunctional labor may produce severe pain that is out of proportion to the stage of labor.
- The initial pain of parturition is localized to the T11 and T12 spinal segments, while later labor pains are referred to a larger nociceptive field.

- There is a dramatic and parallel physiological response to childbirth pain that can produce harmful effects for the mother and fetus.
- Many of the tools used to measure pain in general have significant limitation when applied to parturition.
- Neuraxial analgesia is the most effective method of providing pain relief; non-neuraxial methods, although having a lower efficacy, may be of great benefit in selected populations.

INTRODUCTION

The pain of parturition strikes across ages, races, and cultures.[1] Most women describe the pain of labor as being quite severe. In fact, parturition may produce the worst pain felt by a woman at any time during her life.[2] Parturition has been described as a model of acute pain, producing pain with a finite beginning and ending.[3] However, the stimulus, psychosocial interaction, and subjective perception and expression of pain result in a tremendous variation in the description of childbirth pain among women. This variation has been interpreted in many ways (**Figure 26.1**). To some authors, the varying

degrees of pain during labor are a matter of perception; the stimulus is identical among women, but emotional, psychological, or social conditions lead to varying degrees of expression.[4] To others, the variation in reported pain may be a result of differences in the physical stimulus, neural response, and labor process, which interact with the psychosocial state of the parturient.[5, 6, 7] This divergence of opinions may result from the method of measuring pain.[4] It cannot be denied that psychosocial factors interact with the physical, obstetric stimulus; however, the precise nature of this interaction remains to be defined.

The pain of parturition has an anatomic source, a neurologic transmission, and a proportional physiologic

Source of labor pain   Variation   Modifying factors   Expressed variation

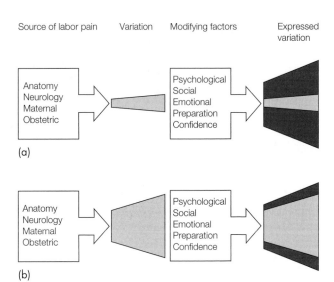

(a)

(b)

Figure 26.1 Models of labor pain variation. This figure is a graphical representation of the two opposing models used to explain the variation in pain during parturition. (a) The amount of labor pain produced by the anatomical, neurological, maternal, and obstetric characteristics (e.g. strength of contractions, pelvic size and shape, fetal size, pain threshold) varies minimally among women. This sensory input is acted upon by the psychological, social, and emotional condition of the parturient, with additional modification with learned preparation and confidence, to produce the wide variation in the expression of pain. Effective preparation and maternal confidence in the ability to control pain will significantly decrease the degree of perceived pain. One possible mechanism is amplification of descending inhibitory pathways by a higher center. (b) The sensory input is depicted as the primary determinant of variation among parturients. This is then influenced to a lesser degree by the modifying factors. The influence of both the source and modifiers may be bidirectional, in that the psychological state of the parturient does appear to influence pain thresholds; likewise, severe pain appears to decrease maternal confidence.

response. Observations of primitive cultures document that most parturients display signs of anguishing pain.[1, 8] Likewise, close observation of various animal species demonstrates that parturition is a painful natural process.[9] Thus, previous claims that childbirth should be painless[10] and the result of culturally derived fear[11] are not supported by the literature. The appreciation of labor pain requires an understanding of the neurobiological nature of parturition.

- What pain may require treatment during pregnancy?
- What is the magnitude of labor pain?
- What is labor and how does the stimulus for pain change throughout labor?
- What are the neural pathways and physiologic responses to labor pain?

Parturition presents a unique form of acute pain in that the process and stimulus for pain evolve throughout the course of childbirth, and the evolution is neither constant throughout labor nor consistent among parturients. Many women start their labor with the expectation that they will not require pain medication, but later change their mind. The treatment of childbirth pain is controversial, mainly stemming from the divergence in opinions over the etiology of pain. To some authors, medications represent a failure of the individual parturient, as all pain is due to fear, anxiety, or lack of confidence. To others, even after accounting for psychological and nonpharmacological therapies, labor remains exquisitely painful for most parturients.

In this chapter, we will review the following questions.

- What are the factors that influence the severity of pain?
- What are the treatment options for the pain of parturition?
- How successful are the treatments?

PAIN DURING PREGNANCY

A number of pain syndromes manifest during pregnancy and may need to be evaluated or treated. The unique nature of these syndromes to pregnancy is that they are caused by the physiological changes in the parturient and are often limited to the duration of the pregnancy. The most common pain syndromes in pregnancy are: lumbosacral back pain, pelvic girdle pain, and pain from nerve compression.

Medication

The pharmacological treatment of pain during pregnancy must take into account two variables. First, consideration must be taken for the effects of the medication on the fetus. Second, pregnancy is associated with an increased circulating level of progesterone. This results in augmented sensitivity to all medications. Thorough descriptions of the risks and benefits of these medications can be found elsewhere; here, we present the general principles of use.

- Paracetamol (acetaminophen)
  - There are no contraindications to the use of paracetamol during pregnancy.
  - Prolonged usage and overdosage may be associated with fetal liver toxicity.
- Nonsteroidal anti-inflammatory drugs (NSAIDs):
  - During early pregnancy, these medications are not associated with adverse effects on fetal development.[12]

- During the third trimester, the use of NSAIDs is associated with constriction of the fetal ductus arteriosis and a reduction in renal blood flow.
  - Use of NSAIDs in the third trimester requires frequent ultrasound evaluations of the ductal flow and of the amniotic fluid volume.
- Opioids:
  - The use of opioids is believed to pose no additional risk to the mother or fetus during pregnancy.
- Steroids:
  - Steroids should be avoided in the first trimester due to teratogenic effects (orofacial).
  - The risk/benefit ratio in the second and third trimesters is undefined, but used extensively for medical diseases.
- Local anesthetics:
  - There are no contraindications to the use of local anesthetics during pregnancy.
  - Progesterone-induced maternal sensitivity to local anesthetics requires a reduced dose compared with nonpregnant adults.

Pain syndromes

LUMBOSACRAL BACK PAIN

Lumbar back pain is common during pregnancy, with an estimated incidence of greater than 50 percent during pregnancy.[13, 14] Approximately 20 percent of pregnant women will report severe pain, and one-third of these will be disabled.[15] The disability from back pain may continue after childbirth. The etiology of back pain in many women relates to the increased lordosis and tension placed on the lumbar spine during gestation. Furthermore, the forward tilt of the pelvis, which is necessary for ideal placement of the pelvis canal for passage of the fetus, causes significant lordosis. Sacroiliac joint dysfunction is also a common cause of pain. The risk factors for back pain during pregnancy include:

- younger or older age;
- previous history of backache;
- obesity;
- lack of physical exercise.

In the postpartum period, approximately 45 percent of women report significant back pain, with 10 percent of women continuing to report pain after one year.[16] A similar set of risk factors has been identified; however, new-onset post partum back pain was found to be associated with greater weight and shorter stature.

The treatment of back pain during pregnancy follows the general principles that are outlined in Chapter 25, Acute low back pain. Physiotherapy and water gymnastics have been reported to reduce pain.[17]

PELVIC GIRDLE PAIN

Pelvic girdle pain is common during pregnancy, with an incidence of 30 percent. Similar to back pain, the incidence of severe pain is close to 10 percent, with a large proportion of these patients having prolonged and severe disability.[15] Typical presentations include pain in the hip, iliosacral region, coccyx, and pubic symphasis. The etiology of pain relates to the increased laxity of the pelvis during pregnancy, rotation of the pelvis, and redistribution of abdominal weight.

The treatment of pelvic girdle pain is with analgesics, bed rest, and physical therapy. Manipulation is effective in a minority of cases. Early delivery is indicated in cases of severe disability. Pain may continue for up to six months in some patients, but delivery is curative in most.[18] Walking support with a cane or other orthotic device is helpful. In general, these patients require epidural analgesia to tolerate labor.

NERVE PAIN

Pregnancy is associated with several forms of nerve-related pain. By far, the most common is carpal tunnel syndrome (CTS), which has an estimated incidence of 2–5 percent.[19] However, investigators have reported a 17 percent incidence of electromyographic evidence of CTS.[20] During pregnancy, the circulating blood volume expands by about 20 percent. In addition, the permeability of the capillary membrane may be increased under the hormonal influence. Thus, pregnancy leads to the development of edema. This is likely to be the etiology of CTS, although a preexisting susceptibility is probably required. Evidence for this is that most women with CTS who are treated conservatively will continue to experience symptoms one year after delivery.[21] Conservative treatment with splinting and elevation is effective in many cases. Surgery is required in a minority of cases of CTS; however, it should be avoided, as the stress of surgery is associated with an increased risk to the pregnancy.

Other forms of pain due to nerve compression include sciatica, meralgia paresthetica, and femoral nerve pain. Sciatica is most likely caused by the altered architecture of the pelvis, induced by the hormonal changes of pregnancy. Compression of the nerve may be at the bony canal, or at the location of the pyriformis muscle. Compression of the femoral nerve commonly occurs at the waist and is accentuated by the expanding abdomen. Pain occurring in the lateral thigh (meralgia paresthetica) or in the anterior thigh is common. A second site of compression can occur in the interior of the pelvis where the lumbar plexus is exposed to the growing uterus. These patients often have hip and thigh pain during pregnancy, significant pain during labor, and occasionally femoral neuropraxia in the postpartum period.

LABOR PAIN

Magnitude

Labor has been described as the most severe pain experienced by many women.[22] Only a minority of parturients describes pain of low intensity; for most, labor is severely or intolerably painful (**Figure 26.2**). Melzack et al.[23] found that 60 percent of primiparas described either severe or extremely severe pain during parturition; an additional 30 percent described moderate pain. Even among multiparas, 75 percent of subjects had at least moderate pain; the majority describing it as severe or extremely severe. Similarly, Ranta et al.,[24] studying Finnish parturients, found that 89 percent of primiparous and 84 percent of multiparous women described their pain as either severe or intolerable. Furthermore, none of the primiparous women had painless labor and only 4 percent of the multiparous women had reported low pain scores. In a study evaluating the effect of psychological factors on pain, Nettelbladt et al.[25] found that 35 percent of parturients described childbirth pain as intolerable, 37 percent severe, and only 28 percent moderate.

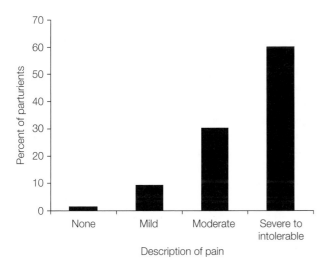

Figure 26.2 Severity of labor pain. The description of the peak labor pain from parturients. These data are retrospective in nature.

In a survey of 1000 mothers, the most common reason for dissatisfaction with the birth experience was inadequate pain relief.[26] In fact, severe pain can darken the experience of childbirth; for example, some women experience posttraumatic stress disorder.[27, 28] Increased risk of psychological trauma may be found with poor pain relief during prolonged, difficult labors, forceps deliveries, and where infant mortality or injury had occurred.

CLINICAL PRESENTATION

Course of normal labor

To a great extent, the pain of parturition parallels the process of labor (**Table 26.1**). The stimulus for pain occurs primarily during the first and second stage of labor. During the first stage, uterine contractions lead to cervical effacement and dilation, producing pain that is visceral in nature. This stage can be subdivided into phases. The latent phase consists of cervical effacement and slow cervical dilation until approximately 3–4 cm of cervical dilation. The active phase consists of a rapid increase in cervical dilation rate until full (10 cm) cervical dilation is reached. During the active phase, the rate of cervical dilation accelerates to a maximum (1 cm/hour in the nulliparas and 1.5 cm/hour in the multiparas parturient), and then decelerates as the cervix reaches full (10 cm) dilation. The end of the first stage is termed the transition stage, during which the fetus begins to descend into the pelvic inlet in preparation for the second stage of labor. This can often be identified by the beginning of somatic pain.[29] The second stage of labor begins with full cervical dilation. Uterine contractions now force the fetus through the bony pelvis, causing significant pressure and stretching and tearing of the cervix, vagina, and perineum. The second stage of labor ends with the birth of the fetus, and with this event, the vast majority of painful stimuli have been removed.

Parturients may continue to feel some pain or discomfort during the passage of the placenta, or contraction of the uterus to its postpartum size; however, this is usually less intense than childbirth. The pain from uterine cramping may persist for days and be uncomfortable.

Table 26.1 Stages of labor and pain.

Stage of labor	First stage			Second stage
	Latent phase	Active phase	Transitional phase	
Nulliparous	<20 hours	<12 hours	2–3 hours	<3 hours[a]
Multiparous	<14 hours	<6 hours	Up to 1 hour	<2 hours[a]
Primary pain type	Visceral	Visceral	Visceral/somatic	Somatic
Pain severity	Mild	Moderate to severe	Severe to intolerable	Severe to intolerable

[a]With epidural analgesia. Two and one hour, respectively, without.

Some evidence suggests that multiparous women have more pain with postpartum uterine cramping.

Visceral pain

Uterine contractions increase the pressure of the amniotic fluid resulting in distention of the lower uterine segment and the cervix.[30] This pain is visceral in nature, diffuse, and poorly characterized, and felt in the abdomen between the pubis and umbilicus, or in the back.[2] Measurements of the pressure in the amniotic fluid generated by the uterine contraction suggest that at least 15–25 mmHg is required for the initiation of pain.[31] The receptors for noxious stimulation are located in the lower uterine segment and cervix, and respond mainly to pressure and stretch. Distention of the cervix in non-pregnant women can elicit discomfort that is similar in nature to uterine contractions during labor.[32] Corli et al.[33] found that the pressure of uterine contraction correlated directly with the amount of pain reported by parturients. The peak intensity of uterine contraction, duration of the contraction, and area under the curve were all found to be predictors of the degree of pain.

Somatic pain

Pain during the second stage of labor is caused by the passage of the fetus through the bony pelvis and birth canal. The presenting part (usually the head) distends the perineum causing stretching and tearing of the skin, subcutaneous tissues, and fascia. This leads to somatic pain in the vaginal and rectal areas, which can be referred to the thighs. Pain during the second stage is often reported to be of the highest intensity; however, some

evidence suggests that pain scores may actually decrease in some women.[23] Active participation in fetal expulsion may improve the perception of pain in some women, compared with the passive tolerance of stimulation during the first stage (**Figure 26.3**).

Variability of experience

The most consistent observation of the pain of labor is the variability of description among women and throughout the course of labor. While some women report mild pain during latent phase or even early active phase, others describe horrible excruciating pain. Similarly, the nature of pain (visceral or somatic) can change during labor and is different among parturients. The latent phase can vary in duration and sensations; some parturients are aware of mild, rhythmic contractions for a brief time, while others may suffer significant distress over a protracted period. A prolonged latent phase is a common occurrence and may persist for days prior to active labor. These women are often exhausted and intolerant of any further stimulation. Severe pain felt during the latent phase is associated with abnormal labor outcomes, including cesarean section, instrumental delivery, and poor cervical dilation.[7]

Most women feel intermittent pain caused by contractions, while some also describe continuous pain. Uterine contraction pain is felt in the abdomen, but most women (75 percent) also feel pain in the back. Melzack et al. reported that 10–30 percent of parturients feel an intense, continuous pain localized to the back.[22, 34] This pain was severe in nature, often the most severe component during the first stage, and was said to "ride upon" the contraction pain. Furthermore, the occurrence of this back pain in parturients was not found to be associated with back pain before or during pregnancy. However, it

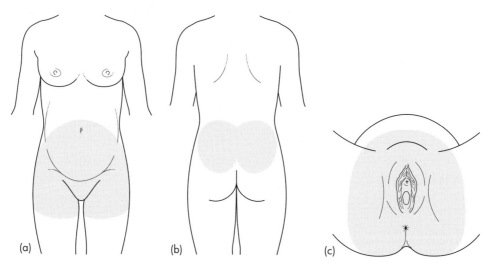

Figure 26.3 Physical location of labor pain. The image represents the idealized dermatomal locations from which labor pain is felt. Parts (a) and (b) represent the first stage of labor. Pain is centered on the lower abdomen and is visceral in nature. Parturients also may report anterior thigh pain and back pain. Part (c) represents the second stage of labor. Pain is somatic in nature and centered around the perineum. Women may also report continued pain from the abdomen and back.

was associated with the degree of pain felt during menstruation, specifically menstrual pain felt in the back.[34] Notably, this continuous back pain is not likely to be caused by the intermittent contraction of the uterus. Theories of its origins include: (1) traction and pressure on the adnexa and parietal peritoneum; (2) pressure and stretch of the bladder, urethra, and rectum; (3) pressure on the roots of the lumbosacral plexus; and (4) reflex muscle spasm.[22] The association between continuous back pain and menstrual pain has led some authors to propose prostaglandins as an etiology.[2, 5]

Some parturients also report a continuous abdominal pain; the incidence (4–13 percent) was lower than that of the continuous back pain.[35, 36] However, Molina *et al.*[37] found that approximately half of their parturients described a continuous abdominal pain. In that investigation, both types of continuous pain (abdominal and lumbar) were of a lesser intensity throughout the first stage than that of the intermittent contraction pain.

PAIN PATHWAYS

Nociceptors sensing pressure and stretch are located in the lateral wall and fornices of the uterus,[2] and are transmitted by Aδ- and C-fibers that travel with the sympathetic efferent nerves (**Figure 26.4**). These fibers then pass through the paracervical region. Local anesthetic blockade at this location can ablate the pain of uterine contractions during early labor.

The nerves then pass through, in sequence, the uterine plexus, pelvic plexus (also termed the inferior hypogastric plexus), middle hypogastric, superior hypogastric, and finally to the lower thoracic and lumbar sympathetic chain. Here, the white rami communicantes enter the spinal cord with the T10, T11, T12, and L1 spinal nerves. Passing through the posterior roots of the spinal nerves, they synapse in the dorsal horns of the spinal cord.[38] The mild to moderate pain of early labor is transmitted to the T11 and T12 spinal cord,[39] whereas the severe pain of late first stage is transmitted to the T10 to L1 spinal cord.[38] It is unclear if this expansion of the nociceptive field is due to the increased pressure generated by the uterus, peripheral sensitization, or central sensitization. However, the pain of uterine contractions may extend above the umbilicus and to the anterior thighs,[23] which are spinal segments that are not known to share nerves with the uterus and cervix, and therefore must be the result of either peripheral or central sensitization.[40]

The descent of the fetal head causes pressure, stretching, and tearing of the cervix and perineum. These noxious stimuli are transmitted by somatic afferents of the pudendal nerve, and synapse within the dorsal horn of the S2, S3, and S4 spinal cord.[38] Pressure on other pelvic structures, such as the lumbosacral plexus, bladder, urethra, rectum, and iliopsoas muscles, are transmitted

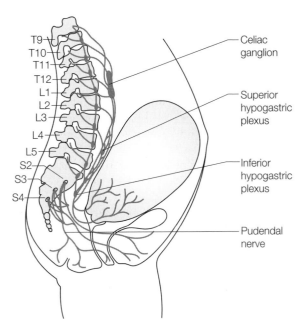

Figure 26.4 Innervation of uterus and perineum. Demonstrating the separate neuronal pathways of visceral and somatic pain during parturition (see text for precise description of pathway). Visceral pain receptors located in the lower uterine segment and cervix extend to the spinal segments of T10 to L1. These nerves can often be blocked in the paracervical region. Somatic pain is received from the perineum, and pelvic structures and is carried to the spinal segments of S2 to S4. These can be blocked at the pudendal nerve.

via the lower lumbar and upper sacral nerves, with pain referred to the lumbar region, thighs, and perineum.[38]

PHYSIOLOGICAL RESPONSE TO PAIN

Childbirth results in physiological changes to both the parturient and fetus. The nature of the stress response is similar to other forms of acute pain; for example, cardiac output and minute ventilation increases, and catecholamines and cortisol are released from the adrenals. Pain stimulates the drive for ventilation. During the first stage of labor, minute ventilation can increase by 75–150 percent of normal. This is further enhanced during the second stage of labor, when maternal expulsion efforts can result in a peak increase of up to 300 percent of normal ventilation. Because arterial carbon dioxide tension is inversely proportional to ventilation, this results in maternal hypocarbia.[41] With the loss of stimulation at the end of a contraction, the absence of respiratory drive due to hypocarbia can lead to maternal and fetal hypoxemia.[42]

Oxygen consumption increases by 40 percent during the first stage of labor, primarily due to the high demands of the uterus. During the second stage, maternal expulsive efforts may increase oxygen consumption by 75 percent of normal.[43] A significant maternal acidosis due to the build up of serum lactate has been demonstrated that increases throughout the course of labor and onset of the second stage.[44, 45] This is accompanied by an acidosis in the fetus.[46, 47] Effective epidural analgesia can ameliorate most of the harmful physiological effects of labor, including a reduction of minute ventilation,[43] oxygen consumption,[43] maternal acidosis,[44, 45] and fetal acidosis during the first stage of labor.[46] During the second stage, fetal acidemia was not affected by analgesia, probably pointing to the severe stress in the fetus during passage through the birth canal.[47] On the other hand, pethidine (meperidine) and nitrous oxide, which are less effective in treating maternal pain (even in combination), do not effectively treat these physiologic alterations.[48]

In normal early labor, catecholamines are not significantly increased from normal values. However, with the onset of pain, the levels of both epinephrine and norepinephrine can increase several fold.[49, 50] The increase in catecholamines can lead to a decrease in uterine blood flow with potentially harmful effects.[51] Pethidine does not significantly decrease the levels of circulating catecholamines during periods of severe pain. Epidural analgesia, on the other hand, has been demonstrated to reduce levels of epinephrine by 56 percent and of norepinephrine by 19 percent.[51]

Pain during parturition results in the release of ACTH, β-endorphins, and cortisol, with levels increasing throughout labor.[52, 53, 54] The levels of these stress response hormones appear to parallel the degree of pain reported by parturients. Effective epidural analgesia decreases levels of β-endorphins to prelabor concentrations.[54] Parenteral pethidine has a small effect on plasma β-endorphins levels, most likely mediated through maternal sedation.[55] Maternal anxiety, such as that found before elective cesarean delivery, can also be a cause of increased plasma β-endorphins.[56] Although plasma β-endorphins are increased, the levels of this hormone in the cerebral spinal fluid remain similar to prelabor values.[57] Plasma β-endorphins at the levels found during labor have no more than a mild analgesic quality, and may provide minimal modulation of pain. The correlation between reported pain and β-endorphin levels suggests that these hormones are a response to, and not a modifier of, maternal pain and anxiety.

FACTORS INFLUENCING LABOR PAIN

Psychological and social factors

The interaction between social and psychological factors and pain during childbirth is complex. The most heavily investigated psychological factors are fear and anxiety. Conceptually, women who are anxious and fearful of their labor will be more likely to interpret their sensory experience as pain or will lack the ability to cope with pain when it arises. Characteristics that are associated with a greater anxiety and fear are reported to be nulliparity, younger age, single parenthood, and lack of a social support structure. A parturient may have considerable pain, but be able to cope with or tolerate that pain with continuous emotional assistance from a spouse or coach.[58] The ability to cope with labor pain may be enhanced with spousal support and assistance by a midwife or others, while being hindered by inexperience, anxiety, and depression. Anxiety can be treated with childbirth preparatory techniques, often utilizing the psychoprophylactic techniques popularized by Lamaze.[59]

The most consistent findings have been that maternal depression and anxiety are associated with reports of increased pain;[60, 61] however, the relationship is very complex. As stated by Reading and Cox:[60]

> The relationship between anxiety and pain is bidirectional, in that in addition to anxiety increasing pain sensitivity, high levels of pain may increase anxiety.

Maternal factors

Studies using the McGill Pain Questionnaire have identified several maternal variables that are associated with increased pain during childbirth, including lesser maternal age, greater maternal weight, nulliparity, greater fetal weight, and a history of painful menstruation.[5, 22, 34] There is considerable agreement in the literature that nulliparas report greater pain than multiparas;[62, 63] however, the timing of the evaluation appears to be important. Nulliparas report greater pain early in labor, but during the active phase multiparas describe pain of equal severity.[64, 65] Even grand multiparas (more than five previous deliveries) experience significant pain once the active phase has commenced, and may feel as much, if not more, pain during delivery.[64] Investigations using scalar measurements, including the visual analog scale (VAS), have not confirmed correlation with younger age,[25, 66] maternal weight,[67] or fetal weight,[67] though this may be due to the lack of discriminative ability of scalar measurements when examining high intensity pain.

Some parturients prefer to walk during early labor and this has raised the question of whether the pain is decreased with vertical positioning. In fact, Roberts et al.[68] found that women in early labor (<6 cm) are more comfortable sitting, whereas in late labor they are more comfortable lying. However, the evaluation was of comfort instead of pain, thus the vertical position might improve coping, not lessen pain. Melzack et al.[36] found that during early labor, women in the vertical position reported a 35 percent decrease in abdominal pain and a 50 percent decrease in lumbar pain. This investigation evaluated parturients very early in labor (2–3-cm dilation). Evaluating parturients throughout labor, Molina *et al.*[37] found that there was little difference between the horizontal and vertical position in early labor, but that most parturients reported less pain with the horizontal position during active labor and beyond. Finally, a study evaluating the effectiveness of walking on the course of labor found no difference in the use of analgesia between those parturients who walked and those who did not, although the average amount of time spent walking was small.[69]

Obstetric factors

FETUS

The position of the fetus within the pelvis has received minimal evaluation as a cause of pain. It is believed that the occiput–posterior (OP) position may cause more pain during the first stage of labor;[7, 32] however, the effect of other positions is unclear. Some authors have disputed the relationship between fetal position and the degree of pain, but it is difficult to interpret these results as the vast majority of subjects in that study received epidural analgesia.[70] Certainly, during the second stage, the OP fetus is unable to flex its neck to decrease the diameter of the presenting part; this will result in greater stretching and tearing of the cervix, vagina, and perineum.

LABOR

The duration of labor has inconsistently been associated with the degree of pain. Some authors have not found a correlation in women with normal labor. Others have found that women with prolonged labor describe severe pain early in the latent phase, and that the degree of pain is correlated with the length of labor.[4, 7] These results suggest that early, severe pain is a characteristic of prolonged labor, but that within normal labor the relationship may be less significant.

Dysfunctional labor is difficult to define, and may have several etiologies including dystocia, poor uterine contractility, or abnormal fetal position. However, the measurable outcomes of dysfunctional labor can be identified as slow cervical dilation, instrumental delivery, and cesarean section. When we focus on these clearly defined outcomes, we find an overwhelming relationship between the severity of pain and dysfunctional labor. In other words, women with dysfunctional labor experience more severe pain than those with a normal course of labor. These women often describe somatic pain in early labor, may be more likely to have continuous pain, and request analgesia early in their labor. It may be that abnormal labor, identified by a slow cervical dilation and the need for an operative delivery, causes an abnormal degree of pain out of proportion to the strength of their uterine contractions. The mechanism of this abnormal pain is not known, but may relate to the size of the fetus in relation to the bony pelvis, uncoordinated uterine activity, or pressure on the pelvic structures. The risk factors for dysfunctional labor correlate with the use of labor epidural analgesia (**Figure 26.5**). The relationship between pain and dysfunctional labor precedes the advent of effective labor analgesia. In 1939, Moir[32] observed that parturients with dysfunctional labor appear to have worse pain than those with normal labor, despite the lesser strength of uterine contractions.

TREATMENT OF LABOR PAIN

Treatment options for the pain of childbirth may be classified as follows:

- nonpharmacologic;
- pharmacologic:
  - systemic:
    - intermittent intramuscular/intravenous;
    - continuous infusion.
  - inhalation;
  - regional;
  - neuraxial:
    - spinal;
    - epidural;
    - combined spinal-epidural (CSE).

The choice of analgesic treatment should be left to the patient, with access to adequate information concerning the local availability, risks and benefits, and alternatives. The care providers should respect the wishes of the

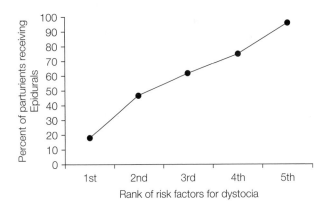

Figure 26.5 Risk for dystocia and epidural use. Demonstrating the association between risk factors for dystocia and the use of epidural analgesia for labor. Parturients are categorized by the number and severity of risk factors for dystocia. The percentage of parturients receiving epidural analgesia is per quintile. There is a linear relationship between the risk for dystocia and epidural use, possibly related to an increase in the severity of pain among parturients with true dystocia.

patient and yet be flexible enough to recognize that labor, and its accompanying pain, is a dynamic process and that the patient may change her mind as labor progresses. To quote from the closing comments of the editorial of Dr Melzack:[3]

> Prepared childbirth training and skillfully administered epidural analgesia are compatible, complimentary procedures that allow recognition of the individuality of each woman.

Nonpharmacological methods

Nonpharmacologic methods of pain control have been practiced for all of human history. The inherent advantages to these methods are that they are noninvasive, there is no pharmacologic effect on the mother or fetus, and some modalities have low or no cost. Fortunately, these methods allow many parturients to tolerate the pain of labor and delivery. These techniques presumably work by increasing the activity of descending inhibitory pathways.[71] The evidence supporting the use of non-pharmacological pain relief tends to compare parturient with a degree of self-selection.[72] While the efficacy of these modalities as labor analgesics may not be nearly as good as that of neuraxial methods, parturients who undergo one of these interventions often report a very satisfying labor experience.

PSYCHOPROPHYLAXIS

The psychoprophylactic method of Lamaze[59] gained considerable interest in the 1970s. This system is based on the belief that most, if not all, of the pain of childbirth is caused by maternal fears. The theories were originally developed by Dick-Read[11] who believed that maternal fear of the labor experience would lead to tensing of the body, labor obstruction, and a sensation that incorrectly was interpreted as pain. Evaluation using the McGill Pain Questionnaire concluded that nulliparous parturients who used techniques learned in childbirth preparation classes had an approximately 10 percent reduction in their pain during labor.[22] There was no reduction among multiparas. A review of the therapeutic effects of childbirth preparatory techniques published in 1978 criticized the literature of that time as having significant methodological shortcomings.[73] Since then, investigations into most psychosocial factors have demonstrated positive,[22] negative,[62] or no effect on the severity of labor pain.[60, 63, 73]

CONTINUOUS LABOR SUPPORT

Continuous labor support describes the presence of a trained practitioner who remains in the constant presence of, and usually continual contact with, the parturient. The

Central American practitioner of this technique is the doula. Traditionally, a doula is a woman who has delivered children of her own and is able to provide support through her experience. The evidence suggesting that this reduced the need for pharmacologic pain control is mixed. Meta-analysis of the multiple trials is challenging due to the heterogeneity of the techniques and medical centers. The use of continuous support (in constant contact, rather than a person coming in and out of the room) is superior to intermittent support.[74] [IV] Continuous labor support decreases the need for parenteral analgesia when compared with standard care; however, the influence of several confounding variables needs to be evaluated.[75]

ACUPUNCTURE

Acupuncture has been used for hundreds, if not thousands, of years. Recent studies have suggested that there may be some improvement in pain perception with some acupuncture techniques. Ramnero et al.[76] [III] showed a significant decrease in the use of epidural analgesia in patients receiving acupuncture versus a control group. Interestingly, although subjects in both groups did not report high pain scores, the circulating beta-endorphin levels of the women who received acupuncture were significantly higher. However, it should be noted that there were only 18 subjects per group in this study. A second study by Skilnand et al.[77] randomly assigned 208 women to either real or sham (needle insertion into incorrect point) acupuncture. They found significantly lower pain scores after real acupuncture compared with the sham group. Furthermore, the women who received real acupuncture had significantly less use of epidural analgesia and intramuscular pethidine. Unfortunately, the analgesia produced with acupuncture has also been described as inconsistent, unpredictable, and incomplete. Importantly, there is dissatisfaction among some with the significant limitations placed on the patient's movement.

MENTAL TRAINING

In evaluation of biofeedback, a study by Duchene[78] showed women using biofeedback during childbirth reported significantly lower pain than control women at admission, delivery, and 24 hours postpartum. Seventy percent of the women in the control group requested and used epidural anesthesia compared with 40 percent of the women of the biofeedback group. Although several trials have been published in the literature, the heterogeneity of methods and evaluations does not support a generalized improvement in pain scores or reduction in requirements for pharmacologic pain control (i.v./i.m. opioids or epidural analgesia).[79] It should be noted that, in these trials, patients were prescreened for hypnotic susceptibility.

INTRADERMAL SALINE INJECTIONS

Intradermal saline injections have been described for persistent back pain during labor.[80] These are simple to administer, inexpensive, and with no known associated risk. While there is no decrease in the use of other pain medications, they appear to provide relief of back pain for 45–90 minutes during the first stage of labor.[81]

ADDITIONAL TECHNIQUES

Several trials have examined the use of water baths, with evidence showing either some improvement in pain, or none at all; only one of the trials demonstrated a decrease in the usage of epidural analgesia.[75] Similarly, the scientific evidence for ambulation or positioning, touch, and massage, while improving maternal mood and decreasing anxiety, do not appear to reduce maternal pain perception.

Pharmacological methods

In the developed world, most women in labor request some form of pharmacologic analgesia. All methods of pain relief have limitations. In addition, no technique can provide continuous comfort at all times. Failure rates for epidural analgesia range from 3–10 percent.[22, 82] Furthermore, as the pain of labor becomes more intense, women frequently have pain that breaks through otherwise effective epidural analgesia. The incidence of breakthrough pain is between 34 and 71 percent.[83, 84, 85, 86] Breakthrough pain during labor analgesia may be an indication of the underlying severity of the pain of childbirth. Recent evidence showing that the amount of medication required for initiating or maintaining labor analgesia confirms the link between dysfunctional labor and severity of labor pain. The amount of bupivacaine required to initiate epidural analgesia is significantly higher among women who proceed to a cesarean delivery than those who delivery vaginally.[87] Others have shown that the amount of medication required to maintain adequate analgesia, whether epidural or intravenous, is greater in women who have dysfunctional labor.[88, 89]

SYSTEMIC ANALGESICS

Parenteral opioids are useful for mild to moderate pain, especially during early labor, but are less effective for the treatment of high intensity pain.[90] Worldwide, pethidine is the most commonly used parenteral opioid, but there does not appear to be any evidence that any other opioid is more or less effective.[91] The partial agonist and agonist–antagonist opioids are popular due to the belief that side effects, especially respiratory depression, are limited. The dose of parenteral opioids is limited by the side effects in the mother and fetus, including maternal sedation, respiratory depression, and nausea/vomiting. Care must be taken as parturients are sensitive to the depressant effects of medications because of elevated levels of circulating progesterone. Undesirable neonatal effects include respiratory depression at birth, abnormal sleep patterns, and poor adaptation to suckling.[72] A unique consideration to pethidine is the potential accumulation in the compromised fetus. This can lead to loss of beat-to-beat variability of the heart rate tracing, which may interfere with interpretation of labor, and may also cause neonatal sedation and depression up to 18 hours after administration, long after the maternal effects have completely worn off.

Lipid-soluble opioids, such as fentanyl, may be more effective at controlling pain due to their rapid onset. An advantage of the lipid-soluble opioids is that they tend to affect the neonate less than the longer-duration opioids. Remifentanil, with its unique pharmacokinetic properties, has also been studied as an intravenous agent for labor analgesia. Results have been variable with some reporting satisfactory results,[92] with others being unable to provide adequate analgesia without significant side effects.[93] Lacassie and Olufolabi[94] found that intravenous remifentanil boluses were superior to a continuous pethidine infusion with lower pain scores and improved patient satisfaction. However, they noted that a continuous infusion caused excessive sedation, and intermittent boluses given at the beginning of each contraction did not work fast enough to provide adequate analgesia.

INHALATIONAL

Inhalational agents used for general anesthesia have also been used for providing analgesia and sedation during labor. Subanesthetic concentrations of these gases allow maintenance of the airway and swallowing reflexes, while providing some level of analgesia. Nitrous oxide is the gas most commonly used, either alone, or in conjunction with other volatile anesthetics, e.g. isoflurane in low concentrations. The risk of inhalational analgesia is aspiration, which is increased in pregnancy due to delayed gastric emptying.

Most commonly used, entonox is a mixture of 50 percent nitrous oxide and 50 percent oxygen in a fixed delivery system. Nitrous oxide can be beneficial for many patients if used correctly and has minimal side effects if limited to 50 percent. The preferred method is intermittent inhalation timed with contractions, as continuous use is associated with greater frequency of side effects.[95] Prolonged use is associated with maternal sedation and nausea and vomiting. The analgesic efficacy of this method is questionable. In a placebo-controlled, randomized study, entonox was shown to be a poor labor analgesic with an efficacy equal to that of compressed air.[96] However, many patients receive benefit from entonox as a method of reducing pain perception, or as a temporizing measure prior to epidural analgesia.[95] Similar lack of effective analgesia has been noted with various halogenated anesthetic agents, unless concentrations high enough to cause sedation are used.[97, 98]

NONNEURAXIAL REGIONAL ANESTHESIA

Paracervical block has been used in the past for analgesia in the first stage of labor. The success of this block is approximately 75 percent.[99] Pain relief lasts for up to 60 minutes after the injection. However, once the local anesthetic wears off, pain returns without abatement. The high incidence of fetal bradycardias (up to 40 percent) and a report of a series of fetal deaths has led to the virtual abandonment of this otherwise technically easy modality.[99, 100, 101, 102]

Bilateral pudendal nerve blocks (S2–S4 roots) provide analgesia for placement of forceps or for the second stage of labor. However, this block is associated with a high failure rate[103] and the dose of local anesthetic needed for a bilateral block may approach produce toxic maternal plasma concentrations.

NEURAXIAL BLOCKADE

Neuraxial analgesia is without doubt the most effective available form of labor pain control. The contraindications to neuraxial analgesia in labor are similar to those for the nonparturient population. They can be divided into absolute and relative contraindications (**Table 26.2**).

Pregnancy is associated with many illnesses that may contraindicate neuraxial analgesia. The most common of these is coagulopathy, which may result from:

- thrombocytopenia of pregnancy;
- preeclampsia;
- HELLP syndrome (hypertension, elevated livery enzymes, low platelets);
- medical anticoagulation – due to the high incidence of deep vein thrombosis in pregnancy.

Spinal analgesia is commonly used when the availability of personnel and equipment is limited. The clear advantage of spinal analgesia is its rapidity of onset and the depth of analgesia. The main disadvantage is that it can only be performed as a single injection; thus, the analgesia may subside. For this reason, spinal analgesia is usually withheld until late in labor (e.g. greater than 7 cm dilation). Repeat injections are possible, but the side effects and complications will increase.

The most frequently described technique is to inject a combination of fentanyl 25 µg and morphine 250 µg. This has been shown to produce analgesia within 15 minutes, with a duration of two to four hours.[104] [II] This dose has been used extensively throughout the world and is the

Table 26.2 Contraindications to neuraxial analgesia.

Absolute	Relative
Patient refusal	Remote infection
Inability to obtain informed consent	Thrombocytopenia
Uncorrected hypovolemia	Obstructive cardiac defect
Coagulopathy	Unstable neurologic injury
Infection at the site of insertion	Spine surgery
Lack of monitoring equipment	
Lack of resuscitative equipment and medications	

most common form of pain control in many countries. Side effects include nausea and pruritus, each with an incidence of 20–40 percent. Analgesia is more effective during early labor and least effective during the second stage.

Lumbar epidural analgesia is the most effective modality of pain control for labor. With the intention of improving efficacy and safety, the techniques of labor epidural analgesia have undergone considerable modifications. It should be emphasized that, given the wide variation in the concentration and type of local anesthetics and narcotic used (with or without additional agents such as α_2 agonists), the term "epidural" should not be used generically. Instead, a clear description of the dose of the various medications and the rate at which they are administered is necessary for making meaningful comparisons of different regimes.

Traditional epidural analgesia uses high concentrations of local anesthetics via intermittent bolus injection to provide complete analgesia at the expense of significant side effects, principally motor blockade, hypotension, and sensory deprivation. This method of analgesia was based on the concept that dense blockade of nerves was necessary for adequate pain control; however, despite successful pain relief, parturients tend to be dissatisfied with the feeling of sensory loss.[105] Furthermore, the intensity of the sympathectomy and resultant hypotension resulted in high rates of fetal bradycardia and maternal complications.

The addition of lipid-soluble opioids allows a reduction of local anesthetic concentration, reducing the side effects of hypotension and dense blockade, but can result in some pruritus, and nausea and vomiting.[86] The development of solutions containing very low concentrations of bupivacaine (**Table 26.3**) makes differential blockade a reality. Using 0.04 percent bupivacaine with fentanyl 2 µg/mL and epinephrine 2 µg/mL, Breen et al.[106] were able to ambulate parturients after hours of successful epidural analgesia. In addition, the side effects are all but negated (**Table 26.4**).

Table 26.3 Medications used for labor epidural analgesia.

Medication	Infusion rate
Local anesthetic	
Bupivacaine 0.04%[a]	15 mL/hour
Bupivacaine 0.0625%	12 mL/hour
Bupivacaine 0.08%	10 mL/hour
Bupivacaine 0.125% (ropivacaine equivalent range of 0.07% to 1.5%)	8 mL/hour
Opioids	
Fentanyl 1–4 μg/mL (equivalent to sufentanil 0.5–1 μg/mL)	Concentration adjusted to delivery 20–25 μg per hour

Epidural analgesia is most effectively performed with a combination of local anesthetic and lipid soluble opioid. The dosage and rate of medications used for labor analgesia are described above. Although individual requirements vary, the typical patient requires approximately 6–10 mg of bupivacaine per hour when combined with 20–25 μg of fentanyl per hour.
[a] The ultralow dose, or walking epidural, described by Breen et al.[106] consists of bupivacaine 0.04%, fentanyl 2 μg/cc, and epinephrine 2 μg/cc.

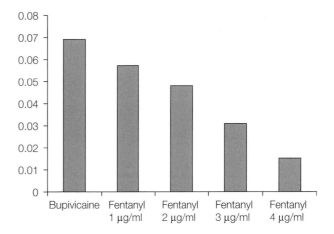

Figure 26.6 The minimum local anesthetic concentration (MLAC) represents the median concentration of epidural local anesthetic required to produce complete pain relief during the first stage of labor (20 mL volume). The MLAC of bupivacaine can be reduced in a dose-dependent manner with the addition of fentanyl.

The minimum local analgesic concentration (MLAC) has been defined as the analgesic concentration in a 20-mL volume required for complete pain relief in the first stage of labor. Determination of MLAC has been used to evaluate the potency of various local anesthetics.[107] Furthermore, it provides a basis for comparison of side effects and toxicities of various medications. The MLAC of bupivacaine is reduced in a dose-dependent manner with the addition of fentanyl (**Figure 26.6**). Investigations determining the MLAC for bupivacaine have found a wide variety of results, ranging from 0.065 percent[107] to 0.104 percent.[108] This variability has been identified for most local anesthetic agents and may be due to the variability in labor pain. For example, the MLAC values

obtained in early versus late labor are 0.048 versus 0.141 percent, respectively.[109] Similarly, variations in MLAC can occur due to underlying dysfunctional labor or maternal factors.[87] Other measures of local anesthetic requirements correlate with the MLAC determination. For example, using the dosing requirements for bupivacaine and levo-bupivacaine via patient-controlled epidural analgesia (PCEA), Hofmann-Kiefer et al.[110] found that bupivacaine PCEA delivery without continuous infusion was 40–50 percent more potent than ropivacaine.

The small therapeutic window for bupivacaine encouraged the development of other local anesthetics, mainly ropivacaine and levobupivacaine, which have less central nervous system (CNS) and cardiac toxicity in animals and humans.[111] However, some investigators have suggested that this lesser toxicity parallels a lesser potency (**Figure 26.7**).[112] Clinically, both medications

Table 26.4 Side effects of neuraxial analgesia.

	Incidence	Treatment
Pruritus	10–20% (labor analgesia)	Small doses of naloxone, nalbuphine
	70–80% (spinal opioid)	Remove opioid from epidural infusion
Nausea and vomiting	2–5% (labor analgesia)	Antiemesis medications (consider effects if mother will breastfeed)
	15–40% (spinal opioid)	
Hypotension	5–10% (labor analgesia)	Uterine displacement
		Fluid administration
		Small doses of vasopressors may be used to temporize
Dural puncture headache	1–2%	Supportive if mild
		Epidural blood patch
Back pain	< 1%	30–40% of women have back pain after childbirth without analgesia
		Supportive
Extensive sensory blockade	10–30%	Reduce concentration of local anesthetic
Motor blockade	5–30%	Reduce concentration of local anesthetic

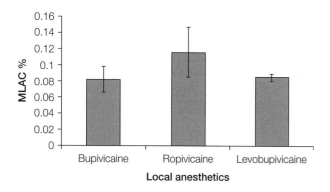

Figure 26.7 Minimum local anesthetic concentration of bupivacaine, ropivacaine, and levobupivacaine. The bars represent the relative potencies of the three local anesthetics for the initiation of labor epidural analgesia in 20 mL volume.

have similar effects when high doses are used. In a meta-analysis comparing bupivacaine and ropivacaine, Writer et al.[113] showed that 0.25 percent bupivacaine caused more motor blockade, higher rates of instrumental deliveries, and lower neonatal adaptive scores than 0.25 percent ropivacaine. Such high concentrations of ropivacaine are not necessary to provide labor analgesia. Halpern et al.[114] showed that 0.1 percent bupivacaine and 0.1 percent ropivacaine both provided comparable analgesia, although motor blockade was higher in the bupivacaine group.

The **combined spinal epidural** technique for labor analgesia was made feasible by the availability of atraumatic spinal needles with a low incidence of postdural puncture headache. Intrathecal administration of opioid results in excellent labor analgesia that lasts for approximately 60 minutes (**Table 26.5**) This duration may be prolonged to about 90–120 minutes by the addition of a small amount of local anesthetic. Insertion of an epidural catheter following the spinal injection permits extension of analgesia beyond that afforded by the intrathecal agents. The CSE may be especially beneficial in situations that require the expeditious administration of profound analgesia, e.g. a multiparous parturient with rapidly progressing labor.

Parturients prefer a low-dose CSE technique to the traditional, higher-dose epidural.[83] Women receiving a CSE achieved effective analgesia faster than with a traditional epidural catheter and were more likely to be satisfied with their analgesia (odds ratio, 5).[115] The main problem with a CSE is an increased incidence of pruritus. However, there is no difference between CSE and epidural techniques with regards to maternal mobility, rescue analgesia requirements, the incidence of postdural puncture headache (PDPH) or blood patch, hypotension, urinary retention, mode of delivery, or admission of the baby to the neonatal unit.[82, 115]

A variety of spinal medications can be used for labor analgesia. Standard solutions often contain a combination of local anesthetic and an opioid. Sia et al.[116] showed that smaller doses of both bupivacaine and sufentanil were as effective as larger doses (sufentanil 10 µg/bupivacaine 2.5 mg versus sufentanil 5 µg/bupivacaine 1.25 µg). Both motor blockade and hypotension were more frequent with higher doses of sufentanil and bupivacaine, but patients receiving a lower dose did not achieve the same level of analgesia. Conversely, the lower doses were less rapid in onset among patients in active labor. In higher doses, morphine may prolong the spinal duration of a CSE, but this may also result in higher rates of nausea and vomiting.[117] Small doses of morphine may also improve the efficacy of subsequent epidural analgesia.[118]

In summary, with respect to CSE:

- spinal injection provides instant relief;
- it can be used as a "walking epidural" prior to administering local anesthetics;
- the epidural catheter provides continuous support;
- complications are identical to standard epidural analgesia;
- it is most useful in advanced or very painful labor.

Table 26.5 Medications used for combined spinal epidural analgesia.

Type	Medication and dose
Opioids	Fentanyl 12.5–25 µg
	Sufentanil 1–5 µg
	Morphine 100 µg
	Pethidine 25 mg
Local anesthetic	Bupivacaine 1–2.5 mg
	Ropivacaine 2.5–4 mg
Epidural infusion	Identical to standard epidural analgesia

The spinal injection used as part of a combined spinal epidural technique consists of an opioid medication, with or without a local anesthetic. The addition of a local anesthetic improves the onset and duration of the pain relief. Side effects of this technique include pruritus and (rare) respiratory depression.

REFERENCES

1. Bonica JJ. The nature of pain in parturition. In: Zundert AV, Ostheimer GW (eds). *Pain relief and anesthesia in obstetrics*. New York: Churchill Livingstone, 1996: 19–52.
2. Brownridge P. The nature and consequences of childbirth pain. *European Journal of Obstetrics, Gynecology, and Reproductive Biology*. 1995; **59** (Suppl): S9–15.
3. Melzack R. Labour pain as a model of acute pain. *Pain*. 1993; **53**: 117–20.
4. Niven C, Gijsbers K. A study of labour pain using the McGill Pain Questionnaire. *Social Science and Medicine*. 1984; **19**: 1347–51.
* 5. Melzack R, Kinch R, Dobkin P et al. Severity of labour pain: influence of physical as well as psychologic variables.

Canadian Medical Association Journal. 1984; **130**: 579–84.

6. Niven CA, Gijsbers KJ. Do low levels of labour pain reflect low sensitivity to noxious stimulation? *Social Science and Medicine.* 1989; **29**: 585–8.

∗ 7. Wuitchik M, Bakal D, Lipshitz J. The clinical significance of pain and cognitive activity in latent labor. *Obstetrics and Gynecology.* 1989; **73**: 35–42.

8. Freedman LZ, Ferguson VS. The question of 'painless childbirth' in primitive cultures. *American Journal of Orthopsychiatry.* 1950; **20**: 363–72.

9. Lefebvre L, Carli G. Parturition in non-human primates: pain and auditory concealment. *Pain.* 1985; **21**: 315–27.

10. Behan RJ. *Pain.* New York: Appleton, 1914.

11. Dick-Read G. *Chilbirth without fear.* New York: Harper, 1944.

12. Nielsen GL, Sorensen HT, Larsen H, Pedersen L. Risk of adverse birth outcome and miscarriage in pregnant users of non-steroidal anti-inflammatory drugs: population based observational study and case-control study. *British Medical Journal.* 2001; **322**: 266–70.

13. Carlson HL, Carlson NL, Pasternak BA, Balderston KD. Understanding and managing the back pain of pregnancy. *Current Women's Health Reports.* 2003; **3**: 65–71.

14. Padua L, Padua R, Bondi R *et al.* Patient-oriented assessment of back pain in pregnancy. *European Spine Journal.* 2002; **11**: 272–5.

∗ 15. Wu WH, Meijer OG, Uegaki K *et al.* Pregnancy-related pelvic girdle pain (PPP). I: Terminology, clinical presentation, and prevalence. *European Spine Journal.* 2004; **13**: 575–89.

16. Breen TW, Ransil BJ, Groves PA, Oriol NE. Factors associated with back pain after childbirth. *Anesthesiology.* 1994; **81**: 29–34.

∗ 17. Young G, Jewell D. Interventions for preventing and treating pelvic and back pain in pregnancy. *Cochrane Database of Systematic Reviews.* 2002; **CD001139**.

∗ 18. Leadbetter RE, Mawer D, Lindow SW. Symphysis pubis dysfunction: a review of the literature. *Journal of Maternal-Fetal and Neonatal Medicine.* 2004; **16**: 349–54.

19. Finsen V, Zeitlmann H. Carpal tunnel syndrome during pregnancy. *Scandinavian Journal of Plastic and Reconstructive Surgery and Hand Surgery.* 2006; **40**: 41–5.

20. Bahrami MH, Rayegani SM, Fereidouni M, Baghbani M. Prevalence and severity of carpal tunnel syndrome (CTS during pregnancy). *Electromyography and Clinical Neurophysiology.* 2005; **45**: 123–5.

∗ 21. Padua L, Aprile I, Caliandro P *et al.* Carpal tunnel syndrome in pregnancy: multiperspective follow-up of untreated cases. *Neurology.* 2002; **59**: 1643–6.

22. Melzack R, Taenzer P, Feldman P, Kinch RA. Labour is still painful after prepared childbirth training. *Canadian Medical Association Journal.* 1981; **125**: 357–63.

∗ 23. Melzack R. The myth of painless childbirth (the John J. Bonica lecture). *Pain.* 1984; **19**: 321–37.

24. Ranta P, Spalding M, Kangas-Saarela T *et al.* Maternal expectations and experiences of labour pain – options of 1091 Finnish parturients. *Acta Anaesthesiologica Scandinavica.* 1995; **39**: 60–6.

25. Nettelbladt P, Fagerstrom CF, Uddenberg N. The significance of reported childbirth pain. *Journal of Psychosomatic Research.* 1976; **20**: 215–21.

26. Paech MJ. The King Edward Memorial Hospital 1,000 mother survey of methods of pain relief in labour. *Anaesthesia and Intensive Care.* 1991; **19**: 393–9.

27. Wijma K, Soderquist J, Wijma B. Posttraumatic stress disorder after childbirth: a cross sectional study. *Journal of Anxiety Disorders.* 1997; **11**: 587–97.

28. Reynolds JL. Post-traumatic stress disorder after childbirth: the phenomenon of traumatic birth. *Canadian Medical Association Journal.* 1997; **156**: 831–5.

29. Cheek TG, Gutsche BB, Gaiser RR. The pain of childbirth and its effects in the mother and fetus. In: Chestnut DH (ed.). *Obstetric anesthesia: principles and practice*, 1st edn. Boston: Mosby, 1994: 314–29.

30. Bonica JJ, Chadwick HS. Labour pain. In: Wall PD, Melzack R (eds). *Textbook of pain*, 2nd edn. New York: Churchill Livingstone, 1989: 482–9.

31. Bonica JJ. *Principles and practice of obstetric analgesia and anesthesia.* Philadelphia: FA Davis, 1967.

32. Moir C. The nature of the pain of labour. *Journal of Obstetrics and Gynaecology of the British Empire.* 1939; **46**: 409–25.

33. Corli O, Grossi E, Roma G, Battagliarin G. Correlation between subjective labour pain and uterine contractions: a clinical study. *Pain.* 1986; **26**: 53–60.

34. Melzack R, Belanger E. Labour pain: correlations with menstrual pain and acute low-back pain before and during pregnancy. *Pain.* 1989; **36**: 225–9.

35. Melzack R, Schaffelberg D. Low-back pain during labor. *American Journal of Obstetrics and Gynecology.* 1987; **156**: 901–05.

36. Melzack R, Belanger E, Lacroix R. Labor pain: effect of maternal position on front and back pain. *Journal of Pain and Symptom Management.* 1991; **6**: 476–80.

37. Molina FJ, Sola PA, Lopez E, Pires C. Pain in the first stage of labor: relationship with the patient's position. *Journal of Pain and Symptom Management.* 1997; **13**: 98–103.

38. Akamatsu TJ, Bonica JJ. Spinal and extradural analgesia–anesthesia for parturition. *Clinical Obstetrics and Gynecology.* 1974; **17**: 183–98.

39. Cleland JGP. Paravertebral anaesthesia in obstetrics. *Surgery, Gynecology and Obstetrics.* 1933; **57**: 51–62.

∗ 40. Lauretti GR. Mechanisms of labor pain. In: Norris MC (ed.). *Obstetric anesthesia*, 2nd edn. New York: Lippincott Williams & Wilkins, 1999: 235–50.

41. Reed PN, Colquhoun AD, Hanning CD. Maternal oxygenation during normal labour. *British Journal of Anaesthesia.* 1989; **62**: 316–18.

42. Miller FC, Petrie RH, Arce JJ *et al.* Hyperventilation during labor. *American Journal of Obstetrics and Gynecology.* 1974; **120**: 489–95.

43. Hagerdal M, Morgan CW, Sumner AE, Gutsche BB. Minute ventilation and oxygen consumption during labor with epidural analgesia. *Anesthesiology*. 1983; **59**: 425–7.

44. Pearson JF, Davies P. The effect of continuous lumbar epidural analgesia on the acid-base status of maternal arterial blood during the first stage of labour. *Journal of Obstetrics and Gynaecology of the British Commonwealth*. 1973; **80**: 218–24.

45. Pearson JF, Davies P. The effect on continuous lumbar epidural analgesia on maternal acid-base balance and arterial lactate concentration during the second stage of labour. *Journal of Obstetrics and Gynaecology of the British Commonwealth*. 1973; **80**: 225–9.

46. Pearson JF, Davies P. The effect of continuous lumbar epidural analgesia upon fetal acid-base status during the first stage of labour. *Journal of Obstetrics and Gynaecology of the British Commonwealth*. 1974; **81**: 971–4.

47. Pearson JF, Davies P. The effect of continuous lumbar epidural analgesia upon fetal acid-base status during the second stage of labour. *Journal of Obstetrics and Gynaecology of the British Commonwealth*. 1974; **81**: 975–9.

48. Deckardt R, Fembacher PM, Schneider KT, Graeff H. Maternal arterial oxygen saturation during labor and delivery: pain-dependent alterations and effects on the newborn. *Obstetrics and Gynecology*. 1987; **70**: 21–5.

49. Shnider SM, Wright RG, Levinson G et al. Uterine blood flow and plasma norepinephrine changes during maternal stress in the pregnant ewe. *Anesthesiology*. 1979; **50**: 524–7.

50. Abboud TK, Artal R, Henriksen EH et al. Effects of spinal anesthesia on maternal circulating catecholamines. *American Journal of Obstetrics and Gynecology*. 1982; **142**: 252–4.

51. Shnider SM, Abboud TK, Artal R et al. Maternal catecholamines decrease during labor after lumbar epidural anesthesia. *American Journal of Obstetrics and Gynecology*. 1983; **147**: 13–15.

52. Houck JC, Kimball C, Chang C et al. Placental beta-endorphin-like peptides. *Science*. 1980; **207**: 78–80.

53. Bacigalupo G, Riese S, Rosendahl H, Saling E. Quantitative relationships between pain intensities during labor and beta-endorphin and cortisol concentrations in plasma. Decline of the hormone concentrations in the early postpartum period. *Journal of Perinatal Medicine*. 1990; **18**: 289–96.

54. Hoffman DI, Abboud TK, Haase HR et al. Plasma beta-endorphin concentrations prior to and during pregnancy, in labor, and after delivery. *American Journal of Obstetrics and Gynecology*. 1984; **150**: 492–6.

55. Raisanen I, Paatero H, Salminen K, Laatikainen T. Pain and plasma beta-endorphin level during labor. *Obstetrics and Gynecology*. 1984; **64**: 783–6.

56. Raisanen I, Paatero H, Salminen K, Laatikainen T. Beta-endorphin in maternal and umbilical cord plasma at elective cesarean section and in spontaneous labor. *Obstetrics and Gynecology*. 1986; **67**: 384–7.

57. Steinbrook RA, Carr DB, Datta S et al. Dissociation of plasma and cerebrospinal fluid beta-endorphin-like immunoactivity levels during pregnancy and parturition. *Anesthesia and Analgesia*. 1982; **61**: 893–7.

58. Kennell J, Klaus M, McGrath S et al. Continuous emotional support during labor in a US hospital. A randomized controlled trial. *Journal of the American Medical Association*. 1991; **265**: 2197–201.

* 59. Lamaze F. *Painless childbirth: psychoprophylactic method*. Chicago: Regnery, 1970.

* 60. Reading AE, Cox DN. Psychosocial predictors of labor pain. *Pain*. 1985; **22**: 309–15.

61. Dannenbring D, Stevens MJ, House AE. Predictors of childbirth pain and maternal satisfaction. *Journal of Behavioral Medicine*. 1997; **20**: 127–42.

62. Brown ST, Campbell D, Kurtz A. Characteristics of labor pain at two stages of cervical dilation. *Pain*. 1989; **38**: 289–95.

63. Sheiner E, Sheiner EK, Shoham-Vardi I. The relationship between parity and labor pain. *International Journal of Gynaecology and Obstetrics*. 1998; **63**: 287–8.

64. Ranta P, Jouppila P, Jouppila R. The intensity of labor pain in grand multiparas. *Acta Obstetrica et Gynecologica Scandinavica*. 1996; **75**: 250–4.

65. Gaston-Johansson F, Fridh G, Turner-Norvell K. Progression of labor pain in primiparas and multiparas. *Nursing Research*. 1988; **37**: 86–90.

66. Cogan R, Henneborn W, Klopfer F. Predictors of pain during prepared childbirth. *Journal of Psychosomatic Research*. 1976; **20**: 523–33.

67. Ranta P, Jouppila P, Spalding M, Jouppila R. The effect of maternal obesity on labour and labour pain. *Anaesthesia*. 1995; **50**: 322–6.

68. Roberts J, Malasanos L, Mendez-Bauer C. Maternal positions in labor: analysis in relation to comfort and efficiency. *Birth Defects Original Article Series*. 1981; **17**: 97–128.

69. Bloom SL, McIntire DD, Kelly MA et al. Lack of effect of walking on labor and delivery. *New England Journal of Medicine*. 1998; **339**: 76–9.

70. Lieberman E, Davidson K, Lee-Parritz A, Shearer E. Changes in fetal position during labor and their association with epidural analgesia. *Obstetrics and Gynecology*. 2005; **105**: 974–82.

71. Oriol NE, Leonard M. Labor pain. In: Warfield CA (ed.). *Manual of pain management*, 1st edn. New York: JB Lippincott, 1991: 220–6.

72. Brownridge P. Treatment options for the relief of pain during childbirth. *Drugs*. 1991; **41**: 69–80.

73. Beck NC, Hall D. Natural childbirth. A review and analysis. *Obstetrics and Gynecology*. 1978; **52**: 371–9.

* 74. Scott KD, Berkowitz G, Klaus M. A comparison of intermittent and continuous support during labor: a meta-analysis. *American Journal of Obstetrics and Gynecology*. 1999; **180**: 1054–9.

∗ 75. Simkin PP, O'Hara M. Nonpharmacologic relief of pain during labor: systematic reviews of five methods. *American Journal of Obstetrics and Gynecology.* 2002; **186**: S131–59.

76. Ramnero A, Hanson U, Kihlgren M. Acupuncture treatment during labour – a randomised controlled trial. *BJOG.* 2002; **109**: 637–44.

77. Skilnand E, Fossen D, Heiberg E. Acupuncture in the management of pain in labor. *Acta Obstetricia et Gynecologica Scandinavica.* 2002; **81**: 943–8.

78. Duchene P. Effects of biofeedback on childbirth pain. *Journal of Pain and Symptom Management.* 1989; **4**: 117–23.

79. Huntley AL, Coon JT, Ernst E. Complementary and alternative medicine for labor pain: a systematic review. *American Journal of Obstetrics and Gynecology.* 2004; **191**: 36–44.

80. Trolle B, Moller M, Kronborg H, Thomsen S. The effect of sterile water blocks on low back labor pain. *American Journal of Obstetrics and Gynecology.* 1991; **164**: 1277–81.

81. Wiruchpongsanon P. Relief of low back labor pain by using intracutaneous injections of sterile water: a randomized clinical trial. *Journal of the Medical Association of Thailand.* 2006; **89**: 571–6.

∗ 82. Norris MC, Grieco WM, Borkowski M *et al.* Complications of labor analgesia: epidural versus combined spinal epidural techniques. *Anesthesia and Analgesia.* 1994; **79**: 529–37.

∗ 83. Collis RE, Davies DW, Aveling W. Randomised comparison of combined spinal-epidural and standard epidural analgesia in labour. *Lancet.* 1995; **345**: 1413–16.

84. Stoddart AP, Nicholson KE, Popham PA. Low dose bupivacaine/fentanyl epidural infusions in labour and mode of delivery. *Anaesthesia.* 1994; **49**: 1087–90.

85. Noble HA, Enever GR, Thomas TA. Epidural bupivacaine dilution for labour. A comparison of three concentrations infused with a fixed dose of fentanyl. *Anaesthesia.* 1991; **46**: 549–52.

86. Chestnut DH, Laszewski LJ, Pollack KL *et al.* Continuous epidural infusion of 0.0625% bupivacaine–0.0002% fentanyl during the second stage of labor. *Anesthesiology.* 1990; **72**: 613–18.

87. Panni MK, Segal S. Local anesthetic requirements are greater in dystocia than in normal labor. *Anesthesiology.* 2003; **98**: 957–63.

88. Hess PE, Pratt SD, Soni AK *et al.* An association between severe labor pain and cesarean delivery. *Anesthesia and Analgesia.* 2000; **90**: 881–6.

89. Alexander JM, Sharma SK, McIntire DD *et al.* Intensity of labor pain and cesarean delivery. *Anesthesia and Analgesia.* 2001; **92**: 1524–8.

90. Olofsson C, Ekblom A, Ekman-Ordeberg G *et al.* Lack of analgesic effect of systemically administered morphine or pethidine on labour pain. *British Journal of Obstetric Gynaecology.* 1996; **103**: 968–72.

∗ 91. Bricker L, Lavender T. Parenteral opioids for labor pain relief: a systematic review. *American Journal of Obstetrics and Gynecology.* 2002; **186**: S94–109.

92. Evron S, Glezerman M, Sadan O *et al.* Remifentanil: a novel systemic analgesic for labor pain. *Anesthesia and Analgesia.* 2005; **100**: 233–8.

93. Olufolabi AJ, Booth JV, Wakeling HG *et al.* A preliminary investigation of remifentanil as a labor analgesic. *Anesthesia and Analgesia.* 2000; **91**: 606–08.

94. Lacassie HJ, Olufolabi AJ. Remifentanil for labor pain: is the drug or the method the problem? *Anesthesia and Analgesia.* 2005; **101**: 1242–3.

95. Rosen MA. Nitrous oxide for relief of labor pain: a systematic review. *American Journal of Obstetrics and Gynecology.* 2002; **186**: S110–26.

96. Carstoniu J, Levytam S, Norman P *et al.* Nitrous oxide in early labor. Safety and analgesic efficacy assessed by a double-blind, placebo-controlled study. *Anesthesiology.* 1994; **80**: 30–5.

97. McLeod DD, Ramayya GP, Tunstall ME. Self-administered isoflurane in labour. A comparative study with Entonox. *Anaesthesia.* 1985; **40**: 424–6.

98. McGuinness C, Rosen M. Enflurane as an analgesic in labour. *Anaesthesia.* 1984; **39**: 24–6.

99. Rosen MA. Paracervical block for labor analgesia: a brief historic review. *American Journal of Obstetrics and Gynecology.* 2002; **186**: S127–30.

100. King JC, Sherline DM. Paracervical and pudendal block. *Clinical Obstetrics and Gynecology.* 1981; **24**: 587–95.

101. LeFevre ML. Fetal heart rate pattern and postparacervical fetal bradycardia. *Obstetrics and Gynecology.* 1984; **64**: 343–6.

102. Rogers RE. Fetal bradycardia associated with paracervical block anesthesia in labor. *American Journal of Obstetrics and Gynecology.* 1970; **106**: 913–16.

103. Scudamore JH, Yates MJ. Pudendal block – a misnomer? *Lancet.* 1966; **1**: 23–4.

∗104. Leighton BL, DeSimone CA, Norris MC, Ben David B. Intrathecal narcotics for labor revisited: the combination of fentanyl and morphine intrathecally provides rapid onset of profound, prolonged analgesia. *Anesthesia and Analgesia.* 1989; **69**: 122–5.

105. Hodnett ED. Pain and women's satisfaction with the experience of childbirth: a systematic review. *American Journal of Obstetrics and Gynecology.* 2002; **186**: S160–72.

∗106. Breen TW, Shapiro T, Glass B *et al.* Epidural anesthesia for labor in an ambulatory patient. *Anesthesia and Analgesia.* 1993; **77**: 919–24.

∗107. Columb MO, Lyons G. Determination of the minimum local analgesic concentrations of epidural bupivacaine and lidocaine in labor. *Anesthesia and Analgesia.* 1995; **81**: 833–7.

108. Polley LS, Columb MO, Wagner DS, Naughton NN. Dose-dependent reduction of the minimum local analgesic concentration of bupivacaine by sufentanil for epidural analgesia in labor. *Anesthesiology.* 1998; **89**: 626–32.

109. Lyons G, Columb M, Hawthorne L, Dresner M. Extradural pain relief in labour: bupivacaine sparing by extradural fentanyl is dose dependent. *British Journal of Anaesthesia*. 1997; **78**: 493–7.

110. Hofmann-Kiefer K, Saran K, Brederode A *et al*. Ropivacaine 2 mg/mL vs. bupivacaine 1.25 mg/mL with sufentanil using patient-controlled epidural analgesia in labour. *Acta Anaesthesiologica Scandinavica*. 2002; **46**: 316–21.

111. McClure JH. Ropivacaine. *British Journal of Anaesthesia*. 1996; **76**: 300–07.

112. Polley LS, Columb MO, Naughton NN *et al*. Relative analgesic potencies of ropivacaine and bupivacaine for epidural analgesia in labor: implications for therapeutic indexes. *Anesthesiology*. 1999; **90**: 944–50.

∗113. Writer WD, Stienstra R, Eddleston JM *et al*. Neonatal outcome and mode of delivery after epidural analgesia for labour with ropivacaine and bupivacaine: a prospective meta-analysis. *British Journal of Anaesthesia*. 1998; **81**: 713–17.

∗114. Halpern SH, Breen TW, Campbell DC *et al*. A multicenter, randomized, controlled trial comparing bupivacaine with ropivacaine for labor analgesia. *Anesthesiology*. 2003; **98**: 1431–5.

∗115. Hughes D, Simmons SW, Brown J, Cyna AM. Combined spinal-epidural versus epidural analgesia in labour. *Cochrane Database of Systematic Reviews*. 2003; **CD003401**.

116. Sia AT, Chong JL, Chiu JW. Combination of intrathecal sufentanil 10 mug plus bupivacaine 2.5 mg for labor analgesia: is half the dose enough? *Anesthesia and Analgesia*. 1999; **88**: 362–6.

117. Yeh HM, Chen LK, Shyu MK *et al*. The addition of morphine prolongs fentanyl-bupivacaine spinal analgesia for the relief of labor pain. *Anesthesia and Analgesia*. 2001; **92**: 665–8.

118. Hess PE, Vasudevan A, Snowman C, Pratt SD. Small dose bupivacaine-fentanyl spinal analgesia combined with morphine for labor. *Anesthesia and Analgesia*. 2003; **97**: 247–52.

27

Acute pain management in children

RICHARD F HOWARD

KEY LEARNING POINTS

- Children of all ages, including premature neonates, are capable of experiencing acute pain.
- Pain should be assessed, using a developmentally appropriate method, in all situations where acute pain is possible.
- Analgesic pharmacology during development is increasingly well understood, and consequently effective and safe analgesic protocols can be developed for the management of acute pain in children of all ages.

- The evidence-base for pediatric acute pain has improved substantially in recent years due to the efforts of researchers, professional organizations, and regulating bodies in many countries of the world.
- Guidelines are available from prominent professional organizations relating to many aspects of pain management in children including acute postoperative and procedural pain.

INTRODUCTION

The obvious difference in physical and cognitive development between a preterm neonate and an adolescent has a profound influence on the way they respond to acute pain and the effects of analgesics. The challenges of pediatric acute pain management are therefore to be able to measure pain as accurately as possible at all ages in this extremely heterogeneous patient group, and to safely and effectively adapt analgesic strategies to meet changing requirements during development.

Today, a great deal is known about how to recognize and manage acute pain in children but, historically, children's pain was often unrecognized and undertreated.

This was especially true of the newborn, as for many years they were thought to be too immature to adequately process nociceptive inputs and therefore not in need of analgesia. This viewpoint was partly sustained by the belief that neonates, infants, and children were more likely to suffer dangerous side effects from potent analgesics such as opioid-induced respiratory depression or even "addiction," and therefore withholding of such treatments was prudent.[1, 2] The study of developmental neurophysiology and pharmacology has changed these views; it is now universally accepted that even the smallest and most premature infant is capable of responding to painful stimulation and that appropriate analgesia should be administered to children of all ages when pain is observed or expected. This chapter will focus on the principles of acute pain management in children and relevant developmental pharmacology. A more detailed account of the developmental neurobiology of pain can be found in Chapter 2, Developmental neurobiology of nociception, and of psychologically based therapies in Chapter 16, Psychological interventions for acute pediatric pain. The assessment of pain, detailed descriptions of techniques and protocols for pain management, and the organization of pain management services are also discussed in the relevant chapters in the *Practical applications and procedures* volume.

THE STUDY OF PAIN IN CHILDREN

Although there have been great advances in recent years, our knowledge of the effects of injury, pain, and analgesia during development still lags far behind what is known about the fully mature human. Currently, the majority of drugs used for pediatric acute pain management are those that have been in more general use for many years. Efficacy and safety are first established in adult populations and new drugs take some time to establish a place in the treatment of children's pain. Particularly worrisome is the fact that many commonly administered analgesics have not been sufficiently investigated in children and therefore are not officially sanctioned or "licensed" for sale or use in pediatric populations. Such "off-label" prescribing of medication is frequent in pediatric practice and can lead to inappropriate withholding of treatment or subjection of children to unnecessary risks.[3, 4, 5] This situation has been recognized as unnecessary and undesirable, resulting in legislative moves and other initiatives initially in the US, and later in the EU, designed to encourage the proper investigation of drugs in children by offering economic advantages to pharmaceutical companies, and requiring that new drugs be at least partly studied in children.[6, 7] Nevertheless, "off-label" use of analgesics and other drugs is still commonplace and a significant cause for concern.[8, 9]

Clinical trials in children are notoriously difficult to conduct. They are particularly subject to methodological problems and complex ethical issues involving recruitment, informed consent, and the use of placebo.[10] In the case of analgesic studies, investigation in children has been further complicated by the lack of widespread adoption of valid, comparable, and reproducible outcome measures. These factors increase costs, have weakened study design, and reduce recruitment rates such that many trials are small and their conclusions difficult to interpret, combine, or compare in meta-analyses and systematic reviews. However, evidence-based guidance is beginning to emerge from a number of sources including the UK Royal College of Nursing, the Australian and New Zealand College of Anaesthetists, and the Association of Paediatric Anaesthetists of Great Britain and Ireland.[11, 12, 13]

Recent advances in pain assessment and better coordination of clinical trials following the establishment of research networks should also go some way to help to redress these problems.

THE DEVELOPMENT OF NOCICEPTION AND THE RESPONSE TO INJURY

The mechanisms of acute pain include both the peripheral and central components of the response to noxious stimulation and injury. From birth to maturity, substantial modifications of these mechanisms take place, which profoundly changes both the immediate and longer-term behavioral response to pain during this period. This process of maturation is known to be at least in part "activity-dependent" in that sensory inputs leading to activation and strengthening of synaptic connections and pain pathways are essential for normal development. It is now also known that excessive or abnormal injury-related activity at critical periods of development can lead to persistent structural and functional changes that are not seen if the same injury occurs in the adult.[14] Clearly, if we are to understand and treat appropriately the response to acute pain in children, a knowledge of the influence of development on nociceptive processes and the effects of analgesia are essential. A detailed account of the underlying biology is given in Chapter 2, Developmental neurobiology of nociception.

PAIN ASSESSMENT

Pain assessment is central to good pain management but the considerable range of psychological development, cognitive and communication abilities, behavioral and physiological responses between the preterm neonate and an adolescent, present enormous problems for valid and reliable measurement. There is a vast literature on pediatric pain assessment and many pain measurement "tools" have been devised and validated for use at different ages and clinical settings; for the neonate alone, at least 14 tools have been described (**Table 27.1**). No single tool or measure has been shown to be accurate at all ages and in all contexts, but consensus is beginning to emerge regarding the best choice for the most frequently encountered circumstances: this is discussed in detail in Chapter 38, Pain assessment in children in the *Practice and Procedures* volume of this series.

Principles of pain assessment

The complexities of measuring pain in children require that heathcare professionals receive suitable education, training, and support in order to implement meaningful assessment. Children are usually part of a wider family

Table 27.1 Neonatal pain assessment tools.

	Pain assessment tool	Age suitability	Acute pain validity
1[a]	CRIES[15]	Full-term neonates	Postoperative
	CRying, Increased vital signs, Expression, and Sleeplessness		
2	LIDS[16]	Full-term neonates	Postoperative
	Liverpool Infant Distress Scale		
3	PAT[17]	Full-term neonates	Postoperative
	Pain Assessment Tool		
4	CHIPPS[18]	Neonate–5 years	Postoperative
	Children's and Infants Postoperative Pain Scale		
5	CSS[19]	1–7 months	Postoperative
	Clinical Scoring System		
6	NAPI[20]	Infants 1–36 months	Postoperative
	Neonatal Assessment of Pain Inventory		
7	NFCS[21]	Preterm–3 months	Procedural pain
	Neonatal Facial Coding System		
8	IBCS[22]	Preterm–full-term neonates	Procedural pain
	Infant Body Coding System		
9	NIPS[23]	Preterm–full-term neonates	Procedural pain
	Neonatal Infant Pain Scale		
10[a]	PIPP[24]	Preterm–full-term neonates	Procedural pain
	Premature Infant Pain Profile		
11	SUN[25]	Preterm–full-term neonates	Procedural pain
	Scale for Use in Newborns		
12	BPS[26]	Preterm–full-term neonates	Procedural pain– ventilated
	Behavioral Pain Score		
13	DSVNI[27]	Preterm–full-term neonates	Procedural pain–ventilated
	Distress Scale for Ventilated Newborn Infants		
14[a]	COMFORT[28]	Full-term–3 years	Postoperative pain
15	Modified COMFORT[29]	Preterm neonate	Procedural pain

Adapted from Refs 18, 28, 29, 30.
[a]Recommended for clinical use.[13]

unit whose values and beliefs will impact on pain assessment and management. As far as possible parents and families should be educated, consulted, and encouraged to participate in this process. In some circumstances parents are expected to supervise analgesia at home, for example following day surgery, and in this case, they should also be given suitable information and support. Acute pain measurement is concerned with both the static and dynamic elements of pain such that tools are generally described as being valid for brief "incident" pain such as that due to procedures, or for more complex situations such as postoperative pain (or both). In general, self-report measures are suitable for both procedural and postoperative pain, whereas observational measures have been specifically validated for age and type of pain.

SELF-REPORT: AGE FIVE YEARS AND ABOVE

Pain is a subjective experience and so self-report is generally considered to be the most accurate method. Clearly, many children do not have sufficient verbal skills or cognitive ability to be able to describe their pain consistently and accurately. Self-report by children is therefore complex, nevertheless it remains the preferred method whenever possible.[31][I] There is no agreement regarding the age threshold for self-report; in practice it is feasible from about five years of age onwards (range three to seven years). It should be combined with effective communication between clinical professionals, children, and their families as this will help considerably in the interpretation of reports.[32] A large number of child-friendly self-report tools have been devised, typically using graphics such as faces as an aid to understanding. Recently, over 30 of such tools have been evaluated in a systematic review, six were found to possess well-established evidence of reliability and validity including visual analog scales (VAS) for older children and adolescents and a number of faces type scales designed for children as young as three years old.[31] These tools are described in detail in Chapter 38, Pain assessment in children in the *Practice and Procedures* volume of this series.

INDIRECT METHODS OF ASSESSMENT: NEONATES, INFANTS, AND CHILDREN

Observations of behavior and physiological parameters are used to provide proxy measurements of pain when self-report is not feasible, for example in the very young, or those with cognitive or communication impairment. There is little evidence to recommend the use of physiological measures alone to assess pain, largely because of wide interindividual variability and the tendency for values to regress with time due to homeostatic mechanisms.[18, 33] Behavior is more reliable but it is subject to modification by developmental age, affect or mood, anxiety, distress, hunger, somnolence, or behavioral state and many drug treatments. Consequently, behavioral tools are generally shown to be valid and reliable for particular patient groups and clinical settings. Facial expression has been found to be one of the most universally reliable behaviors; it is one of five observations identified as providing the most valid information in assessment tools (see **Box 27.1**).[18, 34] In clinical practice, a distinction is usually drawn between the neonatal period and infants and children up to the age of the ability to self-report. **Table 27.1** shows tools validated for use in neonates; of those listed, tools which have been recommended for clinical use are the Premature Infant Pain Profile (PIPP), CRying, Increased vital signs, Expression, and Sleeplessness (CRIES), COMFORT, and Neonatal Facial Coding System (NFCS).[13, 15, 24, 28, 29]

For older children, again there are a large number of behavioral tools available: in a recent systematic review, 20 tools designed for use in children aged over three years were evaluated. Six, listed in **Table 27.2**, were found to have well-established evidence of reliability and validity and they are discussed in detail in Chapter 38, Pain assessment in children in the *Practice and Procedures* volume of this series.[41] [I]

INDIRECT METHODS: NEURODISABILITY AND COMMUNICATION IMPAIRED

Although children with neurodisability who may be cognitively and communication impaired are likely to undergo surgery, there has been little investigation of suitable pain assessment tools. The Face, Legs, Arms, Cry, Consolability (FLACC) tool has been adapted for use in this group of patients, and two new tools specifically developed the Pediatric Pain Profile (PPP) and the Noncommunicating Children's Pain Checklist (NCCPC) (see Chapter 38, Pain assessment in children in the *Practice and Procedures* volume of this series, for a fuller discussion).[42, 43, 44]

PRINCIPLES OF ACUTE PAIN MANAGEMENT

Multimodal or balanced analgesia

Current strategies for the treatment of acute pain in children are centered on the concept of multimodal analgesia which was first proposed in order to increase the efficacy of analgesics whilst reducing their adverse effects.[45] The supporting rationale is that the major pharmacological groups of analgesics act on different components of pain pathways and as such their effects are likely to be complementary. It is therefore logical to give these analgesics, such as paracetamol, nonsteroidal anti-inflammatory drugs (NSAIDs), opioids, and local anesthetics in conjunction in order to achieve the optimum effect whilst keeping the dose of each, and therefore side effects, at a moderate level. Psychological pain management strategies should also be combined with pharmacological analgesia (see Chapter 16, Psychological interventions for acute pediatric pain).

Information and protocols: pain management plan

Training and education for healthcare workers and information for patients, families, and carers are pivotal for successful acute pain management. As acute pain is frequently predictable in its onset, severity, and time course, analgesic regimens can be preplanned and implemented with supporting educational programs, provision of necessary equipment, and management protocols. Pain management protocols must be sufficiently flexible to allow for differences in analgesic requirements due to developmental and other factors and to cater for individual preferences. It should include a pain assessment and reassessment plan, the management of background and incident pain, monitoring for adverse effects and their management, and how and from whom to seek timely help and advice if necessary. A well-designed protocol ensures efficacy and uniformity of

---

Box 27.1 Information for families regarding postoperative pain management at home

- The nature and extent of the planned surgical procedure.
- The site and intensity of expected pain.
- The expected duration of pain.
- How to assess pain: including use of an assessment scale.
- Analgesia and doses, frequency of administration.
- Expected side-effects and their management.
- How and when to seek further advice after discharge from hospital.

Table 27.2 Behavioral tools for infants and older children.

	Pain assessment tool	Acute pain validity
1	FLACC[35]	Postoperative and procedural
	Face, Legs, Arms, Cry, Consolability	
2	CHEOPS[36]	Procedural
	Children's Hospital of E. Ontario Pain Scale	
3	PPPM[37]	Postoperative: at home
	Parents Postoperative Pain Measure	
4	COMFORT[38]	Postoperative and procedural: in critical care
5	PBCL[39]	Procedural: pain-related fear and distress
	Procedure Behavior Check List	
6	PBRS-R[40]	Procedural: pain-related fear and distress
	Procedure Behavioral Rating Scale-Revised	

treatment and will facilitate ongoing evaluation and audit of effectiveness and the incidence of adverse effects. An individual, or group of individuals, must be responsible for the implementation of pain management, and the concept of pain management services has developed from an awareness of this. Such services can be invaluable in the provision and organization of pain management and are discussed in detail in Chapter 50, Organization of pediatric pain services in the *Practice and Procedures* volume of this series.

The role of parents and families

The implementation of family-centered care involving the establishment of a partnership between parents or carers and nursing staff and other healthcare workers has substantially increased parents' role in their child's in-hospital care. An increase in day-stay surgery also means that pain management is frequently devolved to parents at home. Parents may have considerable anxiety about pain and its treatment and have preconceptions, misconceptions, and prejudices about analgesics and their use.[46, 47] If parents are to be expected to initiate therapy and actively participate in management plans, they require considerable support, information, and education (**Box 27.1**).

PHARMACOLOGY OF ANALGESICS FOR PEDIATRIC ACUTE PAIN

In comparison with adults, relatively few analgesics have a clearly established role in pediatric acute pain management. Detailed analgesic clinical pharmacology is discussed in Chapter 3, Clinical pharmacology: opioids; Chapter 4, Clinical pharmacology: traditional NSAIDs and selective COX-2 inhibitors; Chapter 5, Clinical pharmacology: paracetamol and compound analgesics;

Chapter 6, Clinical pharmacology: other adjuvants; and Chapter 7, Clinical pharmacology: local anesthetics.

Systemic analgesics: paracetamol, NSAIDs, opioids

PARACETAMOL (ACETAMINOPHEN)

Paracetamol is an antipyretic and mild analgesic that has been widely used for all ages, including premature neonates, for many years. The precise mechanism of action of paracetamol is unknown but central cyclooxygenase (COX) inhibition is probably important. Other mechanisms have also been proposed including N-methyl-D-aspartate (NMDA) and serotonin antagonism.[48, 49] The efficacy of paracetamol for postoperative pain has been established in the adult, where it is frequently also combined with other analgesics such as codeine to produce modest improvements in analgesia.[50, 51][I] In infants and children, paracetamol has been found to be effective alone or as part of a multimodal analgesic strategy, and to have an opioid-sparing effect when given in conjunction with morphine patient-controlled analgesia (PCA).[52][II], [53][II], [54][II] Paracetamol is used ubiquitously for acute pain indications in pediatrics, where it is considered to be very safe, with few adverse effects provided that dosage recommendations are carefully followed (**Tables 27.3** and **27.4**).

Administration and pharmacokinetics

Paracetamol can be given by the oral, rectal, and intravenous (i.v.) routes. The pharmacokinetics and pharmacodynamics of paracetamol have been relatively well investigated in children; maximum dosage is largely determined by the potential for toxicity and the influence of age on clearance. Antipyretic plasma levels are 10–20 mg/L, levels required for analgesia are thought to be similar and so most dosing regimens aim to maintain

Table 27.3 Paracetamol dosing guide – oral and rectal administration.

Age	Route	Loading dose (mg/kg)	Maintenance dose (mg/kg)	Interval (h)	Maximum daily dose (mg/kg)	Duration at maximum dose (h)
28–32 weeks PCA	Oral	20	10–15	8–12	30	48
	Rectal	20	15	12		
32–52 weeks PCA	Oral	20	10–15	6–8	60	48
	Rectal	30	20	8		
>3 months	Oral	20	15	4	90	72
	Rectal	40	20	6		

PCA, postconceptual age.

Table 27.4 IV Paracetamol/ propacetamol dosing guide.[a]

Age	Drug	Loading dose (mg/kg)	Maintenance dose (mg/kg)	Dose interval (h)	Maximum daily dose (mg/kg)
<32 weeks PCA	Propacetamol	40	20	12	60
	Paracetamol	20	10	12	30
32–36 weeks PCA	Propacetamol	40	20	8	80
	Paracetamol	20	10	8	40
36–52 weeks PCA	Propacetamol	40	20	6	100
	Paracetamol	20	10	6	50
>1 month	Propacetamol	30	30	6	120
	Paracetamol	15	15	6	60

[a] Adapted from Ref. 55.

trough plasma concentrations of 10 mg/L.[56] A higher initial dose followed by maintenance doses not exceeding recommended maxima is generally recommended. Peak plasma levels are rapidly achieved after oral ingestion but there is a one to two hour lag before the maximum therapeutic effect, the onset of analgesia after i.v. administration may be much faster.[57] Rectal bioavailablity is much lower and more variable and so higher initial doses are recommended when this route is used. Rectal absorption is both age and formulation dependent up to the age of six months with relatively greater bioavailability in the premature neonate.[58] There are two i.v. preparations: i.v. paracetamol and propacetamol. Propacetamol is a prodrug which is hydrolyzed to 50 percent paracetamol and is therefore administered in twice the dose, i.e. 1 g propacetamol is equivalent to 500 mg paracetamol, this is a potential source of confusion and error.[55] Propacetamol clearance is reduced below one year of age and lower maintenance doses are therefore required.[59] Histamine release, pain on injection, and contact dermatitis in healthcare workers have been reported with propacetamol, mild platelet dysfunction may also occur.[60, 61] Intravenous paracetamol appears to be devoid of these drawbacks and therefore it has gained widespread acceptance in pediatric practice. See **Table 27.3** for suggested oral and rectal dosing and **Table 27.4** for i.v. dosing.

Side effects and toxicity

When recommended dosage limits are not exceeded, paracetamol is well tolerated. Hepatotoxicity of paracetamol is related to metabolism and excretion of the drug and may be age dependent with neonates being more sensitive, and infants less, than older children and adults.[58, 62] Toxicity has been mainly associated with large single doses of around 150 mg/kg or following chronic use of high doses, particularly in the youngest patients. It is therefore frequently recommended that in routine practice maximum doses only be continued for limited periods, and certainly not longer than five days.[63] Factors associated with liver toxicity include preexisting liver impairment, chronic ingestion in the malnourished, and accidental overdose due to misreading or misinterpretation of package labeling by parents.[64]

NSAIDs

NSAIDs act by inhibition of COX; enzymes that regulate many cellular functions by the production of prostaglandins and other substances. The detailed pharmacology of NSAIDs is discussed in Chapter 4, Clinical pharmacology: traditional NSAIDs and selective COX-2 inhibitors. Ibuprofen, diclofenac, and ketorolac are among the most widely investigated and prescribed for acute pain in children, they are safe and effective and are used interchangeably in clinical practice with the choice of drug largely determined by convenience of formulation (**Table 27.5**). NSAIDs are useful analgesics after minor to intermediate surgery.[65][I] They are often combined with paracetamol and moderate potency opioids such as codeine. Following major surgery they can reduce morphine requirements as part of a multimodal technique.[52][I], [53][II], [66] They are also used extensively where acute pain is associated with inflammation such as in juvenile rheumatoid arthritis (JRA). NSAIDs are not usually used for pain indications in the neonate.[67] Potentially troublesome side effects from NSAIDs include gastrointestinal irritation, renal impairment, exacerbation or precipitation of acute asthma in susceptible individuals, and platelet dysfunction and bleeding. Newer COX-2 selective NSAIDs have been introduced in an attempt to reduce the incidence of these effects but they have not been used widely in children; recent findings of possible increased cardiovascular risk in older adults has resulted in withdrawal of some compounds from the market and a reassessment of their value as a group, which is likely to delay any further introduction into pediatric practice.[68]

Administration and pharmacokinetics

A number of formulations are available: diclofenac is presented in oral and parenteral forms and as a convenient rectal suppository; ketorolac is usually given intravenously. Novel formulations such as eye drops and transdermal patches are also available but have not yet found their place in routine practice. Clearance of NSAIDs increases with age up to about five years old, but there is large interindividual variability in pharmacokinetic parameter estimates due to interaction of age, size, and pharmacogenomic factors such as functional polymorphism in genetic coding for important metabolizing enzymes.[69]

Side effects and toxicity

The most commonly reported adverse effects are bleeding, gastrointestinal symptoms, skin rashes, respiratory, and renal toxicity.[70, 71]

Bleeding

NSAIDs reversibly inhibit the formation of thromboxane A2 and platelet endoperoxides. Platelet dysfunction may lead to increased intraoperative and postoperative blood loss, and if associated with peptic ulceration, gastrointestinal bleeding. Mostly, this is considered a low risk, but significantly increased blood loss has been consistently identified following tonsillectomy; ketorolac has been particularly implicated, but not in other postoperative models.[65][III], [72] A number of meta-analyses have been performed in an attempt to resolve this issue but they have included different trials (including different NSAIDs, populations, and ages) and reached different conclusions.[73, 74, 75, 76] Overall, any risk must be balanced against significant improvements in analgesia and reduction in postoperative nausea and vomiting (PONV) when NSAIDs are used.[75][I], [76][I] Ibuprofen and diclofenac appear to be associated with a very low risk of post-tonsillectomy bleeding, but there is currently insufficient data to assess the risk for individual NSAIDs.[13]

Asthma

Patients with aspirin-induced asthma may be cross-sensitive to NSAIDs. Some caution has also been advised in the use of NSAIDs in the presence of respiratory wheeze in asthmatic patients. Diclofenac did not adversely affect respiratory function in a group of asthmatic children,[77] and in studies of children with fever given paracetamol or ibuprofen, asthma morbidity was in fact relatively reduced by ibuprofen.[78, 79] Risks of exacerbation of respiratory disease by NSAIDs in children may have been somewhat overemphasized. However, it has been suggested that NSAIDs be avoided in a small subgroup of adolescents with severe asthma and chronic rhinosinusitis with nasal polyposis who are likely to be more sensitive.[80]

Nephrotoxicity

NSAID-induced nephrotoxicity is well described. Dose-dependent toxicity induces a functional acute renal failure which resolves on discontinuation of the drug. Prostaglandins regulate renal blood flow in conditions of stress such as hypovolemia or following major surgery. The risk of renal failure is therefore higher in dehydrated, or otherwise hypovolemic patients and in patients with preexisting renal disease. Dose-independent interstitial nephritis with or without nephritic syndrome can also occur, it is treated conservatively or with corticosteroids.

Table 27.5 Dosages and dosage maximae for NSAIDs.

Drug	Class of analgesic	Routes of administration	Maximum doses
Ibuprofen	NSAID	Oral	30 mg/kg/day (5–10 mg/kg qds)
Diclofenac	NSAID	Oral	3 mg/kg/day (1 mg/kg tds)
		Rectal	3 mg/kg/day (1 mg/kg tds)
Ketorolac	NSAID	Oral	0.5–1 mg/kg qds
		Intravenous	0.5 mg/kg qds

MORPHINE

Morphine is the prototype opioid extensively investigated in children and there is considerable clinical experience in its use for the management of severe acute pain.

Administration and pharmacokinetics

Morphine can be given orally, parenterally, and neuraxially. Morphine solutions are well absorbed orally, formulations include a suspension and a slow-release compound. Parenteral morphine is usually given intravenously either by intermittent dosing, continuous infusion, or in a PCA or nurse-controlled analgesia (NCA) regimen. Subcutaneous morphine is also used. Preservative-free (as a precaution against chemical neurotoxicity) morphine is also effective in the epidural space or intrathecally.

The pharmacokinetics and clinical use of morphine in neonates, infants and children has been reviewed.[81, 82, 83, 84][III] The pharmacokinetics of morphine are developmentally regulated, although outside the neonatal period which is characterized by higher interpatient variability and reduced clearance, the effects of morphine are largely predictable. In neonates aged one to seven days, the clearance of morphine is 30 percent of that of older infants and children and elimination half-life is approximately 1.7 times longer.[84, 85] Infusion rates and dose intervals must therefore be adjusted according to both age and weight if accumulation is to be avoided. Although the plasma levels associated with analgesia are not well defined, a mean steady-state serum concentration of 10 ng/mL is a reasonable target. This level was achieved in children in intensive care after noncardiac surgery with a morphine hydrochloride infusion of 5 µg/kg/h at birth (term neonates), 8.5 µg/kg/h at one month, 13.5 µg/kg/h at three months, 18 µg/kg/h at one year, and 16 µg/kg/h for one- to three-year-old children.[83] A common threshold for respiratory depression in neonates, infants, and children has been defined as 20 ng/mL.[86]

Side effects and toxicity

Nausea and vomiting, sedation, and respiratory depression are the most frequently seen adverse effects of morphine (and other opioids), together with itching which is especially common after neuraxial administration. Depression of gastrointestinal motility and constipation also occur, usually with prolonged use. Adverse effects of morphine can be reversed with low doses of the opioid antagonist naloxone. In clinical practice, minor side effects can be managed by reducing the dose of morphine or with appropriate therapy, for example antiemetics, antipruritics, and laxatives.

FENTANYL

Fentanyl is a synthetic, high potency (100× morphine) lipid soluble opioid. Its main use is for intraoperative analgesia where its rapid onset and short initial half-life are an advantage.

Administration and pharmacokinetics

After i.v. administration, a single dose of fentanyl has a duration of 30–45 minutes. As fentanyl is highly lipid soluble, its pharmacokinetic profile is context sensitive such that half-life progressively increases with infusion duration.[87] It can be given parenterally, neuraxially, intranasally, and by oral transmucosal fentanyl citrate (OTFC) and transdermal techniques, the i.v. preparation has also been given orally where its pharmacokinetics resemble OTFC (see below under Administration and pharmacokinetics).[88] Fentanyl can be used for postoperative analgesia and for procedural pain, particularly when morphine is contraindicated. In the epidural space it is used alone or combined with local anaesthetic.[89, 90] A disposable iontophoretic transdermal fentanyl PCA system has been developed recently, which may also be suitable for older children.[91] OTFC has been used for premedication but highly variable bioavailability, PONV, and prolonged postoperative recovery have limited its popularity.[92]

Side effects and toxicity

Opioid-related side effects of sedation, respiratory depression, and itching are to be expected. Higher doses have been associated with chest wall rigidity, especially in the neonate, and such doses are therefore usually only given when respiration is controlled.[93]

HYDROMORPHONE

Hydromorphone is a semisynthetic opioid with high lipid solubility. It has been used widely for acute pain. A systematic review concluded that hydromorphone was similar to morphine in efficacy and side effects when used for both acute and chronic pain indications in adults and children.[94][I]

Administration and pharmacokinetics

The pharmacokinetics and pharmacodynamics of hydromorphone have been studied, including immediate release oral preparations, a variety of slow release oral preparations, as well as administration through intravenous, subcutaneous, epidural, intrathecal, and other routes.[95] It is known to be metabolized to analgesically inactive metabolites. Oral hydromorphone was equivalent to OTFC for procedural pain of burns dressings.[96][II] The efficacy of i.v. PCA hydromorphone was similar to morphine in the management of acute mucositis pain.[97][II] Epidural hydromorphone was similar in efficacy to epidural fentanyl or morphine for postoperative pain (1 µg/kg/h versus 10 µg/kg/h versus 1 µg/kg/h) after orthopedic procedures, but hydromorphone had an improved side-effect profile with less sedation than morphine and less PONV or urinary retention than either alternative.[98][II]

Side effects and toxicity

Opioid-related side effects of sedation, respiratory depression, and itching are to be expected with hydromorphone. Fewer side effects in comparison to morphine or fentanyl were reported when used in the epidural space following lower limb orthopedic surgery.[98][II]

DIAMORPHINE

Diamorphine is a potent opioid analgesic. It is more lipid soluble than morphine and can be used for similar acute pain indications. Diamorphine by the intranasal route has become popular for the management of procedural pain in the emergency department.[99, 100]

Administration and pharmacokinetics

Diamorphine can be given by a variety of routes including the oral, intranasal, parenteral, and for neuraxial analgesia, the epidural or intrathecal. Oral diamorphine has been mostly used for chronic pain. Intranasal diamorphine has a rapid onset and is effective for procedural pain, notably for fracture reduction in emergency departments.[101, 102][II] Intravenous diamorphine caused more rapid sedation and less hypotension than morphine in a group of neonates in the intensive care unit (ICU).[103][II] No age-related differences in the production of active morphine metabolites were found in a pharmacokinetic study of infants receiving intravenous diamorphine.[104] Diamorphine is an effective neuraxial analgesic, it has been used alone and in combination with local anesthetic in the caudal and lumbar epidural space.[105, 106][II], [107]

OXYCODONE AND HYDROCODONE

Oxycodone and hydrocodone are potent opioids that are used for both acute and chronic pain, their high oral bioavailablity has favored this route of administration. They are available in a number of proprietary oral preparations, frequently combined with paracetamol or aspirin (aspirin is unsuitable for children: see Chapter 4, Clinical pharmacology: traditional NSAIDs, and selective COX-2 inhibitors). They are the most frequent opioids of abuse among adults in the US, which is a major public health concern; their efficacy, which is similar to morphine, and wide availability are probably contributing factors.[108] Oxycodone is the better studied of the two, its clinical use has been reviewed recently.[109]

Administration and pharmacokinetics

Oxycodone is usually given by the oral or intravenous route, a long-acting sustained release oral preparation is available and it has also been given by the buccal route. The pharmacokinetics of oral, buccal, sublingual, and parenteral (intramuscular and intravenous) oxycodone have been studied in children.[110, 111, 112] Like morphine, pharmacokinetics are predictable over the age of six months, but marked interpatient variability has been noted in neonates and infants less than two months old.[113] Oxycodone reduced pain scores in children presenting with abdominal pain better than placebo, without masking clinical diagnostic signs of appendicitis.[114][II] The effective use of controlled release oxycodone for postoperative analgesia in children has also been described.[115][III]

Side effects and toxicity

Opioid-related side effects of sedation, respiratory depression, and itching are to be expected with oxycodone and hydrocodone. Hallucinations, an infrequent adverse effect of opioids, have been reported to be less frequent following oxycodone in comparison with morphine.[109][III]

CODEINE

Codeine is a low potency opioid that is popular in pediatric practice, it is used for mild to moderately severe pain, usually in combination with other analgesics such as paracetamol or NSAIDs.[116] Traditionally, codeine has been used where respiratory depression, sedation, or other opioid-related side effects are a particular concern, for example in the neonate and following neurosurgery, but the use of codeine for these indications has been challenged: see below.[116]

Administration and pharmacokinetics

Codeine can be given by the oral and intramuscular routes, it should not be given intravenously. Codeine is a morphine prodrug; approximately 10–15 percent is metabolized to morphine by the cytochrome P450 enzyme CYP2D6 and this metabolite is thought to be responsible for its analgesic effect as analgesia cannot be demonstrated in human volunteers in which the pathway is pharmacologically blocked. CYP2D6 activity is genetically regulated, 5–40 percent of individuals in some populations have reduced, little, or no activity ("slow and intermediate metabolizers") and consequently are less able to produce morphine from codeine, leading to unpredictability of effect.[117] CYP2D6 activity is also developmentally regulated, with lower levels in the very young.[118] Codeine should be avoided when pain assessment is difficult or impossible, and in individuals with reduced enzyme activity.

Side effects and toxicity

Opioid side effects are to be expected with codeine. Dangerous hypotension has been reported following intravenous administration, presumably due to histamine release.[119]

TRAMADOL

The clinical pharmacology of tramadol has been reviewed recently, it is a synthetic opioid analgesic that also inhibits serotonin and norepinephrine reuptake.[120] It is used widely for acute and chronic pain in children, and there is an extensive body of literature describing its efficacy and indications.

Administration and pharmacokinetics

Tramadol is most frequently given by the oral and parenteral routes, it can be given rectally, it has been given epidurally, and has been added to local anesthetics for peripheral nerve blockade and wound infiltration.[121, 122, 123, 124] The pharmacokinetics of parenteral, epidural, and rectal tramadol have been studied in children; values are broadly similar to those obtained in adults above the age of one year.[125, 126] Tramadol is metabolized by the cytochrome enzyme CYP2D6 to its major active metabolite o-desmethyltramadol, which has a 200× increased affinity for the mu opioid receptor. CYP2D6 is genetically and developmentally regulated (see above under Codeine and Administration and pharmacokinetics), which may have implications for the use of tramadol in some individuals and in very young patients. The pharmacokinetics of tramadol in neonates and infants has been investigated, no relationship between postmenstrual age and o-desmethyltramadol production was established, clearance is reduced in the newborn but reaches 80 percent of adult values by one month.[127, 128] The effect of CYP2D6 polymorphism on the efficacy and disposition of tramadol is not known.

Side effects and toxicity

Opioid side effects have been reported as less prominent with tramadol, but this is not confirmed when equianalgesic doses are used.[120, 129] Any potential for neurotoxicity of tramadol when used by the epidural route has not been explored.[124]

KETAMINE, CLONIDINE

These drugs exert their analgesic effects by novel modes of action on transmission in nociceptive pathways. Aside from their systemic use, they have been found to prolong the duration of action of caudal epidural local anesthetics.

KETAMINE

Ketamine is a glutamate NMDA receptor antagonist. It has been used for many years as an intravenous general anesthetic; its principal advantages being profound analgesia, relative preservation of respiration and respiratory reflexes, and cardiovascular stimulation. Ketamine produces a state of "dissociative" anesthesia, a disadvantage is that emergence phenomena including hallucinations and unpleasant dreams have been reported. At low doses (<1 mg/kg), it has been found to be an effective analgesic, in particular it appears to reduce the hypersensitivity due to "central sensitization" following

injury or surgery in both inflammatory and neuropathic conditions. Although there are numerous publications concerning the analgesic effects of ketamine, a recent systematic review concluded that its role in the management of postoperative pain in the adult remains unclear.[130] The NMDA receptor is known to undergo developmental changes in distribution, structure, and function, and is thought to be important in regulating neuronal plasticity during the developmental period.[14] The precise impact of this on the efficacy or toxicity of systemic or neuraxial ketamine (or other NMDA antagonists) during infancy and childhood is still not fully understood.

Administration and pharmacokinetics

Ketamine is a racemic mixture, the S(+) isomer has a faster onset, approximately twice the analgesic potency as the racemate but similar psychomimetic potency, it is available as an intravenous and preservative-free preparation.[131] The principal uses of ketamine in pediatric acute pain practice are as a neuraxial analgesic, principally in caudal epidurals, as an intravenous supplement to postoperative opioid analgesia, and as a sedative-analgesic for painful procedures.[132, 133, 134]

Side effects and toxicity

The side effects of ketamine depend on the dose and route of administration, additionally, the more potent S(+) isomer is associated with fewer unwanted effects for similar levels of analgesia. Hallucinations and dysphoria are not associated with low-dose regimens commonly used for analgesia. The potential for neurotoxicity from systemically or spinally administered NMDA antagonists is a concern, and has been the subject of considerable and ongoing debate.[135] Systemically administered ketamine, and a number of other substances including some sedatives and anesthetic agents, can produce damaging neurodegeneration in the rodent brain if exposure is during a critical period of early postnatal development.[136] The significance of these findings in humans and implications for clinical practice are not known.[137] Early studies in primates indicate that similar histological damage is possible but is critically dependent on age at exposure, drug dose, and duration of treatment, with highest risks being inter-utero and in the first few days of life.[138]

Spinally (epidural) preservative-free ketamine has not been implicated as a cause of neurotoxicity. Although it is presumed to be safe, it has not been directly investigated.[139]

CLONIDINE

Clonidine has analgesic, sedative, and antiemetic properties, it can also cause hypotension and bradycardia. It is an alpha2 adrenergic agonist that is capable of producing neuraxial analgesia and consequently has become popular for caudal analgesia in children, alone or as an adjunct to local anesthesia.[140] Clonidine is also used systemically for premedication, sedation in ICU areas, and for the symptomatic treatment of symptoms due to rapid withdrawal of opioid analgesia.[141]

Administration and pharmacokinetics

Systemic clonidine can be administered orally, parenterally, or rectally. Preservative-free solutions are used in the epidural space. Pharmacokinetic data are limited in children, the pharmacokinetics of epidural clonidine in one to nine year olds was found to be similar to that in adults.[142] Following systemic administration, plasma concentrations within the range of 0.2–2.0 ng/mL are thought to be effective.[143]

Side effects and toxicity

Dose-dependent sedation, hypotension, and bradycardia occurs following systemic clonidine. These effects are not thought to occur in children, outside the neonatal period, at plasma levels below 0.3 ng/mL.[142] Neonates appear to be more susceptible to the adverse effects of clonidine. Since an early description of severe delayed respiratory depression following 2 µg/kg caudal clonidine, there have been a number of similar reports of such events in neonates and caution is advised in this group of patients.[139, 140, 144, 145]

Local anesthetics

Local anesthesia (LA) is very important in pediatric acute pain management, particularly after surgery and for procedural pain. Topical LA, LA infiltration, peripheral, and central regional analgesia are all used extensively for acute pain indications. The detailed pharmacology of local anesthetics is discussed in Chapter 7, Clinical pharmacology: local anesthetics.

LIDOCAINE, BUPIVACAINE, LEVOBUPIVACAINE, AND ROPIVACAINE

Administration and pharmacokinetics

The amide-type LAs lidocaine and bupivacaine have been the most commonly used in children for several decades and there is considerable clinical experience of their efficacy and safety at all ages. Lidocaine has a rapid onset and is of short to intermediate duration, it is used for local infiltration and regional nerve blocks, particularly where a rapid response is required. Lidocaine, with prilocaine are the components of the topical preparation eutectic mixture of local anesthetics (EMLA). Bupivacaine has a slower onset and long duration, four hours analgesia or longer can be expected following single dose central nerve blocks, and consequently it is has been the first choice for postoperative analgesia. Their pharmacology and pharmacokinetics have been well investigated and were reviewed recently.[146] Bupivacaine is a racemic mixture. The

S(+) enantiomer, levobupivacaine, has a slightly improved *in vivo* and *in vitro* safety profile compared to bupivacaine but is otherwise similar.[147, 148] Ropivacaine is an amide LA with similar clinical properties to bupivacaine except that motor block is slower in onset, less intense, and shorter in duration.[139] Ropivacaine may have theoretical advantages during prolonged infusion in neonates and infants as unlike bupivacaine context sensitive half-life does not increase with increased duration of infusion.[139]

Side effects and toxicity

The toxicity of LAs depends on the age of the patient, the drug, absolute dose, and route of administration. Neurotoxicity and cardiotoxicity have been reported in children but provided that dosage recommendations are observed, toxic events are rare.[149] Fatal bupivacaine cardiotoxicity has occurred following intravenous regional analgesia (IVRA), and both bupivacaine and levobupivacaine are contraindicated for this procedure. Neonates may have a lower threshold for toxicity. LAs are extensively protein bound (>90 percent), the free, unbound, fraction is pharmacologically active and therefore important for toxicity. Alpha-acid glycoprotein (AAG) and albumin are the most important plasma proteins. AAG levels are lower in the neonate and increased unbound bupivacaine has been demonstrated in the newborn.[150] Plasma bupivacaine >3 µg/mL is associated with neurotoxicity in the awake adult, cardiotoxicty >4 µg/mL, the equivalent levels for neonates are not known but toxicity has been reported following bupivacaine infusion at "therapeutic" doses, leading to a reduction in recommended doses and infusion durations in the neonatal period.[151] In a study of ropivacaine infusion in children under one year, in contrast to bupivacaine, plasma levels did not continue to rise with infusion duration although absolute levels and free fraction were similarly increased at younger ages.[152]

Topical local anesthetics

Topical local anesthesia has revolutionized the practice of minor needle-related procedures such as venepuncture, venous cannulation, and lumbar puncture.[153] A number of preparations are available, the most frequently studied and used being EMLA and Ametop (amethocaine gel).

EMLA

Lidocaine forms a eutectic mixture with prilocaine such that the combination has a melting point lower than either of the constituents. This mixture, formulated as a cream, can produce local anesthesia when applied to intact skin.

Administration

It should be applied for approximately 60 minutes under an occlusive dressing, the duration of analgesia is several hours. EMLA is suitable for use in the neonate in single doses, multiple doses should be to a maximum of four a day and under close supervision; measurement of blood methemoglobin levels has been advised.[154, 155]

Side effects and toxicity

Transient paleness, redness, and edema of the skin may occur following application.

A metabolite of prilocaine, o-toluidine can lead to the development of methemoglobin, an oxidized form of hemoglobin which has a reduced oxygen carrying capacity. Methemoglobin reductase, the enzyme which catalyzes conversion to hemoglobin, is developmentally regulated, neonates are also susceptible because fetal hemoglobin is more easily oxidized.[156]

AMETOP

Tetracaine is a potent ester-type LA. Due to its high systemic toxicity, it is only used for intrathecal and surface anesthesia, approximately 15 percent bioavailability is expected after application to intact skin.

Administration

Four percent tetracaine gel produces surface anesthesia in approximately 30 minutes, it has an absorption and elimination half-life of about 75 minutes, the duration of analgesia is four to six hours. Ametop therefore produces a more rapid onset and longer lasting effect than EMLA. It has been shown to be effective in the neonate.[157][II]

Side effects and toxicity

Mild erythema at the site of application is seen frequently; edema of the skin, itching, and even blistering have been reported but are rare.

Nitrous oxide

Nitrous oxide is a weak anesthetic gas with analgesic properties, supplied compressed in metal cylinders and administered using specialized equipment. Premixed cylinders with 50 percent N_2O in O_2 are available (Entonox), but it is also sometimes administered in concentrations up to 70 percent. It has been used in dentistry for many years and is also used extensively for brief procedural pain in children who are cooperative and able to self-administer.[158]

ADMINISTRATION AND SIDE EFFECTS

Administration

Nitrous oxide is administered using a face-mask or mouthpiece and a demand-valve system, activated by negative pressure. Patients must be cooperative, willing, and able to use the apparatus unassisted following instruction as a safety feature is that should sedation occur, the patients' arm and hand will relax allowing the apparatus to fall away and prevent further administration.

Side effects and toxicity

Nitrous oxide is a weak general anesthetic and will potentiate the effect of other sedatives and anesthetics. Frequent but usually minor side effects include dizziness, nausea, dry mouth, and disorientation. It is insoluble and readily diffuses into gas-filled enclosed spaces causing them to expand or increase in pressure, nitrous oxide is therefore contraindicated in the presence of pneumothorax. Excessive sedation can occur and is treated by discontinuation of the gas, airway management, and oxygen administration.[158] Prolonged exposure may affect folate metabolism leading to megaloblastosis, anemia, and peripheral neuropathy. Bone marrow depression can occur. Exposure to prolonged high concentrations has been associated with reduced fertility in both men and women. Nitrous oxide should be used in well-ventilated areas which maintain ambient concentrations below national occupational exposure standards (100 ppm in the UK). Patients who are to receive N_2O more frequently than twice every four days should have regular blood examinations for megaloblastic changes and neutrophil hypersegmentation.[158]

Sucrose

Sucrose solutions reduce physiological and behavioral signs of pain in neonates during painful procedures.[159] [I] This effect is thought to be mediated by the activation of descending modulatory pathways, due to activity in brain stem opioid systems in response to the sweet taste.[160]

ADMINISTRATION AND SIDE EFFECTS

Administration

Studies have recommended 0.5–2.0 mL of a 24 percent solution of sucrose administered one to two minutes before a painful stimulus,[161] although studies have found that 0.05–2.0 mL of solutions 12–24 percent are effective.[159][I] It can be given using a pacifier or dripped directly onto the tongue using a syringe, the number of drops should be according to the infant's response.

Side effects and toxicity

Coughing, choking, gagging, and transient oxygen desaturation can occur. The safety of multiple administrations in very small preterm infants has been questioned as changes in neurobehavioral responses were observed after repeated sucrose administration in this group.[162, 163]

POSTOPERATIVE PAIN

Postoperative pain management should be planned prior to the procedure by the pediatric anesthetist in consultation with patients, their families, and other members of the perioperative team.[13] Initiation of postoperative pain relief is usually considered to be part of the plan of anesthesia; patients should not normally be discharged from the postanesthesia recovery unit until they are comfortable and a further pain management plan is established.

Most routine surgery in children is relatively minor and very often undertaken on a day-case or day-stay basis. This is psychologically and economically beneficial to children and their families, and is economically beneficial to providers of health care. Analgesia for such surgery must be effective and not delay discharge from hospital due to immobility, excessive sedation, or PONV. In practice, this means limiting or avoiding the use of opioids and long-acting sedatives whilst encouraging the use of local anesthetic techniques. Pain management will continue to be required at home, parents need information, education, and support (**Box 27.1**) in order to assume this responsibility, see earlier under The role of parents and families. Postoperative pain after day surgery should mostly be treatable with "over the counter" analgesics that are safe and easily obtainable by families. "Take home packs" containing supplies of analgesics and written information and instructions are often supplied prior to discharge from hospital.

Pain management following more major surgery can be required for several days or weeks. High potency analgesics such as parenteral opioids or local anesthetic infusions may be needed as part of a "balanced analgesia" approach. Pain management protocols should include pain assessment, monitoring, criteria for additional analgesia, management of side effects, and criteria for transition to simpler, usually oral, analgesia when appropriate.

LOCAL ANESTHETIC TECHNIQUES

Wound infiltration

Infiltration of the surgical wound is simple, safe, and useful, especially for very superficial surgery. Its utility is limited mainly by the need for large volumes of local anesthetic and dosage constraints. It has been shown to reduce early postoperative pain requirements after a number of procedures.

PROCEDURES

Herniorrhaphy

The quality of analgesia after inguinal hernia repair is comparable with ilioinguinal nerve block or caudal analgesia.[164][II], [165][II], [166][II], [167][II], [168][II] Analgesia after umbilical hernia repair was also good and little improved by supplementary ketorolac in one study.[169][II] Bupivacaine plasma levels were within the nontoxic range after infiltration of 1.25 mg/kg following inguinal herniorraphy.[170]

Squint (strabismus) surgery

Subconjunctival bupivacaine infiltation was as effective as retrobulbar block after strabismus surgery.[171][II] No comparisons with the more favored subtenon's block or peribulbar blocks are currently available.[13]

Dental surgery

Buccal (mandibular) bupivacaine or mepivacaine (an amide-type LA) infiltration was as effective as mandibular block for conservative dental procedures in children, but not extraction or pulpotomies.[172][II], [173][III], [174][II]

Tonsillectomy

The effectiveness of LA infiltration of the tonsillar bed is uncertain, a meta-analysis concluded that efficacy was equivocal and that more trials were required.[175][I] Further studies have shown benefits including increased time to first rescue analgesia, lower pain scores, less referred pain, and earlier oral intake.[176][II], [177][II], [178][III], [179][III], [180][II] Pain after tonsillectomy is a difficult clinical problem and the severity may relate to the technique of surgery and the experience of the surgeon.[181, 182] Pain after tonsillectomy persists for several days; it has also been suggested that children who received LA infiltration experienced less early postoperative pain but more pain later, clearly this requires further investigation.[183]

Simple nerve blocks for minor and intermediate surgery

INGUINAL BLOCK

The ilioinguinal and iliohypogastric nerves supplying the sensory innervation to the groin area are easy to locate and block, ultrasound improves success rates and reduces the dose of LA required.[184][II], [185] Surgical exploration of the inguinal region includes herniorraphy, ligation of patent processus vaginalis, and orchidopexy. The scrotum is also innervated by the genital branch of the genitofemoral nerve and so additional analgesia may be required following a scrotal incision for orchidopexy. Plasma levels of bupivacaine and ropivacaine following ilioinguinal block have been measured, uptake is more rapid with bupivacaine but concentrations were below toxic levels following 1.25–2 and 3 mg/kg, respectively.[170, 186, 187, 188] Reported complications include quadriceps weakness due to femoral nerve block and, rarely, inadvertent colonic perforation.[189, 190] No difference in voiding interval was found between patients who had ilioinguinal block or caudal epidural block.[191][II]

Herniorraphy

Ilioinguinal block is as effective as LA wound infiltration/installation and caudal epidural analgesia.[192, 193, 194][III]

Orchidopexy

Some studies have shown that ilioinguinal block is effective for orchidopexy pain[193][III], [192] but caudal analgesia may be superior.[195][II], [196]

PENILE BLOCK (DORSAL NERVE BLOCK)

The distal one-third of the penis is supplied by the dorsal nerves, which can easily be blocked. Analgesia is suitable for surgery on the urethral meatus, circumcision, and minor hypospadias repair. For pain in the postoperative period, the block has been compared to subcutaneous ring block and caudal epidural block. Penile block has been advocated for the procedural pain of awake neonatal circumcision. Plasma bupivacaine and lidocaine after dorsal nerve block have been compared and found to be well below toxic levels.[197] Reported complication rates are low, but may include bruising or hematoma at the site of injection, occasionally leading to venous compression and swelling.[198, 199] Gangrene of the penis has been reported secondary to a large hematoma, and ischemia was observed following the use of an epinephrine containing solution, which is therefore contraindicated.[200, 201]

Circumcision

Dorsal nerve block is effective for postcircumcision pain.[202, 203][I] It has been shown to be more reliable than subcutaneous ring block,[204][II] and is similar in efficacy to caudal analgesia.[202, 205, 206][II]

Many studies have investigated dorsal block for neonatal circumcision without general anesthesia. It is more effective than topical LA, sucrose, or placebo.[207][I]

INFRAORBITAL NERVE BLOCK

The infraorbital nerve supples the upper lip, lower eyelid, and adjacent skin of the cheek and nose. Unilateral or bilateral infraorbital nerve block can provide analgesia after cleft lip surgery and superficial surgery in the midface.[208][IV] It has been shown to be feasible and effective following cleft lip repair for neonates, infants, and children.[209, 210, 211][II] Two approaches are possible, intraoral and subcutaneous. Intraoral block with 0.125 percent bupivacaine was superior to local infiltration with the same solution in infants and children aged 4–20 months.[210][II]

BRACHIAL PLEXUS BLOCK

Pain after surgery on the hand and forearm can be achieved by block of the brachial plexus using a number of techniques. The brachial plexus is easily and safely accessed by the axillary approach with an acceptable failure rate of 2–6 percent in prospective and retrospective studies.[212][IV], [213, 214][II] Catheter techniques prolong the block and neurological outcome is similar to single injection.[215][IV] This approach has also been used for the procedural pain of forearm fracture reduction.[216][II], [217] Infraclavicular[218][III], [219, 220][IV] approaches are also feasible.

FEMORAL NERVE BLOCK/FASCIA ILIACA COMPARTMENT BLOCK

The upper anterior aspect of the thigh is supplied by the femoral nerve, lateral cutaneous nerve of thigh, and the obturator nerve. Block of the femoral nerve alone or combined with block of the lateral cutaneous nerve has been advocated for superficial procedures of the anterolateral thigh such as skin grafting or muscle biopsy, and also for the pain of fracture of the femur. More complete analgesia in this region is obtained by a single injection as first described in adults, i.e. Winnie's "3 in 1" block. This approach may be less effective in children because of limited spread of the local anesthetic.[221][II] The fascia iliaca "compartment block" reliably blocks the femoral nerve and concurrently achieves lateral cutaneous nerve block in 90 percent of children and obturator nerve block in 75 percent, continuous infusions of bupivacaine 0.01 percent were effective with acceptable plasma levels.[221, 222][IV]

CAUDAL EPIDURAL BLOCK

Caudal analgesia is frequently used in pediatric postoperative pain management with a well-established and extremely important role in postoperative pain relief for surgery in the lower abdomen, perineum, and lower limbs. The caudal approach to the epidural space is technically easy in children, and is described in detail elsewhere. It is also one of the most studied of all local anesthetic techniques in children, where it has been found to be safe and effective in several large series including children of all ages, including neonates.[223, 224, 225][III]

The spread of local anesthetic solution, and hence the extent of analgesia, is related to the volume injected and the age or weight of the patient. Several formulae have been developed: a modification of that suggested by Armitage[226] and given in **Table 27.6** is simple and easy to remember. Of course, such calculations are only estimates and interindividual variation is to be expected. The pharmacokinetics of caudal local anesthetics in children have been studied; plasma concentrations of bupivacaine, levobupivacaine, and ropivacaine remain within safe limits after single caudal injection of 2 mg/kg at all ages.[227, 228][II]

The complications of caudal analgesia can be minimized by meticulous attention to technique: the most

Table 27.6 Caudal local anesthetic block volume versus height of block.

Volume of local anesthetic solution (mL/kg)	Extent of blockade
0.5	Sacral-pelvic
1.0	Lumbar
1.25	Lower thoracic

important are vascular puncture, dural puncture, and inadvertent intravascular or intradural injection. Epidural infection has not been reported following single caudal local anesthetic injections.

Unwanted motor block is greater with bupivacaine, particularly at concentrations of 2.5 mg/mL or greater, both levobupivacaine or ropivacaine 2 mg/mL result in acceptably low incidences.[145, 229][II] Caudal analgesia has been associated with a small but statistically significant delay in the passage of urine after surgery when compared with penile block or subcutaneous "ring block" for circumcision.[202, 230, 231][II] However, in comparison with ilioinguinal block for hernia repair or orchidopexy, caudal analgesia was not associated with a delay in micturition, interestingly some patients in this study did not void for eight hours following surgery.[191][II] Delay in the passage of urine may occur following surgery, and the time to first micturition is very variable. Analgesia is one of many factors that may influence time to first micturition including recent fluid intake, site of surgery, anesthesia, and the duration of the procedure.

Analgesic combinations for caudal analgesia

A number of drugs have been added to the local anesthetic in an attempt to prolong analgesia including opioids, ketamine, clonidine, neostigmine, and midazolam, all these "adjuncts" appear to improve efficacy and prolong the duration of the technique.[232][II], [233, 234, 235][II] Preservative-free solutions of opioids, usually combined with local anesthetic, are frequently infused into the epidural space following major surgery. Single doses of caudal epidural morphine can produce prolonged but modest improvements in analgesia. Small but real risks of early or delayed respiratory depression, and the introduction of higher rates of PONV and itching have limited their use, and so caudal opioids are not now generally recommended following minor procedures or for day-case surgery.[236] S-ketamine and clonidine have been used in a number of studies, alone or in combination with local anesthetic; they are undoubtedly effective but there is insufficient information regarding their potential for adverse effects, particularly possible spinal neurotoxicity, to allow unqualified recommendations for their use, nor for the less studied midazolam and neostigmine.[236, 237][I]

Complex nerve blocks for major surgery

INTERCOSTAL BLOCK

Intercostal nerve blocks have been used extensively in adult practice, particularly following subcostal incisions for cholecystectomy. In children, the use of single and continuous blocks has been described for post-thoracotomy pain and for pain following liver transplantation.[238][II], [239, 240] The pharmacokinetics of intercostal bupivacaine have been studied in infants and children at doses of 1.5 and 2.0 mg/kg, respectively; peak plasma levels are reached after ten minutes but were below those associated with toxicity.[241, 242]

PARAVERTEBRAL BLOCK

Paravertebral block has been suggested as an alternative to intercostal, ilioinguinal, or epidural block.[243, 244, 245][III] The paravertebral space bounded by the vertebral body, costotransverse ligament, and parietal pleura can be accessed percutaneously or a catheter placed under direct vision during surgery. Possible advantages of paravertebral block may include lack of lower limb motor block and reduced incidence of retention of urine.

LUMBAR AND THORACIC EPIDURAL BLOCKADE

Epidural analgesia has been shown to have advantages in both adults and children for postoperative analgesia, including improvements in the quality of analgesia, respiratory function, time to first oral intake, mobilization, and overall recovery and hospital discharge in certain circumstances.[246, 247, 248][III], [249][III] The technique of continuous postoperative epidural infusion has become popular in recent years, and is now used routinely in most pediatric centers around the world. Epidural analgesia is suitable for children of all ages who are to undergo major surgery below the fourth thoracic (T4) dermatome. It is particularly effective after thoracic, spinal, thoracoabdominal and abdominal procedures, and major surgery on the lower limbs.[90, 152, 250][II], [248][III]

Epidural insertion, management, and complications

Epidural block is usually performed percutaneously under general anesthesia either as a single epidural injection or "single-shot," or more commonly a catheter is inserted and its tip situated at the required level of analgesia. The shorter straighter spine and character of the epidural space in young children will allow catheters to be threaded to appropriate levels from low (safer and easier) levels of insertion, for example thoracic epidural catheters can be threaded from caudal insertion sites in neonates for post-thoracotomy pain.[251][IV] Techniques for epidural insertion including location of the epidural space, positioning of catheters, and ongoing care are described elsewhere.

The management of continuous epidural analgesia requires special monitoring and nursing care in order to avoid, diagnose, and treat the many possible complications that can occur.[252, 253] Unfortunately there is no consensus about suitable location, nurse–patient ratio or minimum standards of monitoring for continuous epidural analgesia; decisions on these matters depend on local experience and circumstances, and the characteristics of the patient population. Persistent neurological complications such as isolated nerve palsies, sensory deficits, and motor weakness have been reported following epidural analgesia in adults and children; they are thought to relate to accidental nerve injury by epidural needles or catheters, or pharmacological or technical errors. Overall incidences are apparently very low with estimated rates of 1:10,000 or less in major descriptive series.[226, 253]

DRUGS IN THE EPIDURAL SPACE

Local anesthetics

Bupivacaine is still the most widely used LA in the epidural space, both for "single shot" and infusion techniques, although it is gradually being replaced by the newer levobupivacaine or ropivacaine.[71] Concentrations in the range 2.5–0.625 mg/mL are the most suitable for children; dilute solutions of 1.25–0.625 are most commonly used for infusions. In clinical practice, differences between racemic bupivacaine, levobupivacaine, and ropivacaine are small, but levobupivacaine and ropivacaine may be a little less cardio- and neurotoxic and cause less unwanted motor blockade at equianalgesic doses.[254][II], [139] The pharmacokinetics of epidural bupivacaine, ropivacaine, and levobupivacaine have been studied in children. Infusion of bupivacaine up to 0.4 mg/kg/h for several days in infants and children less than six months of age does not achieve toxic plasma concentrations, but the recommended dose is reduced to 0.2 mg/kg/h in neonates because of lower clearance and less plasma binding which may increase susceptibility to toxicity.[71] Ropivacaine shows different infusion pharmacokinetics in that, unlike bupivacaine, accumulation was not observed over a study period of 72 hours in the neonate, although plasma levels were greater than in older children.[139, 152] Levobupivacaine kinetics have been less investigated, but a 24-hour study of infusion of 1.25 or 0.625 mg/mL solutions in infants and children older than six months showed increasing plasma levels throughout the study period, although remaining well below accepted thresholds for toxicity.[255]

Opioid/local anesthetic

Addition of opioid improves the quality of analgesia in comparison with LA alone but it also introduces a new spectrum of side effects including itching, nausea and vomiting, retention of urine, and respiratory depression. Delayed respiratory depression after (caudal) epidural morphine has been described and depression of the carbon dioxide response curve for 22 hours after administration has also been observed.[256, 257] Despite these drawbacks, opioids are frequently added to LA epidural infusions following major surgery where the benefit of improved analgesic efficacy favors their use.[249, 258][II] In comparison with intravenous opioids, hydrophilic opioids such as hydromorphone and morphine appear to have greater efficacy when used neuraxially than more lipophilic opioids such as fentanyl.[258, 259][II]

SYSTEMIC ANALGESIA

The choice of systemic analgesia will depend on patient characteristics and the expected pain intensity and postoperative course. When LA has been used, analgesic requirements are likely to change once their effects have subsided. Patients and families should be warned that this will occur, and clear instructions on further analgesic management provided.

Opioids, NSAIDS, and paracetamol, usually in combination, form the basis of systemic analgesia after surgery in children. They are also used to supplement LA techniques, although spinal and epidural opioids co-administered with systemic opioids are possibly associated with an increased likelihood of respiratory depression. The oral route is rarely available immediately following surgery, after major procedures oral intake may be delayed for several days and therefore parenteral or rectal routes must be used.

Parenteral analgesia

Parenteral formulations of paracetamol, some NSAIDs, and several opioids are available. Paracetamol and NSAIDs are given by intermittent dosing according to developmental age and physical size (usually estimated by weight), opioids can be given in the same way or more commonly by continuous infusion or using a demand-led system such as PCA or NCA.

PCA

PCA is feasible for children aged five years or older, there is a substantial literature describing its efficacy and use for postoperative pain and many other acute pain situations. Morphine is the most frequently used opioid for PCA, many others including fentanyl and tramadol have also been successfully employed with only minor differences in efficacy and side effects.[129, 260][II] Recently, a novel disposable fentanyl-PCA system using an iontophoretic transdermal delivery system has been described for use in adults, it may also be suitable for older children and adolescents but has not been studied for this indication.[261]

NCA

NCA is a modified continuous morphine infusion using PCA technology, suitable for children who are too young, unwilling, or unable to operate a PCA handset. Nurses can administer supplementary analgesia in prespecified amounts on the basis of pain assessments or prior to painful procedures. NCA is convenient, increases flexibility, total morphine consumption, and parent and nurse satisfaction with analgesia.[105][V]

PONV

Nausea and vomiting is a major cause of morbidity after both major and minor surgery. Its causes are multifactorial, it is more frequent after strabismus correction, tonsillectomy, and other head and neck procedures and when opioids are used intra- or postoperatively.[262] It is not associated with preoperative anxiety, but may be greater in children who suffer from motion sickness.[263][III], [264][III]

Children who are identified as "at risk" should be given prophylactic antiemetic therapy with dexamethasone or a 5HT antagonist.[262] PONV treatment is with either drug in the first instance, unless previously used for prophylaxis, and if this is unsuccessful combination therapy including second-line antiemetics such as dimenhydrinate, cyclizine, or perphenazine should be tried.[262, 265]

PROCEDURAL PAIN

Diagnostic and therapeutic procedures such as venepuncture, insertion of intravascular and other catheters, insertion and removal of drainage tubes, lumbar puncture, bone marrow aspiration, immunization, and injections into joints are painful and potentially difficult to manage. Management of procedural pain in the neonate has been particularly identified as a clinical problem.[266]

Inadequate treatment of pain for a procedure will also have implications for subsequent treatments, and management may become progressively more difficult.[13, 267] Pain management for procedures should include both pharmacological and nonpharmacological strategies whenever possible; developmental differences in the response to pain and analgesia should be taken into account when planning analgesia and sufficient time should be allowed for analgesic drugs and other strategies to be effective.[13, 268] Sedation may also be required in some circumstances and for some children, particularly the very young and uncooperative, there is little

alternative to general anesthesia which is quick, safe, and effective but requires special facilities and personnel.

Psychological and complementary therapies

Psychological interventions have an important place in the management of procedural pain, often in combination with simple measures such as topical LA. Distraction, hypnosis, and cognitive-behavior therapy have all been shown to be effective for needle-related pain in children.[269][I] They are reviewed in Chapter 16, Psychological interventions for acute pediatric pain.

Complementary therapies such as transcutaneous electrical nerve stimulation (TENS), acupuncture, aromatherapy, and massage therapy may also have a role although randomized controlled comparisons with standard treatments in children are not available.[270]

Procedural pain in the neonate

Strategies for the management of procedural pain in the neonate have been relatively well studied, although there are concerns that this has not led to sufficient improvement in clinical practice.[266, 271, 272] A number of guidelines, reviews, and policy statements have been published in recent years providing detailed guidance on this issue.[13, 273, 274]

Breast feeding, sucrose, and to some extent nonnutritive sucking have been shown to be effective for brief painful procedures such as venepuncture.[159, 275, 276][II] Topical LAs such as EMLA and amethocaine gel are also effective for minor needle-related pain including venepuncture and lumbar puncture, but are insufficient to blunt the pain response to heel-lancing when used in isolation.[277, 278][II] Nonpharmacological strategies that may also be beneficial in procedure pain management for neonates include tactile stimulation, swaddling, and "facilitated tucking" for which there is some limited evidence of efficacy.[279, 280][I]

Procedural pain in infants and older children

Painful procedures, particularly needle-related pain such as for blood sampling or suture of lacerations, are often identified by children and their families as one of the most distressing aspects of medical care. Psychological preparation prior to the procedure can help to reduce anxiety, nonpharmacological strategies such as distraction, guided imagery, or hypnosis reduce pain behavior and can be combined with pharmacological analgesic, for example topical LA for many needle-related procedures.[269][I], [281][II]

Nitrous oxide inhalation using a demand-valve self-administration apparatus has become popular for procedural pain in children who are old enough to cooperate.[158, 282] Entonox is supplied as a premixed compressed gas mixture of 50 percent nitrous oxide in oxygen, it has been used for needle-related pain, painful dressing changes, and for removal of chest drains. An important safety aspect of self-administration of Entonox is that should sedation occur, the patients grip on the mouthpiece or facemask is relaxed and inhalation stops. "Free flow" administration of nitrous oxide mixtures and higher concentrations of nitrous oxide are more likely to be associated with loss of consciousness and are not widely recommended or used.

REFERENCES

1. Schechter N, Allen D. Physicians' attitudes toward pain in children. *Journal of Developmental and Behavioral Pediatrics.* 1986; **7**: 350–4.

2. Purcell-Jones G, Dormon F, Sumner E. Paediatric anaesthetists' perceptions of neonatal and infant pain. *Pain.* 1988; **33**: 181–7.

3. Conroy S, Choonara I, Impicciatore P *et al.* Survey of unlicensed and off label drug use in paediatric wards in European countries. European Network for Drug Investigation in Children. *British Medical Journal.* 2000; **320**: 79–82.

4. Banner Jr W. Off label prescribing in children. *British Medical Journal.* 2002; **324**: 1290–1.

5. Conroy S, Peden V. Unlicensed and off label analgesic use in paediatric pain management. *Paediatric Anaesthesia.* 2001; **11**: 431–6.

6. Roberts R, Rodriguez W, Murphy D, Crescenzi T. Pediatric drug labeling: improving the safety and efficacy of pediatric therapies. *Journal of the American Medical Association.* 2003; **290**: 905–11.

7. Schreiner MS. Paediatric clinical trials: redressing the imbalance. *Nature Reviews. Drug Discovery.* 2003; **2**: 949–61.

8. Hill P. Off licence and off label prescribing in children: litigation fears for physicians. *Archives of Disease in Childhood.* 2005; **90** (Suppl 1): i17–8.

9. Shah SS, Hall M, Goodman DM *et al.* Off-label drug use in hospitalized children. *Archives of Pediatrics and Adolescent Medicine.* 2007; **161**: 282–90.

10. Michels KB, Rothman KJ. Update on unethical use of placebos in randomised trials. *Bioethics.* 2003; **17**: 188–204.

* 11. Royal College of Nursing Institute. *Clinical guidelines for the recognition and assessment of acute pain in children.* London: RCNUK, 1999.

* 12. Australian and New Zealand College of Anaesthetists. *Acute pain management: scientific evidence.* Melbourne: ANZCA, 2005.

* 13. Howard RF, Carter B, Curry J *et al.* Good practice in postoperative and procedural pain management. *Pediatric Anesthesia.* 2008; **18** (Suppl. 1): 1–81.

* 14. Fitzgerald M. The development of nociceptive circuits. *Nature reviews. Neuroscience.* 2005; **6**: 507–20.

15. Krechel SW, Bildner J. CRIES: a new neonatal postoperative pain measurement score. Initial testing of validity and reliability. *Paediatric Anaesthesia.* 1995; **5**: 53–61.

16. Horgan M, Choonara I. Measuring pain in neonates: an objective score. *Journal of Pediatric Nursing.* 1996; **8**: 24–8.

17. Hodgkinson K, Bear M, Thorn J. Measuring pain in neonates: Evaluating an instrument and developing a common language. *Australian Journal of Advanced Nursing.* 1994; **12**: 17–22.

18. Buttner W, Fincke W. Analysis of behavioural and physiological parameters for the assessment of postoperative analgesic demand in newborns, infants and young children. *Paediatric Anaesthesia.* 2000; **10**: 303–18.

19. Barrier G, Attia J, Mayer M, Amiel-Tilson C. Measurement of postoperative pain and narcotic administration in infants usind a new clinical scoring system. *Intensive Care Medicine.* 1989; **15S**: 37–9.

20. Schade J, Joyce B, Gerkensmeyer J, Keck J. Comparison of three preverbal scales for postoperative pain assessment in a diverse pediatric sample. *Journal of Pain and Symptom Management.* 1996; **12**: 348–59.

21. Grunau R, Craig K. Pain expression in neonates: facial action and cry. *Pain.* 1987; **28**: 395–410.

22. Craig K, McMahan R, Morison J. Developmental changes in infant pain expression during immunization injections. *Social Science Medicine.* 1984; **19**: 1331.

23. Lawrence J, Alcock D, McGrath P. The development of a tool to assess neonatal pain. *Neonatal Network.* 1993; **12**: 59–66.

24. Ballantyne M, Stevens B, McAllister M *et al.* Validation of the premature infant pain profile in the clinical setting. *Clinical Journal of Pain.* 1999; **15**: 297–303.

25. Blauer T, Gerstmann D. A simultaneous comparion of three neonatal pain scales during common NICU procedures. *Clinical Journal of Pain.* 1988; **14**: 39–47.

26. Pokela M. Pain relief can reduce hypoxaemia in distressed neonates during routine treatment procedures. *Pediatrics.* 1994; **93**: 379.

27. Sparshott M. The development of a clinical distresss scale for ventilated newborn infants: Identification of pain and distress based on validated behavioural scores. *Journal of Neonatal Nursing.* 1996; **2**: 5.

28. van Dijk M, de Boer J, Koot H *et al.* The reliability and validity of the COMFORT scale as a postoperative pain instrument in 0 to 3-year-old infants. *Pain.* 2000; **84**: 367–77.

29. Caljouw MAA, Kloos MAC, Olivier MY *et al.* Measurement of pain in premature infants with a gestational age between 28 to 37 weeks: Validation of the adapted COMFORT scale. *Journal of Neonatal Nursing.* 2007; **13**: 13–8.

30. Franck L, Greenberg C, Stevens B. Pain assessment in infants and children. *Pediatric Clinics of North America.* 2000; **47**: 487–512.

* 31. Stinson J, Kavanagh T, Yamada J *et al.* Systematic review of the psychometric properties, interpretability and feasibility of self-report pain intensity measures for use in clinical trials in children and adolescents. *Pain.* 2006; **125**: 143–57.

32. von Baeyer C. Children's self-reports of pain intensity: scale selection, limitations and interpretation. *Pain Research and Management.* 2006; **11**: 157–62.

33. van Dijk M, de Boer JB, Koot HM *et al.* The association between physiological and behavioral pain measures in 0- to 3-year-old infants after major surgery. *Journal of Pain and Symptom Management.* 2001; **22**: 600–9.

34. Lilley C, Craig K, Grunau R. The expression of pain in infants and toddlers: developmental changes in facial action. *Pain.* 1997; **72**: 161–70.

35. Merkel S, Voepel-Lewis T, Shayevitz J, Malviya S. The FLACC: a behavioral scale for scoring postoperative pain in young children. *Pediatric Nursing.* 1997; **23**: 293–7.

36. McGrath P, Johnson G, Goodman J *et al.* CHEOPS: A behavioral scale for rating postoperative pain in children. In: Fields H, Dubner R, Cervero F (eds). *Advances in pain research and therapy.* New York: Raven Press, 1985: 395–402.

37. Chambers C, Reid G, McGrath P, Finley G. Development and preliminary validation of a postoperative pain measure for parents. *Pain.* 1996; **68**: 307–13.

38. Ambuel B, Hamlett K, Marx C, Blumer J. Assessing distress in pediatric intensive care environments: the COMFORT scale. *Journal of Pediatric Psychology.* 1992; **17**: 95–109.

39. LeBaron S, Zeltzer L. Assessment of acute pain and anxiety in children and adolescents by self-reports, observer reports, and a behavior checklist. *Journal of Consulting and Clinical Psychology.* 1984; **52**: 729–38.

40. Katz ER, Kellerman J, Siegel SE. Behavioral distress in children with cancer undergoing medical procedures: developmental considerations. *Journal of Consulting and Clinical Psychology.* 1980; **48**: 356–65.

* 41. von Baeyer C, Spagrud L. Systematic review of observational (behavioral) measures of pain for children and adolescents aged 3 to 18 years. *Pain.* 2007; **127**: 140–50.

42. Malviya S, Voepel-Lewis T, Burke C *et al.* The revised FLACC observational pain tool: Improved reliability and validity for pain assessment in children with cognitive impairment. *Paediatric Anaesthesia.* 2006; **16**: 258–65.

43. Hunt A, Goldman A, Seers K *et al.* Clinical validation of the paediatric pain profile. *Developmental Medicine and Child Neurology.* 2004; **46**: 9–18.

44. Breau L, Finley G, McGrath P, Camfield C. Validation of the Non-communicating Children's Pain Checklist-Postoperative Version. *Anesthesiology.* 2002; **96**: 528–35.

45. Kehlet H, Dahl JB. The value of "multimodal" or "balanced analgesia" in postoperative pain treatment. *Anesthesia and Analgesia.* 1993; **77**: 1048–56.

46. Gedaly-Duff V, Ziebarth D. Mothers' management of adenoid-tonsillectomy pain in 4- to 8-year-olds: a preliminary study. *Pain.* 1994; **57**: 293–9.

47. P Ikki T, Pietil AM, Vehvil inen-Julkunen K *et al.* Parental views on participation in their child's pain relief measures and recommendations to health care providers. *Journal of Pediatric Nursing.* 2002; **17**: 270–8.

48. Koppert W, Wehrfritz A, Korber N *et al.* The cyclooxygenase isozyme inhibitors parecoxib and paracetamol reduce central hyperalgesia in humans. *Pain.* 2004; **108**: 148–53.

49. Anderson B. What we don't know about paracetamol in children. *Paediatric Anaesthesia.* 1998; **8**: 451–60.

50. Barden J, Edwards J, Moore A, McQuay H. Single dose oral paracetamol (acetaminophen) for postoperative pain. *Cochrane Database of Systematic Reviews.* 2004; **CD004602**.

51. Moore A, Collins S, Carroll D *et al.* Single dose paracetamol (acetaminophen), with and without codeine, for postoperative pain. *Cochrane Database of Systematic Reviews.* 2000; **CD001547**.

52. Hiller A, Meretoja OA, Korpela R *et al.* The analgesic efficacy of acetaminophen, ketoprofen, or their combination for pediatric surgical patients having soft tissue or orthopedic procedures. *Anesthesia and Analgesia.* 2006; **102**: 1365–71.

53. Morton NS, O'Brien K. Analgesic efficacy of paracetamol and diclofenac in children receiving PCA morphine. *British Journal of Anaesthesia.* 1999; **82**: 715–7.

54. Anderson B, Holford N, Woollard G *et al.* Perioperative pharmacodynamics of acetaminophen analgesia in children. *Anesthesiology.* 1999; **90**: 411–21.

55. Allegaert K, Murat I, Anderson BJ. Not all intravenous paracetamol formulations are created equal. *Paediatric Anaesthesia.* 2007; **17**: 811–2.

56. Anderson B, Woollard G, Holford N. Acetaminophen analgesia in children: placebo effect and pain resolution after tonsillectomy. *European Journal of Clinical Pharmacology.* 2001; **57**: 559–69.

57. Murat I, Baujard C, Foussat C *et al.* Tolerance and analgesic efficacy of a new i.v. paracetamol solution in children after inguinal hernia repair. *Paediatric Anaesthesia.* 2005; **15**: 663–70.

58. Anderson B, van Lingen R, Hansen T *et al.* Acetaminophen developmental pharmacokinetics in premature neonates and infants: a pooled population analysis. *Anesthesiology.* 2002; **96**: 1336–45.

59. Anderson B, Pons G, Autret-Leca E *et al.* Pediatric intravenous paracetamol (propacetamol) pharmacokinetics: a population analysis. *Paediatric Anaesthesia.* 2005; **15**: 282–92.

60. Barbaud A, Reichert-Penetrat S, Trechot P *et al.* Occupational contact dermatitis to propacetamol. Allergological and chemical investigations in two new cases. *Dermatology.* 1997; **195**: 329–31.

61. Niemi T, Backman J, Syrjala M *et al.* Platelet dysfunction after intravenous ketorolac or propacetamol. *Acta Anaesthesiologica Scandinavica.* 2000; **44**: 69–74.

62. van der Marel C, Anderson B, van Lingen R et al. Paracetamol and metabolite pharmacokinetics in infants. *European Journal of Clinical Pharmacology.* 2003; **59**: 243–51.

63. Hynson J, South M. Childhood hepatotoxicity with paracetamol doses less than 150 mg/kg per day. *Medical Journal of Australia.* 1999; **171**: 497.

64. Rivera-Penera T, Gugig R, Davis J et al. Outcome of acetaminophen overdose in pediatric patients and factors contributing to hepatotoxicity. *Journal of Pediatrics.* 1997; **130**: 300–4.

65. Rowbotham D. *Guidelines for the use of nonsteroidal anti-inflammatory drugs in the perioperative period.* London: RCA, 1998.

* 66. Anderson B. Comparing the efficacy of NSAIDs and paracetamol in children. *Paediatric Anaesthesia.* 2004; **14**: 201–17.

67. Morris JL, Rosen DA, Rosen KR. Nonsteroidal anti-inflammatory agents in neonates. *Paediatric Drugs.* 2003; **5**: 385–405.

68. Zarraga IG, Schwarz ER. Coxibs and heart disease: what we have learned and what else we need to know. *Journal of the American College of Cardiology.* 2007; **49**: 1–14.

69. Anderson B, Palmer G. Recent developments in the pharmacological management of pain in children. *Current Opinion in Anaesthesiology.* 2006; **19**: 285–92.

70. Kokki H. Nonsteroidal anti-inflammatory drugs for postoperative pain: a focus on children. *Paediatric Drugs.* 2003; **5**: 103–23.

* 71. Lonnqvist P, Morton N. Postoperative analgesia in infants and children. *British Journal of Anaesthesia.* 2005; **95**: 59–68.

72. Forrest J, Heitlinger E, Revell S. Ketorolac for postoperative pain management in children. *Drug Safety.* 1997; **16**: 309–29.

73. Krishna S, Hughes L, Lin S. Postoperative hemorrhage with nonsteroidal anti-inflammatory drug use after tonsillectomy: a meta-analysis. *Archives of Otolaryngology – Head and Neck Surgery.* 2003; **129**: 1086–9.

74. Marret E, Flahault A, Samama C, Bonnet F. Effects of postoperative, nonsteroidal, antiinflammatory drugs on bleeding risk after tonsillectomy: meta-analysis of randomized, controlled trials. *Anesthesiology.* 2003; **98**: 1497–502.

75. Moiniche S, Romsing J, Dahl J, Tramer M. Nonsteroidal antiinflammatory drugs and the risk of operative site bleeding after tonsillectomy: a quantitative systematic review. *Anesthesia and Analgesia.* 2003; **96**: 68–77.

* 76. Cardwell M, Siviter G, Smith A. Non-steroidal anti-inflammatory drugs and perioperative bleeding in paediatric tonsillectomy. *Cochrane Database of Systematic Reviews.* 2005; **CD003591**.

77. Short J, Barr C, Palmer C et al. Use of diclofenac in children with asthma. *Anaesthesia.* 2000; **55**: 334–7.

* 78. Lesko S. The safety of ibuprofen suspension in children. *International Journal of Clinical Practice.* 2003; **135**: 50–3.

* 79. Lesko S, Louik C, Vezina R, Mitchell A. Asthma morbidity after the short-term use of ibuprofen in children. *Pediatrics.* 2002; **109**: E20.

80. Palmer GM. A teenager with severe asthma exacerbation following ibuprofen. *Anaesthesia and Intensive Care.* 2005; **33**: 261–5.

* 81. Kart T, Christrup L, Rasmussen M. Recommended use of morphine in neonates, infants and children based on a literature review: Part 1–Pharmacokinetics. *Paediatric Anaesthesia.* 1997; **7**: 5–11.

* 82. Kart T, Christrup L, Rasmussen M. Recommended use of morphine in neonates, infants and children based on a literature review: Part 2–Clinical use. *Paediatric Anaesthesia.* 1997; **7**: 93–101.

83. Bouwmeester N, Anderson B, Tibboel D, Holford N. Developmental pharmacokinetics of morphine and its metabolites in neonates, infants and young children. *British Journal of Anaesthesia.* 2004; **92**: 208–17.

* 84. Berde CB, Sethna NF. Analgesics for the treatment of pain in children. *New England Journal of Medicine.* 2002; **347**: 1094–103.

85. Anderson BJ, Meakin GH. Scaling for size: some implications for paediatric anaesthesia dosing. *Paediatric Anaesthesia.* 2002; **12**: 205–19.

86. Lynn A, Nespeca M, Opheim K, Slattery J. Respiratory effects of intravenous morphine infusions in neonates, infants, and children after cardiac surgery. *Anesthesia and Analgesia.* 1993; **77**: 695–701.

87. Ginsberg B, Howell S, Glass PS et al. Pharmacokinetic model-driven infusion of fentanyl in children. *Anesthesiology.* 1996; **85**: 1268–75.

88. Wheeler M, Birmingham P, Lugo R et al. The pharmacokinetics of the intravenous formulation of fentanyl citrate administered orally in children undergoing general anesthesia. *Anesthesia and Analgesia.* 2004; **99**: 1347–51.

89. Borland ML, Bergesio R, Pascoe EM et al. Intranasal fentanyl is an equivalent analgesic to oral morphine in paediatric burns patients for dressing changes: a randomised double blind crossover study. *Burns.* 2005; **31**: 831–7.

90. Lejus C, Surbled M, Schwoerer D et al. Postoperative epidural analgesia with bupivacaine and fentanyl: hourly pain assessment in 348 paediatric cases. *Paediatric Anaesthesia.* 2001; **11**: 327–32.

91. Viscusi E, Reynolds L, Chung F et al. Patient-controlled transdermal fentanyl hydrochloride vs intravenous morphine pump for postoperative pain: a randomized controlled trial. *Journal of the American Medical Association.* 2004; **291**: 1333–41.

92. Binstock W, Rubin R, Bachman C et al. The effect of premedication with OTFC, with or without ondansetron, on postoperative agitation, and nausea and vomiting in

pediatric ambulatory patients. *Paediatric Anaesthesia.* 2004; **14**: 759–67.

93. Fahnenstich H, Steffan J, Kau N, Bartmann P. Fentanyl-induced chest wall rigidity and laryngospasm in preterm and term infants. *Critical Care Medicine.* 2000; **28**: 836–9.

94. Quigley C, Wiffen P. A systematic review of hydromorphone in acute and chronic pain. *Journal of Pain and Symptom Management.* 2003; **25**: 169–78.

95. Murray A, Hagen NA. Hydromorphone. *Journal of Pain and Symptom Management.* 2005; **29**: S57–66.

96. Sharar SR, Bratton SL, Carrougher GJ *et al.* A comparison of oral transmucosal fentanyl citrate and oral hydromorphone for inpatient pediatric burn wound care analgesia. *Journal of Burn Care and Rehabilitation.* 1998; **19**: 516–21.

97. Collins J, Geake J, Grier H *et al.* Patient-controlled analgesia for mucositis pain in children: a three-period crossover study comparing morphine and hydromorphone. *Journal of Pediatrics.* 1996; **129**: 722–8.

98. Goodarzi M. Comparison of epidural morphine, hydromorphone and fentanyl for postoperative pain control in children undergoing orthopaedic surgery. *Paediatric Anaesthesia.* 1999; **9**: 419–22.

99. Loryman B, Davies F, Chavada G, Coats T. Consigning "brutacaine" to history: a survey of pharmacological techniques to facilitate painful procedures in children in emergency departments in the UK. *Emergency Medical Journal.* 2006; **23**: 838–40.

100. Davies M, Crawford I. Towards evidence based emergency medicine: best BETs from the Manchester Royal Infirmary. Nasal diamorphine for acute pain relief in children. *Emergency Medicine Journal.* 2001; **18**: 271.

101. Kendall J, Reeves B, Latter V. Multicentre randomised controlled trial of nasal diamorphine for analgesia in children and teenagers with clinical fractures. *British Medical Journal.* 2001; **322**: 261–5.

102. Wilson J, Kendall J, Cornelius P. Intranasal diamorphine for paediatric analgesia: assessment of safety and efficacy. *Journal of Accident and Emergency Medicine.* 1997; **14**: 70–2.

103. Wood C, Rushforth J, Hartley R *et al.* Randomised double blind trial of morphine versus diamorphine for sedation of preterm neonates. *Archives of Disease in Childhood. Fetal and Neonatal Edition.* 1998; **79**: F34–9.

104. Barrett D, Barker D, Rutter N *et al.* Morphine, morphine-6-glucuronide and morphine-3-glucuronide pharmacokinetics in newborn infants receiving diamorphine infusions. *British Journal of Clinical Pharmacology.* 1996; **41**: 531–7.

105. Lloyd-Thomas A, Howard R. A pain service for children. *Paediatric Anaesthesia.* 1994; **4**: 3–15.

106. Kelleher AA, Black A, Penman S, Howard R. Comparison of caudal bupivacaine and diamorphine with caudal bupivacaine alone for repair of hypospadias. *British Journal of Anaesthesia.* 1996; **77**: 586–90.

107. Sanders J. Paediatric regional anaesthesia, a survey of practice in the United Kingdom. *British Journal of Anaesthesia.* 2002; **89**: 707–10.

108. Cicero T, Inciardi J, Munoz A. Trends in abuse of Oxycontin and other opioid analgesics in the United States: 2002-2004. *Journal of Pain.* 2005; **6**: 662–72.

109. Kalso E. Oxycodone. *Journal of Pain and Symptom Management.* 2005; **29**: S47–56.

110. Kokki H, Rasanen I, Lasalmi M *et al.* Comparison of oxycodone pharmacokinetics after buccal and sublingual administration in children. *Clinical Pharmacokinetics.* 2006; **45**: 745–54.

111. El-Tahtawy A, Kokki H, Reidenberg BE. Population pharmacokinetics of oxycodone in children 6 months to 7 years old. *Journal of Clinical Pharmacology.* 2006; **46**: 433–42.

112. Kokki H, Rasanen I, Reinikainen M *et al.* Pharmacokinetics of oxycodone after intravenous, buccal, intramuscular and gastric administration in children. *Clinical Pharmacokinetics.* 2004; **43**: 613–22.

113. Pokela ML, Anttila E, Seppala T, Olkkola KT. Marked variation in oxycodone pharmacokinetics in infants. *Paediatric Anaesthesia.* 2005; **15**: 560–5.

114. Kokki H, Lintula H, Vanamo K *et al.* Oxycodone vs placebo in children with undifferentiated abdominal pain: a randomized, double-blind clinical trial of the effect of analgesia on diagnostic accuracy. *Archives of Pediatrics and Adolescent Medicine.* 2005; **159**: 320–5.

115. Czarnecki M, Jandrisevits M, Theiler S *et al.* Controlled-release oxycodone for the management of pediatric postoperative pain. *Journal of Pain and Symptom Management.* 2004; **27**: 379–86.

116. Williams D, Hatch D, Howard R. Codeine phosphate in paediatric medicine. *British Journal of Anaesthesia.* 2001; **86**: 421–7.

117. Williams D, Patel A, Howard R. Pharmacogenetics of codeine metabolism in an urban population of children and its implications for analgesic reliability. *British Journal of Anaesthesia.* 2002; **89**: 839–45.

118. Williams D, Dickenson A, Fitzgerald M, Howard R. Developmental regulation of codeine analgesia in the rat. *Anesthesiology.* 2004; **100**: 92–7.

119. Shanahan E, Marshall A, Garrett C. Adverse reactions to intravenous codeine phosphate in children. A report of three cases. *Anaesthesia.* 1983; **38**: 40–3.

120. Grond S, Sablotzki A. Clinical pharmacology of tramadol. *Clinical Pharmacokinetics.* 2004; **43**: 879–923.

121. Demiraran Y, Ilce Z, Kocaman B, Bozkurt P. Does tramadol wound infiltration offer an advantage over bupivacaine for postoperative analgesia in children following herniotomy? *Paediatric Anaesthesia.* 2006; **16**: 1047–50.

122. Rose J, Finkel J, Arquedas-Mohs A *et al.* Oral tramadol for the treatment of pain of 7-30 days' duration in children. *Anesthesia and Analgesia.* 2003; **96**: 78–81.

123. Prakash S, Tyagi R, Gogia AR *et al.* Efficacy of three doses of tramadol with bupivacaine for caudal analgesia in

paediatric inguinal herniotomy. *British Journal of Anaesthesia*. 2006; **97**: 385–8.

*124.   Bozkurt P. Use of tramadol in children. *Paediatric Anaesthesia*. 2005; **15**: 1041–7.

125.   Zwaveling J, Bubbers S, van Meurs A *et al.* Pharmacokinetics of rectal tramadol in postoperative paediatric patients. *British Journal of Anaesthesia*. 2004; **93**: 224–7.

126.   Murthy B, Pandya K, Booker P *et al.* Pharmacokinetics of tramadol in children after i.v. or caudal epidural administration. *British Journal of Anaesthesia*. 2000; **84**: 346–9.

127.   Allegaert K, Anderson B, Verbesselt R *et al.* Tramadol disposition in the very young: an attempt to assess in vivo cytochrome P-450 2D6 activity. *British Journal of Anaesthesia*. 2005; **95**: 231–9.

128.   Allegaert K, Van den Anker J, Verbesselt R *et al.* O-demethylation of tramadol in the first months of life. *European Journal of Clinical Pharmacology*. 2005; **61**: 837–42.

129.   Ozalevli M, Unlugenc H, Tuncer U *et al.* Comparison of morphine and tramadol by patient-controlled analgesia for postoperative analgesia after tonsillectomy in children. *Paediatric Anaesthesia*. 2005; **15**: 979–84.

130.   Elia N, Tramer M. Ketamine and postoperative pain–a quantitative systematic review of randomised trials. *Pain*. 2005; **113**: 61–70.

131.   Koinig H, Marhofer P. S(+)-ketamine in paediatric anaesthesia. *Paediatric Anaesthesia*. 2003; **13**: 185–7.

132.   Borker A, Ambulkar I, Gopal R, Advani S. Safe and efficacious use of procedural sedation and analgesia by non-anesthesiologists in a pediatric hematology-oncology unit. *Indian Pediatrics*. 2006; **43**: 309–14.

133.   Martindale S, Dix P, Stoddart P. Double-blind randomized controlled trial of caudal versus intravenous S(+)-ketamine for supplementation of caudal analgesia in children. *British Journal of Anaesthesia*. 2004; **92**: 344–7.

134.   Subramaniam K, Subramaniam B, Steinbrook R. Ketamine as adjuvant analgesic to opioids: a quantitative and qualitative systematic review. *Anesthesia and Analgesia*. 2004; **99**: 482–95.

135.   Haberny KA, Paule MG, Scallet AC *et al.* Ontogeny of the N-methyl-D-aspartate (NMDA) receptor system and susceptibility to neurotoxicity. *Toxicological Sciences*. 2002; **68**: 9–17.

136.   Young C, Jevtovic-Todorovic V, Qin Y *et al.* Potential of ketamine and midazolam, individually or in combination, to induce apoptotic neurodegeneration in the infant mouse brain. *British Journal of Pharmacology*. 2005; **146**: 189–97.

137.   Mellon RD, Simone AF, Rappaport BA. Use of anesthetic agents in neonates and young children. *Anesthesia and Analgesia*. 2007; **104**: 509–20.

138.   Slikker Jr W, Zou X, Hotchkiss CE *et al.* Ketamine-induced neuronal cell death in the perinatal rhesus monkey. *Toxicological Sciences*. 2007; **98**: 145–58.

139.   Dalens B. Some current controversies in paediatric regional anaesthesia. *Current Opinion in Anaesthesiology*. 2006; **19**: 301–8.

140.   Peutrell JM, Lonnqvist PA. Neuraxial blocks for anaesthesia and analgesia in children. *Current Opinion in Anaesthesiology*. 2003; **16**: 461–70.

141.   Bergendahl H, Lonnqvist PA, Eksborg S. Clonidine in paediatric anaesthesia: review of the literature and comparison with benzodiazepines for premedication. *Acta Anaesthesiologica Scandinavica*. 2006; **50**: 135–43.

142.   Ivani G, Bergendahl H, Lampugnani E *et al.* Plasma levels of clonidine following epidural bolus injection in children. *Acta Anaesthesiologica Scandinavica*. 1998; **42**: 306–11.

143.   Lonnqvist PA, Bergendahl HT, Eksborg S. Pharmacokinetics of clonidine after rectal administration in children. *Anesthesiology*. 1994; **81**: 1097–101.

144.   Breschan C, Krumpholz R, Likar R *et al.* Can a dose of 2microg.kg(-1) caudal clonidine cause respiratory depression in neonates? *Paediatric Anaesthesia*. 1999; **9**: 81–3.

145.   Breschan C, Jost R, Krumpholz R *et al.* A prospective study comparing the analgesic efficacy of levobupivacaine, ropivacaine and bupivacaine in pediatric patients undergoing caudal blockade. *Paediatric Anaesthesia*. 2005; **15**: 301–06.

146.   Mazoit J, Dalens B. Pharmacokinetics of local anaesthetics in infants and children. *Clinical Pharmacokinetics*. 2004; **43**: 17–32.

147.   Foster R, Markham A. Levobupivacaine: a review of its pharmacology and use as a local anaesthetic. *Drugs*. 2000; **59**: 551–79.

148.   Morrison S, Dominguez J, Frascarolo P, Reiz S. A comparison of the electrocardiographic cardiotoxic effects of racemic bupivacaine, levobupivacaine, and ropivacaine in anesthetized swine. *Anesthesia and Analgesia*. 2000; **90**: 1308–14.

149.   Dalens B, Mazoit J. Adverse effects of regional anaesthesia in children. *Drug Safety*. 1998; **19**: 251–68.

150.   Luz G, Wieser C, Innerhofer P *et al.* Free and total bupivacaine plasma concentrations after continuous epidural anaesthesia in infants and children. *Paediatric Anaesthesia*. 1998; **8**: 473–8.

151.   Mevorach D, Perkins F, Isaacson S. Bupivacaine toxicity secondary to continuous caudal epidural infusion in children. *Anesthesia and Analgesia*. 1993; **77**: 1305–6.

152.   Bosenberg AT, Thomas J, Cronje L *et al.* Pharmacokinetics and efficacy of ropivacaine for continuous epidural infusion in neonates and infants. *Paediatric Anaesthesia*. 2005; **15**: 739–49.

153.   Eidelman A, Weiss JM, Lau J, Carr DB. Topical anesthetics for dermal instrumentation: a systematic review of randomized, controlled trials. *Annals of Emergency Medicine*. 2005; **46**: 343–51.

154.   Essink-Tjebbes C, Hekster Y, Liem K, van Dongen R. Topical use of local anesthetics in neonates. *Pharmacy World and Science*. 1999; **21**: 173–6.

155. Taddio A, Ohlsson A, Einarson TR *et al.* A systematic review of lidocaine-prilocaine cream (EMLA) in the treatment of acute pain in neonates. *Pediatrics.* 1998; **101**: E1.

156. Nilsson A, Engberg G, Henneberg S *et al.* Inverse relationship between age-dependent erythrocyte activity of methaemoglobin reductase and prilocaine-induced methaemoglobinaemia during infancy. *British Journal of Anaesthesia.* 1990; **64**: 72–6.

157. Jain A, Rutter N. Does topical amethocaine gel reduce the pain of venepuncture in newborn infants? A randomised double blind controlled trial. *Archives of Disease in Childhood. Fetal and Neonatal Edition.* 2000; **83**: F207–10.

158. Bruce E, Franck L. Self-administered nitrous oxide (Entonox) for the management of procedural pain. *Paediatric Nursing.* 2000; **12**: 15–9.

*159. Stevens B, Yamada J, Ohlsson A. Sucrose for analgesia in newborn infants undergoing painful procedures [update of *Cochrane Database of Systematic Reviews.* 2001; **CD001069**]. *Cochrane Database of Systematic Reviews.* 2004; **CD001069**.

160. Anseloni VC, Ren K, Dubner R, Ennis M. A brainstem substrate for analgesia elicited by intraoral sucrose. *Neuroscience.* 2005; **133**: 231–43.

*161. Lefrak L, Burch K, Caravantes R *et al.* Sucrose analgesia: identifying potentially better practices. *Pediatrics.* 2006; **118** (Suppl 2): S197–202.

162. Johnston CC, Filion F, Snider L *et al.* How much sucrose is too much sucrose? *Pediatrics.* 2007; **119**: 226.

163. Johnston CC FF, Snider L, Majnamer A *et al.* Routine sucrose analgesia during the first week of life in neonates younger than 31 weeks post conceptual age. *Paediatrics.* 2002; **110**: 523–8.

164. Suraseranivongse S, Chowvanayotin S, Pirayavaraporn S *et al.* Effect of bupivacaine with epinephrine wound instillation for pain relief after pediatric inguinal herniorrhaphy and hydrocelectomy. *Regional Anesthesia and Pain Medicine.* 2003; **28**: 24–8.

165. Splinter W, Reid C, Roberts D, Bass J. Reducing pain after inguinal hernia repair in children: caudal anesthesia versus ketorolac tromethamine. *Anesthesiology.* 1997; **87**: 542–6.

166. Conroy J, Othersen HJ, Dorman B *et al.* A comparison of wound instillation and caudal block for analgesia following pediatric inguinal herniorrhaphy. *Journal of Pediatric Surgery.* 1993; **28**: 565–7.

167. Casey W, Rice L, Hannallah R *et al.* A comparison between bupivacaine instillation versus ilioinguinal/iliohypogastric nerve block for postoperative analgesia following inguinal herriorrhaphy in children. *Anesthesiology.* 1990; **72**: 637–9.

168. Anatol TI, Pitt-Miller P, Holder Y. Trial of three methods of intraoperative bupivacaine analgesia for pain after paediatric groin surgery. *Canadian Journal of Anaesthesia.* 1997; **44**: 1053–9.

169. Graham S, Wandless J. The effect of ketorolac as an adjuvant to local anaesthetic infiltration for analgesia in

paediatric umbilical hernia surgery. *Paediatric Anaesthesia.* 1995; **5**: 161–3.

170. Mobley K, Wandless J, Fell D. Serum bupivacaine concentrations following wound infiltration in children undergoing inguinal herniotomy. *Anaesthesia.* 1991; **46**: 500–01.

171. Ates Y, Unal N, Cuhruk H, Erkan N. Postoperative analgesia in children using preemptive retrobulbar block and local anesthetic infiltration in strabismus surgery. *Regional Anesthesia and Pain Medicine.* 1998; **23**: 569–74.

172. Anand P, Wilson R, Sheehy EC. Intraligamental analgesia for post-operative pain control in children having dental extractions under general anaesthesia. *European Journal of Paediatric Dentistry.* 2005; **6**: 10–05.

173. Sharaf A. Evaluation of mandibular infiltration versus block anesthesia in pediatric dentistry. *ASDC Journal of Dentistry for Children.* 1997; **64**: 276–81.

174. Oulis C, Vadiakas G, Vasilopoulou A. The effectiveness of mandibular infiltration compared to mandibular block anesthesia in treating primary molars in children. *Pediatric Dentistry.* 1996; **18**: 301–05.

175. Hollis L, Burton M, Millar J. Perioperative local anaesthesia for reducing pain following tonsillectomy (Cochrane review). *Cochrane Database of Systematic Reviews.* 1999; **CD001874**.

176. Akoglu E, Akkurt BC, Inanoglu K *et al.* Ropivacaine compared to bupivacaine for post-tonsillectomy pain relief in children: a randomized controlled study. *International Journal of Pediatrics Otorhinolaryngology.* 2006; **70**: 1169–73.

177. Naja M, El-Rajab M, Kabalan W *et al.* Pre-incisional infiltration for pediatric tonsillectomy: a randomized double-blind clinical trial. *International Journal of Pediatric Otorhinolaryngology.* 2005; **69**: 1333–41.

178. Somdas M, Senturk M, Ketenci I *et al.* Efficacy of bupivacaine for post-tonsillectomy pain: a study with the intra-individual design. *International Journal of Pediatric Otorhinolaryngology.* 2004; **68**: 1391–5.

179. Kaygusuz I, Susaman N. The effects of dexamethasone, bupivacaine and topical lidocaine spray on pain after tonsillectomy. *International Journal of Pediatric Otorhinolaryngology.* 2003; **67**: 737–42.

180. Giannoni C, White S, Enneking FK. Does dexamethasone with preemptive analgesia improve pediatric tonsillectomy pain? *Otolaryngology – Head and Neck Surgery.* 2002; **126**: 307–15.

181. Homer J, Williams B, Semple P *et al.* Tonsillectomy by guillotine is less painful than by dissection. *International Journal of Pediatric Otorhinolaryngology.* 2000; **52**: 25–9.

182. Nordahl S, Albrektsen G, Guttormsen A *et al.* Effect of bupivacaine on pain after tonsillectomy: a randomized clinical trial. *Acta Oto-laryngologica.* 1999; **119**: 369–76.

*183. Warnock F, Lander J. Pain progression, intensity and outcomes following tonsillectomy. *Pain.* 1998; **75**: 37–45.

184. Willschke H, Marhofer P, Bosenberg A *et al.* Ultrasonography for ilioinguinal/iliohypogastric nerve

blocks in children. *British Journal of Anaesthesia*. 2005; **95**: 226–30.

185. Willschke H, Bosenberg A, Marhofer P *et al*. Ultrasonographic-guided ilioinguinal/iliohypogastric nerve block in pediatric anesthesia: what is the optimal volume? *Anesthesia and Analgesia*. 2006; **102**: 1680–4.

186. Ala-Kokko T, Karinen J, Raiha E *et al*. Pharmacokinetics of 0.75% ropivacaine and 0.5% bupivacaine after ilioinguinal-iliohypogastric nerve block in children. *British Journal of Anaesthesia*. 2002; **89**: 438–41.

187. Dalens B, Ecoffey C, Joly A *et al*. Pharmacokinetics and analgesic effect of ropivacaine following ilioinguinal/ iliohypogastric nerve block in children. *Paediatric Anaesthesia*. 2001; **11**: 415–20.

188. Stow P, Scott A, Phillips A, White J. Plasma bupivacaine concentrations during caudal analgesia and ilioinguinal-iliohypogastric nerve block in children. *Anaesthesia*. 1988; **43**: 650–3.

189. Johr M, Sossai R. Colonic puncture during ilioinguinal nerve block in a child. *Anesthesia and Analgesia*. 1999; **88**: 1051–2.

190. Derrick J, Aun C. Transient femoral nerve palsy after ilioinguinal block. *Anaesthesia and Intensive Care*. 1996; **24**: 115.

191. Fisher Q, McComiskey C, Hill J *et al*. Postoperative voiding interval and duration of analgesia following peripheral or caudal nerve blocks in children. *Anesthesia and Analgesia*. 1993; **76**: 173–7.

192. Scott A, Phillips A, White J, Stow P. Analgesia following inguinal herniotomy or orchidopexy in children: a comparison of caudal and regional blockade. *Journal of the Royal College of Surgeons of Edinburgh*. 1989; **34**: 143–5.

193. Markham S, Tomlinson J, Hain W. Ilioinguinal nerve block in children. A comparison with caudal block for intra and postoperative analgesia. *Anaesthesia*. 1986; **41**: 1098–103.

194. Reid M, Harris R, Phillips P *et al*. Day-case herniotomy in children. A comparison of ilio-inguinal nerve block and wound infiltration for postoperative analgesia. *Anaesthesia*. 1987; **42**: 658–61.

195. Findlow D, Aldridge LM, Doyle E. Comparison of caudal block using bupivacaine and ketamine with ilioinguinal nerve block for orchidopexy in children. *Anaesthesia*. 1997; **52**: 1110–3.

196. Somri M, Gaitini LA, Vaida SJ *et al*. Effect of ilioinguinal nerve block on the catecholamine plasma levels in orchidopexy: comparison with caudal epidural block. *Paediatric Anaesthesia*. 2002; **12**: 791–7.

197. Sfez M, Le Mapihan Y, Mazoit X, Dreux-Boucard H. Local anesthetic serum concentrations after penile nerve block in children. *Anesthesia and Analgesia*. 1990; **71**: 423–6.

198. Serour F, Cohen A, Mandelberg A *et al*. Dorsal penile nerve block in children undergoing circumcision in a day-care surgery. *Canadian Journal of Anaesthesia*. 1996; **43**: 954–8.

199. Dalens B, Vanneuville G, Dechelotte P. Penile block via the subpubic space in 100 children. *Anesthesia and Analgesia*. 1989; **69**: 41–5.

200. Sara C, Lowry C. A complication of circumcision and dorsal nerve block of the penis. *Anaesthesia and Intensive Care*. 1985; **13**: 79–82.

201. Berens R, Pontus S. A complication associated with dorsal penile nerve block. *Regional Anesthesia*. 1990; **15**: 309–10.

202. Gauntlett I. A comparison between local anaesthetic dorsal nerve block and caudal bupivacaine with ketamine for paediatric circumcision. *Paediatric Anaesthesia*. 2003; **13**: 38–42.

203. Allan CY, Jacqueline PA, Shubhda JH. Caudal epidural block versus other methods of postoperative pain relief for circumcision in boys. *Cochrane Database of Systematic Reviews*. 2003; **CD003005**.

204. Holder K, Peutrell J, Weir P. Regional anaesthesia for circumcision. Subcutaneous ring block of the penis and subpubic penile block compared. *European Journal of Anaesthesiology*. 1997; **14**: 495–8.

205. Yeoman P, Cooke R, Hain W. Penile block for circumcision? A comparison with caudal blockade. *Anaesthesia*. 1983; **38**: 862–6.

206. Weksler N, Atias I, Klein M *et al*. Is penile block better than caudal epidural block for postcircumcision analgesia? *Journal of Anesthesia*. 2005; **19**: 36–9.

*207. Brady-Fryer B, Wiebe N, Lander JA. Pain relief for neonatal circumcision. *Cochrane Database of Systematic Reviews*. 2004; **CD004217**.

208. Eipe N, Choudhrie A, Pillai AD, Choudhrie R. Regional anesthesia for cleft lip repair: a preliminary study. *Cleft Palate-Craniofacial Journal*. 2006; **43**: 138–41.

209. Bosenberg A, Kimble F. Infraorbital nerve block in neonates for cleft lip repair: anatomical study and clinical application. *British Journal of Anaesthesia*. 1995; **74**: 506–08.

210. Prabhu K, Wig J, Grewal S. Bilateral infraorbital nerve block is superior to peri-incisional infiltration for analgesia after repair of cleft lip. *Scandinavian Journal of Plastic and Reconstructive Surgery and Hand Surgery*. 1999; **33**: 83–7.

211. Nicodemus H, Ferrer M, Cristobal V, de Castro L. Bilateral infraorbital block with 0.5% bupivacaine as post-operative analgesia following cheiloplasty in children. *Scandinavian Journal of Plastic and Reconstructive Surgery and Hand Surgery*. 1991; **25**: 253–7.

212. Fisher W, Bingham R, Hall R. Axillary brachial plexus block for perioperative analgesia in 250 children. *Paediatric Anaesthesia*. 1999; **9**: 435–8.

213. Altintas F, Bozkurt P, Ipek N *et al*. The efficacy of pre- versus postsurgical axillary block on postoperative pain in paediatric patients. *Paediatric Anaesthesia*. 2000; **10**: 23–8.

214. Thornton KL, Sacks MD, Hall R, Bingham R. Comparison of 0.2% ropivacaine and 0.25% bupivacaine for axillary

brachial plexus blocks in paediatric hand surgery. *Paediatric Anaesthesia.* 2003; **13**: 409–12.

215. Bergman BD, Hebl JR, Kent J, Horlocker TT. Neurologic complications of 405 consecutive continuous axillary catheters. *Anesthesia and Analgesia.* 2003; **96**: 247–52.

216. Kriwanek K, Wan J, Beaty J, Pershad J. Axillary block for analgesia during manipulation of forearm fractures in the pediatric emergency department a prospective randomized comparative trial. *Journal of Pediatric Orthopedics.* 2006; **26**: 737–40.

217. Blasier RD. Anesthetic considerations for fracture management in the outpatient setting. *Journal of Pediatric Orthopaedics.* 2004; **24**: 742–6.

218. Fleischmann E, Marhofer P, Greher M *et al.* Brachial plexus anaesthesia in children: lateral infraclavicular vs axillary approach. *Paediatric Anaesthesia.* 2003; **13**: 103–08.

219. de Jose Maria B, Tielens LK. Vertical infraclavicular brachial plexus block in children: a preliminary study. *Paediatric Anaesthesia.* 2004; **14**: 931–5.

220. Pande R, Pande M, Bhadani U *et al.* Supraclavicular brachial plexus block as a sole anaesthetic technique in children: an analysis of 200 cases. *Anaesthesia.* 2000; **55**: 798–802.

221. Dalens B, Vanneuville G, Tanguy A. Comparison of the fascia iliaca compartment block with the 3-in-1 block in children. *Anesthesia and Analgesia.* 1989; **69**: 705–13.

222. Paut O, Sallabery M, Schreiber-Deturmeny E *et al.* Continuous fascia iliaca compartment block in children: a prospective evaluation of plasma bupivacaine concentrations, pain scores, and side effects. *Anesthesia and Analgesia.* 2001; **92**: 1159–63.

223. Veyckemans F, Van Obbergh L, Gouverneur J. Lessons from 1100 pediatric caudal blocks in a teaching hospital. *Regional Anesthesia.* 1992; **17**: 119–25.

224. Dalens B, Hasnaoui A. Caudal anesthesia in pediatric surgery: success rate and adverse effects in 750 consecutive patients. *Anesthesia and Analgesia.* 1989; **68**: 83–9.

∗225. Giaufre E, Dalens B, Gombert A. Epidemiology and morbidity of regional anesthesia in children: a one-year prospective survey of the French-Language Society of Pediatric Anesthesiologists. *Anesthesia and Analgesia.* 1996; **83**: 904–12.

226. Armitage E. Caudal block in children. *Anaesthesia.* 1979; **34**: 396–401.

227. Rapp H, Molnar V, Austin S *et al.* Ropivacaine in neonates and infants: a population pharmacokinetic evaluation following single caudal block. *Paediatric Anaesthesia.* 2004; **14**: 724–32.

228. Ala-Kokko T, Partanen A, Karinen J *et al.* Pharmacokinetics of 0.2% ropivacaine and 0.2% bupivacaine following caudal blocks in children. *Acta Anaesthesiologica Scandinavica.* 2000; **44**: 1099–102.

229. Ivani G, De Negri P, Lonnqvist PA *et al.* Caudal anesthesia for minor pediatric surgery: a prospective randomized comparison of ropivacaine 0.2% vs levobupivacaine 0.2%. *Paediatric Anaesthesia.* 2005; **15**: 491–4.

230. Irwin MG, Cheng W. Comparison of subcutaneous ring block of the penis with caudal epidural block for post-circumcision analgesia in children. *Anaesthesia and Intensive Care.* 1996; **24**: 365–7.

231. Vater M, Wandless J. Caudal or dorsal nerve block? A comparison of two local anaesthetic techniques for postoperative analgesia following day case circumcision. *Acta Anaesthesiologica Scandinavica.* 1985; **29**: 175–9.

232. Gunduz M, Ozalevli M, Ozbek H, Ozcengiz D. Comparison of caudal ketamine with lidocaine or tramadol administration for postoperative analgesia of hypospadias surgery in children. *Paediatric Anaesthesia.* 2006; **16**: 158–63.

233. Yildiz TS, Korkmaz F, Solak M, Toker K. Clonidine addition prolongs the duration of caudal analgesia. *Acta Anaesthesiologica Scandinavica.* 2006; **50**: 501–04.

234. Akbas M, Akbas H, Yegin A *et al.* Comparison of the effects of clonidine and ketamine added to ropivacaine on stress hormone levels and the duration of caudal analgesia. *Paediatric Anaesthesia.* 2005; **15**: 580–5.

235. Kumar P, Rudra A, Pan AK, Acharya A. Caudal additives in pediatrics: a comparison among midazolam, ketamine, and neostigmine coadministered with bupivacaine. *Anesthesia and Analgesia.* 2005; **101**: 69–73.

∗236. de Beer D, Thomas M. Caudal additives in children–solutions or problems? *British Journal of Anaesthesia.* 2003; **90**: 487–98.

∗237. Ansermino M, Basu R, Vandebeek C, Montgomery C. Nonopioid additives to local anaesthetics for caudal blockade in children: a systematic review. *Paediatric Anaesthesia.* 2003; **13**: 561–73.

238. Matsota P, Livanios S, Marinopoulou E. Intercostal nerve block with Bupivacaine for post-thoracotomy pain relief in children. *European Journal of Pediatric Surgery.* 2001; **11**: 219–22.

239. Karmakar MM, Critchley L. Continuous extrapleural intercostal nerve block for post thoracotomy analgesia in children. *Anaesthia and Intensive Care.* 1998; **26**: 115–6.

240. Downs CS, Cooper MG. Continuous extrapleural intercostal nerve block for post thoracotomy analgesia in children. *Anaesthia Intensive Care.* 1997; **25**: 390–7.

241. Bricker S, Telford R, Booker P. Pharmacokinetics of bupivacaine following intraoperative intercostal nerve block in neonates and in infants aged less than 6 months [published erratum appears in *Anesthesiology.* 1989; **71**: 630]. *Anesthesiology.* 1989; **70**: 942–7.

242. Rothstein P, Arthur G, Feldman H *et al.* Bupivacaine for intercostal nerve blocks in children: blood concentrations and pharmacokinetics. *Anesthesia and Analgesia.* 1986; **65**: 625–32.

243. Naja ZM, Raf M, El-Rajab M *et al.* A comparison of nerve stimulator guided paravertebral block and ilio-inguinal nerve block for analgesia after inguinal herniorrhaphy in children. *Anaesthesia.* 2006; **61**: 1064–8.

244. Shah R, Sabanathan S, Richardson J *et al.* Continuous paravertebral block for post thoracotomy analgesia in

children. *Journal of Cardiovascular Surgery.* 1997; **38**: 543–6.

245. Lonnqvist P, Olsson G. Paravertebral vs epidural block in children. Effects on postoperative morphine requirement after renal surgery. *Acta Anaesthesiologica Scandinavica.* 1994; **38**: 346–9.

246. Block B, Liu S, Rowlingson A *et al.* Efficacy of postoperative epidural analgesia: a meta-analysis. *Journal of the American Medical Association.* 2003; **290**: 2455–63.

247. Rodgers A, Walker N, Schug S *et al.* Reduction of postoperative mortality and morbidity with epidural or spinal anaesthesia: results from overview of randomised trials. *British Medical Journal.* 2000; **321**: 1493.

248. McNeely J, Farber N, Rusy L, Hoffman G. Epidural analgesia improves outcome following pediatric fundoplication. A retrospective analysis. *Regional Anesthesia.* 1997; **22**: 16–23.

249. Wilson GA, Brown JL, Crabbe DG *et al.* Is epidural analgesia associated with an improved outcome following open Nissen fundoplication? *Paediatric Anaesthesia.* 2001; **11**: 65–70.

250. Blumenthal S, Borgeat A, Nadig M, Min K. Postoperative analgesia after anterior correction of thoracic scoliosis: a prospective randomized study comparing continuous double epidural catheter technique with intravenous morphine. *Spine.* 2006; **31**: 1646–51.

251. Bosenberg A, Bland B, Schulte-Steinberg O, Downing J. Thoracic epidural anesthesia via caudal route in infants. *Anesthesiology.* 1988; **69**: 265–9.

252. Wood C, Goresky G, Klassen K *et al.* Complications of continuous epidural infusions for postoperative analgesia in children. *Canadian Journal of Anaesthesia.* 1994; **41**: 613–20.

*253. Llewellyn N, Moriarty A. The national pediatric epidural audit. *Paediatric Anaesthesia.* 2007; **17**: 520–33.

254. De Negri P, Ivani G, Tirri T *et al.* A comparison of epidural bupivacaine, levobupivacaine, and ropivacaine on postoperative analgesia and motor blockade. *Anesthesia and Analgesia.* 2004; **99**: 45–8.

255. Lerman J, Nolan J, Eyres R *et al.* Efficacy, safety, and pharmacokinetics of levobupivacaine with and without fentanyl after continuous epidural infusion in children: a multicenter trial. *Anesthesiology.* 2003; **99**: 1166–74.

256. Krane E. Delayed respiratory depression in a child after caudal epidural morphine. *Anesthesia and Analgesia.* 1988; **67**: 79–82.

257. Attia J, Ecoffey C, Sandouk P *et al.* Epidural morphine in children: pharmokinetics and CO2 sensitivity. *Anesthesiology.* 1986; **65**: 590–4.

258. Sucato DJ, Duey-Holtz A, Elerson E, Safavi F. Postoperative analgesia following surgical correction for adolescent idiopathic scoliosis: a comparison of continuous epidural analgesia and patient-controlled analgesia. *Spine.* 2005; **30**: 211–7.

259. O'Hara Jr JF, Cywinski JB, Tetzlaff JE *et al.* The effect of epidural vs intravenous analgesia for posterior spinal fusion surgery. *Paediatric Anaesthesia.* 2004; **14**: 1009–15.

260. Antila H, Manner T, Kuurila K *et al.* Ketoprofen and tramadol for analgesia during early recovery after tonsillectomy in children. *Paediatric Anaesthesia.* 2006; **16**: 548–53.

261. Chelly J. An iontophoretic, fentanyl HCl patient-controlled transdermal system for acute postoperative pain management. *Expert Opinion on Pharmacotherapy.* 2005; **6**: 1205–14.

*262. Gan T, Meyer T, Apfel C *et al.* Consensus guidelines for managing postoperative nausea and vomiting. *Anesthesia and Analgesia.* 2003; **97**: 62–71.

263. Wang S, Kain Z. Preoperative anxiety and postoperative nausea and vomiting in children: is there an association? *Anesthesia and Analgesia.* 2000; **90**: 571–5.

264. Thomas M, Woodhead G, Masood N, Howard R. Motion sickness as a predictor of postoperative vomiting in children aged 1-16 years. *Paediatric Anaesthesia.* 2007; **17**: 61–3.

265. Rose J, Watcha M. Postoperative nausea and vomiting in paediatric patients. *British Journal of Anaesthesia.* 1999; **83**: 104–17.

*266. Walker SM. Management of procedural pain in NICUs remains problematic. *Paediatric Anaesthesia.* 2005; **15**: 909–12.

267. Weisman S, Bernstein B, Schechter N. Consequences of inadequate analgesia during painful procedures in children. *Archives of Pediatrics and Adolescent Medicine.* 1998; **152**: 147–9.

*268. Murat I, Gall O, Tourniaire B. Procedural pain in children: evidence-based best practice and guidelines. *Regional Anesthesia and Pain Medicine.* 2003; **28**: 561–72.

*269. Uman LS, Chambers CT, McGrath PJ, Kisely S. Psychological interventions for needle-related procedural pain and distress in children and adolescents. *Cochrane Database of Systematic Reviews.* 2006; **CD005179**.

*270. Lin Y, Lee A, Kemper K, Berde C. Use of complementary and alternative medicine in pediatric pain management service: a survey. *Pain Medicine.* 2005; **6**: 452–8.

271. Gray PH, Trotter JA, Langbridge P, Doherty CV. Pain relief for neonates in Australian hospitals: a need to improve evidence-based practice. *Journal of Paediatrics and Child Health.* 2006; **42**: 10–3.

272. Anand KJ, Aranda JV, Berde CB *et al.* Summary proceedings from the neonatal pain-control group. *Pediatrics.* 2006; **117**: S9–S22.

*273. Mackenzie A, Acworth J, Norden M, *et al. Guideline statement: Management of procedure-related pain in neonates.* Sydney, NSW, Australia: Paediatrics and Child Health Division RACP, 2005: 24.

274. Batton DG, Barrington KJ, Wallman C. Prevention and management of pain in the neonate: an update. *Pediatrics.* 2006; **118**: 2231–41.

*275. Shah P, Aliwalas L, Shah V. Breastfeeding or breast milk for procedural pain in neonates. *Cochrane Database of Systematic Reviews.* 2006; **CD004950**.

276. Carbajal R, Chauvet X, Couderc S, Olivier-Martin M. Randomised trial of analgesic effects of sucrose, glucose, and pacifiers in term neonates. *British Medical Journal.* 1999; **319**: 1393-7.

277. Jain A, Rutter N. Local anaesthetic effect of topical amethocaine gel in neonates: randomised controlled trial. *Archives of Disease in Childhood. Fetal and Neonatal Edition.* 2000; **82**: F42-5.

278. Kaur G, Gupta P, Kumar A. A randomized trial of eutectic mixture of local anesthetics during lumbar puncture in newborns. *Archives of Pediatrics and Adolescent Medicine.* 2003; **157**: 1065-70.

279. Bellieni C, Bagnoli F, Perrone S *et al.* Effect of multisensory stimulation on analgesia in term neonates: a randomized controlled trial. *Pediatric Research.* 2002; **51**: 460-3.

*280. Cignacco E, Hamers JP, Stoffel L *et al.* The efficacy of non-pharmacological interventions in the management of procedural pain in preterm and term neonates. A systematic literature review. *European Journal of Pain.* 2007; **11**: 139-52.

281. Kolk A, van Hoof R, Fiedeldij Dop M. Preparing children for venepuncture. The effect of an integrated intervention on distress before and during venepuncture. *Child: Care, Health and Development.* 2000; **26**: 251-60.

282. Annequin D, Carbajal R, Chauvin P *et al.* Fixed 50% nitrous oxide oxygen mixture for painful procedures: A French survey. *Pediatrics.* 2000; **105**: E47.

28

Acute pain management in the elderly patient

PAMELA E MACINTYRE AND RICHARD UPTON

KEY LEARNING POINTS

- Older patients may have higher pain thresholds and therefore the early "warning sign" of pain, indicating an underlying pathological process, may be diminished or lost.
- The assessment of pain and the effectiveness of analgesic therapies may be more difficult in the elderly patient due to differences in reporting, measurement, and cognitive impairment.
- The cognitively impaired patient is at greater risk of undertreated acute pain.
- Most of the commonly used unidimensional measures of pain can be used in the elderly patient although the Verbal Descriptor Scale (VDS) and Numerical Rating Scale (NRS) appear to be preferred; the former is probably more reliable in patients with mild to moderate cognitive impairment.

- Compared with younger patients, older patients need less opioid to achieve the same degree of pain relief, although there is still a wide interpatient variation in the dose required. This is probably more related to pharmacodynamic changes in the elderly patient rather than age-related physiological changes.
- Paracetamol is the preferred nonopioid analgesic in the elderly patient; nonsteroidal anti-inflammatory drugs (NSAID) and cyclooxygenase (COX)-2 inhibitors should be used with caution.
- The risk of side effects from tricyclic antidepressant and anticonvulsant agents is higher in the elderly patient.
- The elderly patient may be at increased risk of side effects associated with epidural analgesia; this risk can be reduced with appropriate catheter placement and age-based dose/infusion regimens.

INTRODUCTION

In most countries of the world the proportion of elderly people in the population is increasing. Many will suffer from pain due to trauma, cancer, or surgery, or develop acute pain from other medical conditions, including diseases that disproportionately affect the elderly, such as arthritis, herpes zoster, and atherosclerotic peripheral vascular disease. Advances in anesthetic and surgical techniques have also meant that increasingly older patients now undergo surgery that was once considered to

carry a prohibitive risk (e.g. major orthopedic, thoracic, cardiac).

Up to 75 percent of elderly patients report inadequate pain relief after surgery.[1] Many factors may combine to make effective control of pain more difficult than in the younger patient. These include:

- coexisting diseases and concurrent medications, increasing the risk of disease–drug and drug–drug interactions;
- social and environmental factors;

- diminished functional status and physiological reserve;
- age-related changes in pharmacokinetics and pharmacodynamics;
- altered pain responses;
- difficulties in the assessment of pain, including problems related to cognitive impairment.

Many of these factors also make it more important to treat pain effectively in the older patient. While more likely to suffer from the complications of any pain treatment,[2] the elderly are also at higher risk of adverse consequences from surgery and from undertreated acute pain, including chest infection, myocardial ischemia and infarction, and thromboembolic complications.[2, 3] Given the trend towards ever more aggressive surgery in the elderly, they may be particularly likely to benefit from good pain relief, as better analgesia may reduce the risk of these complications.[4, 5, 6]

Much of the literature concerning acute pain management in the elderly patient centers on the treatment of postoperative pain, but the principles can be applied to the management of acute pain from any cause.

CHANGES IN PHARMACOKINETICS AND PHARMACODYNAMICS

In this section, discussion centers on opioids, in view of their widespread use as analgesic agents in the management of acute pain, although some comments on other analgesic drugs are also included. In all patients, including the elderly, opioids are characterized by considerable inter- and intrapatient variability in their pharmacodynamics and pharmacokinetics.[7] Optimal analgesia can therefore only be obtained by titration to effect for each patient (see below under Titration of opioids).[8]

Dose response in the elderly

Compared with younger patients, older patients need less opioid to achieve the same degree of pain relief. In the clinical setting (reviewed below under Opioid dose), there is evidence of a two- to four-fold decrease in morphine requirements.[9, 10] In a review of the kinetic and dynamic aspects of aging it has also been suggested that doses of fentanyl, alfentanil, sufentanil, and remifentanil should be reduced by up to 50 percent.[11, 12]

Systemic pharmacokinetics

A number of studies have measured the blood concentrations of analgesic drugs in young and elderly patients to test for age-related changes in systemic pharmacokinetics.

After parenteral administration, initial blood concentrations of morphine tend to be higher in the elderly patient,[13, 14] an observation usually interpreted as a reduced central distribution volume but also consistent with a change in cardiac output (see **Table 28.1**). Indeed, general anesthesia with halothane, which lowers cardiac output, has been associated with a trend to increased peak blood concentrations of morphine.[15] In addition, morphine clearance appears to be reduced in the elderly.[13, 14] However, a reduction in apparent distribution volume may mean that this does not result in an increase in the elimination half-life.[14, 16]

For fentanyl, there appear to be few differences in the systemic kinetics in the elderly,[17] although a prolonged elimination phase due to reduced clearance has been reported.[18] Blood concentrations tend to be slightly higher soon after administration in the elderly, suggesting caution with rapid intravenous (i.v.) administration may be warranted.

Remifentanil is unique amongst the clinically used opioids in that it is metabolized by esterase enzymes widely distributed in the body. Its systemic pharmacokinetic properties are therefore little changed by extremes of age or renal or hepatic dysfunction.[19]

The clearance of the local anesthetic lidocaine (lignocaine) is reduced with age,[20] but this change in systemic kinetics may be over-shadowed by age-related changes in absorption rate in typical clinical use (see below under Opioid metabolites). Clearance of bupivacaine[21] and ropivacaine[22] is also reduced in older patients.

ORAL ABSORPTION

Using paracetamol (acetaminophen) as a marker, it has been shown that the rate of gastric emptying and absorption of orally administered drugs does not change substantially with age.[23] Furthermore, there is some evidence to suggest that the active transport system limiting the absorption of some drugs from the gut is not affected by age.[24] However, the bioavailability of drugs may still be changed in the elderly, as it is the net process of both absorption and first-pass metabolism in the liver. Those factors acting to reduce hepatic clearance (see below under Increasing body fat/decreasing muscle mass) will cause corresponding increases in bioavailability leading to relatively higher blood concentrations of some orally administered drugs.[25]

ABSORPTION VIA NON-ORAL ROUTES

Intramuscular (i.m.) and subcutaneous (s.c.) routes of opioid administration are common in acute pain management. The i.m. absorption of drugs of moderate (e.g. morphine) to high (e.g. diazepam) lipophilicity is rapid and complete, and unaffected by age.[26, 27] The s.c. route has been little studied, but s.c. absorption appears to be

Table 28.1 The direction and approximate magnitude of physiological changes apparent in an elderly population (> 70 years) and the effects of individual changes on pharmacokinetic variables.

Physiological process	Magnitude	Likely kinetic/dynamic consequence	Dose strategy
Whole body			
Cardiac output	↓ 0–20%	↓ Central compartment volume	Smaller initial bolus dose
		↑ Peak concentrations after bolus	Slower injection rate
Fat	↑ 10–50% then ↓	Drug specific changes in distribution volume	Drug specific – dose based on total body weight or lean body weight
Muscle mass/blood flow	↓ 20%	↓ Distribution volume (water-soluble drugs)	
Plasma volume	Little change	↑ Free fraction of drug	
Total body water	↓ 10%	↔ Hepatic clearance of high-extraction drugs	Potential for changes in clearance and oral bioavailability
Plasma albumin	↓ 20%	↑ Hepatic clearance of low extraction drugs	Potential for changes in cerebral effects
Alpha-glycoprotein	↑ 30–50%	↑ Cerebral uptake of drug	
Drug binding	Drug specific		
Liver and gut			
Liver size	↓ 25–40%	↓ Hepatic clearance of high-extraction drugs	Minimal effect on i.v. bolus
Hepatic blood flow	↓ 25–40%	↔ Hepatic clearance of low extraction drugs	↓ Maintenance dose
			Potential for changes oral bioavailability
Phase I (e.g. oxidation)	↓ 25%	↓ Hepatic clearance (some low extraction drugs)	Minimal effect on i.v. bolus
Phase II	Little change		↓ Maintenance dose
			Potential for changes in oral bioavailability
Kidney			
Nephron mass	↓ 30%	↓ Clearance (polar drugs)	↓ Maintenance dose (renally cleared drugs)
Renal blood flow	↓ 10% per decade	Little effect on opioids (parent compound)	Assume, and monitor for, accelerated accumulation of polar active (M6G) or toxic (M3G, norpethidine) metabolites
Plasma flow at 80 years	↓ 50%	↓ Clearance of some active metabolites (e.g. M6G).	
Glomerular filtration rate	↓ 30–50%		
Creatinine clearance	↓ 50–70%		
CNS			
Cerebral blood flow and metabolism	↓ 20%	↓ Distribution to the CNS	Little net effect
Cerebral volume	↓ 20%	↓ Apparent volume in the CNS	
Active BBB transport (efflux)	↓ (Drug specific)	↑ Apparent volume in the CNS	↓ Bolus dose during titration
		↑ Apparent increase in CNS sensitivity	↓ Maintenance dose
Pain threshold/sensitivity	Little change		Need for titration unchanged
Concentration response (opioids)	↑ 50% for some opioids	↑ Response to opioids	↓ Bolus dose during titration
			↓ Maintenance dose

Note that the net effect of these changes on drug disposition may be minimal (see text). M6G, morphine-6-glucuronide; M3G, morphine-3-glucuronide.

relatively rapid and complete in the elderly,[28] and contributes no more than other kinetic processes to the variability of the blood concentrations of morphine seen in these patients.[7]

The use of local anesthetics by infiltration, nerve block, epidural, or intrathecal routes is important for pain management. It has been shown that an epidural dose of levobupivacaine produces a higher block and is characterized by faster but less complete absorption in the elderly.[29] In some older patients, epidural injection of bupivacaine produced maximum blood concentrations within five minutes, which may be a consequence of the patient's age. A study of ropivacaine kinetics after epidural administration showed a slight reduction in the initial fraction absorbed, a reduction in clearance and an increase in elimination half-life in older patients. However, the changes in blood concentrations with age were considered unlikely to increase the risk of toxicity.[22]

CEREBRAL DRUG UPTAKE

As most potent analgesics are centrally acting, the rate and extent of their passage from the blood into the central nervous system (CNS) (brain and spinal cord) may influence their clinical behavior.[30] It is now recognized that there are both passive and active components to the cerebral uptake of drugs. With respect to passive uptake, important factors are the lipophilicity of a drug and its protein binding in blood,[31] which affect the distribution volume in the brain. Low distribution volumes imply rapid brain:blood equilibration and relatively less drug in the brain. With age it is known that the size of the brain decreases by up to 20–40 percent and that there is a concomitant decrease in cerebral blood flow. However, if cerebral kinetics are flow limited, as is the case for pethidine (meperidine) and alfentanil,[32] the rate of brain:blood equilibration will be proportional to the ratio of cerebral distribution volume to cerebral blood flow. As both appear to change in unison with age, the cerebral kinetics of these opioids should be relatively unaffected by age. Of more importance may be the changes in plasma protein concentrations in the elderly (see below under Altered protein binding) that could potentially affect the cerebral distribution of drugs that are highly protein bound.

With respect to active processes, it is known that a limited number of drugs (typically endogenous compounds or their analogs) are actively taken into the brain. The activity of these uptake processes may be reduced with age.[33] In contrast, a number of important drugs (e.g. morphine, methadone) are actively removed from the brain by efflux transporter proteins such as P-glycoprotein and multidrug resistance protein (MRP).[34] In theory, the brain concentrations of such transported drugs are subject to the activity of the transporters, their potential inhibition by competing compounds, and disruptions to the blood–brain barrier. There appears to be a modest reduction in P-glycoprotein activity in the elderly leading to higher drug concentrations in the brain,[35] and it has been postulated that some neurodegenerative diseases associated with aging are linked with reductions in efflux transporter activity.[36] However, the implications of these findings for drug therapy in the elderly are largely unknown.

Physiological pharmacokinetics and aging

Aging is associated with a number of physiological changes that have been relatively well documented.[11, 24, 37, 38] These changes are summarized in **Table 28.1**. Pertinent points are, first, that the physiological changes are progressive, but that their rate of onset can be highly variable between individuals. Second, it is important to recognize that the changes in **Table 28.1** are generally those attributable to aging alone, but that these can be compounded by the higher incidence of degenerative and other diseases in the elderly. Therefore, for example, while a decrease in cerebral volume appears to be an inevitable result of aging, recent data would suggest that decreases in cardiac output or fluid volumes reflect concomitant disease. It would be rare to find a cohort of elderly patients whose physiological condition could be attributed to aging alone. This will inevitably complicate the interpretation of kinetic studies comparing young and elderly patient groups. The physiological changes associated with aging that are of most pharmacokinetic significance are as follows.

CARDIAC OUTPUT

Recent studies of drugs other than opioids have shown that cardiac output is itself an important pharmacokinetic parameter, particularly after administration of an i.v. bolus dose. During injection, the i.v. bolus of drug is added to a flowing stream of blood. This is then mixed with other drug-free blood until the dose is effectively diluted in a stream of blood in the pulmonary artery, flowing at a rate determined by the cardiac output. The higher the cardiac output, and therefore the greater the volume of blood per unit time to which the drug has been added, the lower the peak concentration achieved, and vice versa. This dilution effect with cardiac output may be retained in arterial blood, even after first-pass passage of the drug through the lungs. Consequently, the initial high arterial concentrations observed in the first few minutes after administration of a bolus dose of drug is a function of this dilution with cardiac output and the kinetics of its passage through the lungs.[39] This phase of elution of drug from the lungs is traditionally, but erroneously, attributed to the removal of drug from the "central volume."

Given their fundamental basis, these kinetic principles are likely to apply to opioids. Thus, it would be predicted that the 0–20 percent reduction in cardiac output in any group of elderly patients (**Table 28.1**) would lead to higher peak arterial concentrations after administration of a bolus dose and therefore smaller central volumes by compartmental analysis. This is supported by observations in the elderly of higher initial concentrations immediately after i.v. fentanyl administration.[18, 40]

HEPATIC CLEARANCE

The liver decreases in size by 25–40 percent with increasing age and hepatic blood flow decreases in proportion (**Table 28.1**). The activity of hepatic enzymes is unchanged for some phase II pathways, but may be reduced by up to 25 percent for some oxidative pathways.[38] Most opioids have relatively high extraction ratios across the liver. According to the well-stirred model of hepatic clearance, clearance of opioids by the liver would be relatively insensitive to the activity of hepatic enzymes (i.e. they are in excess) but proportional to hepatic blood flow. Thus, for those drugs with predominantly hepatic clearance (e.g. most opioids), a 25–40 percent reduction in clearance could be expected secondary to reduced hepatic blood flow. In practice, the consequences of this would range from small, in the case of administration of a bolus of drug (where peak concentrations and effects are relatively unaffected by hepatic clearance), to very significant, for drugs administered repeatedly or by infusion to pseudo-steady-state concentrations or drugs that are administered orally.

By virtue of the inverse relationship between steady-state blood concentration and clearance, a 25 percent reduction in hepatic clearance would equate to a 33 percent increase in the steady-state blood concentration, while a 40 percent reduction would equate to a 67 percent increase.

RENAL CLEARANCE

The most profound change with age is the reduction in size and functional capacity of the kidneys. Indeed, it has been proposed that elderly patients should be considered renally impaired.[37] While few of the opioids have significant renal clearance, as they are sufficiently lipophilic to be reabsorbed, some (e.g. morphine, hydromorphone, pethidine, tramadol) have relatively polar renally cleared toxic metabolites that they have significant potential for accumulation in the elderly. A 50 percent reduction in the renal clearance of such a metabolite would equate to a two-fold increase in its steady-state blood concentration.

INCREASING BODY FAT/DECREASING MUSCLE MASS

While age itself is a poor predictor of body composition,[41] there are general trends in body composition with age. Lean body mass is generally constant through early adult life, and begins to decline after age 60 years. Fat mass tends to increase during adult life, and also peaks near 60 years of age.[41, 42] There is a tendency for fat in the elderly to be localized in the abdomen.[42] The elderly patient therefore can range from the obese to the very frail.

Dose adjustment for obesity (irrespective of age) is a complex issue[43] and reflects the relative changes in distribution volume of a drug. Drugs that are relatively water-soluble (e.g. morphine) and distribute into lean body tissues have relatively unchanged distribution volumes. Drugs that are lipid soluble (e.g. diazepam, lidocaine, fentanyl) may have relatively increased distribution volumes in the obese subject, although adjustments in dose regimens are drug specific.[24] It could be postulated that this increased uptake into fat could contribute to a more rapid decline in blood concentration after administration of a bolus dose, which may offset any reduced hepatic clearance. Indeed, the kinetics of fentanyl appear to be relatively unaffected by aging.[40]

ALTERED PROTEIN BINDING

There is a readily measurable age-related change in the levels of plasma proteins (**Table 28.1**). Plasma albumin decreases by up to 20 percent and is linked with sarcopenia and poor nutrition,[44] whereas alpha-acid glycoprotein increases by 30–50 percent.[45] The consequences of these changes have been considered by Shafer[11] and depend to which protein the drug is predominantly bound. The major consequences of altered protein binding in the context of pain management are changes in clearance and changes in distribution volumes in target organs such as the CNS. The latter was discussed above under Cerebral drug uptake. The clearances of drugs with high hepatic extraction ratios (e.g. morphine, fentanyl, alfentanil) are relatively unaffected by changes in protein binding. Those with low hepatic extraction ratios (e.g. methadone, diazepam) may have a clearance that is dependent on protein binding and hence age. This has been confirmed for diazepam, which shows an age-related decrease in clearance of free but not total drug.[46]

Pharmacodynamics

There have been relatively few studies of pharmacokinetic–pharmacodynamic relationships for opioids, and most have used a surrogate measure of effect other than clinical pain relief. Scott and Stanski[17] analyzed the effects of fentanyl and alfentanil on the electroencephalogram (EEG) and concluded that the kinetics of these opioids were unaffected by age, but that the sensitivity of the brain to opioids was increased by 50 percent. Similar results have been reported with remifentanil.[12] This is the best available evidence of a substantial pharmacodynamic component to the reduction in opioid dose requirement in the elderly.

It is not clear whether this can be attributed to changes in the number or function of opioid receptors in the CNS, or whether it is due to an increased penetration of opioids in the CNS. Changes to the CNS with age include reductions in the density of neurons, neurotransmitters, and receptors, which may predispose the elderly to increased drug sensitivity (see later under Anti-convulsants).[38, 47]

Simulations

The quantitative consequences of the physiological changes listed in **Table 28.1** are difficult to predict without recourse to physiological models that incorporate drugs kinetics in individual tissues. Such models have been proposed for several opioids, but only Bjorkman *et al.*[48] have used a model to simulate the kinetic consequences of aging. Their simulations predicted that age-related changes in physiological state will have only a minor influence on the kinetics of fentanyl and alfentanil.

To explore this further, we used the simplest physiological model of fentanyl reported by Bjorkman *et al.*[49] and simulated the arterial and CNS concentrations expected in young and old patients based on the physiological changes summarized in **Table 28.1**. This approach is based on the premise that CNS concentrations of opioids are temporally related to the time-course of their clinical effects[30] and that there is (for a given patient at a given time) a minimum effective analgesic concentration (MEAC) in the CNS.

The simulations were of the administration of fentanyl by bolus dose (**Figure 28.1**) and infusion (**Figure 28.2**). In agreement with Bjorkman *et al.*, the time-courses of the arterial blood concentrations, particularly after the bolus dose, did not differ substantially with age. This concurs with studies showing only minor kinetic changes with age for fentanyl.[40] In the above analysis, the cerebral kinetics of opioids were not predicted to differ greatly with age as cerebral blood flow and volume decreased in unison. It is therefore not surprising that there were only minor changes in the predicted time-courses of CNS fentanyl concentrations between young and old patients in these simulations. This analysis assumes that any active transport of fentanyl in the brain of man could be ignored.[50] Thus, in order to account for the 50 percent reduction in dose requirements in the elderly, the MEAC must be reduced.

This was carried out empirically in the simulations, but it is consistent with the 50 percent reduction in brain sensitivity reported by Scott and Stanski.[17] An important corollary is that the time to peak concentrations and effect did not differ between the young and old. This is consistent with the clinical observation that analgesia in elderly patients can be obtained by titration of smaller doses than those required by younger patients, but with the same dose interval.[8]

While the intention is to examine the contribution of age-related kinetic changes to clinical observations, it is important to recognize that such simulations are based on mean physiological data and are not representative of any individual patient. The changes in pharmacokinetics and pharmacodynamics in the elderly can be summarized as:

- a physiological decline with age that is progressive but variable;
- decreases in cardiac output and hepatic and renal drug clearance;
- two- to four-fold reductions in opioid requirements;
- physiological changes associated with aging that may produce higher drug concentrations but are not sufficient to account for the magnitude of these dose reductions;
- a need for reduced doses in the elderly that appears to have a significant pharmacodynamic component.

CHANGES IN PAIN PERCEPTION

A number of structural, neurochemical, and functional changes have been observed in the peripheral and CNSs of elderly patients (**Table 28.2**), including areas involved in nociceptive processing.[51] Some of these changes may place the older patient at greater risk of harm, because the presence of pain as an indicator (a "warning sign") of an underlying pathological process may be reduced. Other changes may make it more difficult for the patient to tolerate pain once it has occurred.

In the experimental setting, changes in pain thresholds and pain tolerance have been reported in the elderly, although the results are inconsistent. This may be partly due to the methodologies used[53] and/or that reported differences in pain can depend on the pain scale used in elderly patients.[54] In general, it seems that thresholds to pain using thermal stimuli are increased; results involving mechanical stimuli are equivocal; and electrical pain thresholds appear not to change[51] unless the stimulus duration is kept short.[53] Increased pain thresholds could mean that there is some deterioration in the early warning function of pain as there is less time between the first perception of pain and tissue damage.[51]

While the significance of these results in the clinical setting remains uncertain, there are a number of clinical reports which are in general agreement with these experimental findings. These reports show that the presentation of some acute disease states that are usually associated with severe pain may differ in the elderly, with pain reported later, less frequently, or not at all.

For example, in patients with angina exercised to produce a 1 mm ST depression, onset of pain was reported later in elderly patients compared with younger patients matched for disease severity and medications.[55, 56]

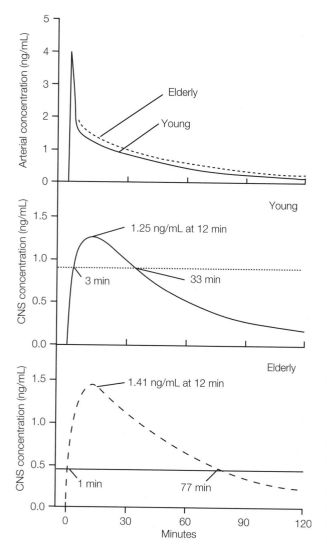

Figure 28.1 An attempt to account for the kinetic and dynamic basis of clinical observations following the bolus administration of 100 µg fentanyl over 0.5 minutes to 20-year-old (young) and 70-year-old (elderly) individuals. The physiological model of Bjorkman *et al.* was used to simulate arterial and CNS fentanyl concentrations. Physiological changes to account for aging were a 20 percent reduction in the size (and flows) to the brain, heart, and muscle mass, a 37.5 percent reduction in liver mass, a 50 percent reduction in kidney mass, and a 30 percent increase in body fat. Together, this produced a 21 percent decrease in cardiac output, and hepatic clearance decreased from 0.8 to 0.54 L/min. It was assumed that the CNS kinetics of fentanyl were flow limited, that the CNS concentrations of opioids were temporally related to the time-course of their clinical effects, and that there was an MEAC in the CNS.[30] (a) The predicted arterial concentrations in the young and the elderly. There were only minor changes in the time-course of arterial concentrations. (b) The time-course of the apparent CNS concentrations of fentanyl in the young with an MEAC of 0.9 ng/mL (dotted line) chosen to be consistent with fentanyl producing 0.5 hours of analgesia. (c) The time-course of the CNS concentrations of fentanyl in the elderly. Peak CNS concentrations occurred at the same time as the younger patient but were slightly higher. A 50 percent reduction in the MEAC (dotted line) was required to produce the two-fold longer duration of action observed in the elderly.

Precordial chest pain and arm pain are also less likely to be presenting complaints in an elderly patient with acute myocardial infarction and "silent" myocardial infarcts are more common.[57, 58, 59, 60]

Similarly, elderly patients are less likely to report abdominal pain, for example with peritonitis, intestinal obstruction, diverticulitis, and gastrointestinal ulceration.[52, 59, 61] Not surprisingly, atypical pain presentations or lack of pain in association with underlying pathology may lead to significant delays in diagnosis.[59]

Similar results have been noted in other acute pain settings. Elderly patients may report less postoperative pain than their younger counterparts when matched for surgical procedure.[54, 62] Thomas *et al.*[62] documented a 10 to 20 percent decrease in pain intensity each decade after the age of 60 years. Procedural pain may also be less, for example on insertion of an i.v. cannula.[63]

Studies looking at age-related changes in pain tolerance are more limited but generally show that tolerance is reduced in elderly people,[51] meaning that they are less able to tolerate severe pain.

ASSESSMENT OF PAIN

While measures of pain are important, pain assessment must start with a basic pain history. The history should also be repeated whenever necessary (for example, if the pain is not well controlled or changing in nature), as changes in treatment may be required. Assessment of other factors that may play a role in the amount of pain experienced or reported are also important (see below under Reporting of pain).

The assessment of pain and evaluation of pain relief therapies in the elderly patient may present problems arising from differences in reporting, cognitive impairment, and difficulties in measurement.

Reporting of pain

Physiological, psychological, and cultural changes associated with aging may result in differences in the reporting of pain. These include fear, anxiety, depression,

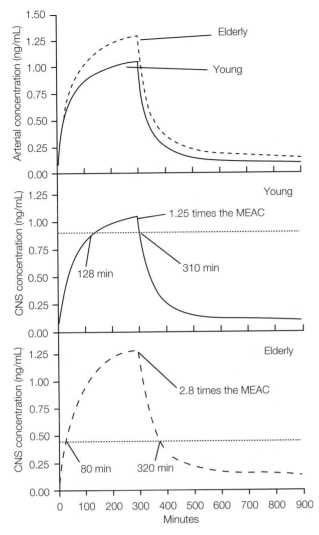

Figure 28.2 An attempt to account for the kinetic and dynamic basis of clinical observations following the infusion (at 1.25 μg/min) of fentanyl for 100 minutes to 20-year-old (young) and 70-year-old (elderly) individuals. Methods were as for **Figure 28.1**. (a) The predicted arterial concentrations after accounting for the physiological changes associated with aging are described in the text. The peak arterial concentrations were 22 percent higher in the elderly after a 300 minute infusion. At steady state, the reduction in clearance from 0.8 to 0.54 L/min would produce concentrations 48 percent higher in the elderly. (b) The time-course of the apparent CNS concentrations of fentanyl in the young with an MEAC of 0.9 ng/mL (dotted line), as used in **Figure 28.1**. (c) The time-course of the CNS concentrations of fentanyl in the elderly after accounting for the physiological changes associated with aging described in the text. Although the concentrations are 23 percent higher in the elderly, an approximate 50 percent reduction in MEAC is required to produce the two-fold increase in analgesia observed in the elderly.

cognitive impairment, the implications of the disease, loss of independence, feelings of isolation, the quality of social support available, culture, and family.[64] The elderly may see pain as a normal part of aging,[65] as will some of their

Table 28.2 Structural, neurochemical, and functional changes associated with aging.[51, 52]

Changes associated with aging
↓ Density of peripheral nerve fibers (unmyelinated > myelinated)
↑ Sensory neuron degeneration (peripheral and spinal cord)
↓ Nerve fiber conduction velocities
↓ Levels of substance P (skin and dorsal root ganglia)
Loss of CNS neurons/dendritic connections
Altered neurotransmitter receptor binding/axonal transport
Neurochemical deterioration of opioid, serotonergic and noradrenergic systems resulting in altered descending inhibitory and endogenous opioid mechanisms

carers. If the situation is potentially painful, the patient should be assumed to be in pain, even though they may not volunteer any complaint of pain.

COGNITIVE IMPAIRMENT

Cognitive function declines with age. Cognitively impaired patients are known to be at greater risk of undertreatment of acute pain.[66, 67, 68] In the studies by Feldt et al.[68][III] and Forster et al.,[66][III] cognitively impaired elderly patients received significantly less opioid analgesia than cognitively intact patients after a hip fracture.

Morrison and Siu,[67][III] in a similar group of elderly patients with hip fractures, also showed that those with advanced dementia received one-third of the amount of opioid given to those patients who were cognitively intact. Of added concern is that 44 percent of the latter group still reported severe to very severe pain after their surgery. In another study, these authors have shown that inadequate pain relief in cognitively intact patients after hip fracture is associated with an increased length of hospital stay, delayed ambulation, and long-term functional impairment.[69][III]

Reported pain intensity and number of pain complaints decrease with increasing cognitive impairment,[70, 71, 72, 73] even though these patients are just as likely as cognitively intact patients of the same age to have painful conditions or illnesses.[70][III] The reasons for this are not clear and could result from a diminished capacity to report or memory impairment.[73] It is not thought that patients with dementia experience less pain.[70] In a study by Cole et al.,[74][III] functional magnetic resonance imaging (MRI) responses following mechanical pressure stimulation showed no evidence of diminished pain-related activity in patients with Alzheimer's disease compared with age-matched controls, indicating that pain perception and processing were not diminished in these patients.

In an interesting study looking at the placebo component of analgesic therapies, Benedetti et al.[75][III] studied the effect of both "overtly applied" and "covertly applied" local anesthetic on pain after venipuncture in patients with Alzheimer's disease. They determined that patients with reduced Frontal Assessment Battery scores (a measure of frontal executive function) had a reduced placebo component to their pain relief which, in turn, reduced treatment efficacy, so that dose increases were required to produce adequate analgesia. They also found that reduced connectivity between prefrontal lobes and the rest of the brain disrupted the placebo component and commented that their results emphasize the active part that cognition and prefrontal lobes play in therapeutic outcome.

DELIRIUM

A common form of acute cognitive impairment in the elderly is delirium or confusion, which is associated with increased postoperative morbidity, impaired postoperative rehabilitation, and prolonged hospital stays.[76] [III], [77][I] Delirium is more common during acute illnesses in the elderly and occurs in up to 80 percent of elderly postoperative patients, depending on the type of surgery.[77] Risk factors for the development of delirium include those listed in **Table 28.3**.[76, 77, 78, 79, 80, 81, 82, 83]

Measurement of pain

Accurate assessment of pain is necessary for effective management of pain. As with the younger patient, the

Table 28.3 Risk factors for delirium.[76, 77, 78, 79, 80, 81, 82, 83]

Nonpharmacologic risk factors	Medications
Old age	Drugs with central anticholinergic activity
Preexisting dementia	Atropine
Depression	Tricyclic antidepressants
Withdrawal from alcohol or sedatives	Major tranquilizers
Infection	Antiparkinsonian drugs
Fluid and electrolyte imbalance	Some antiemetics
Unrelieved pain	Digoxin
Hypoxemia	β-blockers
	H_2 antagonists (e.g. ranitidine)
	Ketamine
	Opioids (especially pethidine)
	Benzodiazepines
	Oral hypoglycemics
	Antihistamines
	NSAIDs
	Anticonvulsants

elderly patient's self-report is the most reliable indicator of pain (see Chapter 8, Assessment, measurement, and history).

PATIENT SELF-REPORT MEASURES OF PAIN

In the acute care setting, unidimensional measures of pain intensity, such as the Visual Analog Scale (VAS), Verbal Numerical Rating Scale (VNRS) and Verbal Descriptor Scale (VDS), Faces Pain Scales (FPS) and Numerical Rating Scale (NRS), a calibrated VAS, are commonly employed measures of pain. All have been used as effective discriminators of pain in this patient group.[84, 85, 86]

In patients using patient-controlled analgesia (PCA) after surgery, the NRS was the preferred pain scale in both younger and older patient groups, with high reliability and validity, although the VDS also had a favorable and similar profile; use of the VAS in the elderly patients resulted in high rates of unscorable data and low validity.[87][III] In this study, patients who were confused were excluded. Similarly, in another comparison of five pain scales (VAS, NRS, VDS, VNRS, and FPS) in younger and older patients, the NRS was the preferred scale, but the VDS was the most sensitive and reliable.[86][III]

Scales such as the VDS, using familiar words such as none, slight, mild, moderate, severe, and extreme, may also be the most reliable in patients with mild to moderate cognitive impairment.[54][III], [65, 70, 84, 85][III], [86][III], [88][III] These patients may need more time to assimilate and respond to questions, and may require repeated questioning in order to obtain an accurate answer.[2, 84] They are able to report pain reasonably reliably at the time when asked (present pain) but the recall of pain experienced over time may be less reliable.[68, 70, 71, 72]

OTHER MEASURES OF PAIN

In noncommunicative patients, behaviors such as restlessness, tense muscles, frowning, or grimacing, and patient sounds such as grunting or groaning, have been used in attempts to assess pain severity. Although some of these behaviors have been shown to correlate reasonably well with patient self-report in cognitively intact adults, this may not be the case in nonverbal adults.[73] While these behaviors may not be able to accurately indicate pain intensity in patients with severe dementia, they are probably a reasonable indicator of the presence of pain.[89, 90] An added complication in patients with dementia is that pain behaviors may not be "typical" – for example, pain may lead to aggression or social withdrawal.[70]

Pain Assessment in Advanced Dementia (PAINAD) is a simple, reliable, and validated five-item observational tool that has been developed to measure pain in patients with moderate or severe dementia.[91, 92][III]

It should not be forgotten that observation of function, such as the ability to take deep breaths and cough, as well as tolerate physiotherapy and ambulation, is also important and may help to assess adequacy of analgesia.

ANALGESIC DRUGS AND THE ELDERLY

Acute pain is commonly nociceptive, as seen after trauma, surgery, or myocardial infarction. However, neuropathic pain may also occur in the acute pain setting, for example, following nerve injury associated with a fracture, amputation of a limb, or compression/invasion by a tumor. As with the younger adult, therefore, a range of analgesic drugs may be required. The list below is not exhaustive and patient age may also need to be taken into consideration before other medications are prescribed and administered.

Opioids and tramadol

Elderly patients require less opioid for the management of acute pain than younger patients.[9][V], [10, 87][V], [93][V] Details of possible age-related changes in pharmacokinetics (see under Systemic pharmacokinetics), pharmacodynamics (see under Pharmacodynamics), and pain perception (see under Assessment of pain) have been discussed above. Also of importance is the enormous interpatient variability in plasma concentrations that follow administration of opioids[7] and the large interpatient variation in the actual blood concentration required for analgesia. These serve only to highlight the need for pain management strategies to be adjusted to suit individual patients.

In general, the safe and effective management of opioid analgesia requires:

- the use of a suitable drug and drug preparation;
- an awareness of potential problems with metabolites of opioids;
- age-related dosage schedules, incorporating flexibility in dose size and dose interval;
- careful titration to effect;
- avoidance of the concurrent use of sedatives;
- recognition and appropriate treatment of opioid-related side effects.

Titration is especially important in the elderly patient. For more details see Chapter 3, Clinical pharmacology: opioids.

SUITABLE OPIOIDS AND OPIOID PREPARATIONS

In general, an opioid with a shorter half-life is preferred as it allows more rapid and safe titration[94][V] and suitable drugs include morphine, oxycodone, hydromorphone, and fentanyl.

Pethidine is best avoided because of potential problems with the metabolite norpethidine[95] and the greater risk of confusion in older patients (**Table 28.3**), agonist-antagonist opioids (e.g. butorphanol and nalbuphine) are generally not recommended because of a higher incidence of delirium in the elderly,[2] and extra caution is required when using methadone as the half-life can be unexpectedly prolonged.[64, 96]

Tramadol is an atypical centrally acting analgesic. It has a weak affinity for the opioid receptor and inhibits norepinephrine (noradrenaline) and serotonin reuptake; the β-elimination phase is increased in patients with renal or hepatic impairment.[97] In elderly patients (over 75 years) the elimination half-life is also slightly prolonged.[98] Daily dose limits of 300 mg are suggested in these patients.[99] It is possible that the lower incidence of constipation[100] and sedation compared with other opioids may be of benefit in the elderly patient.[101][III]

Care is required when preparations designed to allow a slow and sustained release of an opioid are used, such as sustained-release oral morphine or oxycodone preparations and transdermal fentanyl patches. These preparations are not suitable for rapid titration, and the persistent drug concentrations and slow offset can make any side effects difficult to treat. They are not recommended for acute pain management, at least in the initial stages, especially in the elderly patient.[94][V]

OPIOID METABOLITES

Accumulation of active opioid metabolites (for details see Chapter 3, Clinical pharmacology: opioids) can occur in patients with renal impairment or when high doses are used, especially over a prolonged period. Accumulation of morphine-6-glucuronide (M6G), a major metabolite of morphine and a μ agonist more potent than morphine, may contribute to analgesia and μ receptor-related side effects such as sedation. M3G has no affinity for the μ receptor, may antagonize the action of morphine, and may also be responsible for some of the excitatory effects seen after administration of high doses of morphine, such as hyperalgesia, myoclonic jerks, and convulsions.[94] Similar symptoms may be seen with high levels of hydromorphone-3-glucuronide, the major metabolite of hydromorphone.

Pethidine should be avoided in the elderly because significant accumulation of the renally excreted active metabolite, nororpethidine, can occur[64] leading to agitation, tremor, twitching, and convulsions.[95][III]

Accumulation of the metabolites of dextropropoxyphene may lead to confusion, delusions, hallucinations, and cardiotoxicity.[94][V] While it has been suggested that this drug is probably best avoided in older patients,[102] such suggestions have largely been based on expert opinion and good evidence about the safety and tolerability of dextropropoxyphene in the older patient is still lacking.[103][I]

OPIOID DOSE

Age, rather than patient weight, appears to be a better determinant of the amount of opioid an adult is likely to require for effective management of acute pain. Morphine,[9][V], [93][V], [104][V] fentanyl,[11][III], [17][V], and remifentanil[12][V] requirements are known to decrease as patient age increases.

A number of studies have shown that the average parenteral morphine requirements of a 70-year-old are around 70 percent less than the requirements of a 20-year-old patient.[9][V], [93][V], [105][V] Following major surgery in opioid-naive patients aged 20 to 70 years, it was shown that average first-24 hour PCA morphine requirement (mg) was approximately = 100 − age (years), although there was up to a ten-fold variation in dose requirements in each age group.[9] The decrease in opioid requirement is not associated with reports of increased pain.[9, 105]

TITRATION OF OPIOIDS

While opioid dose appears to be best predicted by age, differences in age are not enough to account for the wide interpatient variation seen in total opioid requirement. In the elderly, as with any other patient group, subsequent doses must be titrated to suit individual patient needs.

To enable opioid analgesia to be titrated safely yet effectively, the following are required:

- appropriate age-related doses and dose intervals (see examples in **Table 28.4**);
- measures of pain;
- endpoints that indicate excessive opioid dose, especially respiratory depression.

Detection of early respiratory depression

The risk of respiratory depression is said to be greater in older patients[106][V] and the fear of causing respiratory depression in the elderly patient, especially those with respiratory disease, often leads to inadequate doses of opioid being given. However, as with other patients, significant respiratory depression can generally be avoided if appropriate monitoring is in place.

It is often assumed that respiratory depression will be detected by monitoring a patient's respiratory rate. However, a decrease in respiratory rate is now known to be a late and unreliable sign of respiratory depression. In a review of opioid-related adverse drug reactions before and after the hospital-wide introduction of a numerical pain treatment algorithm, it was noticed that significant oversedation or respiratory depression, which in some cases led to admission to an intensive care unit and/or the death of the patient, was almost inevitably preceded by increasing levels of sedation but, in the vast majority of these patients, respiratory rate remained above 12 breaths per minute.[107][V]

Table 28.4 Suggested initial age-based morphine doses and dose intervals for intermittent s.c./i.m. and i.v. morphine administration.[8, 9]

Age (years)	Initial morphine dose range (mg)
s.c. or i.m. doses, given 1–2 hourly PRN	
15–39	7.5–12.5
40–59	5.0–10.0
60–69	2.5–7.5
70–85	2.5–5.0
>85	2.0–3.0
i.v. doses, given 5 minutely PRN[a]	
15–69	1, 2, or 4
≥70	0.5, 1, or 2

[a]Given in a monitored setting to rapid analgesia and not for routine analgesia in general wards.

This has also been noted in patients given epidural morphine. Ready *et al.*[108][V] reported a series of four patients aged 57 to 69 given epidural morphine, who, despite respiratory rates remaining greater than or equal to eight breaths per minute, developed marked increases in PCO_2. All these patients were noted to be excessively sedated.

Pulse oximetry is sometimes used as a monitor of respiratory depression, but this can also be unreliable. In postoperative patients, hypoxemia is reasonably common. Both persistent hypoxemia (in particular due to decrease in functional residual capacity leading to airway closure, ventilation-perfusion abnormalities and atelectasis) and episodic hypoxemia (thought to be at least partly related to the use of opioids)[109] may be seen even in "healthy" patients and in the absence of any complication,[110] although they are more likely to occur in the elderly.[109, 110]

Supplemental oxygen can help to minimize the risk of significant hypoxemia[111][II] and is therefore recommended for at least the first 48 to 72 hours following major surgery, particularly in the elderly and high risk patient, and regardless of the method of opioid administration.[8][V], [78][V], [94][V]

Clinically, the best indicator of early respiratory depression appears to be sedation.[8, 94, 107] Sedation should be monitored in all patients given opioids, regardless of route, using a simple sedation score (see example in **Table 28.5**).

OTHER SIDE EFFECTS OF OPIOIDS

Nausea and vomiting

Opioids are just one cause of nausea and vomiting in the postoperative period. As the incidence decreases with increasing age,[112][V] routine antiemetics are not recommended. In general, there appears to be little

Table 28.5 Example of a simple sedation score.[8, 108]

Simple sedation score
0 = None
1 = Easy to arouse
2 = Constantly drowsy, easy to arouse, cannot stay awake
3 = Somnolent, difficult to arouse

difference in the side-effect profiles of different opioids at equianalgesic doses.[94, 113][II]

Pruritus

Pruritus also appears to be less common in the elderly.[114] [V] When compared with fentanyl and pethidine, morphine appears to cause more itch.[113][II] Therefore, a simple treatment option, if the itch is of concern to the patient, is to change to another opioid (e.g. from morphine to fentanyl).[8] If itching results from epidural or intrathecal opioids (again, less common in the elderly), small doses of naloxone can be effective.[8]

Cognitive effects

Fentanyl may cause less depression of postoperative cognitive function[115][II] and less confusion[116][II] in elderly patients compared with morphine. In a study comparing patients given PCA tramadol or fentanyl, no difference in cognitive effects were found.[101][II] However, this might not have been a good comparison because the bolus doses used were not equianalgesic (tramadol 20 mg, fentanyl 10 μg) – not surprisingly, patients given tramadol had better pain relief with movement on the first day after surgery.

Local anesthetics

The half-lives of bupivacaine[21] and ropivacaine[22] are significantly increased and clearances significantly decreased in older patients. If repeat doses or continuous infusions are to be used, it might be wise to reduce the total dose in the elderly to avoid possible accumulation. An alternative would be to use a drug reported to have less cardiotoxicity than bupivacaine, such as ropivacaine.[117] In acute pain management practice, epidural infusions using low doses of bupivacaine or ropivacaine combined with low concentrations of an opioid such as fentanyl are commonly used, reducing the total amount of local anesthetic delivered.

Older patients are more sensitive to the effects of local anesthetics because of age-related physiological changes – see above under Opioid metabolites.[118]

Paracetamol

There do not appear to be any age-related reductions in paracetamol clearance in the elderly,[64] and there is

probably no need to reduce the dose given in this patient group.[119, 120] In a group of patients aged 84 to 95 years, a dose regimen of 3 g paracetamol a day did not result in any accumulation of the drug (a dose regimen of 4 g per day was not investigated).[121][V]

For many acutely painful conditions, paracetamol is recommended as an alternative to nonsteroidal anti-inflammatory drugs (NSAID), at least in the first instance.[64, 100, 121, 122] It is well tolerated in elderly patients and, unlike NSAIDs – see below under Nonselective NSAIDs and cyclooxygenase-2 inhibitors – there are few contraindications to its use in this patient group. It has been suggested that paracetamol doses should be reduced in patients with liver disease or a history of heavy alcohol intake.[47, 64] However, it may be that these patients are not at increased risk, as long as recommended doses of paracetamol are used.[94, 123]

Doses may also need to be reduced in patients with renal impairment.[99, 100]

Nonselective NSAIDs and cyclooxygenase-2 inhibitors

Elderly patients are more at risk of gastric and renal side effects of NSAIDs than younger patients and may be more likely to develop cognitive dysfunction.[47, 124][V], [125, 126], [127][V] The incidence of gastrointestinal side effects is lowest with ibuprofen and diclofenac;[123] as with younger patients, the use of routes other than the oral route does not avoid the gastrointestinal side effects.[94][V] Concurrent administration of misoprostol, H_2 antagonists, or proton pump inhibitors may help to reduce the risk of adverse gastrointestinal effects.[64, 123, 127][V]

Renal failure following the administration of an NSAID is of particular concern in the elderly, who are more likely to have preexisting renal impairment, cirrhosis, cardiac failure, or be using diuretic or antihypertensive medications.[124][V] In a survey of elderly (age > 65 years) medical inpatients, use of NSAIDs was shown to be a significant risk factor for renal function decline while in hospital; other risk factors were loop diuretics, hypernatremia, and low serum albumin levels.[128][V] There are also many important potential interactions with other drugs that the older patient in particular may be taking, such as warfarin, low molecular weight heparin, oral hypoglycemic agents, and drugs which are potentially nephrotoxic, for example aminoglycosides.[99, 124]

The analgesic and anti-inflammatory properties of NSAIDs, as well as many of the adverse effects associated with their use, are due to the inhibition of the enzyme cyclooxygenase (COX). Two types of COX have been described, COX-1 and COX-2 (see Chapter 4, Clinical pharmacology: traditional NSAIDs and selective COX-2 inhibitors). While drugs that selectively inhibit COX-2 (coxibs) do not provide more effective analgesia than nonselective COX inhibitors,[129] they have a significantly lower incidence of gastrointestinal complications,[102, 129] which might be of some advantage in the elderly patient. However, the risk of other adverse effects, including effects on renal function and exacerbation of cardiac failure, is similar to nonselective NSAIDs.[102, 129]

Longer-term use of high doses of both coxibs and nonselective NSAIDs (possibly apart from naproxen) appear to increase the risk of cardiovascular and cerebrovascular events.[130, 131][I] In addition, regular use of NSAIDs may interfere with the clinical benefits of low-dose aspirin.[132, 133][V] Extra caution is therefore required in elderly patients. For more detailed information on adverse effects see Chapter 4, Clinical pharmacology: traditional NSAIDs and selective COX-2 inhibitors.

Tricyclic antidepressants

Tricyclic antidepressants (TCAs), which inhibit uptake of both norepinephrine and serotonin, or predominantly norepinephrine, are effective in the treatment of neuropathic pain, while selective serotonin-reuptake inhibitors appear not to be as useful.[94][V], [134, 135][V], [136][I] This analgesic effect is independent of their actions as an antidepressant, is of quicker onset, and requires lower doses.[135]

The elderly may be particularly prone to the side effects of TCAs.[100, 135] Amitriptyline has the highest incidence of adverse effects and nortriptyline, with a lower incidence of adverse effects, may be the better drug to use in this patient group.[102, 134, 135] These side effects, which include anticholinergic symptoms such as sedation, confusion, orthostatic hypotension, dry mouth, constipation, and urinary retention, often lessen with time.[135] Clinical conditions which may require TCAs to be administered with caution are more common in the elderly and include prostatic hypertrophy, narrow angle glaucoma, cardiovascular disease, and impaired liver function; electrocardiogram (ECG) abnormalities may be a contraindication to the use of TCAs in the elderly.[135]

There may be age-related decreases in clearance of TCAs, therefore initial doses of amitriptyline and other TCAs should be decreased in the elderly (starting doses of 10 mg amitriptyline or nortriptyline are recommended) and subsequent doses increased slowly (if needed) with the patient monitored closely.[135]

Anticonvulsants

Anticonvulsant drugs are also useful in the treatment of neuropathic pain.[94, 136][I] The reduced liver function that tends to occur with aging can affect the elimination of anticonvulsants such as carbamazepine and age-related decreases in renal function can reduce the clearance of drugs dependent on the kidney for elimination, for example gabapentin.[135]

As with TCAs, elderly patients are generally more sensitive to anticonvulsant drugs and are more likely to develop side effects, such as drowsiness and unsteadiness.[135] Initial doses should be lower than for younger patients and any increases in dose titrated slowly.[135]

The "second generation" drugs such as gabapentin and topiramate may be preferred in these patients as they are less likely to result in adverse effects.[102] Pregabalin, a structural congener of gabapentin, is also used for neuropathic pain. Studies using this drug in the elderly are limited but the relatively high frequency of side effects such as somnolence and dizziness may be a problem in this group of patients.[137]

N-methyl-D-aspartate receptor antagonists

The N-methyl-D-aspartate (NMDA) receptor is thought to be involved in the development of hyperalgesia, allodynia, and opioid tolerance. As well as having an opioid-sparing effect when used as an adjuvant to opioids for the treatment of acute pain, the NMDA receptor antagonist ketamine has been used in the treatment of neuropathic pain and opioid tolerance.[94][V] While aging has been shown to alter the expression and distribution of NMDA receptors in many areas of the rat brain,[138] there is currently no good information about the effects of age in humans. However, clinical experience suggests that lower doses than those used in younger patients should be used.[8]

Memantine, a noncompetitive NMDA antagonist, is effective in the treatment of moderate to severe Alzheimer's disease[139] but does not appear to be of any benefit in the management of neuropathic pain.[140][II]

ANALGESIC TECHNIQUES AND THE ELDERLY

Many pharmacological and nonpharmacologic treatments may be used in the management of acute pain in the elderly, either alone or in combination. However, differences between elderly and nonelderly patients are more likely to be seen in treatments using analgesic drugs.

Traditional intermittent opioid regimens

It has been suggested that intermittent i.m. injections of opioid are potentially dangerous in the elderly.[2] However, as side effects are dose-dependent, this need not be so if suitable titration regimens are used, with appropriate doses, dose intervals, and monitoring.

Absorption of opioids from a subcutaneous site is often thought to be slower than from an i.m. injection. However, a study using s.c. morphine in elderly postoperative patients showed that times to peak concentration were very similar.[141][V]

Similar consideration with respect to age-adjusted dose, appropriate dose interval, and monitoring apply.

Patient–controlled analgesia

In the general patient population, PCA has been shown to provide better pain relief and greater patient satisfaction than conventional methods of analgesia.[142][I] It can also be a safe and very effective method of pain relief in the elderly, providing they have reasonably normal cognitive function.[93, 143, 144][II]

Elderly patients should not be denied PCA simply on the basis of age; patients in their late 90s have been reported to use PCA successfully.[114, 145][V] In a study comparing PCA use in two groups of general surgical patients: young (mean age 39 years) and old (mean age 67 years), the older group self-administered less opioid than the younger group, there were no differences in pain experienced (at rest or with movement), satisfaction with pain relief and level of control, or concerns about pain relief, adverse drug effects, risks of addiction, or use of the equipment, although older patients expected less intense pain and did not want as much involvement in or information about their medical management.[93][III]

The usual contraindications to PCA still apply, including the absence of trained staff, patient rejection, and inability of the patient to safely comprehend the technique.[8] The patients should be followed closely to ensure that they do understand the concept of self-administration and a change to an alternative method of pain relief made if needed.

In elderly patients, PCA is more effective than intermittent injections of s.c.[146][II] and i.m.[147][II] opioids in this age group.

In patients over 70 years, it may be reasonable to reduce the size of the PCA bolus dose.[8, 148] Recently introduced iontophoretic transdermal fentanyl PCA systems[149][II] have been shown to provide analgesia that is equivalent to standard PCA morphine regimens (1 mg bolus dose). However, care may be needed if this technique is used in elderly patients as the bolus dose of fentanyl that is delivered is fixed at 40 μg (see Chapter 11, Patient-controlled analgesia). The routine use of background infusions should be avoided, especially in older opioid-naive patients.[143, 148]

Epidural analgesia

In the general patient population, epidural analgesia provides better pain relief than parenteral opioids.[150][I], [151][I] This is also true in the elderly. A study by Mann et al.[144][II] compared i.v. PCA with epidural PCA in older patients (average age 76 years) after major abdominal surgery. Those receiving epidural PCA, using a mixture of bupivacaine and sufentanil, had lower pain scores at rest and movement, higher satisfaction scores, more rapid recovery of bowel function and, on the fourth and fifth postoperative days, improved mental status; the incidence of hypotension was increased.

The elderly, because of their age and probable comorbidities, are at higher risk of complications after surgery.[2, 3] Epidural analgesia may reduce the risk of some of these complications.[4, 5][I] This may be of particular benefit in the older patient.

Older patients are more likely to have ischemic heart disease and in such patients coronary blood flow may be reduced rather than increased in response to sympathetic stimulation.[152][V] In a study of patients (average age 67 years) with multivessel ischemic heart disease, high (the epidural catheter was inserted at the T2–T3 interspace) thoracic epidural analgesia (TEA) using 0.5 percent bupivacaine was instituted prior to coronary artery bypass surgery; TEA was able to partly normalize myocardial blood flow in response to sympathetic stimulation.[152][V]

In a group of older patients (median age 81 years), epidural analgesia has been used as part of a multimodal postoperative rapid rehabilitation regimen after laparoscopic colonic resection leading to a median hospital stay of just 2.4 days.[153][V] Perioperative use of epidural analgesia has also led to a reduction in the incidence of severe phantom limb pain after amputation.[154][V]

Many hospitals confine the use of epidural analgesia to intensive care or high dependency settings.[155] However, large audits, which include patients aged over 100 years of age, have shown that when epidural analgesia is closely supervised by an acute pain service with appropriate patient monitoring and staff education, it is a technique that can be safely managed in general surgical wards.[94][V], [114][V], [156][V], [157][V], [158][V] Under these circumstances, even elderly patients with epidural analgesia do not necessarily require admission to an intensive care or high dependency unit.

EPIDURAL LOCAL ANESTHETICS

Age is also a determinant of the spread of local anesthetic in the epidural space and degree of motor blockade. It has been shown that an epidural dose of levobupivacaine produces a higher level of sensory block in the elderly[29][V] and that epidural ropivacaine in older patients also results in a higher block level and more intense motor blockade.[159][V] Thus, smaller volumes will be needed to cover the same number of dermatomes than in a younger patient. Similarly, when the same volume of local anesthetic is given, the concentration of ropivacaine required to produce effective motor blockade decreased as patient age increased.[117][III] Ropivacaine has a lower potential for CNS and cardiovascular toxicity[117] and so may be a better choice than bupivacaine in the elderly patient.

EPIDURAL OPIOIDS

As with parenteral opioids, epidural opioid requirements have been noted to decrease as patient age increases.[160] [V] and itching from epidural opioids is much less common in the elderly.

An extended-release epidural morphine preparation is now available.[161] The recommended doses vary according to the operation type and only for some operations. Where there is a suggested dose range, it is suggested that doses at the lower end of the range be used in elderly patients.[162] The incidence of respiratory depression seems to be quite high using this technique (Viscusi et al.[161] quoted an incidence of 3.7 percent in their study) and it remains to be seen whether older patients will have an even higher risk – although varying definitions were used for respiratory depression and this may have led to an overestimation of the risk.

EPIDURAL LOCAL ANESTHETIC/OPIOID COMBINATIONS

Epidural analgesia using combinations of low concentrations of a local anesthetic and opioid are commonly used in an attempt to provide good analgesia, while minimizing the side effects of either class of drug. As the dose requirements of both classes of drug decrease with increasing patient age (see above under Epidural local anesthetics and Epidural opioids), it would seem reasonable to use age-based doses or infusion rates when this combination is used.[8]

MONITORING ELDERLY PATIENTS WITH EPIDURAL ANALGESIA

Elderly patients need close monitoring as they may be more susceptible to some of the effects of epidural analgesia, including hypotension.[159, 163, 164] Also, they may not voluntarily mention side effects such as motor and sensory block or backache, which may herald a complication such as an epidural hematoma or abscess.

Appropriate segmental placement of the epidural catheter, the use of infusions titrated to provide sufficient analgesia with no motor and sensory block, and careful monitoring should allow minimal hemodynamic changes (including orthostatic hypotension), early ambulation, and the early recognition of any major complication.

EPIDURAL ANALGESIA AND ANTICOAGULANT DRUGS

One of the rare yet potentially disastrous complications of epidural and spinal anesthesia/analgesia is an epidural or spinal hematoma. One of the risk factors for development of this complication is the concurrent use of anticoagulant drugs such as heparin, warfarin, and antiplatelet drugs.[165] All of these drugs are more likely to be required in older, compared with younger, patients.

In the elderly, both dose and duration of effect of anticoagulant drugs can be altered in the elderly and this may be clinically important when these drugs are used in patients receiving epidural analgesia.

In the USA, an alarming frequency of spinal hematomas followed the introduction of low molecular weight heparin (LMWH), particularly enoxaparin, the majority (75 percent) occurred in elderly female orthopedic patients.[165] The high incidence may be partly explained by the larger doses of enoxaparin that were used in the USA at that time, compared with other countries; added risk factors include concurrent use of NSAIDs or other anticoagulants medications,[165] which are more likely to be used in the elderly. It should also be noted that LMWHs are primarily eliminated by the kidney and the half-life is increased in renal impairment.[165]

Warfarin is commonly prescribed for a variety of indications, including those often seen in elderly patients. These include prevention of embolism and stroke in patients with atrial fibrillation and thromboembolism prophylaxis after major joint replacement surgery. There is a wide interpatient variability in dose response with warfarin although, in general, the response is greater in older patients.[165, 166] This difference appears to be primarily pharmacodynamic as the pharmacokinetics of warfarin do not change with age.[166] Concomitant medical problems, including low body weight, low serum albumin (warfarin is 99 percent bound to plasma proteins), significant cardiac, hepatic and renal disease, and interactions with other drugs (including NSAIDs and some herbal medications), are all more likely in the elderly patient and can also lead to an increased sensitivity to warfarin therapy.[165, 166]

If warfarin is given to patients with an epidural catheter in place after surgery, the wide interpatient variability in response and the increased response seen in the elderly may be of considerable importance in relation to the timing of removal of that catheter.

Antiplatelet drugs, including NSAIDs, clopidogrel, and ticlopidine are also more likely to be prescribed in the older patient. NSAIDs (including low-dose aspirin) alone do not appear to increase the risk of hematoma in association with epidural anesthesia/analgesia.[165] The real risk of spinal hematoma in patients taking clopidogrel and ticlopidine is unknown but it is suggested that neuraxial techniques be avoided until platelet function has recovered (see Chapter 13, Epidural and spinal analgesia).[165] However, spinal-epidural hematoma has been reported following combined spinal-epidural analgesia in a patient receiving perioperative LMWH, despite having stopped clopidogrel seven days before surgery.[167]

Intrathecal opioid analgesia

Intrathecal opioids, usually administered as a single dose, are used less commonly than epidural opioids for postoperative pain relief. This is partly because repeat doses cannot be given unless a catheter is inserted (not a common practice in acute pain management) and partly because of a widespread perception that it is a more hazardous technique.[168]

A review of 5969 patients by Gwirtz et al.[168][V] concluded that when managed by adequately trained staff using strict protocols, serial patient assessments, and timely treatment of any side effects that might occur, patients given intrathecal opioids can be managed safely on general hospital wards. The reported incidence of respiratory depression in this survey was 3 percent. Said by the authors to be a "low" incidence, it is considerably higher than that usually reported by others.[169]

Advanced age was considered by this group to be a risk factor for respiratory depression and they suggest that patients over the age of 70 years be monitored in an intensive care setting. However, elderly patients (average age 69 years) given up to 200 μg intrathecal morphine at the time of spinal anesthesia for peripheral vascular and other surgery have been safely nursed on general wards by nursing staff who have received additional education and managed by an acute pain service according to strict guidelines.[169][V]

The "optimal" dose of intrathecal morphine that should be given to elderly patients remains unknown and any evidence for the "best" dose remains inconsistent.

Intrathecal morphine doses of 200 μg given in addition to general anesthesia in elderly patients (average age 70 years) undergoing abdominal aortic surgery led to better postoperative analgesia and reduced postoperative analgesia requirements compared with those given general anesthesia only.[170][II] No respiratory depression was reported, but the total number of patients in the study was small (30 patients only) so no conclusion can be drawn as to relative safety or otherwise of the technique.

In 70 patients having knee replacement surgery, Bowrey et al.[171][II] concluded that intrathecal morphine doses of 500 μg led to better analgesia that doses of 200 μg without any increase in adverse effects.

Murphy et al.[172][II] compared three doses of intrathecal morphine (50, 100, and 200 μg) given to elderly patients after hip surgery and concluded that the 100 μg dose provided the best balance between good pain relief and pruritus; there was no difference seen in the incidences of nausea and vomiting or respiratory depression. However, in general, older patients have a much lower incidence of pruritus following intrathecal opioid administration compared with younger patients.[114, 169]

Other regional analgesic techniques

"Single shot" and continuous regional analgesic techniques (such as continuous brachial plexus or lumbar plexus blockade) may be particularly suited to the elderly patient. Possible advantages include a reduction in the incidence of side effects compared with central neuraxial blockade[173][II] and minimization of opioid doses.

The duration of action of sciatic nerve[174][III] and brachial plexus blocks[175][III] is prolonged in the elderly patient. This may be related to some of the neuroanatomical changes that occur with aging (see before).

In elderly (>65 years) patients undergoing urological surgery via a flank incision, paravertebral blockade of the lumbar plexus using either ropivacaine or bupivacaine has been shown to provide good analgesia with no changes in the patients' heart rate or blood pressure.[176][II]

Unlike epidural analgesia, age did not influence the spread of bupivacaine in the thoracic paravertebral space.[177]

SUMMARY

Elderly patients, particularly those that are cognitively impaired, are at risk of suboptimal management of their acute pain. Adjustments may need to be made to the ways in which pain is assessed, but regular assessments should still be made and analgesia titrated to effect.

The range of analgesic drugs and techniques that can be used in elderly patients is the same as for the younger patient. Age-related changes in pharmacodynamics and pharmacokinetics mean that elderly patients require lower doses of many of the drugs used in pain management and they may be more susceptible to some of the side effects of these drugs and of analgesic techniques such as epidural analgesia.

REFERENCES

1. Karani R, Meier DE. Systemic pharmacologic postoperative pain management in the geriatric orthopaedic patient. *Clinical Orthopaedics and Related Research.* 2004; August: 26–34.

2. Egbert AM. Postoperative pain management in the frail elderly. *Clinics in Geriatric Medicine.* 1996; **12**: 583–99.

3. Liu S, Carpenter RL, Neal JM. Epidural anesthesia and analgesia. Their role in postoperative outcome. *Anesthesiology.* 1995; **82**: 1474–506.

4. Ballantyne JC, Carr DB, deFerranti S et al. The comparative effects of postoperative analgesic therapies on pulmonary outcome: cumulative meta-analyses of randomized, controlled trials. *Anesthesia and Analgesia.* 1998; **86**: 598–612.

5. Beattie WS, Badner NH, Choi P. Epidural analgesia reduces postoperative myocardial infarction: a meta-analysis. *Anesthesia and Analgesia.* 2001; **93**: 853–8.

6. Bulger EM, Edwards T, Klotz P, Jurkovich GJ. Epidural analgesia improves outcome after multiple rib fractures. *Surgery.* 2004; **136**: 426–30.

7. Upton RN, Semple TJ, Macintyre PE, Foster DJR. Population pharmacokinetic modelling of subcutaneous morphine in the elderly. *Acute Pain*. 2006; **8**: 109–16.

8. Macintyre PE, Schug SA. *Acute pain management: a practical guide*, 3rd edn. London: Elsevier, 2007.

* 9. Macintyre PE, Jarvis DA. Age is the best predictor of postoperative morphine requirements. *Pain*. 1996; **64**: 357–64.

10. Coulbault L, Beaussier M, Verstuyft C *et al*. Environmental and genetic factors associated with morphine response in the postoperative period. *Clinical Pharmacology and Therapeutics*. 2006; **79**: 316–24.

11. Shafer SL. Pharmacokinetics and pharmacodynamics of the elderly. In: McKleskey C (ed.). *Geriatric anesthesiology*. Baltimore: Williams & Wilkins, 1997: 123–42.

12. Minto CF, Schnider TW, Egan TD *et al*. Influence of age and gender on the pharmacokinetics and pharmacodynamics of remifentanil. I. Model development. *Anesthesiology*. 1997; **86**: 10–23.

13. Baillie SP, Bateman DN, Coates PE, Woodhouse KW. Age and the pharmacokinetics of morphine. *Age and Ageing*. 1989; **18**: 258–62.

14. Owen JA, Sitar DS, Berger L *et al*. Age-related morphine kinetics. *Clinical Pharmacology and Therapeutics*. 1983; **34**: 364–8.

15. Sear JW, Hand CW, Moore RA, McQuay HJ. Studies on morphine disposition: influence of general anaesthesia on plasma concentrations of morphine and its metabolites. *British Journal of Anaesthesia*. 1989; **62**: 22–7.

16. Berkowitz BA, Ngai SH, Yang JC *et al*. The disposition of morphine in surgical patients. *Clinical Pharmacology and Therapeutics*. 1975; **17**: 629–35.

17. Scott JC, Stanski DR. Decreased fentanyl and alfentanil dose requirements with age. A simultaneous pharmacokinetic and pharmacodynamic evaluation. *Journal of Pharmacology and Experimental Therapeutics*. 1987; **240**: 159–66.

18. Bentley JB, Borel JD, Nenad Jr RE, Gillespie TJ. Age and fentanyl pharmacokinetics. *Anesthesia and Analgesia*. 1982; **61**: 968–71.

19. Beers R, Camporesi E. Remifentanil update: clinical science and utility. *CNS Drugs*. 2004; **18**: 1085–104.

20. Dyck JB, Wallace MS, Lu JQ *et al*. The pharmacokinetics of lignocaine in humans during a computer-controlled infusion. *European Journal of Pain*. 1997; **1**: 141–8.

21. Veering BT, Burm AG, van Kleef JW *et al*. Epidural anesthesia with bupivacaine: effects of age on neural blockade and pharmacokinetics. *Anesthesia and Analgesia*. 1987; **66**: 589–93.

22. Simon MJ, Veering BT, Vletter AA *et al*. The effect of age on the systemic absorption and systemic disposition of ropivacaine after epidural administration. *Anesthesia and Analgesia*. 2006; **102**: 276–82.

23. Gainsborough N, Maskrey VL, Nelson ML *et al*. The association of age with gastric emptying. *Age and Ageing*. 1993; **22**: 37–40.

24. Cusack BJ. Pharmacokinetics in older persons. *American Journal of Geriatric Pharmacotherapy*. 2004; **2**: 274–302.

25. Mangoni AA, Jackson SH. Age-related changes in pharmacokinetics and pharmacodynamics: basic principles and practical applications. *British Journal of Clinical Pharmacology*. 2004; **57**: 6–14.

26. Stanski DR, Greenblatt DJ, Lowenstein E. Kinetics of intravenous and intramuscular morphine. *Clinical Pharmacology and Therapeutics*. 1978; **24**: 52–9.

27. Divoll M, Greenblatt DJ, Ochs HR, Shader RI. Absolute bioavailability of oral and intramuscular diazepam: effects of age and sex. *Anesthesia and Analgesia*. 1983; **62**: 1–8.

28. Roberts MS, Lipschitz S, Campbell AJ *et al*. Modeling of subcutaneous absorption kinetics of infusion solutions in the elderly using technetium. *Journal of Pharmacokinetics and Biopharmaceutics*. 1997; **25**: 1–21.

29. Simon MJ, Veering BT, Stienstra R *et al*. Effect of age on the clinical profile and systemic absorption and disposition of levobupivacaine after epidural administration. *British Journal of Anaesthesia*. 2004; **93**: 512–20.

30. Upton RN, Semple TJ, Macintyre PE. Pharmacokinetic optimisation of opioid treatment in acute pain therapy. *Clinical Pharmacokinetics*. 1997; **33**: 225–44.

31. Parepally JM, Mandula H, Smith QR. Brain uptake of nonsteroidal anti-inflammatory drugs: Ibuprofen, flurbiprofen, and indomethacin. *Pharmaceutical Research*. 2006; **23**: 873–81.

32. Upton RN, Ludbrook GL, Gray EC, Grant C. The cerebral pharmacokinetics of meperidine and alfentanil in conscious sheep. *Anesthesiology*. 1997; **86**: 1317–25.

33. Tang JP, Melethil S. Effect of aging on the kinetics of blood-brain barrier uptake of tryptophan in rats. *Pharmaceutical Research*. 1995; **12**: 1085–91.

34. Loscher W, Potschka H. Role of drug efflux transporters in the brain for drug disposition and treatment of brain diseases. *Progress in Neurobiology*. 2005; **76**: 22–76.

35. Toornvliet R, van Berckel BN, Luurtsema G *et al*. Effect of age on functional P-glycoprotein in the blood-brain barrier measured by use of (R)-[(11)C]verapamil and positron emission tomography. *Clinical Pharmacology and Therapeutics*. 2006; **79**: 540–8.

36. Drozdzik M, Bialecka M, Mysliwiec K *et al*. Polymorphism in the P-glycoprotein drug transporter MDR1 gene: a possible link between environmental and genetic factors in Parkinson's disease. *Pharmacogenetics*. 2003; **13**: 259–63.

37. Turnheim K. Drug dosage in the elderly. *Is it rational? Drugs and Aging*. 1998; **13**: 357–79.

38. Ginsberg G, Hattis D, Russ A, Sonawane B. Pharmacokinetic and pharmacodynamic factors that can affect sensitivity to neurotoxic sequelae in elderly individuals. *Environmental Health Perspectives*. 2005; **113**: 1243–9.

39. Upton RN, Ludbrook G. A physiologically based, recirculatory model of the kinetics and dynamics of propofol in man. *Anesthesiology*. 2005; **103**: 344–52.

40. Singleton MA, Rosen JI, Fisher DM. Pharmacokinetics of fentanyl in the elderly. *British Journal of Anaesthesia.* 1988; **60**: 619–22.

41. Welch GW, Sowers MR. The interrelationship between body topology and body composition varies with age among women. *Journal of Nutrition.* 2000; **130**: 2371–7.

42. Seidell JC, Visscher TL. Body weight and weight change and their health implications for the elderly. *European Journal of Clinical Nutrition.* 2000; **54** (Suppl. 3): S33–9.

43. Cheymol G. Effects of obesity on pharmacokinetics implications for drug therapy. *Clinical Pharmacokinetics.* 2000; **39**: 215–31.

44. Visser M, Kritchevsky SB, Newman AB *et al.* Lower serum albumin concentration and change in muscle mass: the Health, Aging and Body Composition Study. *American Journal of Clinical Nutrition.* 2005; **82**: 531–7.

45. Cals MJ, Bories PN, Blonde-Cynober F *et al.* [Reference intervals and biological profile in a group of healthy elderly population in the Paris region]. *Annales de Biologie Clinique.* 1996; **54**: 307–15.

46. Macklon AF, Barton M, James O, Rawlins MD. The effect of age on the pharmacokinetics of diazepam. *Clinical Science.* 1980; **59**: 479–83.

47. Aubrun F. Management of postoperative analgesia in elderly patients. *Regional Anesthesia and Pain Medicine.* 2005; **30**: 363–79.

48. Bjorkman S, Wada DR, Stanski DR. Application of physiologic models to predict the influence of changes in body composition and blood flows on the pharmacokinetics of fentanyl and alfentanil in patients. *Anesthesiology.* 1998; **88**: 657–67.

49. Bjorkman S, Stanski DR, Verotta D, Harashima H. Comparative tissue concentration profiles of fentanyl and alfentanil in humans predicted from tissue/blood partition data obtained in rats. *Anesthesiology.* 1990; **72**: 865–73.

50. Kharasch ED, Hoffer C, Altuntas TG, Whittington D. Quinidine as a probe for the role of p-glycoprotein in the intestinal absorption and clinical effects of fentanyl. *Journal of Clinical Pharmacology.* 2004; **44**: 224–33.

* 51. Gibson SJ, Farrell M. A review of age differences in the neurophysiology of nociception and the perceptual experience of pain. *Clinical Journal of Pain.* 2004; **20**: 227–39.

* 52. Gibson SJ. Pain and aging: the pain experience over the adult life span. In: Dostrovsky JO, Carr DB, Koltzenburg M (eds). *Proceedings of the 10th World Congress on Pain.* Seattle: IASP Press, 2003: 767–90.

53. Helme RD, Meliala A, Gibson SJ. Methodologic factors which contribute to variations in experimental pain threshold reported for older people. *Neuroscience Letters.* 2004; **361**: 144–6.

54. Gagliese L, Katz J. Age differences in postoperative pain are scale dependent: a comparison of measures of pain intensity and quality in younger and older surgical patients. *Pain.* 2003; **103**: 11–20.

55. Miller PF, Sheps DS, Bragdon EE *et al.* Aging and pain perception in ischemic heart disease. *American Heart Journal.* 1990; **120**: 22–30.

56. Ambepitiya GB, Iyengar EN, Roberts ME. Review: silent exertional myocardial ischaemia and perception of angina in elderly people. *Age and Ageing.* 1993; **22**: 302–7.

57. Mehta RH, Rathore SS, Radford MJ *et al.* Acute myocardial infarction in the elderly: differences by age. *Journal of the American College of Cardiology.* 2001; **38**: 736–41.

58. Tresch DD. Management of the older patient with acute myocardial infarction: difference in clinical presentations between older and younger patients. *Journal of the American Geriatrics Society.* 1998; **46**: 1157–62.

* 59. Gibson SJ, Helme RD. Age-related differences in pain perception and report. *Clinics in Geriatric Medicine.* 2001; **17**: 433–56. v–vi.

60. Gupta M, Tabas JA, Kohn MA. Presenting complaint among patients with myocardial infarction who present to an urban, public hospital emergency department. *Annals of Emergency Medicine.* 2002; **40**: 180–6.

61. Hilton D, Iman N, Burke GJ *et al.* Absence of abdominal pain in older persons with endoscopic ulcers: a prospective study. *American Journal of Gastroenterology.* 2001; **96**: 380–4.

62. Thomas T, Robinson C, Champion D *et al.* Prediction and assessment of the severity of post-operative pain and of satisfaction with management. *Pain.* 1998; **75**: 177–85.

63. Li SF, Greenwald PW, Gennis P *et al.* Effect of age on acute pain perception of a standardized stimulus in the emergency department. *Annals of Emergency Medicine.* 2001; **38**: 644–7.

64. Davis MP, Srivastava M. Demographics, assessment and management of pain in the elderly. *Drugs and Aging.* 2003; **20**: 23–57.

65. McCarberg BH. Managing persistent neuropathic pain in the elderly. *Geriatrics.* 2005; Suppl: 9–14.

66. Forster MC, Pardiwala A, Calthorpe D. Analgesia requirements following hip fracture in the cognitively impaired. *Injury.* 2000; **31**: 435–6.

67. Morrison RS, Siu AL. A comparison of pain and its treatment in advanced dementia and cognitively intact patients with hip fracture. *Journal of Pain and Symptom Management.* 2000; **19**: 240–8.

68. Feldt KS, Ryden MB, Miles S. Treatment of pain in cognitively impaired compared with cognitively intact older patients with hip-fracture. *Journal of the American Geriatrics Society.* 1998; **46**: 1079–85.

69. Morrison RS, Magaziner J, McLaughlin MA *et al.* The impact of post-operative pain on outcomes following hip fracture. *Pain.* 2003; **103**: 303–11.

70. Herr K, Bjoro K, Decker S. Tools for assessment of pain in nonverbal older adults with dementia: a state-of-the-science review. *Journal of Pain and Symptom Management.* 2006; **31**: 170–92.

71. Parmelee PA. Pain in cognitively impaired older persons. *Clinics in Geriatric Medicine.* 1996; **12**: 473–87.

72. Parmelee PA, Smith B, Katz IR. Pain complaints and cognitive status among elderly institution residents. *Journal of the American Geriatrics Society*. 1993; **41**: 517–22.

73. Farrell MJ, Katz B, Helme RD. The impact of dementia on the pain experience. *Pain*. 1996; **67**: 7–15.

74. Cole LJ, Farrell MJ, Duff EP *et al*. Pain sensitivity and fMRI pain-related brain activity in Alzheimer's disease. *Brain*. 2006; **129**: 2957–65.

75. Benedetti F, Arduino C, Costa S *et al*. Loss of expectation-related mechanisms in Alzheimer's disease makes analgesic therapies less effective. *Pain*. 2006; **121**: 133–44.

76. Bitsch MS, Foss NB, Kristensen BB, Kehlet H. Acute cognitive dysfunction after hip fracture: frequency and risk factors in an optimized, multimodal, rehabilitation program. *Acta Anaesthesiologica Scandinavica*. 2006; **50**: 428–36.

77. Fong HK, Sands LP, Leung JM. The role of postoperative analgesia in delirium and cognitive decline in elderly patients: a systematic review. *Anesthesia and Analgesia*. 2006; **102**: 1255–66.

78. Aakerlund LP, Rosenberg J. Postoperative delirium: treatment with supplementary oxygen. *British Journal of Anaesthesia*. 1994; **72**: 286–90.

79. Morrison RS, Magaziner J, Gilbert M *et al*. Relationship between pain and opioid analgesics on the development of delirium following hip fracture. *Journals of Gerontology. Series A, Biological Sciences and Medical Sciences*. 2003; **58**: 76–81.

80. Moore AR, O'Keeffe ST. Drug-induced cognitive impairment in the elderly. *Drugs and Aging*. 1999; **15**: 15–28.

81. Lynch EP, Lazor MA, Gellis JE *et al*. The impact of postoperative pain on the development of postoperative delirium. *Anesthesia and Analgesia*. 1998; **86**: 781–5.

82. Vaurio LE, Sands LP, Wang Y *et al*. Postoperative delirium: the importance of pain and pain management. *Anesthesia and Analgesia*. 2006; **102**: 1267–73.

*83. Alagiakrishnan K, Wiens CA. An approach to drug induced delirium in the elderly. *Postgraduate Medical Journal*. 2004; **80**: 388–93.

84. Gagliese L, Melzack R. Chronic pain in elderly people. *Pain*. 1997; **70**: 3–14.

85. Closs SJ, Barr B, Briggs M *et al*. A comparison of five pain assessment scales for nursing home residents with varying degrees of cognitive impairment. *Journal of Pain and Symptom Management*. 2004; **27**: 196–205.

86. Herr KA, Spratt K, Mobily PR, Richardson G. Pain intensity assessment in older adults: use of experimental pain to compare psychometric properties and usability of selected pain scales with younger adults. *Clinical Journal of Pain*. 2004; **20**: 207–19.

87. Gagliese L, Weizblit N, Ellis W, Chan VW. The measurement of postoperative pain: a comparison of intensity scales in younger and older surgical patients. *Pain*. 2005; **117**: 412–20.

88. Chibnall JT, Tait RC. Pain assessment in cognitively impaired and unimpaired older adults: a comparison of four scales. *Pain*. 2001; **92**: 173–86.

89. Manfredi PL, Breuer B, Meier DE, Libow L. Pain assessment in elderly patients with severe dementia. *Journal of Pain and Symptom Management*. 2003; **25**: 48–52.

90. Cohen-Mansfield J. Pain Assessment in Noncommunicative Elderly persons – PAINE. *Clinical Journal of Pain*. 2006; **22**: 569–75.

91. Warden V, Hurley AC, Volicer L. Development and psychometric evaluation of the Pain Assessment in Advanced Dementia (PAINAD) scale. *Journal of the American Medical Directors Association*. 2003; **4**: 9–15.

92. Leong IY, Chong MS, Gibson SJ. The use of a self-reported pain measure, a nurse-reported pain measure and the PAINAD in nursing home residents with moderate and severe dementia: a validation study. *Age and Ageing*. 2006; **35**: 252–6.

93. Gagliese L, Jackson M, Ritvo P *et al*. Age is not an impediment to effective use of patient-controlled analgesia by surgical patients. *Anesthesiology*. 2000; **93**: 601–10.

*94. ANZCA. *Acute Pain Management: Scientific Evidence*, 2nd edn. Melbourne: Australian and New Zealand College of Anaesthetists, 2005.

95. Simopoulos TT, Smith HS, Peeters-Asdourian C, Stevens DS. Use of meperidine in patient-controlled analgesia and the development of a normeperidine toxic reaction. *Archives of Surgery*. 2002; **137**: 84–8.

96. Lugo RA, Satterfield KL, Kern SE. Pharmacokinetics of methadone. *Journal of Pain and Palliative Care Pharmacotherapy*. 2005; **19**: 13–24.

97. Dayer P, Collart L, Desmeules J. The pharmacology of tramadol. *Drugs*. 1994; **47**: 3–7.

98. Scott LJ, Perry CM. Tramadol: a review of its use in perioperative pain. *Drugs*. 2000; **60**: 139–76.

99. Barkin RL, Barkin SJ, Barkin DS. Perception, assessment, treatment, and management of pain in the elderly. *Clinics in Geriatric Medicine*. 2005; **21**: 465–90, v.

100. Fine PG. Pharmacological management of persistent pain in older patients. *Clinical Journal of Pain*. 2004; **20**: 220–6.

101. Ng KF, Yuen TS, Ng VM. A comparison of postoperative cognitive function and pain relief with fentanyl or tramadol patient-controlled analgesia. *Journal of Clinical Anesthesia*. 2006; **18**: 205–10.

102. Argoff CE. Pharmacotherapeutic options in pain management. *Geriatrics*. 2005; Suppl: 3–9.

103. Goldstein DJ, Turk DC. Dextropropoxyphene: safety and efficacy in older patients. *Drugs and Aging*. 2005; **22**: 419–32.

104. Aubrun F, Bunge D, Langeron O *et al*. Postoperative morphine consumption in the elderly patient. *Anesthesiology*. 2003; **99**: 160–5.

105. Burns JW, Hodsman NBA, McLintock TTC *et al*. The influence of patient characteristics on the requirements for postoperative analgesia. *Anaesthesia*. 1989; **44**: 2–6.

106. Cepeda MS, Farrar JT, Baumgarten M *et al.* Side effects of opioids during short-term administration: effect of age, gender, and race. *Clinical Pharmacology and Therapeutics.* 2003; **74**: 102–12.

∗107. Vila H, Smith RA, Augustyniak MJ *et al.* The efficacy and safety of pain management before and after implementation of hospital-wide pain management standards: is patient safety compromised by treatment based solely on numerical pain ratings? *Anesthesia and Analgesia.* 2005; **101**: 474–80.

108. Ready LB, Oden R, Chadwick HS *et al.* Development of an anesthesiology-based postoperative pain management service. *Anesthesiology.* 1988; **68**: 100–6.

∗109. Jones JG, Sapsford DJ, Wheatley RG. Postoperative hypoxaemia: mechanisms and time course. *Anaesthesia.* 1990; **45**: 566–73.

110. Catley DM, Thornton C, Jordan C *et al.* Pronounced, episodic oxygen desaturation in the postoperative period: its association with ventilatory pattern and analgesic regimen. *Anesthesiology.* 1985; **63**: 20–8.

111. Rosenberg J, Pedersen MH, Gebuhr P, Kehlet H. Effect of oxygen therapy on late postoperative episodic and constant hypoxaemia. *British Journal of Anaesthesia.* 1992; **68**: 18–22.

112. Quinn AC, Brown JH, Wallace PG, Asbury AJ. Studies in postoperative sequelae. Nausea and vomiting-still a problem. *Anaesthesia.* 1994; **49**: 62–5.

113. Woodhouse A, Hobbes AF, Mather LE, Gibson M. A comparison of morphine, pethidine and fentanyl in the postsurgical patient-controlled analgesia environment. *Pain.* 1996; **64**: 115–21.

114. Macintyre PE. Nine years experience in an acute pain service. In: Keneally J, Jones M (eds). *Australasian Anaesthesia.* Melbourne: Australian and New Zealand College of Anaesthetists, 1998: 79–90.

115. Herrick IA, Ganapathy S, Komar W *et al.* Postoperative cognitive impairment in the elderly. Choice of patient-controlled analgesia opioid. *Anaesthesia.* 1996; **51**: 356–60.

116. Narayanaswamy M, Smith J, Spralja A. Choice of opiate and incidence of confusion in elderly postoperative patients. *Annual Scientific Meeting of the Australian and New Zealand Society of Anaesthetists.* Adelaide, Australia, 2006.

117. Li Y, Zhu S, Bao F *et al.* The effects of age on the median effective concentration of ropivacaine for motor blockade after epidural anesthesia with ropivacaine. *Anesthesia and Analgesia.* 2006; **102**: 1847–50.

118. Sadean MR, Glass PS. Pharmacokinetics in the elderly. *Best Practice and Research. Clinical Anaesthesiology.* 2003; **17**: 191–205.

119. Miners JO, Penhall R, Robson RA, Birkett DJ. Comparison of paracetamol metabolism in young adult and elderly males. *European Journal of Clinical Pharmacology.* 1988; **35**: 157–60.

120. Divoll M, Abernethy DR, Ameer B, Greenblatt DJ. Acetaminophen kinetics in the elderly. *Clinical Pharmacology and Therapeutics.* 1982; **31**: 151–6.

121. Bannwarth B, Pehourcq F, Lagrange F *et al.* Single and multiple dose pharmacokinetics of acetaminophen (paracetamol) in polymedicated very old patients with rheumatic pain. *Journal of Rheumatology.* 2001; **28**: 182–4.

122. Whelton A. Clinical implications of nonopioid analgesia for relief of mild-to-moderate pain in patients with or at risk for cardiovascular disease. *American Journal of Cardiology.* 2006; **97**: 3–9.

123. Nikolaus T, Zeyfang A. Pharmacological treatments for persistent non-malignant pain in older persons. *Drugs and Aging.* 2004; **21**: 19–41.

124. RCA. *Guidelines for the use of nonsteroidal antiinflammatory drugs in the perioperative period.* London: Royal College of Anaesthetists, 1998.

125. Peura DA. Prevention of nonsteroidal anti-inflammatory drug-associated gastrointestinal symptoms and ulcer complications. *American Journal of Medicine.* 2004; **117** Suppl 5A: 63S–71S.

126. Juhlin T, Bjorkman S, Hoglund P. Cyclooxygenase inhibition causes marked impairment of renal function in elderly subjects treated with diuretics and ACE-inhibitors. *European Journal of Heart Failure.* 2005; **7**: 1049–56.

127. Pilotto A, Franceschi M, Leandro G *et al.* The risk of upper gastrointestinal bleeding in elderly users of aspirin and other non-steroidal anti-inflammatory drugs: the role of gastroprotective drugs. *Aging Clinical and Experimental Research.* 2003; **15**: 494–9.

128. Burkhardt H, Bruckner D, Gladisch R. Risk factors of worsening renal function in hospitalized elderly patients. *Journal of Nephrology.* 2005; **18**: 166–73.

129. Savage R. Cyclo-oxygenase-2 inhibitors: when should they be used in the elderly? *Drugs and Aging.* 2005; **22**: 185–200.

130. Chan AT, Manson JE, Albert CM *et al.* Nonsteroidal antiinflammatory drugs, acetaminophen, and the risk of cardiovascular events. *Circulation.* 2006; **113**: 1578–87.

∗131. Kearney PM, Baigent C, Godwin J *et al.* Do selective cyclo-oxygenase-2 inhibitors and traditional non-steroidal anti-inflammatory drugs increase the risk of atherothrombosis? Meta-analysis of randomised trials. *British Medical Journal.* 2006; **332**: 1302–8.

132. Kurth T, Glynn RJ, Walker AM *et al.* Inhibition of clinical benefits of aspirin on first myocardial infarction by nonsteroidal antiinflammatory drugs. *Circulation.* 2003; **108**: 1191–5.

133. MacDonald TM, Wei L. Effect of ibuprofen on cardioprotective effect of aspirin. *Lancet.* 2003; **361**: 573–4.

134. McQuay HJ, Tramer M, Nye BA *et al.* A systematic review of antidepressants in neuropathic pain. *Pain.* 1996; **68**: 217–27.

∗135. Ahmad M, Goucke CR. Management strategies for the treatment of neuropathic pain in the elderly. *Drugs and Aging.* 2002; **19**: 929–45.

136. Collins SL, Moore RA, McQuay Hj, Wiffen P. Antidepressants and anticonvulsants for diabetic neuropathy and postherpetic neuralgia: a quantitative systematic review. *Journal of Pain and Symptom Management.* 2000; **20**: 449–58.

137. Guay DR. Pregabalin in neuropathic pain: a more "pharmaceutically elegant" gabapentin? *American Journal of Geriatric Pharmacotherapy.* 2005; **3**: 274–87.

138. Clayton DA, Grosshans DR, Browning MD. Aging and surface expression of hippocampal NMDA receptors. *Journal of Biological Chemistry.* 2002; **277**: 14367–9.

139. Robinson DM, Keating GM. Memantine: a review of its use in Alzheimer's disease. *Drugs.* 2006; **66**: 1515–34.

140. Schifitto G, Yiannoutsos CT, Simpson DM *et al.* A placebo-controlled study of memantine for the treatment of human immunodeficiency virus-associated sensory neuropathy. *Journal of Neurovirology.* 2006; **12**: 328–31.

141. Semple TJ, Upton RN, Macintyre PE *et al.* Morphine blood concentrations in elderly postoperative patients following administration via an indwelling subcutaneous cannula. *Anaesthesia.* 1997; **52**: 318–23.

142. Walder B, Schafer M, Henzi I, Tramer MR. Efficacy and safety of patient-controlled opioid analgesia for acute postoperative pain. A quantitative systematic review. *Acta Anaesthesiologica Scandinavica.* 2001; **45**: 795–804.

143. Mann C, Pouzeratte Y, Eledjam JJ. Postoperative patient-controlled analgesia in the elderly: risks and benefits of epidural versus intravenous administration. *Drugs and Aging.* 2003; **20**: 337–45.

144. Mann C, Pouzeratte Y, Boccara G *et al.* Comparison of intravenous or epidural patient-controlled analgesia in the elderly after major abdominal surgery. *Anesthesiology.* 2000; **92**: 433–41.

145. Tsui SL, Tong WN, Irwin M *et al.* The efficacy, applicability and side-effects of postoperative intravenous patient-controlled morphine analgesia: an audit of 1233 Chinese patients. *Anaesthesia and Intensive Care.* 1996; **24**: 658–64.

146. Keita H, Geachan N, Dahmani S *et al.* Comparison between patient-controlled analgesia and subcutaneous morphine in elderly patients after total hip replacement. *British Journal of Anaesthesia.* 2003; **90**: 53–7.

147. Egbert AM, Parks LH, Short LM, Burnett ML. Randomized trial of postoperative patient-controlled analgesia vs intramuscular narcotics in frail elderly men. *Archives of Internal Medicine.* 1990; **150**: 1897–903.

148. Macintyre PE. Safety and efficacy of patient-controlled analgesia. *British Journal of Anaesthesia.* 2001; **87**: 36–46.

149. Chelly JE, Grass J, Houseman TW *et al.* The safety and efficacy of a fentanyl patient-controlled transdermal system for acute postoperative analgesia: a multicenter, placebo-controlled trial. *Anesthesia and Analgesia.* 2004; **98**: 427–33.

150. Werawatganon T, Charuluxanun S. Patient controlled intravenous opioid analgesia versus continuous epidural analgesia for pain after intra-abdominal surgery. *Cochrane Database of Systematic Reviews.* 2005; **CD004088**.

151. Block BM, Liu SS, Rowlingson AJ *et al.* Efficacy of postoperative epidural analgesia: a meta-analysis. *Journal of the American Medical Association.* 2003; **290**: 2455–63.

152. Nygard E, Kofoed KF, Freiberg J *et al.* Effects of high thoracic epidural analgesia on myocardial blood flow in patients with ischemic heart disease. *Circulation.* 2005; **111**: 2165–70.

153. Bardram L, Funch-Jensen P, Kehlet H. Rapid rehabilitation in elderly patients after laparoscopic colonic resection. *British Journal of Surgery.* 2000; **87**: 1540–5.

154. Gehling M, Tryba M. [Prophylaxis of phantom pain: is regional analgesia ineffective?]. *Schmerz.* 2003; **17**: 11–9.

155. Walton B, Farrow C, Cook TM. A national survey of epidural use and management in elderly patients undergoing elective and emergency laparotomy. *Anaesthesia.* 2006; **61**: 456–61.

156. Scott DA, Beilby DS, McClymont C. Postoperative analgesia using epidural infusions of fentanyl with bupivacaine. A prospective analysis of 1,014 patients. *Anesthesiology.* 1995; **83**: 727–37.

157. Rygnestad T, Borchgrevink PC, Eide E. Postoperative epidural infusion of morphine and bupivacaine is safe on surgical wards. Organisation of the treatment, effects and side-effects in 2000 consecutive patients. *Acta Anaesthesiologica Scandinavica.* 1997; **41**: 868–76.

158. Burstal R, Wegener F, Hayes C, Lantry G. Epidural analgesia: prospective audit of 1062 patients. *Anaesthesia and Intensive Care.* 1998; **26**: 165–72.

159. Simon MJ, Veering BT, Stienstra R *et al.* The effects of age on neural blockade and hemodynamic changes after epidural anesthesia with ropivacaine. *Anesthesia and Analgesia.* 2002; **94**: 1325–30.

160. Ready LB, Chadwick HS, Ross B. Age predicts effective epidural morphine dose after abdominal hysterectomy. *Anesthesia and Analgesia.* 1987; **66**: 1215–8.

161. Viscusi ER, Martin G, Hartrick CT *et al.* Forty-eight hours of postoperative pain relief after total hip arthroplasty with a novel, extended-release epidural morphine formulation. *Anesthesiology.* 2005; **102**: 1014–22.

162. Endo. DepoDur Product Overview [cited October 2006]. Available from: www.depodur.com/depodurmain.html.

163. Crawford ME, Moiniche S, Orbaek J *et al.* Orthostatic hypotension during postoperative continuous thoracic epidural bupivacaine-morphine in patients undergoing abdominal surgery. *Anesthesia and Analgesia.* 1996; **83**: 1028–32.

164. Veering BT. Hemodynamic effects of central neural blockade in elderly patients. *Canadian Journal of Anaesthesia.* 2006; **53**: 117–21.

∗165. Horlocker TT, Wedel DJ, Benzon H *et al.* Regional anesthesia in the anticoagulated patient: defining the risks (the second ASRA Consensus Conference on Neuraxial Anesthesia and Anticoagulation). *Regional Anesthesia and Pain Medicine.* 2003; **28**: 172–97.

166. Jacobs LG. Warfarin pharmacology, clinical management, and evaluation of hemorrhagic risk for the elderly. *Clinics in Geriatric Medicine*. 2006; **22**: 17–32, vii–viii.

167. Tam NL, Pac-Soo C, Pretorius PM. Epidural haematoma after a combined spinal-epidural anaesthetic in a patient treated with clopidogrel and dalteparin. *British Journal of Anaesthesia*. 2006; **96**: 262–5.

168. Gwirtz KH, Young JV, Byers RS *et al.* The safety and efficacy of intrathecal opioid analgesia for acute postoperative pain: seven years' experience with 5969 surgical patients at Indiana University Hospital. *Anesthesia and Analgesia*. 1999; **88**: 599–604.

169. Lim PC, Macintyre PE. An audit of intrathecal morphine analgesia for non-obstetric postsurgical patients in an adult tertiary hospital. *Anaesthesia and Intensive Care*. 2006; **34**: 776–81.

170. Blay M, Orban JC, Rami L *et al.* Efficacy of low-dose intrathecal morphine for postoperative analgesia after abdominal aortic surgery: a double-blind randomized study. *Regional Anesthesia and Pain Medicine*. 2006; **31**: 127–33.

171. Bowrey S, Hamer J, Bowler I *et al.* A comparison of 0.2 and 0.5 mg intrathecal morphine for postoperative analgesia after total knee replacement. *Anaesthesia*. 2005; **60**: 449–52.

172. Murphy PM, Stack D, Kinirons B, Laffey JG. Optimizing the dose of intrathecal morphine in older patients undergoing hip arthroplasty. *Anesthesia and Analgesia*. 2003; **97**: 1709–15.

173. Zaric D, Boysen K, Christiansen C *et al.* A comparison of epidural analgesia with combined continuous femoral-sciatic nerve blocks after total knee replacement. *Anesthesia and Analgesia*. 2006; **102**: 1240–6.

174. Hanks RK, Pietrobon R, Nielsen KC *et al.* The effect of age on sciatic nerve block duration. *Anesthesia and Analgesia*. 2006; **102**: 588–92.

175. Paqueron X, Boccara G, Bendahou M *et al.* Brachial plexus nerve block exhibits prolonged duration in the elderly. *Anesthesiology*. 2002; **97**: 1245–9.

176. Akin S, Aribogan A, Turunc T, Aridogan A. Lumbar plexus blockade with ropivacaine for postoperative pain management in elderly patients undergoing urologic surgeries. *Urologia Internationalis*. 2005; **75**: 345–9.

177. Cheema S, Richardson J, McGurgan P. Factors affecting the spread of bupivacaine in the adult thoracic paravertebral space. *Anaesthesia*. 2003; **58**: 684–7.

29

Acute rehabilitation of sport injury

LOUISE TULLOH, LEO PINCZEWSKI, AND IAN POWER

KEY LEARNING POINTS

- The RICE (rest, ice, compression, elevation) method immediately following acute soft tissue injury is easy, cost-effective and beneficial.
- Limited immobilization (24–72 hours) followed by early controlled mobilization results in optimal functional outcome in soft tissue injuries.

- Short-term use of nonsteroidal anti-inflammatory drugs (NSAIDs) improves pain and speeds recovery.

INTRODUCTION

Sporting injuries are becoming more common with the increased focus of exercise as part of governmental health improvement policies and increased availability of recreational opportunities. Unfortunately, sporting injuries can produce short-term pain and dysfunction, and long-term disability. The ever-increasing demands of professional sport focus our attention upon the correct management of sporting injuries, as the emphasis is on prompt diagnosis, correct management, and rapid rehabilitation of the injured player. This chapter seeks to explain the pathophysiological processes that occur in bones, synovial joints, cartilage, tendons, ligaments, and muscles to aid diagnosis and therapy and to improve rehabilitation after sporting injury.

CLASSIFICATION OF SPORTS INJURIES

Sporting injuries may be classified in various ways. They may result from the cumulative effect of overuse, from acute trauma or the secondary effects of previous injury. An alternative classification is based on the tissue involved. Consideration of each of these categories will help the clinician to arrive at an accurate diagnosis and facilitate effective management.

Acute sporting injuries

DIRECT OR EXTRINSIC MECHANISM

This may result from direct collision with another player or with equipment. The forces involved are often large and may result in head injury, fracture, or dislocation of bone and joints, or muscle contusions.

INDIRECT OR INTRINSIC MECHANISM

These injuries are caused by factors within the individual athlete and include muscle tears and ligament sprains.

Overuse sporting injuries

REPETITIVE FRICTION

This results from apposed structures suffering repetitive frictional wear and includes tenosynovitis, bursitis, and such conditions as iliotibial band friction syndrome.

REPETITIVE MICROFATIGUE

This occurs when a tissue is overloaded in a repetitive fashion beyond its capacity to repair. A mild acute inflammatory response ensues which may progress to chronic inflammation or tissue degeneration. Examples include stress fractures, medial epicondylosis, and Achilles tendinosis.

Secondary sporting injuries

SHORT TERM

This usually follows mismanagement of a primary injury by either inadequate rehabilitation or insufficient rest from activity. Retearing a muscle on premature return to running after injury is a common example of this.

LONG TERM

An injury may eventually lead to a long-term degenerative process. This can be seen where osteoarthrosis develops following joint injury, for example, articular or meniscal injuries of the knee joint.

Classification according to the tissue involved

A tissue-based classification is necessary as different body tissues fail under different circumstances and vary in their capacity to heal (some examples of acute and overuse sporting injuries are listed).

- Soft tissues:
  - skin and fascia (acute: lacerations, abrasions, and punctures; overuse: blister);
  - muscle–tendon units, their tendoperiosteal attachments to the skeleton and synovial sheaths (acute: tears; overuse: fibrosis, tendinosis, paratendinitis, and tenosynovitis);
  - muscle compartments and their enclosing fascia (acute: strains, tears, contusions, cramps, acute compartment syndromes; overuse: chronic compartment syndromes, fibrosis);
  - joints and their associated structures, including ligaments, fibrocartilage, capsule, synovium, and bursae (acute: dislocation, subluxation, traumatic

bursitis, sprains, and tears; chronic: synovitis, osteoarthritis, bursitis, inflammation);
  - intervertebral disk.
- Hard tissues:
  - bone and its periosteal covering (acute: fracture, periosteal contusion; overuse: stress fracture, osteitis, and apophysitis);
  - hyaline articular cartilage (acute: chondral and osteochondral damage; overuse: chondromalacia);
  - epiphysis.
- Special tissues or organs:
  - brain and peripheral nerves (acute: injury, neuropraxia; chronic: entrapment);
  - facial structures;
  - thoracic, abdominal, and pelvic organs.[1]

THE PATHOPHYSIOLOGY OF TISSUE INJURY AND REPAIR

It is important to understand the tissue response to injury in order to rationalize an approach to early management and rapid rehabilitation and to modulate the pain response. The ultimate purpose of the repair process is restoration of tissue continuity, strength, and function, and is produced by an orderly, progressive, and interdependent biological repair process. The three phases of this are summarized here, followed by more specific details of individual musculoskeletal pathophysiology.

The acute inflammatory response

Acute inflammation (**Figure 29.1**) is the immediate and normally occurring protective response to injury. In the case of athletic trauma, it is initiated by disruption of vascularized musculoskeletal tissues that have been exposed to excessive mechanical loads in the form of tensile, compressive, torsional, or shearing forces.

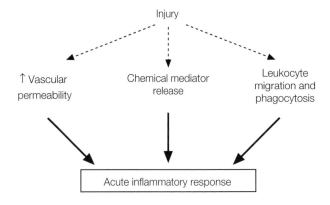

Figure 29.1 The acute inflammatory response to injury.

The repair and regeneration phase

This phase starts approximately 72 hours after injury and continues for up to six weeks. Most soft connective tissues comprising the musculoskeletal system consist largely of highly specialized, permanent cells that do not have the capacity to regenerate a tissue structurally identical to that of the original. The result is the formation of scar tissue, the strength of which can be maximized by the timing and degree of forces applied to it and the avoidance of reinjury. This has obvious implications in the early management of soft tissue injury.

This phase of repair is characterized by the formation of granulation tissue. There are three components to this process:

1. **Angiogenesis**. These immature vessels are leaky, accounting for much of the edema persisting in healing wounds.
2. **Migration and proliferation of fibroblasts**. Growth factors and fibrogenic cytokines trigger the migration, proliferation, and differentiation of fibroblasts to synthesize a matrix of collagen and proteoglycans.
3. **Deposition of extracellular matrix**. This consists of fibrous structural proteins (collagens) and adhesive glycoproteins embedded in a proteoglycan gel. Fibroblasts initially lay down small-diameter type III collagen in large amounts. This is partially converted to larger diameter type I collagen during the next phase of healing.[2]

The remodeling and maturation phase

This phase starts several weeks after injury and continues for several months. Myofibroblasts continue contraction of the collagen framework and reorientate the fibrils in the direction of loading. Collagen maturation also continues with the formation of a larger proportion of type I collagen fibrils. At the same time, collagen is degraded by collagenases secreted by fibroblasts, macrophages, neutrophils, and synovial cells present in the initial cellular part of this phase. Net collagen accumulation depends on the balance between synthesis and degradation, and there are multiple biological checks against the uncontrolled action of the collagenases. Macrophages, present in large numbers in granulation tissue, rid the area of extracellular debris, fibrin, and many of the blood vessels found in the previous phase. The resultant scar is an inactive-looking tissue of mature, spindle-shaped fibroblasts, dense collagen, fragments of elastic tissue, extracellular matrix (ECM), and relatively few vessels. Final tissue strength depends on the orientation and quantity of large diameter collagen fibrils.

THE PATHOPHYSIOLOGY AND EFFECTIVE TREATMENT OF SPORTING INJURIES

The aim of the effective treatment of sporting injuries is to minimize pathophysiological processes and facilitate rapid and optimal healing, in order to return to activity and avoid long-term disability and pain (**Figure 29.2**).[3] Because of the multiple factors involved in the pathophysiological response to sporting injury, treatment must be multifactorial to be effective.

Individual tissue responses to injury

BONE

Bone is essentially a fibrous matrix impregnated with mineral salts that is continuously remodeling according to the mechanical stresses and metabolic demands applied to it. Both cancellous and cortical bone is covered by a layer of periosteum, which is highly vascular and responsible for the nutrition of the underlying bone. The deep layers of periosteum contain the osteoblasts that lay down new bone. Osteoclasts are continually reabsorbing bone, resulting in dynamic balance.

Acute fractures of long limb bones are produced by large direct, torsional, tensile, or compressive forces, and are uncommon injuries in sports. Acute fractures of the cancellous carpal and tarsal bones, and of the metacarpals and metatarsals, are more frequently encountered.

The stages of healing of bone fractures include:

- hematoma;
- inflammation;
- callus formation and appearance of woven bone;
- consolidation of woven bone to lamellar bone;
- remodeling, usually to the point of its premorbid structure.[4]

Bone has the capacity to regenerate to its premorbid form because of the presence of labile cells. This compares favorably with most other musculoskeletal tissues, which heal by scar tissue formation only. However, bone heals more slowly. In general, cancellous bone heals faster than cortical, owing to the large contact area between fractured trabeculae. For the same reason, spiral fractures heal quicker than transverse fractures. The speed of healing of upper limb fractures (firm union taking four to six weeks) exceeds that of lower limb fractures (firm union 8–12 weeks).

The aim of fracture management is anatomical and functional restoration, and the following principles apply:

- Rest, with or without immobilization, for undisplaced or minimally displaced fractures.
- Reduction, open or closed, for displaced fractures, followed by immobilization until the fracture is

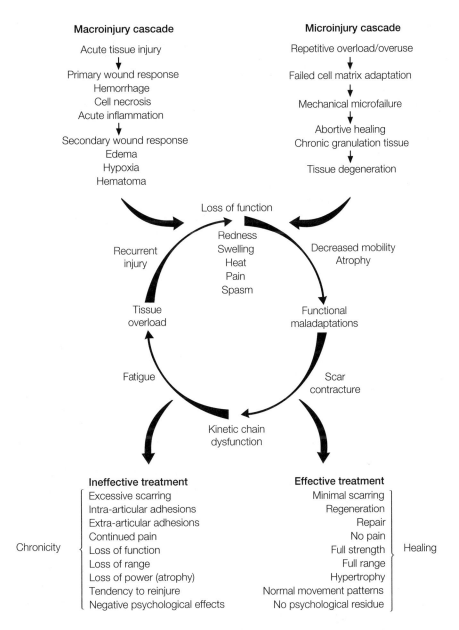

Macroinjury cascade

Acute tissue injury
↓
Primary wound response
Hemorrhage
Cell necrosis
Acute inflammation
↓
Secondary wound response
Edema
Hypoxia
Hematoma

Microinjury cascade

Repetitive overload/overuse
↓
Failed cell matrix adaptation
↓
Mechanical microfailure
↓
Abortive healing
Chronic granulation tissue
↓
Tissue degeneration

Loss of function

Redness
Swelling
Heat
Pain
Spasm

Recurrent injury

Decreased mobility
Atrophy

Tissue overload

Functional maladaptations

Fatigue

Scar contracture

Kinetic chain dysfunction

Ineffective treatment
Excessive scarring
Intra-articular adhesions
Extra-articular adhesions
Continued pain
Loss of function
Loss of range
Loss of power (atrophy)
Tendency to reinjure
Negative psychological effects

Chronicity

Effective treatment
Minimal scarring
Regeneration
Repair
No pain
Full strength
Full range
Hypertrophy
Normal movement patterns
No psychological residue

Healing

Figure 29.2 The outcomes of effective versus ineffective treatment. Reproduced with permission from Leadbetter WB. Soft tissue athletic injury. In: Fu FH, Stone DA (eds). *Sports injuries – mechanisms, prevention and treatment*, © 1994 Lippincott Williams & Wilkins.

clinically united. Removable immobilization devices, e.g. braces, are being increasingly favored above plaster of Paris in order to minimize the negative consequences of immobilization.

- Surgical reduction and fixation for unstable fractures.
- Surgical fixation may otherwise be considered if early mobilization is required.

Avulsion fractures are commonly encountered in sports and are associated with excessive tensile loading of ligament or tendon attachments. Notable examples include the "rugger jersey" finger, where the volar aspect of the base of the distal phalanx is avulsed due to an overload applied by the flexor tendon, while the distal interphalangeal joint is forcibly extended. Avulsion fractures of ligamentous insertions during joint sprains are generally treated as soft-tissue injuries unless the fragment is large and unstable, when surgical reduction and fixation may be considered.

Acute injuries to the periosteum occur with direct blows, causing subperiosteal hematoma with localized swelling and tenderness. These may sometimes ossify due to the involvement of local osteoblasts, but are of little functional consequence.

Overuse injuries of bone are becoming more common because of an ever-increasing participation in recreational running and the heavy training loads of athletes. Bone under loading stress develops increased interstitial calcium, denser trabeculae, and cortical thickening. The mechanism behind the development of stress fractures is incompletely understood, but there is, presumably, a threshold level of mechanical loading above which bone resorption exceeds bone deposition, and failure then occurs. Known associated risk factors include excessive training, rapid increase in training, poor biomechanics, inadequate footwear, muscle fatigue, and hormonal deficiency (such as those associated with athletic amenorrhea[5]). Management consists of rest from offending activities. A period of nonweight-bearing or immobilization may be required if walking causes pain. Certain stress fractures are known to heal poorly, and these should be treated more aggressively with a period of immobilization or internal fixation. These include fractures of the navicular bone, anterior cortex of tibia (transverse), superior neck of femur, base of the fifth metatarsal (Jones type), and base of the second metatarsal.

Epiphyseal injuries occur in the skeletally immature athlete. Pressure epiphyses are found at the end of long bones, and are subject to both shearing and compression forces. Mechanisms of injury that in the adult would cause dislocation or tendon or ligament disruption tend to cause epiphyseal injury in the child. Epiphyseal injuries may also follow overuse, e.g. in young gymnasts performing excessive weight-bearing through their upper limbs. Traction epiphyses (apophyses) occur at the insertion of major muscles and experience tensile forces. They may be acutely avulsed or chronically irritated, for example the common condition of Osgood–Schlatter disease, which occurs at the attachment of the patella tendon to the tibia in 12- to 16-year-olds.

ARTICULAR CARTILAGE

Hyaline articular cartilage is a complex three-dimensional array of type II collagen, embedded in a rich cartilage-specific proteoglycan matrix.[1] Should laceration occur within the more superficial avascular layers, there is no inflammatory response and minimal repair takes place. These lesions do not appear to progress to osteoarthrosis. If, however, the defect extends down to subchondral bone, the acute inflammatory response can proceed, and a new tissue is formed that is composed of both types I and II collagen embedded in a matrix which is mechanically inferior to the original. This eventually breaks down with fibrillation and continued degeneration leads to osteoarthrosis.

Blunt trauma to cartilage, such as a fall on the patella, can cause a change in the proteoglycan matrix and its relationship with the collagen fibrils, a condition termed "chondromalacia."

Loading and joint motion appear to be important in the maintenance of articular cartilage, and prolonged immobilization is associated with cartilage atrophy.

SYNOVIAL JOINTS

Articular hyaline cartilage covering the bone ends is discussed above under Articular cartilage. Fibrocartilage menisci found in the knee are prone to tearing under the high compressive and shearing forces applied to them. If the injury occurs at the periphery where there is a blood supply (outer 25–31 percent), a fibrovascular repair response can ensue. If the tear is in an avascular portion, minimal healing will occur, and surgical meniscectomy may be required to control mechanical symptoms.

Joint capsule has an outer fibrous layer and an inner loose, vascular layer. It is richly innervated for proprioception and nociception and is a source of significant pain when injury results in capsule distension from effusion or hemorrhage. Pain relief may then be afforded by joint aspiration. Prolonged joint immobilization results in capsular shrinkage with fibrous adhesions and restricted range of movement which must be restored to avoid dysfunction.

LIGAMENTS AND TENDONS

Mature ligaments and tendons are composed of large-diameter type I collagen fibrils (with a small amount of type III) embedded in an aqueous gel. The unique feature of these tissues is the collagen "crimp," which is a pattern extending in phase across the width of all ligaments and tendons. It appears to be built into the tertiary structure and is created by cross-linking and an elastic fiber network. Flattening of the collagen crimp is responsible for the initial and physiological lengthening of the tissue under strain. Increasing the strain leads to rupture of the cross-links and eventually failure of the ligament or tendon and either partial or complete tear. Repetitive overloading of tendons can also lead to microfatigue failure.

There is evidence that both immobilization and overly vigorous mobilization within the first three weeks following acute injury is detrimental to collagen orientation. After this time, mobilization probably increases the tensile strength of the repair.[6][II] This information provides a rationale for using early, controlled mobilization of sprained joints, or the use of a limited motion brace, to both minimize eventual joint capsular stiffness and maximize the tensile strength of the repair.

MUSCLE

Contusions, tears, and delayed onset muscle soreness are common occurrences in any sport. Damaged skeletal muscle has the ability to regenerate in the third phase of the healing process and several factors are known to influence this.[7] An intact nerve supply to the muscle is essential. Early muscular contraction will pull torn ends further apart and increase the amount of hematoma, thereby increasing the amount of connective tissue bulk the myotubules have to negotiate to effect a repair.

However, after a few days, the tensile strength in the granulation tissue is probably strong enough to withstand some muscular contraction. If tensile stresses are applied to the granulation tissue at this point, the collagen fibrils will tend to align parallel to the direction of stress, and the myotubules will then grow forward between them in an orderly fashion. Continued muscle contraction during this process results in the regenerating muscle fibers orienting themselves parallel to the direction of tension, thereby maximizing the final strength of the repair.[8]

This has obvious implications for the early management of muscle injuries:

- Minimal muscle activity in the first two to three days after injury allows adequately strong granulation tissue to form.
- Following this, early and gentle contraction and stretching will minimize scar tissue bulk (which is related to stiffness and reinjury), and should result in well-oriented muscle fibers and the quickest return to preinjury tensile strength.

It can be seen from this overview of injury and repair that different musculoskeletal tissues behave differently both in their initial response to injury and in their optimal conditions for repair.

CLINICAL PRESENTATION

It is beyond the scope of this chapter to elaborate on the diagnosis of the wide variety of injuries occurring as a result of sporting activity. It is important to arrive at an accurate diagnosis to ensure the optimal conditions for repair. To aid diagnosis, it is important to elicit certain factors from the history after sporting injury.

- Acute injuries:
  - location of injury;
  - mechanism of injury;
  - previous history of similar or recent injuries;
  - degree of disability or severity of injury;
  - initial management instituted.
- Overuse injuries:
  - site of problem;
  - duration of symptoms;
  - relationship of any symptoms to sporting activity (i.e. occurring at beginning, throughout, or after exercise);
  - intercurrent problems, e.g. the interrelationship of low back pain and hamstring muscle strain;
  - identification of precipitating factors, e.g. the training program, playing surface, footwear;
  - management to date.
- Examination:
  - inspection for swelling, deformity, skin changes;
  - passive and active range of movement;
  - palpation;
  - reproduction of symptoms;
  - stability testing, e.g. of ligament and other joint-stabilizing structures;
  - strength and flexibility;
  - assessment of biomechanics, technique, and equipment;
  - additional tests for
    - neural tension;
    - exclusion of referred pain;
    - local anesthetic blocks to confirm the site of pain origin.

Investigations

In most cases of sporting injuries, clinical assessment is sufficient to provide the diagnosis. Investigations may be used as an adjunct to confirm or exclude a diagnosis, but in some instances, as with many cases of chronic back pain, no amount of investigating will provide an exact tissue cause for the pain. The value of an experienced investigator, using good-quality equipment, cannot be overemphasized.

- Imaging modalities:
  - plain radiographs, including standard, special, and stress views;
  - computed tomography (CT) has a unique ability to display bone detail;
  - magnetic resonance imaging, which can display inflammatory reactions and soft-tissue structure;
  - radioisotopic bone scan to detect areas of increased blood flow and bone turnover;
  - diagnostic ultrasound to image soft tissues and observe dynamic function.
- Other modalities:
  - electromyography and nerve conduction studies;
  - compartment pressure testing and specific muscular strength testing.

MANAGEMENT

The overall management of most sports injuries is based on six principles:

1. Minimize the extent of initial damage.
2. Reduce associated pain and inflammation.
3. Promote healing of damaged tissue.
4. Maintain or restore flexibility, strength, proprioception, and overall cardiovascular fitness during the healing phase.
5. Functionally rehabilitate the athlete to enable a return to sport.
6. Assess and correct any predisposing factors in order to reduce the likelihood of recurrence.[9]

The first three of these will be covered in the context of the information already given on the inflammatory and repair processes, with emphasis on the control of pain in the clinical setting. The fourth, fifth, and sixth are beyond the scope of this text, and involve a thorough knowledge of the biomechanics and physiology of musculoskeletal function, in combination with the specific demands of particular sports.

A variety of treatment modalities is available to manage sporting injuries. However, many traditional methods are not scientifically validated.

Initial treatment

Every effort should be made in the first 24–48 hours following acute soft-tissue injury to minimize bleeding, excessive swelling, and secondary injury. The RICE (rest, ice, compression, elevation) regime is invaluable as a first aid principle owing to its safety and sensibility, and is widely implemented by athletes, coaches, trainers, and health professionals. Additional management not only aims to provide analgesia, but also to speed functional return, whilst remaining low risk and cost-effective.

REST

Wherever possible, the injured part should be rested in relative terms immediately after injury to avoid ongoing hemorrhage. There is also a risk of increasing the severity of primary tissue injury and of injury to other structures should activity be continued.

ICE

This is discussed below under Cryotherapy.

COMPRESSION

The application of a firm elastic bandage may help to reduce bleeding and inflammatory swelling. It should commence just distal to the site of injury and may be applied using a compressive stocking or bandage. It should not be so tight as to cause discomfort or limit venous return, and it should extend at least a hand's breadth proximal to the injury.

ELEVATION

Reduction of blood flow and increased venous and lymphatic return can be assisted by elevating the injured part. A sling can be used for the upper limb, and the lower limb can be rested on a chair or similar object.

During the first 24 hours avoid:

- heat;
- vigorous massage;

- alcohol consumption;
- moderate to intense stretching or contraction (of muscle).

Immobilization

Immobilization was traditionally thought to reduce pain and swelling and to encourage healing, and periods of up to six weeks have been advocated for treatment of severe soft-tissue injuries. It is now known that prolonged immobilization (beyond 72 hours) has detrimental effects on:

- joint stiffness;
- articular cartilage softening;
- muscle disuse atrophy and stiffness;
- suboptimal tendon, ligament, and muscle scar strength;
- bone density;
- deep venous thrombosis formation.

Immobilization is often required for acute, displaced fractures of bone and certain stress fractures. This may be achieved by the application of casts, rigid braces, or air splints. Protected mobilization can be achieved using hinged braces or taping techniques, and prevents excessive stress on the injured structure while allowing others to move, preventing the complications of complete immobilization. Protected mobilization is used to treat ligament injuries, such as medial collateral ligaments of the knee and ankle sprains. Crutches may be used when weight-bearing is contraindicated or painful.

Essentially, soft tissue injuries should receive relative immobilization for 24–72 hours followed by controlled and progressive mobilization.[6, 10][II]

Pharmacological therapy

A small number of drugs have a traditional place in the management of sporting injuries. These predominantly include analgesics and anti-inflammatory drugs. Despite widespread use and apparent clinical efficacy, their long-term effects on tissue function are incompletely understood.

ANALGESICS

In the management of sporting injuries, analgesics are used acutely to alleviate pain. It is rarely necessary to continue their use beyond the acute phase. Acetylsalicylic acid (aspirin), paracetamol (acetaminophen), tramadol, and codeine are the most commonly used analgesics in the sporting setting, with injectable opioids usually only required for very painful displaced fractures. Acetylsalicylic acid in larger doses also has an anti-inflammatory effect. Its effect on platelet adhesiveness suggests that it could be considered a contraindication in acute injuries where hematoma formation is a problem, but this has not been well documented in scientific literature (see Chapter 4, Clinical pharmacology: traditional NSAIDs and selective COX-2 inhibitors).

It is imperative to check the appropriate sporting authority's position regarding the use of prohibited substances before recommending medications to athletes who are subject to drug testing as some are included in the banned list. The World Anti-doping Agency (WADA) was established in 1999 to promote and coordinate the fight against the use of drugs in sport internationally. The WADA list of prohibited substances and methods can be accessed at www.wada-ama.org/rtecontent/document/2006_list.

NONSTEROIDAL ANTI-INFLAMMATORY DRUGS

Nonsteroidal anti-inflammatory drugs (NSAID) are the most commonly used class of drug in the management of both acute and overuse sporting injuries. They are used in the following sports medicine situations to control pain and inflammation:

- early after acute injury;
- in overuse syndromes;
- after surgery;
- during rehabilitation.

Inflammatory stimuli disrupt cell membrane phospholipids, with the eventual production of an array of biologically active substances, including prostaglandins. NSAIDs limit this process by inhibiting the cyclo-oxygenase (COX) pathway, some also inhibit lipoxygenase pathways (**Figure 29.3**).[11] NSAIDs may also have a direct effect on inflammatory cells in modulating cell behavior.[12] Many clinical trials support the observation that modest benefits in pain and function are seen in NSAID-treated patients with acute soft-tissue trauma (ligament sprains, bursitis, synovitis) when compared with placebo.[13][II], [14, 15][II] Weiler,[16][I] in a meta-analysis of 44 studies with respect to the use of NSAIDs in sporting

soft-tissue injuries, concluded that NSAIDs did not seriously delay the healing process when given soon after injury, that healing was slightly more rapid, that inflammation slightly decreased, and that return to practice was occasionally quicker. In general, studies suggest that the improvements most often observed are an earlier decrease in pain, an improved range of motion, and an earlier return to routine and sports activities.[13][II], [15][II], [16][I], [17][II], [18][II], [19] Studies comparing the clinical efficacy of different NSAIDs with each other are inconclusive.

The availability of selective COX-2 inhibitors has held promise for the reduction in the significant incidence of gastrointestinal side effects associated with inhibition of the regulatory role of COX-1 by nonselective NSAIDs. Clinical trials in acute pain, however, are inconclusive as to a consistent class action of COX-2 inhibitors in providing acute analgesia. The early rise of prostaglandin E_2 (PGE_2) levels following soft-tissue trauma (from COX-1 action) is not inhibited and may contribute to this observation.[13][II], [14]

The inflammatory phase is necessary in the healing process to provide a fibrin framework, to mop up necrotic debris, and to provide the necessary vascular and cellular supply for subsequent repair processes. Theoretically, it may be deleterious to inhibit these functions with NSAIDs, and many laboratory studies have attempted to investigate this. There is, however, incredible variability in animal responses to different NSAIDs and in their rates of healing, which must be taken into consideration when extrapolating results to humans. Dahners et al.[20] concluded that piroxicam increased the early strength of healing ligaments (at 14 days) in the rat when it was administered in the first week after injury. There was no recordable difference at 21 days. Kalbhen studied the effects of different anti-inflammatories on articular cartilage in rats following intra-articular injection.[21] He suggested that some (e.g. salicylates, flufenamic acid, indomethacin, ibuprofen, phenylbutazone, and dexamethasone) have catabolic characteristics in regard to connective tissue metabolism with observed degeneration of articular cartilage and subchondral bone. Other NSAIDs had no effect and were classed as noncatabolic (e.g. tiaprofenic acid, diclofenac, ketoprofen). More recent animal research into the tissue effects of

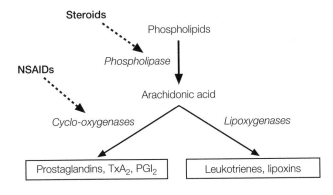

Figure 29.3 The cyclo-oxygenase and lipoxygenase pathways.

COX-2-selective inhibitors also suggests impaired healing of ligament, tendon, and particularly bone; however, the typical use of supratherapeutic doses for long periods and the absence of adequate research tools exploring the *in vivo* consequences of NSAID use following tissue injury limit extrapolation to the clinical setting.[22] This work may have implications in the selection of NSAIDs for sporting injuries; however, clinical data currently do not suggest impaired functional recovery. NSAIDs have little adjuvant role in acute muscular contusions and tears,[19][I], [23][II], [24][I] but may improve the symptoms (but not recovery) of delayed-onset muscle soreness.[19][I]

Peripheral nerve damage demonstrates a true inflammatory response, which suggests that NSAIDs may be useful in this situation, e.g. a herniated disk with a chemical radiculitis or carpal tunnel syndromes.[15][II] Too few well-designed studies evaluating the use of NSAIDs in chronic overuse injuries have been published to draw conclusions regarding their efficacy in these settings.[16][I] NSAIDs are often used in the chronic situation for their analgesic properties, with variable success. The more chronic the injury, the more likely it is that permanent structural damage has been acquired that may be unresponsive to anti-inflammatory medication alone (**Figure 29.4**). The efficacy of medications such as NSAIDs will depend on where the particular injury lies on the spectrum of tissue injury from the early "inflammation-dominant" to the later "degeneration-dominant" states. The focus in overuse injuries, as such, should be to correct the underlying predisposing factors and to restore full function. (Promising new therapeutic treatments for overuse soft tissue injuries include aprotonin, prolotherapy and topical glyceryl trinitrate.)[15][II]

NSAIDs are also available as transdermal preparations. In one systematic review of 37 trials, the relative analgesic benefit of topical NSAID over placebo was found to be 1.7.[25][I] Clinical trials have also demonstrated improved functional capacity against placebo for ligament sprains and acute tendinitis.[26][III] There are obvious advantages of using topical preparations in terms of side-effect

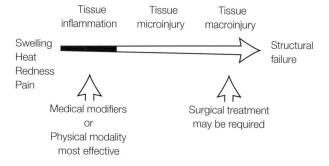

Figure 29.4 The role of nonsteroidal anti-inflammatory drugs (NSAIDs) during the inflammatory stage. Reproduced with permission from Leadbetter WB. Soft tissue athletic injury. In: Fu FH, Stone DA (eds). *Sports injuries – mechanisms, prevention and treatment*, © 1994 Lippincott Williams & Wilkins.

profile, with the most notable reaction being minor skin irritation. Their efficacy may be improved by concurrent massage and iontophoresis (the electrical current-mediated transfer of ionic molecules through the skin).[27][II]

Recommendations for the clinical use of NSAIDs in sporting injuries are based on the balance between short-term gains in function and pain relief and potential side effects and possible healing impairment. Athletes will often have an urgency to return to training and competition, ever more so with the increase in professionalism of recent decades. It is imperative that the treating physicians reassess progress and efficacy and monitor side effects if NSAIDs are to be used in the management of athletic injuries. It must always be remembered that the most crucial factor in rehabilitation is not simply the relief of symptoms but the return to maximal function. Current practice suggests that NSAIDs should be prescribed as soon as possible following acute injury and maintained at recommended doses for three to ten days. Caution should be exercised in the use beyond three days of NSAIDs for muscular injuries, where healing may be prolonged.[19][I]

CORTICOSTEROIDS

Corticosteroids are one of the most potent anti-inflammatory medications available to the clinician. This is partly due to their action on phospholipase A_2, which reduces membrane phospholipid breakdown and decreases the amount of arachidonic acid available as a substrate for both the cyclo-oxygenase and lipoxygenase pathways (**Figure 29.3**) (see Chapter 6, Clinical pharmacology: other adjuvants). Corticosteroids also exert a direct suppressive effect on cellular components of inflammation and immunity.[28] Their broad mode of action underlies their potential to impair wound healing, induce tissue catabolism, and disrupt normal tissue maintenance. Although they were welcomed enthusiastically by clinicians treating inflammatory arthropathies, the same characteristics limit the use of steroids in the sporting context.

Corticosteroids may be given by injection, taken orally, or delivered by iontophoresis. Oral corticosteroid use is banned by many sporting bodies, and in any case is seldom indicated in the sporting context owing to potential side effects and interference with collagen synthesis. Most research into the efficacy of corticosteroids is carried out using local injection, and, even then, a great deal of the information in the sports medicine setting is anecdotal or of poor statistical value.[12]

In the absence of an animal model for overuse injury, studies on the effects of corticosteroid injection on normal tissues that are commonly injured in sports (tendon, ligament, and articular cartilage) reveal conflicting and often deleterious effects. Sharing characteristics of hypovascularity and a highly differentiated parenchymal cell population, these tissues lack the ideal requirements for tissue healing. Injection studies of ligament and tendon have revealed retardation of the normal processes of acute wound healing[29] by inhibiting both the inflammatory and proliferative phases. In a large study on rhesus knees by Noyes et al.,[30] a dose-dependent, significant, and long-lasting deterioration in the mechanical properties of the anterior cruciate ligament was noted after a single intraligamentous, or two intra-articular injections, of methylprednisolone acetate. While useful in inflammatory synovitis, the effects of corticosteroids on articular cartilage are primarily catabolic.[12, 21] In an extensive review of the use of anti-inflammatory therapy in sports injury, Leadbetter[12] concluded that the most reliable effect of corticosteroid use is in the setting of excessive inflammatory activity. An inadvertent injection into a dense connective tissue, such as ligament or tendon, is of concern in sports medicine as cystic spaces and collagen necrosis can be seen as early as 48 hours later and may predispose to tissue rupture.[29] Despite the concern over impaired healing and weakening of normal tissue, injectable corticosteroids have an accepted role in the management of some sports-related conditions:

- bursitis;
- paratendinitis;
- tenosynovitis;
- joint synovitis;
- vertebral facet joints.

Corticosteroids demonstrate short-term efficacy in symptom relief for degenerative tendinopathies e.g. lateral epicondylosis ("tennis elbow").[15][I] They can decrease pain sufficiently to allow a rehabilitation program to proceed, but should rarely be the sole form of therapy.

Corticosteroid preparations vary in their water solubility. As a result, the duration of action differs. Triamcinolone is the least water soluble and therefore a good choice for achieving long-term effects in joints and bursae. Betamethasone has a short duration of action and is thus valuable in bathing tendons, or injecting into tendon sheaths, where there is a concern for tendon strength.

It is common practice to mix local anesthetic (e.g. 1 or 2 percent lidocaine) with the steroid to reduce the pain produced upon injection, although it should be noted that the product information cautions against this practice because of changes in solubility and drug distribution. Combining a local anesthetic also allows diagnostic confirmation of the site of pain and success of placement by immediate pain ablation.

Corticosteroid injection commonly causes an exacerbation of symptoms for one to three days, the so-called "postinjection flare," due to crystal-induced inflammation. Local complications also include subcutaneous fat necrosis, overlying depigmentation, osteolysis, and possible increased risk of tendon rupture. Systemic complications are rare, but include transient hyperglycemia in diabetics and an allergic reaction (perhaps due to sodium metabisulfate present in some preparations as a preservative).

Corticosteroids can also be delivered transdermally via iontophoresis, which has the advantages of avoiding injection and its complications and local tissue necrosis effect of bolus injection. Dexamethasone and methylprednisolone are both suitable for delivery in this fashion, and this method has been advocated in superficial inflammatory conditions, such as tendinitis and fasciitis. Clinical studies have shown earlier relief of pain and return to function compared with placebo in shoulder tendinitis and plantar fasciitis.[31][III] The ideal variables for depth of penetration are a current of 4 mA applied for ten minutes with 4 percent lidocaine solution.[32] The main complications are those of skin irritation, either chemical or thermal, due to inappropriately applied electrodes.

Cryotherapy

The application of ice or cold for the treatment of soft-tissue injury was first recorded by Hippocrates around 400BC. It remains a cheap, readily available tool in common usage for sporting injuries that effectively reduces pain and swelling.[22][II], [33] Transfer of heat energy away from body tissues using a local cold application depends on:

- the temperature difference between the coolant and the tissues;
- the thermal conductivity of the tissues. (Tissues with high water content, such as muscle, have a high thermal conductivity compared with skin and fat. Subcutaneous fat may act to insulate heat loss to the environment.)
- the length of time coolant is applied. (Temperature will fall until equilibrium is reached.)
- the size of the area being cooled;
- the vascularity of the area.

While skin temperature may drop from 30 to 14°C using ice massage, the temperature of muscles only 30–50 mm below the skin may be lowered by as little as 4°C.[34] This lowering of local tissue temperature persists for up to 45 minutes.

PHYSIOLOGICAL EFFECTS OF CRYOTHERAPY

Cold application is followed by immediate vasoconstriction of cutaneous blood vessels as an autonomic reflex to stimulation of skin thermoreceptors. Increased blood viscosity also contributes to slowed blood flow. By causing vasoconstriction, cold therapy attempts to limit edema and painful mediators resulting from the inflammatory response. A study on ankle volume in sprained ankles showed a significant decrease following application of a cold gel pack for 20 minutes when compared with no treatment.[35][III] The slowing of the metabolic rate induced by lowering the temperature affects all tissues. In conjunction with vasoconstriction, which should minimize the release of active inflammatory mediators, secondary hypoxic tissue damage can be limited, and this provides the rationale for the early use of cryotherapy in acute sporting injury.

The response of muscle has been well studied using the experimental model of eccentrically induced delayed onset muscle soreness. Cryotherapy results in improved range of motion and reduced pain;[27][II] however, field studies of muscular injuries, such as strain and contusion, are lacking. Muscle strength can be diminished in accordance with the lowered metabolic rate. When combined with decreased neuromuscular activity, the clinical result is a loss of motor skill and strength. As mentioned above, muscle temperature changes persist after the coolant has been removed. This may possibly be due to the insulating effect of overlying fat, and is a warning against the use of ice during a sporting competition when an immediate return to play is being considered.

Local effects of cooling include a decrease in motor and sensory nerve conduction velocity, a decrease in the rate of firing of muscle spindle afferents and stretch reflex responses, and therefore a decrease in nociception and muscle spasm.[36]

Much attention has been given to the role of cryotherapy in the postoperative setting. Results of clinical trials indicate some evidence of improved pain relief, swelling, range of motion, or time to weight-bearing with cryotherapy compared with placebo.[37][II], [27, 38, 39, 40][II]

There is no evidence-based consensus as to the optimal frequency of cryotherapy.

POSSIBLE THERAPEUTIC USES OF CRYOTHERAPY

The following uses of cryotherapy are based on the pathophysiological observations discussed above under The pathophysiology of tissue injury and repair:

- acute injury;
- pain control;
- relief of muscle spasm;
- chronic edema and joint effusions;
- in the rehabilitation of chronic injury;
- postoperative pain management.

TECHNIQUES OF ADMINISTERING CRYOTHERAPY

Local immersion

This involves immersing the body part in a container of iced water. At a temperature of 16–18°C, immersion can be tolerated for 15–20 minutes. Whole body immersion is increasingly used by professional athletes to aid post-match recovery. Its usefulness, however, has not been strongly supported by research.

Ice packs

These consist of crushed ice wrapped in a moist towel or cloth, which molds directly on to the skin of the involved area. These can be tolerated for 15–20 minutes and care should be taken to avoid skin damage by frequent inspection. Application of oil to the skin may provide some insulation to control the rate of skin cooling and also causes a rapid run-off of water from the melting ice to maintain the temperature at the pack–skin interface.

Commercial cold packs

These are plastic or vinyl bags filled with water and a substance to lower the freezing point. They are stored in the freezer and remain flexible to enable molding. It should be remembered that these packs are colder than ice, and extra care is needed to prevent skin damage during early application. As a precaution, it is wise to place a moist towel between the pack and the skin.

Cooling packs may also contain chemicals that are mixed by breaking a container within the pack to result in an exothermic reaction. These are obviously for single use, but are useful in first-aid application.

Ice massage

Ice massage has advantages over ice pack in that it reaches peak temperature change (in muscle) more rapidly.[34][III] An ice block can be made by freezing a water-filled Styrofoam cup, which can be partially torn off once frozen. The painful or swollen area is massaged with the ice block. The massage initially produces a burning sensation, followed by aching, then numbness. The time to reach peak cooling at the level of muscle is 15–20 minutes.[34] [III] When the pain has been reduced by the massage, mobilization techniques or exercises can follow.

CONTRAINDICATIONS

Cryotherapy should be used with caution in the following situations:

- peripheral vascular disease;
- neurological sensory impairment;
- cold urticaria;
- cryoglobulinemia;
- skin wounds.

Other nonpharmacological transdermal modalities

A multitude of electrotherapeutic modalities are used in clinical practice for the treatment of sporting injuries, including:

- ultrasound;
- transcutaneous electrical nerve stimulation (TENS);
- inferential stimulation;

- high-voltage galvanic stimulation;
- laser;
- extracorporeal shock wave therapy;
- magnetic field therapy.

Their use varies widely among physical therapists and depends more on empirical clinical experience than scientific evidence. Meta-analyses of clinical trials fail to conclude that any modality is beneficial in the use of musculoskeletal pain, acute injury, or rehabilitation.[41][III], [27, 42, 43, 44, 45, 46, 47, 48][II], [49][I] Despite the number of laboratory and clinical studies, results remain inconclusive as to the benefit of these techniques, and further well-designed research is required.[41][III]

HYPERBARIC OXYGEN THERAPY

The promise of faster recovery by increasing oxygen concentration at the site of injured soft tissue has led many professional sporting organizations to use hyperbaric oxygen therapy (HBOT). This typically involves the administration of 100 percent oxygen at ambient pressures of 1.5–3.0 atmospheres, once or twice daily for 60–120 minutes. Adverse effects include barotrauma, oxygen toxicity, and visual deterioration. Trials in ankle sprains, knee ligament injury, and experimental models of delayed onset muscle soreness do not show any benefit in pain scores or functional outcome. At this stage, there does not appear to be an indication for the use of HBOT in sports injury where barotrauma is not involved.[50][I], [51, 52]

PROGNOSIS

The prognosis regarding sporting injuries depends largely on the tissue damaged, its degree of injury, and the level of functional activity expected of it. For example, acute, uncomplicated fractures can heal to their functional premorbid level, but acute or degenerative tendon ruptures, despite optimal primary repair, hold a low expectation of return to preinjury levels of activity. A small rotator cuff tear in a recreational tennis player may not result in any symptoms once rehabilitated, but the same injury in a professional baseball pitcher may mark the end of his career. Other sporting injuries have recognized long-term sequelae, such as the relationship between meniscal tears and the later development of osteoarthrosis of the knee joint.

REFERENCES

* 1. Oakes BW. The classifications of injuries and mechanisms of injury, repair and healing. In: Bloomfield J, Fricker PA, Fitch KD (eds). *Textbook of science and medicine in sport*. Melbourne: Blackwell Scientific, 1992: 200–17.

2. Mitchell RN, Cotran RS. Acute and chronic inflammation. In: Kumar V, Cotran R, Robbins S (eds). *Basic pathology*. Philadelphia, PA: WB Saunders, 1992: 25–46.

* 3. Leadbetter WB. Soft tissue athletic injury. In: Fu FH, Stone DA (eds). *Sports injuries – mechanisms, prevention and treatment*. Baltimore, MD: Williams & Wilkins, 1994: 733–80.

4. Apley AG, Solomon I (eds). Principles of fractures. In: *Apley's system of orthopaedics and fractures*. London: Butterworths, 1987: 333–68.

5. Drinkwater BL, Nilson K, Chesmur CH et al. Bone mineral content of amenorrheic athletes. *New England Journal of Medicine*. 1984; **311**: 277–21.

6. Hart DP, Danhers LE. Healing of the medial collateral ligament in rats. *Journal of Bone and Joint Surgery*. 1987; **69A**: 1194–9.

* 7. Lennox CME. Muscle injuries. In: McLatchie GR, Lennox CME (eds). *The soft tissues*. Oxford: Butterworth-Heinemann, 1993: 83–103.

* 8. Carlson BM. The regeneration of skeletal muscle – review. *American Journal of Anatomy*. 1973; **137**: 119.

* 9. Brukner P, Khan K (eds). Principles of treatment. In: *Clinical sports medicine*. Sydney: McGraw-Hill, 1994: 103–51.

* 10. Kannus P, Parkkari J, Jarvinen TLN et al. Basic science and clinical studies coincide: active treatment approach is needed after a sports injury. *Scandinavian Journal of Medicine and Science in Sports*. 2003; **13**: 150–4.

11. Berger RG. Non-steroidal anti-inflammatory drugs: making the right choices. *Journal of the American Academy of Orthopaedic Surgeons*. 1994; **2**: 255–60.

* 12. Leadbetter WB. Anti-inflammatory therapy in sports injury. *Clinics in Sports Medicine*. 1995; **14**: 353–410.

13. Petri M, Hufman S, Waser G et al. Celexocib effectively treats patients with acute shoulder tedinitis/bursitis. *Journal of Rheumatology*. 2004; **31**: 1614–20.

14. Dionne RA, Khan AA, Gordon SM. Analgesia and COX-2 inhibition. *Clinical and Experimental Rheumatology*. 2001; **19** (Suppl. 25): S63–70.

* 15. Paoloni J, Orchard J. The use of therapeutic medications for soft-tissue injuries in sports medicine. *Medical Journal of Australia*. 2005; **183**: 384–8.

* 16. Weiler JM. Medical modifiers of sports injury: the use of NSAIDs in sports soft tissue injury. *Clinics in Sports Medicine*. 1992; **11**: 635–44.

17. Lereim P, Gabor I. Piroxicam and naproxen in acute sporting injuries. *American Journal of Medicine*. 1988; **84**: 50–55.

18. Heere LP. Piroxicam in acute musculoskeletal disorders and sports injuries. *American Journal of Sports Medicine*. 1988; **16**: 641–79.

19. Almekinders LC. Anti-inflammatory treatment of muscular injuries in sport. *Sports Medicine*. 1999; **28**: 383–8.

20. Dahners LE, Gilbert JA, Lester GE et al. The effect of non-steroidal anti-inflammatory drugs on the healing of ligaments. *American Journal of Sports Medicine*. 1988; **16**: 641–6.

21. Kalbhen DA. The influence of non-steroidal anti-inflammatory drugs on morphology of articular cartilage. *Scandinavian Journal of Rheumatology. Supplement.* 1988; **17**: 13–22.

* 22. Warden S. Cyclo-oxygenase-2 inhibitors: beneficial or detrimental for athletes with acute musculoskeletal injuries? *Sports Medicine.* 2005; **35**: 271–83.

23. Reyolds JF, Noakes TD, Schwellnus MP *et al.* Non-steroidal anti-inflammatory drugs fail to enhance the healing of acute hamstring injuries treated with physiotherapy. *South African Medical Journal.* 1995; **85**: 517–22.

24. Almekinders LC, Gilbert JA. Healing of experimental muscle strains and the effects of non-steroidal anti-inflammatory medications. *American Journal of Sports Medicine.* 1986; **14**: 303–08.

25. Moore RA, Tramer MR, Carroll D *et al.* Quantitative systematic review of topically applied non-steroidal anti-inflammatory drugs. *British Medical Journal.* 1998; **316**: 333–8.

26. Heyneman CA. Topical non-steroidal anti-inflammatory drugs for acute soft tissue injury. *Annals of Pharmacotherapy.* 1995; **29**: 780–2.

* 27. Bolin DJ. Transdermal approaches to pain in sports injury management. *Current Sports Medicine Reports.* 2003; **2**: 303–09.

28. Goodwin JS. Mechanism of action of corticosteroids. In: Goodwin JS (ed). *Mediguide to inflammatory diseases.* New York: Pfizer Laboratories, 1987: 1–5.

29. Kennedy JC, Willis RB. The effects of local corticosteroid injections on tendons: a biomechanical and microscopic correlative study. *American Journal of Sports Medicine.* 1976; **4**: 11–21.

30. Noyes FR, Grood ES, Nussbaum NS. Effect of intra-muscular corticosteroids on ligament properties: a biomechanical and histological study in rhesus knees. *Clinical Orthopaedics and Related Research.* 1977; **123**: 197–209.

31. Bertolucci LE. Introduction of anti-inflammatory drugs by iontophoresis: a double blind study. *Journal of Orthopaedic and Sports Physical Therapy.* 1982; **4**: 103–08.

32. Costello CT, Jeske AH. Iontophoresis; applications in transdermal medication delivery. *Physical Therapy.* 1995; **75**: 554–63.

33. MacAuley DC. Ice therapy-how good is the evidence? *International Journal of Sports Medicine.* 2001; **22**: 379–84.

34. Zemke JE, Andersen JC, Guion K *et al.* Intramuscular temperature response in the human leg in two forms of cryotherapy: ice massage and ice bag. *Journal of Orthopaedic and Sports Physical Therapy.* 1998; **27**: 301–07.

35. Weston M, Taber C, Casagranda I, Cornwall M. Changes in local blood volume during cold gel pack application to traumatised ankles. *Journal of Orthopaedic and Sports Physical Therapy.* 1994; **19**: 197–9.

36. Low J, Reed A (eds). Cold therapy. In: *Electrotherapy explained: principles and practice.* Oxford: Butterworth-Heinemann, 1990: 202–20.

37. Konrath GA, Lock T, Goitz HT, Schneidler T. The use of cold therapy after anterior cruciate ligament reconstruction: a prospective, randomised study and literature review. *American Journal of Sports Medicine.* 1996; **24**: 629–33.

38. Lessard LA, Scudds RA, Amendola A, Vaz MD. The efficacy of cryotherapy following arthroscopic knee surgery. *Journal of Orthopaedic and Sports Physical Therapy.* 1997; **26**: 14–22.

39. Edwards DJ, Rimmer M, Keene GC. The use of cold therapy in the post-operative management of patients undergoing arthroscopic anterior cruciate ligament reconstruction. *American Journal of Sports Medicine.* 1996; **24**: 193–5.

40. Speer KP, Warren RF, Horowitz L. The efficacy of cryotherapy in the post-operative shoulder. *Journal of Shoulder and Elbow Surgery.* 1996; **5**: 62–8.

41. Fedorczyk J. The role of physical agents in modulating pain. *Journal of Hand Therapy.* 1997; **10**: 110–21.

42. Wadsworth H, Chanmugam APP (eds). Low frequency currents. In: *Electrotherapeutic agents in physiotherapy.* Marrickville: Science Press, 1988: 264–7.

43. Fourie JA, Bowerbank P. Stimulation of bone healing in new fractures of the tibial shaft using interferential currents. *Physiotherapy Research International.* 1997; **2**: 255–68.

44. Taylor K, Newton RA, Personius WJ, Bush FM. Effects of interferential current stimulation for the treatment of patients with recurrent jaw pain. *Physical Therapy.* 1987; **67**: 346–50.

45. Robinson AJ. Transcutaneous electrical nerve stimulation for the control of pain in musculoskeletal disorders. *Journal of Orthopaedic and Sports Physical Therapy.* 1996; **24**: 208–26.

* 46. Carroll D, Tram'er M, McQuay H *et al.* Randomization is important in studies with pain outcomes: systematic review of transcutaneous electrical nerve stimulation in acute post-operative pain. *British Journal of Anaesthesia.* 1996; **77**: 798–803.

* 47. Riet G, Kleijnen J, Knipschild P. Acupuncture and chronic pain: a criteria-based meta-analysis. *Journal of Clinical Epidemiology.* 1990; **43**: 1191–9.

48. Gam AN, Johannsen F. Ultrasound therapy in musculoskeletal disorders: a meta-analysis. *Pain.* 1995; **63**: 85–91.

49. Van der Windt DAWM, Van der Heijden GJMG, Van deb Berg SGM *et al.* Therapeutic ultrasound for acute ankle sprains. *Cochrane Database of Systematic Reviews.* 2006; **CD001250**.

50. Bennett M, Best TM, Babul S *et al.* Hyperbaric oxygen therapy for delayed onset muscle soreness and closed soft tissue injury. *Cochrane Database of Systematic Reviews.* 2006; **CD00471353**.

51. Babul S, Rhodes EC, Taunton JE, Lepawsky M. Effects of intermittent exposure to hyperbaric oxygen for the treatment of an acute soft tissue injury. *Clinical Journal of Sport Medicine.* 2003; **13**: 138–47.

52. Bleakley CM, McDonough SM, MacAuley DC. The use of ice in the treatment of acute soft tissue injury: a systematic review of randomized controlled trials. *American Journal of Sports Medicine.* 2004; **32**: 251–61.

30

The opioid-tolerant patient, including those with a substance abuse disorder

LINDY J ROBERTS

KEY LEARNING POINTS

- Opioid tolerance occurs in a variety of settings, often in patients who are predisposed to the development of acutely painful conditions. Despite this, opioid-tolerant subjects are most often excluded from acute pain studies; thus there is little evidence to guide management.
- A collaborative interdisciplinary approach to the assessment and management of these patients is essential.
- Goals include optimization of analgesia, management of psychiatric and behavioral disorders, and prevention of withdrawal syndromes.
- Opioid requirements are increased two- to three-fold. The usual opioid should be viewed as the baseline requirement and, where possible, continued. Patient-

controlled analgesia (PCA) with larger than usual bolus doses is the technique of choice for moderate to severe pain.
- Buprenorphine and naltrexone provide particular challenges and specialist advice may need to be sought.
- Adjuvant agents, particularly ketamine, decrease opioid requirements, may reduce tolerance, and are effective for neuropathic pain.
- The role of nonpharmacological therapies is poorly studied, although they would be expected to be useful.
- Follow up must include communication with the usual treatment provider with monitored return to the preexisting opioid regimen, and, where indicated, referral for ongoing specialist management.

OVERVIEW

Acute pain in the setting of opioid tolerance provides substantial assessment and management challenges.[1] Opioid tolerance may be seen in patients with:

- persistent noncancer pain;
- persistent cancer pain;

- substance abuse disorder (SAD);
- acute tolerance.

There may be overlap between these groups. For example, some patients with noncancer pain exhibit aberrant drug-taking behaviors; those with SAD may also have persistent pain; and cancer pain may occur in those with a history of SAD or persistent noncancer pain. Patients with SAD who are in remission and drug-free present particular challenges for pain management;[2] however, it would not be expected that this would include opioid tolerance.

Systematic investigation of opioid-tolerant patients is potentially confounded by complexity and heterogeneity. As a result, these patients are almost always excluded from studies of acute pain. The influence of psychological factors such as anxiety, depression and the meaning of surgery has been investigated in opioid-naive patients,[3] and although these issues would be expected to be extremely important in the opioid-tolerant, they have been far less studied in this group.

There is little high-level evidence to guide assessment and management recommendations. Evidence-based acute pain management guidelines published by the Australian and New Zealand College of Anaesthestists in 2005 contain no level 1 citations and only one level 2 citation in the section on the opioid-tolerant patient;[1] thus, of necessity, reliance is placed upon case series,[4, 5, 6, 7, 8] case reports,[9, 10] and expert opinion.[11, 12, 13, 14, 15, 16, 17, 18, 19, 20, 21, 22, 23, 24, 25]

DEFINITIONS

To avoid misconceptions and mislabeling, it is essential that uniform definitions are employed. In particular, it is important to differentiate "addiction" from the common consequences of long-term opioid administration, particularly tolerance and physical dependence.

Tolerance is "a state of adaptation in which exposure to a drug induces changes that result in a diminution of one or more of the drug's effects over time."[26] This occurs for both desired and adverse effects, often at different rates or in some cases not at all.[26] Pseudotolerance has been used to indicate that the requirement for increased opioid dosing is due to other causes, for example disease progression, rather than true tolerance.[19]

Cross-tolerance is tolerance to the effects of agents within the same drug class.[16] For example, methadone-maintained patients are cross-tolerant to the effects of high concentrations of morphine.[27]

Physical dependence is "a state of adaptation that is manifested by a drug class-specific withdrawal syndrome that can be produced by abrupt cessation, rapid dose reduction, decreasing blood level of the drug, and/or administration of an antagonist."[26]

Addiction is "a primary chronic neurobiologic disease with genetic, psychosocial, and environmental factors affecting its development and manifestations. It is characterized by behaviors that include one or more of the following: impaired control over drug use, compulsive use, continued use despite harm, and craving."[26] Although some favor the use of the term "addiction,"[28] the stigma associated with this label has led to the use of other terms such as substance misuse or even substance use. Regardless, this is not a predictable drug effect,

but rather occurs in susceptible individuals with the appropriate environmental and other triggers.[26]

The American Psychiatric Association (DSM-IV[29]) uses the terms substance dependence and substance abuse. Substance dependence disorder involves three of the following over a 12-month period: tolerance, withdrawal, higher doses or longer duration of therapy than intended, unsuccessful attempts at cessation, excessive time spent obtaining the substance, reduced activities because of the substance, and ongoing use despite adverse physical or psychological consequences. Substance abuse disorder involves at least one of the following over a 12-month period: failure to fulfill major role obligations, use in physically hazardous situations, substance-related legal problems, and ongoing use despite social or interpersonal problems caused by the substance. It is notable that abuse may occur in the absence of physical dependence or tolerance.

The term "pseudoaddiction" has been used to describe the phenomenon whereby there are the behavioral hallmarks of addiction, but these aberrant behaviors resolve with the provision of adequate pain relief.[30] This condition is identified retrospectively and may be difficult to differentiate from addiction.[19]

OPIOID–TOLERANT PATIENTS IN ACUTE SETTINGS

Opioid consumption and adverse effects

Postoperatively, opioid-tolerant patients using patient-controlled analgesia (PCA) administer on average two to three times more opioid than do matched opioid-naive controls undergoing similar surgery.[4, 6, 7, 8][III] The explanation is probably multifactorial and may include psychosocial issues such as levels of trait anxiety, depression,[31] and the amount of social support,[32] which are known to predict PCA use. Opioid-tolerant patients are more likely to become sedated, possibly due to greater administration of anxiolytics,[4, 33] but less likely to experience adverse effects such as nausea and vomiting.[7]

Pain scores

Despite higher opioid consumption, opioid-tolerant patients report consistently higher rest and dynamic pain scores.[4, 7, 8][III] Persistent pain is an independent predictor for the presence of severe postoperative pain,[31, 34] particularly in those with noncancer pain.[4] High pain scores may represent part of a learned response to validate pain experience or to obtain assistance, including more analgesia,[4] or may reflect pathological states such as opioid-induced hyperalgesia (OIH). Staff tend not to rely on pain scores, instead using functional measures such as ability to cough and ambulate.[33]

Workload impact

Opioid-tolerant patients increase the workload for attending clinicians, requiring greater time for assessment and management. Compared with matched opioid-naive patients, those with persistent pain and opioid-tolerance require more PCA opioid prescription changes, more frequent nonroutine review, and longer duration of care, increasing the workload of an acute pain service.[8][III] Greater workload demand has been demonstrated in a labor ward setting.[5][V] PCA with background infusion is perceived by staff as the least labor-intensive method of providing analgesia.[33][V]

Staff knowledge and attitudes

These patient groups may invoke strong feelings in attending staff. In the acute setting, patients with non-cancer pain are perceived as "manipulative," "not congenial," and "not cooperative,"[33] and as having high levels of anxiety.[4] There is apprehension regarding the large opioid doses required,[33] which may reflect unjustified concern about exacerbating "addiction," or causing adverse events, particularly respiratory depression. Nursing and medical staff may have limited understanding of opioid pharmacology, particularly regarding the differences between tolerance, physical dependence, and SAD. The consequences of the rising abuse of prescription opioids may include stigmatization of those treated with opioids, and "opiophobia" in healthcare providers.[35] These factors may lead to undertreatment of pain. This has been shown in ambulatory AIDS patients, where a history of SAD reduces the likelihood of strong opioid prescription, even for severe pain.[36]

In a small study of public teaching hospital inpatients with active SAD and treating internists,[37] some important themes emerge. The doctors are concerned about deception and being manipulated into opioid prescribing. There is a variable and inconsistent approach to assessment and management, and a tendency to avoid addressing pain and its treatment.

Patient concerns

There may be fear of inadequate treatment of pain, acute withdrawal, disrespectful treatment by staff, and, for those on methadone maintenance treatment (MMT), the possibility that methadone replacement will not be given.[21] Concern about stigmatization may lead to denial of drug use and impede identification.[21] It is known that pain expectations are influenced by past experiences of pain;[38] patients who encounter judgmental attitudes may be afraid of future undertreatment.[21]

Patients may interpret medical behavior, and even systems delays, as evidence of stigmatization and inadequate treatment.[37] Interestingly, individuals with SAD express the same skepticism (as the medical staff) about others with SAD and feel that this leads to stigmatization and undertreatment of their own "legitimate" pain.[37]

Patients and prescribers may be concerned that opioid prescription will trigger a relapse of SAD. Triggers for relapse include states of stress (such as inadequately treated pain and anxiety[2]), availability, and exposure to cues that were previously associated with drug taking.[39] Inadequately treated pain may be a greater risk for relapse than is the rational use of opioids for acute management.[16, 19][V]

PATIENT GROUPS AND CLINICAL FEATURES

Patients with persistent noncancer pain

Persistent noncancer pain is a significant global disease burden.[40, 41, 42] Opioids are one treatment option,[43] ideally prescribed in the context of a multidisciplinary assessment and management paradigm. Over the past two decades, the prescription of opioids for noncancer pain has increased significantly, as shown by data from North America,[44, 45] Europe,[46] and Australia.[47] An exception is the use of pethidine (meperidine), which has declined.[45] In seven US states from 1998 to 2003, despite only a 31 percent increase in eligible individuals, total numbers of Medicaid opioid prescriptions almost doubled and related costs tripled.[48] It is expected that increasing numbers of opioid-tolerant patients with noncancer pain will be seen in acute settings.

The experience of persistent pain is multidimensional,[49, 50] and patient presentation in acute settings is influenced by the factors described below.[3]

- **Psychological factors**, cognitive (memory including previous pain experiences, learning, attention, discrimination, the meaning of pain, expectations, coping ability and strategies, control) and affective (anxiety, depression, anger, fear).
- **Psychiatric comorbidities**, including mood and anxiety disorders.
- **Sociocultural factors**, for example, social support and cultural beliefs.
- **Pathophysiological factors**. It is hypothesized that the patient with long-standing cancer or noncancer pain with central sensitization is predisposed to the exacerbation of preexisting pain syndromes or the development of new ones.[13][V]

The outward manifestation of this complex mix is pain behaviors. The contribution of the above factors and hence the behaviors will vary from one individual to the next, and over time in the same individual.[50]

Estimated rates of aberrant drug-taking behaviors[51] in patients with persistent noncancer pain treated with opioids vary from 3 to 35 percent.[52, 53, 54] This is due to variation in study populations, definitions of aberrant behaviors, and detection methods. Predictors of drug misuse in those with persistent pain include younger age, personal or family history of SAD, anxiety, and legal problems including drug- or alcohol-related conviction.[54, 55, 56] Those with aberrant behaviors are more likely to have coexisting psychiatric illness[55] and to endorse opioid efficacy while acknowledging the addictive potential.[56]

Patients with persistent cancer pain

Opioids are integral to the management of background and breakthrough pain in patients with cancer, with most experiencing relief with administration according to published guidelines.[57] Acute pain may occur as a result of the malignancy, the effects of treatment (for example, mucositis following chemotherapy), or unrelated conditions. The acute presentation may be influenced by:

- psychological factors, such as anxiety, anger and fear;
- psychiatric comorbidities, for example depression;
- spiritual, including existential issues, grieving and end-of-life concerns;[58]
- sociocultural issues, including spouse/family grieving, other caregiver issues, cultural perspectives, and social support;
- physical symptoms related to malignancy and/or treatment. This may include delirium which has significant consequences for pain assessment and management.

Patients with substance abuse disorder

Substance abuse disorder, particularly injecting drug use, predisposes to the development of particular types of acute pain, including traumatic injury, infections (for example, subacute bacterial endocarditis, epidural abscess, septic arthritis, AIDS-related), ischemia from inadvertent intra-arterial injection or embolism, and pancreatitis. In a Canadian study of illicit drug users outside treatment programs, approximately half had presented to an Emergency Room in the previous 6 months.[59]

SAD is a disease with both genetic[60] and environmental determinants, and presentation may be at any stage of the disease, from active untreated polysubstance abuse to stable remission.[19] Identification and management may be hampered by urgent presentations, particularly if a history of drug use is denied or is not available, for example when mental state is altered by intoxication or withdrawal.

EPIDEMIOLOGY

The 2001 National Household surveys in the USA and Australia demonstrated lifetime prevalence of heroin use

of 1.4 and 1.6 percent, respectively, with 0.2 percent of community subjects in both countries reporting heroin use within the previous 12 months.[61] In young adults in the USA, previous 12-month prevalence of substance abuse or dependence was 24.7 percent for all substances, 5.1 percent if alcohol and marijuana were excluded, and 8.5 percent met the criteria for at least one SAD and one other psychiatric diagnosis.[62]

Since the early 1990s there has been growing awareness of prescription opioid abuse, the prevalence of which is increasing.[35, 45, 59, 63] For example, since its introduction to the United States in 1995, abuse of the sustained-release opioid oxycodone (Oxycontin®) has steadily grown.[64] Internet sites now provide no-prescription access to prescription drugs in an unregulated manner.[65] The National Epidemiologic Survey on Alcohol and Related Conditions in 43 093 adults, reported a lifetime prevalence of nonmedical use of opioids of 4.7 percent, with abuse in 1.4 percent of cases.[66] In those on MMT, prescription opioid abuse is widespread.[67]

Polysubstance abuse, often involving both illicit agents and legal substances such as alcohol[68] and tobacco,[69] is common in SAD,[67] including in those undergoing treatment.[68] Pharmacotherapies, particularly naltrexone[17] and buprenorphine,[23] increase the complexity of acute pain management (see below under Specific therapies).

COMORBID DIAGNOSES

Substance abuse disorder commonly coexists with other psychiatric diagnoses, so called dual-diagnosis.[70] Associations include personality disorders,[71, 72, 73, 74] particularly of the antisocial, borderline or dependent types, mood disorders,[59, 73, 75] anxiety disorders,[59, 73] post-traumatic stress disorder,[76] eating disorders, and schizophrenia-spectrum disorders.[77]

Risk-taking behaviors associated with SAD, such as needle sharing, increase the prevalence of hepatitis B and C, and HIV/AIDS.[5, 59, 78] Resultant end-organ dysfunction may contraindicate some interventions, for example, using paracetamol (acetaminophen) in hepatic disease or neuraxial blockade in the presence of coagulopathy.

There is a significant overlap with persistent pain.[59, 79] In a US study of 248 MMT participants, 61.3 percent reported persistent pain with almost half reporting that treatment of pain had led to addiction.[80] Comorbid pain in SAD is associated with more psychiatric illness, greater difficulty controlling violent behavior, impaired concentration, and greater healthcare utilization.[79] Self-medication for pain may determine the choice of substance,[79] for example prescription opioids,[67] and interfere with management of SAD.[81]

PSYCHOSOCIAL ISSUES

Substance abuse disorder is independently associated with social disruption, including problems related to employment, housing, finances, access to healthcare services, involvement in crime and with the legal system;[77] social problems are more common in those with a dual diagnosis. In a Canadian study of 679 illicit opioid users, half did not have permanent housing, a similar proportion had been arrested in the previous year, and a majority were under some form of legal restraint.[59]

DRUG-SEEKING BEHAVIOR

Clinicians are aware of the potential for drug-seeking behavior with acute pain as a presenting feature.[82] This raises ethical and regulatory concerns in relation to the potential for drug diversion and behavioral reinforcement.[1] A balance needs to be obtained between addressing this concern and potential undertreatment of pain. While prescribers should be aware of scams used to obtain opioids for diversion,[35] it should also be appreciated that so-called "drug-seeking" may represent "pain-relief seeking."[16] A careful history and examination is important, as is liaising with the patient's usual treatment providers and consulting with local drug and alcohol and psychiatric services.[16] It may be better to err on the side of treating the occasional patient who is drug-seeking, rather than delaying treatment of some with legitimate pain.

Acute opioid tolerance

Tolerance, or at least the appearance of tolerance, may develop surprisingly quickly, with a time course as short as days or even hours. Relevant settings include those where high doses are administered, for example in an intensive care unit, or following use of particular opioids, such as remifentanil by infusion.[83]

Animal studies confirm that tolerance is more likely with low potency opioids like morphine than it is with high potency ones like sufentanil, and the degree of tolerance is dose related.[84] Human studies examining the development of acute tolerance yield conflicting results. Some show that intraoperative remifentanil[85][II] or high-dose fentanyl[86][II] induce tolerance resulting in increased postoperative opioid requirements, whereas others report no such effect.[87, 88, 89][II] Likewise, volunteer studies show both positive[90][IV] and null effect.[91, 92][II] The clinical significance of acute tolerance is not known.

Opioid-induced hyperalgesia

Opioids may result in paradoxical excitatory effects, such as myoclonus, seizures, and hyperalgesia.[93] Circumstances associated with hyperalgesia include chronic dosing, high or rapidly escalating doses, opioid withdrawal, and ultra-low doses.[93, 94, 95] Human and animal evidence for OIH has been comprehensively reviewed elsewhere.[93]

In a volunteer model an area of capsaicin-induced hyperalgesia and allodynia was increased following cessation of remifentanil.[92] Comparison of intraoperative low- and high-dose remifentanil shows that the latter results in greater wound hyperalgesia and postoperative opioid requirements, and that this is reversed by the coadministration of ketamine.[96][II]

It is uncertain whether so-called acute tolerance represents tolerance or OIH. Additionally, the requirement for increased opioid doses to treat acute pain in those with opioid tolerance may be a manifestation of OIH.[93, 97] There is no clear guidance about how to differentiate these phenomena clinically, although this has management implications. Quantitative sensory testing may be helpful.[97] Management of OIH may include opioid dose reduction, rotation to a different opioid class, and the use of nonopioid analgesics,[97] particularly N-methyl-D-aspartate (NMDA)-receptor antagonists.[94][II]

Pain tolerance

Patients on long-term opioid therapy exhibit greater pain sensitivity than do controls.[27, 98, 99, 100] In subjects receiving MMT (dose range 12–100 mg/day orally) and buprenorphine (range 8–12 mg/day sublingually), compared with matched opioid-naive controls, withdrawal latencies for cold pressor pain are reduced.[98] Likewise, a small number of patients with persistent noncancer pain had reduced cold pressor threshold and tolerance within one month of commencing sustained-release morphine.[101] This may be a manifestation of OIH.

PATHOPHYSIOLOGY

Opioid tolerance

The mechanisms of opioid tolerance are complex, incompletely understood and may vary for different opioid effects.[102, 103] Adaptations at multiple levels involve interplay between opioid receptors, postreceptor intracellular signaling mechanisms, NMDA receptors, and excitatory amino acids.[102] There is overlap with mechanisms of hyperalgesia and pathological pain.[97, 104, 105] Elucidation of these processes may lead to the development of novel therapies to prevent the development of tolerance or to improve analgesia in those with established tolerance.

Activation of the μ-opioid receptor (MOR) promotes receptor phosphorylation by a G protein-coupled receptor kinase (GRK)[106] initiating binding by β-arrestin.[107] This leads to uncoupling of the receptor from G proteins (G_i/G_o) with blunting of receptor signaling (desensitization) and also to receptor internalization and trafficking within the cell. Some receptors are degraded, for example within lysosomes, and others are recycled.[107] The precise role of internalization and its relationship to the development of tolerance is unclear. Internalization may represent a means for receptor resensitization.[107] Less MOR internalization is seen with morphine[106] than with agonists of higher intrinsic efficacy such as fentanyl, and this may explain why tolerance is more likely to develop with morphine.[107]

Other receptors are implicated. Activation of NMDA-receptors by glutamate leads to increased intracellular calcium, protein kinase C (PKC) activation, production of nitric oxide, and neuronal apoptosis.[12] NMDA-receptors are regulated by PKC with its phosphorylation leading to removal of the blocking magnesium ion. Nitric oxide increases the release of excitatory neurotransmitters.[12] Tolerance is inhibited in animal models by NMDA-receptor antagonists MK801, dextrometorphan, and ketamine.

Excitatory neurotransmitters, including calcitonin gene-related peptide (CGRP), colocated L-glutamate and substance P,[108] neurokinins, glycine, and more recently discovered transmitters such as orexin, are involved.[107] Activation of CGRP, NK-1, and NMDA-receptors on the postsynaptic membrane leads to the generation of prostaglandins and lipoxygenase metabolites which results in release of more excitatory neurotransmitters.[108] In patients with cancer pain treated with intrathecal opioids, loss of analgesic effectiveness is associated with higher cerebrospinal fluid (CSF) levels of glutamate and aspartate than those measured during periods of pain control.[109]

Physical dependence

Following cessation of opioids, neuronal hyperexcitability is associated with superactivation of cAMP and increased levels of adenyl cyclase with protein kinase A activation.[107] Alterations in neurotransmitter release include enhanced GABA-ergic transmission and hyperexcitability of neurones in the peri-aqueductal gray.[107] Elevation of CGRP in the medulla oblongata and corpus striatum mediates increased cAMP levels with induction of cFOS.[108] Endocannabinoids may be involved in physical dependence possibly via modulation of CGRP.[108]

Addiction

Mesocorticolimbic dopaminergic pathways are part of the common reward system for drugs of addiction.[2, 60, 110] There is an interaction between the endogenous cannabinoid system and the opioid system in terms of drug reward and abuse,[111] although the details of this remain to be clarified. The endogenous opioid system is involved in the rewarding effects of nonopioid drugs, for example alcohol.[60] Long-term neurophysiological changes support the conceptualization of SAD as a chronic, potentially

relapsing, disease.[2] These adaptations include transcription factor induction, glutaminergic activation, and increased spinal dynorphin.[12]

Opioid–induced hyperalgesia

Chronic opioid treatment results in system adaptations in both negative (desensitization, tolerance) and positive (sensitization, OIH) senses.[93, 97] Mechanisms of OIH include sensitization in the periphery, enhanced descending pronociceptive pathways,[104] increased release of excitatory neurotransmitters, and sensitization of second-order neurons to neurotransmitters.[93] NMDA-receptor activation, cAMP up-regulation, release of spinal dynorphin,[104] increased expression of Gs-coupled opioid receptors, and, in some cases, the action of opioid metabolites (for example, morphine-3-glucuronide) are also involved.[103, 112] Resolution of OIH probably occurs due to up-regulation of inhibitory pathways including endogenous opioid mechanisms.[93, 113] This may render the animal vulnerable to reactivation of OIH with subsequent opioid exposure.[113]

Hyperalgesia may occur as a result of nonopioid mechanisms, including those involving the NMDA-receptor and impaired glycinergic inhibition.[93] This may resolve with switching from a phenanthrene (for example, morphine) to a piperadine (for example, sufentanil or fentanyl).[93]

Learning and conditioning may play a role in both OIH and tolerance, although the contribution of these processes is not well understood.[12, 93]

PATIENT ASSESSMENT AND MANAGEMENT PLANNING

General principles

- Identification is important. In the management of persistent pain, it has been suggested that a universal precautions approach, that is, a careful assessment of all patients in relation to drug use, allows stratification according to risk, reduces stigma, and improves patient care.[39][V] In the acute setting, for many reasons this is not always possible, but drug users may not fit a stereotype and a high index of suspicion should be maintained. The following triad is predictive of opioid tolerance: higher pain scores, greater opioid requirements, and lower opioid side effects than expected.[7][V]
- It is likely that more time will be needed than in the opioid-naive patient.
- An open, honest, nonjudgmental approach with maintenance of privacy and confidentiality promotes patient trust[18][V] and is likely to facilitate assessment. The patient should be reassured that a

history of SAD or previous bad experiences of pain management will not preclude the provision of analgesia.[18, 21][V]

- A detailed pain history is required to make a diagnosis, inform treatment aimed at the primary disease process, infer whether the pain is likely to be opioid-sensitive, and determine the role of non-opioid (including nonpharmacological) therapies.[19] [V] In particular, nociceptive and neuropathic pain should be differentiated as treatment modalities differ (see below under Adjuvants).
- Assessment (and management) requires an integrated approach, which includes liaison with the usual healthcare providers and knowledge of local resources.[20][V] Relevant services include the primary care physician, pain management specialist/clinic, drug and alcohol services, consultation-liaison psychiatry, clinical psychology, and social work.
- The patient should be included in the development of the management plan.[15][V] This must include reassurance about the aims of treatment, in particular that pain management is a high priority.[21] However, realistic goals should be identified,[1][V] expectations clearly outlined and limits on behaviors set. It is easier if one physician (or service) has overall responsibility for pain management decisions. Staff members should demonstrate consistency in relation to the management plan; this reduces the potential for dysfunctional interactions within the team, and between the patient and staff.[114][V]
- Assessment may be difficult. In general terms, pain scores are unreliable and it is more useful to use functional measures, for example ability to cooperate with postoperative rehabilitation.[33][V] Postoperatively, persistently high pain scores may mask or delay the diagnosis of surgical complications or result in unnecessary reoperation.
- The clinician should be mindful of appropriate labeling and consider the stigma associated with particular terminologies (for example, "addict").[12][V]

The patient with persistent pain (noncancer and cancer)

In addition to the general principles outlined above, a pain-related history should identify:

- pain diagnosis or diagnoses;
- comorbid diagnoses, including anxiety, depression, and SAD;
- medically prescribed opioid and nonopioid medications, including doses and routes (in a small proportion of cases, this may involve intrathecal opioid administration (see below under Specific therapies);
- current healthcare providers;

- experiences and expectations of acute pain management – in particular, what has been effective in the past;[22]
- drug allergies and reactions.

The patient with SAD

Apart from the general issues already listed, the following are important.

- Usual treatment providers and current management of SAD, including maintenance therapies, such as naltrexone, buprenorphine, and methadone, should be identified.
- Take a complete drug history, defining all substances used, whether medically prescribed or illicit, remembering that polysubstance abuse is common. Dose estimates should be made, although this may be difficult for illicitly acquired agents. A urine drug screen may be helpful,[22][V] although limitations should be recognized.
- For prescribed medications, an attempt should be made to verify doses with the usual provider.[19][V] If this is unable to be done, for example with methadone, it has been recommended that the reported amount is given in two to four divided doses and the response observed.[1, 21, 22][V]
- Attempt to determine whether the problem is primarily pain or addiction, or a combination.[19][V]
- Define comorbid pathologies, for example, blood-borne viruses, hepatic disease, other infections, persistent pain, and the presence of or potential for abstinence and intoxication syndromes. The specific features of intoxication and withdrawal syndromes for different drug classes are described elsewhere.[29]
- Assess the patient's social situation including associates and supports.
- Identify behaviors including drug seeking or using, unacceptable interactions with staff (for example, aggression, manipulation, or lying[114]), and risk taking (for example, unsafe injecting techniques, injection into medically placed intravenous lines). Be mindful that ongoing drug-taking behaviors may occur in an inpatient setting and result in cardiopulmonary arrest calls.[5][V]

GENERAL PRINCIPLES OF MANAGEMENT

Management goals

- Optimisation of analgesia through the use of a multimodal approach that includes adequate opioid doses. Maximize nonopioid analgesia, including, where indicated, regional blocks and adjuvants. Consider the use of nonpharmacological strategies addressing the cognitive and affective aspects of the pain experience,[3] including for example to increase the patient's sense of control over pain.

- Management of psychiatric and behavioral disorders.[1]
- Prevention of abstinence syndromes. Opioid-tolerant patients are at risk of opioid withdrawal syndromes, if administered by a completely nonopioid technique. Nonopioid substances, including nicotine, benzodiazepines, and alcohol, may be overlooked. A careful history, withdrawal protocols, and judicious replacement are important.

Importance of a collaborative approach

There is great value in collaboration with those having special expertise, for example, drug and alcohol services, pain management and palliative care specialists, and consultation-liaison psychiatrists. Advantages include:

- the patient may be known to the other provider;
- access to skilled specialist assessment, as well as expertise in negotiation with and support for the patient;
- advice regarding opioid dosing and the use of adjuvants;
- in the case of SAD, specialist management of drug-related issues such as withdrawal, intoxication, and overdose;
- behavioral management (see below under Management of psychiatric and behavioral disorders);
- discharge planning and follow up;[12][V]
- collaborative guideline development and education.

Management of psychiatric and behavioral disorders

- Where required, seek specialist advice. Advantages for the individual physician or acute pain service include skilled assessment, patient support, withdrawal regimens and protocols, contracts, appropriate pharmacotherapy, and discharge planning.
- Promote a team approach,[115] with clearly defined roles, a unified management plan, and avoidance of dysfunction, for example, where the patient pits one part of the team against the rest. Ensure adequate communication, including, for example, team meetings.[114, 115]
- Set appropriate limits.[23] At times a written behavioral contract, as is widely used for opioid therapy in an outpatient setting,[21] may be required to formalize expectations,[22] minimize disruption for ward staff, and promote patient safety.
- It is important to be aware of institutional policies regarding the management of unsanctioned drug-taking on the ward or in the Emergency Room.

Additional security measures, such as security staff surveillance or involvement of the police, may be required.

Issues in SAD

- It is helpful to distinguish between pain management and the treatment of addiction. The former includes anxiety reduction, a nonjudgmental approach, higher opioid doses, and avoidance of antagonists and mixed agonists–antagonists (for example, pentazocine, nalbuphine, and butorphanol).[16, 21][V] The latter requires verification of doses with the usual prescriber, administration of the usual opioid where indicated, and notification (on discharge) of medications prescribed in hospital as these will appear in urine drug screens.[16][V]
- Drug security may be an issue and locked PCA and infusion devices should be used.[18][V]
- Venous access is often difficult and central venous cannulation may be required.[5][V] This carries the risk of unsanctioned access and the potential for bacterial infection or other complications, such as air embolism.
- During an episode of acute pain is not the optimal time to attempt detoxification or rehabilitation management.[19][V] However, it may represent an opportunity to refer the patient for ongoing SAD management.[21][V]

OPIOID MANAGEMENT

Usual opioid

Full-agonist opioids should be continued, even if the patient is fasting preoperatively.[12, 22][V] Where this is not possible, parenteral replacement should be provided. Long-term tramadol should be continued as withdrawal associated with cessation has been described.[116][V] Management of partial agonists and antagonists is more complex (see below under Specific therapies).

Additional opioid

The usual opioid should be regarded as the baseline requirement with extra analgesia provided for acute pain.[22][V] Some would advocate a 50 percent increase in the dose of the usual long-acting agent.[13][V] It has been suggested that patients with SAD may be better managed with a time-contingent dose, rather than an as-needed schedule,[18, 21][V] as this may decrease potential conflicts with staff and provide more stable serum drug levels.

The addictive potential of medications is known to be influenced by dose, route of administration, coadministration with other drugs, context, and expectations; in particular, more rapid rate of onset is associated with greater reinforcement.[28] As a general rule, less addictive medications and the oral route should be considered whenever practicable, although parenteral administration may be required for initial stabilization[18] [V] or if the patient is "nil per oral." There is no indication for the use of pethidine, even in those with allergies. The high opioid requirement may increase the risk of norpethidine (normeperidine) toxicity including seizures,[21][V] and alternatives are available. Due to the risk of opioid withdrawal, a technique solely using tramadol is not recommended.[1][V]

Opioid-tolerant patients undergoing surgery are at increased risk of intraoperative awareness,[117][II] and management should address this. In the ventilated patient, it may be useful to induce spontaneous ventilation towards the end of the surgery and titrate the opioid to achieve a respiratory rate of 14–16 per minute before emergence from anesthesia.[12, 13][V]

Patient-controlled analgesia

Intravenous PCA is frequently the mainstay of treatment and is widely regarded as the technique of choice.[22][V] It allows individual dose titration and reduces workload for ward staff. Where the patient is able to continue the usual opioid, this is given along with a bolus-only PCA. Otherwise, the PCA is programmed with a larger than usual bolus dose plus a background infusion to replace the usual opioid.

Davis and colleagues propose the following regimen to estimate PCA requirements.[15, 118][III] Before anesthesia induction and with oxygen therapy and full monitoring, an intravenous infusion of fentanyl at 2 μg/kg per minute is titrated until respiratory rate is less than 5 per minute.

Pharmacokinetic simulation software is used to calculate the fentanyl effect site concentration (C_e) near the onset of respiratory depression. Intraoperatively, an hourly infusion rate to produce a fentanyl C_e that is 30 percent of that associated with respiratory depression is programmed. Postoperatively, 50 percent of this rate is given as a background infusion, with the remainder given as PCA bolus doses aiming to maintain a demand dose rate of two to three per hour. At four-hourly intervals, the background infusion is altered (± 20 percent) to maintain the target bolus dose rate.

Opioid rotation

Opioid rotation, that is replacement of the usual opioid with a different one, may prove a useful strategy. Evidence for this practice comes from the management of cancer pain, generally in the setting of inadequate analgesia or intolerable adverse effects, and most frequently rotating from morphine to methadone.[119][III] Pain control may improve and side effects decrease.[119, 120][III] The effectiveness of opioid rotation may be explained by loss of the adverse effects of metabolites, particularly in the presence of renal impairment, and differing receptor affinity.[119] Opioid rotation may be particularly useful in patients treated with high-dose opioids where there is concern about OIH.

A common approach is to calculate the previous 24-hour opioid requirement in morphine equivalents, convert this to an equianalgesic dose of the new agent (see **Table 30.1**), and then reduce this by 30–50 percent.[123][V] It should be noted that conversion from one opioid to another is complicated by conflicting data about equianalgesic dosing, differences in single dose compared with chronic dosing studies, opioid receptor diversity, and variation depending upon the direction of switch.[121, 124]

Table 30.1 Estimated[a] equianalgesic doses of opioids (after Ref. 121).

Opioid	Dose
Morphine (M)	10 mg intravenously (i.v.), 20–30 mg oral (p.o.), 1 mg epidural, 0.1 mg intrathecal[122]
Fentanyl	150 μg i.v. or transdermal
Hydromorphone (HM)	2 mg i.v.[b] or 4–6 mg p.o.
Oxycodone	7–10 mg i.v.[c] or 10–15 mg p.o.[d]
Methadone (ME)	2–4 mg parenteral or 5–8 mg p.o.[e]
Buprenorphine[f]	0.3 mg i.v.[25] or 0.8 mg sublingually[12]
Tramadol	100 mg i.v. or 100–150 mg p.o.[g]

[a]See text for discussion of the difficulties regarding equianalgesic estimation.
[b]Direction of switch is important (M to HM 5:1, HM to M 3.5:1, overall potency ratio HM:M 4.3:1).[121]
[c]Potency of oral is 70% of i.v. administration.
[d]Wide ranges of bioavailability reported.[121]
[e]Conversion is dose-dependent:[121] morphine dose: 30–90 mg M:ME 3.7:1; 90–300 mg M:ME 7.75:1; >300 mg M:ME 12.25:1.
[f]Buprenorphine 0.8 mg is equivalent to 20 mg oral methadone;[12] potency 25–50 times that of morphine.[25]
[g]Conversion ratios may be different in neuropathic pain.

Cross-tolerance between opioids may be incomplete and asymmetric.[125] Changing to an opioid with higher intrinsic activity, for example from epidural morphine to sufentanil in opioid-tolerant patients with cancer pain undergoing laparotomy, improves analgesic efficacy.[126][III]

Step-down analgesia

Conversion from parenteral to oral analgesia requires provision of information and reassurance, dosing based upon the previous 24-hour opioid use,[15][V] and often more time than in the average patient. One approach is to convert the last 24-hour opioid use to oral-dose equivalents, give half to two-thirds as a time-contingent long-acting agent, and then give additional immediate-release opioid for breakthrough pain.[13][V] At the time of discharge, usual opioid doses may not be sufficient for pain control.[13] A time-limited prescription may be required,[19] with doses tapered over a week or more.[12][V] Some patients will require daily or second-daily dispensing.[22][V] Liaison with the usual prescriber is essential.[16][V]

REGIONAL ANALGESIA

Although regional analgesic techniques reduce opioid requirements in the opioid-naive,[127, 128][II] this has not been well studied in patients with opioid tolerance. Catheter techniques may be preferable.[13][V] Greater doses of epidural opioids may be required[6, 13][III] and higher potency agents are more effective.[126][III] As neuraxial opioids may not be sufficient to prevent opioid withdrawal, some systemic opioid administration may be required.[12][V] Fifty percent of the usual opioid dose by the regular route, where feasible, or otherwise parenterally has been recommended.[13, 15][V] Some patients require opioid to treat persistent pain in a site not covered by the regional block.[13][V]

ADJUVANTS

As for all acute pain, the emphasis should be on a multimodal analgesic regimen. Opioids vary in their effectiveness and this is due to opioid receptor diversity, some of it genetically determined, and variability in the opioid responsiveness of particular types of pain.

Paracetamol and nonsteroidal anti-inflammatory agents

Simple analgesics, such as paracetamol and nonsteroidal anti-inflammatory agents, should be used except as contraindicated by the presence of end-organ dysfunction.

Due to the potential for hepatic toxicity, paracetamol use should be accompanied by monitoring in those with mild liver disease and avoided in those with more severe dysfunction.[1, 129]

NMDA-receptor antagonists

In the opioid-naive, ketamine decreases perioperative opioid requirements and pain scores[130, 131, 132][I] in both adults and children. Compared with placebo, PCA morphine consumption is reduced by a median of 32 percent or a weighted mean difference of -15.7 mg in the first 24 hours, and pain scores by an average of 10 mm on a 100-mm scale.[131][I] This is accompanied by an increased incidence of psychomimetic side effects, including hallucinations (odds ratio (OR) 2.28 (95 percent CI 1.19–4.40) numbers-needed-to-harm (NNH) 27); nightmares (OR 2.64 (95 percent CI 0.76–9.12), NNH 62); and visual disturbances (OR 2.34 (95 percent CI 1.09–5.04) NNH 28).[131][I] However, the incidence of opioid-related side effects, particularly nausea and vomiting, is reduced.[130, 132][I] In the postanesthesia care unit, for those with high pain levels despite prior morphine administration, bolus ketamine (0.25 mg/kg) and morphine has been shown to be more effective than morphine alone with greater pain reduction, lower total opioid requirements, and few side effects.[133][II]

Ketamine also has a role in preventative analgesia, that is analgesia beyond the expected clinical duration of effect of the drug. In a recent systematic review, 14 of 24 studies (58 percent) found a positive effect on preventative analgesia, at doses ranging from 0.15 to 1 mg/kg.[134][I] Reduced hyperalgesia has been shown in experimental pain settings,[95, 135][II] and around wounds following open nephrectomy[136][II] and major abdominal surgery performed with remifentanil infusion.[96][II] Ketamine doses in the latter study were an intraoperative bolus of 0.5 mg/kg with intraoperative infusion of 5 μg/kg per minute and postoperative infusion of 2 μg/kg per minute for 48 hours.[96] Intravenous, but not epidural, ketamine reduces wound hyperalgesia for up to six months following rectal surgery for carcinoma.[137][II]

In general, randomized trials of ketamine have excluded opioid-tolerant patients. However, for this group, ketamine may be of particular value because of its potential to reverse or decrease opioid tolerance.[138][V] For those with persistent pain, other potential benefits include reduced central sensitization and efficacy in neuropathic pain. Animal models of opioid tolerance confirm the value of both noncompetitive and competitive NMDA-receptor antagonists in inhibiting the development of tolerance and reducing OIH.[113, 139, 140] A number of case reports confirm that ketamine improves pain control in opioid-tolerant patients, particularly those receiving high opioid doses where OIH may be present.[141, 142, 143][V]

In all patients,[105][II] but particularly in those who are opioid-tolerant and thus likely to require larger doses of opioids, ketamine should not be given in a fixed dosing ratio with an opioid (for example, mixed with the opioid in a PCA solution); this is likely to result in high ketamine doses with the potential for adverse effects.[13][V]

As yet, there is no clear benefit of S(+) ketamine over racemic ketamine.[105][V] Other NMDA-receptor antagonists, such as dextromethorphan[134][I] and amantadine, may have similar benefits, but these agents have not been as widely studied.

Anxiolytics

Long-term benzodiazepines should be continued perioperatively to avoid an abstinence syndrome. Treating staff report that anxiolytics are useful for managing patients with persistent pain in the acute setting.[4][III] Coadministration of anxiolytics and opioids increases the risk of oversedation and respiratory depression, and is a hypothesized mechanism for out-of-hospital fatal overdose in SAD.[16][V]

α-2 Adrenergic agonists

Clonidine is useful for the symptomatic management of opioid withdrawal.[144] Opioids and clonidine have synergistic analgesic actions,[122, 145] although the disadvantages of clonidine, particularly when administered parenterally, include sedation and hypotension.[146][II] Dexmedetomidine significantly reduces opioid requirements in the early postoperative recovery phase.[147][II] Intrathecal clonidine has been used for management of persistent neuropathic pain, for example associated with spinal cord injury.[122][II] In a volunteer study of remifentanil-induced withdrawal hyperalgesia and allodynia, coadministration of clonidine reduced postinfusion pain ratings and hyperalgesia, but not allodynia.[95][II] Clonidine may be a useful adjunctive agent in the patient with opioid tolerance, particularly in the presence of neuropathic pain or opioid withdrawal, but side effects may be limiting.

Anticonvulsants

In opioid-naive patients, gabapentin reduces opioid requirements,[148][I] may have anxiolytic properties,[149][II] and is effective in neuropathic pain;[150][I] each of these effects may benefit those with opioid tolerance. Additionally, in a rat model of thermal and mechanical nociception, intrathecal gabapentin has been shown to prevent the development of opioid tolerance,[151] even in doses that do not enhance antinociception in opioid-naive animals.[152] In animals with preexisting opioid tolerance, gabapentin partially restores opioid effectiveness.[153] The mechanism may be inhibition of opioid-induced increases in aspartate and glutamate.[152] It is unclear how these preclinical findings will translate into clinical practice. Pregabalin may have similar effects but has been less well studied.[154]

Antidepressants

These may be required for treatment of neuropathic pain, affective disorders, or, in low dose, to improve sleep. A major disadvantage is limited parenteral formulations.

Opioid receptor antagonists

In animal models, very low doses of opioid antagonists attenuate excitatory but not inhibitory effects of morphine, thereby reducing OIH[155] and preventing the development of morphine-induced tolerance.[156] Clinical studies in both adults and children demonstrate that low-dose naloxone (for example, 0.25 μg/kg/hour by continuous intravenous infusion) reduces postoperative opioid side effects, such as pruritus and nausea, without compromising analgesia.[157, 158][II] Compared with a higher-dose infusion or placebo, a continuous infusion of 0.25 μg/kg/hour reduces opioid requirements.[158][II] The effect of opioid antagonists in opioid-tolerant patients has not been explored. However, conceivably the quality of analgesia might be improved.

NONPHARMACOLOGICAL TECHNIQUES

Nonpharmacological treatments are well established and validated for management of persistent noncancer pain.[49] For example, psychological treatments, mainly cognitive-behavioral therapy and relaxation, are effective at reducing persistent headache-related pain in children and adolescents.[159][I] However, whether patients transfer these strategies to acute pain settings is unclear.

There is evidence for the efficacy of nonpharmacological management of acute pain, but this is mostly in opioid-naive subjects. For example, brief procedure-related pain in children is reduced by distraction and hypnosis.[160][I] Simple maneuvers, such as hot or cold application and repositioning, should be considered. Other therapies that may be of benefit include transcutaneous electrical nerve stimulation (TENS), relaxation, and meditation. The effectiveness of these treatments in the opioid-tolerant patient with acute pain is uncertain.

SPECIFIC THERAPIES

Long-term neuraxial opioids

A small number of patients with persistent cancer or noncancer pain will be treated with long-term intrathecal or epidural opioid therapy via exteriorized or fully implanted drug administration systems. The neuraxial opioid should be viewed as the background requirement,[12, 18][V] and additional opioids and nonopioids given as required for the acutely painful condition.

Methadone

Methadone is a racemic synthetic μ-receptor agonist which also has noncompetitive NMDA-receptor antagonism, and inhibition of 5-hydroxytryptamine and norepinephrine reuptake.[22, 161] It has a long history of use as maintenance therapy in SAD,[162] where a single dose blocks craving for 24 to 36 hours.[21] Reduction in illicit opioid use is more likely with replacement doses above 50 mg.[163][I] Recently, methadone has had a resurgence in use for both cancer and noncancer pain,[161, 164] where it may be particularly effective as a second-line agent in opioid rotation and for neuropathic pain.

It has high oral bioavailability, but a long and variable elimination half-life of 15 to 60 hours.[21, 161] For MMT in SAD, it is given as a once-daily dose. For analgesia, it is typically given three to four times daily.[21, 22, 119, 164] When oral administration is not possible, it may be given rectally (equivalent to oral dose) or parenterally (30–50 percent dose reduction compared with the oral route[16, 21]). Relevant drug interactions may include antivirals, tricyclic antidepressants, and selective serotonin reuptake inhibitors.[161, 164]

As methadone is a drug with which many physicians have poor familiarity,[22][V] it may be easier to continue the usual dose and give an alternative agent for pain.[21, 22][V] It is also important to be aware of jurisdictional regulations governing supply and to liaise with the usual prescriber.[22]

Methadone has been advocated as a useful agent for acute pain in the opioid-tolerant patient when more commonly used opioids have been ineffective.[165][V] Reasons for this may include methadone activity at nonopioid receptors. Conversion from morphine to methadone is dose dependent (see **Table 30.1**).[121]

Levo-alpha-acetylmethadol

Levo-alpha-acetylmethadol is a μ-agonist with a long duration of effect largely due to two active metabolites.[166] Two- to three-daily dosing is used for maintenance in SAD,[167] where it has lower retention rates than MMT.[163] [I] General principles of management are similar to those in MMT.

Naltrexone

Naltrexone, a competitive μ-receptor antagonist, is used for maintenance therapy in alcoholism and SAD (following detoxification to avoid precipitating an opioid withdrawal syndrome). It is administered orally, usually as a once daily dose of 25–50 mg.[1, 17, 168] The effective duration of action of this formulation is 72 hours. With the aim of improving compliance, sustained release formulations have been developed. These include a subcutaneous implant,[169] which has a dose-dependent effective duration of three to six months,[170] and a long-acting injectable formulation which is effective for one month.[171]

Management should be planned in consultation with the usual treatment provider or local drug and alcohol services.[17][V] In an elective setting, oral naltrexone may be ceased for 48 to 72 hours before an anticipated painful episode such as surgery.[1, 17][V] Chronic naltrexone therapy results in up-regulation of receptors with the potential for increased opioid sensitivity once the drug is ceased. Inadvertent opioid overdose may occur and, if administration of opioids is required, consideration should be given to careful titration and monitoring for sedation or respiratory depression.[12][V]

In the nonelective setting, oral naltrexone may be ceased, but it will take 48 to 72 hours after the last dose for the effect to abate. Competitive opioid antagonism may be overcome by high-dose opioids, but very large amounts may be required. Nonopioid analgesia, including regional analgesia where feasible, should be maximized. For patients with a naltrexone implant, when it is expected that pain is likely to be moderate to severe and ongoing (for example, multiple trauma), consideration may be given to surgical removal of the implant.[17][V]

Full opioid agonists should be weaned before naltrexone is reintroduced, otherwise opioid withdrawal may be precipitated.

Buprenorphine

Buprenorphine has μ-agonist activity and weak κ-receptor antagonism.[25, 172] Its maximum effect at the μ-receptor is less than a full agonist producing a ceiling effect for respiratory depression[25, 173] and analgesia.[19] Binding to the μ-opioid receptor is not easily reversed by other opioids or naloxone.[25, 174] In the presence of a full agonist, it may behave as an antagonist, including precipitating opioid withdrawal,[172, 175] although this is thought unlikely at doses equivalent to or less than 30 mg/day of oral methadone.[176][III]

Buprenorphine is used as a replacement in SAD, with typical sublingual maintenance doses ranging from 4 to 32 mg.[172, 177] The terminal elimination phase is 20–25 hours.[178] Doses greater than 8 mg/day have similar efficacy to MMT.[163][I] High doses have similar maximum efficacy but with a more prolonged duration of effect,[178] allowing second- or third-daily dosing.[23] Withdrawal from buprenorphine is of mild to moderate intensity.[25] Abuse of buprenorphine is well recognized.[25, 178] Buprenorphine is also formulated as a sublingual preparation combined with naloxone (Suboxone®). Naloxone has no effect when administered sublingually, but antagonizes opioid action if the combination is diverted to intravenous use.[172]

In both persistent noncancer and cancer pain, buprenorphine may be administered transdermally via a polymer matrix.[179, 180] However, the doses used (up to 70 μg/hour, that is 1.68 mg/24 hours) are unlikely to interfere significantly with the use of full-agonist opioids for acute pain; thus transdermal buprenorphine may be continued and acute pain treated using conventional approaches.

In the case of buprenorphine maintenance in SAD, the treatment plan should be determined in consultation with the patient, the usual treatment provider and local drug and alcohol services. For acute pain in the patient maintained on sublingual buprenorphine, management options include:[16][V]

- Continue the usual buprenorphine dose and provide analgesia with a combination of nonopioids and high-dose full-agonist opioids titrated to effect.
- Divide the buprenorphine into 6–8-hourly doses, perhaps with an overall increase in daily dose to a maximum of 32 mg.[23][V]
- Discontinue the buprenorphine for at least 48 hours before an anticipated painful episode and give conventional opioids.
- Discontinue buprenorphine, change the patient to methadone or another sustained release full-agonist and use conventional analgesic techniques. Guidelines for this conversion have been suggested.[23]

The first two options are suitable for elective minor surgery and other elective or nonelective conditions which are readily treated with nonopioid analgesics. However, for major elective surgery, recommendations have included ceasing the buprenorphine at least 48 hours preoperatively and converting to methadone[23, 172][V] or continuing the buprenorphine at the usual dose in the perioperative period. The latter avoids the challenges of converting the patient to methadone.

A major challenge arises in nonelective presentations with conditions associated with moderate to severe pain. Management is guided by the time and amount of the last dose, and the usual dosing interval. The latter reflects the duration of effect[23] and hence the likely efficacy of full-agonist opioids. Nonopioid, including non-pharmacological, techniques should be maximized; regional analgesia may be particularly useful. Conventional full agonists may be titrated to effect, but this often requires high doses and is most safely performed with close monitoring.[23][V] In extreme cases, general anesthesia may be required to achieve pain control. Opioid requirements will decrease as the effect of buprenorphine declines. The patient should preferably be discharged on the usual dose of buprenorphine along with simple

analgesics.[16, 23][V] Switching from methadone (or another full agonist) to buprenorphine is easier at lower doses of methadone and if there are 24 hours between the last dose of methadone and the first of buprenorphine.[178] [V] It is recommended to wait 8–24 hours (depending on the duration of effect of the full agonist) or until mild opioid withdrawal symptoms are experienced.[16, 23] [V] It is important to communicate with the usual prescriber/program to ensure continuity of maintenance prescribing.[23][V]

THE OPIOID-TOLERANT OBSTETRIC PATIENT

Principles of assessment and management are as previously outlined. Specific issues in the parturient include difficulties with antenatal identification; the effects of substance abuse, overdose, withdrawal, and prescribed drugs on the mother and fetus; comorbid SAD complications including infectious diseases, increased risk of obstetric emergencies, and increased perinatal mortality/morbidity; unstable social situation and poor nutrition; and often inadequate antenatal care leading to suboptimal planning for delivery, including analgesia.[5, 11, 24]

Where possible, antenatal referral for analgesia planning is recommended.[5][V] Regional techniques are useful, including in patients with HIV/AIDS, but may be contraindicated by the presence of infection.[11][V] Systemic opioid administration may be required to prevent withdrawal. PCA is an effective means of allowing the patient to titrate to requirement.[10][V] The presence of liver disease may contraindicate the use of paracetamol or neuraxial blocks. Pain control following cesarean section may be difficult.[5][V]

Planning must include involvement of a neonatologist for management of opioid and other withdrawal syndromes in the neonate. The pharmacokinetics of methadone are altered in pregnancy with increased elimination.[161] This changes in the first few weeks after delivery and may necessitate dose adjustment.[19]

REFERENCES

* 1. Australian and New Zealand College of Anaesthetists and Faculty of Pain Medicine. Acute pain management: scientific evidence, 2nd edn. Melbourne: Australian and New Zealand College of Anaesthetists and Faculty of Pain Medicine, 2005. Available from: www.anzca.edu.au/resources/books-and-publications

* 2. May JA, White HC, Leonard-White A et al. The patient recovering from alcohol or drug addiction: special issues for the anesthesiologist. *Anesthesia and Analgesia*. 2001; 92: 1601–8.

* 3. Williams DA. Acute pain (with special emphasis on painful medical procedures). In: Gatchel RJ, Turk DC (eds).

Psychosocial factors in pain: critical perspectives.
New York: The Guilford Press, 1999: 151–63.

4. Rapp SE, Ready LB, Nessly ML. Acute pain management in patients with prior opioid consumption: a case-controlled retrospective review. *Pain.* 1995; **61**: 195–201.

* 5. Cassidy B, Cyna AM. Challenges that opioid-dependent women present to the obstetric anaesthetist. *Anaesthesia and Intensive Care.* 2004; **32**: 494–501.

6. de Leon-Casasola OA, Myers DP, Donaparthi S *et al.* A comparison of postoperative epidural analgesia between patients with chronic cancer taking high doses of oral opioids versus opioid-naive patients. *Anesthesia and Analgesia.* 1993; **76**: 302–7.

7. Ready LB. Acute pain: lessons learned from 25,000 patients. *Regional Anesthesia and Pain Medicine.* 1999; **24**: 499–505.

8. Roberts LJ, Hellier L, Croy H. Opioid tolerance and perioperative pain management. *Proceedings of the International Association for the Study of Pain 11th World Congress.* Sydney: IASP Press, 2005.

9. Rogers AG. Management of postoperative pain in patients on methadone maintenance. *Journal of Pain and Symptom Management.* 1989; **4**: 161–2.

10. Boyle RK. Intra- and postoperative anaesthetic management of an opioid addict undergoing caesarean section. *Anaesthesia and Intensive Care.* 1991; **19**: 276–9.

* 11. Kuczkowski KM. Anesthetic implications of drug abuse in pregnancy. *Journal of Clinical Anesthesia.* 2003; **15**: 382–94.

* 12. Mitra S, Sinatra RS. Perioperative management of acute pain in the opioid-dependent patient. *Anesthesiology.* 2004; **101**: 212–27.

* 13. Carroll IR, Angst MS, Clark JD. Management of perioperative pain in patients chronically consuming opioids. *Regional Anesthesia and Pain Medicine.* 2004; **29**: 576–91.

14. de Leon-Casasola OA. Cellular mechanisms of opioid tolerance and the clinical approach to the opioid tolerant patient in the post-operative period. *Best Practice and Research Clinical Anaesthesiology.* 2002; **16**: 521–5.

15. Swenson JD, Davis JJ, Johnson KB. Postoperative care of the chronic opioid-consuming patient. *Anesthesiology Clinics of North America.* 2005; **23**: 37–48.

* 16. Alford DP, Compton P, Samet JH. Acute pain management for patients receiving maintenance methadone or buprenorphine therapy. *Annals of Internal Medicine.* 2006; **144**: 127–34.

17. Vickers AP, Jolly A. Naltrexone and problems in pain management. *British Medical Journal.* 2006; **332**: 132–3.

18. Mehta V, Langford RM. Acute pain management for opioid dependent patients. *Anaesthesia.* 2006; **61**: 269–76.

* 19. Jovey RD. Managing acute pain in the opioid-dependent patient. In: Flor H, Kalso E, Dostrovsky JO (eds). *Proceedings of the 11th World Congress on Pain.* Seattle: IASP Press, 2006: 469–79.

20. American Society for Pain Management Nursing. Position statement: Pain management in patients with addictive disease. *Journal of Vascular Nursing.* 2004; **22**: 99–101.

* 21. Scimeca MM, Savage SR, Portenoy R, Lowinson J. Treatment of pain in methadone-maintained patients. *Mount Sinai Journal of Medicine.* 2000; **67**: 412–22.

* 22. Peng PW, Tumber PS, Gourlay D. Review article: perioperative pain management of patients on methadone therapy. *Canadian Journal of Anaesthesia.* 2005; **52**: 513–23.

* 23. Roberts DM, Meyer-Witting M. High-dose buprenorphine: perioperative precautions and management strategies. *Anaesthesia and Intensive Care.* 2005; **33**: 17–25.

* 24. Birnbach DJ, Stein DJ. The substance-abusing parturient: implications for analgesia and anaesthesia management. *Baillière's Clinical Obstetrics and Gynaecology.* 1998; **12**: 443–60.

* 25. Johnson RE, Fudala PJ, Payne R. Buprenorphine: considerations for pain management. *Journal of Pain and Symptom Management.* 2005; **29**: 297–326.

26. American Academy of Pain Medicine, APS, and the American Society of Addiction Medicine. Definitions related to the use of opioids for the treatment of pain. www.ampainsoc.org/advocacy/opioids.

27. Athanasos P, Smith CS, White JM *et al.* Methadone maintenance patients are cross-tolerant to the antinociceptive effects of very high plasma morphine concentrations. *Pain.* 2006; **120**: 267–75.

* 28. Compton WM, Volkow ND. Abuse of prescription drugs and the risk of addiction. *Drug and Alcohol Dependence.* 2006; **83** (Suppl. 1): S4–7.

29. American Psychiatric Association. *Diagnostic and statistical manual of mental disorders DSM-IV,* 4th edn. Washington: American Psychiatric Association, 1995.

30. Weissman DE, Haddox JD. Opioid pseudoaddiction – an iatrogenic syndrome. *Pain.* 1989; **36**: 363–6.

31. Caumo W, Schmidt AP, Schneider CN *et al.* Preoperative predictors of moderate to intense acute postoperative pain in patients undergoing abdominal surgery. *Acta Anaesthesiologica Scandinavica.* 2002; **46**: 1265–71.

32. Gil KM, Ginsberg B, Muir M *et al.* Patient-controlled analgesia in postoperative pain: the relation of psychological factors to pain and analgesic use. *Clinical Journal of Pain.* 1990; **6**: 137–42.

33. Rapp SE, Wild LM, Egan KJ, Ready LB. Acute pain management of the chronic pain patient on opiates: a survey of caregivers at University of Washington Medical Center. *Clinical Journal of Pain.* 1994; **10**: 133–8.

34. Thomas T, Robinson C, Champion D *et al.* Prediction and assessment of the severity of post-operative pain and of satisfaction with management. *Pain.* 1998; **75**: 177–85.

* 35. Zacny J, Bigelow G, Compton P *et al.* College on Problems of Drug Dependence taskforce on prescription opioid non-medical use and abuse: position statement. *Drug and Alcohol Dependence.* 2003; **69**: 215–32.

36. Breitbart W, Rosenfeld BD, Passik SD et al. The undertreatment of pain in ambulatory AIDS patients. *Pain.* 1996; **65**: 243–9.

∗ 37. Merrill JO, Rhodes LA, Deyo RA et al. Mutual mistrust in the medical care of drug users: the keys to the "narc" cabinet. *Journal of General Internal Medicine.* 2002; **17**: 327–33.

38. Walmsley PN, Brockopp DY, Brockopp GW. The role of prior pain experience and expectations on postoperative pain. *Journal of Pain and Symptom Management.* 1992; **7**: 34–7.

39. Gourlay DL, Heit HA, Almahrezi A. Universal precautions in pain medicine: a rational approach to the treatment of chronic pain. *Pain Medicine.* 2005; **6**: 107–12.

40. Eriksen J, Jensen MK, Sjogren P et al. Epidemiology of chronic non-malignant pain in Denmark. *Pain.* 2003; **106**: 221–8.

41. Blyth FM, March LM, Brnabic AJ et al. Chronic pain in Australia: a prevalence study. *Pain.* 2001; **89**: 127–34.

42. Elliott AM, Smith BH, Penny KI et al. The epidemiology of chronic pain in the community. *Lancet.* 1999; **354**: 1248–52.

∗ 43. Furlan AD, Sandoval JA, Mailis-Gagnon A, Tunks E. Opioids for chronic noncancer pain: a meta-analysis of effectiveness and side effects. *Canadian Medical Association Journal.* 2006; **174**: 1589–94.

44. Caudill-Slosberg MA, Schwartz LM, Woloshin S. Office visits and analgesic prescriptions for musculoskeletal pain in US: 1980 vs. 2000. *Pain.* 2004; **109**: 514–9.

45. Gilson AM, Ryan KM, Joranson DE, Dahl JL. A reassessment of trends in the medical use and abuse of opioid analgesics and implications for diversion control: 1997–2002. *Journal of Pain and Symptom Management.* 2004; **28**: 176–88.

46. Groth Clausen T, Eriksen J, Borgbjerg FM. Legal opioid consumption in Denmark 1981–1993. *European Journal of Clinical Pharmacology.* 1995; **48**: 321–5.

47. Bell JR. Australian trends in opioid prescribing for chronic non-cancer pain, 1986–1996. *Medical Journal of Australia.* 1997; **167**: 26–9.

48. Brixner DI, Oderda GM, Roland CL, Rublee DA. Opioid expenditures and utilization in the Medicaid system. *Journal of Pain and Palliative Care Pharmacotherapy.* 2006; **20**: 5–13.

∗ 49. Bond MR. Psychological issues in cancer and non-cancer conditions. *Acta Anaesthesiologica Scandinavica.* 2001; **45**: 1095–9.

∗ 50. Chapman CR, Nakamura Y, Flores LY. Chronic pain and consciousness: a contructivist perspective. In: Gatchel RJ, Turk DC (eds). *Psychosocial factors in pain: critical perspectives.* New York: The Guildford Press, 1999: 35–55.

∗ 51. Portenoy RK. Opioid therapy for chronic nonmalignant pain: a review of the critical issues. *Journal of Pain and Symptom Management.* 1996; **11**: 203–17.

∗ 52. Fishbain DA, Rosomoff HL, Rosomoff RS. Drug abuse, dependence, and addiction in chronic pain patients. *Clinical Journal of Pain.* 1992; **8**: 77–85.

53. Manchikanti L, Damron KS, McManus CD, Barnhill RC. Patterns of illicit drug use and opioid abuse in patients with chronic pain at initial evaluation: a prospective, observational study. *Pain Physician.* 2004; **7**: 431–7.

54. Ives TJ, Chelminski PR, Hammett-Stabler CA et al. Predictors of opioid misuse in patients with chronic pain: a prospective cohort study. *BMC Health Services Research.* 2006; **6**: 46.

55. Michna E, Ross EL, Hynes WL et al. Predicting aberrant drug behavior in patients treated for chronic pain: importance of abuse history. *Journal of Pain and Symptom Management.* 2004; **28**: 250–8.

56. Schieffer BM, Pham Q, Labus J et al. Pain medication beliefs and medication misuse in chronic pain. *Journal of Pain.* 2005; **6**: 620–9.

∗ 57. Hanks GW, Conno F, Cherny N et al. Morphine and alternative opioids in cancer pain: the EAPC recommendations. *British Journal of Cancer.* 2001; **84**: 587–93.

∗ 58. Sinclair S, Pereira J, Raffin S. A thematic review of the spirituality literature within palliative care. *Journal of Palliative Medicine.* 2006; **9**: 464–79.

59. Fischer B, Rehm J, Brissette S et al. Illicit opioid use in Canada: comparing social, health, and drug use characteristics of untreated users in five cities (OPICAN study). *Journal of Urban Health.* 2005; **82**: 250–66.

∗ 60. Mayer P, Hollt V. Genetic disposition to addictive disorders – current knowledge and future perspectives. *Current Opinion in Pharmacology.* 2005; **5**: 4–8.

61. Maxwell JC. Update: comparison of drug use in Australia and the United States as seen in the 2001 National Household Surveys. *Drug and Alcohol Review.* 2003; **22**: 347–57.

62. Turner RJ, Gil AG. Psychiatric and substance use disorders in South Florida: racial/ethnic and gender contrasts in a young adult cohort. *Archives of General Psychiatry.* 2002; **59**: 43–50.

63. Sigmon SC. Characterizing the emerging population of prescription opioid abusers. *American Journal on Addictions.* 2006; **15**: 208–12.

64. Cicero TJ, Inciardi JA, Munoz A. Trends in abuse of Oxycontin and other opioid analgesics in the United States: 2002–2004. *Journal of Pain.* 2005; **6**: 662–72.

65. Forman RF, Woody GE, McLellan T, Lynch KG. The availability of web sites offering to sell opioid medications without prescriptions. *American Journal of Psychiatry.* 2006; **163**: 1233–8.

66. Huang B, Dawson DA, Stinson FS et al. Prevalence, correlates, and comorbidity of nonmedical prescription drug use and drug use disorders in the United States: Results of the National Epidemiologic Survey on Alcohol and Related Conditions. *Journal of Clinical Psychiatry.* 2006; **67**: 1062–73.

67. Brands B, Blake J, Sproule B et al. Prescription opioid abuse in patients presenting for methadone maintenance treatment. *Drug and Alcohol Dependence.* 2004; **73**: 199–207.

68. Dobler-Mikola A, Hattenschwiler J, Meili D et al. Patterns of heroin, cocaine, and alcohol abuse during long-term methadone maintenance treatment. *Journal of Substance Abuse Treatment*. 2005; **29**: 259–65.

69. Kalman D, Morissette SB, George TP. Co-morbidity of smoking in patients with psychiatric and substance use disorders. *American Journal on Addictions*. 2005; **14**: 106–23.

70. Farrell M, Howes S, Taylor C et al. Substance misuse and psychiatric comorbidity: an overview of the OPCS National Psychiatric Morbidity Survey. *Addictive Behaviors*. 1998; **23**: 909–18.

71. Skodol AE, Oldham JM, Gallaher PE. Axis II comorbidity of substance use disorders among patients referred for treatment of personality disorders. *American Journal of Psychiatry*. 1999; **156**: 733–8.

72. Grant BF, Stinson FS, Dawson DA et al. Co-occurrence of 12-month alcohol and drug use disorders and personality disorders in the United States: results from the National Epidemiologic Survey on Alcohol and Related Conditions. *Archives of General Psychiatry*. 2004; **61**: 361–8.

73. Merikangas KR, Mehta RL, Molnar BE et al. Comorbidity of substance use disorders with mood and anxiety disorders: results of the International Consortium in Psychiatric Epidemiology. *Addictive Behaviors*. 1998; **23**: 893–907.

74. Fassino S, Daga GA, Delsedime N et al. Quality of life and personality disorders in heroin abusers. *Drug and Alcohol Dependence*. 2004; **76**: 73–80.

75. Teesson M, Havard A, Fairbairn S et al. Depression among entrants to treatment for heroin dependence in the Australian Treatment Outcome Study (ATOS): prevalence, correlates and treatment seeking. *Drug and Alcohol Dependence*. 2005; **78**: 309–15.

76. Mills KL, Lynskey M, Teesson M et al. Post-traumatic stress disorder among people with heroin dependence in the Australian Treatment Outcome Study (ATOS): prevalence and correlates. *Drug and Alcohol Dependence*. 2005; **77**: 243–9.

77. Compton MT, Weiss PS, West JC, Kaslow NJ. The associations between substance use disorders, schizophrenia-spectrum disorders, and Axis IV psychosocial problems. *Social Psychiatry and Psychiatric Epidemiology*. 2005; **40**: 939–46.

78. Shapatava E, Nelson KE, Tsertsvadze T, del Rio C. Risk behaviors and HIV, hepatitis B, and hepatitis C seroprevalence among injection drug users in Georgia. *Drug and Alcohol Dependence*. 2006; **82** (Suppl 1): S35–8.

79. Trafton JA, Oliva EM, Horst DA et al. Treatment needs associated with pain in substance use disorder patients: implications for concurrent treatment. *Drug and Alcohol Dependence*. 2004; **73**: 23–31.

80. Jamison RN, Kauffman J, Katz NP. Characteristics of methadone maintenance patients with chronic pain. *Journal of Pain and Symptom Management*. 2000; **19**: 53–62.

81. Rosenblum A, Joseph H, Fong C et al. Prevalence and characteristics of chronic pain among chemically dependent patients in methadone maintenance and residential treatment facilities. *Journal of the American Medical Association*. 2003; **289**: 2370–8.

82. Sim MG, Hulse GK, Khong E. Acute pain and opioid seeking behaviour. *Australian Family Physician*. 2004; **33**: 1009–12.

83. Paech M, Gharbi R, Oh T. Postoperative pain management after intravenous remifentanil. *Anaesthesia and Intensive Care*. 2004; **32**: 288.

84. Stevens CW, Yaksh TL. Potency of infused spinal antinociceptive agents is inversely related to magnitude of tolerance after continuous infusion. *Journal of Pharmacology and Experimental Therapeutics*. 1989; **250**: 1–8.

85. Guignard B, Bossard AE, Coste C et al. Acute opioid tolerance: intraoperative remifentanil increases postoperative pain and morphine requirement. *Anesthesiology*. 2000; **93**: 409–17.

86. Chia YY, Liu K, Wang JJ et al. Intraoperative high dose fentanyl induces postoperative fentanyl tolerance. *Canadian Journal of Anaesthesia*. 1999; **46**: 872–7.

87. Cortinez LI, Brandes V, Munoz HR et al. No clinical evidence of acute opioid tolerance after remifentanil-based anaesthesia. *British Journal of Anaesthesia*. 2001; **87**: 866–9.

88. Schraag S, Checketts MR, Kenny GN. Lack of rapid development of opioid tolerance during alfentanil and remifentanil infusions for postoperative pain. *Anesthesia and Analgesia*. 1999; **89**: 753–7.

89. Hansen EG, Duedahl TH, Romsing J et al. Intra-operative remifentanil might influence pain levels in the immediate post-operative period after major abdominal surgery. *Acta Anaesthesiologica Scandinavica*. 2005; **49**: 1464–70.

90. Vinik HR, Kissin I. Rapid development of tolerance to analgesia during remifentanil infusion in humans. *Anesthesia and Analgesia*. 1998; **86**: 1307–11.

91. Gustorff B, Nahlik G, Hoerauf KH, Kress HG. The absence of acute tolerance during remifentanil infusion in volunteers. *Anesthesia and Analgesia*. 2002; **94**: 1223–8.

92. Hood DD, Curry R, Eisenach JC. Intravenous remifentanil produces withdrawal hyperalgesia in volunteers with capsaicin-induced hyperalgesia. *Anesthesia and Analgesia*. 2003; **97**: 810–5.

* 93. Angst MS, Clark JD. Opioid-induced hyperalgesia: a qualitative systematic review. *Anesthesiology*. 2006; **104**: 570–87.

94. Angst MS, Koppert W, Pahl I et al. Short-term infusion of the mu-opioid agonist remifentanil in humans causes hyperalgesia during withdrawal. *Pain*. 2003; **106**: 49–57.

95. Koppert W, Sittl R, Scheuber K et al. Differential modulation of remifentanil-induced analgesia and postinfusion hyperalgesia by S-ketamine and clonidine in humans. *Anesthesiology*. 2003; **99**: 152–9.

96. Joly V, Richebe P, Guignard B et al. Remifentanil-induced postoperative hyperalgesia and its prevention with small-dose ketamine. *Anesthesiology*. 2005; **103**: 147–55.

∗ 97. Mao J. Opioid-induced abnormal pain sensitivity: implications in clinical opioid therapy. *Pain.* 2002; **100**: 213–7.

∗ 98. Compton P, Charuvastra VC, Ling W. Pain intolerance in opioid-maintained former opiate addicts: effect of long-acting maintenance agent. *Drug and Alcohol Dependence.* 2001; **63**: 139–46.

99. Compton P, Charuvastra VC, Kintaudi K, Ling W. Pain responses in methadone-maintained opioid abusers. *Journal of Pain and Symptom Management.* 2000; **20**: 237–45.

100. Doverty M, White JM, Somogyi AA et al. Hyperalgesic responses in methadone maintenance patients. *Pain.* 2001; **90**: 91–6.

101. Chu LF, Clark DJ, Angst MS. Opioid tolerance and hyperalgesia in chronic pain patients after one month of oral morphine therapy: a preliminary prospective study. *Journal of Pain.* 2006; **7**: 43–8.

∗102. Gintzler AR, Chakrabarti S. Post-opioid receptor adaptations to chronic morphine; altered functionality and associations of signaling molecules. *Life Science.* 2006; **79**: 717–22.

∗103. South SM, Smith MT. Analgesic tolerance to opioids. International Association for the Study of Pain. *Pain: Clinical Updates.* 2001; **9**: 1–4.

∗104. Vanderah TW, Ossipov MH, Lai J et al. Mechanisms of opioid-induced pain and antinociceptive tolerance: descending facilitation and spinal dynorphin. *Pain.* 2001; **92**: 5–9.

∗105. Himmelseher S, Durieux ME. Ketamine for perioperative pain management. *Anesthesiology.* 2005; **102**: 211–20.

∗106. Connor M, Osborne PB, Christie MJ. Mu-opioid receptor desensitization: is morphine different? *British Journal of Pharmacology.* 2004; **143**: 685–96.

∗107. Bailey CP, Connor M. Opioids: cellular mechanisms of tolerance and physical dependence. *Current Opinion in Pharmacology.* 2005; **5**: 60–8.

∗108. Trang T, Quirion R, Jhamandas K. The spinal basis of opioid tolerance and physical dependence: Involvement of calcitonin gene-related peptide, substance P, and arachidonic acid-derived metabolites. *Peptides.* 2005; **26**: 1346–55.

109. Wong CS, Chang YC, Yeh CC et al. Loss of intrathecal morphine analgesia in terminal cancer patients is associated with high levels of excitatory amino acids in the CSF. *Canadian Journal of Anaesthesia.* 2002; **49**: 561–5.

∗110. Wise RA. Dopamine, learning and motivation. *Nature Reviews. Neuroscience.* 2004; **5**: 483–94.

∗111. Fattore L, Deiana S, Spano SM et al. Endocannabinoid system and opioid addiction: behavioural aspects. *Pharmacology, Biochemistry, and Behavior.* 2005; **81**: 343–59.

∗112. Wilder-Smith OH, Arendt-Nielsen L. Postoperative hyperalgesia: its clinical importance and relevance. *Anesthesiology.* 2006; **104**: 601–7.

113. Celerier E, Laulin JP, Corcuff JB et al. Progressive enhancement of delayed hyperalgesia induced by repeated heroin administration: a sensitization process. *Journal of Neuroscience.* 2001; **21**: 4074–80.

114. Gabbard GO. Splitting in hospital treatment. *American Journal of Psychiatry.* 1989; **146**: 444–51.

∗115. Mickan S, Rodger S. Characteristics of effective teams: a literature review. *Australian Health Review.* 2000; **23**: 201–8.

116. Thomas AN, Suresh M. Opiate withdrawal after tramadol and patient-controlled analgesia. *Anaesthesia.* 2000; **55**: 826–7.

117. Myles PS, Leslie K, McNeil J et al. Bispectral index monitoring to prevent awareness during anaesthesia: the B-Aware randomised controlled trial. *Lancet.* 2004; **363**: 1757–63.

∗118. Davis JJ, Swenson JD, Hall RH et al. Preoperative "fentanyl challenge" as a tool to estimate postoperative opioid dosing in chronic opioid-consuming patients. *Anesthesia and Analgesia.* 2005; **101**: 389–95.

119. Mercadante S, Casuccio A, Fulfaro F et al. Switching from morphine to methadone to improve analgesia and tolerability in cancer patients: a prospective study. *Journal of Clinical Oncology.* 2001; **19**: 2898–904.

∗120. Quigley C. Opioid switching to improve pain relief and drug tolerability. *Cochrane Database of Systematic Reviews.* 2004; **CD004847**.

∗121. Pereira J, Lawlor P, Vigano A et al. Equianalgesic dose ratios for opioids. A critical review and proposals for long-term dosing. *Journal of Pain and Symptom Management.* 2001; **22**: 672–87.

122. Siddall PJ, Molloy AR, Walker S et al. The efficacy of intrathecal morphine and clonidine in the treatment of pain after spinal cord injury. *Anesthesia and Analgesia.* 2000; **91**: 1493–8.

123. Gammaitoni AR, Fine P, Alvarez N et al. Clinical application of opioid equianalgesic data. *Clinical Journal of Pain.* 2003; **19**: 286–97.

∗124. Lipkowski AW, Carr DB. Rethinking opioid equivalence. International Association for the Study of Pain. *Pain: Clinical Updates.* 2002; **10**: 1–4.

125. Nielsen CK, Ross FB, Smith MT. Incomplete, asymmetric, and route-dependent cross-tolerance between oxycodone and morphine in the Dark Agouti rat. *Journal of Pharmacology and Experimental Therapeutics.* 2000; **295**: 91–9.

∗126. de Leon-Casasola OA, Lema MJ. Epidural bupivacaine/sufentanil therapy for postoperative pain control in patients tolerant to opioid and unresponsive to epidural bupivacaine/morphine. *Anesthesiology.* 1994; **80**: 303–9.

127. Klein SM, Grant SA, Greengrass RA et al. Interscalene brachial plexus block with a continuous catheter insertion system and a disposable infusion pump. *Anesthesia and Analgesia.* 2000; **91**: 1473–8.

128. White PF, Issioui T, Skrivanek GD et al. The use of a continuous popliteal sciatic nerve block after surgery

involving the foot and ankle: does it improve the quality of recovery? *Anesthesia and Analgesia*. 2003; **97**: 1303–9.

129. Murphy EJ. Acute pain management pharmacology for the patient with concurrent renal or hepatic disease. *Anaesthesia and Intensive Care*. 2005; **33**: 311–22.

*130. Bell RF, Dahl JB, Moore RA, Kalso E. Peri-operative ketamine for acute post-operative pain: a quantitative and qualitative systematic review (Cochrane review). *Acta Anaesthesiologica Scandinavica*. 2005; **49**: 1405–28.

*131. Elia N, Tramer MR. Ketamine and postoperative pain – a quantitative systematic review of randomised trials. *Pain*. 2005; **113**: 61–70.

*132. Bell RF, Dahl JB, Moore RA, Kalso E. Perioperative ketamine for acute postoperative pain. *Cochrane Database of Systematic Reviews*. 2006; **CD004603**.

133. Weinbroum AA. A single small dose of postoperative ketamine provides rapid and sustained improvement in morphine analgesia in the presence of morphine-resistant pain. *Anesthesia and Analgesia*. 2003; **96**: 789–95.

*134. McCartney CJ, Sinha A, Katz J. A qualitative systematic review of the role of *N*-methyl-D-aspartate receptor antagonists in preventive analgesia. *Anesthesia and Analgesia*. 2004; **98**: 1385–400.

135. Warncke T, Stubhaug A, Jorum E. Ketamine, an NMDA receptor antagonist, suppresses spatial and temporal properties of burn-induced secondary hyperalgesia in man: a double-blind, cross-over comparison with morphine and placebo. *Pain*. 1997; **72**: 99–106.

136. Stubhaug A, Breivik H, Eide PK *et al*. Mapping of punctuate hyperalgesia around a surgical incision demonstrates that ketamine is a powerful suppressor of central sensitization to pain following surgery. *Acta Anaesthesiologica Scandinavica*. 1997; **41**: 1124–32.

137. De Kock M, Lavand'homme P, Waterloos H. 'Balanced analgesia' in the perioperative period: is there a place for ketamine? *Pain*. 2001; **92**: 373–80.

138. Sator-Katzenschlager S, Deusch E, Maier P *et al*. The long-term antinociceptive effect of intrathecal S(+)-ketamine in a patient with established morphine tolerance. *Anesthesia and Analgesia*. 2001; **93**: 1032–4.

139. Laulin JP, Maurette P, Corcuff JB *et al*. The role of ketamine in preventing fentanyl-induced hyperalgesia and subsequent acute morphine tolerance. *Anesthesia and Analgesia*. 2002; **94**: 1263–9.

140. Kissin I, Bright CA, Bradley Jr EL. The effect of ketamine on opioid-induced acute tolerance: can it explain reduction of opioid consumption with ketamine-opioid analgesic combinations? *Anesthesia and Analgesia*. 2000; **91**: 1483–8.

141. Bell RF. Low-dose subcutaneous ketamine infusion and morphine tolerance. *Pain*. 1999; **83**: 101–3.

142. Duncan MA, Spiller JA. Analgesia with ketamine in a patient with perioperative opioid tolerance. *Journal of Pain and Symptom Management*. 2002; **24**: 8–11.

143. Haller G, Waeber JL, Infante NK, Clergue F. Ketamine combined with morphine for the management of pain in an opioid addict. *Anesthesiology*. 2002; **96**: 1265–6.

144. Gold MS, Pottash AC, Sweeney DR, Kleber HD. Opiate withdrawal using clonidine. A safe, effective, and rapid nonopiate treatment. *Journal of the American Medical Association*. 1980; **243**: 343–6.

145. Plummer JL, Cmielewski PL, Gourlay GK *et al*. Antinociceptive and motor effects of intrathecal morphine combined with intrathecal clonidine, noradrenaline, carbachol or midazolam in rats. *Pain*. 1992; **49**: 145–52.

146. Marinangeli F, Ciccozzi A, Donatelli F *et al*. Clonidine for treatment of postoperative pain: a dose-finding study. *European Journal of Pain*. 2002; **6**: 35–42.

147. Arain SR, Ruehlow RM, Uhrich TD, Ebert TJ. The efficacy of dexmedetomidine versus morphine for postoperative analgesia after major inpatient surgery. *Anesthesia and Analgesia*. 2004; **98**: 153–8.

*148. Ho KY, Gan TJ, Habib AS. Gabapentin and postoperative pain – a systematic review of randomized controlled trials. *Pain*. 2006; **126**: 91–101.

149. Menigaux C, Adam F, Guignard B *et al*. Preoperative gabapentin decreases anxiety and improves early functional recovery from knee surgery. *Anesthesia and Analgesia*. 2005; **100**: 1394–9.

*150. Wiffen PJ, McQuay HJ, Edwards JE, Moore RA. Gabapentin for acute and chronic pain. *Cochrane Database of Systematic Reviews*. 2005; **CD005452**.

*151. Hansen C, Gilron I, Hong M. The effects of intrathecal gabapentin on spinal morphine tolerance in the rat tail-flick and paw pressure tests. *Anesthesia and Analgesia*. 2004; **99**: 1180–4.

152. Lin JA, Lee MS, Wu CT *et al*. Attenuation of morphine tolerance by intrathecal gabapentin is associated with suppression of morphine-evoked excitatory amino acid release in the rat spinal cord. *Brain Research*. 2005; **1054**: 167–73.

153. Gilron I, Biederman J, Jhamandas K, Hong M. Gabapentin blocks and reverses antinociceptive morphine tolerance in the rat paw-pressure and tail-flick tests. *Anesthesiology*. 2003; **98**: 1288–92.

*154. Dahl JB, Mathiesen O, Moiniche S. 'Protective premedication': an option with gabapentin and related drugs? A review of gabapentin and pregabalin in the treatment of post-operative pain. *Acta Anaesthesiologica Scandinavica*. 2004; **48**: 1130–6.

*155. Crain SM, Shen KF. Acute thermal hyperalgesia elicited by low-dose morphine in normal mice is blocked by ultra-low-dose naltrexone, unmasking potent opioid analgesia. *Brain Research*. 2001; **888**: 75–82.

156. Wang HY, Friedman E, Olmstead MC, Burns LH. Ultra-low-dose naloxone suppresses opioid tolerance, dependence and associated changes in mu opioid receptor-G protein coupling and Gbetagamma signaling. *Neuroscience*. 2005; **135**: 247–61.

157. Maxwell LG, Kaufmann SC, Bitzer S *et al*. The effects of a small-dose naloxone infusion on opioid-induced side effects and analgesia in children and adolescents treated with intravenous patient-controlled analgesia: a

double-blind, prospective, randomized, controlled study. *Anesthesia and Analgesia.* 2005; **100**: 953–8.

158. Gan TJ, Ginsberg B, Glass PS *et al.* Opioid-sparing effects of a low-dose infusion of naloxone in patient-administered morphine sulfate. *Anesthesiology.* 1997; **87**: 1075–81.

159. Eccleston C, Yorke L, Morley S *et al.* Psychological therapies for the management of chronic and recurrent pain in children and adolescents. *Cochrane Database of Systematic Reviews.* 2003; **CD003968**.

160. Uman L, Chambers C, McGrath P, Kisely S. Psychological interventions for needle-related procedural pain and distress in children and adolescents. *Cochrane Database of Systematic Reviews.* 2006; **CD005179**.

*161. Davis MP, Walsh D. Methadone for relief of cancer pain: a review of pharmacokinetics, pharmacodynamics, drug interactions and protocols of administration. *Supportive Care in Cancer.* 2001; **9**: 73–83.

*162. Amato L, Davoli M, Ferri M *et al.* Effectiveness of interventions on opiate withdrawal treatment: an overview of systematic reviews. *Drug and Alcohol Dependence.* 2004; **73**: 219–26.

163. Farre M, Mas A, Torrens M *et al.* Retention rate and illicit opioid use during methadone maintenance interventions: a meta-analysis. *Drug and Alcohol Dependence.* 2002; **65**: 283–90.

*164. Brown R, Kraus C, Fleming M, Reddy S. Methadone: applied pharmacology and use as adjunctive treatment in chronic pain. *Postgraduate Medical Journal.* 2004; **80**: 654–9.

165. Sartain JB, Mitchell SJ. Successful use of oral methadone after failure of intravenous morphine and ketamine. *Anaesthesia and Intensive Care.* 2002; **30**: 487–9.

166. Walsh SL, Johnson RE, Cone EJ, Bigelow GE. Intravenous and oral L-alpha-acetylmethadol: pharmacodynamics and pharmacokinetics in humans. *Journal of Pharmacology and Experimental Therapeutics.* 1998; **285**: 71–82.

167. Johnson RE, Chutuape MA, Strain EC *et al.* A comparison of levomethadyl acetate, buprenorphine, and methadone for opioid dependence. *New England Journal of Medicine.* 2000; **343**: 1290–7.

168. Tucker T, Ritter A, Maher C, Jackson H. Naltrexone maintenance for heroin dependence: uptake, attrition and retention. *Drug and Alcohol Review.* 2004; **23**: 299–309.

169. Hulse GK, Tait RJ. A pilot study to assess the impact of naltrexone implant on accidental opiate overdose in 'high-risk' adolescent heroin users. *Addiction Biology.* 2003; **8**: 337–42.

170. Hulse GK, Arnold-Reed DE, O'Neil G *et al.* Blood naltrexone and 6-beta-naltrexol levels following naltrexone implant: comparing two naltrexone implants. *Addiction Biology.* 2004; **9**: 59–65.

171. Comer SD, Sullivan MA, Yu E *et al.* Injectable, sustained-release naltrexone for the treatment of opioid dependence: a randomized, placebo-controlled trial. *Archives of General Psychiatry.* 2006; **63**: 210–8.

*172. Sporer KA. Buprenorphine: a primer for emergency physicians. *Annals of Emergency Medicine.* 2004; **43**: 580–4.

173. Dahan A, Yassen A, Romberg R *et al.* Buprenorphine induces ceiling in respiratory depression but not in analgesia. *British Journal of Anaesthesia.* 2006; **96**: 627–32.

174. van Dorp E, Yassen A, Sarton E *et al.* Naloxone reversal of buprenorphine-induced respiratory depression. *Anesthesiology.* 2006; **105**: 51–7.

175. Clark NC, Lintzeris N, Muhleisen PJ. Severe opiate withdrawal in a heroin user precipitated by a massive buprenorphine dose. *Medical Journal of Australia.* 2002; **176**: 166–7.

176. Strain EC, Preston KL, Liebson IA, Bigelow GE. Acute effects of buprenorphine, hydromorphone and naloxone in methadone-maintained volunteers. *Journal of Pharmacology and Experimental Therapeutics.* 1992; **261**: 985–93.

*177. Ling W, Smith D. Buprenorphine: blending practice and research. *Journal of Substance Abuse Treatment.* 2002; **23**: 87–92.

*178. Davids E, Gastpar M. Buprenorphine in the treatment of opioid dependence. *European Neuropsychopharmacology.* 2004; **14**: 209–16.

179. Griessinger N, Sittl R, Likar R. Transdermal buprenorphine in clinical practice – a post-marketing surveillance study in 13,179 patients. *Current Medical Research and Opinion.* 2005; **21**: 1147–56.

180. Sorge J, Sittl R. Transdermal buprenorphine in the treatment of chronic pain: results of a phase III, multicenter, randomized, double-blind, placebo-controlled study. *Clinical Therapeutics.* 2004; **26**: 1808–20.

31

Preventing chronic pain after surgery

WILLIAM A MACRAE, ALISON E POWELL, AND JULIE BRUCE

KEY LEARNING POINTS

- Chronic pain after surgery is common.
- Surgery is widely performed, therefore the population at risk is large.
- There are many types of chronic postoperative pain syndromes.
- There is no single definition, although a working definition has been proposed.
- The mechanisms for the development of chronic pain after surgery are complex.
- Avoid blame culture – the surgeon is seldom to blame.
- Multiple risk factors associated with onset of chronic postsurgical pain (CPSP): demographic, genetic, and medical.

- The precise role of risk factors associated with chronic pain is unknown, although the evidence base is growing.
- There is a need for prospective studies with pre- and postoperative assessment of demographic, genetic, and medical factors.
- Further research is needed to assess the role of analgesic interventions in reducing the incidence of chronic pain after surgery.
- The long-standing organizational, cultural, and technical barriers to effective management of perioperative pain need to be addressed.
- Unnecessary surgery should be avoided.

INTRODUCTION

An alarmingly high number of patients develop chronic pain after routine surgery.[1]

This chapter will review the evidence on preventing chronic pain after surgery. It complements Chapter 30, Chronic pain after surgery in the *Chronic Pain* volume of this series, which looks at the general topic of chronic pain after surgery. Some of these general topics will be

briefly reviewed, risk factors and strategies for prevention discussed, and future directions suggested.

The role of surgery as an etiological factor in the development of chronic pain was first acknowledged less than ten years ago.[2] At that time, there were several hundred papers on pain after individual operations, but no publications on the topic in general. Several review articles followed[1, 3, 4, 5] and the problem is now acknowledged by those working in the field of pain medicine, but other specialties and the general public are less well informed. Much work remains to be done and there is a need for clarity in the terminology and interpretation of the research. Existing studies suggest that various factors are associated with a greater risk of chronic pain after surgery, but their precise role and impact is unknown; the association between surgery and chronic pain may not necessarily mean causation, and we need to understand more about these factors before they can inform clinical practice.

What is now clear is that chronic pain after surgery is common. **Table 31.1** shows the approximate incidence of chronic pain after surgery following a range of common operations, aggregated across many studies. The wide variation in the figures is an indication of the lack of uniformity in study design, definitions, patients, and operations. Also shown are approximate figures for the number of operations performed in the USA in 1994 taken from Rutkow.[6] Rutkow's paper[6] reported that the ten most frequently performed operations in the USA had increased by 38 percent between 1983 and 1994, from about 5.7 million to almost 8 million. There is no reason to suppose that it has not continued to increase, although the pattern of surgery may have changed. Assuming that not all these operations are associated with persistent postsurgical pain (for example, cataract surgery), the overall population at risk might be about five million people. Taking a conservative figure of 10 percent of patients suffering persistent pain, this amounts to approximately half a million people a year in the USA. This is clearly a major public health issue: it affects large numbers of people, has a significant impact on quality of life,[7, 8, 9] and has considerable economic consequences.[10, 11] Chronic pain after surgery is challenging to treat, therefore prevention becomes of paramount importance.

DEFINITION

The problem of definition is covered in greater detail in Chapter 30, Chronic pain after surgery in the *Chronic Pain* volume of this series, and only a summary will be given here. Chronic pain after surgery is a term that is often used loosely in published studies and clinical practice to cover a diverse range of conditions. Surgery may be responsible for several different types of chronic pain syndrome, even after a single operation. For example, after thoracotomy, patients may suffer musculoskeletal pain from rib resection or spreading the ribs, in order to gain access to the chest. Neuropathic pain may result from damage to the intercostal nerves and damage to organs may cause visceral pain. Chest drains can be a source of pain.[12] After breast surgery, patients may experience phantom breast pain,[13, 14] neuropathic pain caused by damage to the intercostobrachial nerve,[15] or scar pain.[13, 16] In addition to pain, patients report a wide diversity of symptoms including numbness, tingling, swelling, or sensitivity which they report as unpleasant and distressing.[17, 18] These symptoms also cause morbidity and disability. It is obvious therefore that even after a single operation, there may be a diverse group of problems.

The difficulty of definition is compounded because pain may have been one of the symptoms that the patient experienced prior to surgery, and in fact may have been the main reason for seeking medical help. For example, in patients with right upper quadrant pain, the preexisting pain will confound measurement as many patients continue to complain of pain after cholecystectomy.[19] This does not necessarily mean the surgery was responsible. In practice, some patients present with chronic pain which they attribute to an operation, but on further questioning at the pain clinic, it transpires that the pain predates surgery. Many patients have inappropriate surgery; for example, those with irritable bowel syndrome or those undergoing surgery for chronic back pain. Most of these patients will continue to have the same pain after the operation, as these are not conditions that usually respond well to surgery, and in many cases their pain will be worse. It is then very hard to tease apart the current chronic pain and the original chronic pain. It is clearly not possible to attribute escalating pain solely to the surgery as natural deterioration cannot be ruled out.

A working definition of chronic postsurgical pain has been proposed,[3] which suggests the following criteria:

- the pain developed after a surgical procedure;
- the pain is of at least two months duration;
- other causes for the pain should have been excluded (e.g. continuing malignancy or chronic infection);
- the possibility that the pain is continuing from a preexisting problem must be explored and exclusion attempted. (There is an obvious gray area here in that surgery may simply exacerbate a preexisting condition, but attributing escalating pain to the surgery is clearly not possible as natural deterioration cannot be ruled out.)

Table 31.1 Approximate incidence of chronic pain after operations and approximate numbers of operations performed in the USA in 1994.

	Incidence of chronic pain (%)	No. of operations in USA (1994)
Mastectomy	20–50	131,000
Thoracotomy	5–65	660,000
Lower limb amputation	50–85	132,000
Open cholecystectomy	10–50	667,000
Hernia	5–35	689,000
Cesarean section	15	858,000
Cardiac surgery	30–55	501,000

MECHANISMS AND IMPLICATIONS

The mechanisms leading to chronic pain after surgery are complex and not fully understood. Chapter 30, Chronic pain after surgery in the *Chronic Pain* volume of this series reviews current knowledge on mechanisms in more detail and makes it clear that both the syndromes and mechanisms are diverse, but that changes in the nervous system play a central role. Injury of any sort changes the nervous system.[20] The pain experienced after an injury does not bear a simple relationship to the extent of the injury. Minimally traumatic operations, such as vasectomy, can cause chronic pain in the same way as major surgery, such as total hip replacement. As stated by Brandsborg et al.,[21] "Several studies, however, have shown that surgery *per se* carries a significant risk for chronic or long-lasting pain. This is not only after major surgery such as amputation and thoracotomy, but also after minor procedures …"

It is not possible to perform surgery without some damage to tissues, and therefore a hyperalgesic state will be induced after any operation, regardless of how it is done. This should revert to normal as healing occurs, but not always. Whether a patient experiences chronic pain after surgery or not, is therefore more likely to depend on the "set" of their nervous system than on precisely what the surgeon did. Although the patient complains of pain, in reality they may have a hyperalgesic or allodynic pain syndrome. Whether these postinjury pain syndromes are true neuropathic pain syndromes is a matter of debate, and they may be more accurately called "mixed pain syndromes".

Understanding the mechanisms that lead to chronic pain after surgery is important for many reasons. If the pain has a neuropathic basis, then further surgery may make it worse, by further winding up the nervous system.[22] Simplistic notions about treatment, such as nerve blocks, should be discouraged in favor of a more multidimensional approach. Reaching a more rational understanding of the cause of their pain may help patients come to terms with it. Patients who believe that someone was to blame for their chronic pain report more distress and behavioral disturbance, as well as poor response to treatments and lower expectations of future benefits.[23] Cognitive mechanisms of symptom perception in chronic pain may be affected by a patient's belief that they were injured,[24] leading to lower pain threshold and tolerance, decreased activity, and general deconditioning. It is therefore clear that removing the climate of blame would help both patients and surgeons. By accepting that chronic pain is, for a proportion of patients, an inevitable consequence of surgery, like a wound infection, and openly discussing it prior to surgery, much subsequent grief could be avoided. If surgery has the potential to cause chronic pain, then patients should be warned about this prior to consenting for surgery. This is particularly important in operations performed out of choice rather than necessity, for example cosmetic surgery or where there is a poor evidence base for benefit, such as some operations performed for back pain.[25] Lastly, research into chronic pain after surgery should be guided by an understanding of the complexity of the mechanisms.

This complex etiology makes the issue of prevention more complicated and challenging. It suggests that we need to be careful not to draw simplistic conclusions about the causes of chronic pain after surgery. Each patient will bring their own genotype, past experiences, beliefs, medical history, and psychosocial circumstances to the problem. The environmental and clinical factors which then act on the patient will include type of surgery and anesthesia, perioperative analgesia, and other treatments given.

RISK FACTORS FOR THE DEVELOPMENT OF CHRONIC PAIN AFTER SURGERY

An ideal model for studying the development of chronic pain in surgical patients, and establishing predictive factors for the condition, would include preoperative and postoperative assessment of psychological and neuro-physiological factors, detailed intra-operative data on handling of tissue and nerves, and detailed early and late postoperative pain data, as well as a thorough clinical investigation to exclude other causes of the chronic pain state. No such study has been reported.[1]

There are a range of factors that appear to be associated with a greater risk of developing chronic pain after surgery:[1, 26]

- age;
- patients' beliefs about their pain;
- psychological factors;
- preoperative pain;
- type of surgery;
- type of anesthesia (e.g. general or local);
- severity of acute postoperative pain;
- reason for surgery;
- concomitant treatments (e.g. radiotherapy and chemotherapy).

The complexity of these risk factors reflects the complexity of the etiology and mechanisms of chronic pain as mentioned above under Mechanisms and implications. The factors can be broadly grouped into demographic factors, genetic factors, and medical factors.

Demographic factors

Many studies have reported higher rates of chronic pain and other symptoms after breast cancer surgery in younger women. Tasmuth *et al.*[27] found that younger patients tended to have larger tumors, as well as more postoperative and long-term pain. Smith *et al.*[28] found that the incidence of chronic pain following mastectomy was 65 percent in those between 30 and 49 years of age, 40 percent in those between 50 and 69, and 26 percent in those over 70 years. Poleshuck *et al.*[29] were the first to perform adjusted models of risk of chronic pain after breast cancer surgery; they found the probability of developing chronic pain decreased by 5 percent with each one-year increase in age (odds ratio (OR), 0.95; 95 percent confidence interval (CI) 0.91–0.99). This is remarkably similar to the probability of developing chronic pain after hernia surgery, reported by Poobalan *et al.*[30] (5 percent reduction in risk per one year increase in age). Other demographic and clinical factors related to age (e.g. marital status, housing, and employment) may also be influential.[28] Age has a significant effect on prognosis in breast cancer, with younger women (under 35 years) having the worst histopathological features, a poorer prognosis, and more likelihood of relapse than older women.[31, 32] The reasons for this may be because of rapid tumor proliferation related to over-expression of the gene *c-erbB-2* and changes in the p53 protein, which allow proliferation of damaged DNA and a reduced response to chemotherapy and radiotherapy.[33] The combination of more severe pathology and resistance to treatment may be related to the increased incidence of pain.

For hernia surgery, the risk of chronic pain decreases with increasing age, with younger patients experiencing more severe pain.[30, 34] Those in work are also more at risk, but marital and household status is not a factor.[30] Age and work status may influence the level of physical activity, thus confounding pain reporting. Demographic factors do not seem to be of importance in phantom pain after upper or lower limb amputation.[35, 36, 37]

Genetic factors

Why only certain people develop chronic pain after surgery is a puzzle. Clearly many factors determine susceptibility and it is probable that some of these will be genetic. To date, there are no studies that examine genetic risk factors for chronic pain after surgery, but it is obvious from the research published on genetic influences on chronic pain in general that this will be an important area for future work.[38, 39, 40, 41, 42]

Animal research has shown that genetic factors influence whether mice will develop chronic pain after nerve injury.[39, 40] In 2005, Diatchenko *et al.*[38] published the first paper showing an association between pain sensitivity, the risk of developing a chronic pain syndrome, and a genetic polymorphism. In this study, having a specific haplotype of the gene for catecholamine-O-methyltransferase (COMT) diminished the risk of developing temporomandibular joint dysfunction by as much as 2.3-fold.

In an interesting commentary on a study of chronic pain after cardiac surgery,[43] Devor[42] observes that these patients often develop pain at two operative sites, the chest, where the cardiac operation was performed, and the leg, where the vein was harvested for grafting. Devor highlights that if the chances of developing pain at the two sites were independent, and the chances were 0.12 for chest pain and 0.09 for the leg pain, then the odds of pain at both sites should be $0.12 \times 0.09 = 0.01$ (1.1 percent). In fact chronic pain occurred at both sites in 18 percent of patients. This suggests a predisposition to develop chronic pain in these patients. It seems likely that part of this predisposition will be genetic.

Several pain syndromes have a genetic component and many working in this field anecdotally suspect that the presence of these conditions may increase the risk of developing chronic pain after injury. These conditions include migraine headaches, fibromyalgia syndrome, irritable bowel syndrome, irritable bladder, and Raynaud's syndrome, especially bipolar Raynaud's – excessively cold extremities in cold weather, but also burning hot feet, usually at night (erythromelalgia). There are no studies on this topic specifically, but two studies of chronic pain after hernia have found that in patients with severe chronic postsurgical pain there was a previous history of conditions such as backache, irritable bowel, or headache.[44, 45] An excellent study of risk factors for chronic pain after hysterectomy found that women with pain problems elsewhere (head, neck, shoulder, or lower back) had an increased risk of having chronic postsurgical pain.[21]

However, many patients have bilateral operations and yet only develop a chronic postsurgical pain syndrome on one side, while others have several operations, but only develop chronic pain after one. Clearly, genetic factors are only one aspect of a complex chain of causation. The interactions between our genotype, our upbringing, and the environment are complex and interdependent.[46] This fascinating subject will probably provide us with as many interesting questions as answers in the next few years.

Medical factors

PREOPERATIVE PAIN

Several studies have found an association between preoperative pain and the incidence of chronic pain after surgery. In an excellent study of pain after amputation, Nikolajsen *et al.*[47] found that significant preamputation pain increased the risk of stump and phantom pain postoperatively and of phantom pain at three months. This study also showed that patients tend to overestimate the severity of their preamputation pain six months after amputation. This emphasizes the need to measure and record the pain preoperatively rather than rely on patients' memories of the pain at a later date. In a study of pain after mastectomy, Kroner *et al.*[13] interviewed patients three weeks after the operation and then at one and six years. They found a correlation between breast pain prior to mastectomy and long-term phantom breast pain and nonpainful phantom breast sensations. A study of postthoracotomy pain in patients with cancer[48] reported that 48 percent of those taking opioid analgesics prior to surgery suffered chronic postthoracotomy pain, but only 5 percent of those not taking opioids did so. It is possible that this was a continuation of the pre-operative pain, rather than postsurgical pain.

Some studies on hernia suggest that preoperative pain is a risk factor, although in most studies the data were collected retrospectively.[30, 44, 49] The well-designed prospective study by Page *et al.*[50] interviewed patients before the operation about the pain from their inguinal hernia. About a quarter of patients had no pain from their hernia at rest, half had mild pain, and the remainder had moderate or severe pain at rest. Understandably the numbers were higher for pain on movement. Older patients were more likely to have pain from their hernia. The type of hernia (direct or indirect) was not a significant risk factor. A year after the operation, 25 percent of patients had no pain at rest and only 22 percent no pain on moving. Unfortunately, some patients who had no pain before the hernia repair reported pain after the operation and 5 percent said that their day-to-day life was worse one year after the operation. The authors raised the question of whether surgery was appropriate in asymptomatic patients.

TYPE OF SURGERY AND EXPERIENCE OF SURGEONS

The type of operation and how it is performed influences the incidence of chronic postsurgical pain, although as stated above there is no simple correlation with the size of the operation and the risk of developing chronic pain or its severity. Having said that, one study found that longer, more complex operations had a higher incidence of postoperative problems. Peters *et al.*[51] found that operations lasting more than three hours were associated with more chronic pain, increased functional limitation, poor global recovery, and poorer quality of life at six months postoperatively. Fear of surgery and severe postoperative pain were also associated with a worse outcome. The authors suggest that the prolonged and intense nociceptive barrage may increase central sensitization. Recent work on the role of the brainstem in influencing spinal cord amplification may help to explain the role of emotions and psychological factors.[52]

Different types of breast surgery were studied using similar methodology by Wallace *et al.*[53] Breast reduction had an incidence of chronic postsurgical pain of 22 percent, augmentation from 22–50 percent depending on technique, mastectomy 31 percent, but mastectomy with reconstruction by implant 53 percent. Open cholecystectomy seems to result in a higher incidence of chronic pain than laparoscopic cholecystectomy.[54] The evidence on thoracotomy is contradictory.[12, 55] In a study of pain after hernia repair, Callesen and Kehlet[56] found no difference between the various types of open hernia repair, but less pain and shorter convalescence after laparoscopic repair. This difference between open and laparoscopic herniorraphy is confirmed by the systematic reviews of over 100 publications conducted by Aasvang and Kehlet[34] and Poobalan *et al.*[57] Dividing the ilioinguinal nerve during the operation increases the risk of chronic pain.[49] Ravindran *et al.*[58] surveyed over 1000 UK surgeons to investigate usual surgical practice of handling nerves in the inguinal canal during herniorrhaphy. There was considerable variation in routine surgical practice, although surgeons performing high volumes of hernia surgery were more likely to preserve than transect nerve structures.

There is evidence that surgical experience can affect outcomes in terms of morbidity and mortality.[59, 60] A study from Finland found that women who had breast surgery for cancer in high volume surgical units, thus experienced in breast cancer surgery, were less likely to suffer chronic pain than women who had their operations in lower volume units with less experience.[61] However, a study of pain after hernia repair found no association between grade of operating surgeon and severe pain after surgery.[45] The evidence on day case versus inpatient surgery for hernias is contradictory.[30, 45]

REASON FOR SURGERY AND ROLE OF CONCOMITANT TREATMENTS

The relationship between the reason for surgery, for example for benign or malignant disease, and the risk of chronic pain after surgery is difficult to study, as different operations are performed for different conditions. For thoracotomy, one study has shown a higher incidence of chronic pain after operations for benign esophageal disease than for lung cancer,[12] but other studies have shown no difference in rates of pain.[62, 63] Studies of lower limb amputation have shown no influence from cause.[36, 64] The type of hernia does not influence the prevalence of postherniorraphy pain in groin hernias.[45, 50] Some studies report an increased incidence of chronic pain after surgery for recurrent hernias,[56] while others have shown no difference.[45] Poobalan *et al.*[30] found a doubling in risk of chronic postsurgical pain in patients having subsequent surgery for recurrence compared to those having primary repair (OR 2.16, 95 percent CI 1.03, 4.52). The evidence on the influence of concomitant treatments such as radiotherapy and chemotherapy is conflicting. Some studies have shown an increase in chronic pain,[18, 27, 61, 65] while others showed no difference.[12, 13] The recent study by Poleshuck *et al.*[29] is the most scientifically rigorous study published to date, with detailed pre- and post-operative assessment of multiple factors. Surgery type and use of radiation therapy were found to independently increase the risk of chronic pain after breast cancer surgery; this finding persisted after adjustment for age, preoperative pain, acute postoperative pain, and other factors.

ANESTHESIA AND ANALGESIA

A study of chronic pain after cesarean section reported a lower incidence of chronic pain in patients who had had a spinal rather than general anesthetic,[66] and patients with chronic pain had a higher recall of severe postoperative pain. Similarly, patients having a spinal anesthetic for hysterectomy had a lower incidence of chronic pain than those having a general anesthetic.[21] However, in a well-designed study, McCartney et al.[67] compared general and regional anesthesia for ambulatory hand surgery and found that although patients who had regional anesthesia had reduced pain in the short term, there was no long-term benefit.

SEVERITY OF ACUTE POSTOPERATIVE PAIN

There is a correlation between acute postoperative pain and long-term chronic pain. Katz et al.[68] found that acute pain following thoracic surgery predicts chronic postthoracotomy pain. Several other studies have confirmed this finding.[12, 69] Postoperative pain seems to be a risk factor for chronic pain after hernia repair[34] and after surgery for breast cancer.[29] Whether the effect is causal or not is impossible to say at present, although the basic science would strongly support the assertion that severe pain around the time of surgery will sensitize the nervous system, making long-term pain more likely.

PSYCHOSOCIAL FACTORS

Much research has focused on the role of affect, in particular anxiety, on surgical recovery, although mostly investigating the relationship with recovery in the acute postoperative period. Munafo and Stevenson[70] reviewed studies that assessed the relationship between anxiety, surgical recovery, and response to surgery, restricting variability by only including papers where anxiety was measured using the State-Trait Anxiety Inventory (STAI). Consistent associations between preoperative measures of anxiety and postoperative pain were found across 12 studies. However, no details were provided on timing of pain assessment and these studies have predominantly focused on acute postoperative pain, rather than any longer-term follow up, see Chapter 15, Psychological therapies – adults, for further details.

Similarly, in 1993, Johnston and Vogele[71] published an influential review and meta-analysis of the benefits of psychological preparations for surgery, comparing levels of negative affect, pain, pain medication, and other outcomes from 35 clinical trials. There was strong evidence of benefit from provision of procedural information and behavioral instructions and this was consistent across all postoperative outcomes. As with the Munafo and Stevenson review,[70] however, studies were limited in terms of pain assessment, with most studies failing to record pain status beyond several weeks. There is a need to repeat these systematic reviews to include more recent publications, many of which report longer patient follow up.

Psychosocial distress has been found to be both a consequence of chronic pain and a risk factor for its development.[72, 73] Katz et al.[74] found that greater preoperative anxiety independently predicted clinically meaningful pain up to day 30 after breast cancer surgery. While younger age and being unmarried were also independently associated with persisting acute pain, these were postulated to reflect the psychosocial effects of reduced social support.

More recently, interest in psychological characteristics has widened from measurement of affect to include another construct of distress, "pain catastrophizing," defined as a tendency to exaggerate negative responses and perceived inability to control pain.[75, 76] Most developmental work using the Pain Catastrophizing Scale has been conducted on acute pain conditions or chronic nonsurgical pain.[77, 78] However, one recent large surgical cohort study found that pain catastrophizing was predictive of chronic postoperative pain.[51] Fear of long-term consequences of surgery and optimism were associated with poor recovery and good quality of life, respectively.

In summary, there is a range of demographic, genetic, clinical, and psychosocial factors that appear to be associated with a greater risk of chronic pain after surgery. These factors are clearly not discrete, but rather are overlapping and interconnected, underlining how more research is needed to tease out the nature and impact of these associations and their implications for clinical practice. In particular, clinical and epidemiological studies are required. Animal studies may be able to investigate individual factors and inform future human studies, but it is evident that they can never address the true complexity of this multifactorial condition. However, the universal risk factor is already clear: chronic pain after surgery only occurs when the patient has had a surgical procedure. We discuss the policy and clinical implications of this in the next section.

PREVENTION

Chronic postsurgical pain syndromes are usually difficult to treat and therefore prevention is important. Unfortunately, we only have limited evidence about effective strategies for preventing chronic postsurgical pain. As we have shown in this chapter, considerable further research is needed about the etiology, mechanisms, and risk factors for chronic postsurgical pain before we can determine effective strategies for preventing it. In the meantime, there are two areas that we can consider.

Reducing the use of surgery as an intervention

The universal risk factor for chronic pain after surgery is having had a surgical procedure. Preventing unnecessary surgery is therefore an obvious and important strategy. There are two approaches which may achieve this goal, first preventing diseases that often require surgery and second preventing patients from having operations that are ineffective, unnecessary, or inappropriate for their condition.

Many surgical procedures are performed for diseases which are preventable. For example, the two most common reasons for lower limb amputation are peripheral vascular disease and diabetes.[79] In order to prevent phantom pain therefore, addressing the problems of smoking and obesity in the population are measures that could be effective. Obesity increases the risk for many other conditions which often result in surgery as well, including gallbladder disease, osteoarthritis, some types of cancer, and heart disease.[80] For many types of cancer, screening can detect early tumors, resulting in less radical treatments.

Some patients have what might be described as "inappropriate operations" for diseases where there is no evidence to support surgical treatment, for example some types of back pain[81] or irritable bowel syndrome.[82] Patients who are considering undergoing a surgical procedure for cosmetic reasons need to be aware of the risk of persistent pain after surgery.

It is well recognized that interventions provided by health services are prey to errors of over-use, misuse, and under-use,[83, 84, 85, 86] and that striking variations are found in surgical practice as in other specialties.[84, 87] It is not possible here to explore the very complex issues around the provision of surgery and of other nonsurgical interventions in detail, but it is clear that these are important areas to address in taking a realistic and broad view of prevention of chronic pain after surgery.

Managing perioperative pain effectively

Good perioperative analgesia should be part of a comprehensive program of perioperative care[88] for several reasons, including ethical, humanitarian, and medical. It may lead to a reduction of complications in the immediate postoperative period as well as in the long term. We referred above to studies that show an association between acute postoperative pain and chronic pain after surgery. This association would suggest that

effective treatment of perioperative pain may also have the important benefit of reducing the incidence of chronic pain after surgery.

The choice of anesthetic and analgesic technique influences pain in the immediate postoperative period, but there are few good studies on different types of anesthesia and analgesia and chronic pain after surgery. The impetus for research in this area is the hope that by preventing the afferent barrage of signals from the periphery at the time of surgery and during the postoperative period, and by giving drugs that affect the mechanisms responsible for sensitizing the nervous system, chronic pain may be prevented.

Studies in this area are challenging and many have methodological problems. For example, controlling for all other variables is almost impossible. The further problem of recall bias is illustrated in a paper by the Helsinki group in a study of women with breast cancer.[73] They found that the memory of the intensity of the postoperative pain increased with time in those who had chronic pain, but decreased in those who did not have chronic postsurgical pain.[73] As with preoperative pain, this underlines the importance of collecting data in the perioperative period, and calls into question the validity of pain scores based on patients' recall of past pain. The importance of rigorous methodology is illustrated by the case of cryoanalgesia for postthoracotomy pain. A study which described the technique in some detail but was short on other details recommended the method.[89] It was widely used at one time, but a subsequent randomized controlled trial[90] showed no benefit, with a suggestion that it made the problem worse, a finding confirmed by Richardson et al.[12]

Several studies have examined the link between perioperative analgesic techniques and chronic postsurgical pain. The results are contradictory, with many studies showing no benefit.[67, 91] Paxton et al.[92] studied the effect of a local anesthetic block in vasectomy and concluded that it could prevent chronic testicular discomfort. However, this optimistic finding is not borne out by other studies of vasectomy.[93]

Some studies are encouraging. Local anesthesia at the time of the operation can reduce pain for up to ten days in tonsillectomy[94, 95] and herniorrhaphy.[96] The local anesthetic will clearly have worn off after a few hours, so such a prolonged effect is presumably caused by reducing central sensitization. There is evidence that regional anesthetic techniques confer benefit in the perioperative period for thoracotomy[97] and this may give long-term benefit. A study of thoracotomy patients found that those who had epidural analgesia that was initiated before surgery and continued into the postoperative period had less pain at six months compared to those who had received i.v. patient-controlled analgesic opioids.[98] Tiippana et al.[99] also found a decreased incidence of chronic pain when thoracic epidural analgesia was used for analgesia after thoracotomy. However, technical problems can limit the effectiveness of interventions.[69, 99]

A study of 60 patients undergoing cervical spinal fusion using bone from the ilium found that those who received morphine injected into the site of iliac bone harvest were much less likely to have pain at one year after surgery than those who had either the same dose of morphine intramuscularly or those who had saline infiltrated into the harvest site.[100] A study comparing patients who had ropivacaine infusion into the site of iliac crest bone graft harvest against a placebo group (all patients had an intravenous morphine patient-controlled analgesia device) found that patients in the ropivacaine group had significantly less pain at the iliac crest on movement at three months after surgery than patients in the placebo group.[101]

Early studies on the use of adjuvant drugs around the time of surgery, such as anticonvulsants like gabapentin,[102, 103, 104, 105, 106] or *N*-methyl-D-aspartic acid (NMDA) antagonists, such as ketamine,[107, 108] have shown contradictory results (see also Chapter 6, Clinical pharmacology: other adjuvants). More recent studies using combinations of local anesthesia and gabapentin have shown encouraging results.[109, 110] Good quality long-term studies are needed to investigate whether using combinations of drugs around the time of surgery can be effective in reducing postoperative pain and chronic pain after surgery.

Preemptive analgesia: early promising signs?

There is evidence from animal work that giving analgesic drugs prior to injury is more effective in reducing the hyperexcitability that occurs in the spinal cord than giving the same drugs after the injury.[111] This finding led to many papers on the subject of preemptive analgesia, a term first used by Wall in 1988.[112] The subject was reviewed by Woolf and Chong in 1993,[113] who expressed the view that preempting pain must be the goal of all those involved in the postoperative care of patients (see also Chapter 9, Preventive analgesia and beyond: current status, evidence, and future directions for a discussion of the differentiation between, and evidence for, preemptive and preventive analgesia).

One of the early clinical studies by Bach *et al.*[114] reported that the incidence of phantom pain at one year was reduced in patients having lower limb amputations, who were given analgesia by epidural local anesthetic and opioid for 72 hours preoperatively. There were methodological problems with this study, however, and a later randomized, controlled, double-blind trial showed no benefit.[115] There was also no difference in hyperalgesia, allodynia nor wind up-like pain[116] between those given preemptive treatment and the controls. Despite many subsequent studies there is still no convincing evidence that treating pain prior to amputation or other forms of surgery prevents chronic pain after surgery.

Despite the fact that no consistent clinical benefit has yet been shown from preemptive analgesia, we should not give up hope that preemptive analgesia may prove to have a role in reducing chronic postsurgical pain. The animal work is robust and we have to ask why it has not translated into clinical benefit. In a thoughtful article on the subject, Aida[117] points out that there are many important differences between the animal studies and the reality of clinical work. Experimental animals have no preexisting pain and the pain stimulus is normally to an extremity, with segmental innervation only. The animal procedure is normally short and circumscribed, whereas in human surgical operations the operation may be prolonged, over a large area of the body, with complex innervation. The pain may persist into the postoperative period. As Aida points out, if pain breaks through at any point during the patient's surgical episode, even for a short while, then sensitization of the nervous system may occur, leading to long-term changes and persistent pain. It may be that the methods used in previous clinical studies of preemptive analgesia were inadequate to reduce afferent input sufficiently. Perhaps by using combinations of drugs it may be possible to reduce both acute postoperative pain and chronic pain after surgery.

Research needs to continue to further our understanding of the role of anesthesia and analgesia in reducing chronic pain after surgery and to determine the best methods of achieving this. In the meantime, controlling pain in the perioperative period is something over which we have some control and about which there is a great deal of evidence.[118] Applying this knowledge of acute postoperative pain management is important in its own right and it appears that it may also be important because of the apparent association between intensity of acute postoperative pain and chronic pain after surgery. Thus, in comparison to many of the other risk factors, there is existing knowledge that we can bring to bear on the problem of chronic pain after surgery while we wait for the further research that we need. However, using this knowledge in routine clinical practice is not straightforward.

Achieving effective postoperative pain management: organizational barriers

Despite its importance, it has long been recognized that postoperative pain management is not well managed in hospitals in many countries.[119, 120, 121, 122] Problems continue despite the introduction of acute pain services and the considerable efforts made by many individuals and teams, and it has proved hard in many settings to embed lasting changes in routine postoperative pain management for all surgical patients.[123, 124, 125, 126] There is therefore a gap between the current knowledge about effective practice in postoperative pain management and the service that patients routinely receive.[127] As Chapter

48, Acute pain services and organizational change in the *Practice and Procedures* volume of this series explores, the reasons for this are complex and include technical problems, lack of resources, conflicting organizational priorities, and the need to change attitudes and practices around pain management. Tackling the deficits in postoperative pain management will require clinicians, policymakers, and researchers to address a range of challenges.

CONCLUSIONS

In the past ten years, much work has been published on chronic pain after surgery, and some of the recent work has focused on risk factors. There are many methodological problems in this area and future research needs to take account of the complexity of the mechanisms and multifactorial nature of the causes. Chronic pain after surgery is common and hard to treat, so prevention is important. At present, the options are limited, but providing the best possible pain relief around the time of surgery and preventing unnecessary operations are two worthwhile strategies.

REFERENCES

* 1. Kehlet H, Jensen TS, Woolf C. Persistent postsurgical pain: risk factors and prevention. *Lancet.* 2006; **367**: 1618–25.

2. Crombie IK, Davies HTO, Macrae WA. Cut and thrust: antecedent surgery and trauma among patients attending a chronic pain clinic. *Pain.* 1998; **76**: 167–71.

3. Macrae WA, Davies HTO. Chronic postsurgical pain. In: Crombie IK, Linton S, Croft P *et al.* (eds). *Epidemiology of pain.* Seattle: International Association for the Study of Pain, 1999: 125–42.

* 4. Perkins FM, Kehlet H. Chronic pain as an outcome of surgery. *Anesthesiology.* 2000; **93**: 1123–33.

* 5. Macrae WA. Chronic pain after surgery. *British Journal of Anaesthesia.* 2001; **87**: 88–98.

6. Rutkow IM. Surgical operations in the United States. Then (1983) and now (1994). *Archives of Surgery.* 1997; **132**: 983–90.

* 7. Lame IE, Peters ML, Vlaeyen JWS *et al.* Quality of life in chronic pain is more associated with beliefs about pain, than with pain intensity. *European Journal of Pain.* 2005; **9**: 15–24.

8. Smith BH, Torrance N, Bennett MI, Lee AJ. Health and quality of life associated with chronic pain of predominantly neuropathic origin in the community. *Clinical Journal of Pain.* 2007; **23**: 143–9.

9. Galvez R, Marsal C, Vidal J *et al.* Cross-sectional evaluation of patients functioning and health-related quality of life in patients with neuropathic pain under standard care conditions. *European Journal of Pain.* 2007; **11**: 244–55.

10. Smith BH, Hopton L, Chambers WA. Chronic pain in primary care. *Family Practice.* 1999; **16**: 475–82.

11. Blyth FM, March LM, Cousins MJ. Chronic pain-related disability and use of analgesia and health services in a Sydney community. *Medical Journal of Australia.* 2003; **179**: 84–7.

12. Richardson J, Sabanathan S, Mearns AJ *et al.* Post-thoracotomy neuralgia. *The Pain Clinic.* 1994; **7**: 87–97.

13. Kroner K, Knudsen UB, Lundby L, Hvid H. Long term phantom breast syndrome after mastectomy. *Clinical Journal of Pain.* 1992; **8**: 346–50.

14. Dijkstra PU, Rietman JS, Geertzen JHB. Phantom breast sensations and phantom breast pain: A 2-year prospective study and a methodological analysis of literature. *European Journal of Pain.* 2007; **11**: 99–108.

15. Vecht CJ, Van der Brand HJ, Wajer OJM. Post-axillary dissection pain in breast cancer due to a lesion of the intercostobrachial nerve. *Pain.* 1989; **38**: 171–6.

* 16. Jung BF, Ahrendt GM, Oaklander AL, Dworkin RH. Neuropathic pain following breast cancer surgery: proposed classification and research update. *Pain.* 2003; **104**: 1–13.

17. Polinsky ML. Functional status of long-term breast cancer survivors. *Health and Social Work.* 1994; **19**: 165–73.

18. Tasmuth T, von Smitten K, Hietanen P *et al.* Pain and other symptoms after different treatment modalities of breast cancer. *Annals of Oncology.* 1995; **6**: 453–9.

19. Bates T, Mercer JC, Harrison M. Symptomatic gall stone disease: before and after cholecystectomy. *Gut.* 1984; **24**: 579–80.

20. Villanueva L, Dickenson AH, Ollat H. *The pain system in normal and pathological states.* Seattle: IASP Press, 2004.

21. Brandsborg B, Nikolajsen L, Hansen CT *et al.* Risk factors for chronic pain after hysterectomy: a nationwide questionnaire and database study. *Anesthesiology.* 2007; **106**: 1003–12.

22. Wilder-Smith OH, Tassonyi E, Senly C *et al.* Surgical pain is followed not only by spinal sensitization but also by supraspinal antinociception. *British Journal of Anaesthesia.* 1996; **76**: 816–21.

23. DeGood DE, Kiernan B. Perception of fault in patients with chronic pain. *Pain.* 1996; **64**: 153–9.

24. Turk DC, Okifuji A. Perception of traumatic onset, compensation status, and physical findings: impact on pain severity, emotional distress, and disability in chronic pain patients. *Journal of Behavioural Medicine.* 1996; **19**: 435–53.

25. Turner JA, Ersek M, Herron L *et al.* Patient outcomes after lumbar spinal fusions. *Journal of the American Medical Association.* 1992; **268**: 907–11.

* 26. Macrae WA. Can we prevent chronic pain after surgery? In: Shorten G, Carr DB, Harmon D *et al.* (eds). *Postoperative pain management.* Philadelphia: Saunders Elsevier, 2006: 259–64.

27. Tasmuth T, von Smitten K, Hietanen P et al. Pain and other symptoms after different treatment modalities of breast cancer. *Annals of Oncology*. 1995; **6**: 453–9.

28. Smith WCS, Bourne D, Squair J et al. A retrospective cohort study of post mastectomy pain syndrome. *Pain*. 1999; **83**: 91–5.

∗ 29. Poleshuck EL, Katz J, Andrus CH et al. Risk factors for chronic pain following breast cancer surgery: a prospective study. *Journal of Pain*. 2006; **7**: 626–34.

∗ 30. Poobalan AS, Bruce J, King PM et al. Chronic pain and quality of life following open inguinal hernia repair. *British Journal of Surgery*. 2001; **88**: 1122–6.

31. Yildirim E, Dalgic T, Berberoglu U. Prognostic significance of young age in breast cancer. *Journal of Surgery and Oncology*. 2000; **74**: 267–72.

32. Kroman N, Jensen MB, Wohlfahrt J et al. Factors influencing the effect of age on prognosis in breast cancer: population based study. *British Medical Journal*. 2000; **320**: 474–8.

33. Tutt A, Ross G. Commentary: much still to learn about relations between tumour biology, prognosis, and treatment outcome in early breast cancer. *British Medical Journal*. 2000; **320**: 478–9.

∗ 34. Aasvang E, Kehlet H. Chronic postoperative pain: the case of inguinal herniorrhaphy. *British Journal of Anaesthesia*. 2005; **95**: 69–76.

35. Kooijman CM, Dijkstra PU, Geertzen JH et al. Phantom pain and phantom sensations in upper limb amputees: an epidemiological study. *Pain*. 2000; **87**: 33–41.

36. Jensen TS, Krebs B, Nielsen J, Rasmussen P. Immediate and long-term phantom limb pain in amputees: incidence, clinical characteristics and relationship to pre-amputation limb pain. *Pain*. 1985; **21**: 267–78.

37. Wartan SW, Hamann W, Wedley JR, McColl I. Phantom pain and sensation among British veteran amputees. *British Journal of Anaesthesia*. 1997; **78**: 652–9.

∗ 38. Diatchenko L, Slade GD, Nackley AG et al. Genetic basis for individual variations in pain perception and the development of a chronic pain condition. *Human Molecular Genetics*. 2005; **14**: 135–43.

39. Devor M, Raber P. Heritability of symptoms in an experimental model of neuropathic pain. *Pain*. 1990; **42**: 51–67.

40. Seltzer Z, Wu T, Max MB, Diehl SR. Mapping a gene for neuropathic pain-related behaviour following peripheral neurectomy in the mouse. *Pain*. 2001; **93**: 101–06.

41. Mogil JS, Wilson SG, Bon K et al. Heritability of nociception I: responses of 11 inbred mouse strains on 12 measures of nociception. *Pain*. 1999; **80**: 67–82.

42. Devor M. Evidence for heritability of pain in patients with traumatic neuropathy. *Pain*. 2004; **108**: 200–1; author reply *Pain*. 2004; **108**: 202.

43. Bruce J, Drury N, Poobalan AS et al. The prevalence of chronic chest and leg pain following cardiac surgery: a historical cohort study. *Pain*. 2003; **104**: 265–73.

44. Wright D, Paterson C, Scott N et al. Five-year follow-up of patients undergoing laparoscopic or open groin hernia repair: a randomized controlled trial. *Annals of Surgery*. 2002; **235**: 333–7.

45. Courtney CA, Duffy K, Serpell MG, O'Dwyer PJ. Outcome of patients with severe chronic pain following repair of groin hernia. *British Journal of Surgery*. 2002; **89**: 1310–14.

46. Ridley M. *Nature via nurture*. London: Harper Perennial, 2004.

47. Nikolajsen L, Ilkjaer S, Kroner K et al. The influence of preamputation pain on postamputation stump and phantom pain. *Pain*. 1997; **72**: 393–405.

48. Keller SM, Carp NZ, Levy MN, Rosen SM. Chronic post thoracotomy pain. *Journal of Cardiovascular Surgery*. 1994; **35**: 161–4.

49. Liem MS, van Duyn EB, van der Graaf Y, van Vroonhoven TJ. Recurrences after conventional anterior and laparoscopic inguinal hernia repair: a randomized comparison. *Annals of Surgery*. 2003; **237**: 136–41.

50. Page B, Paterson C, Young D, O'Dwyer PJ. Pain from primary inguinal hernia and the effect of repair on pain. *British Journal of Surgery*. 2002; **89**: 1315–18.

∗ 51. Peters ML, Sommer M, Rijke JM et al. Somatic and psychologic predictors of long-term unfavourable outcome after surgical intervention. *Annals of Surgery*. 2007; **245**: 487–94.

52. Suzuki R, Rygh LJ, Dickenson AH. Bad news from the brain: descending 5-HT pathways that control spinal pain processing. *Trends in Pharmacological Sciences*. 2004; **25**: 613–17.

53. Wallace MS, Wallace AM, Lee J, Dobke MK. Pain after breast surgery: a survey of 282 women. *Pain*. 1996; **66**: 195–205.

54. Stiff G, Rhodes M, Kelly A et al. Long-term pain: less common after laparoscopic than open cholecystectomy. *British Journal of Surgery*. 1994; **81**: 1368–70.

55. Landreneau RJ, Mack MJ, Hazelrigg SR et al. Prevalence of chronic pain after pulmonary resection by thoracotomy or video-assisted thoracic surgery. *Journal of Thoracic and Cardiovascular Surgery*. 1994; **107**: 1079–86.

56. Callesen T, Kehlet H. Postherniorraphy pain. *Anesthesiology*. 1997; **87**: 1219–30.

∗ 57. Poobalan AS, Bruce J, Smith WC et al. A review of chronic pain after inguinal herniorrhaphy. *Clinical Journal of Pain*. 2003; **19**: 48–54.

58. Ravindran R, Bruce J, Debnath D et al. A United Kingdom survey of surgical technique and handling practice of inguinal canal structures during hernia surgery. *Surgery*. 2006; **139**: 523–6.

59. Flum DR, Salem L, Elrod JA et al. Early mortality among Medicare beneficiaries undergoing bariatric surgical procedures. *Journal of the American Medical Association*. 2005; **294**: 1903–08.

60. Begg CB, Riedel ER, Bach PB et al. Variations in morbidity after radical prostatectomy. *New England Journal of Medicine*. 2002; **346**: 1138–44.

61. Tasmuth T, Blomqvist C, Kalso E. Chronic post-treatment symptoms in patients with breast cancer operated in

different surgical units. *European Journal of Surgery and Oncology*. 1999; **25**: 38–43.

62. Perttunen K, Tasmuth T, Kalso E. Chronic pain after thoracic surgery: a follow-up study. *Acta Anaesthesiologica Scandinavica*. 1999; **43**: 563–7.

63. Kalso E, Perttunen K, Kaasinen S. Pain after thoracic surgery. *Acta Anaesthesiologica Scandinavica*. 1992; **36**: 96–100.

64. Houghton AD, Saadah E, Nicholls G *et al*. Phantom pain: natural history and association with rehabilitation. *Annals of the Royal College of Surgeons of England*. 1994; **76**: 22–5.

65. Smith J, Thompson JM. Phantom limb pain and chemotherapy in pediatric amputees. *Mayo Clinic Proceedings*. 1995; **70**: 357–64.

66. Nikolajsen L, Sorensen HC, Jensen TS, Kehlet H. Chronic pain after Caesarean section. *Acta Anaesthesiologica Scandinavica*. 2004; **48**: 111–16.

67. McCartney CJL, Brull R, Chan VWS *et al*. Early but not long-term benefit of regional compared with general anesthesia for ambulatory hand surgery. *Anesthesiology*. 2004; **101**: 461–7.

68. Katz J, Jackson M, Kavanagh BP, Sandler AN. Acute pain after thoracic surgery predicts long-term post-thoracotomy pain. *Clinical Journal of Pain*. 1996; **12**: 50–5.

69. Pluijms WA, Steegers MA, Verhagen AF *et al*. Chronic post-thoracotomy pain: a retrospective study. *Acta Anaesthesiologica Scandinavica*. 2006; **50**: 804–08.

70. Munafo MR, Stevenson J. Anxiety and surgical recovery. Reinterpreting the literature. *Journal of Psychosomatic Research*. 2001; **51**: 589–96.

* 71. Johnston M, Vogele C. The benefits of psychological preparation for surgery: A meta-analysis. *Annals of Behavioural Medicine*. 1993; **15**: 245–56.

72. Akechi T, Okuyama T, Imoto S *et al*. Biomedical and psychosocial determinants of psychiatric morbidity among postoperative ambulatory breast cancer patients. *Breast Cancer Research and Treatment*. 2001; **65**: 195–202.

73. Tasmuth T, Estlanderb AM, Kalso E. Effect of present pain and mood on the memory of past postoperative pain in women treated surgically for breast cancer. *Pain*. 1996; **68**: 343–7.

* 74. Katz J, Poleshuck EL, Andrus CH *et al*. Risk factors for acute pain and its persistence following breast cancer surgery. *Pain*. 2005; **119**: 16–25.

75. Sullivan MJ, Bishop S, Pivic J. The Pain Catastrophizing Scale: development and validation. *Psychological Assessment*. 1995; **7**: 524–32.

76. Granot M, Ferber SG. The roles of pain catastrophizing and anxiety in the prediction of postoperative pain intensity: a prospective study. *Clinical Journal of Pain*. 2005; **21**: 439–45.

77. Pavlin DJ, Sullivan MJ, Freund PR, Roesen K. Catastrophizing: a risk factor for postsurgical pain. *Clinical Journal of Pain*. 2005; **21**: 83–90.

78. Sullivan MJ, Adams H, Rhodenizer T, Stanish WD. A psychosocial risk factor – targeted intervention for the prevention of chronic pain and disability following whiplash injury. *Physical Therapy*. 2006; **86**: 8–18.

79. Chaturvedi N, Abbott CA, Whalley A *et al*. Risk of diabetes related amputation in South Asians vs Europeans in the UK. *Diabetic Medicine*. 2002; **19**: 99–104.

80. Bray GA. Risks of obesity. *Endocrinology and Metabolism Clinics of North America*. 2003; **32**: 787–804, viii.

81. Turner JA, Ersek M, Herron L *et al*. Patient outcomes after lumbar spinal fusions. *Journal of the American Medical Association*. 1992; **268**: 907–11.

82. Cole JA, Yeaw JM, Cutone JA *et al*. The incidence of abdominal and pelvic surgery among patients with irritable bowel syndrome. *Digestive Diseases and Sciences*. 2005; **50**: 2268–75.

83. Berwick D, Davidoff F, Hiatt H, Smith R. Refining and implementing the Tavistock principles for everybody in health care. *British Medical Journal*. 2001; **323**: 616–20.

84. Charatan F. US report blames poor quality care for soaring healthcare costs. *British Medical Journal*. 2002; **324**: 1478.

85. Wennberg JE. Unwarranted variations in healthcare delivery: implications for academic medical centres. *British Medical Journal*. 2002; **325**: 961–4.

86. Davis D, Evans M, Jadad A *et al*. The case for knowledge translation: shortening the journey from evidence to effect. *British Medical Journal*. 2003; **327**: 33–5.

87. Jennett B. Variations in surgical practice: welcome diversity of disturbing differences. *British Journal of Surgery*. 1988; **75**: 630–1.

88. Kehlet H. Multimodal approach to control postoperative pathophysiology and rehabilitation. *British Journal of Anaesthesia*. 1997; **78**: 606–17.

89. Maiwand MO, Makey AR, Rees A. Cryoanalgesia after thoracotomy. Improvement of technique and review of 600 cases. *Journal of Thoracic and Cardiovascular Surgery*. 1986; **92**: 291–5.

90. Roxburgh JC, Markland CG, Ross BA, Kerr WF. Role of cryoanalgesia in the control of pain after thoracotomy. *Thorax*. 1987; **42**: 292–5.

91. Katz J, Schmid R, Snijdelaar DG *et al*. Pre-emptive analgesia using intravenous fentanyl plus low-dose ketamine for radical prostatectomy under general anesthesia does not produce short-term or long-term reductions in pain or analgesic use. *Pain*. 2004; **110**: 707–18.

92. Paxton LD, Huss BK, Loughlin V, Mirakhur RK. Intra-vas deferens bupivacaine for prevention of acute pain and chronic discomfort after vasectomy. *British Journal of Anaesthesia*. 1995; **74**: 612–13.

93. McMahon AJ, Buckley J, Taylor A *et al*. Chronic testicular pain following vasectomy. *British Journal of Urology*. 1992; **69**: 188–91.

94. Jebeles JA, Reilly JS, Gutierrez JF *et al*. Tonsillectomy and adenoidectomy pain reduction by local bupivacaine

infiltration in children. *International Journal of Pediatric Otorinolaryngology*. 1993; **25**: 149–54.

95. Naja MZ, El-Rajab M, Kabalan W *et al*. Pre-incisional infiltration for pediatric tonsillectomy: a randomized double-blind clinical trial. *International Journal of Pediatric Otorhinolaryngology*. 2005; **69**: 1333–41.

96. Tverskoy M, Cozacov C, Ayache M *et al*. Postoperative pain after inguinal herniorraphy with different types of anaesthesia. *Anesthesia and Analgesia*. 1990; **70**: 29–35.

97. Davies RG, Myles PS, Graham JM. A comparison of the analgesic efficacy and side-effects of paravertebral vs epidural blockade for thoracotomy – a systematic review and meta-analysis of randomized trials. *British Journal of Anaesthesia*. 2006; **96**: 418–26.

98. Senturk M, Ozcan PE, Talu GK *et al*. The effects of three different analgesia techniques on long-term postthoracotomy pain. *Anesthesia and Analgesia*. 2002; **94**: 11–15.

99. Tiippana E, Nilsson E, Kalso E. Post-thoracotomy pain after thoracic epidural analgesia: a prospective follow-up study. *Acta Anaesthesiologica Scandinavica*. 2003; **47**: 433–8.

100. Reuben SS, Vieira P, Faruqi S *et al*. Local administration of morphine for analgesia after iliac bone graft harvest. *Anesthesiology*. 2001; **95**: 390–4.

101. Blumenthal S, Dullenkopf A, Rentsch K, Borgeat A. Continuous infusion of ropivacaine for pain relief after iliac crest bone grafting for shoulder surgery. *Anesthesiology*. 2005; **102**: 392–7.

102. Fassoulaki A, Patris K, Sarantopoulos C, Hogan Q. The analgesic effect of gabapentin and mexilitene after breast surgery for cancer. *Anesthesia and Analgesia*. 2002; **95**: 985–91.

103. Dirks J, Fredensborg BB, Christensen D *et al*. A randomised study of the effects of single-dose gabapentin versus placebo on postoperative pain adn morphine consumption after mastectomy. *Anesthesiology*. 2002; **97**: 560–4.

104. Rorarius MGF, Mennader S, Suominen P *et al*. Gabapentin for the prevention of postoperative pain after vaginal hysterectomy. *Pain*. 2004; **110**: 175–81.

105. Dierking G, Duedahl TH, Rasmussen ML *et al*. Effects of gabapentin on postoperative morphine consumption and pain after abdominal hysterectomy: a randomised, doule blind study. *Acta Anaesthesiologica Scandanavica*. 2004; **48**: 322–7.

106. Nikolajsen L, Finnerup NB, Kramp S *et al*. A randomized study of the effects of gabapentin on postamputation pain. *Anesthesiology*. 2006; **105**: 1008–15.

107. Katz J, Scmid R, Snijdelaar DG *et al*. Pre-emptive analgesia using intravenous fentanyl plus low-dose ketamine for radical prostatectomy under general anesthesia does not produe short-term or long-term reductions in pain or analgesic use. *Pain*. 2004; **110**: 707–18.

108. De Kock M, Lavand'homme P, Waterloos H. 'Balanced analgesia' in the perioperative period: is there a place for ketamine? *Pain*. 2001; **92**: 373–80.

109. Fassoulaki A, Triga A, Melemeni A, Sarantopoulos C. Multimodal analgesia with gabapentin and local anesthetics prevents acute and chronic pain after breast surgery for cancer. *Anesthesia and Analgesia*. 2005; **101**: 1427–32.

110. Fassoulaki A, Melemeni A, Stamatakis E *et al*. A combination of gabapentin and local anaesthetics attenuates acute and late pain after abdominal hysterectomy. *European Journal of Anaesthesiology*. 2007; **24**: 521–8.

111. Woolf CJ, Wall PD. Morphine-sensitive and morphine-insensitive actions of C-fibre input on the rat spinal cord. *Neuroscience Letters*. 1986; **64**: 221–5.

112. Wall PD. The prevention of postoperative pain. *Pain*. 1988; **33**: 289–90.

113. Woolf CJ, Chong M. Preemptive analgesia-treating postoperative pain by preventing the establishment of central sensitisation. *Anesthesia and Analgesia*. 1993; **77**: 362–79.

114. Bach S, Noreng MF, Tjellden NU. Phantom limb pain in amputees during the first 12 months following limb amputation, after preoperative lumbar epidural blockade. *Pain*. 1988; **33**: 297–301.

115. Nikolajsen L, Ilkjaer S, Christensen JH *et al*. Randomised trial of epidural bupivacaine and morphine in prevention of stump and phantom pain in lower limb amputation. *Lancet*. 1997; **350**: 1353–7.

116. Nikolajsen L, Ilkjaer S, Jensen TS. Effect of preoperative extradural bupivacaine and morphine on stump sensation in lower limb amputees. *British Journal of Anaesthesia*. 1998; **81**: 348–54.

117. Aida S. The challenge of preemptive analgesia. *Pain Clinical Updates*. 2005; **XIII**: 1–4.

*118. Australian and New Zealand College of Anaesthetists and Faculty of Pain Medicine. *Acute pain management: scientific evidence*, 2nd edn. Melbourne: ANZCA, 2005.

119. Wallace PGM, Norris W. The management of postoperative pain. *British Journal of Anaesthesia*. 1975; **47**: 113–20.

120. Spence AA. Relieving acute pain. *British Journal of Anaesthesia*. 1980; **52**: 245–6.

121. Weis O, Sriwatanakul K, Alloza J *et al*. Attitudes of patients, housestaff, and nurses toward postoperative analgesic care. *Anesthesia and Analgesia*. 1983; **62**: 70–4.

122. Armitage EN. Postoperative pain – prevention or relief? *British Journal of Anaesthesia*. 1989; **63**: 136–8.

*123. Rawal N. 10 years of acute pain services – achievements and challenges. *Regional Anesthesia and Pain Medicine*. 1999; **24**: 68–73.

*124. Clinical Standards Advisory Group. *Services for patients with pain*. London: Department of Health, 2000.

125. Nagi H. Acute pain services in the United Kingdom. *Acute Pain*. 2004; **5**: 89–107.

*126. Powell AE, Davies HTO, Bannister J, Macrae WA. Rhetoric and reality on acute pain services in the NHS: a national postal questionnaire survey. *British Journal of Anaesthesia*. 2004; **92**: 689–93.

127. National Institute of Clinical Studies. *Evidence-practice gaps report*. Adelaide: National Institute of Clinical Studies, 2003.

Index

This index covers the chapters in this volume only. A combined index covering all four volumes in the *Clinical Pain Management* series is available as a pdf on the accompanying website: www.clinicalpainmanagement.co.uk

An *F* following a page reference indicates that the reference is to a figure; a *T* indicates that the reference is to a table.

Notes
To save space in the index, the following abbreviations have been used:
    CBT – cognitive-behavioral therapy
    ICU – intensive care unit
    NSAIDs – nonsteroidal anti-inflammatory drugs
    PCA – patient-controlled analgesia
    TENS – transcutaneous electrical nerve stimulation